Practical Anatomic Pathol

Series Editors

Fan Lin
Geisinger Health System
Danville, PA, USA

Ximing J. Yang
Feinberg School of Medicine
Northwestern University
Chicago, IL, USA

This Book Series is designed to provide a comprehensive, practical and state-of-the-art review and update of the major issues and challenges specific to each subspecialty field of surgical pathology in a question and answer (Q&A) format. Making an accurate diagnosis especially from a limited sample can be quite challenging, yet crucial to patient care. This Book Series, using the most current and evidence-based resources 1) focuses on frequently asked questions in surgical pathology in day-to-day practice; 2) provides quick, accurate, terse, and useful answers to many practical questions encountered in daily practice; 3) emphasizes the importance of a triple test (clinical, radiologic, and histologic correlation); 4) delineates how to appropriately utilize immunohistochemistry, in situ hybridization and molecular tests; and 5) minimizes any potential diagnostic pitfalls in surgical pathology. These books also include highly practical presentations of typical case scenarios seen in an anatomic pathology laboratory. These are in the form of case presentations with step-by-step expert analysis. Sample cases include common but challenging situations, such as evaluation of well-differentiated malignant tumors vs. benign/reactive lesions; distinction of two benign entities; sub-classification of a malignant tumor; identification of newly described tumor and non-tumor entities; workup of a tumor of unknown origin; and implementation of best practice in immunohistochemistry and molecular testing in a difficult case. The Q&A format is well accepted, especially by junior pathologists, for several reasons: 1) this is the most practical and effective way to deliver information to a new generation of pathologists accustomed to using the Internet as a resource and, therefore, comfortable and familiar with a Q&A learning environment; 2) it's impossible to memorialize and digest massive amounts of new information about new entities, new and revised classifications, molecular pathology, diagnostic IHC, and the therapeutic implications of each entity by reading large textbooks; 3) sub-specialization is a very popular practice model highly demanded by many clinicians; and 4) time is very precious for a practicing pathologist because of increasing workloads in recent years following U.S. health care reforms. This Book Series meets all of the above expectations. These books are written by established and recognized experts in their specialty fields and provide a unique and valuable resource in the field of surgical pathology, both for those currently in training and for those already in clinical practice at various skill levels. It does not seek to duplicate or completely replace other large standard textbooks; rather, it is a new, comprehensive yet concise and practical resource on these timely and critical topics.

More information about this series at http://www.springer.com/series/13808

Endi Wang • Anand Shreeram Lagoo
Editors

Practical Lymph Node and Bone Marrow Pathology

Frequently Asked Questions

Springer

Editors
Endi Wang
Department of Pathology
Duke University School of Medicine
and Duke Health System
Durham, NC
USA

Anand Shreeram Lagoo
Department of Pathology
Duke University School of Medicine
and Duke Health System
Durham, NC
USA

Practical Anatomic Pathology
ISBN 978-3-030-32188-8 ISBN 978-3-030-32189-5 (eBook)
https://doi.org/10.1007/978-3-030-32189-5

This Springer imprint is published by the registered company Springer Nature Switzerland AG
The registered company address is: Gewerbestrasse 11, 6330 Cham, Switzerland

Dedicated with love to my wife Frances F. Wang

Endi Wang

Dedicated with love to my wife Sandhya, with respect to my teachers, and with gratitude to all the patients in whose care I could contribute but who contributed much more to my learning.

Anand Shreeram Lagoo

Preface

Among the subspecialties of surgical pathology, hematopathology occupies a rather unique place due to the convergence of histopathology and cytopathology, particularly when diagnosing conditions involving the bone marrow, and the ever-increasing repertoire of diagnostic and prognostic ancillary tests. Hematopathology was an "early adopter" of immunological and molecular techniques and continues to embrace the advances in the ancillary testing modalities. The diagnostic certainty offered by the objective results obtained from the ancillary studies attracts some pathologists (including us) to this field. Paradoxically it is also the reason why many surgical pathologists shun hematopathology!

The multi-pronged approach to classification of hematopoietic and lymphoid neoplasms, combining morphology, immunophenotype, cytogenetic and molecular genetic findings, and clinical features espoused in the Revised European and American Lymphoma (REAL) classification (1993), was more successful in predicting outcomes in each entity as compared to its predecessors. The success of the REAL classification led to the WHO (2001) classification based on the same principles, which additionally incorporated the classification of myeloid neoplasms. The WHO classification has gained worldwide recognition as *the* classification of hematolymphoid neoplasia. The recognition of subtle differences in immunophenotypic, molecular, and biological properties of previously recognized entities which dictate optimal therapy and/or outcome, was used to subdivide some common entities, in the second edition published in 2008 and even more so in the recent revision published in 2017*. This book follows this recent revision of the WHO classification in essence, but the material is organized in a fashion which will be most useful to a practicing surgical pathologist. This is achieved by focusing on the morphological findings as the starting point. Using this morphological "backbone" and several frequently asked questions (FAQs), the reader is guided to a list of differential diagnoses and a rational final diagnosis.

The unprecedented success of tyrosine kinase inhibitor Gleevec in treating chronic myeloid leukemia and the rapidly accumulating knowledge of the molecular processes involved in controlling the growth, maturation, division, and death of various hematolymphoid cells have started a race to discover similar "magic bullets" for other leukemias and lymphomas. Many novel therapies have been introduced particularly in the past decade, which aim to replace or complement existing therapies to induce deeper and lasting remissions in previously incurable hematolymphoid malignancies. The clinicians expect pathological guidance not only with accurate diagnosis but also about disease progression, minimal residual disease, disease susceptibility to a particular therapy, effects of prior therapy on prognosis and subsequent therapy, etc. This book provides brief but to the point guidance about the prognostic and therapeutic implications of key ancillary studies so that the pathologist is comfortable to answer clinician's questions over the entire arc of manifestations and management of the disease.

---

*NOTE: The recent revision to the 4th (2008) edition of the WHO Classification of Tumours of Haematopoietic and Lymphoid Tissues was originally slated for publication in 2016. Several papers published around that time refer to the revision as "WHO (2016) classification" or "WHO (2016) revision". However, the monograph was actually published in the second half of 2017. Therefore, in the present volume, we have referred to this revision as the "WHO (2017) classification" or "WHO (2017) revision".

The authors have been fortunate to practice hematopathology in a tertiary care center providing advanced treatments for hematolymphoid malignancies, including an active stem cell transplant program. A close collaboration and daily face-to-face meetings with the clinical team have allowed us to understand the issues crucial to the management of these patients with multimodality treatments, including many trials of novel agents. We have recruited expert hematopathologists who have academic and/or practical interest in a subtype of myeloid or lymphoid neoplasm. We are grateful for the valuable contribution of these scholars, who volunteered their time and energy to provide up-to-date material on the topic in the unique FAQ format of this book. Like the editors, most of the authors mentor pathology residents and hematopathology fellows and know which points are difficult to understand. Together we have carefully revised each chapter so that the practically important and directly applicable information is available in an easy-to-find and easy-to-grasp format.

We want to thank the series editors for entrusting this task on us; the developmental editor, Ms Connie Walsh, for her patient and careful collection and organization of contributions from authors; and above all the contributing authors, without whose input this endeavor would not have been possible. We hope that this book will serve as a practical introduction and handbook for pathology trainees and hematopathology fellows and will remain a useful reference to practicing pathologists when they are signing out lymph nodes or bone marrow specimens.

Durham, NC, USA

Endi Wang
Anand Shreeram Lagoo

Contents

Contributors

Le Aye, DO Department of Hematopathology, University of Southern California, Children's Hospital Los Angeles, Los Angeles, CA, USA

Sharathkumar Bhagavathi, MD Pathology and Laboratory Medicine, University of Iowa Carver College of Medicine, Iowa City, IA, USA

Parul Bhargava, MD Department of Laboratory Medicine, University of California, San Francisco, San Francisco, CA, USA

Jason X. Cheng, MD, PhD Department of Pathology, University of Chicago, Chicago, IL, USA

Siraj M. El Jamal, MD The Department of Pathology, Molecular and Cell-Based Medicine, Icahn School of Medicine at Mount Sinai, Mount Sinai Hospital, New York, NY, USA

Juehua Gao, MD, PhD Department of Pathology, Northwestern University Feinberg School of Medicine, Chicago, IL, USA

Juan Camilo Gómez-Gélvez, MD Department of Pathology and Laboratory Medicine, Henry Ford Health System, Detroit, MI, USA

Jerald Z. Gong, MD Department of Pathology, Anatomy and Cell Biology, Thomas Jefferson University, Philadelphia, PA, USA

Shunyou Gong, MD, PhD Hematology and Hematopathology, Department of Pathology, Ann & Robert H. Lurie Children's Hospital, Northwestern University Feinberg School of Medicine, Chicago, IL, USA

David D. Grier, MD Division of Pathology & Laboratory Medicine, Cincinnati Children's Hospital Medical Center, Cincinnati, OH, USA

Rohit Gulati, MBBS Department of Pathology and Laboratory Medicine, Indiana University School of Medicine, Indianapolis, IN, USA

Ashley S. Hagiya, MD Department of Pathology, Keck Medical Center of the University of Southern California, Los Angeles, CA, USA

Kathryn M. Hogan, MD Department of Pathology, Henry Ford Hospital, Detroit, MI, USA

Qin Huang, MD, PhD Pathology and Laboratory Medicine, Cedars-Sinai Medical Center, Los Angeles, CA, USA

Shimin Hu, MD, PhD Department of Hematopathology, The University of Texas MD Anderson Cancer Center, Houston, TX, USA

Kedar V. Inamdar, MD, PhD Department of Pathology, Henry Ford Hospital, Detroit, MI, USA

Lina Irshaid, MD Departments of Pathology and Laboratory Medicine, Yale University School of Medicine, New Haven, CT, USA

Matthew E. Keeney, MD Pathology, University of Iowa Hospitals and Clinics, Iowa City, IA, USA

Anand Shreeram Lagoo, MD, PhD Department of Pathology, Duke University School of Medicine and Duke Health System, Durham, NC, USA

Shiyong Li, MD, PhD Hematopathology, Pathology and Laboratory Medicine, Emory University School of Medicine, Atlanta, GA, USA

Chuanyi Mark Lu, MD Department of Laboratory Medicine, University of California San Francisco and San Francisco VA Healthcare System, San Francisco, CA, USA

Chad M. McCall, MD, PhD Department of Pathology, Duke University School of Medicine, Durham, NC, USA

Hematology Laboratory Services, Duke University Health System, Durham, NC, USA

Durham VA Medical Center, Durham, NC, USA

L. Jeffrey Medeiros, MD Department of Hematopathology, The MD Anderson Cancer Center, Houston, TX, USA

Jadee Neff, MD, PhD Department of Pathology, Duke University School of Medicine, Durham, NC, USA

Zenggang Pan, MD, PhD Department of Pathology, Yale University School of Medicine, New Haven, CT, USA

Nancy S. Rosenthal, MD Department of Pathology, Wake Forest School of Medicine, Winston-Salem, NC, USA

Rosemary She, MD Clinical Pathology, Department of Pathology, Keck School of Medicine of USC (University of Southern California), Los Angeles, CA, USA

Yang Shi, MD, PhD Department of Pathology, Montefiore Medical Center, Albert Einstein College of Medicine, Bronx, NY, USA

Imran N. Siddiqi, MD, PhD Department of Pathology, Keck School of Medicine, University of Southern California, Los Angeles, CA, USA

Jinming Song, MD, PhD Department of Hematopathology and Laboratory Medicine, Moffitt Cancer Center, Tampa, FL, USA

Guldeep Uppal, MD Department of Pathology, Anatomy and Cell Biology, Thomas Jefferson University, Philadelphia, PA, USA

Bethany D. Vallangeon, MD Pathologists Diagnostic Services, PLLC, Winston Salem, NC, USA

James W. Vardiman, MD Department of Pathology, University of Chicago, Chicago, IL, USA

Maria (Ria) Vergara-Lluri, MD Clinical Pathology, Hematopathology Service, Department of Pathology, LAC+USC Medical Center, Keck School of Medicine of USC (University of Southern California), Los Angeles, CA, USA

Endi Wang, MD, PhD Department of Pathology, Duke University School of Medicine and Duke Health System, Durham, NC, USA

Huan-You Wang, MD, PhD Department of Pathology, University of California San Diego Health System, La Jolla, CA, USA

Jun Wang, MD Pathology and Laboratory Medicine, Loma Linda University Medical Center, Loma Linda, CA, USA

Linlin Wang, MD, PhD Lab Medicine, University of California San Francisco, San Francisco, CA, USA

Wei Wang, MD, PhD Department of Hematopathology, The MD Anderson Cancer Center, Houston, TX, USA

Xiaoqiong Wang, MD, PhD Robert J. Tomisch Pathology and Laboratory Medicine Institute, Cleveland Clinic, Cleveland, OH, USA

Jeffrey D. Whitman, MD, MS Department of Laboratory Medicine, University of California, San Francisco, San Francisco, CA, USA

Cleandrea Williams, MD Department of Pathology, Keck Medical Center of the University of Southern California, Los Angeles, CA, USA

Wenbin Xiao, MD, PhD Department of Pathology, Memorial Sloan Kettering Cancer Center, New York, NY, USA

Yi Xie, MD, PhD Department of Laboratory Medicine, University of California San Francisco, San Francisco, CA, USA

Mina L. Xu, MD Departments of Pathology and Laboratory Medicine, Yale University School of Medicine, New Haven, CT, USA

Linsheng Zhang, MD, PhD Department of Pathology and Laboratory Medicine, Emory University School of Medicine, Atlanta, GA, USA

Chen Zhao, MD, PhD Department of Pathology, Carver College of Medicine, University of Iowa, Iowa City, IA, USA

Yue Zhao, MD, PhD Department of Pathology, College of Basic Medical Sciences and the First Affiliated Hospital, China Medical University, Shenyang, P. R. China

Department of Pathology, Duke University School of Medicine, Durham, NC, USA

Jiehao Zhou, MD, PhD Department of Pathology and Laboratory Medicine, Indiana University School of Medicine, Indianapolis, IN, USA

Ting Zhou, MD, PhD Pathology & Immunology, Baylor College of Medicine, Houston, TX, USA

Yi Zhou, MD, PhD Pathology and Laboratory Medicine, University of Miami Miller School of Medicine, Miami, FL, USA

Essentials of the Immune Response and Immunophenotyping

1

Chad M. McCall, Bethany D. Vallangeon, and Anand Shreeram Lagoo

List of Frequently Asked Questions

1. What are the basic divisions of the immune response?
2. How does the immune system distinguish self from nonself?
3. How does the acquired immune system respond to antigens?
4. What are pathologic immune reactions?
5. How do the cellular components of the immune system develop, and how are they distributed in the body?
6. What is an "immunophenotype"? How is it determined in hematopathology?
7. What is the immunophenotype of maturing myeloid and lymphoid cells at various stages in maturation?
8. What is the role of immunophenotyping in the classification of acute leukemias?
9. How are the compartments of the immune system and normal lymphoid architecture related to the classification of lymphomas?
10. How can immunohistochemistry (IHC) be used optimally for diagnosis and differential diagnosis in hematopathology?
11. How can a panel of antibodies be used to differentiate among the common B-cell neoplasms?
12. How can a panel of antibodies be used to differentiate among the common T-cell neoplasms?
13. How can a basic panel of antibodies be used to distinguish common neoplasms from reactive lymphoid hyperplasia?
14. How does the immunophenotype of normal thymus differ from T-lymphoblastic leukemia/lymphoma?
15. How does the immunophenotype of normal B-cell precursors (hematogones) differ from B-lymphoblastic leukemia/lymphoma (B-ALL)?
16. Which antibodies are most useful for determining the immunophenotype of myeloid neoplasms?
17. How are antigens expressed by various lymphoid and myeloid malignancies being targeted by immune-based therapies in hematologic oncology?

1. What are the basic divisions of the immune response?

- Immunity literally means a protection or exemption from something onerous, and the term was used in ancient times to denote exemption from paying taxes or protection from adverse legal action. In medicine the term is used to denote the body's ability to protect itself from infectious microorganisms as well as from cancer and related conditions. The immune response is the sum of cellular and molecular interactions involved in this protective activity [1].
- The immune response can be divided according to key functional properties into innate/natural immunity and acquired/adaptive/specific immunity. Or, it can be divided based on effectors of the immune response into humoral immunity and cell-mediated immunity. While convenient for conceptual understanding, these divisions are not absolute and have many critically important interactions in both directions [2].

C. M. McCall
Department of Pathology, Duke University School of Medicine, Durham, NC, USA

Hematology Laboratory Services, Duke University Health System, Durham, NC, USA

Durham VA Medical Center, Durham, NC, USA
e-mail: chad.mccall@duke.edu

B. D. Vallangeon
Pathologists Diagnostic Services, PLLC, Winston Salem, NC, USA
e-mail: vallangeonb16@ecu.edu

A. S. Lagoo (✉)
Department of Pathology, Duke University School of Medicine and Duke Health System, Durham, NC, USA
e-mail: anand.lagoo@duke.edu

E. Wang, A. S. Lagoo (eds.), *Practical Lymph Node and Bone Marrow Pathology*, Practical Anatomic Pathology,
https://doi.org/10.1007/978-3-030-32189-5_1

- The innate immune response does not require prior exposure to the offending agent by the individual. These responses have evolved in multicellular organisms to quickly combat common threats, such as pathogenic organisms, to all members of the species [3]. These responses are relatively stereotypical but available immediately after an encounter with the offending agent. The innate immune response also facilitates the development of the acquired immune response.
- The acquired immune response, also known as adaptive or specific immune response, involves prior interaction between an individual's immune cells and the offending antigen.
  - An *antigen* is a key concept in acquired immunity. It refers to any molecule or part of molecule which is recognized due to its unique physicochemical structure by the antibodies produced by B-cells and/or by T-cell antigen receptors (TCRs).
- B- and T-lymphocytes mediate the acquired immune response through the great diversity in their specialized cell surface receptor, surface immunoglobulin (sIg), and TCR, respectively.
  - Further divisions of adaptive immune response: auto- versus alloimmune (based on source of antigen); active versus passive (antibodies made by patient versus passively transferred); and natural versus artificial (mother to fetus antibody transfer versus injected immunoglobulin).
- Humoral immunity is mediated by antibodies produced by B-cells and plasma cells, and cellular immunity is mediated by T-cells, NK-cells, and T/NK-cells.

2. How does the immune system distinguish self from non-self?

- What are self and nonself?
  - In specific immunity: Fine structural differences due to genetic polymorphisms producing alleles of molecules present in all members of a species.
  - In innate immunity: Structural "patterns" present in molecules produced by microorganisms, but absent from eukaryotes, and some products of tissue injury and cell death ("damage-associated molecular patterns") are recognized by "pattern recognition molecules" as "nonself" and evoke an immune response.
- The proteins coded by the major histocompatibility complex (MHC) and expressed on the surface of virtually all cells in the body are primarily responsible for the distinction between "self" and "nonself." In humans the MHC is called the human leukocyte antigen (HLA) system. The genetic locus is on the short arm of chromosome 6 between 6p21.1 and 6p21.3. It contains 224 genes; about half are involved in the immune response.
- The MHC genes are divided into Class I genes (in humans, *HLA-A*, *HLA-B*, and *HLA-C*), Class II genes (in humans, *HLA-DR*, *HLA-DP*, *HLA-DQ*, and others), and MHC Class III genes (including complement components). According to recent estimates, there are about 13,000 HLA Class I alleles and 7500 Class II alleles [4]. Due to this enormous polymorphism, the MHC alleles expressed in any individual are nearly unique (except in identical twins), and the two sets of HLA alleles (the maternal and paternal "haplotypes") constitute the "self" MHC for the individual.
- Class I genes are expressed on nearly all human cells (including platelets) but not on red blood cells. In contrast, Class II genes are expressed on restricted cell types—mainly antigen-presenting cells such as dendritic cells, macrophages, and B-cells.
- During maturation in the thymus ("thymic education"), T-cells undergo a complex process of positive and negative selection to generate a broad repertoire of T-cells capable of recognizing nonself peptide antigens in the context of self-MHC while being tolerant to a wide array of self-antigens [5]. Some TCRs can recognize nonself MHC molecules encountered on transplanted or transfused cells and mount an immune response [6].

3. How does the acquired immune system respond to antigens?

- Specificity and memory characterize the acquired immune response. Specificity derives from the ability to generate a large repertoire of antigen receptors (sIg on B-cells and TCRs on T-cells) containing thousands of unique antigen binding sites [7]. The diversity in both Ig and TCR is the result of genetic recombination of gene fragments termed V, D, and J, additional point mutations, variations during and after the recombination, and the multimeric nature of the antigen receptor.
- Classical T-cells respond to peptide antigens only in the context of self-MHC molecules (except when they encounter cells expressing nonself MHC molecules, as in organ transplantation). CD4+ T-cells primarily respond to antigenic peptides presented in the peptide binding groove of MHC Class II molecules, while CD8+ cells respond to antigens displayed on Class I MHC molecules. The peptide in the binding groove on Class I and Class II molecule, along with the surrounding parts of the MHC molecule itself, is recognized together by the T-cell antigen receptor (TCR).
- Before cell surface expression, MHC molecules are "loaded" with antigenic peptides in a complex event orchestrated by chaperone molecules [4].
  - Class I molecules are loaded with peptides derived from proteins synthesized by the cell, while Class II molecules get peptides derived from external proteins taken up by the cell and hydrolyzed in the phagolysosome.

- Non-classical T-cells respond to non-peptide antigens (glycolipids and others) in the context of the five members of CD1 family of molecules [8, 9] expressed on "professional" antigen-presenting cells such as Langerhans cells. These cells are important in defense against lipid-rich bacteria and have the major characteristics (specificity, memory, etc.) of the adaptive immune response.
- T-cells require accessory signals mediated through coreceptors on T-cells interacting with ligands on antigen-presenting cells and soluble molecules (e.g., cytokines). The results vary from activation of the T-cell to produce other cytokines to transformation into an effector or memory cell [10].
- B-cells can be activated by soluble antigens without MHC-restricted antigen presentation. However, the requirement and extent of help from T-cells vary depending on the nature of antigen and other factors such as the inflammatory microenvironment [11–13].

4. What are pathologic immune reactions?

- Broadly, these can be divided into (a) hypersensitivity reactions (excessive or deleterious immune response to antigens); (b) autoimmunity (immune response to self-antigens); (c) immunodeficiency conditions (inadequate or insufficient immune response in quantity or quality); (d) immune dysregulation (inappropriate immune response); and (e) pathological effects of nonself, immunologically competent cells or molecules.
  (a) The traditional classification of hypersensitivity reactions into four major types, proposed over 55 years ago [14], has proved to be a useful scheme to categorize the basic mechanisms underlying pathologic immune reactions to exogenous antigens in most cases, but is also applicable to other situations. The four categories include types I (immediate, atopic or anaphylactic, IgE mediated), II (cytotoxic, IgG or IgM mediated), III (immune complex mediated), and IV (delayed type, T-cell mediated). Type II can be further divided into IIa (cytotoxic) and IIb (cell stimulating). Similarly type IV can be subdivided into four subtypes, each mediated by a different subset of T-cells [15, 16].
  (b) Autoimmune processes arise when humoral and/or cell-mediated adaptive immune reactions are directed against self-antigens. Over 80 well-defined autoimmune clinical entities are currently recognized [17]. Taken together, these diseases are quite common (overall prevalence of 2.7%), occur most frequently in the fourth and fifth decades of life, and affect females more than twice as often as men. The autoantigens are clearly identified in 45 diseases, and 19 of these have germline mutations. A complex interplay between genetic, epigenetic, and environmental factors (including microbiomes, external microbial and nonmicrobial antigens, diet, etc.) causes susceptibility to autoimmunity [18].
  (c) Immunodeficiency conditions: These may be primary or secondary and show great variation in clinical severity and the component(s) of the immune system which is (are) deficient. Over 230 genetic mutations causing immunodeficiency have been identified [19]. Secondary immunodeficiencies are far more common and may arise from natural aging processes, retroviral (e.g., HIV) and other infections, or iatrogenic causes. These conditions lead to significant morphological changes in the lymphoid tissues, and selected conditions will be discussed more fully in Chaps. 10 and 11.
  (d) Immune dysregulation is a term used for unbalanced immune responses with overlapping features of immunodeficiency associated with autoimmunity and/or enlargement of lymphoid tissue. This may arise due to mutations in genes which control immune responses [20] or is due to viral- [21] or age-induced [22] imbalances in innate or acquired immunity.
  (e) Foreign antibodies detrimental to the subject can be introduced naturally, e.g., from a previously sensitized Rh-negative mother to an Rh-positive fetus, or artificially, due to a mismatched blood transfusion. Immunocompetent foreign lymphocytes are introduced primarily during allogeneic stem cell transplantation, but can also be introduced through blood transfusion in certain situations. The common pathological effect is graft versus host disease, which accompanies the desired, beneficial "graft versus tumor" effect.

5. How do the cellular components of the immune system develop and how are they distributed in the body?

- The lymphoid lineages (except NK-cells) arise from bone marrow HSCs but complete their development in lymphoid tissues. Early T-cell precursors migrate to the thymus where T-cells develop, while naïve mature B-cells populate the peripheral lymphoid organs and develop further after antigen exposure.
- B-cells: Since the functional molecules of humoral immunity (antibodies or immunoglobulins) can be carried by blood to the site of immune reactions, B-cells remain concentrated in the peripheral lymphoid organs.
  - B-cell precursors develop through the early stages of maturation in the bone marrow, where they sequentially undergo rearrangement of the immunoglobulin heavy and light chain genes and eventually express IgM (and IgD) antibodies on the cell surface.

- Allelic exclusion: All immunoglobulin molecules expressed by a B-cell express only one type of light chain, kappa or lambda. Even in a B-cell expressing IgM and IgD simultaneously, the same light chain is used in both isotypes of immunoglobulin.
- These antigen-naïve B-cells migrate to the primary follicles of lymph nodes, spleen, and mucosa-associated lymphoid tissue, including tonsils and Peyer's patches. The subset of naïve B-cells with surface IgM/IgD molecules, which react to antigens presented by dendritic cells, proliferate and form the germinal center. These activated B-cells undergo somatic hypermutation in the rearranged immunoglobulin genes, followed by "affinity maturation"—a process in which subclones with highest affinity receptors for the antigen survive and others undergo apoptosis.
- Germinal center B-cells also undergo class switching to produce smaller but more efficient IgG or IgA molecules, instead of IgM, while maintaining their antigen specificity. Some B-cells mature into plasma cells which are specialized to produce large quantities of the specific immunoglobulin molecule. Long-lived plasma cells migrate to the bone marrow. After the initial immune response winds down, some long-lived memory B-cells are produced and reside in the marginal zones of the lymphoid follicles.

• T-cell precursors from the marrow pass through the thymus. They rearrange the four *TCR* genes (alpha, beta, gamma, and delta) and eventually express either alpha/beta or gamma/delta heterodimeric TCRs on their surface.
  - T-cells are selected for their ability to recognize antigenic peptides in the context of self-MHC antigens ("MHC restriction"). This "positive selection" is followed by a "negative selection" in which T-cells with strong interaction with self-MHC or self-antigens are eliminated.
  - Mature T-cells constantly recirculate through blood, lymphoid organs, and tissues to ensure the presence of appropriately reactive T-cells at the site of an immune reaction. T-cells are also concentrated in peripheral lymphoid organs to provide help in the "germinal center reaction" of antigen-activated B-cells.

6. What is an "immunophenotype"? How is it determined in hematopathology?

The immunophenotype, also called "immunoprofile" or simply "phenotype," is a descriptive list of antigens expressed by a uniform population of normal or abnormal cells. These antigens are predominantly cell surface molecules, but others are present in the cytoplasm and/or nucleus.

Two methods are used to determine the immunophenotype in diagnostic hematopathology—flow cytometry and immunohistochemistry.

• Flow cytometry: Antibodies conjugated to a fluorescent molecule are used to examine the presence or absence of the corresponding antigen on fresh (unfixed) cells in suspension using light scatter and fluorescence emitted by these "stained" cells. Modern clinical flow cytometry is multiparametric, allowing simultaneous evaluation of multiple antigens on each of the thousands of cells analyzed. Flow cytometers also provide an estimation of cell size and cytoplasmic complexity for each cell. Data analysis software permits accurate identification of cell populations and subpopulations from a complex mixture of cells.
• Immunohistochemistry (IHC): Antibodies conjugated to enzymes are used to identify the presence of the corresponding antigen in various cellular components of a tissue section. Unlike flow cytometry, IHC can be performed on formalin-fixed paraffin-embedded (FFPE) sections of tissues. Double (and more recently three to five) stains with two (or more) different enzyme-antibody conjugates can be helpful in situations with limited tissue, such as fine needle aspiration biopsies.
• See Table 1.1 for a comparison of pros and cons of the two methods used for immunophenotyping.
• Questions 11 to 18 provide more details about the typical immunophenotypes observed in various types of hematologic and lymphoid neoplasms and how to distinguish them from normal counterparts.

7. What is the immunophenotype of myeloid and lymphoid cells at various stages in maturation?

• Both the myeloid and lymphoid cell lineages arise from hematopoietic stem cells (HSCs) normally resident only in the bone marrow in adults.
• Normally in adults, the myeloid lineages (granulocytes, monocytes, red blood cells, and megakaryocytes) develop entirely within the bone marrow. The most immature cells committed to each of these myeloid lineages can be identified by their morphology and immunophenotype as myeloblasts, monoblasts, proerythroblasts, and megakaryoblasts, respectively. Each lineage matures through various intermediate stages which are best characterized cytologically.
• The immunophenotype of the various immature and mature cells in these lineages is summarized below [23]:
• Myeloid lineage.
  - Myeloblasts express CD34, CD117, CD13, and HLA-DR on their surface. CD33 expression is usually

Table 1.1 Comparative advantages and disadvantages of flow cytometry and immunohistochemistry as phenotyping methods

	Flow cytometry	Immunohistochemistry
Advantages	Higher sensitivity (~2–3 logs better than IHC) Easy to quantify Multiple antigens evaluated on each cell Wider array of antibodies available Rapid analysis High sensitivity and specificity to detect abnormal populations mixed with normal population of similar cells	Can be performed on FFPE[a] tissue Tissue architecture intact Cytoplasmic and nuclear antigens equally accessible and cellular localization of stain verifiable Antibodies can be selected after evaluating histology and other results Routine light microscopic readout, no special equipment
Disadvantages	Requires fresh tissue Viability lost rapidly in some cells (e.g., plasma cells) A suitable sample may not be obtainable due to pathological changes (fibrosis, necrosis, etc.) Specialized equipment and expertise needed Usually a large antibody panel tested with high cost The antibody panel must be selected based largely on clinical suspicion Evaluation of cytoplasmic antigens requires cellular permeabilization, which may cause cell loss Impossible to ascertain subcellular localization (cytoplasmic versus nuclear)	Routinely only single antibody (or at most 2 antibodies) tested per section Not suitable to identify very small number of phenotypically abnormal cells without morphological atypia Fewer antibodies available than for flow cytometry Difficult to quantify

[a]Formalin-fixed, paraffin-embedded

dim, and cytoplasmic myeloperoxidase is often negative. As the myeloid lineage matures, there is sequential loss of CD34, followed by CD117 and HLA-DR. Concurrently, sequential gain of CD15, CD11b, and CD16 expression occurs from promyelocyte to myelocyte to metamyelocyte. CD13 expression follows a biphasic pattern: becomes dim in myelocytes and then is regained later in maturation. Myeloperoxidase is expressed throughout myeloid differentiation.

  - Monoblasts have a similar expression pattern to myeloblasts but are always negative for myeloperoxidase and express dim CD4. Maturing monocytes gain CD64 and CD11b and then CD14.
  - Proerythroblasts express CD117 and dim CD235a (glycophorin A). During further maturation they lose CD117, increase CD235a expression, and gain hemoglobin and CD71.
  - Megakaryoblasts express dim CD41 and CD61 but are negative for CD42. They increase expression of CD41 and CD61 and gain expression of CD42, as megakaryocytes mature.
- T-cells acquire antigens in an orderly fashion during development.
  - The earliest T-cell precursors (pro-T-cells), which migrate from the bone marrow to the thymic cortex, express CD2, CD7, and CD34, but do not express CD3, CD4, CD5, or CD8.
  - Alpha/beta pre-T-cells in the thymic cortex express TdT, cytoplasmic (but not surface) CD3, as well as CD1a, CD5, and both CD4 and CD8.
  - Medullary pre-T-cells then express either CD4 or CD8 and typically lose expression of CD1a.
  - Mature alpha/beta T-cells express surface CD3 and either CD4 or CD8, and do not express TdT or CD1a.
- As with T-cells, B-cells acquire antigens in an orderly fashion during development:
  - Pro-B-cells express CD19, CD22, CD79a, CD34, CD38, and TdT but do not express CD10.
  - Pre-B-cells acquire CD10.
  - TdT and CD34 expression is lost in further maturation, and cytoplasmic mu heavy chain expression is detected.
  - Finally, CD10 and CD38 expression is lost, while CD20 expression begins along with cell surface expression of fully assembled immunoglobulins M and D along with kappa or lambda light chains, creating the mature naïve B-cells. Some naïve B-cells (called B1 cells) show dim CD5 expression.
  - Germinal center B-cells lose expression of IgD and regain expression of CD10.
  - Post-germinal center B-cells (marginal zone, memory, plasma cells) do not express CD10 (Table 1.2).

8. What is the role of immunophenotyping in the classification of acute leukemias? (See also Chap. 21)

- In the latest WHO classification (2017 revision), acute myeloid leukemia (AML) is classified into prognostically and therapeutically relevant categories based on specific cytogenetic and molecular abnormalities, the presence of dysplasia, and a history of prior chemo- or

Table 1.2 Common antigens evaluated in hematopathology

Antigen	Expressed on
CD1a	Cortical thymocytes, Langerhans cells
CD2	T-cells NK-cells
CD3	T-cells (surface)a; pre-T cells (cytoplasmic), NK-cells
CD4	Subset of T-cells (strong); monocytes/macrophages (weak)
CD5	T-cells (strong), mantle zone B-cells (weak)
CD8	Subset of T-cells
CD7	T-cells, NK-cells
CD10	Pre-B cells, germinal center B-cells, mature neutrophils
CD13	Neutrophils and monocytes
CD14	Mature monocytes [a]
CD15	More mature myeloid precursors, monocytes
CD16	NK-cells, Neutrophils, subset of monocytes
CD19	B-cells,[a] reactive plasma cells
CD20	Mature B-cells
CD33	Neutrophils and precursors (weak), monocytes (strong), basophils (weak)
CD34	Hematopoietic stem cells, myeloblasts, monoblasts, pro-B cells, pro-T cells.
CD38	Plasma cells, hematogones, subset of B-cells.
CD41	Megakaryocytes and platelets
CD56	NK-cells, small subset of T-cells
CD61	Megakaryocytes and platelets
CD64	Monocytes
CD71	Erythroid precursors, dividing lymphocytes
CD79a	B-cells, plasma cells.
CD117	Myeloblasts/promyelocytes, early stages of erythroid maturation, mast cells.
CD123	Basophils, blasts, plasmacytoid dendritic cells
CD138	Plasma cells, many epithelial cells
CD235a (glycophorin A)	Erythroid precursors (increased expression with maturation)
E-cadherin	Erythroid precursors (decreased expression with maturation)
HLA-DR	B-cells, myeloblasts, monoblasts, mature monocytes/macrophages, activated neutrophils and T-cells.
Myeloperoxidase	Myeloid lineage (neutrophils)a
PAX5	B-cells except plasma cells
TdT	Immature B and T cells.

Color coding to emphasize major cell types
[a]Lineage defining

radiation therapy. When none of the above conditions are present, which occurs in 30–40% of newly diagnosed cases, the AML is designated as AML-NOS. Morphologic and phenotypic characteristics are used for further subtyping these AML cases analogous to the categories in the earlier French-American-British (FAB) classification [24, 25]. See Table 1.3 for the most important distinguishing features of subtypes of AML-NOS.

- B-lymphoblastic leukemia is also typically classified according to cytogenetics or molecular abnormalities but may also be divided into morphologic/phenotypic subsets [23]. See Table 1.4 for the phenotypic features of each subset.
- T-lymphoblastic leukemia may also be divided into phenotypic subtypes (see Table 1.5) [23].
- These morphologically and phenotypically defined subcategories in the acute leukemias appear to have limited prognostic significance, and the primary clinical value in subclassifying these cases is to:
  - Distinguish AML from ALL and between B- and T-ALL
  - Alert the fluorescence in situ hybridization (FISH) lab if acute promyelocytic leukemia (APML) is suspected based on the immunophenotype

Table 1.3 Key immunophenotypic features of different categories of acute myeloid leukemia without recurrent genetic abnormalities

WHO 2017	FAB	Key immunophenotypic features
AML with minimal differentiation	M0	<3% of blasts are positive for myeloid or monocytic markers (myeloperoxidase (MPO), Sudan black B (SBB), or chloroacetate esterase (CAE)). By flow cytometry, blasts express at least two myeloid markers, do not show evidence of monocytic differentiation and are negative for cytoplasmic lymphoid markers (cCD3, cCD79a, and cCD22)
AML without maturation	M1	<10% of nucleated bone marrow cells are maturing myeloid precursors and > 3% of blasts positive for MPO or SBB (or Auer rods identified)
AML with maturation	M2	≥10% of nucleated bone marrow cells are maturing myeloid precursors
Acute myelomonocytic leukemia	M4	Maturing myeloid and monocytic cells each account for ≥20% of bone marrow nucleated cells
Acute monoblastic leukemia	M5a	≥20% of blasts/promonocytes, ≥80% of leukemic cells are of monocytic lineage, ≥80% of leukemic cells are monoblasts
Acute monocytic leukemia	M5b	Similar to M5a but most of the leukemic cells are promonocytes or monocytes
Pure erythroid leukemia	M6b	>80% of bone marrow cells are erythroid with ≥30% of proerythroblasts
Acute megakaryoblastic leukemia	M7	Blasts negative for MPO and monocytic markers, positive for at least one megakaryocytic marker (CD41, CD61, CD42b)

Table 1.4 Key immunophenotypic features in major categories of B-ALL without recurrent genetic abnormalities

Category	Positive markers	Negative markers
Early precursor/pro-B-ALL	CD19, cytoplasmic CD79a, cytoplasmic CD22, TdT	CD10
Intermediate stage/"common" B-ALL	As above, plus CD10	N/A
Precursor/pre-B-ALL	As above, plus cytoplasmic mu chain	N/A
Transitional pre-B-ALL	As above, plus surface heavy chain	N/A

Table 1.5 Key immunophenotypic features in various categories of T-lymphoblastic leukemia/lymphoma

Category	Positive markers	Negative markers
Early T-cell precursor ALL	One or more myeloid/stem cell markers (CD34, CD117, HLA-DR, CD13, CD33, CD11b) Cytoplasmic or rarely surface CD3	CD5 (or positive on <75% of blasts), MPO
Cortical	CD4, CD8, CD1a (analogous to normal cortical thymocytes)	N/A
Medullary	CD4 or CD8 (analogous to normal medullary thymocytes)	CD8 or CD4

  - Identify cases of acute leukemia with ambiguous lineage
  - Provide a detailed immunophenotype of leukemic cells, as a reference for future possible analyses of minimal residual disease

9. How are the compartments of the immune system and normal lymphoid architecture related to the classification of lymphomas?

- Most common B-cell neoplasms can be correlated to the pattern of maturation of B-cells in the bone marrow and lymphoid tissue (Fig. 1.1) [23, 26].
  - B-lymphoblastic leukemia/lymphoma arises from B-cell precursors in the bone marrow, which is reflected in its usual phenotype: the immunoglobulin genes are typically clonally rearranged, but surface immunoglobulins are not yet expressed.
  - Mantle cell lymphoma and a subset of chronic lymphocytic leukemia/small lymphocytic lymphoma arise from mature, naïve B-cells that are found circulating in the peripheral blood, as well as in primary follicles and germinal center mantle zones. This is reflected in their expression of CD5 and in their unmutated immunoglobulin heavy chain variable (IGV) regions.
  - Many lymphomas arise from cells undergoing the germinal center reaction, which is reflected in their IGV somatic hypermutation and expression of germinal center markers: CD10 and BCL6. These include follicular lymphoma, Burkitt lymphoma, and the germinal center B-cell subtype of diffuse large B-cell lymphoma. Hodgkin lymphomas also fall under this category despite their unusual immunophenotype.
  - Post-germinal center memory B-cells are negative for CD10 and BCL6 and express IRF4/MUM1. They also home to sites of antigen stimulation, such as mucosa-associated lymphoid tissue and the spleen, as well as to the germinal center marginal zones of the lymph node. Marginal zone lymphomas (all types), lymphoplasmacytic lymphoma, the activated B-cell subtype of diffuse large B-cell lymphoma, and the IGV hypermutated subset of CLL/SLL fall under this category.
  - Plasma cells express IRF4/MUM1 but also CD138 and lack expression of surface immunoglobulins and CD20. Plasma cell neoplasms (monoclonal gammopathy of undetermined significance, plasma cell myeloma, plasmacytoma) arise from these cells.
- T-cell lymphomas have a similar relationship to normal T-cell distribution and development.
  - T-lymphoblastic lymphoma/leukemia arises from progenitor T-cells in the bone marrow or immature T-cells in the thymus, as reflected in their immunophenotype (lacking surface CD3 in most cases and expressing CD4 and/or CD8 in a pattern reflective of the stage of

Fig. 1.1 Putative origin of B-cell neoplasms. Stages of B-cell differentiation from which specific lymphoid tumors may emerge are shown

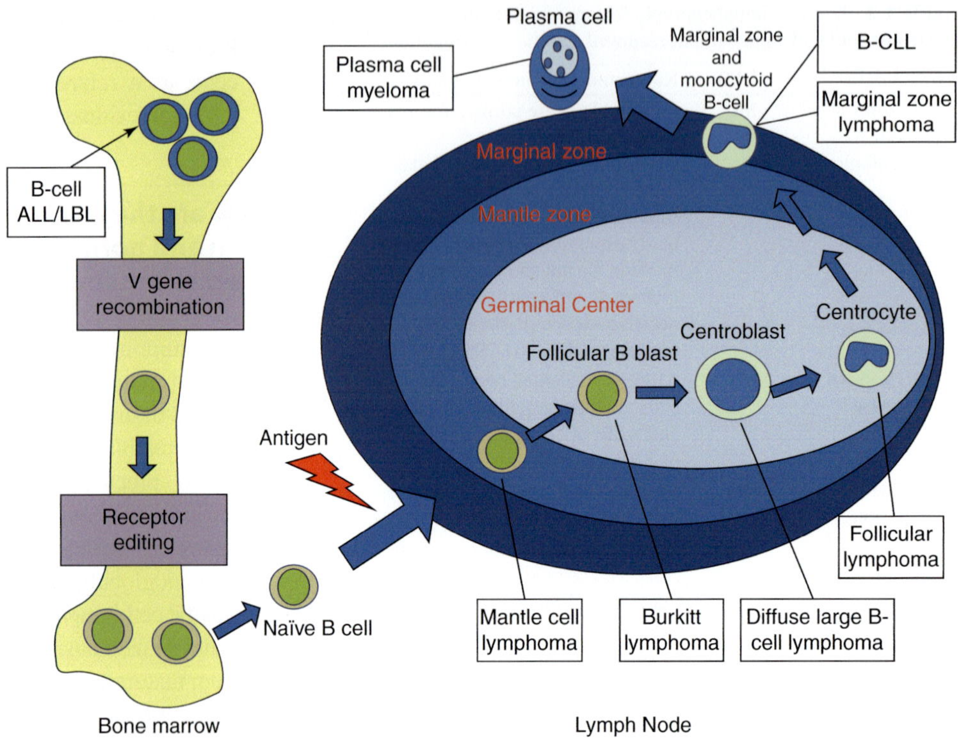

T-cell development from which they arose) (see Question 5).

- Lymphomas arising from cells of the innate immune system (NK-cells and gamma/delta T-cells) have a predominantly extranodal distribution. NK-cell lymphomas have a predilection for the sinonasal tract (extranodal NK/T-cell lymphoma, nasal type), liver, spleen, and bone marrow (aggressive NK-cell leukemia). Gamma/delta T-cells are normally involved predominantly in mucosal/epithelial defense, and their corresponding lymphomas have a similar distribution (intestinal epithelium, skin, and liver/spleen).
- Alpha/beta (adaptive immune system) T-cell lymphomas reflect the nodal origin of these cells. Some T-cell lymphomas arise from specific subsets of alpha/beta T-cells. Angioimmunoblastic T-cell lymphoma, for instance, arises from T-follicular helper (TFH) cells, which function within germinal centers, reflected in its phenotype. Adult T-cell leukemia/lymphoma (ATLL) arises from regulatory T-cells (Tregs), which dampen the immune response, which may explain the unusual immunosuppression seen in this disease [26].

10. How can immunohistochemistry be used optimally for diagnosis and differential diagnosis in hematopathology?

- Diagnosis based on limited tissue biopsies requires careful utilization of available material. A careful differential diagnosis based on H&E morphology, cytology, and clinical and ancillary findings is absolutely essential in such cases. Judicious use of double staining techniques (e.g., combined CD3 and CD20), performing stains in steps and choosing subsequent stains on first results, as well as preparing sufficient unstained sections to avoid refacing the tissue blocks repeatedly are helpful (see also Chap. 4).
- Development of panels of immunohistochemical stains for common differential diagnoses can aid in reaching the final diagnosis in a cost-effective and expeditious manner. Examples of such panels are given in Table 1.6.

11. How can a panel of antibodies be used to differentiate among the common B-cell neoplasms?

- All lymphomas are clonal proliferations. In case of most mature B-cell lymphomas expressing surface immunoglobulins, this monoclonality is translated into monotypic expression of kappa *or* lambda immunoglobulin light chain. This is due to the molecular phenomenon of allelic exclusion described in Question 5. Consequently, all cells comprising a mature B-cell lymphoma express the same immunoglobulin light chain, while a reactive lymphoid infiltrate typically shows a mixture of kappa-positive and lambda-positive B-cells, with a ratio of about 2:1 in favor of kappa-expressing cells.
- In general, the phenotype of neoplastic B-cells resembles that of a specific stage of normal lymphocyte differentiation (see Question 9), which is exploited by

utilizing a combination of immunohistochemical stains, flow cytometric analysis, fluorescence in situ hybridization (FISH), and molecular analysis in both the diagnosis and classification of B-cell lymphomas (Fig. 1.1) [26].
- Additionally, certain B-cell neoplasms also demonstrate aberrant expression of specific markers which may reflect disease-defining translocations. For example, immunohistochemical staining for cyclin D1/BCL-1 is present in >95% of cases of mantle cell lymphoma due to the characteristic t(11;14)(q13;q32) translocation between an *IgH* gene and *CCND1* (encoding cyclin D1) [28].
- Table 1.7 lists the common B-cell neoplasms and their immunophenotypic profiles.

Table 1.6 Example of immunohistochemical stain panels for common hematologic malignancy indications

Differential diagnosis or indication	Stains
Reactive follicular hyperplasia versus follicular lymphoma	CD3, CD20, CD10, BCL6, BCL2, Ki-67
Small and mature B-cell lymphomas	CD3, CD20, CD5, CD10, CD23, cyclin D1, Ki-67
Subtyping and prognosis of diffuse large B-cell lymphoma	CD10, BCL6, MUM1, Ki-67, BCL2, MYC, consider CD5, and *EBV*
Limited tissue with possible lymphoma	1. CD3, CD20, Ki-67 2. Additional stains as needed to refine classification
Bone marrow plasmacytosis	CD138, kappa, lambda, CD56, cyclin D1
Bone marrow myeloid neoplasm without adequate bone marrow aspirate	CD34, CD117, E-cadherin, CD71 or glycophorin A, myeloperoxidase
Peripheral T-cell lymphoma subtypes	CD3, CD2, CD4, CD5, CD7, CD8, PD1, CD10, BCL6, CXCL13, CD20, CD21, *EBV*

12. How can a panel of antibodies be used to differentiate among the common T-cell neoplasms?

- As with B-cell neoplasms, the phenotype of the neoplastic T-cells also resembles that of a specific stage of normal lymphocyte differentiation and can be used to diagnose and classify T-cell lymphomas [23].
- T-cell neoplasms are generally defined as clonal proliferations of morphologically and immunophenotypically mature T-cells of either helper (CD4+) or cytotoxic/suppressor (CD8+) type. However, in contrast to B-cell neoplasms in which analysis of surface immunoglobulins can determine clonality, no such corresponding flow cytometric marker of T-cell clonality is yet in routine clinical use. Therefore, the identification of T-cell neoplasms requires using a broad panel of antibodies/markers.
- Criteria that are helpful in the diagnosis of T-cell neoplasms include T-cell subset antigen restriction, aberrant T-cell subset antigen expression, loss or attenuation of one of the pan T-cell antigens, or expression of additional markers.
- However, correlation with morphologic features, clinical and laboratory data, and molecular studies for T-cell receptor gene rearrangement [30] are often required to establish the diagnosis.

13. How can a basic panel of antibodies be used to distinguish common neoplasms from reactive lymphoid hyperplasia?

- Activation of immune cells via antigenic stimulation causes morphologic changes which are fairly predictable depending on the particular stimulus. The most common reactive patterns seen include follicular and/or paracortical hyperplasia, which are caused by activation of the humoral immune response and T-cell-mediated immune response, respectively.

Table 1.7 Classic immunophenotypic profile of common B-cell neoplasms

Disorder	sIg	CD19	CD20	CD22	CD5	CD10	CD23	FMC-7	Cyclin D1	Annexin A1
CLL/SLL	w	+	w	w	+	–	+	–	–	–
B-PLL	+	+	+	+	v	–	–/w	+	–	–
MCL	+	+	+	+	+	–	–/w	+	+	–
FL	+	+	+	+	–	+	v	+	–	–
SMZL	+	+	+	+	v	v	–/w	+	–	–
HCL	+	+	+	+	–	+s	–/w	+	+s	+
LPL	v, cIg+	+	+	+	–	–	–	–	–	–

Modified from [29]

CLL/SLL chronic lymphocytic leukemia/small lymphocytic lymphoma, *B-PLL* B-cell prolymphocytic leukemia, *MCL* mantle cell lymphoma, *FL* follicular lymphoma, *SMZL* splenic marginal zone lymphoma, *HCL* hairy cell leukemia, *LPL* lymphoplasmacytic lymphoma

v variable expression, *w* weakly expressed, *+s* subset of cases positive

- Depending on the size of the submitted tissue (needle core biopsy or excisional lymph node biopsy), availability of flow cytometry analysis, and which architectural and/or cytological features deviate from a "normal" lymph node, immunohistochemical stains can be performed to aid in the distinction. A small panel of antibodies (CD3, CD20, CD10, CD21/CD23, BCL2, and Ki-67) is often helpful, or only selected antibodies can be used to address specific concerns. See Chap. 4 for special considerations for diagnosis of lymphomas in limited tissue biopsies and Chap. 18 for distinguishing features of reactive lymphoid hyperplasia and lymphoma.

14. How does the immunophenotype of normal thymus differ from T-lymphoblastic leukemia/lymphoma?

- T-acute lymphoblastic leukemia/ lymphoma (T-ALL), normal thymic lymphocytes, and lymphocytes in thymomas can show the same immature T-cell phenotype. Differentiating either normal thymus or thymoma from T-ALL can be challenging and requires careful review of the immunophenotype obtained by flow cytometry (e.g., see Fig. 1.2) [31]. On the other hand, detection of immature T-cells (showing simultaneous expression of

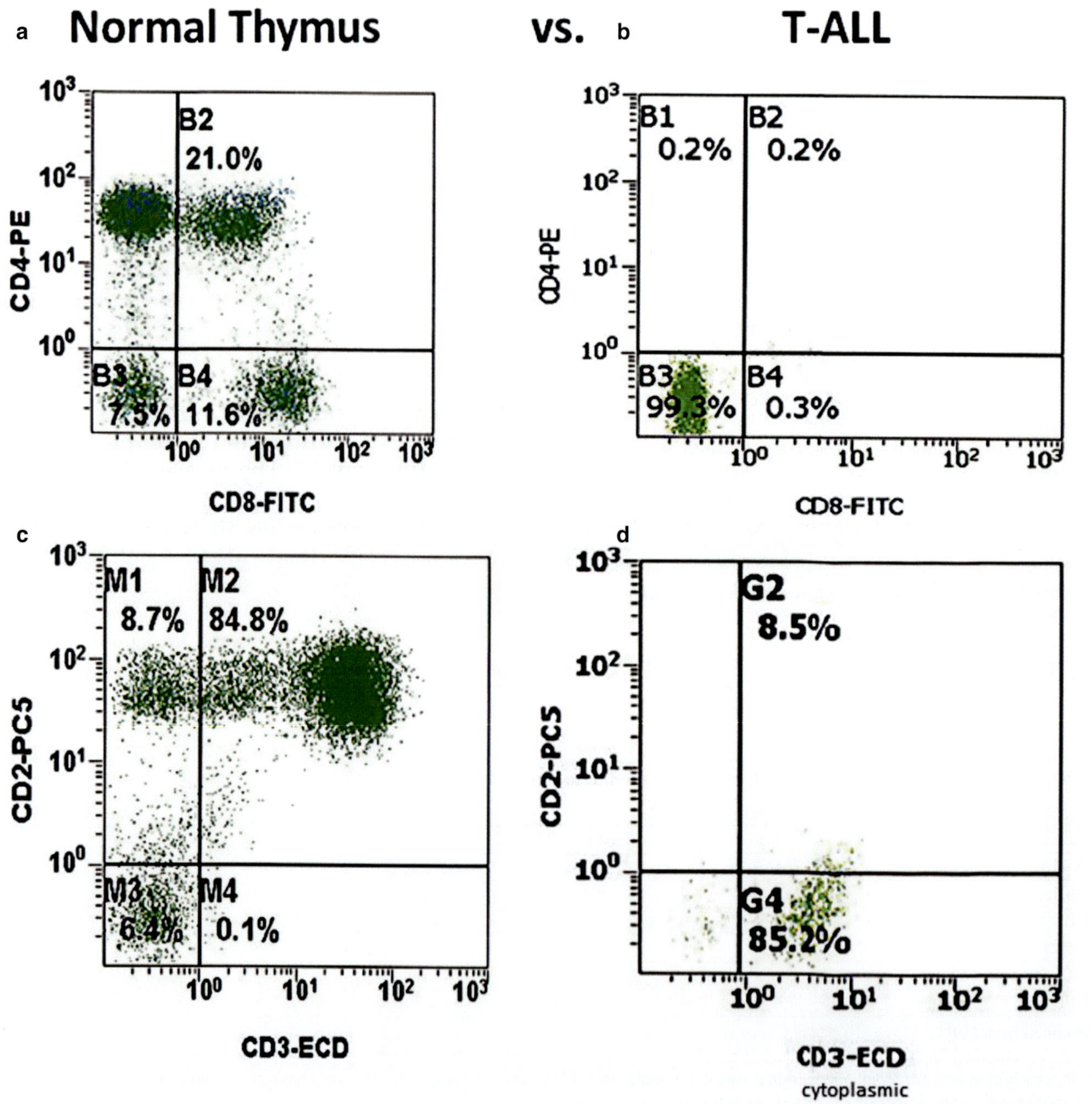

Fig. 1.2 Differentiation of normal and abnormal lymphocytes in thymus: **(a)** Smear pattern of CD4/CD8 characteristic of thymus/thymoma. **(b)** Pre-thymocyte immunophenotype of T-ALL. **(c)** Strong/uniform expression of surface CD3 and CD2 in normal thymus. **(d)** Cytoplasmic expression of CD3 in T-ALL without expression of CD2 (surface CD3 was negative in this case)

terminal deoxynucleotidyl transferase [TdT] and CD3) in the blood or bone marrow is sufficient evidence of disease [32].
- Features characteristic of normal thymus and/or thymoma can include:
  - A heterogeneous pattern of CD3 and TdT expression
  - Lack of pan T-cell antigen deletion (aside from partial CD3 expression)
- Features characteristic of T-ALL:
  - Variable but relatively uniform expression of CD4 or CD8—can be double-negative or double-positive depending on stage of differentiation
  - Significant loss of pan T-cell antigens
  - Absence of a heterogeneous TdT or CD3 pattern

15. How does the immunophenotype of normal B-cell precursors (hematogones) differ from B-lymphoblastic leukemia/lymphoma?

- Hematogones are defined as normal immature B-cells that are a normal component of the bone marrow cell population and are often present in large numbers in healthy infants and young children. Therefore, detecting immature B-cells alone is not sufficient evidence of disease; B-lymphoblasts must be distinguished from normal B-cell progenitors when diagnosing B-lymphoblastic leukemia/lymphoma (B-ALL).
- Hematogones exhibit a typical but complex pattern of antigen expression that follows the normal phenotypic evolution of B-cell precursors and lacks aberrant antigenic expression. In contrast, B-lymphoblasts demonstrate maturational arrest at a certain stage of maturation and exhibit variable number of immunophenotypic aberrancies.
- Markers that are utilized in typical flow cytometric assays for diagnosis and follow-up (minimal residual disease) of B-ALL include CD10, CD19, CD34, CD38, CD58, CD45, and CD9 [32]. Table 1.8 compares the expression patterns of hematogones and abnormal B-lymphoblasts. See case studies in Chap. 31 for examples.

16. Which antibodies are most useful in the analysis of myeloid neoplasms?

- Myeloid neoplasms are divided into four broad categories: (1) acute myeloid leukemias (Chap. 21), (2) myelodysplastic syndromes (Chap. 24), (3) myeloproliferative neoplasms (Chaps. 22 and 23), and myelodysplastic/myeloproliferative neoplasms (Chap. 25).
- The goal of determining the immunophenotype of a suspected myeloid neoplasm is to establish the lineage of neoplastic cells, determine the proportion of blasts, determine if blasts are neoplastic, characterize the blasts for future identification of residual disease after treatment, and investigate if the maturation of various cell lineages is normal or abnormal. The antibodies used are derived from the normal differentiation antigens that appear at various stages of development [23] and can be demonstrated by flow cytometric analysis [33]. See Question 7.
- Identification of a neoplastic process is based upon increased or decreased expression of normal antigens, asynchronous maturational expression, and aberrant antigen expression [33].
- Typically, flow cytometric analysis of a new acute leukemia will include evaluation for the myeloid markers mentioned above to assign a lineage (myeloid, monocytic, megakaryocytic, etc.) and evaluate for asynchronous antigen expression [34], abnormal intensity of normally expressed antigens [35], or lineage infidelity (cross-lineage antigen expression) as compared to normally developing myeloid blasts (Fig. 1.3) [34].
- Multiparameter flow cytometric immunophenotyping in cases of suspected myelodysplastic syndrome can be informative where morphology and cytogenetics are indeterminate [36]. Expression patterns of various antigen combinations on maturing bone marrow subpopulations of myeloid, monocytic, and erythroid precursors which deviate from normal appear to correlate with myelodysplasia [37].
  - Common abnormalities that may be seen in MDS include abnormal intensity of normally expressed antigens (CD34, CD117, and HLA-DR), aberrant antigen expression (CD7 or CD56), or abnormal patterns of expression on granulocytes and monocytes (CD13, CD14, CD15, and CD16) [38]. However, due to lack of a consensus method of analysis and agreement about the minimum number and nature of abnormalities required for diagnosis of MDS, flow cytometry is not considered essential in the workup of MDS.

Table 1.8 Immunophenotype of hematogones versus malignant B-lymphoblasts

Antibody	Hematogones	B-lymphoblasts
CD19	Normal expression	Variable, often brightly positive
CD10	More immature forms have brighter CD10; more mature forms have moderate CD10	Lack a maturational pattern; often uniformly bright expression
CD20	Early hematogones are CD20 negative	Negative or variable more often than bright
TdT	Positive	Positive
CD34	Lose CD34 as they mature	Lack maturational pattern if positive
CD58	Variable, lower intensity	Frequently overexpressed, higher intensity with narrow, prominent peak
CD38	Heterogeneous	Abnormally underexpressed

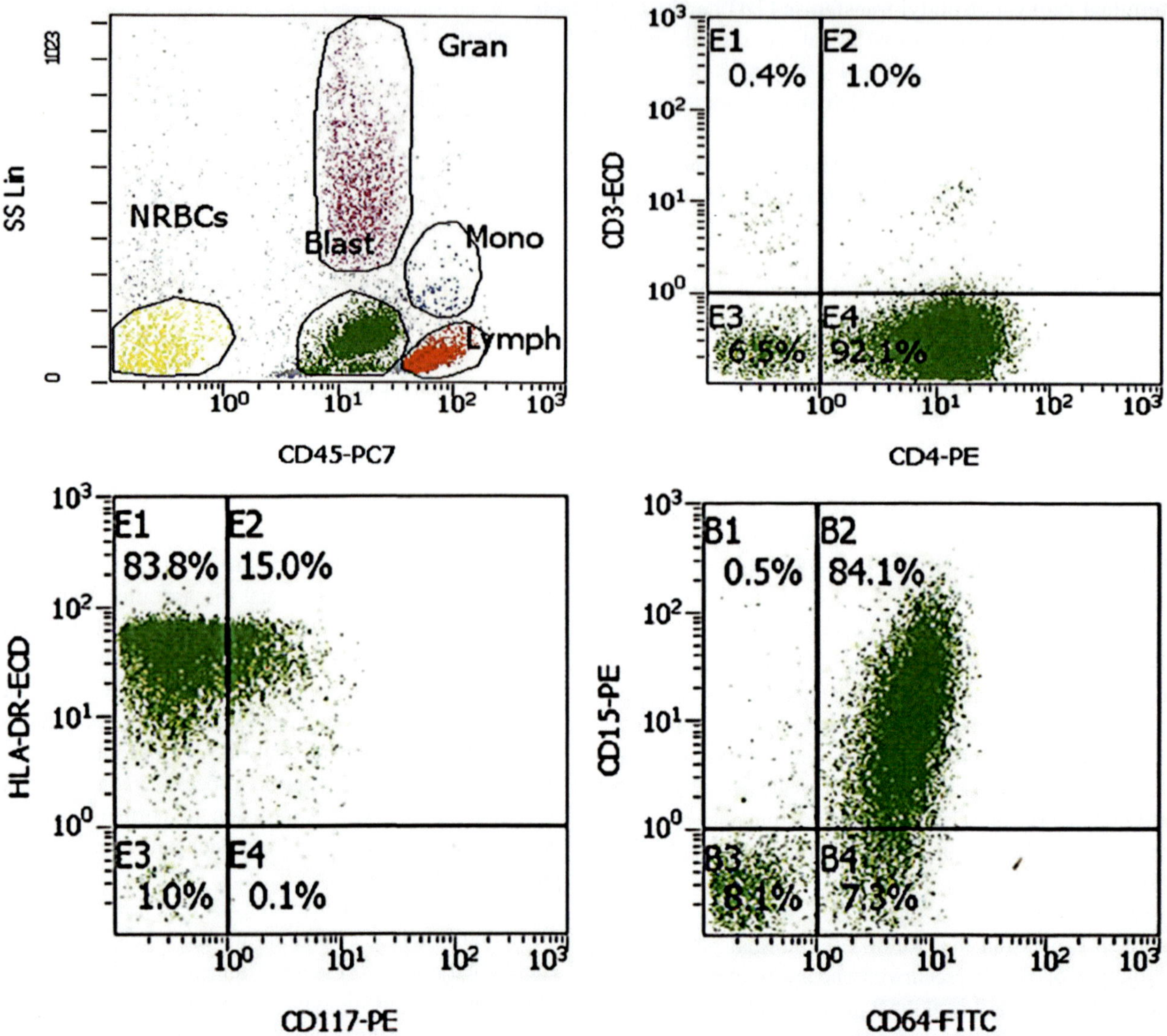

Fig. 1.3 Acute leukemia. The neoplastic population is identified in green; maturing granulocytes are pink, and lymphocytes are red. In this example, there is aberrant expression of both CD4 and CD64 indicating monocytic differentiation

17. How are antigens expressed by various lymphoid and myeloid malignancies being targeted by immune-based therapies?

- Many novel treatments for hematologic malignancies target antigens on the cell surface of these malignancies; therefore, understanding and properly reporting the status of these antigens is essential for optimal therapeutic management.
- The mechanisms of action of these therapies include:
  - Direct induction of apoptosis
  - Complement-mediated cytotoxicity
  - Antibody-dependent, cell-mediated cytotoxicity (ADCC)
  - Delivery of conjugated cytotoxic drugs
  - Direct recruitment of cytotoxic T-cells
  - Release from immune checkpoint inhibition
- Table 1.9 lists the currently available immune-based therapies, their target antigens, and likely mechanisms of action.

Table 1.9 Common immune-based therapies used in treatment of hematologic malignancies

Antigen	Therapy	Mechanism(s) of action
CD20	Rituximab [39]	CDC, direct apoptosis, ADCC
	Ocrelizumab [40]	ADCC, direct apoptosis, CDC
	Obinutuzumab [40]	Direct apoptosis, ADCC, CDC
CD19	Blinatumomab [41]	BiTE
	CAR-T-cells	Direct cytotoxicity
CD22	Inotuzumab ozogamicin [41]	Delivery of cytotoxin
CD30	Brentuximab vedotin [41]	Delivery of cytotoxin
CD38	Daratumumab [42]	ADCC, CDC
CD52	Alemtuzumab [41]	ADCC
CD33	Gemtuzumab ozogamicin [43]	Delivery of cytotoxin
PD1	Pembrolizumab [44]	Immune checkpoint inhibition
SLAMF7 (CD319)	Elotuzumab [45]	Immune checkpoint inhibition

CDC complement-dependent cytotoxicity, *ADCC* antibody-dependent, cellular-mediated cytotoxicity, *BiTE* bi-specific T-cell engagement, *CAR-T* chimeric antigen receptor T-cells

References

1. Stephen B, Hajjar J. Overview of basic immunology for clinical investigators. Adv Exp Med Biol. 2017;995:1–31.
2. Schenten D, Medzhitov R. The control of adaptive immune responses by the innate immune system. Adv Immunol. 2011;109:87–124.
3. McCoy KD, Ronchi F, Geuking MB. Host-microbiota interactions and adaptive immunity. Immunol Rev. 2017;279(1):63–9.
4. Natarajan K, Jiang J, May NA, Mage MG, Boyd LF, McShan AC, et al. The role of molecular flexibility in antigen presentation and T cell receptor-mediated signaling. Front Immunol. 2018;9:1657.
5. Klein L, Kyewski B, Allen PM, Hogquist KA. Positive and negative selection of the T cell repertoire: what thymocytes see (and don't see). Nat Rev Immunol. 2014;14(6):377–91.
6. Wang Y, Singh NK, Spear TT, Hellman LM, Piepenbrink KH, McMahan RH, et al. How an alloreactive T-cell receptor achieves peptide and MHC specificity. Proc Natl Acad Sci U S A. 2017;114(24):E4792–E801.
7. Dare R, Sykes PJ, Morley AA, Brisco MJ. Effect of age on the repertoire of cytotoxic memory (CD8+CD45RO+) T cells in peripheral blood: the use of rearranged T cell receptor gamma genes as clonal markers. J Immunol Methods. 2006;308(1–2):1–12.
8. De Libero G, Mori L. Recognition of lipid antigens by T cells. Nat Rev Immunol. 2005;5(6):485–96.
9. Singhal A, Mori L. De Libero G. T cell recognition of non-peptidic antigens in infectious diseases. Indian J Med Res. 2013;138(5):620–31.
10. den Haan JM, Arens R, van Zelm MC. The activation of the adaptive immune system: cross-talk between antigen-presenting cells, T cells and B cells. Immunol Lett. 2014;162(2 Pt B):103–12.
11. Degauque N, Brosseau C, Brouard S. Regulation of the immune response by the inflammatory metabolic microenvironment in the context of allotransplantation. Front Immunol. 2018;9:1465.
12. Heinzel S, Marchingo JM, Horton MB, Hodgkin PD. The regulation of lymphocyte activation and proliferation. Curr Opin Immunol. 2018;51:32–8.
13. Seda V, Mraz M. B-cell receptor signalling and its crosstalk with other pathways in normal and malignant cells. Eur J Haematol. 2015;94(3):193–205.
14. Gell PGH, Cooms RRA. The classification of allergic reactions underlying disease. Clinical aspects of immunology. Oxford: Blackwell; 1963.
15. Sell S. Immunopathology of experimental models of syphilis, influenza, and asthma. Immunopathol Dis Therap. 2016;7(3–4):225–36.
16. Uzzaman A, Cho SH. Chapter 28: classification of hypersensitivity reactions. Allergy Asthma Proc. 2012;33(Suppl 1):96–9.
17. Hayter SM, Cook MC. Updated assessment of the prevalence, spectrum and case definition of autoimmune disease. Autoimmun Rev. 2012;11(10):754–65.
18. Chen B, Sun L, Zhang X. Integration of microbiome and epigenome to decipher the pathogenesis of autoimmune diseases. J Autoimmun. 2017;83:31–42.
19. Al-Herz W, Bousfiha A, Casanova JL, Chatila T, Conley ME, Cunningham-Rundles C, et al. Primary immunodeficiency diseases: an update on the classification from the international union of immunological societies expert committee for primary immunodeficiency. Front Immunol. 2014;5:162.
20. Azizi G, Pouyani MR, Abolhassani H, Sharifi L, Dizaji MZ, Mohammadi J, et al. Cellular and molecular mechanisms of immune dysregulation and autoimmunity. Cell Immunol. 2016;310:14–26.
21. Epeldegui M, Vendrame E, Martinez-Maza O. HIV-associated immune dysfunction and viral infection: role in the pathogenesis of AIDS-related lymphoma. Immunol Res. 2010;48(1–3):72–83.
22. Shaw AC, Goldstein DR, Montgomery RR. Age-dependent dysregulation of innate immunity. Nat Rev Immunol. 2013;13(12):875–87.
23. WHO Classification of Tumours of Haematopoietic and Lymphoid Tissues. Revised 4th ed. Lyon: International Agency for Research on Cancer; 2017.
24. Bennett JM, Catovsky D, Daniel MT, Flandrin G, Galton DA, Gralnick HR, et al. Proposals for the classification of the acute leukaemias. French-American-British (FAB) co-operative group. Br J Haematol. 1976;33(4):451–8.
25. Bene MC, Castoldi G, Knapp W, Ludwig WD, Matutes E, Orfao A, et al. Proposals for the immunological classification of acute leukemias. European Group for the Immunological Characterization of Leukemias (EGIL). Leukemia. 1995;9(10):1783–6.
26. Robbins SL, Kumar V. Robbins and Cotran pathologic basis of disease. 8th ed. Philadelphia: Saunders/Elsevier; 2010.
27. Karube K, Ohshima K, Tsuchiya T, Yamaguchi T, Kawano R, Suzumiya J, et al. Expression of FoxP3, a key molecule in CD4CD25 regulatory T cells, in adult T-cell leukaemia/lymphoma cells. Br J Haematol. 2004;126(1):81–4.
28. Wang Y, Li Q, Zhu L, Mao X, Zhang H, Huang L, et al. Cytogenetics with flow cytometry in lymph node/extranodal tissue biopsies is sensitive to assist the early diagnosis of suspected lymphomas. Ann Hematol. 2017;96(10):1673–80.
29. Foucar K, Reichard K, Czuchlewski D. Bone marrow pathology. 3rd ed. Chicago: ASCP Press; 2010.

30. Gorczyca W, Weisberger J, Liu Z, Tsang P, Hossein M, Wu CD, et al. An approach to diagnosis of T-cell lymphoproliferative disorders by flow cytometry. Cytometry. 2002;50(3):177–90.
31. Dunphy CH. American Society for Clinical Pathology. Integrated hematopathology: morphology and FCI with IHC. Chicago: American Society for Clinical Pathology; 2010.
32. Gaipa G, Basso G, Biondi A, Campana D. Detection of minimal residual disease in pediatric acute lymphoblastic leukemia. Cytometry B Clin Cytom. 2013;84(6):359–69.
33. Wood B. Multicolor immunophenotyping: human immune system hematopoiesis. Methods Cell Biol. 2004;75:559–76.
34. Peters JM, Ansari MQ. Multiparameter flow cytometry in the diagnosis and management of acute leukemia. Arch Pathol Lab Med. 2011;135(1):44–54.
35. Wood BL. Flow cytometric monitoring of residual disease in acute leukemia. Methods Mol Biol. 2013;999:123–36.
36. Stetler-Stevenson M, Arthur DC, Jabbour N, Xie XY, Molldrem J, Barrett AJ, et al. Diagnostic utility of flow cytometric immunophenotyping in myelodysplastic syndrome. Blood. 2001;98(4):979–87.
37. Wells DA, Benesch M, Loken MR, Vallejo C, Myerson D, Leisenring WM, et al. Myeloid and monocytic dyspoiesis as determined by flow cytometric scoring in myelodysplastic syndrome correlates with the IPSS and with outcome after hematopoietic stem cell transplantation. Blood. 2003;102(1):394–403.
38. McPherson RA, Pincus MR, Henry JB. Henry's clinical diagnosis and management by laboratory methods. 22nd ed. Philadelphia: Elsevier/Saunders; 2011.
39. Cerny T, Borisch B, Introna M, Johnson P, Rose AL. Mechanism of action of rituximab. Anti-Cancer Drugs. 2002;13(Suppl 2):S3–10.
40. van Meerten T, Hagenbeek A. CD20-targeted therapy: the next generation of antibodies. Semin Hematol. 2010;47(2):199–210.
41. Suresh T, Lee LX, Joshi J, Barta SK. New antibody approaches to lymphoma therapy. J Hematol Oncol. 2014;7:58.
42. Palumbo A, Chanan-Khan A, Weisel K, Nooka AK, Masszi T, Beksac M, et al. Daratumumab, bortezomib, and dexamethasone for multiple myeloma. N Engl J Med. 2016;375(8):754–66.
43. Godwin CD, Gale RP, Walter RB. Gemtuzumab ozogamicin in acute myeloid leukemia. Leukemia. 2017;31(9):1855–68.
44. Hu B, Jacobs R, Ghosh N. Checkpoint inhibitors Hodgkin lymphoma and non-Hodgkin lymphoma. Curr Hematol Malig Rep. 2018;13:543.
45. Radhakrishnan SV, Bhardwaj N, Steinbach M, Weidner J, Luetkens T, Atanackovic D. Elotuzumab as a novel anti-myeloma immunotherapy. Hum Vaccin Immunother. 2017;13(8):1751–7.

Molecular Genetics and Cell Biology for Hematopathology

2

Linsheng Zhang

List of Frequently Asked Questions

1. What is molecular genetics, and why is understanding molecular genetics and cellular biology critical for the pathological diagnosis of lymph node and bone marrow?
2. Why are some molecular features (like *PML-RARA*) used to classify a disease, while others (like *FLT3-ITD* and *TP53*) are not?
3. What is a clonal process, and how is it related to a neoplastic process?
4. What is clonal evolution and how is it related to disease progression?
5. With fluorescence in situ hybridization (FISH) and all the molecular methods including next-generation sequencing (NGS) available in the clinical laboratories, why is chromosome analysis (conventional karyotyping) still necessary?
6. What are the advantages and disadvantages of fluorescence in situ hybridization (FISH) test?
7. If we have conventional karyotyping and FISH test available, is microarray test still useful?
8. What are the typical applications of polymerase chain reaction (PCR)-based tests in the clinical laboratory?
9. What are the indications of conventional sequencing (first-generation Sanger sequencing and pyrosequencing) in the lymph node and bone marrow pathology?
10. Testing for *IGH/BCL2* can be performed by a PCR-based method or a FISH method. Are there any differences in the indications of these two methods?
11. What are the indications of FISH test for *BCR-ABL1* fusion when there is a quantitative PCR test available?
12. How do I choose a method to test for *PML-RARA* when blood smear review suspects acute promyelocytic leukemia?
13. What are the principles of B-cell (immunoglobulin gene) and T-cell (T-cell receptor gene) clonality tests?
14. What are the indications of B-cell (immunoglobulin gene) and T-cell (T-cell receptor gene) clonality tests, and what are the pitfalls in interpreting the test results?
15. Can I use clonal immunoglobulin (Ig) or T-cell receptor (TCR) gene rearrangement as an evidence to prove the B-cell or T-cell lineage of lymphoma?
16. What are the key concepts required to understand the clinical next-generation sequencing (NGS)?
17. What is the benefit of performing clonality test by next-generation sequencing, and when should I consider it for clinical samples?
18. When is a NGS-based mutation profiling test indicated for hematopoietic and lymphoid disorders?
19. What are the limitations of current clinical NGS mutation profiling tests?

1. What is molecular genetics, and why is understanding molecular genetics and cellular biology critical for the pathological diagnosis of lymph node and bone marrow?

- Molecular genetics is the application of molecular methods to study the structure and function of genes, improving our understanding of the genetic basis of biology.
- Due to the complexity of the pathologic processes and our limited knowledge about the fundamental mechanisms leading to tumors of hematopoietic and lymphoid tissues, currently their diagnosis and classification do not always reflect the pathobiology of the diseases, but rather a consensus opinion based on all the information that can be obtained with available clinical and laboratory methods [1]. The cellular and molecular genetic features are of critical importance to provide objective evidence to formulate a final diagnosis and refine the classification.

L. Zhang (✉)
Department of Pathology and Laboratory Medicine, Emory University School of Medicine, Atlanta, GA, USA
e-mail: linsheng.zhang@emory.edu

E. Wang, A. S. Lagoo (eds.), *Practical Lymph Node and Bone Marrow Pathology*, Practical Anatomic Pathology,
https://doi.org/10.1007/978-3-030-32189-5_2

- In daily pathology practice, the approach to lymph node and bone marrow pathology is usually a stepwise workup. Understanding the basic principles used in the classification of hematolymphoid neoplasms facilitates the process in a cost-effective way.
- Molecular methods available for clinical diagnosis have different performance characteristics; the requirements for specimens also vary (Table 2.1). A well-planned approach is critical to save correct sample for appropriate diagnostic tests.

2. Why are some molecular features (like *PML-RARA*) used to classify a disease, while others (like *FLT3-ITD* and *TP53*) are not?

- Currently, the primary principle of classification for hematopoietic and lymphoid neoplasms is the "cell of origin" or corresponding normal counterpart [2]. Therefore the cellular differentiation or phenotype, whenever detectable, defines an entity. When a molecular genetic feature determines or affects the phenotype of the cells harboring the abnormality, the specific abnormality may be used to define a disease entity. The six classes of genes frequently involved in hematopoietic and lymphoid neoplasms and their disease associations are listed in Table 2.2.
- Some genetic abnormalities (e.g., mutations in class 1 and 2 genes in Table 2.2) are present in many entities. Although they may play an important role in disease pathobiology and affect the prognosis, they are not "disease defining" [3–5].
- In recent years, there have been significant advances in developing novel therapeutic agents targeting molecular/genetic abnormalities. Molecular tests are requested to identify the treatment targets regardless whether they change disease classification or not [6].
- As new molecular signatures and markers or new evidence of their clinical significances are discovered and clarified, molecular genetic alterations may become more important in diagnosis or classification [3, 7].

3. What is a clonal process, and how is it related to a neoplastic process?

- A clone refers to a group of cells produced from one ancestor cell. Theoretically, the cell population in one clone is genetically identical.
- In clinical practice, clonality is determined by a unique molecular signature present in all cells tested, for example, a cell population that harbors *TET2* mutation can be practically referred to as a clonal population.

Table 2.1 Comparison of different molecular/genetic methods

Method	Advantages	Disadvantages
Chromosome analysis (conventional karyotyping)	Whole-genome view of genetic alterations Particularly good to detect unknown/unexpected abnormalities	Labor intensive; long turnaround time Need fresh tissue and cell culture Need cell proliferation; less useful for neoplasm with low proliferation index Low sensitivity (routinely 20 cells are examined) Cannot detect alterations <10 Mb
FISH	More sensitive than conventional karyotyping Specific for the targeted abnormalities (deletion, duplication/amplification, translocation) Works for both smear and FFPE Less labor intensive; shorter turnaround time	Only detects alterations covered by the probe design May not always have satisfactory hybridization
CN-SNP array	Broad to whole-genome coverage Detecting small copy number changes Works for both fresh and FFPE tissue	Cannot detect alterations in <20% of alleles Cannot detect balanced translocations
PCR	Sensitive and specific Works for fresh and FFPE tissue Can be multiplexed for a variety of targets Quick turnaround time Can be designed for quantitative test	Need to know the exact target sequence of the abnormal gene for primer design Detects only the abnormalities targeted by the primers Mutation at the primer binding site may cause false-negative result Can be "too sensitive" for clinical purpose
Next-generation sequencing	Broad coverage of many genes and alterations in one test. Excellent sensitivity and specificity Detects unknown/unexpected abnormalities with in the designed scope Has the potential to cover the whole genome and detects all kinds of alterations	Relatively expensive and longer turnaround time Currently only for targeted genes/hotspots in clinical laboratory Not yet suitable for large insertions/deletions Detecting translocation (especially those without fusion RNA product) is challenging

Abbreviations: *FISH* fluorescence in situ hybridization, *FFPE* formalin-fixed paraffin-embedded, *CN-SNP* copy number and single-nucleotide polymorphism, *PCR* polymerase chain reaction

Table 2.2 Types of genetic abnormalities in hematopoietic and lymphoid neoplasms

Types of alteration	Representative genes	Disease association
Receptor signal transduction: proliferation and/or survival advantage; not affecting differentiation	*CALR, FLT3, KIT, RAS, JAK2*	Usually not specific for any entity
Tumor suppressor, apoptosis	*TP53, CDKN2A/B, RB*	Usually not disease specific
Cell differentiation, transcription factors	*PML-RARA, RUNX1, CBFB, MLL, CEBPA, NPM1, GATA2*	Acute myeloid leukemia, defining subclassification
Epigenetic regulators	*ASXL1, BCORL1, EZH2, DNMT3A, IDH1/2, TET2*	MDS, MDS/MPN
RNA spliceosome	*SF3B1, SRSF2, U2AF1, ZRSR2*	MDS, MDS/MPN
Chromosome-level alterations	Multiple genes involved: del(5q)/-5, del(7q)/-7	MDS, other myeloid neoplasms, not very specific

- In lymphoid cells, the clonality is readily recognized by the unique rearrangements of their antigen receptor genes: T-cell receptor genes or immunoglobulin heavy and light chain genes.
- A neoplastic process is usually a clonal process [8]. However, a clonal process does not equal to a neoplastic or malignant process. Some clonal processes have variably low potential of progressing to malignant neoplasm (see next question).

4. What is clonal evolution and how is it related to disease progression?

- A neoplasia tends to contain relatively unstable genome; therefore the clonal process of a neoplasia may evolve and diverge to subclones. A multistep tumorigenesis is widely accepted in cancers of various organs [8].
- Clonal processes with the potential to gradually progress to malignancies have been confirmed in several hematolymphoid neoplasms:
  - Monoclonal gammopathy of undetermined significance (MGUS) in plasma cell neoplasm [9]
  - In situ follicular neoplasia, in situ mantle cell lymphoma (MCL) [10], and monoclonal B-cell lymphocytosis [11, 12] in mature B-cell neoplasms
  - Clonal hematopoiesis of indeterminate potential (CHIP) in myeloid cells [13]
- Molecular genetic tests have the potential to detect clonal diversity in a population of cells based on the different allele frequency of the genetic abnormalities [14]. Next-generation sequencing (NGS) has the ability to reveal multiple genetic alterations with relatively accurate allele frequency, demonstrating the clonal diversity within a neoplastic population [15].
- Follow-up or repeat testings of one disease process at different time points provide information on the clonal evolution [15, 16]. Clonal evolution has been well characterized in leukemia [17].
- Clonal evolution is usually associated with disease progression, with later-stage disease harboring more complex mutations [14, 15].

5. With fluorescence in situ hybridization (FISH) and all the molecular methods including next-generation sequencing (NGS) available in the clinical laboratories, why is chromosome analysis (conventional karyotyping) still necessary?

- Chromosome analysis is a labor-intensive "old" method and requires fresh tissue to separate single cells for in vitro culture. It also requires the cells to be actively proliferating to generate metaphase karyotype. However, this is not an outdated technology.
- Chromosome analysis has a whole-genome coverage capable of detecting genetic lesions including copy number (CN) and structural abnormalities above 10 Mb [18, 19]. It is especially useful in capturing unknown and relatively complex abnormalities [20].
- In most cases of myelodysplastic syndrome and acute myeloid leukemia (AML), conventional cytogenetic study can reliably detect chromosomal abnormalities [21, 22].
- Some abnormalities detected by conventional karyotyping but not usually associated with a specific entity can be used to follow up treatment response if a FISH test is available for that abnormality [18].
- Conventional karyotyping is less practical for neoplasms with low proliferation rate, such as chronic lymphocytic leukemia and multiple myeloma.
- Routinely only 20 cells are counted for conventional karyotyping; therefore the analytic sensitivity of detecting abnormalities is poor compared with molecular genetic methods (see Table 2.1).

6. What are the advantages and disadvantages of fluorescence in situ hybridization (FISH) test?

- Compared to conventional karyotyping, FISH method has significantly improved sensitivity and specificity in detecting specific copy number changes and structural aberrations [23].
- FISH can detect genotypic abnormalities with a resolution of 1–3 Mb. Usually 200 cells are observed routinely,

increasing the analytic sensitivity to 5% or lower depending on the probe design and test validation, 10–100-fold higher than conventional karyotyping.

- If neoplastic cells can be enriched (e.g., plasma cells enriched with CD138-labeled magnetic beads), the detection sensitivity can be further increased.
- FISH can also detect cryptic translocations frequently not visible by conventional karyotyping such as inv(16);*CBFB-MYH11* [24] and t(12;21)(p13;q22)(*ETV6-RUNX1*) [25].
- FISH is particularly useful to determine the level of gene amplification, such as intrachromosomal amplification of chromosome 21 (iAMP21) [26].
- Based on the probe design, FISH tests have the ability to detect copy number changes as small as 100 kb. Smaller insertions and deletions (indels) such as internal deletion of *IKZF1* gene are not detectable by FISH test.
- By counting the percentage of abnormal cells, FISH may reveal clonal diversity based on the different alterations present in subpopulations of cells.
- Most clinical laboratories use a set of probes (panels) for a specific disease to increase the probability of detecting recurrent abnormalities associated with that entity; for example, a typical chronic lymphocytic leukemia/small lymphocytic lymphoma (CLL/SLL) FISH test panel includes probes for chromosomes 6q, 11q (*ATM*), 12, 13q, and 17p (*TP53*); and t(11;14);*CCND1-IGH* may also be included routinely to rule out mantle cell lymphoma [18].
- FISH test only detects what the probes are designed for. Abnormalities not affecting the regions covered by the probes will not be identified [23]. Therefore it cannot replace chromosome analysis (see Table 2.1).

7. If we have conventional karyotyping and FISH test available, is microarray test still useful?

- The microarray tests available for clinical laboratories are usually copy number (CN) and single nucleotide polymorphism (SNP) arrays. Due to the technical complexity, the arrays used to detect RNA expression (expression profile arrays) are only used in limited reference laboratories or for research purposes.
- The CN-SNP array has the ability to interrogate whole genome for copy number changes and loss of heterozygosity at a resolution as small as 10 kb, a significant improvement over conventional karyotyping [18, 27] (see Table 2.1).
- It is most useful when the genetic alterations in a disease are limited to chromosome gains and losses, such as CLL/SLL, for which CN-SNP array can essentially replace a FISH panel.
- SNP array is the only method currently available in clinical laboratories to detect copy neutral loss of heterozygosity (CN-LOH). Studies have confirmed that CN-LOH is significantly associated with the prognosis of myelodysplastic syndrome and acute myeloid leukemia [28–30]. Detecting CN-LOH also provides clonal evidence for the "cytogenetic normal" myeloid neoplasms.
- CN-SNP array has also been proven useful for B-lymphoblastic leukemia/lymphoma in detecting copy number changes and loss of heterozygosity too small for conventional karyotyping to uncover, and these are not routinely covered by FISH probes either.
- The detection sensitivity of CN-SNP array is approximately 20% allele frequency, which means the tumor cell percentage needs to be relatively high in the sample for CN-SNP array to reliably uncover alterations associated with the neoplastic process [14].
- The major disadvantage of CN-SNP array test is the method cannot identify balanced chromosome translocations if there is no loss or gain of genetic material at the break points. This is where FISH test cannot be replaced by array method.

8. What are the typical applications of polymerase chain reaction (PCR)- based tests in the clinical laboratory?

- PCR methods amplify targeted DNA (or RNA with reverse transcription PCR, RT-PCR) template millions of times in a short period of time by thermocycling.
- PCR tests with real-time fluorescent detection (real-time PCR) can not only be quantitative (Q-PCR) but also run in a closed tube system to avoid contamination.
- Of all molecular methods available in the clinical diagnostic laboratories, PCR is the most sensitive method in detecting point mutations [31]. Quantitative allele-specific PCR can detect mutation frequency down to 0.01%. A typical example is the detection of *JAK2* V617F mutation [32, 33].
- Quantitative reverse transcription PCR (Q-RT-PCR) is routinely used to monitor the treatment response of chronic myeloid leukemia (CML) (*BCR-ABL1*) and acute promyelocytic leukemia (*PML-RARA*).
- PCR method is also the basis for many other molecular genetic tests:
  1. Fragment size analysis to detect small insertions and deletions (indels) such as seen in *FLT3-ITD*, *NPM1*, and *CALR* mutations [34].
  2. Multiplex PCR is a method including many primers in one single reaction. This method has the ability to amplify multiple targeted DNA or RNA sequences. Coupled with fragment size analysis, it is commonly used in the analysis of T-cell receptor or immunoglobulin gene rearrangements (see Question 13) [35].

3. Multiplex PCR method is also used to detect many different fusion genes in one reaction [36].

- PCR methods only amplify the targeted sequence(s) flanked by the primers. Therefore similar to the FISH methods, PCR can only detect known abnormalities with well-characterized sequences.
- Mutations or sequence variants occurring at the primer binding site will variably affect the PCR efficiency, rendering a negative result or inaccurate quantitation [37].

9. What are the indications of conventional sequencing (first- generation Sanger sequencing and pyrosequencing) in the lymph node and bone marrow pathology?

- Sequencing is the best method to look for mutations in a gene where the mutated nucleotides are not precisely known and the mutation types are variable (point mutation, insertion, or deletion). For example, *TP53* mutations can happen at many hotspots along the gene, and *CEBPA* also has multiple mutation spots; both genes have small insertion, deletion, or point mutations with clinical significance. Only a sequencing method can uncover all of these abnormalities.
- Due to significant background noise, the analytic sensitivity of Sanger sequencing is usually 15–20% allele frequency [38]. It is therefore unsuitable for samples with low tumor cell content.
- In the clinical laboratory, pyrosequencing is a cost-effective method to read through a short fragment of DNA sequences to interrogate well-characterized mutations in the hotspot region, for example, *BRAF* codon V600 [39], *MYD88* L265P [40], and *KRAS* mutation in codons 12 and 13 [41].
- Pyrosequencing has a better analytic sensitivity, detecting as low as 5% of mutant alleles [38]. However, pyrosequencing is challenging when sequencing through a homopolymer, i.e., a continuous sequence of the same nucleotide, for example, a repeat of adenosine (A) for more than three times [42].

10. Testing for *IGH/BCL2* can be performed by a PCR- based method or a FISH method. Are there any differences in the indications of these two methods?

- The t(14;18)(q32;q21);*IGH/BCL2* translocation juxtaposes the *BCL2* oncogene on 18q21 to an enhancer of the *IGH* gene on 14q32 [43]. It is detected in approximately 80% of follicular lymphoma (FL) and 20–30% of large B-cell lymphoma.
- The translocation generates no fusion RNA product and only upregulates the expression of *BCL2*. Therefore a PCR-based method to detect the translocation can only use DNA as template [43].
- Because the potential break points in the *BCL2* gene span a large region, clinical PCR test will not detect all the possible translocations. FISH method has better overall sensitivity in detecting *IGH/BCL2* than PCR method for the initial diagnostic sample [44, 45].
- Similarly, due to the variable break points in DNA and lack of fusion RNA product, FISH is better than PCR test for t(11;14);*IGH/CCND1* translocation found in mantle cell lymphoma (MCL) at the time of initial diagnosis [46].
- If a translocation is detectable by PCR, it can be detected at much lower level than FISH. Therefore PCR method is more appropriate when monitoring treatment response or detection of minimal residual disease is clinically indicated.

11. What are the indications of FISH test for *BCR-ABL1* fusion when there is a quantitative PCR test available?

- The t(9;22);*BCR-ABL1* translocation is the molecular signature of chronic myeloid leukemia (CML). It is also present in a fraction of B lymphoblastic leukemia/lymphoma and rarely in acute myeloid leukemia.
- This translocation creates a fusion gene with RNA and protein expression. Depending on the break point at *BCR* gene, the fusion RNA may translate to protein of three different molecular weights, named p190, p210, or p230 [47].
- Although chromosome analysis by conventional karyotyping can identify the Philadelphia chromosome in the majority of cases, FISH- and RNA-based RT-PCR have better sensitivity in detecting the fusion.
- Due to the variable break points in *BCR* gene, it is essentially impossible to design primers to cover all the potential fusions at the DNA level for clinical laboratories. Currently available PCR tests for *BCR-ABL1* use RNA as template (RT-PCR) [48].
- Q-RT-PCR using international scale (IS) is recommended at the initial diagnosis and to monitor treatment response of CML. International scale is developed from the p210 fusion variant, although most laboratories also report p190 with the same calculation [49].
- For initial diagnosis, FISH method has better overall sensitivity in detecting *BCR-ABL1* fusion than PCR method [50].
- Q-RT-PCR test for p230 is not standardized [51] and not routinely included in the PCR-based *BCR-ABL1* tests. Therefore this rare variant is usually only detected by FISH, not PCR; and the p230 variant of *BCR-ABL1* is usually monitored with FISH test.

12. How do I choose a method to test for *PML-RARA* when blood smear review suspects acute promyelocytic leukemia (APL)?

- Testing for *PML-RARA* translocation to confirm the diagnosis of APL is a unique situation where the clinical team would want the molecular/genetic result available as soon as possible to make a major treatment decision [52, 53].
- Most oncologists will start all-trans retinoic acid (ATRA) treatment when there is a reasonable suspicion of APL [54]. A definitive diagnosis would be required to decide whether to continue ATRA or start standard chemotherapy for acute myeloid leukemia. Therefore molecular genetic testing for an initial diagnosis of APL is usually an emergency (STAT) test.
- Fast hybridization fluorescence in situ hybridization (FISH) and rapid RT-PCR for *PML-RARA* fusion transcript [55] both can provide reasonable turnaround time for a STAT test. FISH test may be more cost-effective because PCR test needs separate controls for each run.
- Alternatively, an immunofluorescent method using antibodies directed against the PML protein is also available in some clinical laboratories for the rapid diagnosis of APL [56].
- Each clinical laboratory reviewing blood and bone marrow samples needs to find the best solution for an emergency *PML-RARA* test based on the availability and cost [52].
- Regardless of which rapid method is used for APL diagnosis, a Q-RT-PCR method for *PML-RARA* is still needed to quantify the fusion transcript in order to establish a base line to monitor the treatment response and minimal residual disease [53].

13. What are the principles of B- cell (immunoglobulin gene) and T- cell (T- cell receptor gene) clonality tests?

- In the development of lymphoid system, B-cells and T-cells go through a series of recombination processes in their "antigen receptor" genes (B-cells use the surface immunoglobulin as antigen receptor), creating the final receptor coding sequences (Fig. 2.1).
- The recombination process uses one of the many building blocks to assemble a complete coding sequence for the antigen binding region of the receptor. The combinations of different building blocks correspond to billions of different clones of B-cells and T-cells.
- At the recombination interface of the "building blocks," nucleotides are added on by terminal deoxynucleotidyl transferase (TdT) to further increase the diversity of the coding sequences.
- When B-cells or T-cells encounter foreign antigens, they go through somatic mutation to refine the antigen binding affinity. This process further enhances the diversity of lymphocytes.
- The clonality tests take advantage of the fact that each lymphocyte clone has a unique coding sequence for the antigen receptor. The receptor DNA sequences are amplified by multiplex PCR reactions that contain primers binding to the conserved regions (see Fig. 2.1). Due to the size difference of the "building blocks" in a diversified lymphoid population, the PCR products (amplicons) will have a variety of sizes in the Gaussian distribution pattern when running through size differentiating electrophoresis (Fig. 2.2a, c).

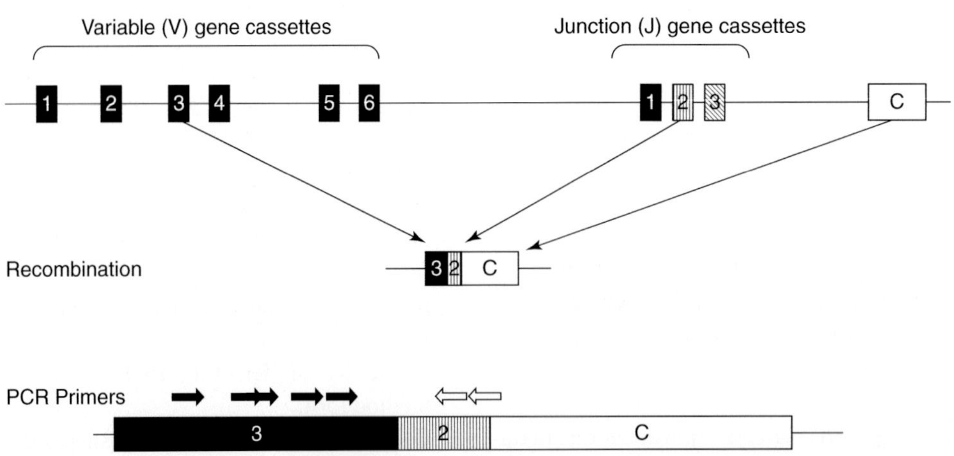

Fig. 2.1 V-J gene rearrangement and PCR primers. A simplified illustration of V-J rearrangement (D region omitted for simplified purpose; this illustration is close to the primer design of *TRG* gene). One of the gene cassettes from V and J loci is rearranged into the final coding sequence (V-J-C). For the multiplex polymerase chain reaction (PCR), several forward primers are designed based on the relatively conserved sequences in the V region and a couple of reverse primers based on the J region, to increase the sensitivity

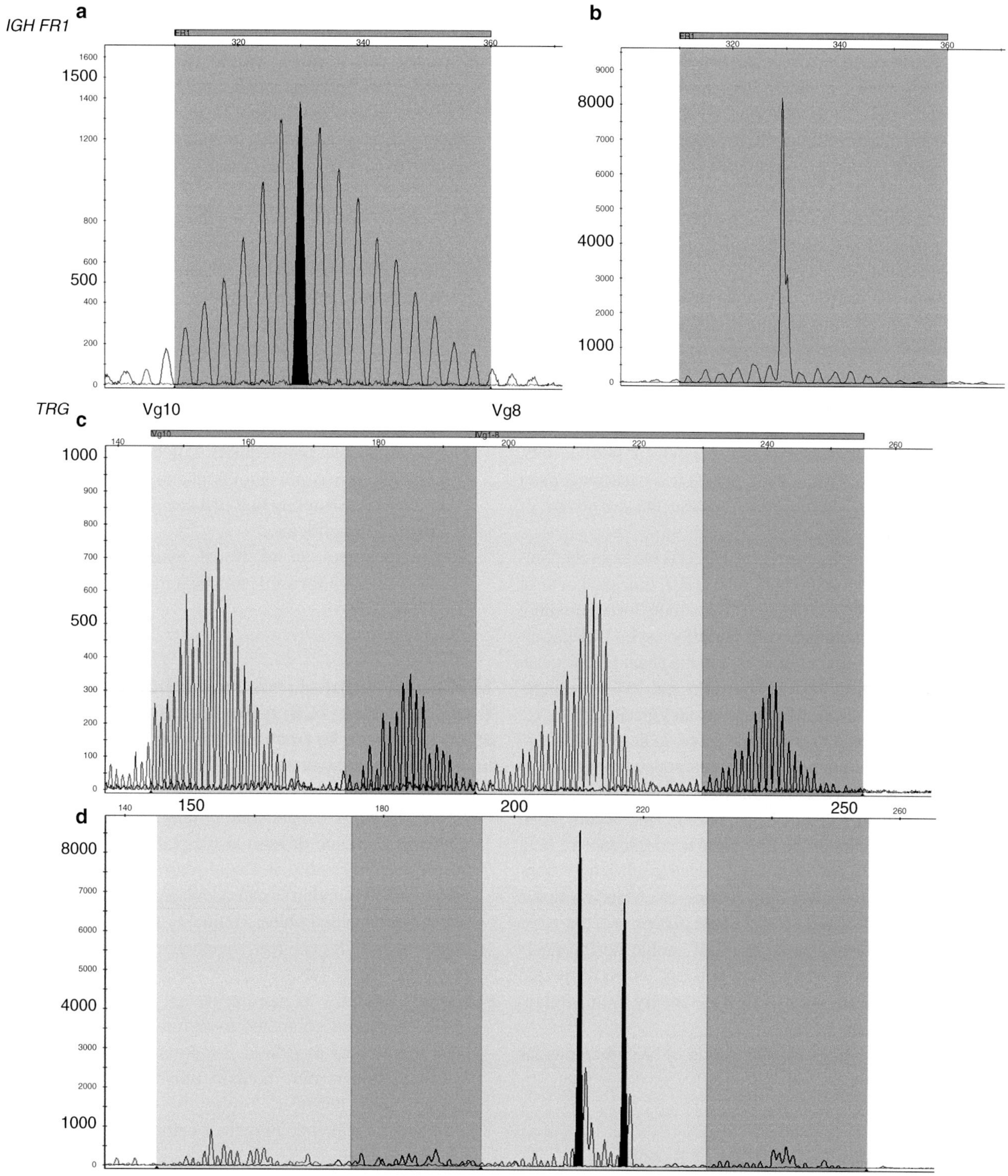

Fig. 2.2 Electropherogram of clonality tests. Polyclonal (**a**, **c**) and monoclonal (**b**, **d**) pattern of *IGH* framework 1 (FR1, **a** and **b**) and *TRG* reaction tube 1 (**c**, **d**). The polyclonal pattern shows amplified fragments as peaks of different sizes in bell-shaped normal distribution. In contrast, one or two peaks stand out in the background low peaks when a monoclonal population is present

- Whenever there is a clonal proliferation, the amplicon corresponding to the clonal population becomes predominant and can be recognized as "clonal rearrangement" (Fig. 2.2b, d).
- Currently most clinical laboratories use the primer designed and standardized by BIOMED2 for clonality tests [35]. The multiplex PCR performs reasonably well for DNA templates extracted from formalin-fixed paraffin-embedded (FFPE) tissue, which makes it an invaluable ancillary study for lymph node samples, especially when flow cytometric analysis was not performed due to lack of fresh tissue.
- Clonality test for B-cells usually includes Ig heavy chain gene (*IGH*) and kappa light chain gene (*IGK*). Adding kappa light chain gene rearrangement to the test increases the detection sensitivity especially for the post-germinal center type B-cells that have accumulated somatic mutations in the variable region. Because *IGK* is rearranged in the lambda light chain expressing B-cells or plasma cells, adding lambda light chain gene (*IGL*) rearrangement study does not significantly increase the sensitivity of B-cell clonality test.
- T-cell receptor alpha chain gene (*TRA*) is too large for clinical PCR test. The delta chain gene (*TRD*) is deleted in most T-cells with *TRA* rearrangement due to its location within the *TRA* loci. Therefore T-cell clonality test by PCR is performed on beta chain (*TRB*) or gamma chain (*TRG*) gene. Some laboratories include both *TRB* and *TRG* rearrangement tests to increase the sensitivity and specificity.
- It should be noted that in some cases, molecular analysis of a true monoclonal B-cell or T-cell population can show two clonal peaks (or bands) instead of one peak (or band) for the antigen receptor being tested. This occurs when the rearrangement of the first allele is nonproductive (i.e., the rearranged gene does not produce a full-length transcript due to premature stop codons, etc.), leading to the rearrangement of the second allele. Therefore, the presence of two clonal peaks by itself should not be interpreted as evidence of a biclonal process, unless supported by other evidence such as flow cytometry, immunofixation electrophoresis, etc.
- See also Question 17 for application of NGS methods for clonality testing.

14. What are the indications of B- cell (immunoglobulin gene) and T- cell (T- cell receptor gene) clonality tests, and what are the pitfalls in interpreting the test results?

- The clonality tests are indicated whenever there is a need to obtain molecular evidence of clonal proliferation of lymphocytes. However, when morphologic and immunophenotypic features are sufficient for a lymphoma diagnosis, clonality test is not required.
- Clonality test is also a useful tool to clarify whether lesions from different location and time originate from the same clonal population.
- There are several pitfalls in interpreting clonality test results based on the examination of the electropherogram of the PCR amplicons [57]:
  1. A positive clonal rearrangement does not equal to malignancy. Many reactive conditions can have predominant clones that may be interpreted as clonal rearrangement, although oligoclonal pattern is more commonly seen [58, 59].
  2. When the sample contains relatively few lymphocytes, the PCR reaction may create artifact called pseudoclonality. This is especially common in cutaneous specimens with relatively sparse lymphocytes [60].
  3. Not all clonal proliferation will be detected. Some populations may not amplify due to somatic hypermutation [35]. Sampling bias and sample quality can also affect the amplification.
  4. The interpretation of clonal rearrangement is not always straightforward, and the judgment is subjective [57, 61, 62].

15. Can I use clonal immunoglobulin (Ig) or T- cell receptor (TCR) gene rearrangement as an evidence to prove the B- cell or T- cell lineage of lymphoma?

- Neoplastic lymphoid populations may not follow the rearrangement scheme of normal lymphoid development. It has been confirmed that clonal rearrangements of *TCR* genes can be found in B-cell neoplasms and vice versa, a phenomenon called lineage infidelity [63]. Therefore the clonal *Ig* or *TCR* gene rearrangement can support but not prove the lineage [58].
- Lineage infidelity is more prevalent in precursor lymphoid neoplasms compared to mature neoplasms. It has been reported up to 70% of B-cell lymphoblastic leukemias/lymphomas may contain monoclonal *TRG* rearrangements; however, only 5–10% of chronic lymphocytic leukemia harbors T-cell receptor gene rearrangement [63].
- Clonal *IGH/IGK* gene rearrangement is also frequently present in angioimmunoblastic T-cell lymphoma [64]. Without morphologic evidence of a neoplastic B-cell proliferation, the evidence of a clonal B-cell or plasma cell population should not lead to a diagnosis of B-cell lymphoproliferative disorder, although some cases may eventually progress to B-cell lymphoma [65].

16. What are the key concepts required to understand the clinical next- generation sequencing (NGS)?

- Next-generation sequencing (NGS) is also known, and more appropriately described, as "massive parallel sequencing." The basic principle is to have a very large number of sequencing reactions running at the same time (in parallel), usually within a very tiny space. NGS tests have the potential to detect almost all kinds of genetic abnormalities [66].
- Currently two major NGS platforms are used in clinical laboratories: sequencing by synthesis (Illumina®) and semiconductor sequencing (Ion Torrent™, ThermoFisher). Both methods share a clonal amplification of barcoded DNA templates, followed by massive parallel sequencing of the templates on beads or a solid surface (flow cell).
- The chemical reaction of sequencing by synthesis is similar to the traditional chain termination Sanger sequencing, except that the chain termination is reversible; therefore the synthesis continues on the same template molecule after the signal of incorporating one nucleotide is captured.
- The process of semiconductor sequencing is similar to the pyrosequencing method. When a nucleotide (the substrate is nucleoside triphosphate) is added to the DNA chain, pyrophosphate and hydrogen ions are released. In pyrosequencing, the energy from the pyrophosphates is captured to generate a detectable light signal, whereas in Ion Torrent™ semiconductor sequencing, the alteration of pH caused by the hydrogen ions released from nucleotide incorporation is detected and converted into digital information (0, 1) by the semiconductors.
- The Ion Torrent™ sequencing, like pyrosequencing, is prone to error reads and noise calls in homopolymer tracts [42]. For example, while incorporation of three consecutive adenines (AAA) to a DNA template can be read precisely as three signals, a homopolymer of ten adenines (AAAAAAAAAA) may not be read exactly as ten signals and thus could be inaccurately converted to deletions or insertions in the base-calling results.
- The basic steps of NGS, from library preparation, clonal amplification, sequencing reaction, to data analysis, are illustrated and described in Fig. 2.3.
- There are two concepts critical to understanding and interpreting the clinical NGS results: sequencing quality and read depth (or sequencing depth).
  1. Sequencing quality is the quality of the signal generated by the chemical reaction, defined by the chance of error reads when converting the raw signal to bases (base calling). The current standard of sequencing quality is the Q score, calculated as $Q = -10 \log_{10}P$ where P is the error probabilities. For example, if the error probability is 1 in 1000 (0.001), the Q score is 30. A Q score no less than 20 is required for Ion Torrent™ platform and 30 is required for Illumina® platform for the sequencing data to be included in the subsequent analysis. When sequencing quality of a sample is low, a large fraction of data may be discarded, reducing the test sensitivity and specificity.
  2. The read depth or sequencing depth is defined by how many times a specific nucleotide sequence in the sample DNA is identified/read. Generally speaking, higher read depth corresponds to better sensitivity and specificity in detecting low-frequency variants by NGS and a sequencing panel with more genes will have less sequencing depth.
- In most clinical laboratories, NGS for cancer mutation profiling is performed on a group of targeted hotspot genes (targeted panel) with a limited number of DNA or RNA fragments, allowing high read depth to enable sufficient sensitivity and specificity in detecting sequence variants associated with neoplastic components.
- With the capacity to simultaneously sequence a massive amount of DNA (or cDNA reverse transcribed from RNA), NGS methods can be used to sequence all coding regions of the genome (whole-exome sequencing, WES) or the entire genome including coding and noncoding regions (whole-genome sequencing, WGS), as well as all mRNA transcripts (whole-transcriptome sequencing, WTS).
- WGS requires very complex bioinformatics tool due to enormous amount of data generated. It is not currently employed in clinical laboratories. WES, which requires less complex bioinformatics analysis, has been validated in some clinical laboratories for germline mutation testing and rarely used for cancer mutation profiling.
- Because PCR is performed to amplify the DNA fragments during the library preparation process (Fig. 2.3, step 3), even though the NGS is in effect a single molecule sequencing, the read depth reflects the collective reads from all the molecules after PCR, instead of reads from the original DNA fragments. If one DNA fragment contains a variant that is amplified preferentially by the PCR during library preparation, the percentage of this specific variant will be skewed to a higher number in all the sequencing reads.
- If an artifact (mismatch) is generated at the early stage of PCR, the artifactual variant may be amplified to a significant number/frequency, causing false-positive results and/or noise.
- To avoid the biases and noise created by PCR reaction, molecular barcodes (unique nucleotide sequences) can be added to the DNA molecules before the PCR amplification, in addition to patient-specific barcodes (added after PCR).

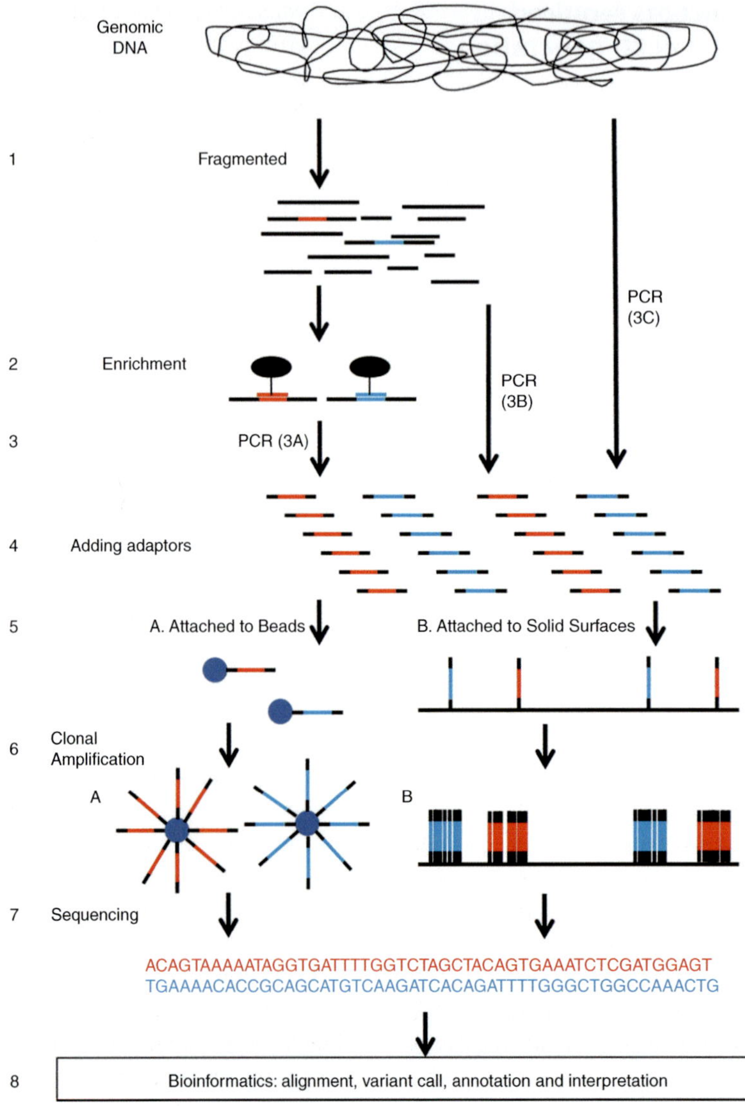

Fig. 2.3 The work flow of NGS. (**1**) A DNA sample is fragmented by using restriction enzyme(s) or physical methods. Because NGS can only sequence through relatively short fragments of DNA, the genomic DNA needs to be fragmented before preparing library for WGS or WES reaction. For targeted panel sequencing, the color bars in the fragments represent the targets of interest. (**2**) Target enrichment. Enrichment can be achieved by selectors. Probes of specific sequences attached to magnetic beads are illustrated. Enrichment can also be achieved by PCR (amplicon-based target enrichment; see 3C). (**3**) Multiplex PCR amplification of DNA fragments. The concentration of DNA fragments from genomic DNA (or cDNA from mRNA) is usually not sufficient for sequencing reactions. Therefore all the NGS library preparation methods include a PCR amplification step to generate enough molecules for the subsequent reactions. In this step, the captured fragments are amplified in a multiplex PCR. Note that for WGS, there is no enrichment (3B); for amplicon-based enrichment, genomic DNA is used as template of multiplex PCR, and there is no need for fragmentation (3C). Molecular barcodes used to label each single molecule, if considered for the NGS protocol, are added before PCR reaction. (**4**) Adding adaptors and patient barcodes. The adaptors and patient barcodes (unique sequences of several nucleotides) are attached to each end of each PCR product to facilitate clonal amplification and sequencing reactions. Adding patient barcode allows sequencing different patient samples in a single chip or flow cell. (**5**) Attaching single DNA fragments to beads or solid surface. The PCR products are separated into single strands and bound to beads in limiting dilutions, resulting in one unique fragment per bead (A). In the Illumina platform, this process is replaced by attachment of single-stranded DNA fragments to the probes anchored on the solid surface (B). (**6**) Clonal amplification. The beads are clonally amplified in droplets of an oil-emulsion-based PCR, resulting in beads carrying millions of target sequences (A). In Illumina platform, this is replaced by onboard cluster generation (B). This step is critical for the sequencing reaction to generate signal strong enough for detection. (**7**) Sequencing reaction and base calling. The beads are finally deposited into picoliter-sized wells, one bead per well, where solid-phase pyrosequencing is performed and signal captured by the semiconductors. For Illumina platform, the solid-phase sequencing by synthesis is performed in a flow cell, and the signals are captured by a high-resolution camera. The captured signals are then converted to A, T, C, and G base reads (base calling). Summarized data can be viewed in formats such as FASTQ. Because each clone is sequenced separately and the sequencing signal generated from each molecule is recorded separately, NGS is not only massive and parallel but also a signal molecule sequencing. This allows recognition of cis variants when two or more variants are detected in the same molecular read. (**8**) Bioinformatics analysis and reporting. Sequence data are then aligned with known reference sequences, and variants are identified through different algorithm with bioinformatics pipelines. The resulting output is a variant call file (VCF) and binary alignment/map files (BAM), among others. The variants will usually need to be confirmed, annotated, and interpreted by bioinformatics pipeline and/or manual inspection before pathologists create a molecular test report

Prior to the alignment of sequencing reads to the reference, the reads that belong to a unique molecule with the same molecular barcode are recognized by informatics analysis. This process is called deduplication. The variant frequency can then be correctly calculated based on the reads from unique molecules. Using molecular barcodes can significantly increase the specificity of variant calls and accuracy of variant allele frequency; it is therefore essential for the NGS method used for minimal residual disease detection.

- Of note, the sequencing reaction is a chemical reaction of DNA synthesis that may in itself create artifacts and result in low-frequency "variants" or noise signals. A conventional NGS test has an estimated noise level of 0.5–2% [67]. Therefore, protocols to reduce noise (error correction) together with an ultra-deep sequencing are usually required to detect low-allele-frequency variants with high confidence [68].

17. What is the benefit of performing clonality test by next- generation sequencing, and when should I consider it for clinical samples?

- In recent years, sequencing TCR or Ig genes as a method for clonality analysis is available for clinical samples. By reading through the unique clonal rearrangement sequence, the NGS method provides better analytic sensitivity and specificity than the PCR-based fragment size analysis method.
- By recognizing the unique clonal DNA sequence, NGS-based clonality test provides accurate information on the clonal relation between different space (anatomic location) and time.
- The unique sequence obtained at the initial diagnosis can be used to search for residual clonal population; therefore it is a sensitive method for MRD detection [69].
- The analytic precision of NGS-based clonality test is related to the sequencing read depth; it is also affected by sampling, sequencing error, and bias introduced by PCR steps prior to sequencing.
- The unique index clonal sequences may not be stable after treatment; study on the clonal evolution may provide insights into this phenomenon [70].

18. When is a NGS-based mutation profiling test indicated for hematopoietic and lymphoid disorders?

- Next-generation sequencing (NGS) is a high-throughput method that can generate a huge amount of data by reading through numerous nucleotide fragments at the same time [71].
- With the significant decrease in sequencing costs, it is estimated that when testing for mutations in more than three genes is required; it is cost-effective to use NGS than to perform the single-gene mutation tests separately.
- As more and more clinically significant hotspot mutations are discovered and characterized, NGS-based mutation profiling is gradually gaining popularity for certain neoplasms [72]. There is a desire from both oncologists and patients to identify as many abnormalities as possible; however, there are also practical considerations in the clinical laboratories to decide the scope of mutation profiling.
- Currently, most clinical laboratories sequence a panel of most relevant genes instead of performing whole-exome or whole-genome sequencing for mutational profiling [73].
- Requesting NGS-based mutation profiling could be considered as the routine ancillary study for the diagnosis and classification of myeloid neoplasms [74, 75].
  (a) Approximately 90% of MDS patients harbor at least one myeloid-related mutation [76]. Although some myeloid neoplasm-related mutations, such as mutations in *TET2*, *DNMT3A*, *ASXL1*, and *JAK2*, have also been seen in elderly individuals without overt hematological abnormalities (CHIP) [77], some mutations, especially when present at a relatively high allele frequency, predict high risk of progressing to overt MDS, and the "mutation-defined" MDS cases appear to have the same clinical course with low-grade MDS diagnosed with traditional criteria [78, 79].
  (b) If clinical suspicion of MDS is high, but the morphologic and immunophenotypic features are not sufficient for a diagnosis of MDS, mutation profiling may be useful as a supporting evidence for low-grade MDS [78].
  (c) More and more targeted therapies are becoming available for AML. Mutation profiling is also of key importance to guide management decision of AML after induction chemotherapy. Therefore NGS tests may be desirable for AML patients in some institutions [3].
- For selected cases of B lymphoblastic leukemia/lymphoma (B-ALL), NGS mutation profiling and fusion gene test may have unique value. Deregulation of targetable tyrosine kinases was found in *BCR-ABL1*-like B-ALL. No single method except NGS can reveal all the abnormalities pointing to *BCR-ABL1*-like B-ALL [80].

19. What are the limitations of current clinical NGS mutation profiling tests?

- Several limitations yet to be overcome before NGS-based tests can replace other molecular methods to cover all the needs of molecular/genetic diagnosis for hematopoietic and lymphoid neoplasms [81].
- Large insertions and deletions are usually not recognized by NGS-based methods due to the limited sequencing

length and/or imperfect bioinformatics algorithms currently used in NGS data analysis [82].

- Large amount of sequencing resources is required if NGS is used to detect chromosome rearrangements at DNA level, predominantly due to the variable break points scattered along long regions of DNA fragments [83, 84].
- RNA-based NGS will detect fusion transcripts with reasonable sequencing cost [85]; however, it can only be used for translocations that create fusion RNA. For translocations like *IGH/BCL2* that only upregulates *BCL2* expression instead of forming an *IGH/BCL2* fusion RNA, RNA-based NGS tests will not be able to detect the translocation.
- It is still challenging to sequence a large number (>500) of genes to a reasonable read depth for somatic mutation profiling with the current NGS method. Large panel whole-exome or whole-genome sequencing not only is cost-prohibiting but also generates difficulty for the analysis and interpretation of the sequencing data [75].
- Detecting low-level mutant alleles is a special challenge because of the need to generate tremendous amount of data in ultra-deep sequencing. In addition, there is also noise from sequencing methods and the bias created by the library preparation process to enrich target regions before the samples are loaded into the sequencing machine [86].

Case Presentations

Case 1

Learning Objective

1. Chromosome analysis (conventional karyotyping) can reveal complex karyotype leading to a refined final diagnosis.
2. Clonal diversity demonstrated by karyotyping may provide information for disease progression.

Case History

A 25-year-old male had fever, body aches, and insomnia as well as night sweats for a few days. He developed calf swelling and was sent to the emergency department for evaluation of "blood clotting disorder."

Laboratory Findings

- Blood cell counts: WBC 270 K/uL; hemoglobin 8.5 g/dL; platelets 361 K/uL.
- A picture of the blood smear is shown in Fig. 2.4a. The bone marrow was hypercellular with sheets of blasts (Fig. 2.4b).
- Flow cytometric analysis: a population of blasts expressing CD7 (subset), CD13, CD33, CD34, CD117, HLA-DR, and myeloperoxidase and negative for CD19, cytoplasmic CD3, and terminal deoxynucleotidyl transferase (TdT).

Genetic Study

Chromosome analysis revealed abnormal karyotype: 46,XY,t(9;22)(q34.1;q11.2)[4]/45,sl,-Y,inv(3)(q21q26.2)[8]/48,sdl,+8,+14,+19[8]

Final Diagnosis

Acute myeloid leukemia, consistent with myeloid blast phase of chronic myeloid leukemia.

Follow-Up

Patient received tyrosine kinase inhibitor imatinib and combined chemotherapy. Posttreatment bone marrow showed features consistent with chronic phase of chronic myeloid leukemia, *BCR-ABL1* positive (confirmed by FISH).

Discussion

This case demonstrates that conventional karyotyping is still a valuable method for genetic analysis. The blood and bone marrow findings of this case are characteristic for acute

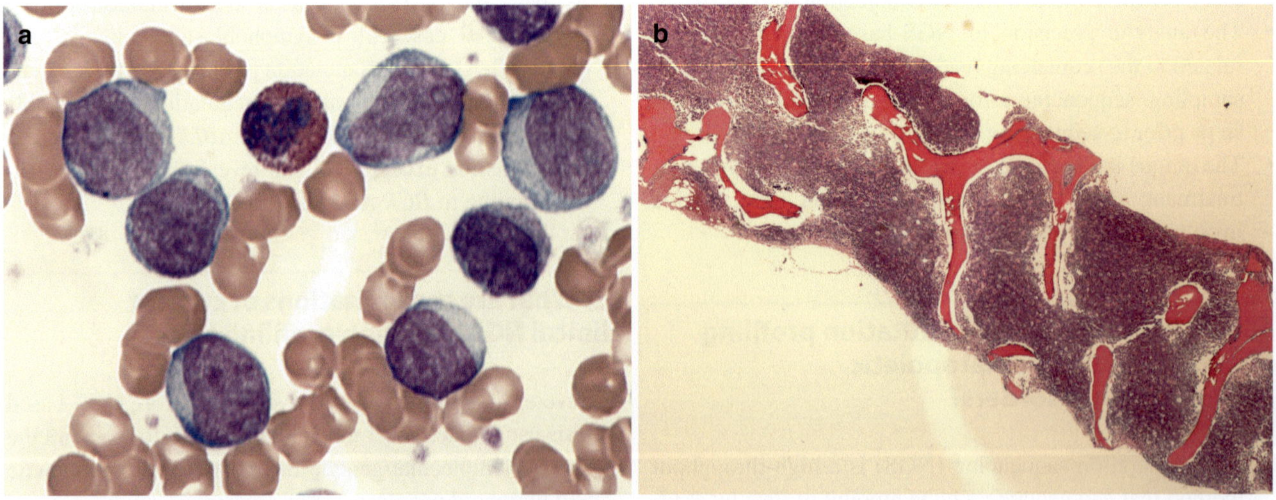

Fig. 2.4 Blood smear (**a**) shows frequent blasts, and bone marrow biopsy (**b**) is hypercellular with sheets of blasts

myeloid leukemia (AML). Chromosome analysis revealed all cells were positive for Philadelphia chromosome; a large fraction of the cells also harbor inv(3), and a smaller fraction harbors yet some more abnormalities. The genetic features indicate a clonal diversity in the blast population [87]. Because only Philadelphia chromosome is present in all cells, it is most consistent with CML with secondary inv(3) at blast phase.

FISH test as a panel for AML would be routinely performed in most laboratories for cases like this one. However, due to the rarity of AML with inv(3) or t(3;3), this abnormal chromosome change is not usually included in the FISH panel for AML. If chromosome analysis was not performed in this case, it would be difficult to distinguish a blast phase of CML from de novo AML with *BCR-ABL1*.

Case 2

Case History

A 39-year-old female incidentally noted a painless mass in the right groin. Excisional biopsy was performed and was diagnosed as CD5-positive diffuse large B-cell lymphoma (DLBCL). Patient had no constitutional symptoms. PET-CT showed no other sites of disease. Bone marrow biopsy revealed no lymphoma involvement.

Histologic Features

- The histomorphology and representative immunohistochemical stains are shown in Fig. 2.5.
- The large cells in the nodular areas stain positive for CD20, PAX5, CD5, BCL6, and MUM-1 and negative for CD3, CD10, cyclin D1, and BCL2 with no CD21-positive dendritic cell meshwork.
- Ki-67 proliferation index is approximately 60–70%.

Genetic Study

- FISH for *IRF4/MUM1* translocation was positive.

Final Diagnosis

Large B-cell lymphoma with *IRF4* rearrangement

Discussion

This case represents a typical situation when only genetic study is performed and the lymphoma can be correctly classified. Large B-cell lymphoma with *IRF4* rearrangement has excellent outcome with treatment (chemotherapy or chemotherapy with local radiation). A correct diagnosis is critical for the management of the patient.

Case 3

Learning Objective

1. Understand the limitations of fluorescence in situ hybridization test and the application and advantages of CN-SNP array test.

Case History

A 39-year-old male had back pain for a month; imaging revealed a sacral soft tissue mass. He gradually developed weakness in his lower extremities and underwent a sacral S1, S2, S3 laminectomy and subtotal excision of the dural mass. Pathological examination of the mass revealed "inflammatory tissue" with numerous eosinophils. The patient continued to develop increasing numbness and decreased proprioception in lower extremities. He subsequently underwent T10 hemilaminectomy with an epidural biopsy and T7 through T10 laminectomy with epidural mass excision.

Histologic Features and Other Laboratory Findings

- The epidural mass showed fibrous tissue with extensive infiltration of eosinophils.
- Review of the blood cell counts found that patient had eosinophilia approximately 6 months prior to the time he developed back pain. The eosinophil counts ranged from 3000 to 4000 per microliter.
- Bone marrow aspirate and biopsy were performed. The aspirate was hemodiluted.
- The biopsy core was paucicellular with focal areas of eosinophils and rare scattered pockets of trilineage hematopoiesis.

Molecular Genetic Tests

- Fluorescence in situ hybridization (FISH) for *PDFGRA*, *PDGFRB*, and *FGFR1* performed on the marrow aspirate smear revealed no abnormality.
- Next-generation sequencing for a panel of 56 genes associated with myeloid neoplasms was performed on blood cells (at the time of testing, eosinophil count was approximately 600 per microliter), and no clinically significant mutation was detected.
- FISH analysis was attempted on the formalin-fixed paraffin-embedded (FFPE) epidural mass sections but failed due to poor hybridization.
- CN-SNP analysis was performed on the FFPE epidural mass. The test clearly showed deletion of *CHIC2*, resulting in *FIP1L1-PDGFRA* fusion (Fig. 2.6).

Final Diagnosis

Myeloid neoplasm with eosinophilia and *FIP1L1-PDGFRA*

Follow-Up

Patient started treatment with imatinib and had remarkable improvement of neurologic symptoms with no new lesions developed.

Discussion

This unusual case illustrates the utility of CN-SNP array analysis in the diagnosis of hematolymphoid neoplasms. The *FIP1L1-PDGFRA* [88] fusion is cryptic for conventional

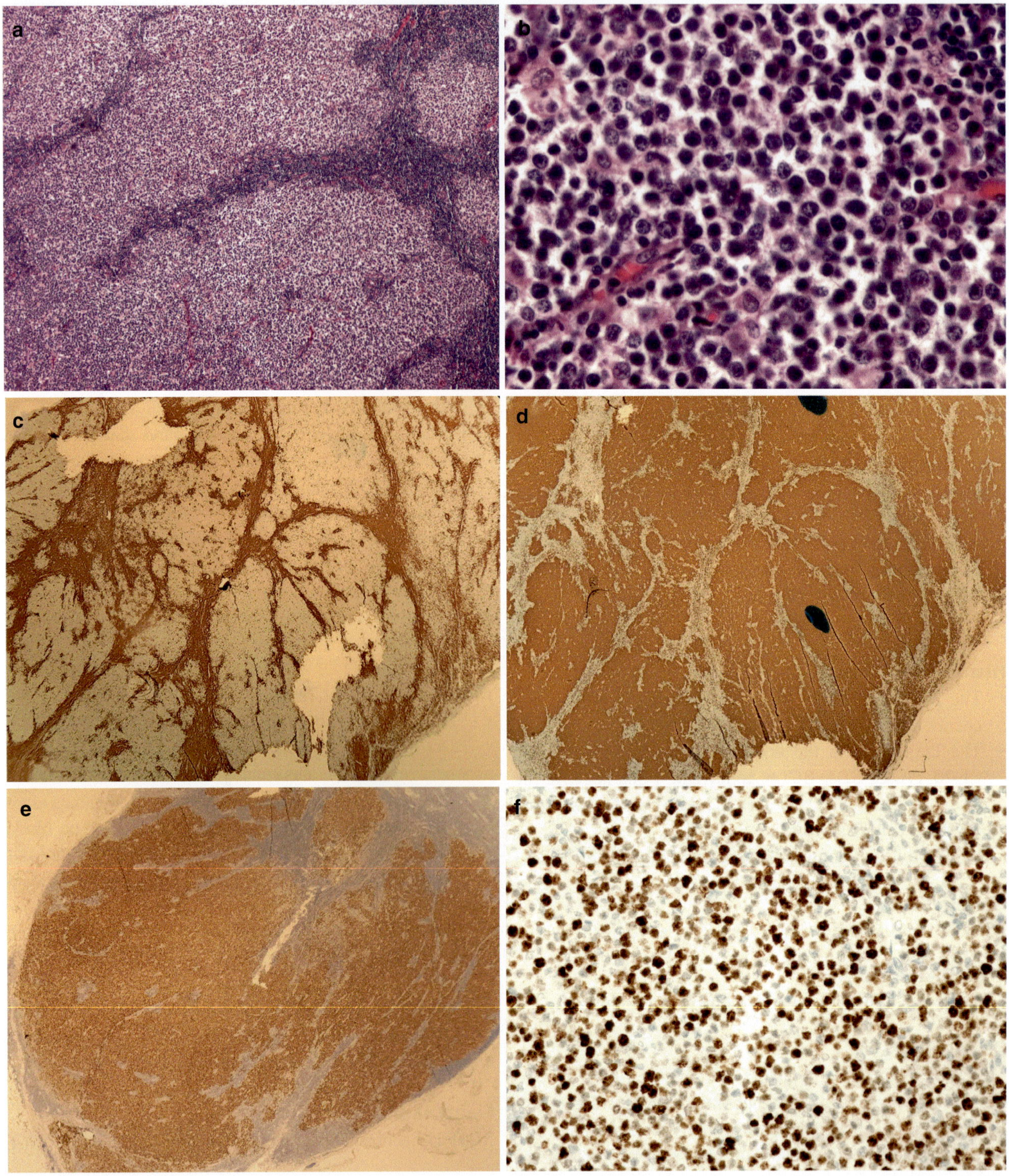

Fig. 2.5 Lymph node biopsy. (**a**, **b**) H&E stain low and high power; immunohistochemical stains: (**c**) CD3, (**d**) CD20, (**e**) MUM1, and (**f**) Ki-67

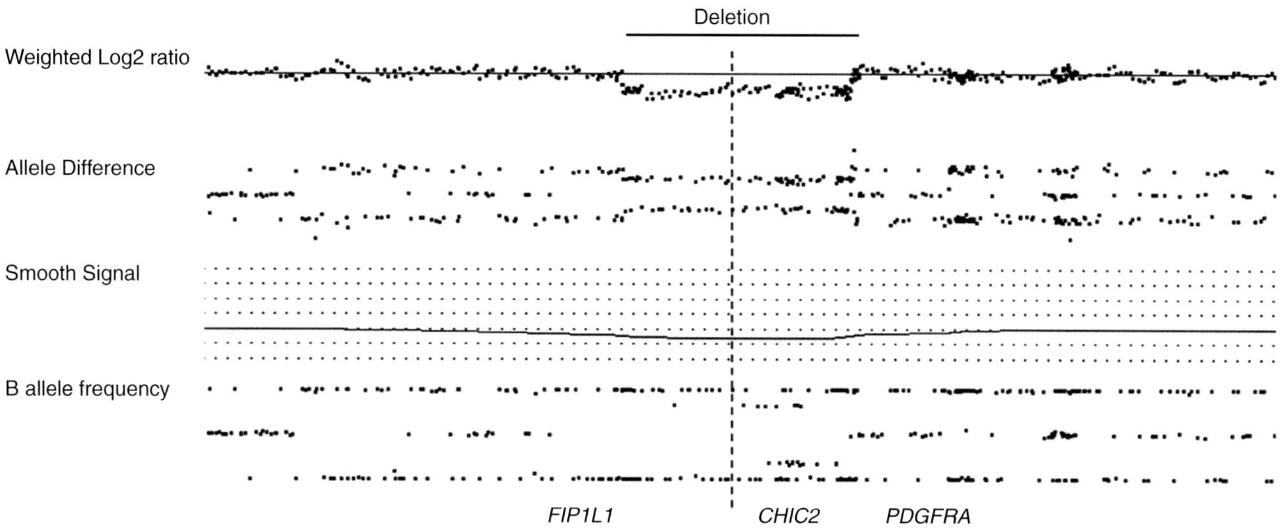

Fig. 2.6 CN-SNP array detected a small deletion including the *CHIC2* gene locus. The CN-SNP array shows some tracks based on the signal detected by the probes that are displayed as dots in the graph. The "weighted Log2 ratio" clearly reveals the internal deletion, which is displayed in a different way in the "allele difference" track, although only slightly lowered in the "smooth signal." The "B allele frequency" track shows split of the middle dotted line indicating loss of one allele in a high percentage of cells

cytogenetic analysis [88]. This fusion is usually detectable by FISH using a probe for the *CHIC2* gene (which is uniformly deleted) or in combination with probes for *FIP1L1* and *PDGFRA*. In this case, FISH test was negative in marrow aspirate likely due to low percentage of neoplastic cells in the hemodiluted sample. FISH also failed in FFPE epidural mass sample due to sample quality issue, and the deletion of *CHIC2* gene was only detected by CN-SNP array analysis. The recently improved array technology has enabled detection of small copy number changes in FFPE tissue. As confirmed in this case, it could have invaluable application in samples with high suspicion of neoplastic process.

Case 4

Case History

A 75-year-old female presented with mediastinal, paratracheal, and axillary lymphadenopathy. Immediately prior, she had a history of autoimmune hemolytic anemia (IgG and complement) and was on prednisone and rituximab treatment. Later she also developed generalized rash. PET-CT from the skull base to the mid-thigh demonstrated multiple hypermetabolic enlarged lymph nodes in bilateral cervical, axillary, inguinal, and right external iliac regions. A right inguinal lymph node was biopsied.

Histologic Features

- The lymph node architecture is largely effaced.
- The morphologic features and immunohistochemical and in situ hybridization for *EBV* (*EBER*) are shown in Fig. 2.7.

Laboratory Results

- *EBV* viral load 1300 IU/mL (ref: 0–299).
- Flow cytometric analysis failed to detect definitive monotypic B-cell or aberrant T-cell population.

Molecular Study

- Clonality testing for *IGH/IGK* and *TRG* genes both positive for clonal rearrangement.

Final Diagnosis

Angioimmunoblastic T-cell lymphoma with *EBV*-associated monotypic plasma cells proliferation

Discussion

Diagnosis of angioimmunoblastic T-cell lymphoma (AITL) can be challenging at the early stage of disease [89], especially when complicated with other immunologic disorders like in this case. At the early stage, AITL is difficult to distinguish from reactive changes by morphologic examination and immunohistochemical staining pattern, and it is not

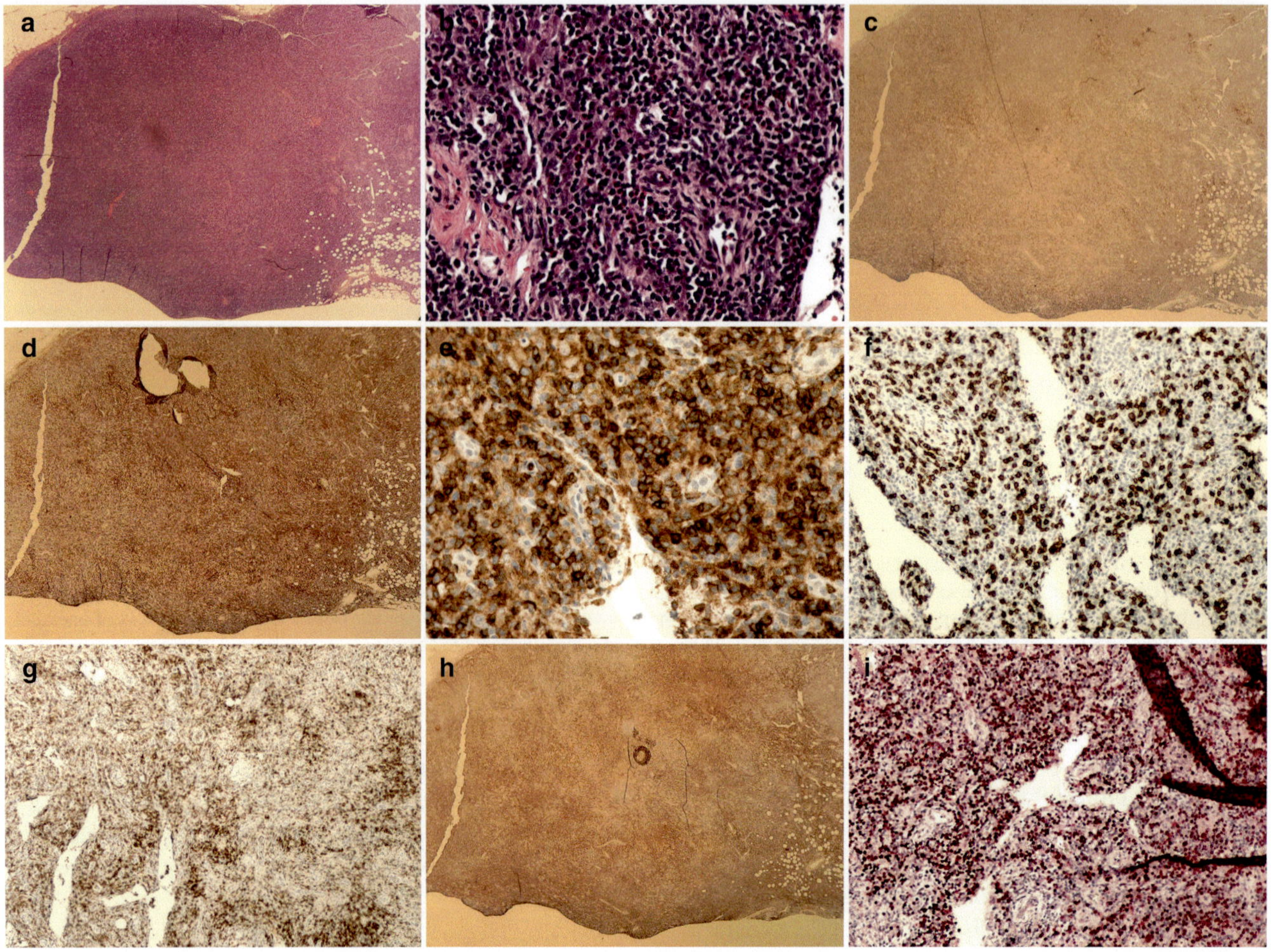

Fig. 2.7 Lymph node biopsy. (**a**, **b**) H&E stain shows effaced architecture with dense lymphoplasmacytic infiltrate. Lymphocytes with mildly atypical nuclear features are present. (**c**) CD20 shows focal disrupted distribution. (**d**) T-cells are mildly increased with CD3 stain; they are mostly CD4 positive (**e**) and less CD8 positive (**f**); many are PD1 positive (**g**). Plasma cells are focally increased with CD138 stain (**h**), and B-cells and plasma cells are diffusely positive for Epstein-Barr virus (*EBV*). (**i**) In situ hybridization of *EBV*-encoded small RNAs, (*EBER*). The plasma cells show kappa light chain restriction (not shown)

uncommon to be misdiagnosed as reactive lymphadenopathy. The clonality tests are very helpful for a definitive diagnosis. Interestingly, clonal immunoglobulin gene rearrangements are frequently detected in AITL, reported in about 25–30% of cases. The clonal B-cell and plasma cell populations are related to *EBV* infection [90]. The flow cytometric analysis did not provide definitive evidence of an abnormal T-cell population or a monotypic B-cell population and made the diagnosis of AITL challenging without clonality evidence. This case also showed exuberant *EBV*-positive clonal plasma cell proliferation, likely associated with the patient's compromised immune function.

Case 5

Case History

A 20-year-old female with no significant past medical history presented with pancytopenia persistent for several months.

Laboratory Findings

- Blood cell counts: WBC 1.6 K/uL with segmented neutrophils 30% (0.49 K/uL); lym phocytes 68% (1.1 K/uL); monocytes 0% (0); eosinophils 2% (40/uL); RBC 2.78 M/uL; Hb 8.8 g/dL; MCV 94.2 fL; and platelets 93 K/uL.
- Bone marrow aspirate and biopsy core photos are shown in Fig. 2.8. Flow cytometry analysis reported no increase of myeloblasts, B-cells were polyclonal, and no abnormal phenotype was detected in T-cells (CD4/CD8 ratio = 0.63).
- Chromosome analysis showed normal female karyotype. The case was reported as "features suggest primary or secondary marrow insufficiency."

Molecular Study

- A NGS test for myeloid neoplasm-related mutations was requested by the oncologist. *GATA2* c.1187G > A, p. Arg396Gln detected at 48.2% of alleles.
- The flow cytometric analysis was reviewed again in light of the NGS finding; the following findings were confirmed: (1) very low monocyte count; (2) low percentage of B-cells (<2%); (3) low NK-cells (<1%); (4) absent hematogones; (5) relatively increased T-cells (86% of all lymphocytes); (6) inverted CD4:CD8 ratio (0.63).

Final Diagnosis

Bone marrow failure syndrome with *GATA2* mutation (likely germline)

Discussion

The revised fourth edition of WHO classification of hematopoietic and lymphoid neoplasms (WHO 2017) added a new category in the myeloid neoplasms: myeloid neoplasms with germline predisposition. Myeloid neoplasm with germline *GATA2* mutation is one of the relatively frequent entities in this new category [91]. It is of critical importance to look for subtle features that may be associated with germline mutations and perform next-generation sequencing test in order to correctly diagnose cases in this new category. The flow cytometric analysis demonstrated some characteristic features for *GATA2* deficiency in this case [92]. However, the diagnosis of *GATA2* mutation would not be rendered without NGS test that detected a well-defined *GATA2* mutation c.1187G > A, p.Arg396Gln [93].

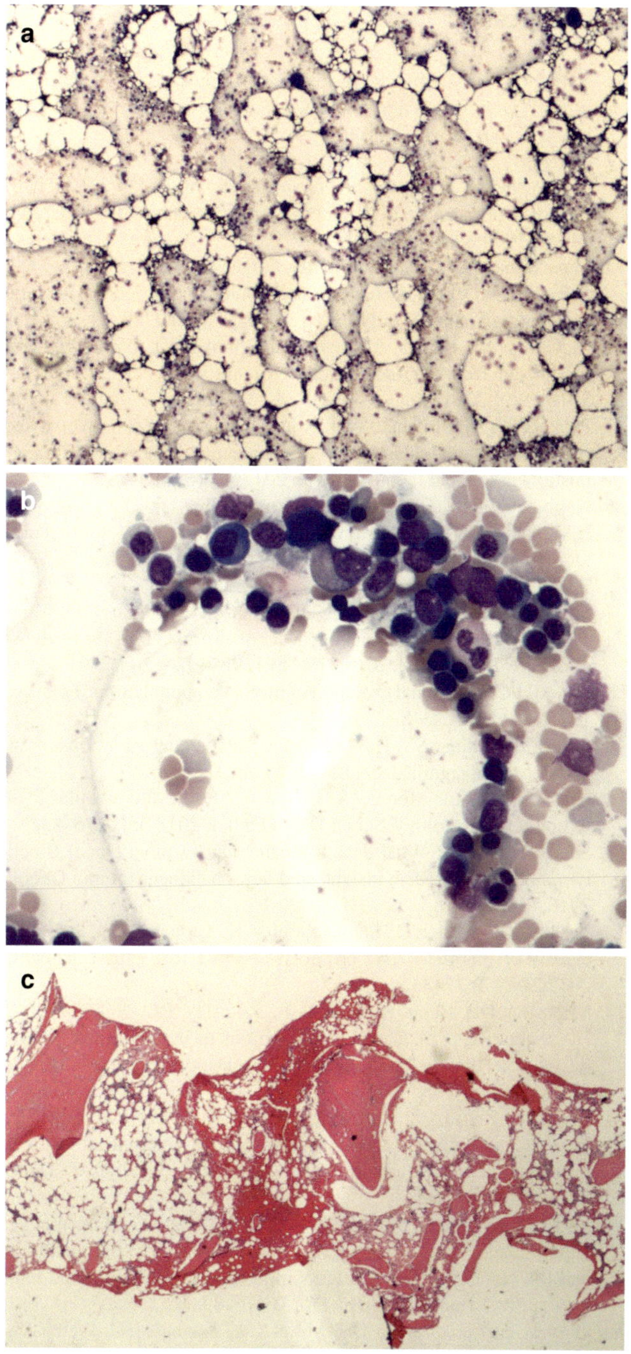

Fig. 2.8 Bone marrow aspirate is hypocellular (**a**, 20×) with decreased myeloid population (**b**, 400×), and the biopsy core confirms hypercellular marrow for patient's age (**c**, 20×)

References

1. Swerdlow SH, Campo E, Harris NL, Jaffe ES, Pileri SA, Stein H, et al. WHO classification of tumours of haematopoietic and lymphoid tissues. Revised 4th ed. Lyon: IARC Press; 2017.
2. Harris NL, Jaffe ES, Stein H, Banks PM, Chan JK, Cleary ML, et al. A revised European-American classification of lymphoid neoplasms: a proposal from the International Lymphoma Study Group. Blood. 1994;84(5):1361–92.
3. Papaemmanuil E, Gerstung M, Bullinger L, Gaidzik VI, Paschka P, Roberts ND, et al. Genomic classification and prognosis in acute myeloid leukemia. N Engl J Med. 2016;374(23):2209–21.
4. McCurdy SR, Levis MJ. Emerging molecular predictive and prognostic factors in acute myeloid leukemia. Leuk Lymphoma. 2018;59(9):2021–39.
5. Prokocimer M, Molchadsky A, Rotter V. Dysfunctional diversity of p53 proteins in adult acute myeloid leukemia: projections on diagnostic workup and therapy. Blood. 2017;130(6):699–712.
6. Nebbioso A, Benedetti R, Conte M, Iside C, Altucci L. Genetic mutations in epigenetic modifiers as therapeutic targets in acute myeloid leukemia. Expert Opin Ther Targets. 2015;19(9):1187–202.
7. Schmitz R, Wright GW, Huang DW, Johnson CA, Phelan JD, Wang JQ, et al. Genetics and pathogenesis of diffuse large B-cell lymphoma. N Engl J Med. 2018;378(15):1396–407.
8. Nowell PC. The clonal evolution of tumor cell populations. Science. 1976;194(4260):23–8.
9. Go RS, Rajkumar SV. How I manage monoclonal gammopathy of undetermined significance. Blood. 2018;131(2):163–73.
10. Oishi N, Montes-Moreno S, Feldman AL. In situ neoplasia in lymph node pathology. Semin Diagn Pathol. 2018;35(1):76–83.
11. Scarfo L, Ghia P. What does it mean I have a monoclonal B-cell lymphocytosis? Recent insights and new challenges. Semin Oncol. 2016;43(2):201–8.
12. Xochelli A, Oscier D, Stamatopoulos K. Clonal B-cell lymphocytosis of marginal zone origin. Best Pract Res Clin Haematol. 2017;30(1–2):77–83.
13. Steensma DP, Bejar R, Jaiswal S, Lindsley RC, Sekeres MA, Hasserjian RP, et al. Clonal hematopoiesis of indeterminate potential and its distinction from myelodysplastic syndromes. Blood. 2015;126(1):9–16.
14. Zhang L, Znoyko I, Costa LJ, Conlin LK, Daber RD, Self SE, et al. Clonal diversity analysis using SNP microarray: a new prognostic tool for chronic lymphocytic leukemia. Cancer Genet. 2011;204(12):654–65.
15. Shiba N, Yoshida K, Shiraishi Y, Okuno Y, Yamato G, Hara Y, et al. Whole-exome sequencing reveals the spectrum of gene mutations and the clonal evolution patterns in paediatric acute myeloid leukaemia. Br J Haematol. 2016;175(3):476–89.
16. Ding L, Ley TJ, Larson DE, Miller CA, Koboldt DC, Welch JS, et al. Clonal evolution in relapsed acute myeloid leukaemia revealed by whole-genome sequencing. Nature. 2012;481(7382):506–10.
17. Ferrando AA, Lopez-Otin C. Clonal evolution in leukemia. Nat Med. 2017;23(10):1135–45.
18. Li S, Jaye DL, Bradley KT, Zhang L, Saxe D, Deeb G, et al. Multimodality technologies in the assessment of hematolymphoid neoplasms. Arch Pathol Lab Med. 2017;141(3):341–54.
19. Martin CL, Warburton D. Detection of chromosomal aberrations in clinical practice: from karyotype to genome sequence. Annu Rev Genomics Hum Genet. 2015;16:309–26.
20. Bi W, Borgan C, Pursley AN, Hixson P, Shaw CA, Bacino CA, et al. Comparison of chromosome analysis and chromosomal microarray analysis: what is the value of chromosome analysis in today's genomic array era? Genet Med. 2013;15(6):450–7.
21. Lang BJ, Minyon C, Dhiman N, Gupta S, Wenceslao S, Vuica-Ross M, et al. Does supplemental interphase FISH analysis to standard chromosome analysis improve the detection of myelodysplastic syndrome? J Clin Oncol. 2017;35(15_suppl):7060–7060.
22. Fröhling S, Skelin S, Liebisch C, Scholl C, Schlenk RF, Döhner H, et al. Comparison of cytogenetic and molecular cytogenetic detection of chromosome abnormalities in 240 consecutive adult patients with acute myeloid leukemia. J Clin Oncol. 2002;20(10):2480–5.
23. Wolff DJ, Bagg A, Cooley LD, Dewald GW, Hirsch BA, Jacky PB, et al. Guidance for fluorescence in situ hybridization testing in hematologic disorders. J Mol Diagn. 2007;9(2):134–43.
24. Ritter M, Thiede C, Schäkel U, Schmidt M, Alpen B, Pascheberg U, et al. Underestimation of inversion (16) in acute myeloid leukaemia using standard cytogenetics as compared with polymerase chain reaction: results of a prospective investigation. Br J Haematol. 1997;98(4):969–72.
25. Raynaud SD, Dastugue N, Zoccola D, Shurtleff SA, Mathew S, Raimondi SC. Cytogenetic abnormalities associated with the t(12;21): a collaborative study of 169 children with t(12;21)-positive acute lymphoblastic leukemia. Leukemia. 1999;13(9):1325–30.
26. Harrison CJ. Blood Spotlight on iAMP21 acute lymphoblastic leukemia (ALL), a high-risk pediatric disease. Blood. 2015;125(9):1383–6.
27. Song J, Shao H. SNP array in hematopoietic neoplasms: a review. Microarrays (Basel). 2015;5(1):1–23.
28. Hemmat M, Chen W, Anguiano A, Naggar ME, Racke FK, Jones D, et al. Submicroscopic deletion of 5q involving tumor suppressor genes (CTNNA1, HSPA9) and copy neutral loss of heterozygosity associated with TET2 and EZH2 mutations in a case of MDS with normal chromosome and FISH results. Mol Cytogenet. 2014;7:35.
29. Yeung CCS, McElhone S, Chen XY, Ng D, Storer BE, Deeg HJ, et al. Impact of copy neutral loss of heterozygosity and total genome aberrations on survival in myelodysplastic syndrome. Mod Pathol. 2018;31(4):569–80.
30. Jerez A, Sugimoto Y, Makishima H, Verma A, Jankowska AM, Przychodzen B, et al. Loss of heterozygosity in 7q myeloid disorders: clinical associations and genomic pathogenesis. Blood. 2012;119(25):6109–17.
31. Macintyre EA. The use of the polymerase chain reaction in haematology. Blood Rev. 1989;3(3):201–10.
32. Frantz C, Sekora DM, Henley DC, Huang CK, Pan Q, Quigley NB, et al. Comparative evaluation of three JAK2V617F mutation detection methods. Am J Clin Pathol. 2007;128(5):865–74.
33. Zapparoli GV, Jorissen RN, Hewitt CA, McBean M, Westerman DA, Dobrovic A. Quantitative threefold allele-specific PCR (QuanTAS-PCR) for highly sensitive JAK2 V617F mutant allele detection. BMC Cancer. 2013;13:206.
34. Maier CL, Fisher KE, Jones HH, Hill CE, Mann KP, Zhang L. Development and validation of CALR mutation testing for clinical diagnosis. Am J Clin Pathol. 2015;144(5):738–45.
35. van Dongen JJ, Langerak AW, Bruggemann M, Evans PA, Hummel M, Lavender FL, et al. Design and standardization of PCR primers and protocols for detection of clonal immunoglobulin and T-cell receptor gene recombinations in suspect lymphoproliferations: report of the BIOMED-2 Concerted Action BMH4-CT98-3936. Leukemia. 2003;17(12):2257–317.
36. Iijima-Yamashita Y, Matsuo H, Yamada M, Deguchi T, Kiyokawa N, Shimada A, et al. Multiplex fusion gene testing in pediatric acute myeloid leukemia. Pediatr Int. 2018;60(1):47–51.
37. Lefever S, Pattyn F, Hellemans J, Vandesompele J. Single-nucleotide polymorphisms and other mismatches reduce performance of quantitative PCR assays. Clin Chem. 2013;59(10):1470–80.
38. Tsiatis AC, Norris-Kirby A, Rich RG, Hafez MJ, Gocke CD, Eshleman JR, et al. Comparison of Sanger sequencing, pyrosequencing, and melting curve analysis for the detection of KRAS

mutations: diagnostic and clinical implications. J Mol Diagn. 2010;12(4):425–32.
39. Lennerz JK, Klaus BM, Marienfeld RB, Möller P. Pyrosequencing of BRAF V600E in routine samples of Hairy Cell Leukaemia identifies CD5+ variant Hairy Cell Leukaemia that lacks V600E. Br J Haematol. 2012;157(2):267–9.
40. Gebauer N, Bernard V, Röhner C, Krokowski M, Merz H, Feller AC, et al. Pyrosequencing as a fast and reliable method in detecting the MYD88 p.L265P mutation in decalcified formalin-fixed and paraffin-embedded tissues. Ann Lab Med. 2014;34(2):170–3.
41. Ogino S, Kawasaki T, Brahmandam M, Yan L, Cantor M, Namgyal C, et al. Sensitive sequencing method for KRAS mutation detection by Pyrosequencing. J Mol Diagn. 2005;7(3):413–21.
42. Fakhrai-Rad H, Pourmand N, Ronaghi M. Pyrosequencing: an accurate detection platform for single nucleotide polymorphisms. Hum Mutat. 2002;19(5):479–85.
43. Hsi ED, Tubbs RR, Lovell MA, Braziel RM, Gulley ML. Detection of bcl-2/JH translocation by polymerase chain reaction. Arch Pathol Lab Med. 2002;126(8):902–8.
44. Espinet B, Bellosillo B, Melero C, Vela MC, Pedro C, Salido M, et al. FISH is better than BIOMED-2 PCR to detect IgH/BCL2 translocation in follicular lymphoma at diagnosis using paraffin-embedded tissue sections. Leuk Res. 2008;32(5):737–42.
45. Belaud-Rotureau MA, Parrens M, Carrere N, Turmo M, Ferrer J, de Mascarel A, et al. Interphase fluorescence in situ hybridization is more sensitive than BIOMED-2 polymerase chain reaction protocol in detecting IGH-BCL2 rearrangement in both fixed and frozen lymph node with follicular lymphoma. Hum Pathol. 2007;38(2):365–72.
46. Remstein ED, Kurtin PJ, Buno I, Bailey RJ, Proffitt J, Wyatt WA, et al. Diagnostic utility of fluorescence in situ hybridization in mantle-cell lymphoma. Br J Haematol. 2000;110(4):856–62.
47. Advani AS, Pendergast AM. Bcr-Abl variants: biological and clinical aspects. Leuk Res. 2002;26(8):713–20.
48. Press RD, Kamel-Reid S, Ang D. BCR-ABL1 RT-qPCR for monitoring the molecular response to tyrosine kinase inhibitors in chronic myeloid leukemia. J Mol Diagn. 2013;15(5):565–76.
49. Foroni L, Wilson G, Gerrard G, Mason J, Grimwade D, White HE, et al. Guidelines for the measurement of BCR-ABL1 transcripts in chronic myeloid leukaemia. Br J Haematol. 2011;153(2):179–90.
50. Cox MC, Maffei L, Buffolino S, Del Poeta G, Venditti A, Cantonetti M, et al. A comparative analysis of FISH, RT-PCR, and cytogenetics for the diagnosis of bcr-abl-positive leukemias. Am J Clin Pathol. 1998;109(1):24–31.
51. Gabert J, Beillard E, van der Velden VH, Bi W, Grimwade D, Pallisgaard N, et al. Standardization and quality control studies of 'real-time' quantitative reverse transcriptase polymerase chain reaction of fusion gene transcripts for residual disease detection in leukemia – a Europe against cancer program. Leukemia. 2003;17(12):2318–57.
52. O'Connor SJ, Evans PA, Morgan GJ. Diagnostic approaches to acute promyelocytic leukaemia. Leuk Lymphoma. 1999;33(1–2):53–63.
53. Tallman MS, Altman JK. How I treat acute promyelocytic leukemia. Blood. 2009;114(25):5126–35.
54. Sanz MA, Grimwade D, Tallman MS, Lowenberg B, Fenaux P, Estey EH, et al. Management of acute promyelocytic leukemia: recommendations from an expert panel on behalf of the European LeukemiaNet. Blood. 2009;113(9):1875–91.
55. Shigeto S, Matsuda K, Yamaguchi A, Sueki A, Uehara M, Sugano M, et al. Rapid diagnosis of acute promyelocytic leukemia with the PML-RARA fusion gene using a combination of droplet-reverse transcription-polymerase chain reaction and instant-quality fluorescence in situ hybridization. Clin Chim Acta. 2016;453:38–41.
56. Dimov ND, Medeiros LJ, Kantarjian HM, Cortes JE, Chang KS, Bueso-Ramos CE, et al. Rapid and reliable confirmation of acute promyelocytic leukemia by immunofluorescence staining with an antipromyelocytic leukemia antibody: the M. D. Anderson Cancer Center experience of 349 patients. Cancer. 2010;116(2):369–76.
57. Langerak AW, Groenen PJ, Bruggemann M, Beldjord K, Bellan C, Bonello L, et al. EuroClonality/BIOMED-2 guidelines for interpretation and reporting of Ig/TCR clonality testing in suspected lymphoproliferations. Leukemia. 2012;26(10):2159–71.
58. Evans PA, Pott C, Groenen PJ, Salles G, Davi F, Berger F, et al. Significantly improved PCR-based clonality testing in B-cell malignancies by use of multiple immunoglobulin gene targets. Report of the BIOMED-2 Concerted Action BHM4-CT98-3936. Leukemia. 2007;21(2):207–14.
59. Langerak AW, Molina TJ, Lavender FL, Pearson D, Flohr T, Sambade C, et al. Polymerase chain reaction-based clonality testing in tissue samples with reactive lymphoproliferations: usefulness and pitfalls. A report of the BIOMED-2 Concerted Action BMH4-CT98-3936. Leukemia. 2007;21(2):222–9.
60. Boer A, Tirumalae R, Bresch M, Falk TM. Pseudoclonality in cutaneous pseudolymphomas: a pitfall in interpretation of rearrangement studies. Br J Dermatol. 2008;159(2):394–402.
61. Langerak AW, van Dongen JJM. Multiple clonal Ig/TCR products: implications for interpretation of clonality findings. J Hematop. 2012;5(1):35–43.
62. Groenen P, Langerak AW, van Dongen JJM, van Krieken J. Pitfalls in TCR gene clonality testing: teaching cases. J Hematop. 2008;1(2):97–109.
63. Bagg A. Immunoglobulin and T-cell receptor gene rearrangements: minding your B's and T's in assessing lineage and clonality in neoplastic lymphoproliferative disorders. J Mol Diagn. 2006;8(4):426–9.
64. Huppmann AR, Roullet MR, Raffeld M, Jaffe ES. Angioimmunoblastic T-cell lymphoma partially obscured by an Epstein-Barr virus-negative clonal plasma cell proliferation. J Clin Oncol. 2013;31(2):e28–30.
65. Skugor ND, Peric Z, Vrhovac R, Radic-Kristo D, Kardum-Skelin I, Jaksic B. Diffuse large B-cell lymphoma in patient after treatment of angioimmunoblastic T-cell lymphoma. Coll Antropol. 2010;34(1):241–5.
66. Dahl F, Stenberg J, Fredriksson S, Welch K, Zhang M, Nilsson M, et al. Multigene amplification and massively parallel sequencing for cancer mutation discovery. Proc Natl Acad Sci U S A. 2007;104(22):9387–92.
67. Wong TN, Ramsingh G, Young AL, Miller CA, Touma W, Welch JS, et al. Role of TP53 mutations in the origin and evolution of therapy-related acute myeloid leukaemia. Nature. 2015;518(7540):552–5.
68. Young AL, Wong TN, Hughes AE, Heath SE, Ley TJ, Link DC, et al. Quantifying ultra-rare pre-leukemic clones via targeted error-corrected sequencing. Leukemia. 2015;29(7):1608–11.
69. Ladetto M, Bruggemann M, Monitillo L, Ferrero S, Pepin F, Drandi D, et al. Next-generation sequencing and real-time quantitative PCR for minimal residual disease detection in B-cell disorders. Leukemia. 2014;28(6):1299–307.
70. Jiang Y, Nie K, Redmond D, Melnick AM, Tam W, Elemento O. VDJ-Seq: deep sequencing analysis of rearranged immunoglobulin heavy chain gene to reveal clonal evolution patterns of B cell lymphoma. J Vis Exp. 2015;106:e53215.
71. Klee EW, Hoppman-Chaney NL, Ferber MJ. Expanding DNA diagnostic panel testing: is more better? Expert Rev Mol Diagn. 2011;11(7):703–9.
72. Meldrum C, Doyle MA, Tothill RW. Next-generation sequencing for cancer diagnostics: a practical perspective. Clin Biochem Rev. 2011;32(4):177–95.

73. Hagemann IS, Cottrell CE, Lockwood CM. Design of targeted, capture-based, next generation sequencing tests for precision cancer therapy. Cancer Genet. 2013;206(12):420–31.
74. Kuo FC, Dong F. Next-generation sequencing-based panel testing for myeloid neoplasms. Curr Hematol Malig Rep. 2015;10(2):104–11.
75. Kuo FC, Mar BG, Lindsley RC, Lindeman NI. The relative utilities of genome-wide, gene panel, and individual gene sequencing in clinical practice. Blood. 2017;130(4):433–9.
76. Haferlach T, Nagata Y, Grossmann V, Okuno Y, Bacher U, Nagae G, et al. Landscape of genetic lesions in 944 patients with myelodysplastic syndromes. Leukemia. 2014;28(2):241–7.
77. Jaiswal S, Fontanillas P, Flannick J, Manning A, Grauman PV, Mar BG, et al. Age-related clonal hematopoiesis associated with adverse outcomes. N Engl J Med. 2014;371(26):2488–98.
78. Valent P, Orazi A, Steensma DP, Ebert BL, Haase D, Malcovati L, et al. Proposed minimal diagnostic criteria for myelodysplastic syndromes (MDS) and potential pre-MDS conditions. Oncotarget. 2017;8(43):73483–500.
79. Malcovati L, Galli A, Travaglino E, Ambaglio I, Rizzo E, Molteni E, et al. Clinical significance of somatic mutation in unexplained blood cytopenia. Blood. 2017;129(25):3371–8.
80. Yap KL, Furtado LV, Kiyotani K, Curran E, Stock W, McNeer JL, et al. Diagnostic evaluation of RNA sequencing for the detection of genetic abnormalities associated with Ph-like acute lymphoblastic leukemia (ALL). Leuk Lymphoma. 2017;58(4):950–8.
81. Sheikine Y, Kuo FC, Lindeman NI. Clinical and technical aspects of genomic diagnostics for precision oncology. J Clin Oncol. 2017;35(9):929–33.
82. Thomas M, Sukhai MA, Zhang T, Dolatshahi R, Harbi D, Garg S, et al. Integration of technical, bioinformatic, and variant assessment approaches in the validation of a targeted next-generation sequencing panel for myeloid malignancies. Arch Pathol Lab Med. 2017;141(6):759–75.
83. Koboldt DC, Larson DE, Chen K, Ding L, Wilson RK. Massively parallel sequencing approaches for characterization of structural variation. Methods Mol Biol. 2012;838:369–84.
84. Abel HJ, Duncavage EJ. Detection of structural DNA variation from next generation sequencing data: a review of informatic approaches. Cancer Genet. 2013;206(12):432–40.
85. Stengel A, Nadarajah N, Haferlach T, Dicker F, Kern W, Meggendorfer M, et al. Detection of recurrent and of novel fusion transcripts in myeloid malignancies by targeted RNA sequencing. Leukemia. 2018;32(5):1229–38.
86. Scherer F, Kurtz DM, Diehn M, Alizadeh AA. High-throughput sequencing for noninvasive disease detection in hematologic malignancies. Blood. 2017;130(4):440–52.
87. Wang W, Cortes JE, Lin P, Beaty MW, Ai D, Amin HM, et al. Clinical and prognostic significance of 3q26.2 and other chromosome 3 abnormalities in CML in the era of tyrosine kinase inhibitors. Blood. 2015;126(14):1699–706.
88. Cools J, DeAngelo DJ, Gotlib J, Stover EH, Legare RD, Cortes J, et al. A tyrosine kinase created by fusion of the PDGFRA and FIP1L1 genes as a therapeutic target of imatinib in idiopathic hypereosinophilic syndrome. N Engl J Med. 2003;348(13):1201–14.
89. Mourad N, Mounier N, Briere J, Raffoux E, Delmer A, Feller A, et al. Clinical, biologic, and pathologic features in 157 patients with angioimmunoblastic T-cell lymphoma treated within the Groupe d'Etude des Lymphomes de l'Adulte (GELA) trials. Blood. 2008;111(9):4463–70.
90. Tan BT, Warnke RA, Arber DA. The frequency of B- and T-cell gene rearrangements and epstein-barr virus in T-cell lymphomas: a comparison between angioimmunoblastic T-cell lymphoma and peripheral T-cell lymphoma, unspecified with and without associated B-cell proliferations. J Mol Diagn. 2006;8(4):466–75.
91. Mir MA, Kochuparambil ST, Abraham RS, Rodriguez V, Howard M, Hsu AP, et al. Spectrum of myeloid neoplasms and immune deficiency associated with germline GATA2 mutations. Cancer Med. 2015;4(4):490–9.
92. Ganapathi KA, Townsley DM, Hsu AP, Arthur DC, Zerbe CS, Cuellar-Rodriguez J, et al. GATA2 deficiency-associated bone marrow disorder differs from idiopathic aplastic anemia. Blood. 2015;125(1):56–70.
93. Cortes-Lavaud X, Landecho MF, Maicas M, Urquiza L, Merino J, Moreno-Miralles I, et al. GATA2 germline mutations impair GATA2 transcription, causing haploinsufficiency: functional analysis of the p.Arg396Gln mutation. J Immunol. 2015;194(5):2190–8.

Evaluation of Excised Lymph Nodes

3

Zenggang Pan, Le Aye, Imran N. Siddiqi, and Endi Wang

List of Frequently Asked Questions

1. What are the major clinical indications for excisional biopsy of lymph node?
2. What are the important instructions to the surgeons prior to excision of lymph node?
3. What intraoperative assessments (e.g., frozen section, touch prep/imprints) may be indicated when a fresh lymph node is obtained?
4. What are the important instructions for transportation of lymph node sample?
5. How should the lymph node excisional sample be grossed properly?
6. When should fresh lymphoid tissue be apportioned for additional studies (e.g., flow cytometry, cytogenetics, gene expression analysis) prior to fixation?
7. What are the likely differences in clinical presentations between reactive lymphadenopathy and nodal involvement by lymphoma?
8. What are the likely differences in clinical presentations between Hodgkin lymphoma and non-Hodgkin lymphoma?
9. Which types of lymphoid neoplasms often present with splenomegaly?
10. Which types of lymphoid neoplasms often present with neutropenia, anemia, thrombocytopenia, or pancytopenia?
11. Which lymphomas and non-leukemic hematolymphoid neoplasms can sometimes present as leukemia or have a leukemic phase?
12. What are the differential diagnoses in a patient who presents with an anterior/superior mediastinal mass?
13. Which types of hematolymphoid neoplasms tend to present with skin lesions, besides extracutaneous or nodal involvement?
14. Which anatomical sites (head/neck, axillary, thoracic, abdominal, retroperitoneal, inguinal, etc.) are more likely to be involved by particular lymphoid neoplasms or other hematolymphoid neoplasms?
15. How should the lymph node sections be examined microscopically?
16. What are the major morphological patterns of reactive lymphadenopathy?
17. Which clinical diagnoses are likely associated with a reactive follicular pattern in the lymph node?
18. What is the initial workup for the reactive appearing lymph node with dominant follicular pattern?
19. Which diagnoses are commonly associated with a paracortical pattern in reactive lymphadenopathy?
20. Which diagnoses are commonly associated with a sinus pattern in reactive lymphadenopathy?
21. Which diagnoses are commonly associated with a granulomatous pattern in reactive lymphadenopathy?
22. What are the major morphological patterns of lymphoma involvement in lymph node?
23. What are the major differential diagnoses and initial workup for lymphomas with follicular or nodular pattern?
24. What are the major differential diagnoses and initial workup for the lymph node with a diffuse infiltration by small cell lymphoma?

Z. Pan (✉)
Department of Pathology, Yale University School of Medicine, New Haven, CT, USA
e-mail: zenggang.pan@yale.edu

L. Aye
Department of Hematopathology, University of Southern California, Children's Hospital Los Angeles, Los Angeles, CA, USA

I. N. Siddiqi
Department of Pathology, Keck School of Medicine, University of Southern California, Los Angeles, CA, USA
e-mail: Imran.Siddiqi@med.usc.edu

E. Wang
Department of Pathology, Duke University School of Medicine and Duke Health System, Durham, NC, USA
e-mail: endi.wang@duke.edu

E. Wang, A. S. Lagoo (eds.), *Practical Lymph Node and Bone Marrow Pathology*, Practical Anatomic Pathology,
https://doi.org/10.1007/978-3-030-32189-5_3

25. What are the major differential diagnoses and initial workup for the lymph node with an interfollicular growth pattern?
26. What are the major differential diagnoses and initial workup for the lymph node with a diffuse infiltration by blastoid cells?
27. What are the major differential diagnoses and initial workup for the lymph node with a diffuse infiltration by large tumor cells?
28. What are the major differential diagnoses and initial workup for the lymph node with a prominent sinus infiltration of tumor cells?
29. What is the initial workup for lymph node cases with morphologic features suggestive for classic Hodgkin lymphoma (CHL)?

1. What are the major clinical indications for excisional biopsy of lymph node?

- An excisional biopsy of a lymph node is indicated when there is a clinical or radiologic concern for malignancy, for persistent or progressive lymphadenopathy of unknown cause, with nondiagnostic infectious workup and lack of response to conservative treatment. Risk factors for malignancy are [1, 2]:
  - Age older than 40 years
  - Immunocompromised status
  - Systemic signs: night sweats, fever, weight loss, and hepatosplenomegaly
  - Physical exam findings: firm or hard in consistency, fixed nodes, lack of tenderness, rapid increase in size, nodal diameter >2 cm, and generalized lymphadenopathy (two or more regions involved)
  - Supraclavicular, mediastinal, or posterior cervical chain location
  - Persistent lymphadenopathy greater than 4–6 weeks without a documented infectious cause and lack of response to conservative treatment
- In children, criteria for performing biopsy of an enlarged lymph node include age >8 years, generalized lymphadenopathy, supraclavicular or lower cervical node involvement, and fixation to the overlying skin regardless of size. Likelihood of malignancy for lymphadenopathy in the supraclavicular or lower cervical regions is higher compared to the other sites [3–8].
- Other indications for excisional biopsy include findings from a preceding fine needle aspiration biopsy, including:
  - Nondiagnostic fine needle aspiration results
  - Features of follicular lymphoma but to exclude a component of diffuse large B-cell lymphoma (DLBCL)
  - Insufficient neoplastic cells for a definitive diagnosis of a specific subtype of lymphoma
  - Discordant cytomorphologic features and clinical signs (e.g., findings of a predominance of small lymphoid cells by cytomorphology with clinical signs of high-grade lymphoma/transformation) (to exclude a large cell component)
  - Evaluating for an initial diagnosis of classic Hodgkin lymphoma with any unusual features raising the possibility of composite or "gray-zone" lymphoma (e.g., B-cell lymphoma, unclassifiable, with features intermediate between DLBCL and classic Hodgkin lymphoma)
  - Presence of necrosis and polymorphous cells in the evaluation of recurrent non-Hodgkin lymphoma

2. What are the important instructions to the surgeons prior to excision of lymph node?

- An intact specimen should be submitted fresh and on saline-soaked gauze or in a sealed jar containing saline or tissue culture media.
- The largest, most suspicious and most accessible node should be sampled. In general, the inguinal nodes display the lowest yield, and the supraclavicular nodes have the highest yield, followed by those from the deep nodes [9].
- The lymph node should be excised completely with the capsule intact to maintain the lymph node architecture.
- A specimen requisition should include a relevant history with pertinent results of the clinical presentation, physical exam, imaging studies, and lab values.
- If there is a clinical concern for an infectious process, it is most appropriate to submit the fresh tissue at the time of procedure in a sterile manner and in appropriate medium for microbiology culture.

3. What intraoperative assessments (e.g., frozen section, touch prep/imprints) may be indicated when a fresh lymph node is obtained?

- Frozen section has a very limited role in the evaluation of a lymph node biopsy. It may be useful if (1) there is a clinical suspicion for metastatic malignancy and (2) the patient has a prior history or strong suspicion for a non-hematolymphoid malignancy. See Fig. 3.1 for algorithm on processing an excisional biopsy of lymph node.
- Touch imprints should be made from a section of the fresh specimen and results used to guide lymphoma workup. Benefits of imprints are:
  - They are free from frozen section artifacts, and they can preserve sampled tissue [10].
  - They can be used to assess adequacy and risk stratify lymph node specimens (e.g., infectious, Hodgkin

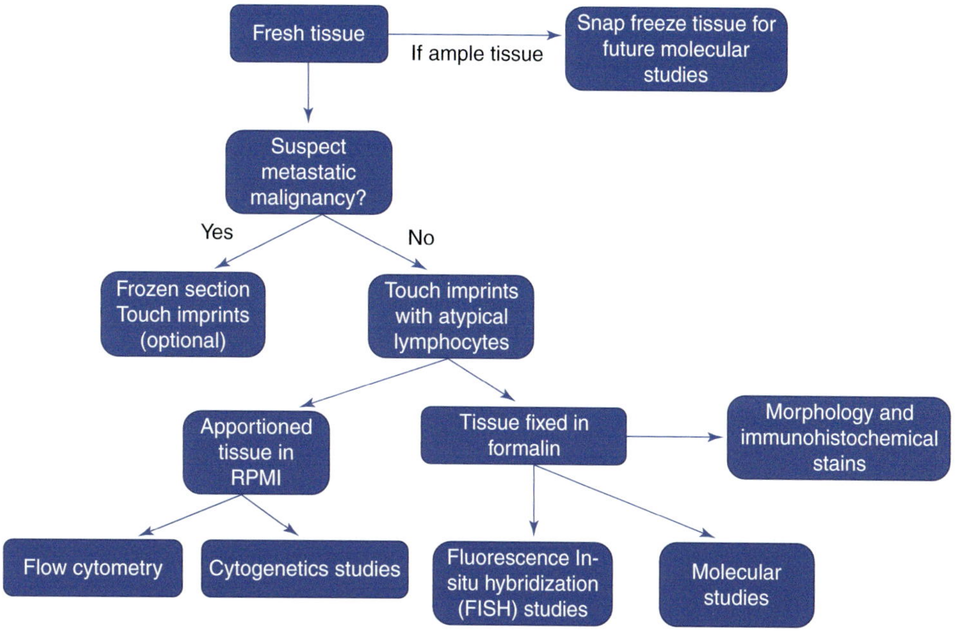

Fig. 3.1 Algorithm for excisional biopsy of lymph node processing. Refer to the answer text for Question 3

vs non-Hodgkin lymphoma, low-grade, reactive versus high-grade, non-hematolymphoid neoplasm, etc.) [11].
  - They can help guide the need for ancillary studies such as flow cytometry (see Question 6 for details).
  - Thoroughly air-dried imprint preparations can retain most antigens for immunohistochemical staining or fluorescence in situ hybridization (FISH) analysis up to 1 week if stored at 20 °C and up to many months or years if stored at −80 °C [12, 13].
- To perform a touch imprint:
  - Gently blot the fresh tissue to remove blood or saline.
  - Press a clean slide to the cut surface at least 2–3 times on adjacent areas of the slide.
  - Prepare a total of 5 or 6 slides in this manner.
  - Air-dry one slide and stain with Diff-Quik stain for rapid assessment. The remaining slides can be air-dried or fixed in alcohol and stained with Wright-Giemsa stain.

4. What are the important instructions for transportation of lymph node sample?

- To avoid irreversible drying artifacts, biopsy specimens should be submitted on saline-soaked gauze or in a specimen container and immersed in saline or culture medium.
- Tissue should not be transported on dry towels or surgical sponges.
- Separating adhered delicate tissue from dry gauze fibers causes architectural damage.
- Surface desiccation due to drying during transport results in irreversible dehydration of cellular proteins and causes morphologic distortion such as "dark-edge" staining on hematoxylin and eosin (H&E)-stained sections. In addition, it can affect antigen preservation for immunoreactivity [14].
- When a delay in transport is expected, the specimen should be refrigerated at 4 °C to delay autolysis. Storage at 4 °C is satisfactory for morphology, immunoreactivity for most markers, and nucleic acid preservation for cytogenetic and molecular studies.

5. How should the lymph node excisional sample be grossed properly?

- The biopsy tissue should be processed promptly upon receipt. See Table 3.1 for common errors in transport and grossing [13, 15].
- The fresh specimen size, color, and consistency should be recorded.
- For lymph nodes less than 1 cm in diameter, a single cut along the long axis is recommended.
- Small specimens may be crushed when attempting to perform cross sections perpendicular to the long axis.
- For lymph nodes greater than 1 cm, the lymph node can be sectioned into 2–3 mm slices perpendicular to the long axis of the node with a sharp knife.
- Sections should not be greater than 3 mm in thickness to allow adequate fixation and processing.
- After sectioning, grossly examine for the presence or absence of any visible nodularity, hemorrhage, or necrosis and then place promptly into fixative. See Table 3.2 for commonly used fixatives for hematolymphoid malignancy and their formulations [16–19].

Table 3.1 Common errors in transport and grossing

Error	Artifacts	Correction
Specimen transported in dry towel	"Dark-edge" on H&E sections due to tissue desiccation	Submit tissue on saline-soaked gauze or in a sealed jar containing saline or tissue culture medium
Thick sections (>3 mm)	Fragmented tissue (loss of architecture) on H&E sections	2–3 mm thickness is ideal
Inadequate fixation or overfixation in mercuric fixative	Homogenous fragmentation of sections	Tissue should be fixed in 10% buffered formalin for at least 6–8 hours, but no more than 24 hours in formalin and no more than 4 hours in mercuric fixatives

Table 3.2 Fixatives for hematolymphoid malignancy and their formulations

Fixatives	Formulation
10% neutral-buffered formalin	Tap water (900 mL), concentrated formalin (=37% formaldehyde solution, 100 mL) sodium phosphate, monobasic, monohydrate (4 g), sodium phosphate, dibasic, anhydrous (6.5 g); adjust pH to 7.2–7.4
B5 fixative (mercuric based)	Stock solution: Mercuric chloride: 12 g Sodium acetate anhydrous: 2.5 g Distilled water: 200 g Working solution: prepare immediately before use B5 stock solution: 20 mL 37% formaldehyde: 2 mL
Wright-Giemsa stain	Wright stain Giemsa stain in methyl alcohol Phosphate buffer (pH 6.4)
Zinc formalin	Zinc sulfate: 1 g Deionized water: 900 ml Stir until dissolved and then add 37% formaldehyde: 100 ml

- Fascia and capsules are naturally occurring physical barriers to fixatives and can decrease penetration. They should be incised prior to fixation.
- Fixation:
  - It is important to record fixative(s) used for individual slices of the specimen since fixatives impact nuclear preservation for molecular studies.
  - 10% neutral buffered formalin is preferred when the tissue is limited since it is suitable for molecular studies, in situ hybridization, and immunohistochemical evaluation.
  - If tissue is abundant, one or two slices of tissue can be fixed in zinc formalin or B5, as available in the laboratory, for superior cytologic detail. However, these fixatives are suboptimal for DNA extraction. B5 also requires proper hazardous-material disposal.
  - Underfixation (less than 6 hours in 10% neutral buffered formalin, alcoholic formalin, and zinc formalin) should be avoided for optimal immunophenotypic reactivity and molecular studies [20].

6. When should fresh lymphoid tissue be apportioned for additional studies (e.g., flow cytometry, cytogenetics, gene expression analysis) prior to fixation?

Flow Cytometry

- Flow cytometry is helpful to immunophenotype and quantify the cell population of interest.
- If the submitted specimen is sufficient for morphologic and immunohistochemical analysis, a touch prep should be performed to evaluate the specimen for the utility of flow cytometry. See Table 3.3 for limited and extended flow cytometry panel [21, 22]. See Fig. 3.2 for algorithm for flow cytometry.
- If the touch prep shows predominantly small lymphoid cells (low-grade morphology), then flow cytometric analysis should be prioritized.
- If the touch prep demonstrates large cells with necrosis (high-grade morphology), flow cytometry may not be necessary. Morphologic evaluation and immunohistochemical phenotyping should be favored.
- If the touch prep shows granulomas and necrosis, flow cytometry is not indicated unless touch preparations demonstrate abnormal lymphoid cells suspicious for lymphoma.
- If the specimen shows a polymorphous lymphoid population, correlate with clinical information. If the clinical information favors reactive, flow cytometry may not be necessary. If there is a clinical suspicion for a particular subtype of lymphoma, especially T- or NK-cell neoplasm such as angioimmunoblastic T-cell lymphoma (AITL) (widespread lymphadenopathy, constitutional symptoms, skin rash), enteropathy-associated T-cell lymphoma (EATCL) (GI mass), or large granular lymphocytic leukemia (LGL) (autoimmune disorder and neutropenia), flow cytometry may be helpful.

Table 3.3 Flow cytometric reagents for evaluation of hematopoietic neoplasia

Lineage	Limited panel	Extended panel
B-cells	CD5, CD10, CD19, CD20, CD45, kappa, and lambda surface	CD9, CD11c, CD22, CD23, CD25, CD13, CD33, CD34, CD38, CD43, CD58, CD79a and b, CD103, FMC-7, kappa and lambda cytoplasmic, TdT
T-cells and NK-cells	CD2, CD3 surface, CD4, CD5, CD7, CD8, CD45, CD56	CD1a, CD3 cytoplasmic, CD10, CD16, CD25, CD30, CD34, CD57, TdT
Myeloid cells	CD13, CD33, CD34, CD45, CD117	CD11b, CD14, CD15, CD16, CD56, CD2, CD4, CD7, CD36, CD41, CD61, CD64, CD71, MPO cytoplasmic, CD123
Plasma cells	CD19, CD38, CD45, CD56	CD10, CD117, CD138, kappa and lambda cytoplasmic

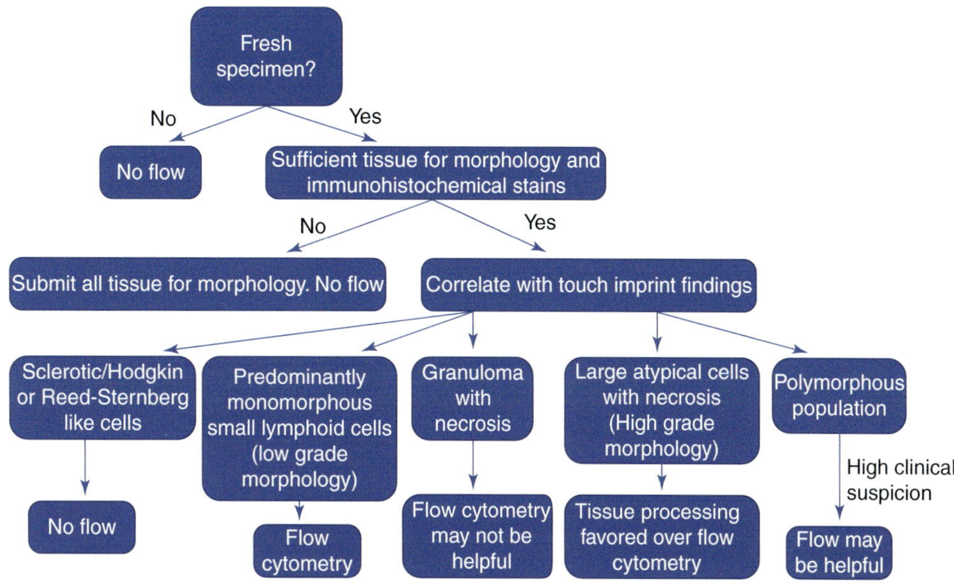

Fig. 3.2 Algorithm for flow cytometry. Refer to the answer text for Question 6

Cytogenetics and Gene Expression Analysis

- Cytogenetic studies such as karyotype and FISH analysis, RNA/gene expression profiling, and mutational analyses by next-generation sequencing or PCR can play important roles in diagnosis and prognosis.
- However, morphology and immunohistochemical stains remain essential for a diagnosis. If the specimen is small (<1 cm), the entire specimen should be fixed in formalin for histologic evaluation. As necessary, FISH studies can be performed on fixed tissue and DNA and RNA can be recovered for molecular studies [23–26].
- If tissue is abundant, optimal recovery for DNA and RNA can be achieved by snap freezing small portions of fresh tissue.
- To snap freeze fresh tissue:
  - Place fresh tissue in aluminum foil or cover in OCT (optimal cutting temperature) medium.
  - Immerse in dry ice or liquid nitrogen.
  - Store at −80 ° C until needed.

Table 3.4 Clinical features in reactive lymphadenopathy and lymphoma

	Reactive lymphadenopathy	Lymphoma
Fever	Sometimes	Often
Night sweat	Usually not	Often
Weight loss	Usually not	Often
Associated pain	Often	Painless
Tenderness on palpation	Often	Non-tender
Other features on palpation	Soft and moveable node	Firm and fixed node
Onset	Acute, fluctuate in size	Progressive, persistent
PET/CT	Not avid	Avid
Sites frequently involved	Axillary, inguinal	Mediastinal, supraclavicular

PET/CT positron emission tomography/computed tomography

7. What are the likely differences in clinical presentations between reactive lymphadenopathy and nodal involvement by lymphoma?

Age is a critical factor for differentiating a benign from a malignant lymphadenopathy. While lymphadenopathy in adult or old individual has high chance of lymphoma or another malignancy, some lymphomas, such as Hodgkin lymphoma, large B-cell lymphoma, and high-grade B-cell lymphoma, can occur in children and young adults. See Table 3.4 for clinical features which distinguish between reactive lymphadenopathy and lymphoma.

8. What are the likely differences in clinical presentations between Hodgkin lymphoma and non-Hodgkin lymphoma?

While Hodgkin lymphoma is mainly defined by its morphologic features and immunophenotypic profile of its malignant cells, it has clinical presentations distinct from the majority of non-Hodgkin lymphomas. See Table 3.5 for a summary of major differences in clinical presentations between Hodgkin lymphoma and non-Hodgkin lymphoma.

Table 3.5 Major differences in clinical presentations between Hodgkin lymphoma and non-Hodgkin lymphoma

	Hodgkin lymphoma	Non-Hodgkin lymphoma
Age of occurrence	Bimodal peaks	Later life for most types
B-symptoms	Majority	Varied with types
Lymphadenopathy	1–2 nodes in majority	>1 nodes in majority
Sites of lymph nodes	Cervical, mediastinal	Varied with types
Extranodal involvement	Rare	Often in most types
Clinical stage	Usually low, I or II	Varied with types
Prognosis	Usually good	Varied with types; poor for majority

9. Which types of lymphoid neoplasms often present with splenomegaly?

- Essentially, all types of lymphoma/lymphoid leukemia can involve spleen except for a few types of tissue-specific lymphoma, including cutaneous lymphoma and extranodal marginal zone lymphoma of mucosa-associated lymphoid tissue. Below are several types of lymphoma that arise in spleen or primarily involve the spleen and present with splenomegaly which can be detected by physical examination or radiological imaging:
  - Splenic marginal zone lymphoma
  - Hairy cell leukemia
  - Splenic diffuse red pulp small B-cell lymphoma
  - Hairy cell leukemia variant
  - Hepatosplenic T-cell lymphoma
- Below are several systemic leukemias/lymphomas that frequently involve spleen:
  - B-cell prolymphocytic leukemia
  - Chronic lymphocytic leukemia/small lymphocytic lymphoma
  - Mantle cell lymphoma, leukemic non-nodal variant
  - T-cell prolymphocytic leukemia
  - T-cell large granular lymphocytic leukemia
  - Aggressive NK-cell leukemia
  - *EBV*-positive T-cell and NK-cell lymphoproliferative disease of childhood
  - Adult T-cell leukemia/lymphoma

10. Which types of lymphoid neoplasms often present with neutropenia, anemia, thrombocytopenia, or pancytopenia?

- Essentially any lymphoma, when involving bone marrow, can cause anemia, neutropenia, thrombocytopenia, or pancytopenia. These include entities primarily involving bone marrow, such as:
  - B-cell prolymphocytic leukemia
  - Chronic lymphocytic leukemia
  - B-lymphoblastic leukemia/lymphoma
  - Hairy cell leukemia
  - Hairy cell leukemia variant
  - Lymphoplasmacytic lymphoma
  - Plasma cell myeloma
  - T-cell prolymphocytic leukemia
  - Aggressive NK-cell leukemia
  - Adult T-cell leukemia/lymphoma
  - T-cell large granulocytic leukemia
  - Hepatosplenic T-cell lymphoma
  - T-lymphoblastic leukemia/lymphoma
- A few types of lymphoma with primary splenic involvement often present with peripheral thrombocytopenia and/or anemia due to bone marrow involvement, autoimmunity, or sequestration in the spleen. These include splenic marginal zone lymphoma, splenic diffuse red pulp small B-cell lymphoma, and hairy cell leukemia.
- A few types of T-cell lymphoma, such as angioimmunoblastic T-cell lymphoma and peripheral T-cell lymphoma, can present with cytopenia due to immune dysregulation or cytokine-mediated mechanisms.

11. Which lymphomas and non-leukemic hematolymphoid neoplasms can sometimes present as leukemia or have a leukemic phase?

Besides a few B-cell and T/NK-cell leukemias, a few types of lymphoma or hematolymphoid neoplasm can present as leukemic phase, which need to be distinguished from certain types of leukemia. See Table 3.6 for several common leukemic phases of lymphomas.

Table 3.6 Leukemic phases of lymphomas and mimics

Lymphoma with leukemic presentation	Need to be distinguished from
Mantle cell lymphoma, non-nodal variant	CLL, B-cell prolymphocytic leukemia
Splenic marginal zone lymphoma	Hairy cell leukemia or its variant, lymphoplasmacytic lymphoma, atypical CLL
Lymphoplasmacytic lymphoma	CLL, splenic marginal zone lymphoma
Mycosis fungoides/Sezary syndrome	T-cell prolymphocytic leukemia, adult T-cell leukemia/lymphoma
Blastic plasmacytoid dendritic cell neoplasm	Acute myeloid leukemia, T-lymphoblastic leukemia

12. What are the differential diagnoses in a patient who presents with an anterior/superior mediastinal mass?

- Lymphoid neoplasms presenting as anterior mediastinal mass include:
  - Classic Hodgkin lymphoma
  - Primary mediastinal large B-cell lymphoma
  - T-lymphoblastic lymphoma
  - Mediastinal lymph node involvement by lymphoma
- Non-lymphoid neoplasms presenting as anterior mediastinal mass include:
  - Thymoma/thymic carcinoma
  - Thymic carcinoid
  - Germ cell tumor
  - Involvement by lung carcinoma
  - Thyroid tumor
  - Metastatic tumor
- Nonneoplastic lesions include:
  - Sclerosing mediastinitis
  - Sarcoidosis
  - Thymic hyperplasia
  - Thymic cyst
  - Goiter

13. Which types of hematolymphoid neoplasms tends to present with skin lesions, besides extracutaneous or nodal involvement?

Besides a few types of primary cutaneous lymphoma, other hematolymphoid lesions could involve the skin and initially present as cutaneous lesions that may potentially be confused with primary cutaneous lymphoma or other hematolymphoid neoplasms. See Table 3.7 for several hematolymphoid neoplasms that often involve the skin and their differentials.

Table 3.7 Hematolymphoid neoplasms that often involve skin and their differentials

Nodal or systemic neoplasm	To be distinguished from
BPDCN	Leukemia cutis, CTCL
AITL	CTCL
MN	BPDCN, CTCL
ATLL	MF/Sezary syndrome, T-PLL
Sezary syndrome	MF, ATLL, T-PLL
EBV + DLBCL	PCDLBCL-leg type
Hydroa vacciniforme-like LPD	Infection, dermatosis

BPDCN blastic plasmacytoid dendritic cell neoplasm, *AITL* angioimmunoblastic T-cell lymphoma, *MN* myeloid neoplasm, including myeloid sarcoma or acute myeloid leukemia, *ATLL* adult T-cell leukemia/lymphoma, *EBV+ DLBCL EBV*-positive diffuse large B-cell lymphoma, *CTCL* cutaneous T-cell lymphoma, mainly mycosis fungoides, *T-PLL* T-cell prolymphocytic leukemia/lymphoma, *PCDLBCL-leg type* primary cutaneous diffuse large B-cell lymphoma, leg type, *LPD* lymphoproliferative disorder

14. Which anatomical sites (head/neck, axillary, thoracic, abdominal, retroperitoneal, inguinal, etc.) are more likely to be involved by particular lymphoid neoplasms or other hematolymphoid neoplasms?

Except for a few tissue-specific lymphomas and several precursor lesions, essentially all hematolymphoid neoplasm can involve any tissue site, when become disseminated. However, certain tissues or organs do have some predisposition for certain types of hematolymphoid neoplasms (Table 3.8).

Table 3.8 Common locations of primary involvement by hematolymphoid neoplasms

Sites involved	Types of hematolymphoid neoplasm
Anterior mediastinal mass	CHL, PMBCL, T-ALL
Cervical node	CHL, NLPHL
Tonsils	FL, DLBCL
Nasal sinuses	NK/T-cell lymphoma, PBL
Axillary node	CHL, NLPHL
Inguinal node	NLPHL
Retroperitoneal node	FL, DLBCL, Burkitt, HGBCL
Brain parenchyma	DLBCL
Meninges	MALT lymphoma, DLBCL
Orbits of the eye	MALT lymphoma, DLBCL
Splenic white pulp	SMZL, FL
Splenic red pulp	HCL, CLL, MN, SRPBCL, HSTCL, MCL-non-nodal variant, DLBCL
Liver	HSTCL, DLBCL
Gastric mucosa or wall	MALT lymphoma, DLBCL, HGBCL
Small bowel mucosa or wall	EATL, HGBCL, DLBCL, MCL, FL
Skin (primary lesions)	PCMZL, PCFCL, PCLBCL-leg type, MF, C-ALCL, other CTCL, BPDCN, LyP
Primary osseous lesion	DLBCL, PCN

DLBCL diffuse large B-cell lymphoma, *CHL* classic Hodgkin lymphoma, *FL* follicular lymphoma, *MZL* marginal zone lymphoma, *HGBCL* high-grade B-cell lymphoma, including Burkitt lymphoma, *MALT lymphoma* extranodal marginal zone lymphoma of mucosa-associated lymphoid tissue, *PMBCL* primary mediastinal B-cell lymphoma, *T-ALL* T-lymphoblastic lymphoma, *PBL* plasmablastic lymphoma, *SMZL* splenic marginal zone lymphoma, *HCL* hairy cell leukemia, *CLL* chronic lymphocytic leukemia, *MN* myeloid neoplasms, including acute myeloid leukemia, myeloproliferative neoplasm, and myelodysplastic neoplasm, *MCL* mantle cell lymphoma, *EATL* enteropathy-associated T-cell lymphoma, *SRPBCL* splenic red pulp B-cell leukemia/lymphoma, *CMZL* cutaneous marginal zone lymphoma, *CFCL* cutaneous follicle center lymphoma, *PCDLBCL* primary cutaneous diffuse large B-cell lymphoma, leg type, *MF* mycosis fungoides, *C-ALCL* cutaneous anaplastic large cell lymphoma, *LyP* lymphomatoid papulosis, *CTCL* cutaneous T-cell lymphoma, *BPDCN* blastic plasmacytoid dendritic cell neoplasm, *PCN* plasma cell neoplasm

15. How should the lymph node sections be examined microscopically?

- It is important to follow an established approach consistently to effectively and systemically examine the different compartments of a lymph node at lower- and higher-power magnifications.
- At low power, first evaluate the overall architecture to determine if it is preserved, distorted, or effaced.
- Next determine the pattern(s) of proliferating cells. See list of patterns in Q 16.
- When possible, try to identify areas likely to have major pathological changes during the low power examination.
- Focus on the selected areas first with higher power.
- Nest, carefully and systematically examine the cells within the perinodal soft tissue, capsule, lymphoid follicles, paracortex, and sinuses, with alternating lower- and higher-power magnifications.
- Prepare a list of differential diagnoses on morphologic grounds, and select necessary ancillary studies, such as immunohistochemistry, special stains for microorganisms, and molecular genetic analyses.

16. What are the major morphological patterns of reactive lymphadenopathy?

- Reactive lymph nodes have many different and unique patterns.
- The lymph node may show a dominant or mixed patterns since multiple nodal compartments may be involved in a single process.
- In addition, reactive conditions in the lymph node are dynamically active, and the dominant pattern may differ, depending on the stages of disease.
- Primary proliferative patterns of reactive lymphadenopathy:
  - Follicular pattern
  - Paracortical pattern
  - Sinus pattern
  - Granulomatous pattern
  - Mixed patterns
  - Miscellaneous

17. Which clinical diagnoses are likely associated with a reactive follicular pattern in the lymph node?

Follicular hyperplasia is defined as an increase in the number and size of secondary lymphoid follicles, which is one of the most common reactive patterns encountered by the pathologists. Reactive follicular hyperplasia is commonly seen as the dominant pattern or part of the processes below:

- Usual follicular hyperplasia (Fig. 3.3a)
- Human immunodeficiency virus lymphadenitis: typically florid follicular hyperplasia in the acute phase of infection (Fig. 3.3b, c)
- Progressive transformation of germinal centers (Fig. 3.3d)
- Toxoplasmosis lymphadenitis: follicular hyperplasia, small aggregates of epithelioid histiocytes impinging germinal centers, and paracortical monocytoid B-cell hyperplasia
- Kimura disease: follicular hyperplasia, marked eosinophilic infiltration, and vascular proliferation in the paracortex
- Castleman disease: often accompanied with paracortical expansion
- Systemic lupus erythematosus
- Rheumatoid arthritis
- IgG4-related lymphadenopathy, type II
- Syphilitic lymphadenitis (luetic lymphadenitis)

18. What is the initial workup for the reactive appearing lymph node with dominant follicular pattern?

- If an excised lymph node does not show obvious lymphoma based on morphologic and flow cytometric findings, but clinical suspicion of malignancy is high, immunoperoxidase stains may be warranted:
  - CD3: confirm positive staining T-cells are in paracortical areas and scattered follicular T-helper cells (Fig. 3.3e)
  - CD20: B-cells should be mostly in the lymphoid follicles (Fig. 3.3f)
  - BCL2: moderately positive in paracortical T-cells and mantle zone B-cells; negative in germinal center B-cells (Fig. 3.3g). May highlight in situ follicular neoplasia when scattered or small clusters of cells are brightly positive in the germinal centers
  - CD30: used to rule out a subtle involvement by anaplastic large cell lymphoma, classic Hodgkin lymphoma, and other CD30+ lymphomas. Also variably positive in reactive immunoblasts
  - CD10 and BCL6: normally germinal center B-cells positive, abnormal T-cells may stain
  - CD21and CD23: Useful to see the size, shape and distribution of follicular dendritic cell meshworks
  - Cytokeratin: to rule out subtle metastatic carcinomas, eg breast or head/neck primary
  - CD138, kappa, and lambda: for cases with marked plasmacytosis
  - IgG4: for all cases with PTGC and cases with persistent lymphadenopathy and increased plasma cells, but no other identifiable causes
  - Cyclin D1: for cases with expanded mantles or cytologic atypia in the mantles

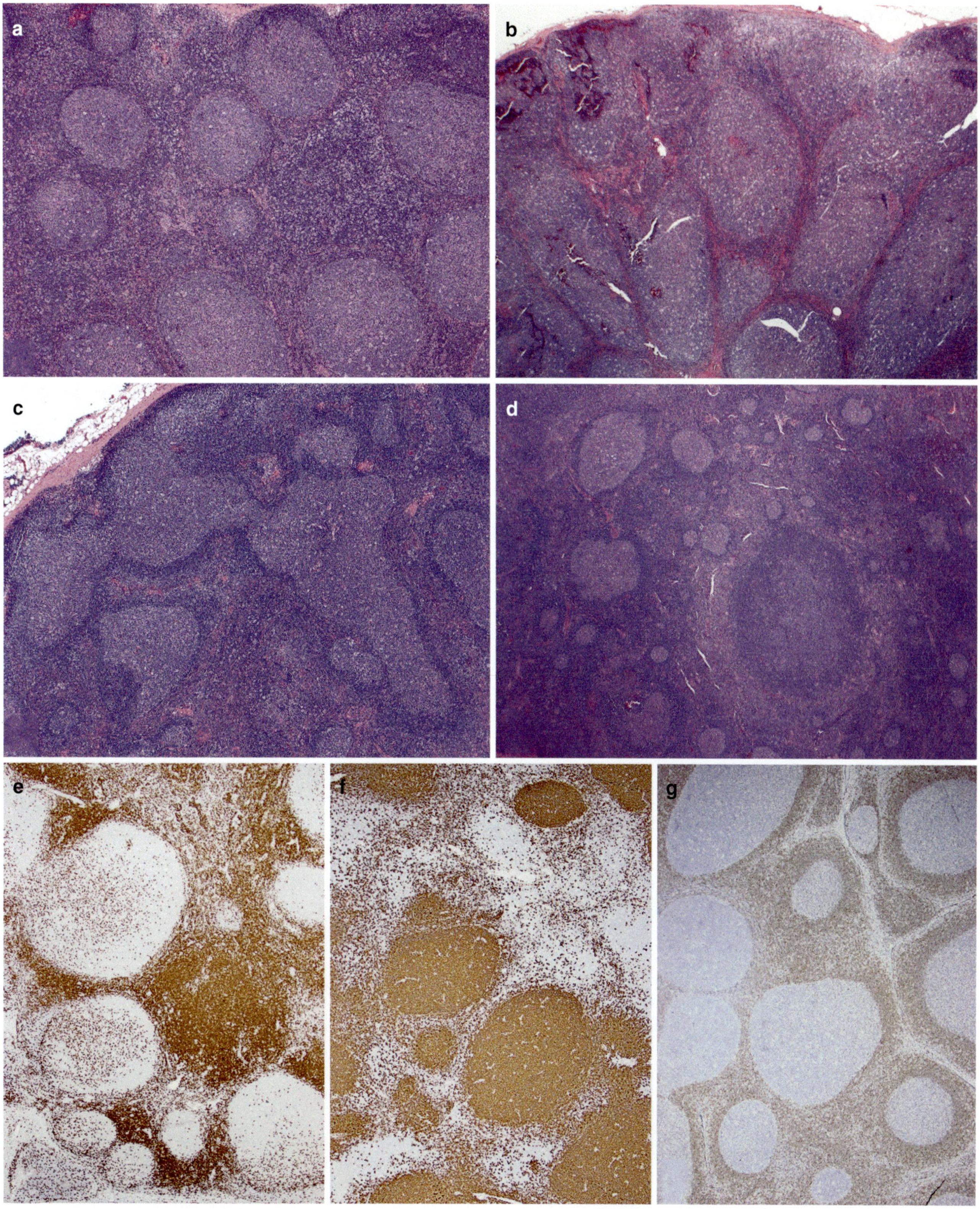

Fig. 3.3 Reactive follicular hyperplasia. (**a**) Usual follicular hyperplasia. The lymph node architecture is well preserved with frequent reactive lymphoid follicles and mild paracortical expansion. (**b**) Acute phase of HIV lymphadenopathy with many large and expansile lymphoid follicles. (**c**) A reactive lymph node with florid follicular hyperplasia containing serpiginous germinal centers. (**d**) The follicle of progressive transformation of germinal center is at least twice the size of a usual secondary follicle and consists mostly of small lymphocytes. (**e–g**) In a reactive lymph node, T-cells are mostly located in the paracortex (**e**, CD3), and B-cells are mostly in the lymphoid follicles (**f**, CD20). BCL2 (**g**) highlights reactive T-cells and mantle cells, whereas the germinal center B-cells are negative. (**a–g**) × 40

19. Which diagnoses are commonly associated with a paracortical pattern in reactive lymphadenopathy?

- The paracortex in a normal lymph node consists predominantly of small lymphocytes (mostly T-cells), scattered larger lymphocytes, plasma cells, granulocytes, histiocytes, dendritic cells, and high endothelial venules (HEVs).
- The paracortex of a reactive lymph node may be expanded by proliferation of a dominant population and/or mixed cell types, including:
  - Nonspecific paracortical T-cell proliferation
  - Reactive immunoblastosis
  - Reactive monocytoid B-cell hyperplasia
  - Prominent plasmacytosis
  - Proliferation of histiocytes, Langerhans cells, and interdigitating dendritic cells
  - Marked proliferation of HEVs
  - Plasmacytoid dendritic cell nodules
- The common and/or specific diagnoses associated with reactive paracortical expansion include:
  - Nonspecific paracortical hyperplasia
  - Acute infectious mononucleosis: marked paracortical expansion with immunoblastosis (Fig. 3.4a)
  - Castleman disease: often accompanied with follicular hyperplasia (Fig. 3.4b)
  - Cytomegalovirus infection: often accompanied with follicular hyperplasia
  - Kikuchi-Fujimoto lymphadenitis (Fig. 3.4c)
  - Dermatopathic lymphadenitis (Fig. 3.4d)
  - Post-vaccinial lymphadenitis
  - IgG4-related lymphadenopathy
  - Drug-induced lymphadenopathy

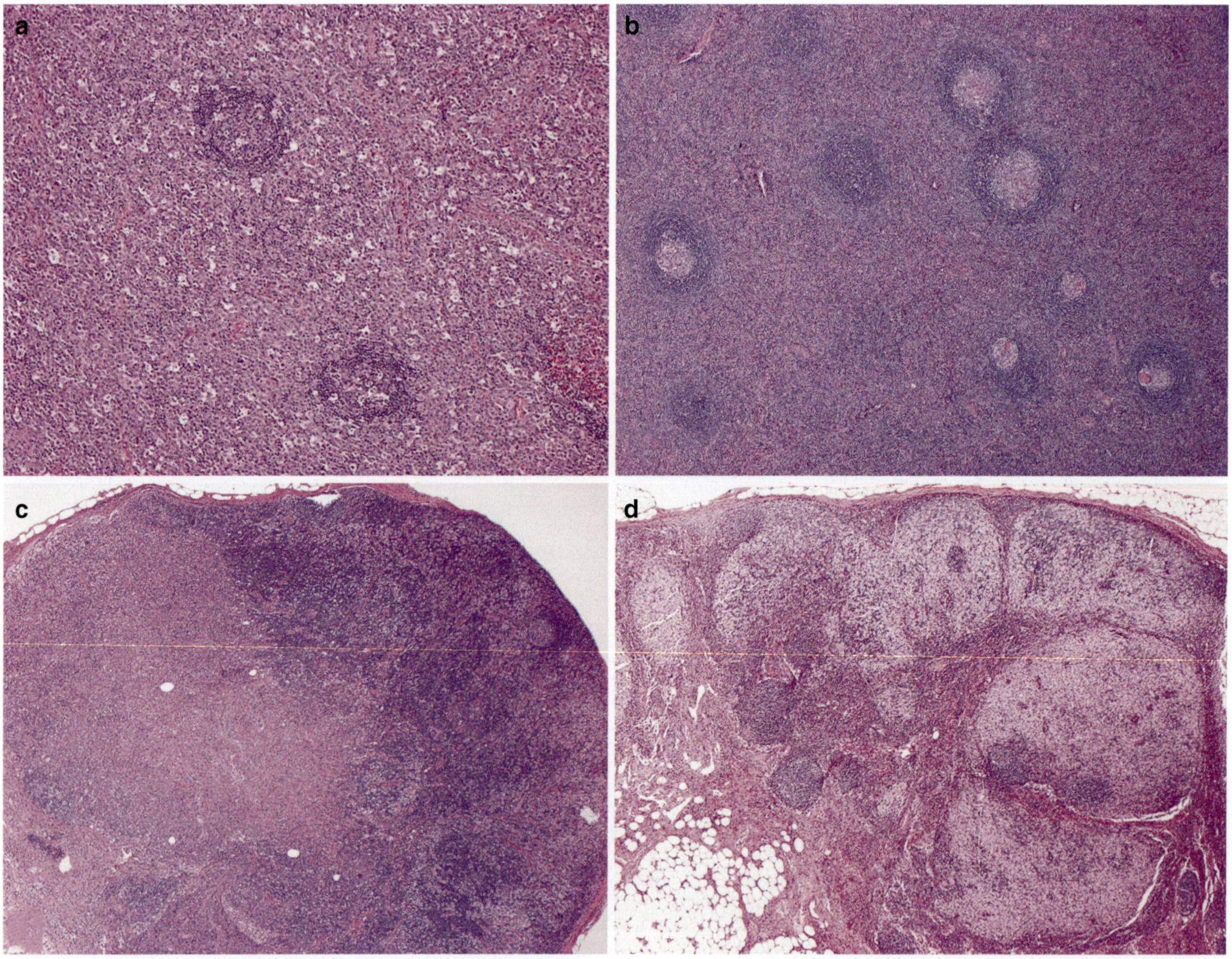

Fig. 3.4 Reactive lymph node with paracortical expansion. (**a**) Acute infectious mononucleosis. The markedly expanded paracortex contains mixed lymphocytes and abundant immunoblasts. H&E stain, ×200. (**b**) The paracortex in a hyaline vascular-type Castleman disease is significantly expanded by mixed inflammatory cells and vascular proliferation. H&E stain, ×100. (**c**) In a case of Kikuchi-Fujimoto disease, there is a focal and patchy paracortical expansion with mixed lymphocytes and histiocytes. H&E stain, ×40. (**d**) A case of dermatopathic lymphadenopathy reveals characteristic paracortical expansion by mixed histiocytes and Langerhans cells. H&E stain, ×40

20. Which diagnoses are commonly associated with a sinus pattern in reactive lymphadenopathy?

- Reactive sinus histiocytosis (Fig. 3.5a)
- Whipple disease (Fig. 3.5b)
- Rosai-Dorfman disease (Fig. 3.5c, d)
- Hemophagocytic syndrome
- Histiocytic lymphadenopathy after joint prosthesis (Fig. 3.5e, f; reaction to polyethylene and medal wear particles)
- Exogenous or endogenous lipids
- Vascular transformation

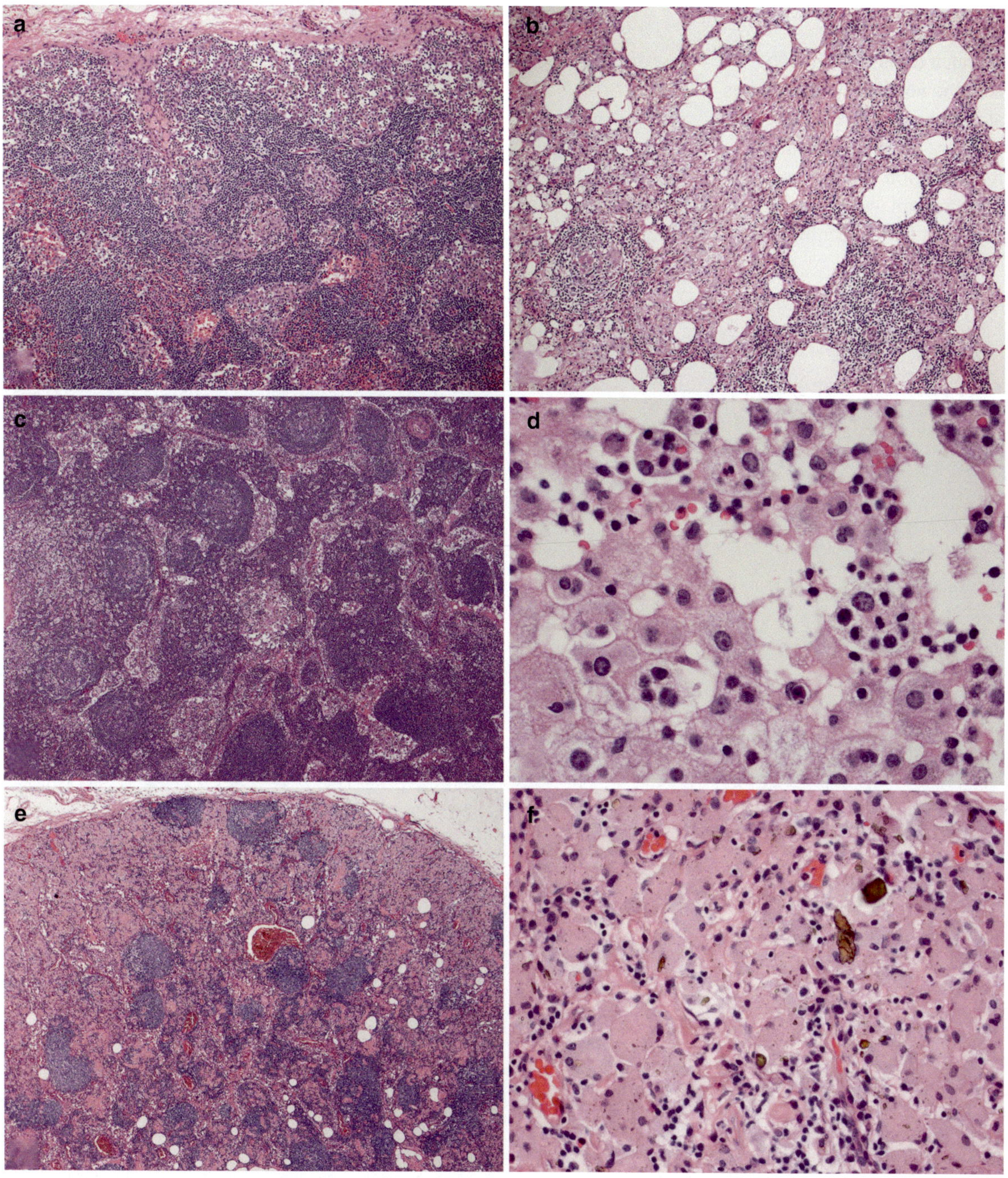

Fig. 3.5 Reactive lymph node with sinus dilation. (**a**) A case with reactive sinus histiocytosis. ×40. (**b**) A Whipple disease shows marked dilated sinuses containing abundant histiocytes and frequent large empty spaces. ×40. (**c**, **d**) In Rosai-Dorfman disease, there are abundant large histiocytes in the expanded sinuses with characteristic emperipolesis. **c**, ×40; **d**, ×400. (**e**, **f**) A para-aortic lymph node from a patient with joint prosthesis reveals abundant large histiocytes in the sinuses. **e**, ×40; **f**, ×200

21. Which diagnoses are commonly associated with a granulomatous pattern in reactive lymphadenopathy?

There are different types of reactive granulomas in lymph node, including non-necrotizing, suppurative, and necrotizing with coagulative necrosis, which are associated with different etiologies:

- Sarcoidosis (Fig. 3.6a)
- Cat-scratch disease (Fig. 3.6b)
- Mesenteric yersinia lymphadenitis
- Viral lymphadenitis (Fig. 3.6c, d)
- Lymphogranuloma venereum
- Fungal infection
- Mycobacterium avium-intracellulare lymphadenitis
- Tuberculous lymphadenitis

22. What are the major morphological patterns of lymphoma involvement in lymph node?

- **Follicular or nodular pattern**
  - Well-defined follicular pattern: follicular lymphoma
  - Vague follicular pattern: nodal marginal zone lymphoma with colonization of lymphoid follicles
  - Pseudofollicles (proliferation centers): seen in small lymphocytic lymphoma and usually poorly demarcated
  - Vague nodular pattern: mantle cell lymphoma
  - Macronodular pattern: well or poorly demarcated, in nodular lymphocyte predominant Hodgkin lymphoma (NLPHL)
  - Classic Hodgkin lymphoma (CHL), nodular variant of lymphocyte-rich subtype
  - Rarely follicular T-cell lymphoma

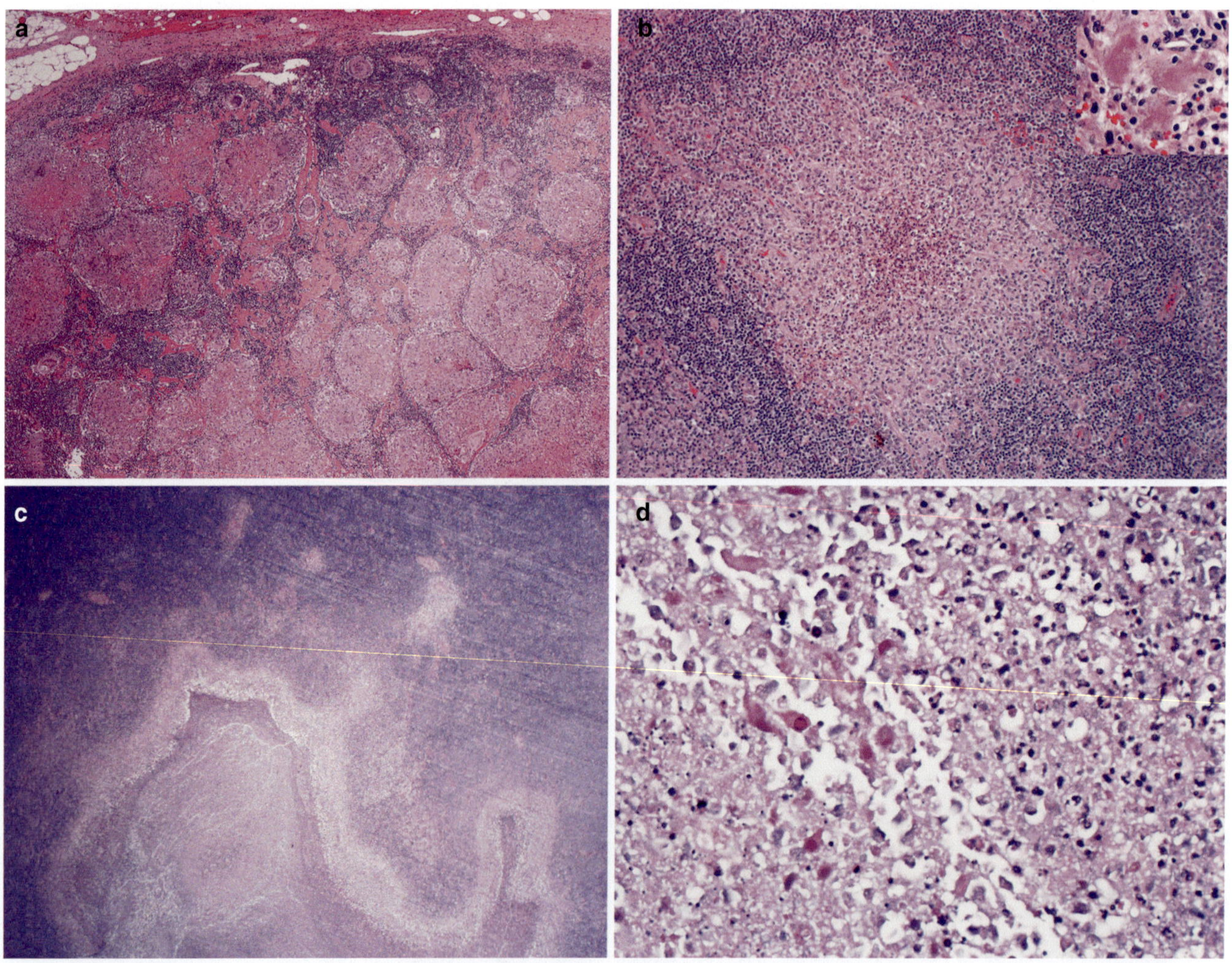

Fig. 3.6 Granulomatous reactive in the lymph node. (**a**) Sarcoidosis. The lymph node is replaced by numerous non-necrotizing granulomas. ×40. (**b**) A case of cat-scratch disease contains suppurative granulomas. ×100. Insert: areas of pink amorphous extracellular material containing bacteria. ×400. (**c**) A case of HSV lymphadenitis shows geographic necrotizing granulomas with peripheral palisading histiocytes (×40), and (**d**) scattered cells with viral inclusions are noted (×400)

- Diffuse pattern: entire architectural effacement by a diffuse infiltration of lymphoma cells
- Paracortical pattern: including early stage of low-grade B-cell neoplasm (i.e., marginal zone lymphoma, lymphoplasmacytic lymphoma), peripheral T-cell lymphoma, anaplastic large cell lymphoma, and cutaneous T-cell lymphoma with nodal involvement
- Sinusoidal pattern: anaplastic large cell lymphoma, ALK+ large B-cell lymphoma, CD30+ sinus large B-cell lymphoma, Langerhans cell histiocytosis, and histiocytic sarcoma
- Mantle zone pattern: rare cases of mantle cell lymphoma present with a pure mantle zone growth pattern, which is best highlighted with cyclin D1 staining

23. What are the major differential diagnoses and initial workup for lymphomas with follicular or nodular pattern?

- Major differential diagnosis:
  - Follicular lymphoma (Fig. 3.7a, b)
  - Follicular hyperplasia, florid follicular hyperplasia
  - Nodal marginal zone lymphoma with colonization of lymphoid follicles
  - Nodular lymphocyte predominant Hodgkin lymphoma (NLPHL) (Fig. 3.7c)
  - Progressive transformation of germinal centers (PTGC)
  - Classic Hodgkin lymphoma (CHL), nodular variant of lymphocyte-rich subtype
  - Mantle cell lymphoma with follicular, nodular, or mantle zone growth pattern
- Initial workup, if morphology is suggestive for follicular lymphoma and flow cytometry is unavailable/inconclusive/discrepant.
  - CD3: stains T-cells and highlights the follicular architecture
  - CD20: positive in B-cells in the follicles
  - BCL2: typically brightly positive in follicular lymphoma cells and may show reversed staining pattern in nodal marginal zone lymphoma with follicular colonization
  - CD10 and BCL6: positive in reactive and neoplastic follicular cells
  - Ki-67: lower in neoplastic than reactive follicles
  - CD43: negative in follicular lymphoma cells
- Initial workup if suspicious for NLPHL and CHL: CD3, CD15, CD20, CD21, CD30, CD45, CD57, PAX5, PD1, and EBER-ISH

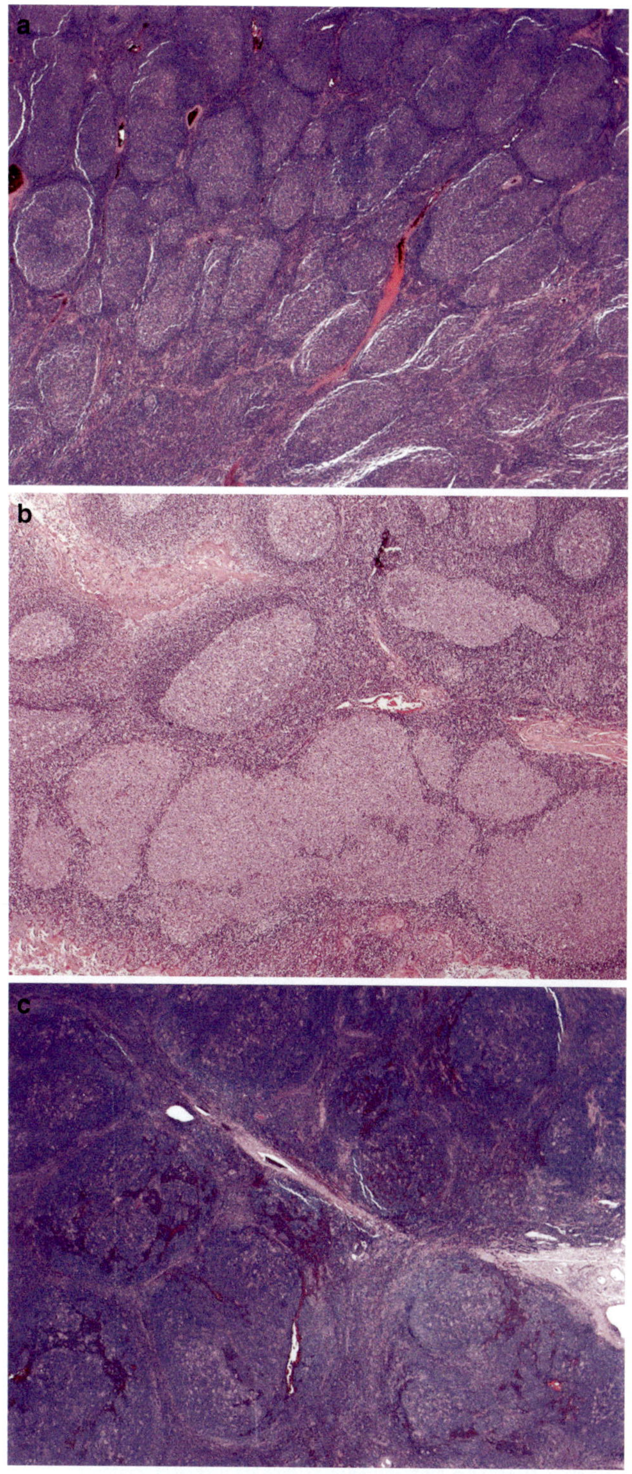

Fig. 3.7 Examples of follicular and nodular infiltration of lymphoma. (**a**) A case of follicular lymphoma contains many neoplastic follicles. (**b**) Florid follicular pattern in a pediatric follicular lymphoma. (**c**) Macronodular pattern in a nodular lymphocyte predominant Hodgkin lymphoma. (**a**–**c**), ×40

24. What are the major differential diagnoses and initial workup for the lymph node with a diffuse infiltration by small cell lymphoma?

- Major differential diagnosis:
  - Small lymphocytic lymphoma: pseudofollicles, small round nuclei, condensed chromatin, scant cytoplasm, and scattered prolymphocytes (Fig. 3.8a)
  - Mantle cell lymphoma: small to medium sized, angulated nuclei with moderately condensed chromatin, scattered epithelioid histiocytes, and hyaline vessels
  - Nodal marginal zone lymphoma: irregular nuclei, scant to moderate amount of cytoplasm, and plasmacytic differentiation
  - Lymphoplasmacytic lymphoma: patent sinuses; mixed populations of lymphocytes, plasmacytoid cells, and plasma cells; *MYD88* mutation
  - Follicular lymphoma: rare cases with diffuse pattern; mostly centrocytes and scattered centroblasts
- Initial workup: CD3, CD5, CD10 (or BCL6), CD20, CD23, cyclin D1, SOX11, Ki-67, and LEF1

25. What are the major differential diagnoses and initial workup for the lymph node with an interfollicular growth pattern?

- Differential diagnosis:
  - Marginal zone lymphoma
  - Lymphoplasmacytic lymphoma
  - Peripheral T-cell lymphoma (Fig. 3.8b)
  - Angioimmunoblastic T-cell lymphoma, pattern 2
  - Immunoblastic hyperplasia
  - Rare classic Hodgkin lymphoma
  - Rare small lymphocytic lymphoma, interfollicular pattern
- Suggested initial workup: CD20, CD3, CD5, CD23, CD10, BCL2, and Ki-67

26. What are the major differential diagnoses and initial workup for the lymph node with a diffuse infiltration by blastoid cells?

- Blastoid cytology: medium cell size, high N/C ratio, round or irregular nuclei, fine chromatin, inconspicuous or prominent nuclei, and rich in mitoses and apoptotic cells
- Major differential diagnosis: B-cell or T-cell lymphoblastic lymphoma, blastoid mantle cell lymphoma, Burkitt lymphoma, myeloid sarcoma, and diffuse large B-cell lymphoma
- Suggested initial workup: CD3, CD10, CD20, CD34, CD45, cyclin D1, Ki-67, MPO, and TdT

27. What are the major differential diagnoses and initial workup for the lymph node with a diffuse infiltration by large tumor cells?

- Differential diagnosis: diffuse large B-cell lymphoma (Fig. 3.8c), blastoid or pleomorphic mantle cell lymphoma, peripheral T-cell lymphoma, anaplastic large cell lymphoma, and metastatic carcinoma or sarcoma
- Initial workup: CD3, CD20, CD30, CD45 (or CD43), cyclin D1, CK AE1/AE3, and S100

28. What are the major differential diagnoses and initial workup for the lymph node with a prominent sinus infiltration of tumor cells?

- Hematopoietic neoplasms in the lymph node may show a prominent sinusoidal infiltration, including anaplastic large cell lymphoma, ALK+ large B-cell lymphoma (Fig. 3.8e, f), and CD30+ sinusoidal large B-cell lymphoma (Fig. 3.8g, h). Hepatosplenic T-cell lymphoma also shows a similar pattern although lymph node involvement is not common. Langerhans cell histiocytosis and histiocytic sarcoma often have a sinusoidal pattern, particularly in the early stage of disease.
- Metastatic tumor in the lymph node may reveal a focal or prominent sinusoidal infiltration, including carcinoma (Fig. 3.8d), melanoma, and soft tissue sarcoma.
- Initial workup: ALK, CD3, CD20, CD30, CD45 (or CD43), CK AE1/3, and S100.
- Initial workup if morphology suggestive for Langerhans cell histiocytosis: CD1a, S100, and langerin.

29. What is the initial workup for lymph node cases with morphologic features suggestive for classic Hodgkin lymphoma?

- CD3: positive in many T-cells as a feature of microenvironment.
- CD20: mostly negative, 20–30% of cases focally and weakly positive; if diffuse and strong expression, rule out

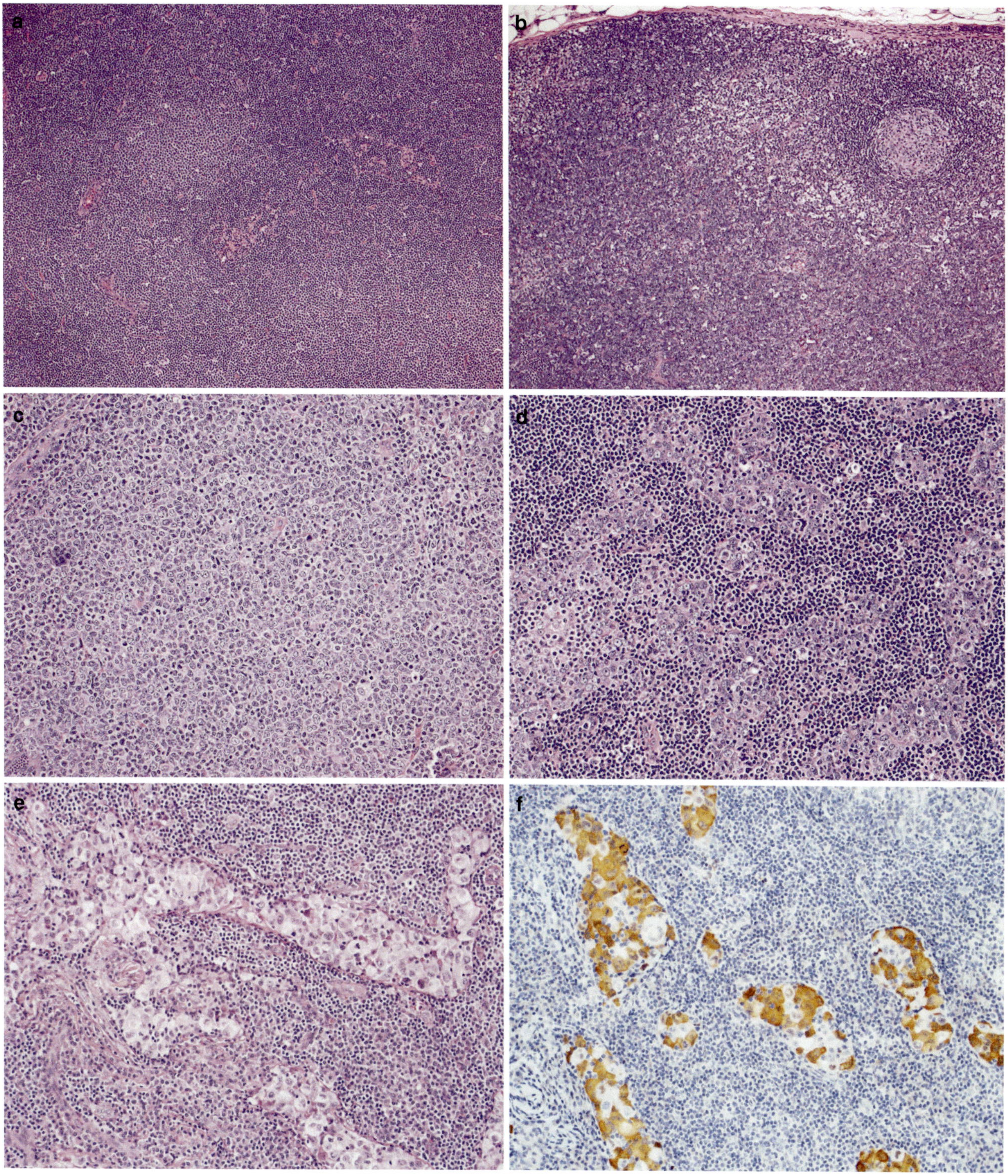

Fig. 3.8 Other examples of lymph node involvement. (**a**) Diffuse infiltration of small lymphocytic lymphoma with scattered proliferative centers. ×40. (**b**) Interfollicular infiltration of a T-cell lymphoblastic lymphoma. ×40. (**c**) Diffuse involvement of a diffuse large B-cell lymphoma. ×100. (**d**) Sinusoidal pattern of a metastatic undifferentiated nasopharyngeal carcinoma. ×100. (**e**) Sinusoidal pattern of anaplastic large cell lymphoma, ALK-positive (**f**, ALK, ×100)

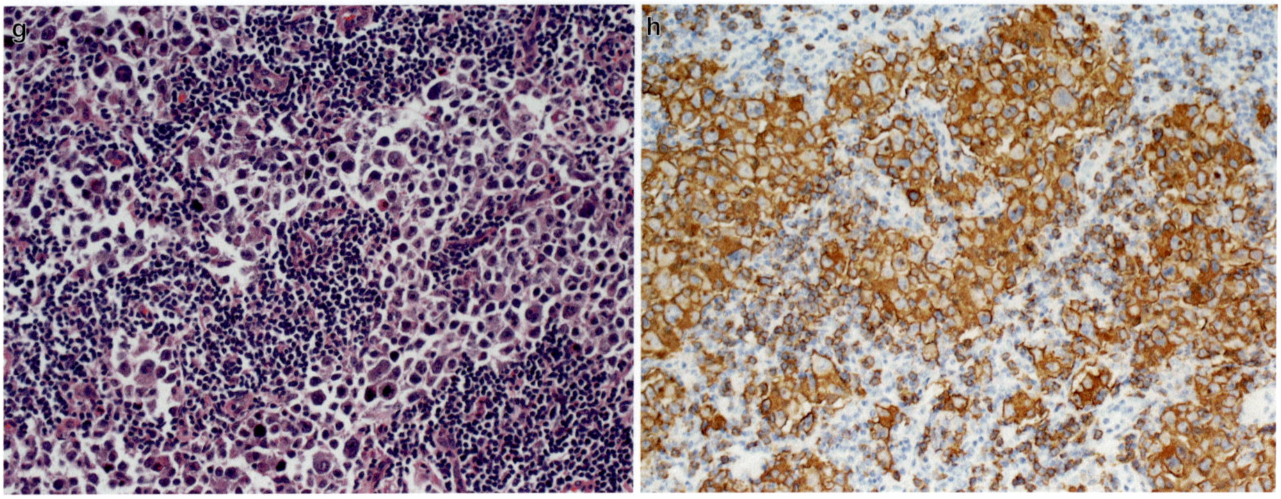

Fig. 3.8 (continued) (**g**) Sinusoidal pattern of a large B-cell lymphoma (×100), highlighted by CD20 immunostaining (**h**) CD20 (×100)

T-cell/histiocyte-rich large cell lymphoma and nodular lymphocyte predominant Hodgkin lymphoma.

- CD45: mostly negative, 5% of cases focally and weakly positive.
- CD30: almost always positive, strong, and diffuse, with membrane and Golgi zone pattern.
- CD15: mostly positive in CHL, typically with membrane and Golgi zone pattern.
- PAX5: mostly weakly positive in CHL.
- EBER-ISH: if positive, support the diagnosis over ALCL, NLPHL, and T/HRLBCL.

References (Questions 1–6): [1–26]; References (Questions 7–28): [27–32]

References

1. Salzman BE, Lamb K, Olszewski RF, Tully A, Studdiford J. Diagnosing cancer in the symptomatic patient. Prim Care. 2009;36(4):651–70.
2. Gaddey HL, Riegel AM. Unexplained lymphadenopathy: evaluation and differential diagnosis. Am Fam Physician. 2016;94(11):896–903.
3. King D, Ramachandra J, Yeomanson D. Lymphadenopathy in children: refer or reassure? Arch Dis Child Educ Pract Ed. 2014;99(3):101–10.
4. Locke R, Comfort R, Kubba H. When does an enlarged cervical lymph node in a child need excision? A systematic review. Int J Pediatr Otorhinolaryngol. 2014;78(3):393–401.
5. Nolder AR. Paediatric cervical lymphadenopathy: when to biopsy? Curr Opin Otolaryngol Head Neck Surg. 2013 Dec;21(6):567–70.
6. Esra AÖ, Ceren CG, Zeynep TÖ, Serdar Y, Nuri EG, Meryem D, et al. Evaluation of peripheral lymphadenopathy with excisional biopsy: six-year experience. Int J Clin Exp Pathol. 2015;8(11):15234–9.
7. Chiappini E, Camaioni A, Benazzo M, Biondi A, Bottero S, De Masi S, et al. Development of an algorithm for the management of cervical lymphadenopathy in children: consensus of the Italian Society of Preventive and Social Pediatrics, jointly with the Italian Society of Pediatric Infectious Diseases and the Italian Society of Pediatric Otorhinolaryngology. Expert Rev Anti-Infect Ther. 2015;13(12):1557–67.
8. Karadeniz C, Oguz A, Ezer U, Oztürk G, Dursun A. The etiology of peripheral lymphadenopathy in children. Pediatr Hematol Oncol. 1999;16(6):525–31.
9. Steel BL, Schwartz MR, Ramzy I. Fine needle aspiration biopsy in the diagnosis of lymphadenopathy in 1,103 patients. Role, limitations and analysis of diagnostic pitfalls. Acta Cytol. 1995;39(1):76–81.
10. Desciak EB, Maloney ME. Artifacts in frozen section preparation: how I do it/back to basics. Dermatol Surg. 2000;26:500–4.
11. Rakha EA, Haider A, Patil S, et al. Evaluation of touch preparation cytology during frozen-section diagnoses of pulmonary lesions. J Clin Pathol. 2010;63:675–7.
12. Brunner C, Brunner-Herglotz B, Ziegler A, Frech C, Amann G, Ladenstein R, et al. Tumor touch imprints as source for whole genome analysis of neuroblastoma tumors. PLoS One. 2016;11(8):e0161369.
13. Loo E, Siddiqi IN. Processing the lymph node biopsy. In: Day C, editor. Histopathology: methods in molecular biology (methods and protocols). New York: Humana Press; 2014. p. 271–82.
14. Pelstring RJ, Allred DC, Esther RJ, et al. Differential antigen preservation during tissue autolysis. Hum Pathol. 1991;22:237–41.
15. Prakash S, Banks PM. Technical factors in the preparation and evaluation of lymph node biopsies. In: Orazi A, Knowles DM, Foucar K, Weiss LM, editors. Knowles' neoplastic hematopathology. Philadelphia: LWW; 2014. p. 286–92.
16. Grizzle WE, Fredenburgh JL, Myers RB. Fixation of tissues. In: Bancroft JD, Gamble M, editors. Theory and practice of histological techniques. 6th ed. Philadelphia: Churchill Livingstone/Elsevier; 2008. p. 53–74.
17. Rolls G. Fixation and fixatives – popular fixative solutions. Leica Biosyst. https://www.leicabiosystems.com/pathologyleaders/fixation-and-fixatives-4-popular-fixative-solutions/#c22930/. Accessed Dec 24 2018.
18. Qidwai K, Afkhami M, Day C. The pathologist's guide to fixatives. In: Day C, editor. Histopathology: methods in molecular biology (methods and protocols). New York: Humana Press; 2014. p. 21–30.
19. Brynes RK. LAC+USC Medical Center, clinical hematology laboratory, procedure manual. Los Angeles; 2018.

20. Babic A, Loftin IR, Stainslaw S, Wang M, Miller R, Warren SM, et al. The impact of pre-analytical processing on staining quality for H&E, dual hapten, dual color in situ hybridization and fluorescent in situ hybridization assays. Methods. 2010;52:287–300.
21. Wood BL, Arroz M, Barnett D, DiGiuseppe J, Greig B, Kussick SJ, Oldaker T, Shenkin M, Stone E, Wallace P. 2006 Bethesda International Consensus recommendations on the immunophenotypic analysis of hematolymphoid neoplasia by flow cytometry: optimal reagents and reporting for the flow cytometric diagnosis of hematopoietic neoplasia. Cytometry B Clin Cytom. 2007;72(Suppl 1):S14–22.
22. Craig FE, Foon KA. Flow cytometric immunophenotyping for hematologic neoplasms. Blood. 2008;111(8):3941–67.
23. Zeka F, Vanderheyden K, De Smet E, Cuvelier CA, Mestdagh P, Vandesompele J. Straightforward and sensitive RT-qPCR based gene expression analysis of FFPE samples. Sci Rep. 2016;6:21418.
24. Iddawela M, Rueda OM, Klarqvist M, Graf S, Earl HM, Caldas C. Reliable gene expression profiling of formalin-fixed paraffin-embedded breast cancer tissue (FFPE) using cDNA-mediated annealing, extension, selection, and ligation whole-genome (DASL WG) assay. BMC Med Genet. 2016;9:54.
25. Lefrançois P, Tetzlaff MT, Moreau L, Watters AK, Netchiporouk E, Provost N, Gilbert M, Ni X, Sasseville D, Duvic M, Litvinov IV. TruSeq-based gene expression analysis of formalin-fixed paraffin-embedded (FFPE). Cutaneous T-cell lymphoma samples: subgroup analysis results and elucidation of biases from FFPE sample processing on the TruSeq platform. Front Med. 2017;4:153.
26. Kim SJ, Sohn I, Do IG, Jung SH, Ko YH, Yoo HY, Paik S, Kim WS. Gene expression profiles for the prediction of progression-free survival in diffuse large B cell lymphoma: results of a DASL assay. Ann Hematol. 2014;93(3):437–47.
27. Jaffe ES, Arber DA, Campo E, et al. Hematopathology. 2nd ed. Philadelphia: Elsevier; 2017.
28. Orazi A, Foucar K. Knowles neoplastic hematopathology. 3rd ed. Philadelphia: Wolters Kluwer Health/Lippincott Williams & Wilkins; 2014.
29. His ED. Hematopathology. 2nd ed. Philadelphia: Elsevier/Saunders.
30. Swerdlow SH, Campo E, Harris NL, et al. WHO classification of tumors of hematopoietic and lymphoid tissues. Revised 4th ed. Lyon: World Health Organization; International Agency for Research on Cancer. International Agency for Research on Cancer; 2017.
31. O'Malley DP, George TI, Orazi A, et al. Benign and reactive conditions of the lymph node and spleen. Atlas of nontumor pathology. 7th ed. Washington, D.C.: ARP PRESS; 2009.
32. Ioachim HL, Medeiros LJ. Ioachim's lymph node pathology. 4th ed. Philadelphia: Wolters Kluwer Health/Lippincott Williams & Wilkins; 2009.

Lymphoid Pathology on Small Biopsies (FNA and Small Core) – Advantages and Limitations: Guidelines for Ancillary Studies According to Clinical Scenario and Morphology

4

Kathryn M. Hogan, Anand Shreeram Lagoo, and Kedar V. Inamdar

List of Frequently Asked Questions

1. What are the "small biopsy" alternatives to an excisional lymph node biopsy, and what is the optimal procedure for handling each?
2. What are the advantages and drawbacks of these techniques?
3. What is the difference in approach to small biopsies which are performed for initial diagnosis versus those performed in patients with previously treated disease? How are clinical findings used to guide interpretation of "small biopsy" of lymphoid tissue?
4. What are the diagnostic challenges using FNA for lymphoma diagnosis? What is the clinical relevance of misinterpretation between the true diagnosis and mimics with reference to mistreatment and/or wrong prognosis?
5. What are the advantages and limitations of core needle biopsy (CNB) for lymphoma diagnosis?
6. For small biopsies performed for initial diagnosis, which ancillary test results are diagnostic, are suggestive of diagnosis, are unreliable for diagnosis, or rule out the diagnosis?
7. What is the workup appropriate in patients with prior diagnosis of B-cell lymphomas? What are the special considerations to evaluate disease progression, secondary effects of prior treatment, presence of therapeutic targets for additional treatment, etc. in these cases?
8. What are the major pitfalls when diagnosing recurrent B-cell lymphomas on small biopsy?
9. What is the workup of a small biopsy in patients with prior diagnosis of T-/NK-cell lymphomas? What are the special considerations to evaluate disease progression, secondary effects of prior treatment, presence of therapeutic targets for additional treatment, etc. in these cases?
10. What are the pitfalls in the diagnosis of HL with a small biopsy? What steps should be taken to avoid these pitfalls?

K. M. Hogan · K. V. Inamdar (✉)
Department of Pathology, Henry Ford Hospital, Detroit, MI, USA
e-mail: khogan3@hfhs.org; kinamda1@hfhs.org

A. S. Lagoo
Department of Pathology, Duke University School of Medicine and Duke Health System, Durham, NC, USA
e-mail: anand.lagoo@duke.edu

1. What are the "small biopsy" alternatives to an excisional lymph node biopsy and what is the optimal procedure for handling each?

Fine needle aspiration (FNA) cytology and core needle biopsy (CNB) are the two main techniques used to obtain tissue material when a surgical excisional biopsy (SEB) is not possible or is not desired. In a minority of patients, exfoliated cytology in tissue fluids such as cerebrospinal fluid, urine, or pleural or peritoneal fluid may be submitted to rule out lymphoma.

FNA Cytology

- Optimally a rapid morphologic review of the aspirate at the time of collection should be performed, in order to assess specimen adequacy and to screen for a lymphoid proliferation. The latter is particularly useful in the setting of an FNA of an extranodal mass, where a lymphoma may not be suspected. One can assess the likely quantity of lymphoid tissue available and perform additional FNA passes if necessary. Depending on the quantity of lymphoid tissue avaialble, one can choose the type (e.g., mature B panel vs. lymphoblastic) and extent of flow cytometric immunophenotyping.

E. Wang, A. S. Lagoo (eds.), *Practical Lymph Node and Bone Marrow Pathology*, Practical Anatomic Pathology,
https://doi.org/10.1007/978-3-030-32189-5_4

- A rapid Romanowsky-stained FNA smear or cytospin preparation is a helpful complement to the Papanicolaou stain. The cytomorphology on the air-dried smears resembles the more familiar bone marrow aspirate and peripheral blood smear cytology. This and the flow immunophenotypic profiles together maximize the overall diagnostic sensitivity for lymphoma and enhance the ability to classify the type of lymphoma.
- If sufficient quantity of aspirate is obtained, then air-dried smears or formalin-fixed paraffin-embedded cell block sections may also be used for:
  - Immunocytochemical (ICC) or immunohistochemical (IHC) analysis of antigen expression
  - Molecular tests (e.g., PCR for *IGH* or *TCR* gene clonality; FISH cytogenetic tests)

CNB

- Ideally, obtain two to three cores for formalin-fixed paraffin embedded (FFPE) tissue for histopathologic exam and one core (submitted in saline) for flow cytometric immunophenotyping.
  - These should be obtained with a core needle of 18 gauge or larger, and each core should be at least 1 cm in length. Multiple touch imprints (three to five) from the unfixed core biopsy should be obtained for potential molecular tests, and one should be Giemsa-stained for cytological examination. The individual cores for FFPE should be submitted in separate blocks, in order to maximize the availability of tissue for ancillary exams. This may be modified to one block if there is minimal quantity and/or extreme fragmentation of the biopsy.
  - Each block should be serially sectioned with multiple blanks for potential IHC and/or molecular studies. An example would be sections 1 and 11 being H&E stained for routine histopathologic exam and sections 2 through 10 being blanks.
- If the unfixed core is deemed quantitatively sufficient for flow cytometry, then it should be immediately minced and placed in tissue culture media, or wrapped in saline-soaked gauze and placed in container with saline, and then immediately sent to the flow cytometry laboratory. The choice of panel is dictated by the likely differential diagnosis (e.g., relapsed disease in a patient previously diagnosed with leukemia/lymphoma vs. de novo presentation; clinical features favoring a T-cell neoplasm, etc.).

Given the robust nature of IHC of FFPE lymphoma sections, a reasonable minimal panel would include kappa and lambda immunoglobulin light chains with one specific pan B- (e.g., CD19) and pan T-cell (e.g., CD3) marker. While not as specific for T lineage as CD3, CD5 antigen combined with CD19 allows a clear separation of CD5+/CD19+ B cells from CD5+/CD19-negative T lymphocytes.

2. What are the advantages and drawbacks of these techniques?

FNA

Advantages

- Least complicated of the three techniques (FNA, CNB, and SEB), with the least comorbidity in the hands of experienced operators. The diagnostic advantage offered by FNA as a procedure depends on:
  - The ability of the provider (cytopathologist or clinician) to obtain a good specimen.
  - The location of the lesion (superficial versus deep; proximity to a vital structure, etc.).
  - Choice of technique (non-image- versus image-guided FNA). Image-guided FNAs in general offer better precision and diagnostic accuracy compared to non-image-guided FNAs [1].
- FNA can be performed on an outpatient basis and does not require admission and scheduling for surgery.
- FNA is of particular value in patients in whom biopsy may be relatively contraindicated, for example, in old patients with multiple comorbidities or patients on anticoagulants. In patients where lesion(s) or lymph nodes are in locations not amenable to surgery and are close to or involve a vital organ or a major blood vessel, FNA is of particular value in preventing the risks associated with a surgical procedure such as incision or excision biopsy.
- FNA specimens are easier to process, thus allowing for quicker results, and are relatively inexpensive to perform. In the setting of the differential diagnosis of localized lymphadenopathy, this technique has excellent diagnostic sensitivity and specificity for a wide range of neoplasms (e.g., carcinomas; melanomas).
- While a multitude of variables including the clinical situation, location of lesion, technical difficulty, and accessibility of lesion can affect the cost of a procedure, FNA is generally more cost-effective compared to surgically performed core needle or excision biopsies [2].
- When specifically performed for suspected lymphoma, FNA combined with flow immunophenotyping is quite sensitive and reasonably specific for most lymphomas. Numerous studies have evaluated the efficacy of FNA in lymphoma diagnosis over the past decade.
  - When diagnosed using cytomorphology alone, Hodgkin lymphoma (HL) is more likely to be diagnosed correctly (approx. 87% accuracy) than non-Hodgkin lymphoma (NHL) (approx. 70% accuracy) [3]. The WHO classification scheme for tumors of hematopoietic and lymphoid tissues and especially the

2017 revision [4] incorporates data from ancillary studies including flow cytometry, immunohistochemistry, cytogenetics, and molecular assays in the diagnosis and classification of lymphoid neoplasms. When these techniques are incorporated, the diagnosis of lymphoid neoplasms using FNA achieves high levels of sensitivity, specificity, and accuracy. Using FNA for first-time diagnosis in a previously undiagnosed patient, the diagnostic sensitivity (between 61% and 100%), specificity (88–100%), and accuracy (on average greater than 80%) are much higher for NHL when compared to HL (sensitivity and accuracy between 40% and 80%). The value of FNA is much higher in patients with a previous history of lymphoma where the diagnostic sensitivity, specificity, and accuracy are even higher for both groups.

Drawbacks

- One of the biggest disadvantages of FNA is its limited ability to accurately classify lymphomas and differentiate between benign and malignant lymphoid proliferations due to lack of architectural context available in tissue biopsy. The European Society of Medical Oncology (ESMO), the WHO system for lymphoma classification, the British Committee for Standards in Haematology, and the National Comprehensive Cancer Network (NCCN) recommend excisional biopsy for lymphoma diagnosis and subtyping. In fact, the current NCCN clinical practice guidelines in oncology specifically state that FNA or core needle biopsy is insufficient in the diagnosis of follicular lymphoma (FL), diffuse large B-cell lymphoma (DLBCL), mantle cell lymphoma (MCL), and marginal zone lymphoma (MZL). Furthermore, FNAs are not ideal specimens for grading of follicular lymphoma [5].
- Few lymphomas have very characteristic immunocytological (IC) profiles that would allow a full diagnosis (e.g., CLL/SLL, MCL, T or B-lineage lymphoblastic lymphomas). Others have suggestive IC profiles (follicular lymphoma; Burkitt lymphoma) that often allow a general diagnosis of lymphoma. FNA has a lesser sensitivity for detection of cytological transformation.
- Clonal B-lymphoproliferative disorders (B-LPDs) may be detected by flow cytometric immunophenotyping in the clinical and histopathologic setting of lymphoid hyperplasia.
- FNA in particular has low diagnostic yield in lesions that are fibrotic or necrotic and a high rate of false-negative results compared to CNB or SEB.
  - FNAs involving lesions with higher-grade lymphomas (e.g., diffuse large B-cell lymphoma) and lymphomas with neoplastic cells confined to focal areas [e.g., HL; T-cell−/histiocyte-rich diffuse large B-cell lymphoma (T/HCRLBCL)] frequently yield false-negative results. This is mainly because higher-grade lymphomas often have tumor necrosis with subsequent lack of viable tumor cells for cytological exam and/or flow cytometric immunophenotyping.

3. What is the difference in approach to small biopsies which are performed for initial diagnosis versus those performed in patients with previously treated disease? How are clinical findings used to guide interpretation of "small biopsy" of lymphoid tissue?

- Assessment of lymphoid pathology generally begins with morphologic evaluation to determine whether morphologic features indicate a neoplastic or nonneoplastic etiology as possible cause for clinical symptoms, lymph node enlargement, organomegaly, and/or extranodal masses. Ancillary studies are guided primarily by cytomorphologic determination of possible etiology.
- Certain diagnoses such as infections or metastatic malignancies do not need flow cytometry and/or molecular tests, and a diagnosis can be generally rendered in such cases with the use of special stains or targeted IHC panels. Special stains, such as Gomori methenamine silver (GMS) and periodic acid Schiff (PAS) stains for fungal microorganisms, Ziehl-Neelsen stain for mycobacterial organisms, Warthin-Starry stain for spirochetes, and Gram stain for bacilli and cocci and certain virus-specific stains (HSV, CMV, etc.) to characterize viral inclusions, are generally applied. In cases of metastatic malignancies, morphologic clues may guide the selection of targeted IHC markers to determine the site of primary cancer. These studies can be performed in cell block preparations or CNB, and a final diagnosis can be reached in majority of cases with a fairly high degree of accuracy (at least in metastatic malignancies).
- Once infections or metastatic malignancy is excluded, the next step in assessment is to distinguish benign reactive hyperplasia from NHL. Whether this is achievable in an FNA specimen is debatable for the reasons discussed earlier in this chapter. In a CNB or SEB, reactive hyperplasia generally shows preservation of nodal architecture. The follicles are well-spaced from one another, and mantle zones are well-demarcated. Polarity is maintained and tingible body macrophages are readily observed. Cytologically, reactive proliferations exhibit minimal or no atypia and comprise of mixed populations of small lymphocytes, plasmacytoid lymphocytes, centrocytes, centroblasts, immunoblasts, tingible body macrophages, and dendritic cells. In contrast to reactive hyperplasia, NHLs typically distort or efface nodal architecture in a nodular, diffuse, or a mixed pattern. Neoplastic proliferations, particularly the small-cell/low-grade lymphomas (FL, CLL/SLL, MZL, and LPL) with the exception of mantle cell lymphoma, may not exhibit much cytologic

atypia but, in contrast to reactive hyperplasia, exhibit a rather monotonous proliferation.

- High-grade/large-cell lymphoid proliferations (high-grade FL, DLBCL, Burkitt lymphoma, ALCL, PTCLs) exhibit frank cytologic atypia with enlarged nuclei, nuclear irregularities, nucleoli, karyorrhexis, and/or necrosis. In these cases, immunocytochemistry or immunohistochemistry is more useful than flow cytometry in differentiating lymphoid from other neoplasms (carcinoma, melanoma, and sarcoma). High-grade lymphomas have a high rate of false-negative results by flow cytometry as the lymphoma cells in most cases do not survive flow cytometric processing. Besides, flow cytometric immunoanalysis is not quite useful in entities such as anaplastic large cell lymphoma (ALCL), T/HCRLBCL, and HL, and these entities are better characterized by immunohistochemistry.
- While cytomorphologic features can provide clues to differentiate benign from malignant entities, a diagnosis of NHL and its subclassification according to the WHO scheme cannot be achieved without combining morphology with flow cytometry and/or immunocytochemistry (immunohistochemistry in case of CNB).

4. What are the diagnostic challenges using FNA for lymphoma diagnosis? What is the clinical relevance of misinterpretation between the true diagnosis and mimics with reference to mistreatment and/or wrong prognosis?

FNA

- Challenge for CD10-positive lymphomas:
  - Distinction between high-grade (grade 3) follicular lymphomas (FL), diffuse large B-cell lymphoma (DLBCL), Burkitt lymphoma (BL), and non-Burkitt-type high-grade B-cell lymphoma may not be possible with some limited tissue biopsies that may be insufficient for ancillary tests such as FISH for high-grade B-cell lymphoma panel.
  - CD10+ small B-cell lymphomas may contain variable proportion of large cells. Grading of FL is preferentially done in excisional biopsies per the WHO recommendations. Furthermore, FL pattern (predominantly follicular, follicular and diffuse, or predominantly diffuse) cannot be assessed on FNA. Finally, CD10 is known to be aberrantly expressed in other small B-NHLs and may cause diagnostic confusion without assessment of morphology either in CNB or SEB.
- Challenges for B- and T-cell lymphomas lacking characteristic cytological and/or immunophenotypic features:
  - Marginal zone lymphomas (MZL) have nonspecific cytological or immunophenotypic features and thus are difficult to classify on FNA or CNB.
  - Peripheral T-cell lymphoma, not otherwise specified (PTCL, NOS), is a diagnosis of exclusion and generally requires careful exclusion of specific entities in the realm of T-NHLs that can show immunophenotypic overlap with this entity. This is challenging even in well-sampled tissue biopsies.
- Challenges for diagnosis of HL: Even more challenging given the paucity of tumor cells, the abundance of reactive lymphocytes in the milieu of HL, fibrosis of involved nodes especially in nodular sclerosis type of HL, limited value of flow cytometry, and presence of cells resembling Hodgkin/Reed-Sternberg (HRS) cells in a number of NHL types, metastatic melanoma, metastatic carcinoma, and reactive immunoblastic proliferations [6–8].
- Two NHL entities, anaplastic large-cell lymphoma (ALCL) and T-cell–/histiocyte-rich large B-cell lymphoma (T/HCRLBCL), have significant morphologic and immunophenotypic overlap with HL creating diagnostic confusion [9–14]. T/HCRLBCL has morphologic similarities to lymphocyte predominant subtype of HL (NLPHL) but has vastly different clinical outcome. Architectural context provided by CNB or SEB is required to differentiate between CHL, NLPHL and T/HCRLBCL.
- A number of morphologic attributes of HL related to cell morphology and cellular composition, as well as immunophenotype of abnormal cells, are found with equal frequency in ALCL cases [15].

5. What are the advantages and limitations of Core Needle Biopsy for lymphoma diagnosis?

- CNB provides histological context lacking in FNA smears, but an excisional biopsy is optimal if a definitive diagnosis, with correct subclassification, is required.
- On the other hand, if there is urgency of diagnosis, or questions about accessibility of lesion, patient compliance, and excessive operative risk, CNB is relatively a simpler procedure with minimal risks of hemorrhage or damage to vital structures.
  - It generally requires local anesthesia and can be performed on an outpatient basis.
  - In lesions that are deep-seated or located in the vicinity of vital organs or major blood vessels where a SEB may be relatively or absolutely contraindicated, CNB or FNA is particularly useful in obtaining material for diagnosis [16, 17].
  - Architectural assessment is necessary for differentiating reactive or benign entities from malignant lesions. Also, diagnosis of in-situ lymphomas (follicular and mantle) is only possible with the use of immunohistochemistry (IHC) on an excisional or incisional biopsy.

- CNB permits an integrated approach involving assessment of complex architectural patterns and use of various ancillary studies including IHC, cytogenetics, and molecular studies and has a higher diagnostic yield over FNA specimens in lymphomas with complex architectural patterns, lesions with paucity of tumor cells, and lesions with fibrosis or sclerotic background.

  CNB as a stand-alone technique in first-time lymphoma diagnosis has a reported sensitivity ranging from 70% to 100% [16, 18].

  In a study of cervical lymph nodes comparing the value of CNB to FNA, sensitivity and negative predictive value (NPV) for critical disease (lymphoma, carcinoma, and tuberculosis) were significantly higher with CNB ($p = 0.006$, $p = 0.001$, respectively) than with FNA. When analyzed specifically for lymphoma diagnosis, CNB proved to have greater sensitivity, requiring open biopsy for confirmatory diagnosis less frequently than FNA [19].

  When a specific lymphoma diagnosis and subclassification according to WHO classification is required, several studies have shown than CNB has relatively better diagnostic yield compared to FNA [20–22]. In a prospective study comparing CNB to FNA in head and neck lesions, CNB was found to be superior to FNA in providing a specific diagnosis (90% vs. 66%) and achieved a higher accuracy in identifying true neoplasms (100% vs. 93%) and detecting malignancy (99% vs. 90%). There was however no statistically significant difference in the two methods with respect to sensitivity and specificity [23]. Other studies have demonstrated statistically significant differences in sensitivity, negative predictive value, and accuracy for CNB over FNA [20–22].

6. For small biopsies performed for initial diagnosis, which ancillary test results are diagnostic, suggestive of diagnosis, unreliable for diagnosis, or rule out the diagnosis?

The use of FNA and/or CNB for initial lymphoma diagnosis and classification continues to grow largely due to advances in flow cytometry, cytogenetic analysis, and molecular diagnostic techniques.

Flow Cytometry

In routine practice, morphologic assessment combined with immunophenotypic analysis (by flow cytometry and/or immunohistochemistry) is adequate in a majority of suspected lymphoma cases.

- Flow cytometry is useful in determination of clonality in B-cell lymphomas by assessment of immunoglobulin light chain restriction as well as simultaneous assessment of multiple surface or cytoplasmic antigen markers to provide a comprehensive immunophenotypic profile for lymphoma diagnosis and subclassification.
- The technique has high sensitivity in identifying a low number of clonal lymphoid cells in a predominantly polyclonal background.
- More recently flow cytometry has found utility in the assessment of markers of prognostic or therapeutic relevance [5, 24].
- The 2006 Bethesda International Consensus Conference on Flow Cytometry Immunophenotyping of Hematolymphoid Neoplasia consensus recommendations endorse flow cytometry as a useful tool for staging previously diagnosed lymphomas, monitoring response to treatment including detection of MRD, and documenting relapse or progression [25].
- In several reported series in literature, cytomorphologic evaluation with FNA alone in the diagnosis and classification of NHL has diagnostic sensitivity, specificity, and accuracy ranging between 61–100%, 88–100%, and greater than 80%, respectively. Combined with immunophenotyping by flow cytometry, the sensitivity and specificity for diagnosis and classification of NHL is even higher with sensitivity ranging from 75% to 100% and specificity from 87% to 100% [26–33].

Immunohistochemistry (IHC)

Advances in cell block preparation techniques over the years allow for assessment of some architectural clues (although not to the extent allowed by CNB or SEB) as well as offer an opportunity to perform immunohistochemical studies.

- IHC is particularly useful in selected cases with paucity of tumor cells (HL, T/HCRLBCL).
- T-cell lymphomas are better characterized by IHC than by flow cytometry.
- Certain diagnostic and prognostic markers (cyclin D1, ALK, BCL2, BCL6, P53, MYC, Ki-67, etc.) are better assessed by IHC than flow cytometry.

Combined use of FNA with flow cytometry and cell block/CNB with IHC remarkably improves diagnostic sensitivity, specificity, and diagnostic accuracy of lymphoid neoplasms, often mitigating the need for SEB.

Molecular Genetic Methods

See Chap. 2 for the application of molecular genetic methods in diagnosis of lymphomas. As is true for flow cytometry and

IHC, careful selection and prioritization of appropriate molecular tests is important. Purifying DNA from the initial sections when "facing" a tissue blocks is a valid option and it is a good practice to request the histology laboratory to save these initial sections for potential use later.

Small Biopsies in Patients with Previously Diagnosed and Treated Disease

With that background, the rest of this chapter will attempt to provide some basic guidelines for the optimal use of ancillary studies in the context of cytomorphologic characteristics to provide diagnosis based on small biopsies (FNA, NCB) of different lymphoma types. The reader is directed to relevant chapters in this book for comprehensive discussion of these lymphomas. Published reviews referenced in this section provide additional guidelines for using ancillary techniques in specific lymphoma diagnoses [34–36].

Small biopsy has almost completely replaced an excisional biopsy for pathological diagnosis of suspected recurrence or disease progression in a patient with prior diagnosis of a lymphoid malignancy. In these cases, information about the type of original lymphoma, the nature of treatment given, and current clinical and radiographic findings is essential in order to triage the limited specimen appropriately and to interpret the morphological findings correctly. The following section highlights the best approach for handling a small biopsy for the common types of lymphomas. For a detailed description and primary diagnosis of each of these lymphomas, please see the subsequent chapters in this book. Here, we emphasize the optimal ancillary workup, elucidate key findings which help in differential diagnosis of closely related entities, and point out the main diagnostic pitfalls in each case, such as the reactive and degenerative changes induced by treatment, possible emergence of treatment-related second malignancy, and the occurrence of an unrelated second lymphoma.

7. What is the work-up appropriate in patients with prior diagnosis of B-cell lymphomas? What are the special considerations to evaluate disease progression, secondary effects of prior treatment, and presence of therapeutic targets for additional treatment etc. in these cases?

Flow cytometry is most valuable in the diagnosis of B-cell NHLs and should be prioritized over saving material for a cell block, especially in cases of small B-cell lymphomas (CLL/SLL, MCL, FCL, MZL, LPL), in which the lymphoma cells lack sufficient cytological atypia to definitively exclude reactive lymphoid populations.

- Surface kappa and lambda immunoglobulin light chain expression distinguishes mature B-cell neoplasms from precursor B cells and between monotypic and polytypic B cells.
- Majority of B-NHLs can be divided into three broad groups based on expression of CD5 and CD10 [36] – NHLs with CD5 co-expression, CD10 co-expression, and NHLs which lack expression of both CD5 and CD10.
- Rare B-cell NHLs co-express both CD5 and CD10. This is not a distinct group, but a small proportion of DLBCL, FL, MCL, CLL/SLL, and BL can show this phenotype [37].
- Multiparameter flow cytometry is essential to optimize the diagnostic information from a small number of cells. The following antibody combinations are suggested in which the antibodies are listed in this order to accommodate for varying capabilities of commonly used flow cytometers (from 4 to 10 color): CD19, CD20, kappa, lambda, CD5, CD10, CD23, CD45, CD123, and CD38.
  - Treatment with anti-CD20 antibodies is almost universal in B-NHLs and can lead to prolonged downregulation of CD20 expression.
  - Anti-CD19 antibody is now introduced to treat refractory B-NHLs. Flow cytometry can be used to determine if the lymphoma cells express the therapeutic target molecules to guide further therapy.

CD5+/CD10- B-NHLs

Small B-cell neoplasms that express CD5 without CD10 usually represent CLL or MCL. Other B-NHLs such as MZL, FL, and LPL can aberrantly express CD5 [38–40] and may be more likely to present as a disseminated disease requiring a second biopsy. Aberrant co-expression of CD5 by MZL of mucosa associated lymphoid tissue (MALT) lymphoma is extremely rare at initial diagnosis [41]. The cases of MALT lymphoma with aberrant CD5 expression are predominantly non-gastric and tend to have disseminated disease [42]. In these cases, correlation with the initial diagnostic immunophenotype is crucial to avoid diagnostic pitfalls even though morphologic evaluation can provide significant diagnostic clues. See also Chap. 5 for detailed description of these entities.

- Both CLL/SLL and MCL are composed of monotonous small lymphoid cells with mature clumped chromatin, inconspicuous nucleoli, and scant cytoplasm. In CLL/SLL, cells have rounded nuclear contours, while in MCL they exhibit more irregularities of their nuclear outlines (see Case 1 Figs. 4.1, 4.2, and 4.3). The centrocytes in a low-grade CD5+ FL are somewhat larger, and their nuclei are more irregular than MCL cells, and variable numbers of centrocytes are always present in FL. CD5+ MZL and LPL can be identified by the presence of variable number of plasmacytoid lymphocytes and plasma cells. In blastoid MCL, the cells are medium-sized with scant cytoplasm, rounded nuclei containing fine chromatin, and inconspicuous nucleoli.

- In CLL/SLL, scattered medium-sized cells with variable amount of cytoplasm and nuclei demonstrating single prominent nucleolus (prolymphocytes or paraimmunoblasts) are usually present, while in MCL large transformed cells are conspicuously absent (except in blastoid or pleomorphic variants).
  - Mitoses, apoptosis, and necrosis are absent except for the cases with Richter transformation in CLL or blastoid variant of MCL. In blastoid variant of MCL, up to 20–30 mitoses per 10 high power fields can occur. The pleomorphic variant mimics DLBCL and contains large pleomorphic lymphoid cells with oval to irregular nuclear contours, pale cytoplasm, and prominent nucleoli.
  - In tissue biopsy, CLL/SLL usually shows a diffuse pattern or alternating dark and light zones imparting a vaguely nodular pattern may be seen, indicating the presence of proliferation centers. MCL can present in mantle zone, nodular, diffuse, or mixed patterns, but most cases of relapsed/refractory MCL show a diffuse pattern. Scattered epithelioid histiocytes and hyalinized vessels are commonly encountered which serve as useful diagnostic clues to the diagnosis of MCL (see Case 1 Fig. 4.2).
  - Characteristically, CD20 and immunoglobulin light chain are expressed at low intensity, and CD23 is usually moderate to strong on CLL cells. In contrast, a typical MCL has bright CD20 and/or immunoglobulin light chain expression, absent CD23 expression, or positivity for FMC7. This phenotype can however also be seen in "atypical CLL" [43, 44]. However, if the immunophenotype at initial diagnosis is not available, such "atypical" immunophenotype can lead to a mis-diagnosis of MCL since CD23 can be dimly expressed in a subset of MCL [45, 46].
  - In addition, large-cell ("Richter") transformation of CLL/SLL may alter the original "typical" CLL/SLL immunophenotype to an atypical one. In such cases, assessment of cyclin D1 and Ki-67 by IHC or *CCND1* by FISH must be performed for confirmation.
  - Rare cases of MCL-like Richter transformation of CLL have been reported [47] as are cases of composite SLL and MCL affecting lymph nodes simultaneously [48].

CD10+/CD5- B-NHLs (See also Chap. 5 for a detailed description of these entities)

- The CD10+/CD5- group of B-lymphoid neoplasms includes mature low-grade (grade 1 and grade 2 FLs) and high-grade B-NHLs (grade 3 FL, DLBCL, BL, and non-Burkitt high-grade B-cell lymphomas), as well as precursor B- and T-cell lymphomas (lymphoblastic lymphoma). Few cases of lymphoplasmacytic lymphoma cells co-expressing CD10+ are described [40].
- While aberrant expression of CD10 by marginal zone lymphoma at initial diagnosis appears to be extremely rare, it is described in large-cell transformation of MALT lymphomas [41].
- The biological diversity of CD10+ B-cell lymphomas is usually reflected in the cytomorphology of lymphoma cells. Therefore, examination of well-prepared, air-dried cytology smears stained with a Romanowsky stain is especially important in these cases. Identification of following patterns is especially important:
  - Presence of centrocytes intermixed with increasing numbers of centroblasts seen in FL. Centrocytes are small lymphocytes with irregular nuclear contours (often angulated or twisted), coarsely condensed chromatin, inconspicuous nucleoli, and scant cytoplasm. Centroblasts are large cells, 3–4 times the size of normal lymphocytes with rounded or irregular nuclear contours, vesicular chromatin, and prominent membrane-bound nucleoli and basophilic or amphophilic cytoplasm (see Case 2 Figs. 4.4, 4.5, and 4.6).
  - As the proportion of centroblasts increases, the boundaries between a DLBCL and a grade 3 FL become indistinct on cytology and need correlation with histology.
  - Grade of FL can be different from original disease at relapse. The change is usually, but not invariably, to a higher grade.
  - Grading of FL on FNA smears is difficult because the proportion of centrocytes and centroblasts cannot be assessed without the context of follicle structures. The latter can be achieved by examination of cell block or tissue biopsy (CNB or SEB) immunostained for CD21+ to identify follicular dendritic cell (FDC) networks to distinguish follicular, follicular and diffuse, or predominantly diffuse growth.
  - Evidence of *BCL2* rearrangement, resulting from translocation t(14;18)(q32;q21), is particularly useful when there are immunophenotypic variations such as lack of or dim expression of CD10 [49, 50] or BCL2 negativity due to mutations in the *BCL2* gene [51].
- Presence of frank cytological atypia associated with necrosis, karyorrhexis, and abundant cellular debris in the background indicates a high-grade process.

- DLBCL can have centroblastic morphology. These are large neoplastic cells with rounded or irregular nuclear contours, vesicular chromatin, and one or more membrane-bound nucleoli (see Case 3 Figs. 4.7 and 4.8). Alternatively, in immunoblastic variant, the cells are large with variable amount of amphophilic cytoplasm, rounded nuclei, vesicular chromatin, and single prominent nucleolus.
- The anaplastic variant of DLBCL contains markedly pleomorphic tumor cells with bizarre nuclear shapes. These neoplastic cells can be round, oval, or polygonal and multinucleated. Differential diagnosis is quite broad when this subtype is encountered and includes non-hematolymphoid malignancies such as melanoma, germ cell tumors, and poorly differentiated carcinoma. Among lymphoid neoplasms, it most closely resembles anaplastic large cell lymphoma (ALCL) or HL, syncytial variant.
- Diagnosis of grade 3 follicular lymphoma and its distinction from DLBCL is not possible on aspirate smears as recognition of follicular/nodular versus diffuse architecture is critical in differentiating the two entities from one another (see Case 4 Figs. 4.9, 4.10, and 4.11).
- A monotonous population of intermediate-sized cells with multiple indistinct nucleoli, scant basophilic cytoplasm, and small cytoplasmic vacuoles favors BL, but distinction from a CD10+ "double hit" lymphoma or high-grade B-cell lymphoma not otherwise specific (NOS) may be impossible without additional IHC stains and/or FISH (see Case 6 Fig. 4.15).

  BL lacks BCL2 staining by IHC, unlike grade 3 FL, DLBCL, and other HGBLs.

  When morphologic and immunophenotypic features overlap, further characterization can be achieved by genetic studies. In these cases, it is usually necessary to perform FISH for rearrangements involving *MYC*, *BCL2*, and *BCL6*. (See Chap. 6 for additional details to distinguish between DLBCL and related high-grade B-cell lymphomas.)

  CD10+ lymphomas with blastoid morphology: Precursor B-cell neoplasms (B-ALL/LBL) by definition lack surface immunoglobulin light chain expression, but a small proportion of mature B-cell neoplasms may also lack light chain expression [52]. If necessary, IHC staining for CD34 and TdT on cell block or CNB can be used to demonstrate an immature phenotype in ALL/LBL.

CD5-/CD10- B-NHLs (See also Chap. 5, for a detailed descriptions of these entities)

B- NHLs which lack expression of both CD5 and CD10 include small-cell as well as large-cell NHL. The entities diagnosed primarily with blood and bone marrow examination (B-PLL, HCL, aCLL) are considered elsewhere (see Chap. 27). The small-cell group comprises of the subtypes of marginal zone lymphoma (MALT lymphoma, NMZL, and SMZL) and lymphoplasmacytic lymphoma (LPL).

- While specific subtype of MZL can be diagnosed in FNA depending on site (although spleen is not a feasible site for FNA), FNAs are not ideal specimens to distinguish between different MZL types or between MZL and LPL due to cytomorphologic overlap.
  - All subtypes of MZL and LPL show a heterogeneous cell population comprising of small-to-intermediate sized lymphocytes, plasma cells, scattered large centroblastic or immunoblastic cells, histiocytes, follicular dendritic cells and/or lymphohistiocytic aggregates.
  - The phenotype is usually CD5–/CD23–/CD10–/BCL6–/cyclin D1– and BCL2+, but a proportion of cases can be CD5+ or rarely CD10+ [38–40, 42, 53].
  - The histologic features characteristic of MZL such as marginal zone growth pattern, lymphoepithelial lesions, follicular colonization by neoplastic cells, and disruption of follicular dendritic meshworks demonstrated by anti-CD21 or CD23 immunohistochemical staining cannot be elucidated in FNAs and require examination of tissue biopsy.
  - MZLs can have a variable proportion of large transformed cells. Even in tissue biopsies, criteria for transformation of MZL to DLBCL are not well defined.
  - Cytogenetically, while presence of t(11;18)(q21;q21) favors MALT lymphoma [54], other chromosomal aberrations including total or partial trisomies of chromosomes 3, 18, and X, aberrations of chromosomes 1q21 and 1p34, or partial or total deletions of chromosomes 17p and 9p are found in all MZL types [55–57].
  - *MYD88* mutation is present in most cases of LPL but also can be seen rarely in MZL [58].

8. What are the major pitfalls when diagnosing recurrent B-cell lymphomas on small biopsy?

- MCL can lack CD5 expression in approx. 10% of cases (see Case 1 Figs. 4.1, 4.2, and 4.3) and can be a potential diagnostic pitfall if one is not aware of this aberrancy [59]. Immunohistochemistry for cyclin D1 or cytogenetics for t(11;14)(q13;q32) can avoid this diagnostic pitfall.
- Among the high-grade CD5-/CD10- B- NHLs, approximately 60–70% of DLBCL lack expression of CD10 and constitute the non-germinal center subtype in the currently proposed algorithms for prognostication of DLBCL [60].

- Grade 3 FLs can be negative for CD10, and therefore lack of CD10 expression [61] may not entirely exclude the diagnosis of FL. Furthermore, due to overlap of grade 3 FL with DLBCL, lack of CD10 expression in high-grade NHLs may erroneously lead to the diagnosis of DLBCL on small biopsy if one is not careful in considering the possibility of CD10-negative FL [50].

9. What is the work-up of a small biopsy in patients with prior diagnosis of T/NK-cell lymphomas? What are the special considerations to evaluate disease progression, secondary effects of prior treatment, and presence of therapeutic targets for additional treatment etc. in these cases? (See also Chap. 8 for a detailed description of these entities)

The diagnosis, and even more so the classification, of this group of lymphoid neoplasms on small specimens is more challenging compared to B-NHLs due to several factors:

- Most T- and NK-cell malignancies lack defined marker of clonality by flow cytometry.
- Most T-cell NHLs do not have consistent, well-defined immunophenotypic signatures. Furthermore, the immunophenotypic aberrations manifested by T-cell NHLs overlap with normal phenotypic variations seen in nonneoplastic T cells.
- Even demonstration of a T-cell clone by T-cell receptor gene rearrangement studies does not equate to malignancy.
- Clonality assessment for V-beta expression by flow cytometry or T-cell receptor gene rearrangement by PCR is not useful in the diagnosis of NK-cell neoplasms as they lack expression of TCR and their *TCR* genes are theoretically in germline configuration.
- Cell size, cytologic atypia, and anaplasia are not always correlated with aggressiveness of these neoplasms. However, cytological examination of FNA or a limited tissue biopsy is important for primary distinction between a mature and precursor T-/NK-cell lymphoma. Immature neoplasms (T-lymphoblastic lymphoma/leukemia or blastic NK-cell neoplasms) comprise of a monotonous population of medium-sized cells with finely dispersed chromatin and small nucleoli (blastoid cytomorphology). Mitotic figures are plenty, and tingible body macrophages may impart a starry-sky pattern.
- Among mature T-/NK-cell neoplasms, with the exception of some entities, majority lack characteristic morphologic features.
  - ALCL (except for its small-cell variant) is characterized by presence of "hallmark" cells which are large lymphoid cells with abundant cytoplasm and a horseshoe or wreath shaped nucleus (Wreath cells are not exclusive to ALCL and other characteristics listed in a subsequent section must also be present).
  - Angioimmunoblastic T-cell lymphoma (AITL), a neoplasm of T-follicular helper (TFH) cell origin, in its classic form (pattern 3), is characterized by marked proliferation of high endothelial venules (HEVs) in an arborizing network effacing the nodal architecture and presence of atypical neoplastic lymphocytes with abundant pale/clear cytoplasm that form clusters adjacent to the HEVs. While these features offer important clues to possible diagnosis, they by themselves are not specific to this entity. Multinucleated cells as well as vascular proliferation and polymorphous cellular infiltrates can be found in other neoplasms such as HL or peripheral T-cell lymphoma, not otherwise specified (PTCL NOS).

Many T-/NK-cell neoplasms rather characteristically involve particular tissues and/or extranodal sites, at least in initial stages. Progressive or relapsed disease may be disseminated to nodal and extranodal sites in any of these T-/NK-cell lymphomas, but in many cases lymph nodes may not be involved and only FNA (soft tissue lesions) or CNB (e.g., skin, GI tract, other mucosal sites, or liver) may be available. While a consistent, well-defined immunophenotypic signature is not available in most T-/NK-cell NHLs, an algorithmic approach to immunophenotyping and additional genetic/molecular testing can provide definitive diagnosis when combined with clinical and morphological findings even with small biopsies. Thus, diagnosis of T- or NK-cell malignancies requires diligent combination of clinical presentation, morphology, immunophenotypic features, cytogenetics, and molecular studies for T-cell receptor gene rearrangement in most if not all cases. For an algorithmic approach to the use of immunophenotyping in the diagnosis of T-/NK-cell lymphomas, see the review by Soo [62]. See Table 4.1 for characteristic immunophenotype of some common T-/NK-lymphomas.

- General approach to immunophenotyping T-/NK-cell lymphomas: A broad antigen panel is required for initial diagnosis and classification of these lymphomas, including pan-T-cell antigen markers, immature markers, NK markers, T_{FH} markers, activation markers, T-cell antigen receptor subtype, and additional markers for prognosis or therapeutic targets such as CD30, CD52, and ALK. In the absence of prior diagnosis or very strong clinical suspicion of a T-/NK-cell lymphoma, a limited specimen such as FNA is likely to be first examined to rule out a B-cell lymphoma, since these are vastly more common. The FNA specimen submitted for flow cytometry is often exhausted with the initial screen, and further immunophenotyping must be performed by IHC in many cases.
- Flow cytometry: If specimen for flow cytometry is available

- In case of a previously characterized T-/NK-cell lymphoma, a custom panel of antibodies can be assembled to examine antigens which were aberrantly expressed as well as aberrantly lost in the original diagnostic sample.
- In case of lymphomas without previously defined immunophenotype, the following points are worth noting:
  Unlike precursor B-cell neoplasms, precursor T-cell neoplasms are not necessarily negative for surface expression of TCR.
  Flow cytometric immunoanalysis is better than IHC in distinguishing T- from NK-cell neoplasms as FC can demonstrate expression of fully assembled TCR-CD3 complex, which is present on the surface of T cells and absent from NK cells. In contrast, the epsilon chain of the CD3 complex detected by IHC is expressed in both T and NK cells. Furthermore, flow cytometry is superior to IHC in separating NK cells from aberrant T cells with NK-cell antigen expression.
  Flow cytometry is particularly useful to assess expression of TCR-α/β versus TCR-γ/δ, CD103 (by lymphoma cells in EATL), and CD10 in AITL.
- Depending on the instrumentation available (from 4 to 10 colors), the following antibodies should be used in the order given here to maximize the diagnostic yield in a limited flow cytometry analysis: CD1a, CD3, CD4, CD5, CD7, CD8, CD10, CD56, CD103, TCR-α/β and TCR-γ/δ.

• Immunohistochemistry: Since the tissue available for IHC stains is limited, a judicious, stepwise approach is prudent when prior definitive diagnosis and immunophenotype of the lymphoma is not available. We suggest starting with CD3, CD7, CD30, CD56, and chromogenic in-situ hybridization (CISH) for *EBV* encoded mRNA (EBER) along with preparation of 10 to 15 additional unstained sections.

• CD30: A strong and uniform expression of CD30 with a characteristic membrane and Golgi distribution with dot-like Golgi accentuation suggests possibility of ALCL and ALK expression by IHC confirms the diagnosis of ALK+ ALCL.
  - In the absence of ALK expression by the CD30+ neoplastic cells, the differential diagnostic considerations are primarily between ALK-negative ALCL and CD30+ PTCL when the disease has predominantly nodal presentation. Strong CD30 expression of equal intensity in all neoplastic cells is an important feature that distinguishes ALK-ALCLs from PTCLs with CD30 expression. ALK-negative ALCL cells are more frequently CD3+, express EMA less frequently, and are frequently positive for cytotoxic markers TIA1-1, granzyme B, and/or perforin. In an extranodal setting, CD30 expression in T-LPDs is common in cutaneous ALCL, lymphomatoid papulosis, transformed mycosis fungoides, and enteropathy-associated T-cell lymphoma (EATL).
  - ALK+ ALCL are associated with characteristic translocations, while ALK-negative cases show recurrent activating mutations of *JAK1* and/or *STAT3* [63], and a subset (approximately 30%) of ALK-negative ALCL show rearrangements of *DUSP22-IRF4* locus on chromosome 6p25.3 and a smaller subset (approximately 8%) harbors *TP63* rearrangements [64].
  - PTCL, NOS is a heterogeneous entity that occurs in both nodal and extranodal locations. This remains a diagnosis of exclusion after carefully excluding other well-defined entities. They frequently show loss of one or more T-cell antigens and can be CD4 or CD8 positive as well as double negative for CD4 and CD8.
    The "double negative" phenotype can create confusion with precursor T-NHLs or gamma-delta T-NHLs. Expression of T-cell receptor beta (TCR-beta F1) by the neoplastic cells excludes the latter but not necessarily the former.
    CD30 positivity is seen in approximately half of PTCL, NOS cases [65]. The frequency of CD30 expression among lymphoma cells and subcellular staining pattern provide important diagnostic clues [66, 67]. Cytotoxic granule expression is uncommon in PTCL, NOS. Genetically, they demonstrate complex karyotypes with frequent chromosomal gains or losses but lack the ALK+ ALCL-specific translocations or *DUSP22* and *TP63* rearrangements associated with ALK- ALCL [64].
  - CD30+ LPDs involving the skin include large-cell transformation of mycosis fungoides (MF), primary cutaneous CD30+ LPDs (lymphomatoid papulosis (LyP) and primary cutaneous ALCL), and cutaneous involvement by systemic ALCL (ALK+ or ALK-negative) and PTCL, NOS. These entities are discussed more fully in Chap. 12.
  - Enteropathy associated T-cell lymphoma (EATL) is also frequently positive for CD30 [68]. While CD103 expression is characteristically present in EATL, flow cytometry is required for its demonstration. In contrast, the frequent expression of cytotoxic granule-associated proteins in EATL [69] is demonstrated by IHC. This entity is discussed in more detail in Chap. 12.

• CD56: CD30-negative T/NK lymphomas can be further characterized based on the expression status of cytotoxic granules and CD56. CD56 expression is seen in NK-cell and some NK-like T-cell malignancies, mainly extranodal, nasal-type, or extranasal NK/T-cell lymphoma (ENKTL) and aggressive NK/T-cell leukemia. See also Chap. 8.

- Immunophenotype is almost identical in NK/T-cell lymphoma and aggressive NK/T-cell leukemia. NK/T-cell lymphoma often exhibits angiocentricity/angioinvasion, angiodestruction, mucosal ulceration, and coagulative necrosis, which are important clues in the diagnosis of this entity.
- Both entities also show strong association with *EBV* which can be demonstrated by in situ hybridization for *EBV*-encoded mRNA (EBER).
- Bone marrow and peripheral blood involvement is uncommon in extranodal or nasal NK/T-cell lymphomas, but when involved, these can mimic aggressive NK-cell leukemia and distinction can be quite challenging.
- CD52 is expressed in essentially all T-cell neoplasms but variably on NK-cell neoplasms. Expression of CD52 is therapeutically important.

• CD56+ and *EBV*-negative T-/NK-cell neoplasms include hepatosplenic T-NHL (HSTCL), non-hepatosplenic (cutaneous) gamma-delta T-NHL, and monomorphic epitheliotropic intestinal T-NHL (MEITL). These are usually site-specific diseases, and excisional biopsies are unlikely, and FNA is not helpful in their diagnosis.
  - Additional IHC staining for CD4, CD8, CD5, cytotoxic molecules (TIA1, granzyme B, perforin), and TCR-α/β is required to differentiate between these entities. See Table 4.1 for the typical immunophenotype expected in these lymphomas.
  - HSTCL by definition presents with hepatosplenomegaly. Bone marrow involvement is present in nearly all cases. Histologically, the neoplasm has predilection to involve the sinuses and shows a non-activated cytotoxic phenotype [70] and frequently demonstrates presence of isochromosome 7q.
  - Primary cutaneous gamma-delta T-NHL and mucosal gamma-delta T-NHLs have identical immunophenotype, except the mucosal types are *EBV*+.
  - Monomorphic epitheliotropic intestinal T-NHL (MEITL), previously designated as EATL type II, is more common in Asian or Hispanic populations and is not associated with celiac disease. MEITL tumor cells are positive for CD3, CD8, and CD56 but negative for CD4, CD30, CD103, and EBER and are usually TCR-gamma-delta positive. Recently, a novel marker, megakaryocyte-associated tyrosine kinase (*MATK*), was shown to be highly expressed in MEITL and is useful in its distinction from EATL [71]. MEITL also demonstrates high incidence of *MYC* abnormalities [72]. Whole-exome sequencing has demonstrated *STAT5B* and *SETD2* mutations in a large number of cases [73, 74].

• CD30 negative, CD56 negative, and *EBV*-negative cytotoxic T-cell NHLs include T-large granular lymphocytic leukemia (T-LGL) and subcutaneous panniculitis-like T-NHL (SPTCL).
  - Diagnosis of T-LGL is established in peripheral blood and/or bone marrow. A tissue biopsy is highly unlikely as lymphadenopathy or skin involvement is uncommon. See Chap. 8 for more details.
  - SPTCL is a cutaneous T-NHL presenting primarily in the form of subcutaneous plaques or nodules without evidence of systemic disease. The characteristic histologic features and disease localization are often diagnostic of this entity in the setting of an appropriate phenotype with expression of CD8, TCR-beta F1, cytotoxic molecules TIA1, granzyme B, and perforin and absence of CD56, CD30, and *EBV*.

• T-/NK-cell neoplasms of T-follicular helper (T_{FH}) phenotype: These should be considered in T-/NK-cell lymphomas lacking CD30, CD56, and cytotoxic molecule expression but showing a significant number of intermixed B cells and/or EBER+ cells. T_{FH} phenotype is defined by the expression of at least two (preferably three) of the following markers: CD10, BCL6, PD1, CXCL13, CXCR5, ICOS, and SAP by the neoplastic cells [75, 76].
  - Angioimmunoblastic T-cell lymphoma (AITL) is the prototype lymphoma in this group of neoplasms, along with follicular T-cell lymphoma (FTH) and a small subset of PTCL-NOS that exhibits T_{FH} phenotype. There is a significant clinical, immunophenotypic, and genetic overlap between AITL and FTH, and distinction between these entities largely depends on architectural features. Thus, in the assessment of T-NHLs with T_{FH} phenotype, FNA or needle biopsies are likely to be of limited utility to differentiate between these two entities, and only a more general diagnosis of T-cell LPD with TFH phenotype may be appropriate. Genetic studies (conventional karyotyping, comparative genomic hybridization, or next-generation sequencing) are less likely to be useful and seldom performed in limited samples.

Table 4.1 Immunophenotypic profiles of selected T-/NK-cell lymphomas

Lymphoma	Location	sCD3	cCD3	CD30	ALK1	CD56	*EBV*	CD4	CD8	CD7	CD5	CD1a	GrnzB	TIA1	Perf
ALK+ ALCL	LN	−/+	+	+++	+	−	−	+	−	+	+	−	+	+	+
ALK− ALCL	LN	−/+	+	+++	−	−	−	+	−	+/−	+/−	−	+	+	+
Cutaneous CD30+ LPD	Skin	−/+	+	+++	−	−	−	+	−	+	−/+	−	+	+	+
PTCL	LN	+	+	−/+	−	−	−	+	−/+	−/+	−/+	−	−	−	−
EATL	GI T	+	+	+	−	−	−	−	−	+	−	−	+	+	+
MF	Skin	+	+	−*	−	−	−	−	+	−	+/−	−	−	−	−
ENKTL	Nasal, upper RS	−	+	−/+	−	+	+	−	−	+	−	−	+	+	+
Aggre NK leuk	PB, BM	−	+	−	−	+	+	−	−	+	−	−	+	+	+
HSTCL	Liver, spleen	+	+	−	−	−/+	−	−	−/+		−	−	−	+	−
CGDTCL	Skin	+	+	−	−	+	−	−	−	+/−	−	−/+	++	++	++
MEITL	GI Tract	+	+	−	−	+	−	−	+	+/−	−	−	−/+	+	−/+

*Partial expression of CD30 can be found in neoplastic cells of MF at all stages but more commonly in tumor stage

10. What are the pitfalls in the diagnosis of HL with a small biopsy? What steps should be taken to avoid these pitfalls? (See also Chap. 9 for the basic classification and a detailed description of the subtypes of HL)

The diagnosis of HL by FNA/core biopsy may appear straightforward by visualization of Hodgkin/Reed Sternberg cells (HRS cells) in an appropriate polymorphous cellular milieu (see Case 5 Figs. 4.13 and 4.14); however, it can be a potential minefield due to a variety of issues [77].

- HRS-like cells can be found in a number of reactive conditions including viral lymphadenitis, infectious mononucleosis, immunodeficiency-related lymphoproliferative disorders, and some acute lymphadenitis [78–80].
- Non-hematolymphoid malignancies such as metastatic carcinoma or melanoma can harbor tumor cells that resemble HRS cells [63, 81, 82].
- A number of B- and T-NHLs including CLL/SLL, FL, NLPHL, ALCL, TCRBCL, AITL, and PTCL, NOS can harbor HRS-like cells posing a diagnostic challenge to the pathologists [64, 66, 67, 83].
- FNA without a needle core biopsy does not provide tissue materials for IHC and lacks architectural context and thus is suboptimal for diagnosis of HL [68, 69, 84–86].
- In general, flow cytometry is less useful in immunophenotypic characterization of HL due to relative scarcity of tumor cells in the background of an abundant inflammatory microenvironment [21] (see Case 4 Fig. 4.10), although some recent studies report high sensitivity and specificity of flow cytometry in the diagnosis of CHL. Immunohistochemical evidence of CD15 and CD30 expression in HRS cells (see Case 4 Fig. 4.11), with lack of CD20 and CD45 combined with flow cytometric expression of bright CD40 and CD95 expression, has been demonstrated with high specificity and sensitivity in a great majority of cHL [87–90]. Nevertheless, in routine practice, flow cytometry is not commonly used in the diagnosis of cHL or its mimics (NLPHL).
- IHC is the diagnostic tool of choice in characterization of HRS cells. At a minimum, the basic panel in the workup of HL and its mimics should include cytokeratin, CD45, CD20, CD3, CD15, CD30, EMA, and PAX5. Tumor cells of classic HL commonly express CD15, CD30, and dim PAX5 and are negative for CD20, CD3, CD45, EMA, and cytokeratin (see Case 4 Fig. 4.12).
- Deviation from this classic immunophenotype is frequently observed, and one must be aware of immunophenotypic variations to avoid misdiagnosis. For example, CD15 can be absent in up to 20% of cHL; conversely, it can be detected in some B- and T-cell lymphomas as well as some non-hematolymphoid tumors [91–93]. CD20 can be positive in Hodgkin cells in up to 40% of cases, but in contrast to B-cell NHL, it is expressed by only a small subset of tumor cells, and the intensity is usually variable [94, 95]. Infrequently, HRS cells may show aberrant expression of T-cell markers (CD2, CD3, CD4, CD5, and/or CD8) which can cause confusion with T-NHLs [96]. Nodular lymphocyte predominant HL (NLPHL) shows some morphological overlap with cHL, demonstrating scattered large cells in a lymphocyte predominant mixed inflammatory background. Its distinction from cHL is primarily based on demonstration of a distinct immunophenotype of the large abnormal cells (called LP or "popcorn" cells) which differs from HRS cells of cHL. LP cells are positive for CD45, CD20, PAX5, OCT2, BOB1, and CD79a, and they are negative for CD15 and CD30 although the latter can be weakly expressed in a subset of tumor cells.
  - In contrast to HRS cells, LP cells typically show strong expression of PAX5, and they are positive for both OCT2 and BOB1.
  - They are rimmed by CD3+/CD57+/PD1+ T-cell rosettes.
  - NLPHL demonstrates a variety of histologic patterns, and in its most diffuse T-cell-rich pattern, it is practically indistinguishable from TCRLBCL. Identification of different histologic patterns and its distinction from TCRLBCL has therapeutic and prognostic implications, and thus in routine practice neither FNA nor CNB are preferred specimen types in rendering a diagnosis of NLPHL and its distinction from TCRLBCL. Thus, an excision biopsy is preferred when clinically feasible.

Case Presentations

Case 1 (Figs. 4.1, 4.2, and 4.3)

Learning Objectives

1. Become familiar with the cytology, tissue histology, and immunohistochemistry of mantle cell lymphoma.
2. Generate a differential diagnosis based on FNA and use tissue biopsy to further characterize lymphoma.
3. Understand the limitations of FNA in characterizing malignant lymphomas and appreciate the value of tissue biopsy for accurate diagnosis.
4. Understand immunophenotypic variations that can lead to misdiagnosis.

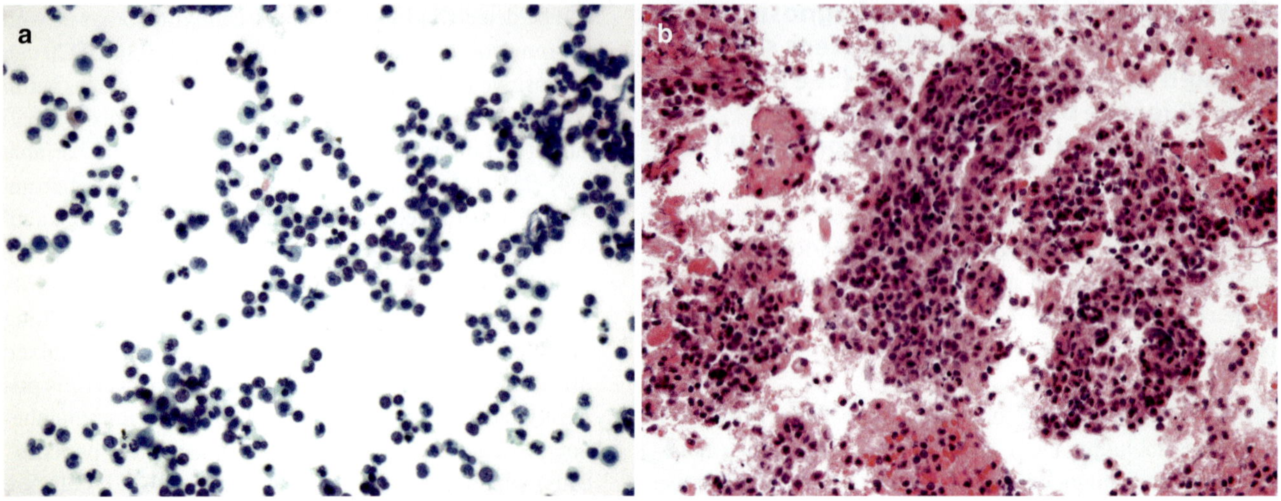

Fig. 4.1 Mantle cell lymphoma, FNA cytology. Cytologic features (**a**) magnification, 600×. Cell block histology (**b**) H&E, magnification 400×

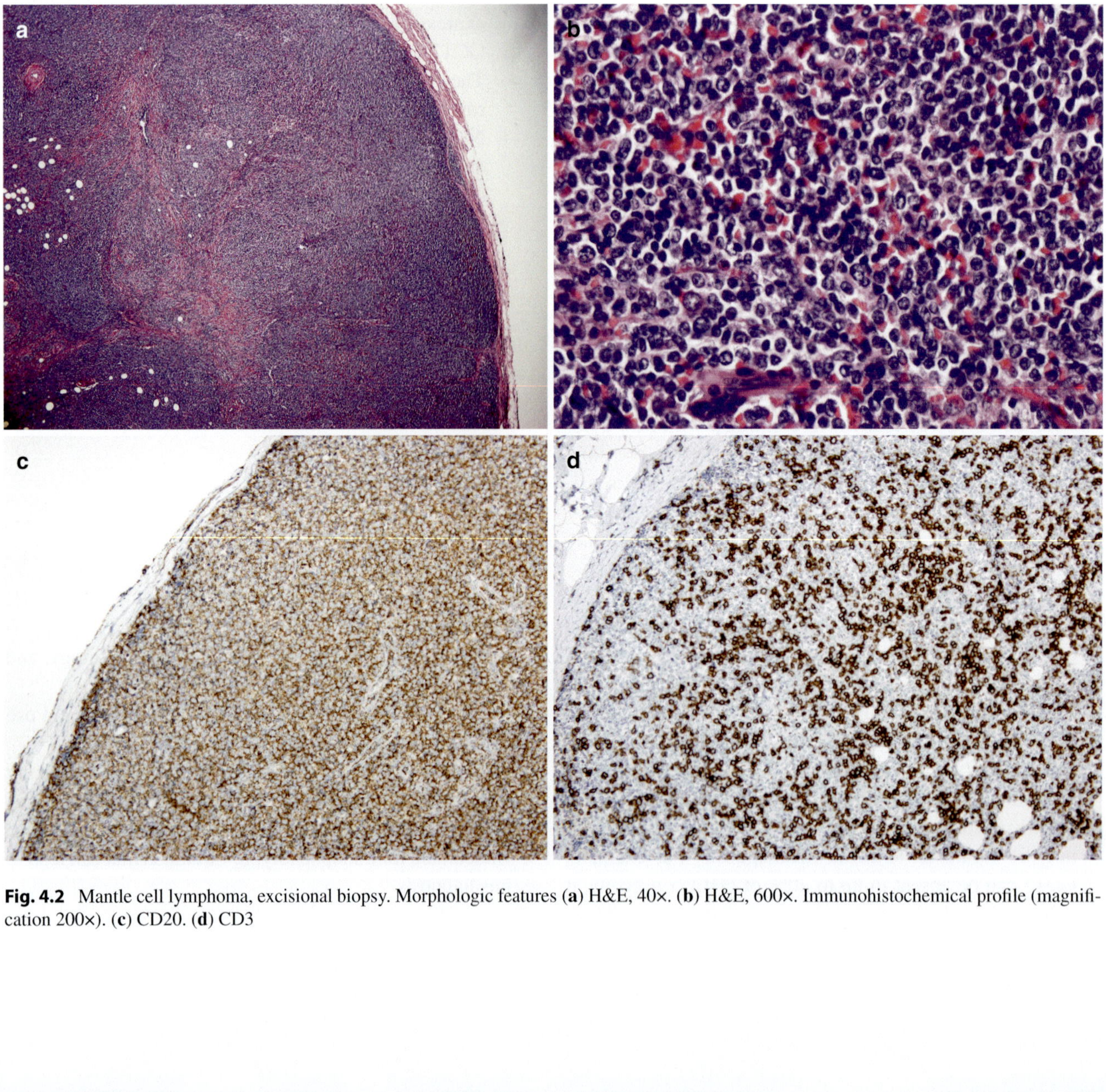

Fig. 4.2 Mantle cell lymphoma, excisional biopsy. Morphologic features (**a**) H&E, 40×. (**b**) H&E, 600×. Immunohistochemical profile (magnification 200×). (**c**) CD20. (**d**) CD3

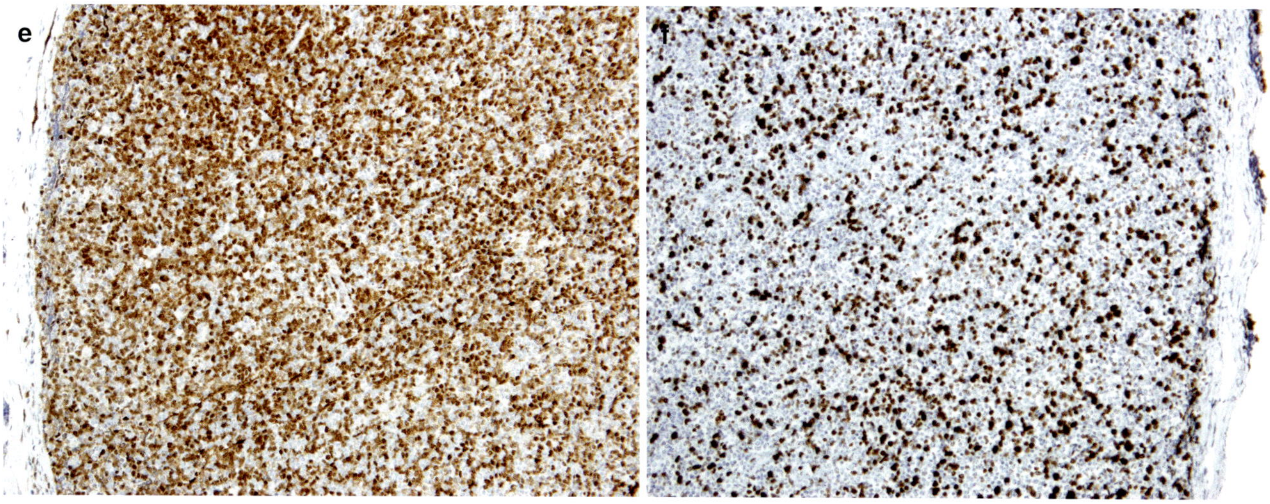

Fig. 4.2 (continued) (**e**) Cyclin D1 (**f**) Ki-67

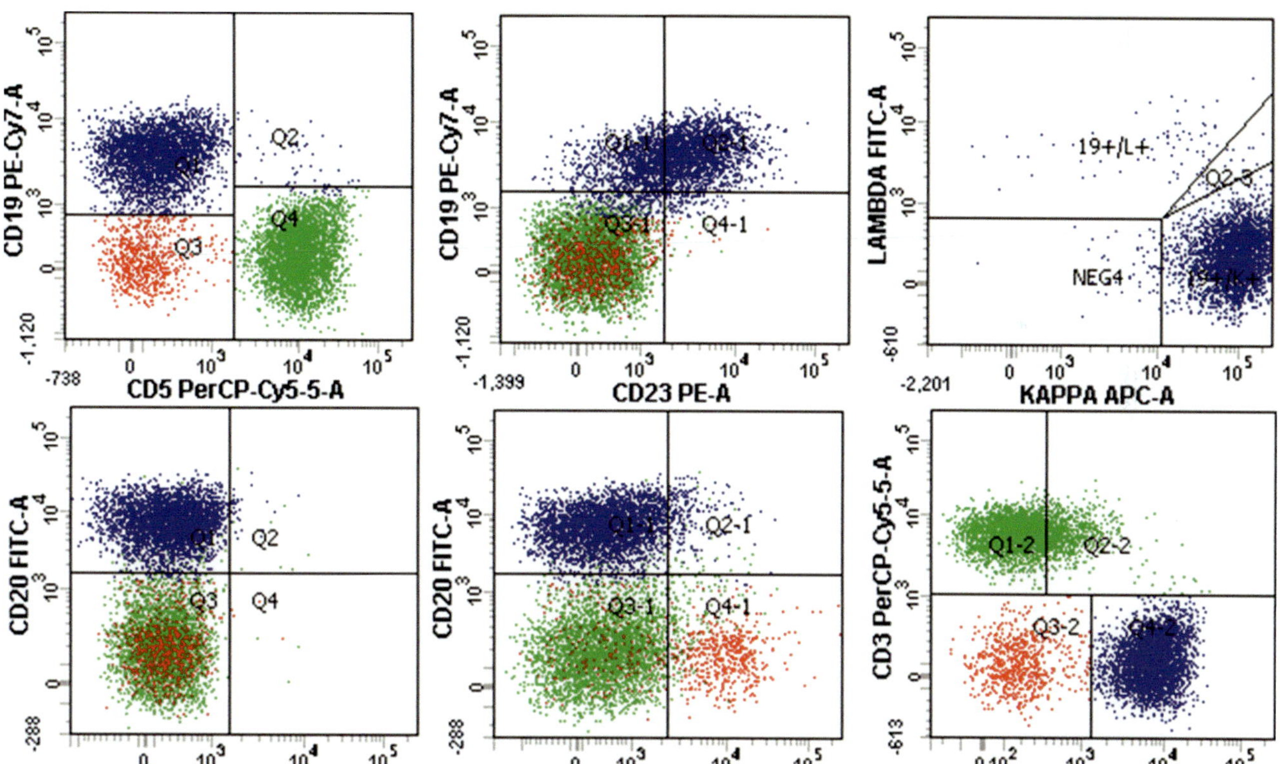

Fig. 4.3 Mantle cell lymphoma, flow cytometry. There is a mix of predominantly monoclonal B cells (in blue) with a minor population of mature T cells. The monoclonal B cells have a composite antigen profile of CD19+, CD20+, CD5 Neg., CD23+, CD10 Neg., CD11c Neg., CD38+ (subset), and immunoglobulin kappa light chain + (bright). (Note: *in this particular case of mantle cell lymphoma, CD5 is aberrantly negative. Flow cytometric immunoprofile alone can lead to diagnostic confusion with CD5 Neg., CD10 Neg. entities and mantle cell lymphoma, and the correct diagnosis will be missed without immunohistochemistry for cyclin D1*)

Case History
A 61-year-old male presents with massive splenomegaly, anemia, and enlarged lymph nodes.

Histologic Findings
- FNA of an enlarged lymph node – small- to intermediate-sized lymphocytes with irregular nuclear contours

Differential Diagnosis
- Follicular lymphoma
- Mantle cell lymphoma
- Marginal zone lymphoma

Diagnosis
Probably small mature B-cell lymphoma. Because flow cytometry was not performed in this FNA sample, excisional biopsy was recommended to further characterize and classify the process.

Further Workup and Other Ancillary Studies
- Excisional biopsy
  - Lymph node architecture is effaced by a proliferation of small- to medium-sized atypical lymphocytes in a vaguely nodular-to-diffuse pattern.
  - Neoplastic cells are positive for CD20, cyclin D1, CD21, and BCL2.
  - They are negative for CD10, BCL6, and CD3; Ki-67 proliferation rate is 40%.
  - Flow cytometry (population of interest in blue): There is a mix of predominantly monoclonal B cells with a minor population of mature T cells. The monoclonal B cells have a composite antigen profile of CD19+, CD20+, CD5 Neg., CD23+, CD10 Neg., CD11c Neg., CD38+ (subset), and immunoglobulin kappa light chain + (bright).
- This antigen profile is consistent with a CD5 Neg., CD10 Neg. B-cell lymphoma.

Final Diagnosis
Mantle cell lymphoma

Take-Home Messages
1. FNA without immunophenotyping may not optimally characterize small B-cell lymphoma.
2. Immunophenotypic variations can further create challenges in accurate diagnosis without proper architectural context.
3. Assessment of cyclin D1 is essential in the diagnosis of mantle cell lymphoma and can be performed by immunohistochemistry and not flow cytometry; otherwise, *CCND1/IGH* fusion gene can be confirmed by interphase FISH analysis on paraffin-embedded tissue section.
4. Tissue biopsy is required to accurately diagnose and classify mantle cell lymphomas. This may also include small core needle biopsy or FNA cell block, besides excisional biopsy.

Case 2 (Figs. 4.4, 4.5, and 4.6)

Learning Objectives
1. Become familiar with cytology, histology, and immunohistochemistry of low-grade follicular lymphoma.
2. Generate a differential diagnosis based on cytologic findings and narrow differential based on histology and immunohistochemistry on excision.
3. Understand the limits of FNA in diagnosis and further characterization of lymphoma over tissue biopsy.

Case History
A 72-year-old male with slow growing left neck adenopathy for 2 months

Histologic Findings
- FNA
  - Small- to medium-sized lymphocytes with irregular nuclear contours, coarse chromatin; no significant proportion of large cells.
  - IHC: predominantly CD20+ B cells that co-express CD10, BCL2, and BCL6, and are negative for cyclin D1; Ki-67 proliferation rate is 50%.

Differential Diagnosis
- CD10+ B-cell lymphoma.
- Preferred diagnosis: Follicular lymphoma. However, because of unexpected high proliferative index, an excisional biopsy was recommended to rule out high-grade follicular lymphoma or focal diffuse large B-cell lymphoma.

Further Workup and Other Ancillary Studies
- Excisional biopsy
  - Lymph node architecture is effaced by proliferation of atypical back-to-back follicles with no discernible mantle zones, lack of polarization, and tingible body macrophages in the germinal centers and atypical lymphoid cells consistent with centrocytes and scattered centroblasts.
  - Morphologic features support low grade: centroblasts less than 15/hpf.
  - Increased proliferation index is indicative of probable increased aggressive course of disease, possibly behaving similar to grade 3.
- Flow cytometry (blue represents population of interest):

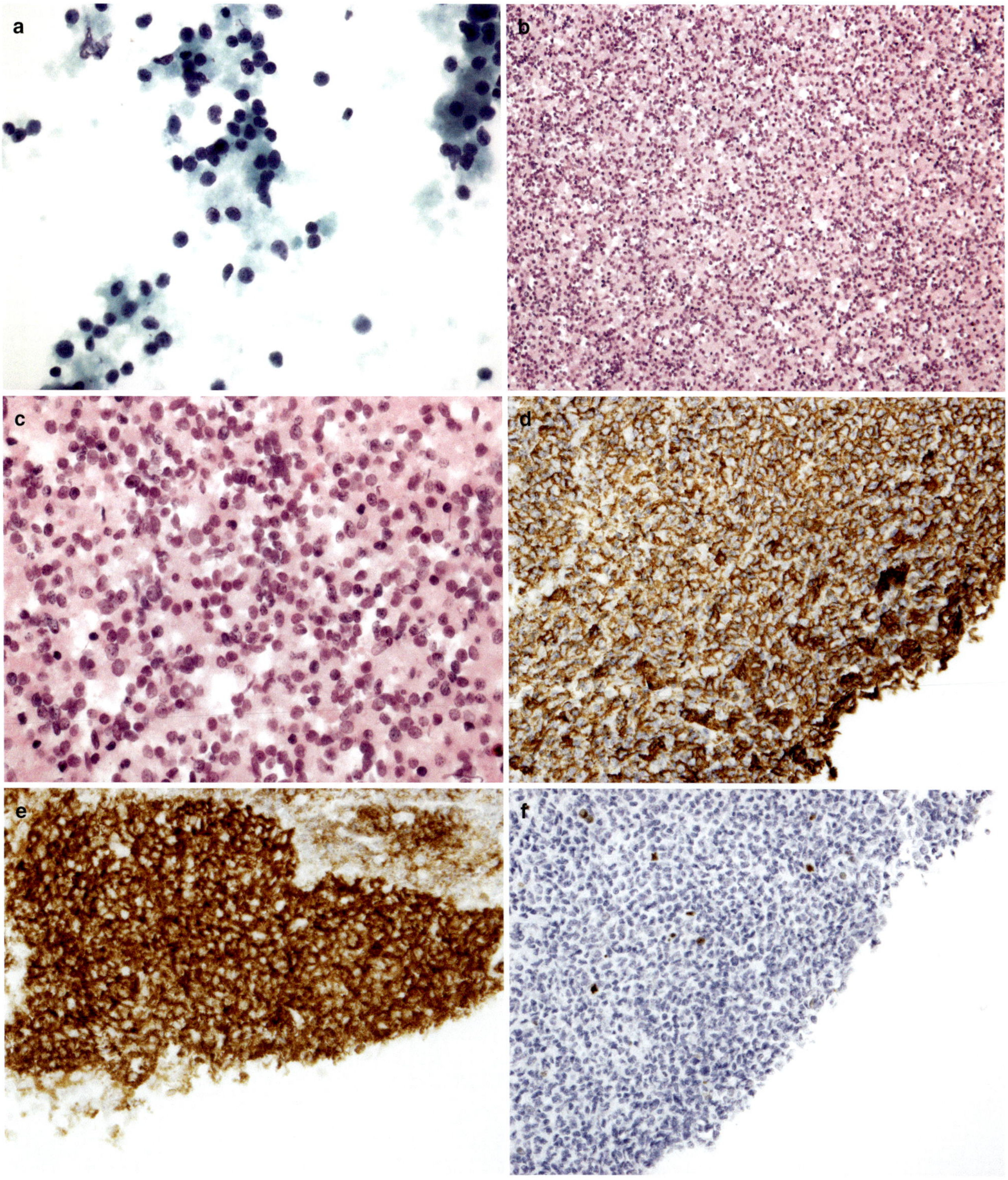

Fig. 4.4 Low-grade follicular lymphoma FNA cytology. Cytologic features (**a**) magnification, 600×. Cell block histology (**b**) H&E, magnification 200×. (**c**) H&E, magnification 600×. Immunohistochemical profile (magnification 400×). (**d**) CD20. (**e**) CD10. (**f**) Cyclin D1

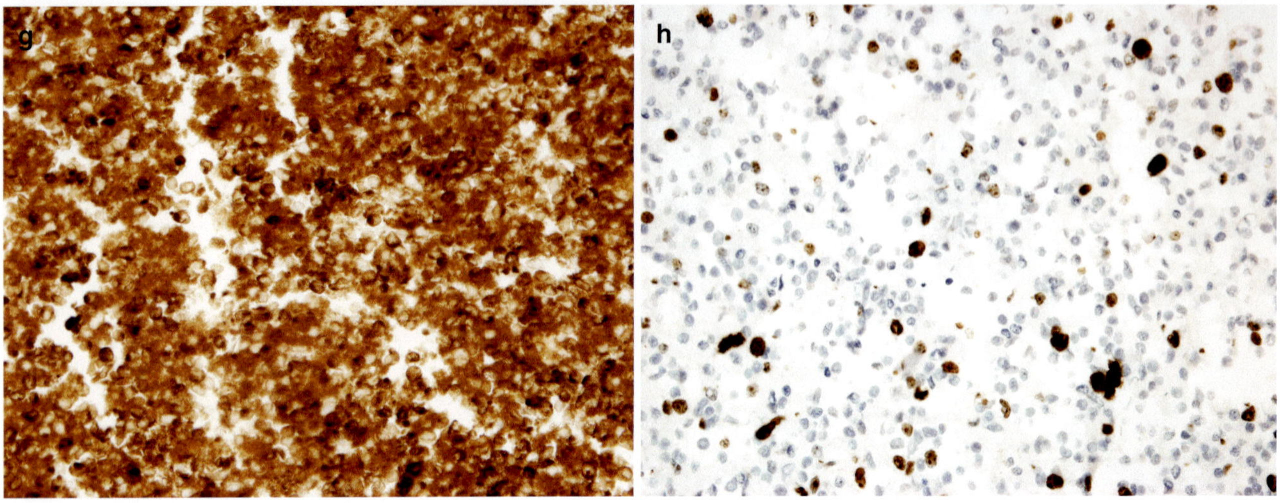

Fig. 4.4 (continued) (**g**) BCL2 (**h**) Ki-67

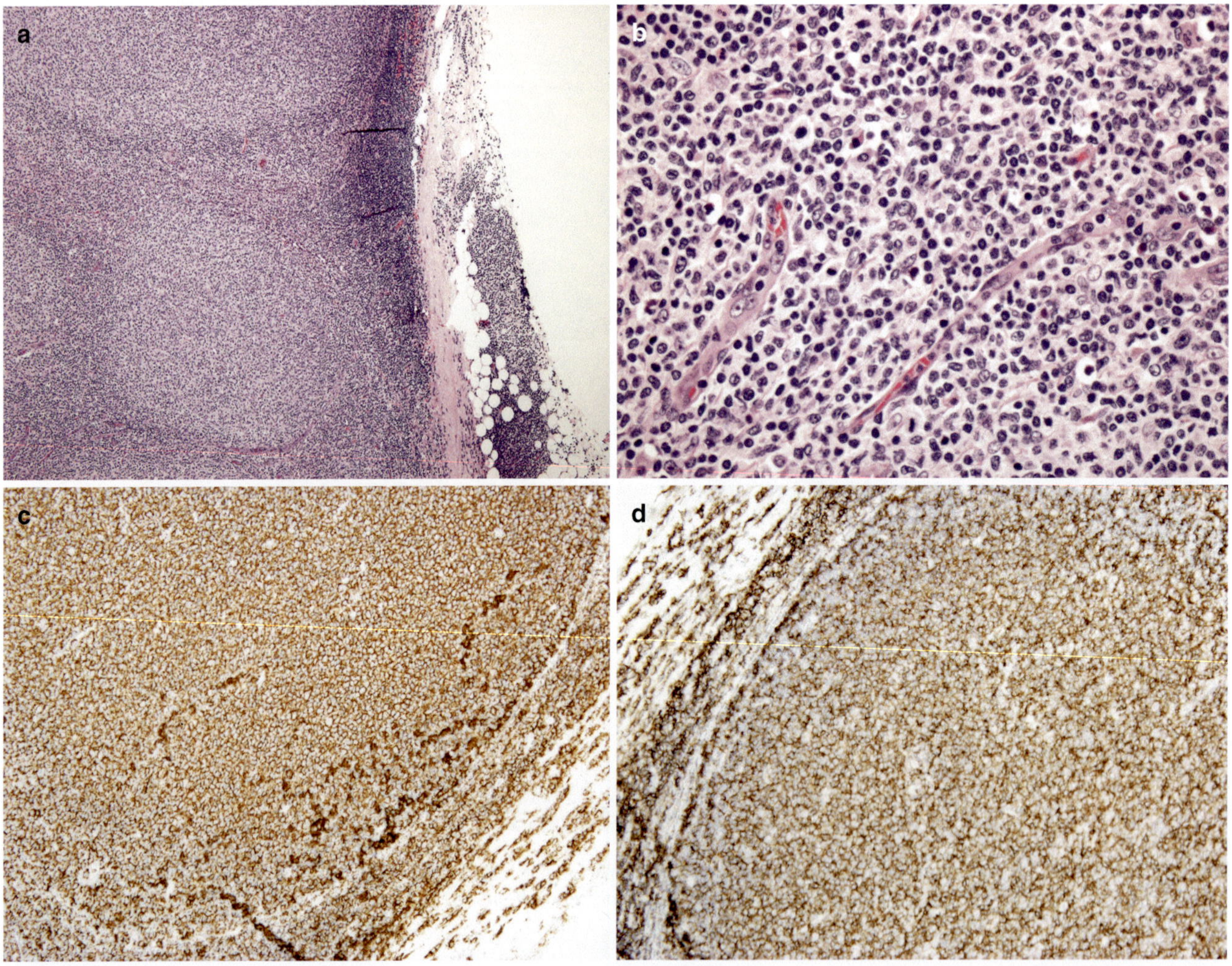

Fig. 4.5 Low-grade follicular lymphoma, excisional biopsy. Morphologic features (**a**) H&E, magnification 100×. (**b**) H&E, magnification 600×. Immunohistochemical profile (magnification 200×). (**c**) CD20. (**d**) CD10

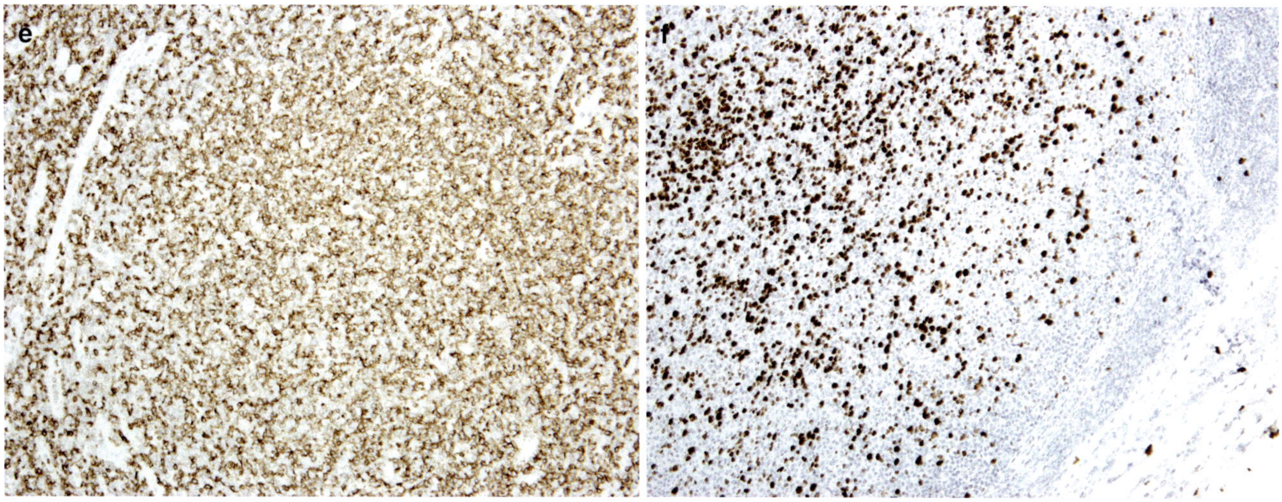

Fig. 4.5 (continued) (**e**) BCL2 (**f**) Ki-67

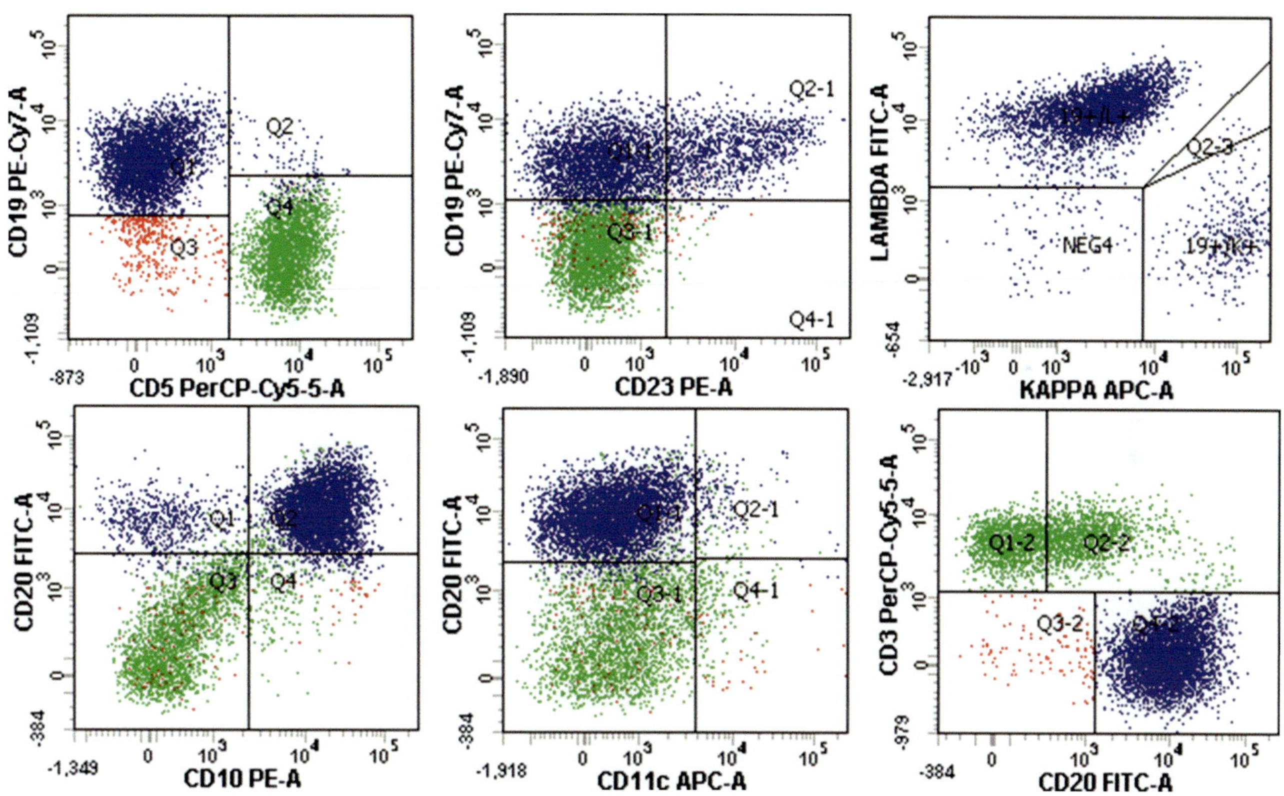

Fig. 4.6 Follicular lymphoma, flow cytometry. The B cells (*in blue*) are monoclonal/monotypic with a composite antigen profile of CD19+, CD5 Neg., CD23+, CD3 Neg., CD20+, CD10+, CD11c Neg., CD38+ (minor subset), with lambda light chain restriction

- The B cells are monoclonal/monotypic with a composite antigen profile of CD19+, CD5 Neg., CD23+, CD3 Neg., CD20+, CD10+, CD11c Neg., and CD38+ (minor subset), with lambda light chain restriction.

Final Diagnosis

Low-grade follicular lymphoma, grades 1–2 out of 3 with high proliferation index

Take-Home Messages

1. Patterns and grade of follicular lymphoma are challenging to assess on FNA alone.
2. FNA cannot reliably assess the proliferation rate of follicular lymphomas.
3. Tissue biopsy is required for pattern assessment, histologic grading, and determination of proliferation rate.

Case 3 (Figs. 4.7 and 4.8)

Learning Objectives

1. Become familiar with cytology, tissue biopsy histology, and immunohistochemistry of DLBCL.
2. Generate broad differential diagnosis based on FNA cytology and immunohistochemistry.
3. Understand the limits of FNA when diagnosing large B-cell lymphomas and that tissue biopsy is required for further characterization.

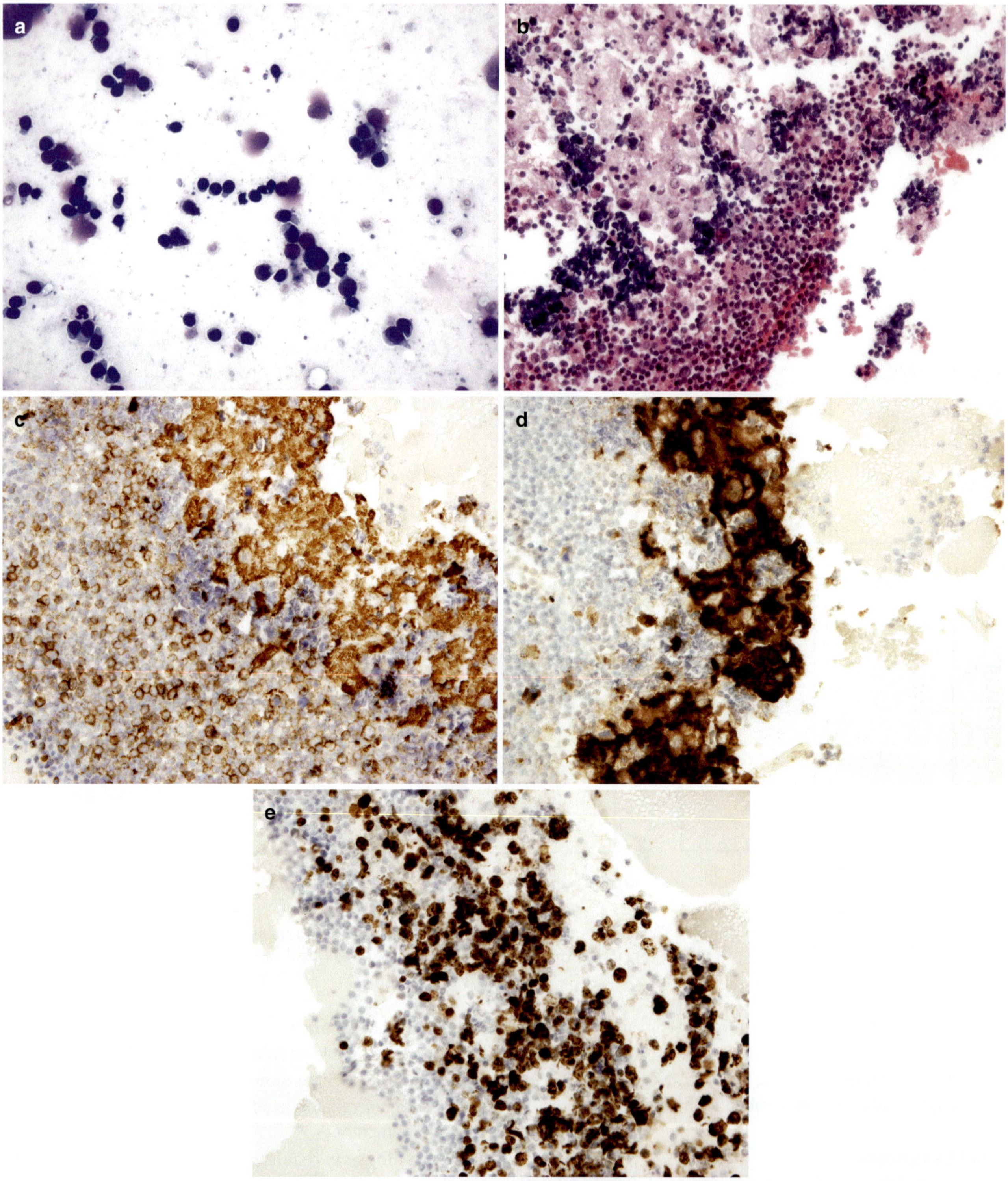

Fig. 4.7 Diffuse large B-cell lymphoma, FNA cytology. Cytologic features (**a**) magnification 600×. Cell block histology (**b**) magnification 400×. Immunohistochemical profile (magnification 400×). (**c**) CD20. (**d**) CD30. (**e**) Ki-67

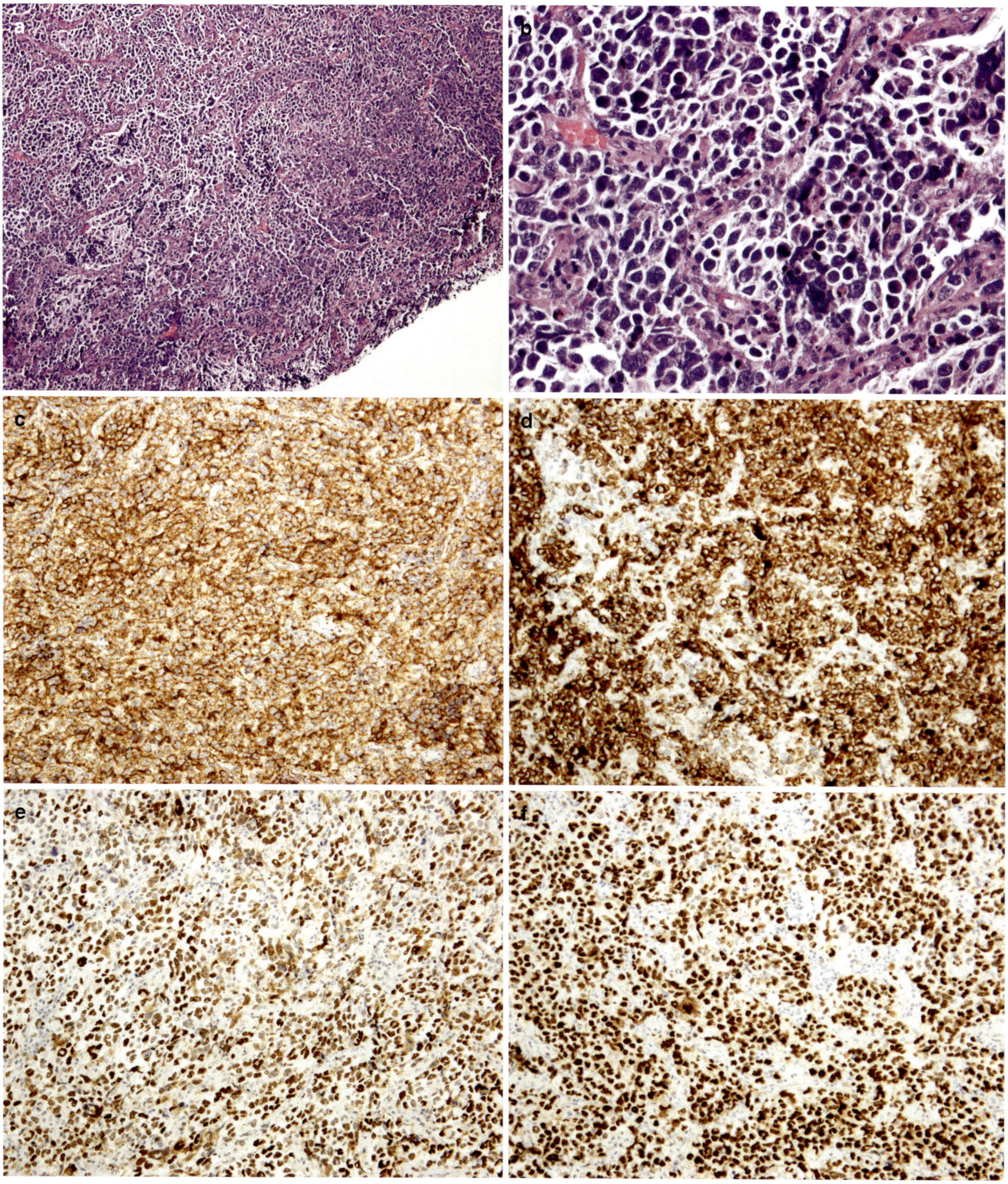

Fig. 4.8 Diffuse large B-cell lymphoma, excisional biopsy. Morphologic features (**a**) H&E, magnification 100×. (**b**) H&E, magnification 400×. Immunohistochemical profile (magnification 200×). (**c**) CD20. (**d**) BCL2. (**e**) BCL6. (**f**) MUM1

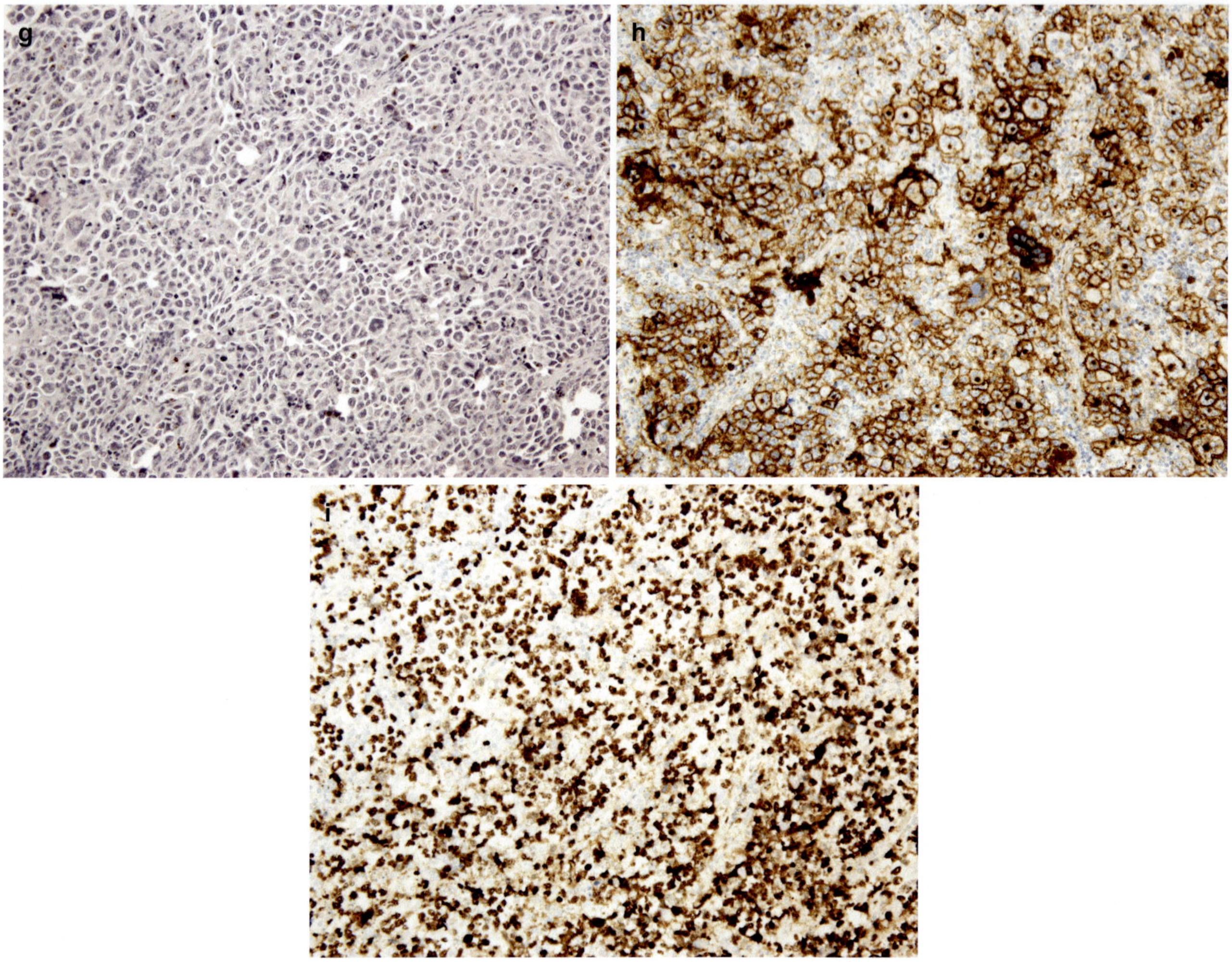

Fig. 4.8 (continued) (**g**) CD15. (**h**) CD30. (**i**) Ki-67

Case History

A 59-year-old male with a left submandibular mass for 1 month with no associated symptoms

Histologic Findings

- FNA
  - Small and large lymphoid cells (confirmed by +LCA, negative cytokeratin).
  - Large lymphoid cells are atypical.
  - Large cells are positive for CD20 consistent with B cells. They are negative for CD3, CD5, CD10, CD15, and cyclin D1. They also express CD30. Ki-67 proliferation rate is high (>80% of the total B cells).

Differential Diagnosis

- B-cell HNL (high-grade follicular lymphoma or DLBCL)
- Preferred diagnosis: DLBCL, recommend tissue for further classification

Further Workup and Other Ancillary Studies

- Excisional biopsy
  - Diffuse proliferation of large cells that were positive for B-cell antigens
  - Non-germinal center subtype: CD10 negative, BCL6+ MUM1+
  - MYC+ (>40% cells) and BCL2 + (>50% cells), Ki-67 proliferation rate 80–90%
- *EBV* by in situ hybridization: negative for *EBV*-encoded mRNA (EBER)
- FISH: gains of chromosome 14 and chromosome 18
- Flow cytometry
  - The B cells have slight decrease in CD19 intensity but polyclonal expression of immunoglobulin kappa and

lambda light chains. There is no abnormal dimming or loss of pan B-cell antigens nor atypical co-expression of CD5 on B cells. There is no immunophenotypic evidence of B-lymphoid neoplasia by flow cytometry.

Final Diagnosis

DLBCL, non-germinal center subtype

Take-Home Messages

1. Full characterization of B-cell lymphoma with medium-sized to large cells is challenging on FNA alone.
2. Flow cytometry can be false negative as aggressive lymphoma cells often do not survive flow processing.
3. Distinction between DLBCL and high-grade (grade 3) FL or other mimics can be challenging in FNA specimens due to lack of architectural context.
4. Tissue biopsy is required for accurate morphologic and immunohistochemical characterization of B-cell lymphoma with medium to large size.

Case 4 (Figs. 4.9, 4.10, 4.11, and 4.12)

Learning Objectives

1. Become familiar with cytology, tissue histology, and immunohistochemistry of follicular lymphoma and DLBCL.
2. Understand that DLBCL can progress from follicular lymphoma and both entities can occur simultaneously.
3. Acknowledge that FNA may not be sufficient to diagnose DLBCL and FL in the same specimen due to lack of spatial context and sampling bias.

Case History

A 65-year-old male who has a past medical history of follicular lymphoma and DLBCL presented with abdominal pain and a pancreatic mass approximately 1 year after his initial diagnosis.

Histologic Findings

- FNA of pancreas body mass

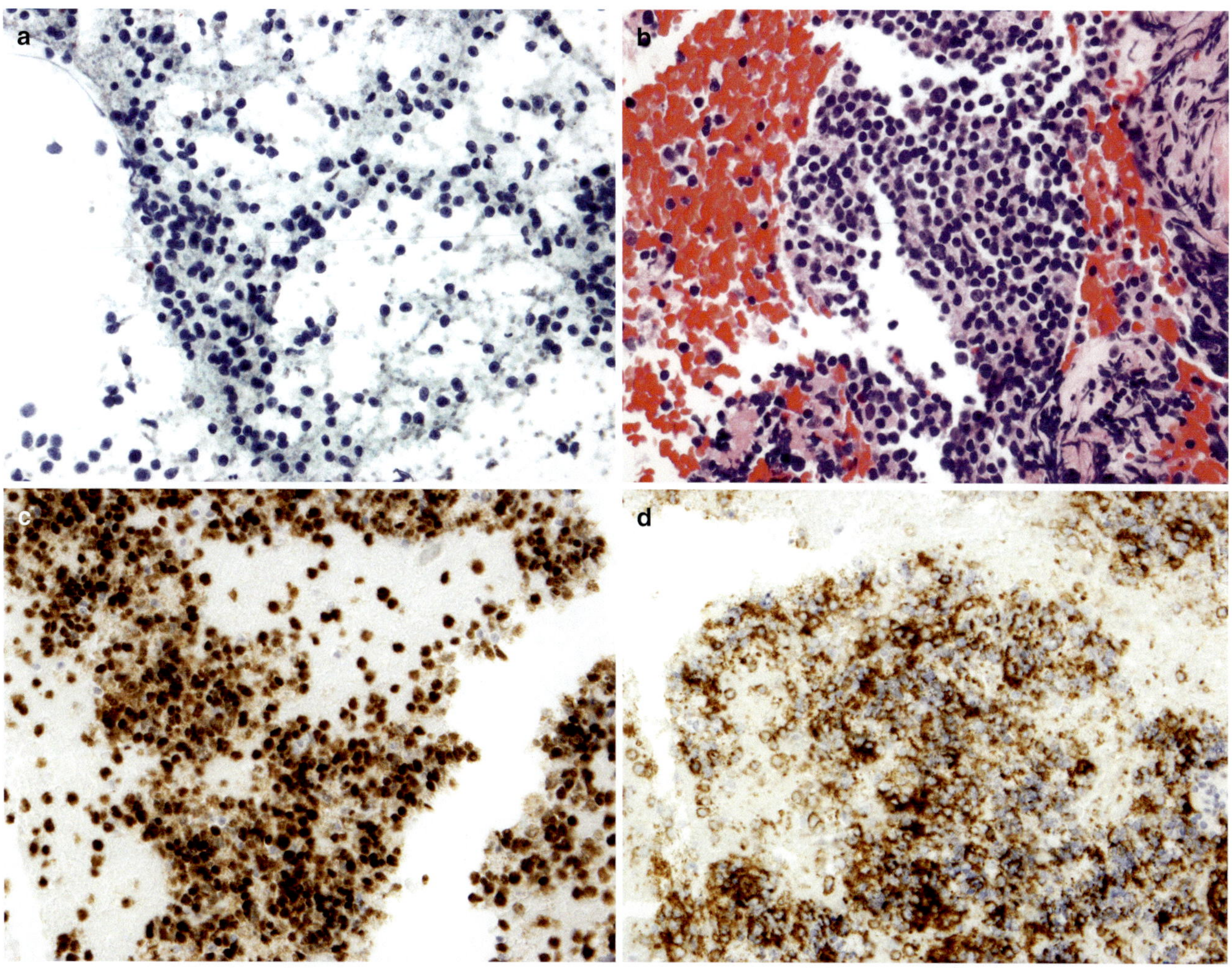

Fig. 4.9 Diffuse large B-cell lymphoma and follicular lymphoma FNA cytology. Cytologic features (**a**) magnification, 400×. Cell block histology (**b**) H&E, magnification 600×. Immunohistochemical profile (magnification 400×). (**c**) PAX5. (**d**) CD10

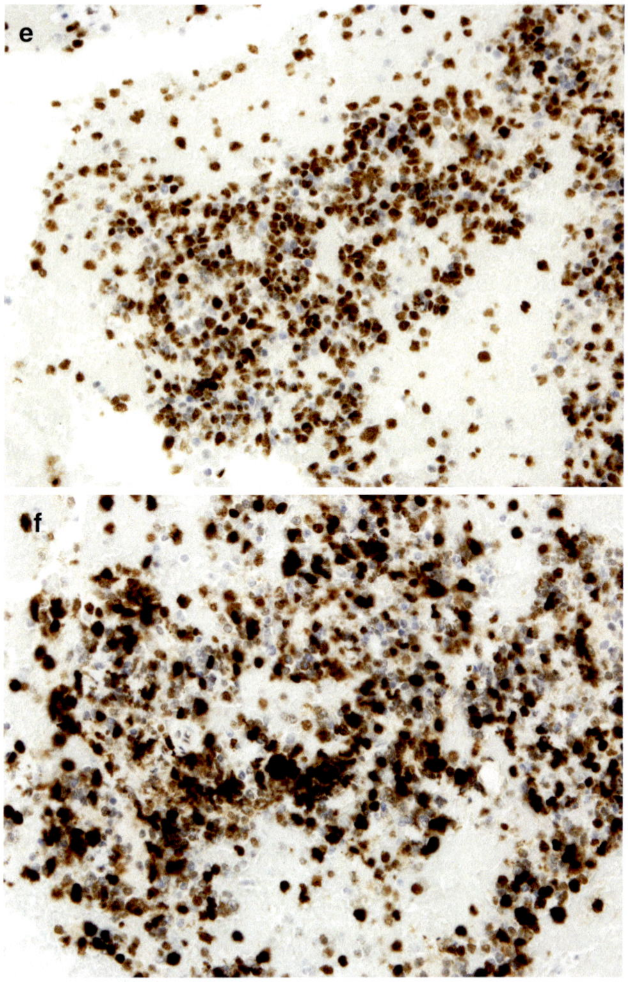

Fig. 4.9 (continued) (**e**) BCL6. (**f**) Ki-67

– Malignant lymphoma
– Medium- to large-sized lymphoid cells positive for CD20, PAX5, CD10, and BCL6
– Scattered CD3+ T cells in background
– Ki-67 proliferation rate 60%

Differential Diagnosis

- Follicular lymphoma, DLBCL
- Proposed diagnosis: Favor recurrent follicular lymphoma

Further Workup and Other Ancillary Studies

- Excisional biopsy
  – DLBCL in the background of grade 3 FL.
  – Sheets of large pleomorphic cells effacing approximately 60% of nodal parenchyma.

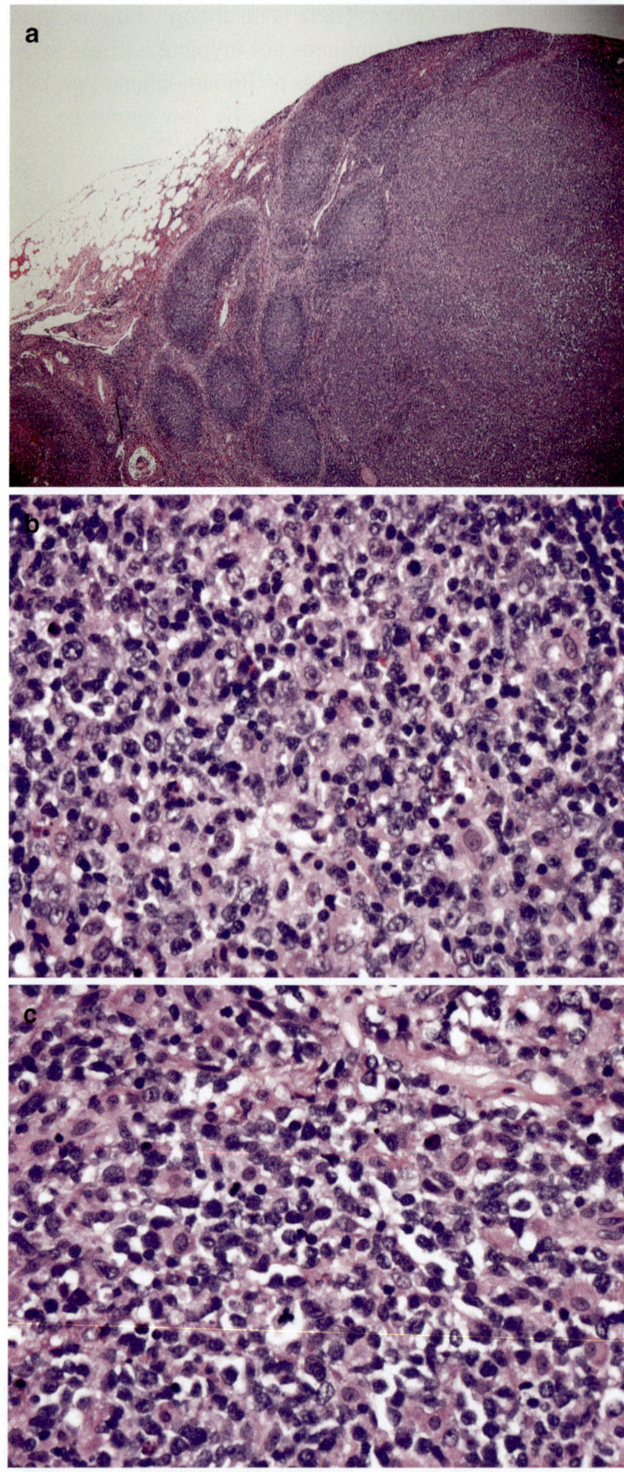

Fig. 4.10 Follicular lymphoma and diffuse large B-cell lymphoma excisional biopsy. Morphologic features follicular area of lymph node (**a**) H&E, 40×. (**b**) H&E, 600×. Diffuse area of lymph node. (**c**) H&E, 600×

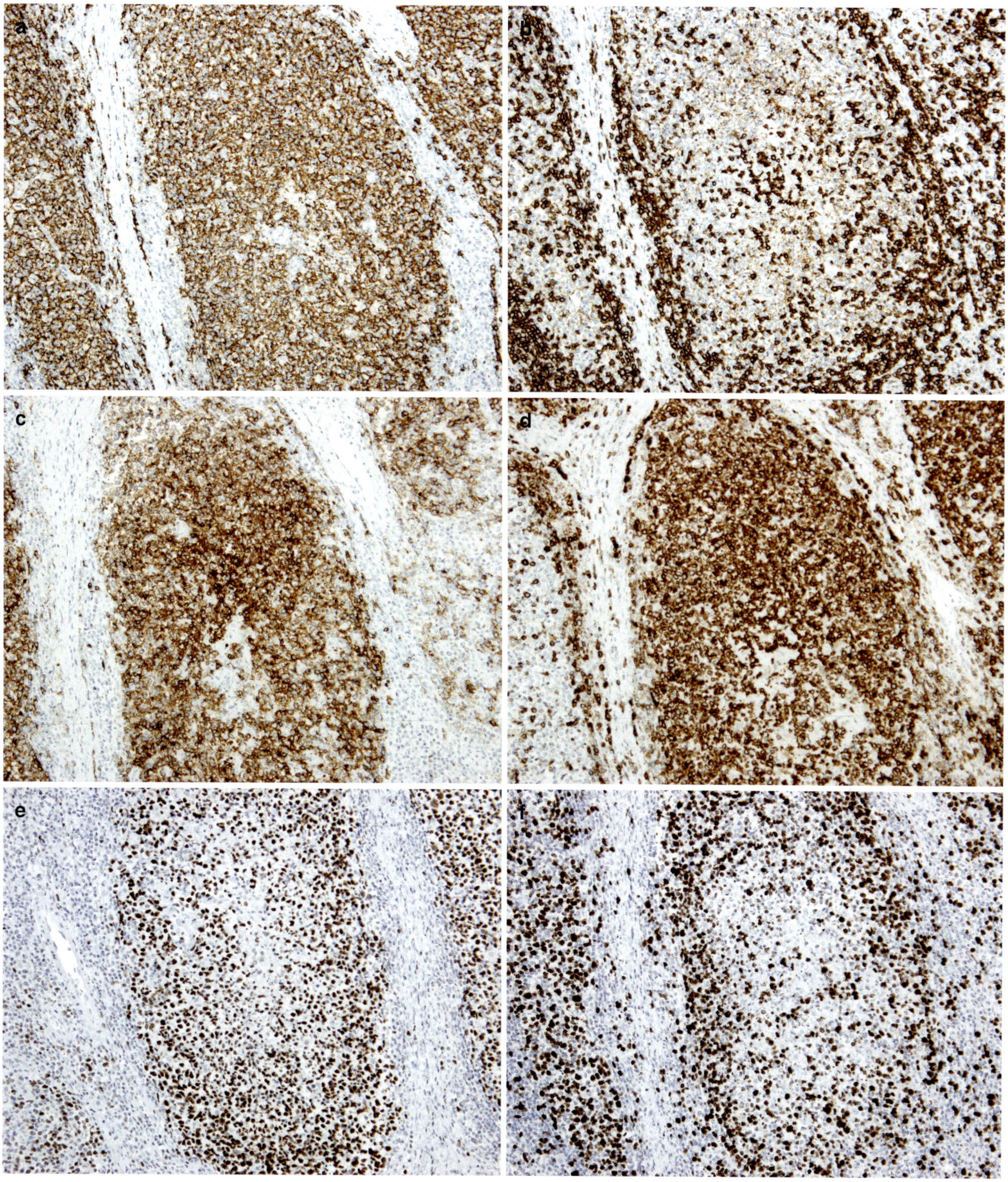

Fig. 4.11 Follicular lymphoma and diffuse large B-cell lymphoma excisional biopsy. Follicular area, immunohistochemical profile (magnification 200×). (**a**) CD20. (**b**) CD3. (**c**) CD10. (**d**) BCL2 (**e**) BCL6 (**f**) Ki-67

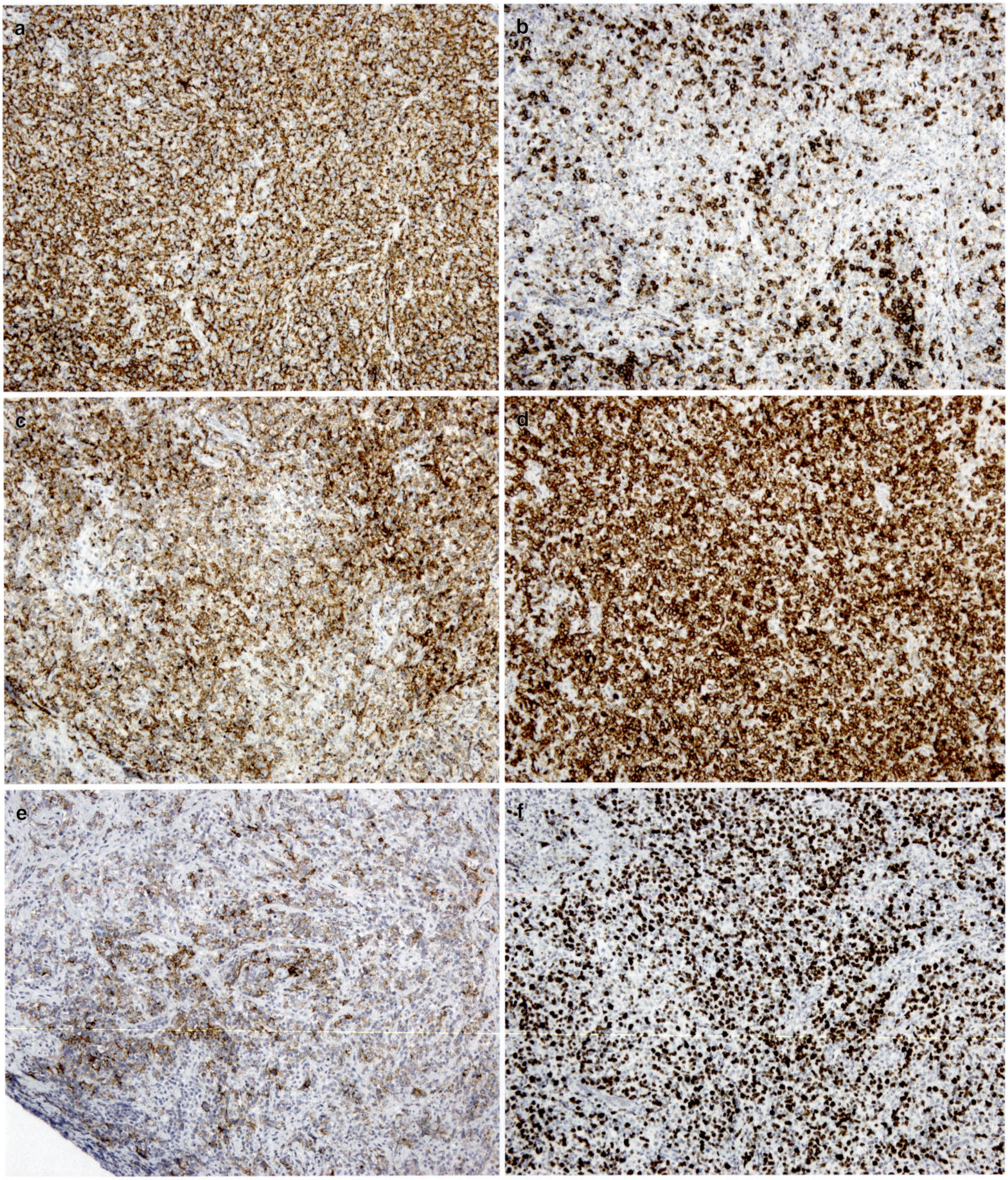

Fig. 4.12 Follicular lymphoma and diffuse large B-cell lymphoma excisional biopsy. Diffuse area, immunohistochemical profile (magnification 200×). (**a**) CD20. (**b**) CD3. (**c**) CD10. (**d**) BCL2. (**e**) CD21. (**f**) Ki-67

  - In approximately 40% of the node, atypical follicles with grade 3A or 3B pattern.
  - DLBCL component has germinal center phenotype, consistent with transformation, proliferative index by MIB-1 = 40–50%.
- Flow cytometry (not shown):
  - Lymphoid cells are predominantly B cells (approximately 51%) admixed with T cells (approximately 34.8%). B cells have a composite antigen profile of CD19+ (dim), CD5 Neg., CD23 Neg., CD10+ (bright), CD20+ (bright), CD11c Neg., and CD38+/−, and they are lambda light chain restricted monotypic B cells.
  - Positive for a CD10+ B-lymphoproliferative disorder/lymphoma.

Final Diagnosis

DLBCL, germinal center subtype (60%), and high-grade follicular lymphoma (40%), likely representing DLBCL transformed from high-grade follicular lymphoma

Take-Home Messages

1. FNA is not adequate to assess progression of a high-grade follicular lymphoma to DLBCL.
2. FNA cannot adequately grade follicular lymphoma; tissue biopsy is required to assess centroblasts and proliferation index.
3. Tissue biopsy is required to further characterize high-grade lymphomas diagnosed initially by FNA to rule out focal DLBCL.

Case 5 (Figs. 4.13 and 4.14)

Learning Objectives

1. Become familiar with cytology, tissue biopsy histology, and immunohistochemistry of cHL.
2. Generate a differential diagnosis based on FNA findings.
3. Understand the limits of FNA in the diagnosis of cHL.
4. Recognize that tissue biopsy is required for definitive diagnosis of cHL and exclusion of its morphologic and immunophenotypic mimics.

Clinical History

A 30-year-old male presented with mediastinal mass causing airway compression as well as 8-month history of fatigue, anorexia, 50 lb. weight loss, and night sweats.

Histologic Findings

- FNA:
  - Crushed biopsy, rare large cells with large nucleoli, suspicious for Hodgkin/Reed-Sternberg (HRS) cells

Differential Diagnosis

- cHL
- DLBCL such as primary mediastinal large B-cell lymphoma

Further Workup and Other Ancillary Studies

- Recommend excision
- Core needle biopsy

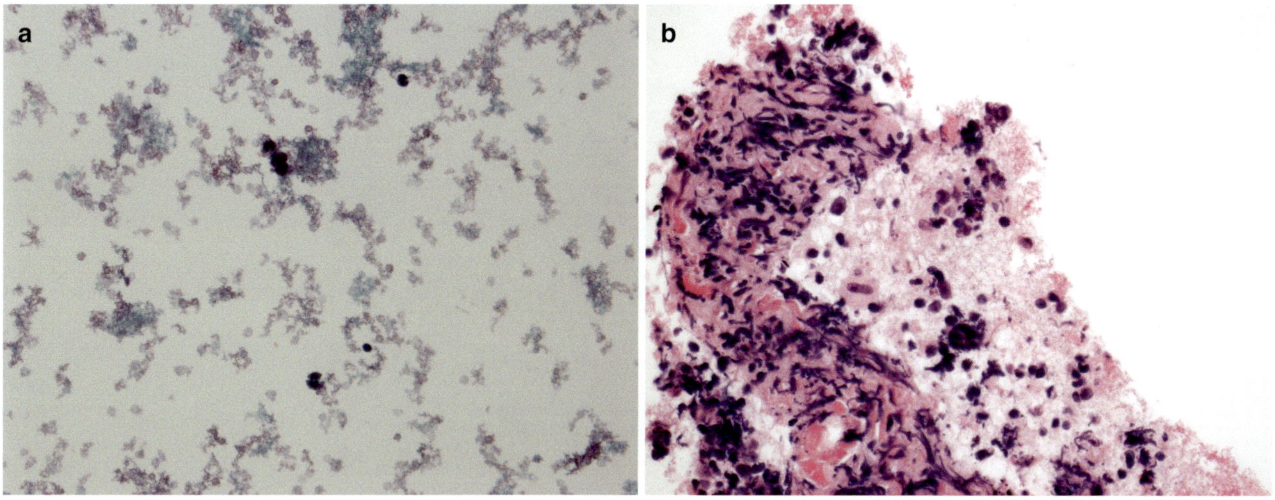

Fig. 4.13 Classic HL, FNA cytology. Cytologic features (**a**) magnification 400×. Cell block histology. (**b**) H&E, magnification 600×

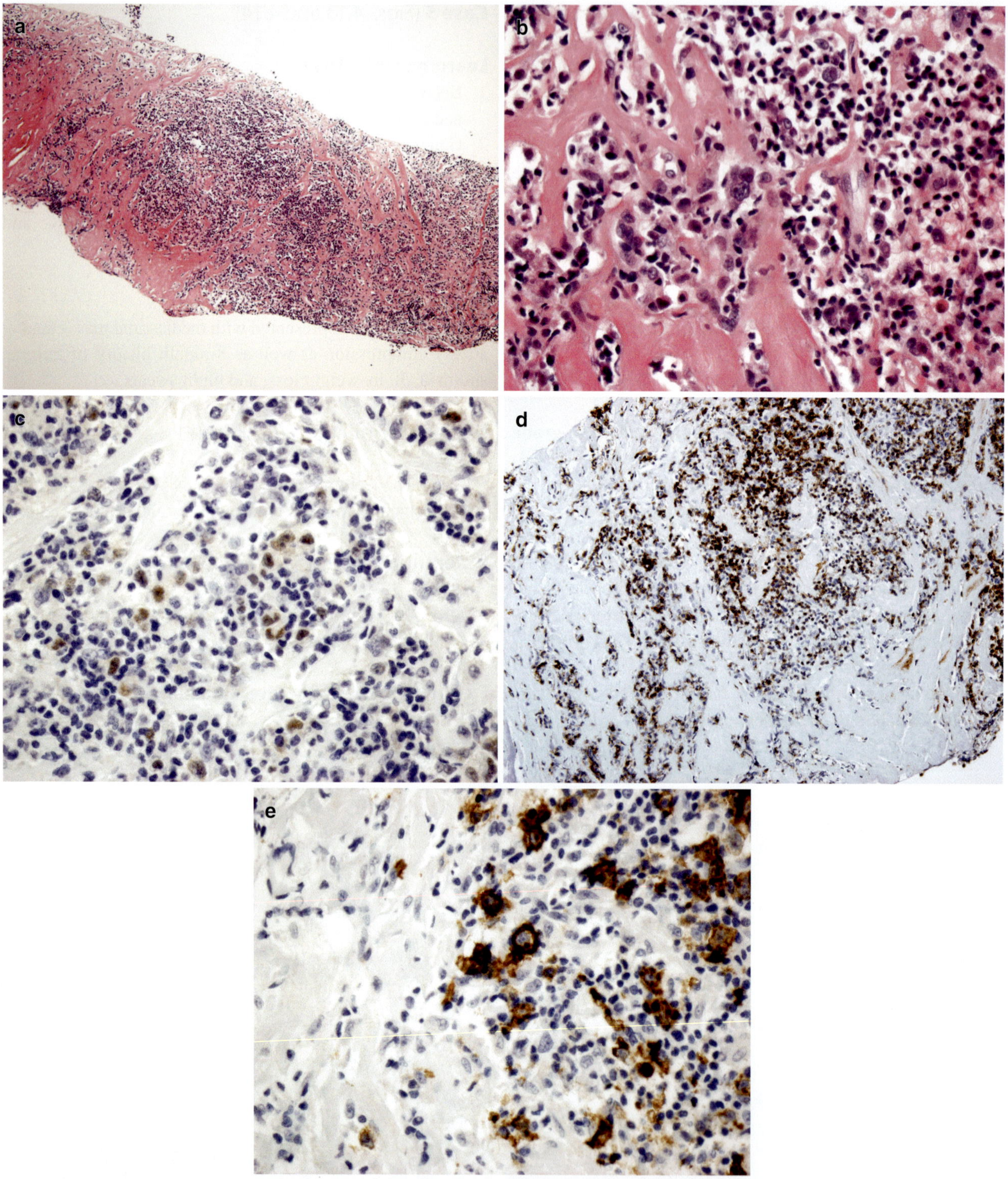

Fig. 4.14 Classic HL, core needle biopsy. Morphologic features (**a**) H&E, magnification 100×. (**b**) H&E, magnification 600×. Immunohistochemical profile (magnification 200×). (**c**) PAX5, magnification 600×. (**d**) CD3. (**e**) CD30 (magnification 400×)

  - Atypical lymphoid infiltrate in the background of extensive stromal fibrosis.
  - Lymphoid infiltrate is composed mainly of small lymphocytes with scattered larger cells showing Hodgkin/Reed-Sternberg (HRS) cytomorphology.
  - CD20 highlights few small B cells, PAX5 weakly positive on HRS cells, highlights small B cells in the background, CD30 strong + on HRS cells, CD15 negative on HRS cells, highlights few scattered background cells, CD3 highlights T cells as majority of small lymphocytes, BCL6 and ALK negative, cytokeratin negative.
- Flow cytometry
  - The specimen shows low viability and cellularity with insufficient B cells for adequate analysis of clonality by light chain distribution. Lymphoid cells represent less than 1% of cells in the flow specimen.

Final Diagnosis

Classic HL, probably nodular sclerosis subtype

Take-Home Messages

1. HRS cells can be found in entities other than cHL.
2. Flow cytometry is not useful in the diagnosis.
3. Tissue biopsy is required for correct diagnosis and avoiding diagnostic pitfalls.
4. Characteristic cytomorphology and immunophenotype, along with typical clinical presentation, may be helpful for the diagnosis of cHL, even with small needle core biopsy or cell block tissue fragments.

Case 6 (Fig. 4.15)

Learning Objectives

1. Become familiar with cytology, tissue biopsy histology, and immunohistochemistry of high-grade B-cell lymphoma.
2. Generate a differential diagnosis based on FNA/CNB findings.
3. Recognize that tissue biopsy is required for definitive diagnosis of high-grade B-cell lymphoma, particularly application of ancillary tests, including cytogenetic analysis, to classify this category of the B-cell lymphoma.

Case History

A 72-year-old female with weight loss and left lower extremity lymphadenopathy. Ultrasound-guided core needle biopsy and touch preps of left groin lymph node. No prior history of malignancy

Histologic Findings

- Core needle biopsy
  - Touch imprint showed monotonous population of medium-sized lymphoid cells with high nuclear/cytoplasmic ratio, indented nuclei, and scant basophilic cytoplasm, some with small vacuoles.
  - Core section showed monomorphic lymphoid cells that are small to medium in size with clear cytoplasm (contraction artifact).
  - By immunohistochemistry, the lymphoid cells were positive for CD20, PAX5, CD10, BCL6, BCL2, and MYC. They are negative for CD3, CD5, CD23, and cyclin D1. Proliferative index was >95% by Ki-67 stain.

- Flow cytometry
  - Monoclonal B-cell population with expression of CD10
  - Molecular cytogenetic analysis (interphase FISH):
  - Rearrangement of *MYC* gene
  - Rearrangement of *BCL2* gene (*IGH/BCL2*)
  - No rearrangement of *BCL6* gene

Final Diagnosis

High-grade B-cell lymphoma with *MYC* and *BCL2* rearrangements (double hit lymphoma)

Take-Home Messages

1. FNA/NCB is effective in evaluating high-grade B-cell lymphoma.
2. Monotonous small- to medium-sized lymphocytes with high proliferative index raises a possibility of high-grade B-cell lymphoma.
3. Most common immunophenotypic profile is CD10+/BCL6+/MUM1-.
4. Double expresser phenotype predicts a double "hit" genotype but is not necessarily equivalent to.
5. Molecular cytogenetic analysis is needed to classify this category of mature B-cell lymphoma.
6. The prognosis is poor.

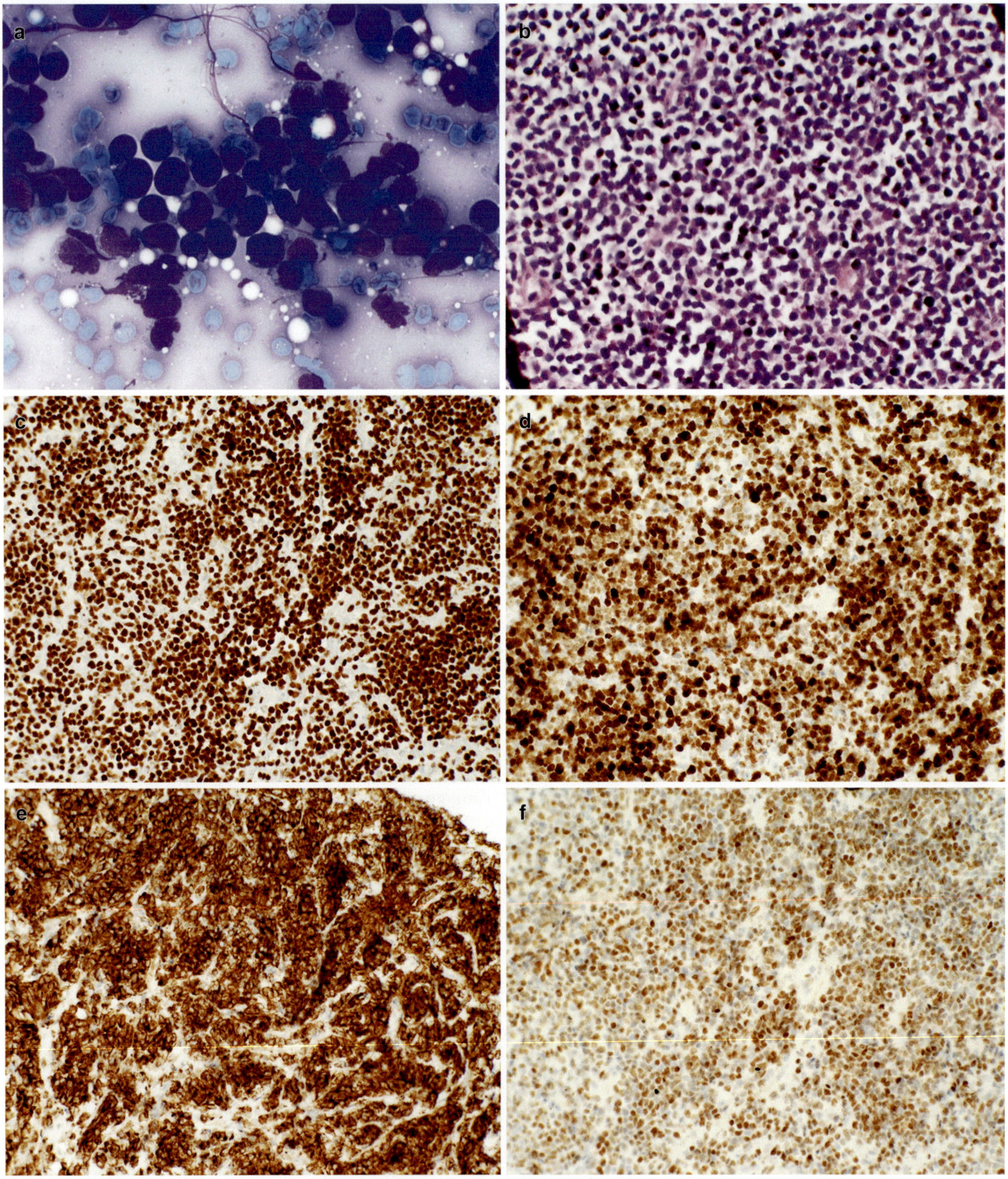

Fig. 4.15 High-grade B-cell lymphoma with *MYC* gene and *BCL2* gene rearrangement. (**a**) Touch imprint showing monotonous population of lymphoid cells with medium to large size. Modified Wright Giemsa stain, ×400. (**b**) Section of needle core biopsy. Note a monomorphic lymphoid population that is small to medium in size. H&E stain, ×200. (**c**) The lymphoid cells are positive for PAX5. ×200. (**d**) Lymphoid cells demonstrate high proliferative index (>90%). Ki-67 stain, ×200. (**e**) The lymphoid cells are strongly positive for BCL2 ×200. (**f**) Expression of cMyc protein in lymphoid cells. MYC stain, ×200

References

1. Lieu D. Cytopathologist-performed ultrasound-guided fine-needle aspiration and core-needle biopsy: a prospective study of 500 consecutive cases. Diagn Cytopathol. 2008;36(5):317–24.
2. Florentine BD, Staymates B, Rabadi M, Sarda N, Barstis J, Black A. Cost savings associated with the use of fine-needle aspiration biopsy (FNAB) for the diagnosis of palpable masses in a community hospital-based FNAB clinic. Cancer. 2006;107(9):2270–81.
3. Young NA, Moriarty AT, Haja JC, Wilbur DC. Fine-needle aspiration biopsy of lymphoproliferative disorders–interpretations based on morphologic criteria alone: results from the College of American Pathologists Interlaboratory Comparison Program in Nongynecologic Cytopathology. Arch Pathol Lab Med. 2006;130(12):1766–71.
4. Swerdlow SH, O. World Health, and C. International Agency for Research on, WHO classification of tumours of haematopoietic and lymphoid tissues: Lyon, International Agency for Research on Cancer; 2017.
5. Scallon BJ, Snyder LA, Anderson GM, Chen Q, Yan L, Weiner LM, et al. A review of antibody therapeutics and antibody-related technologies for oncology. J Immunother. 2006;29(4):351–64.
6. Das DK, Gupta SK, Pathak IC, Sharma SC, Datta BN. Burkitt-type lymphoma. Diagnosis by fine needle aspiration cytology. Acta Cytol. 1987;31(1):1–7.
7. Yazdi HM, Burns BF. Fine needle aspiration biopsy of Ki-1-positive large-cell "anaplastic" lymphoma. Acta Cytol. 1991;35(3):306–10.
8. Frizzera G. The distinction of Hodgkin's disease from anaplastic large cell lymphoma. Semin Diagn Pathol. 1992;9(4):291–6.
9. Das DK, Francis IM, Sharma PN, Sathar SA, John B, George SS, et al. Hodgkin's lymphoma: diagnostic difficulties in fine-needle aspiration cytology. Diagn Cytopathol. 2009;37(8):564–73.
10. Butler JJ. The histologic diagnosis of Hodgkin's disease. Semin Diagn Pathol. 1992;9(4):252–6.
11. Pai RR, Khadilkar UN, Pai MR, Dinesh M. T-cell rich B-cell lymphoma–a case report. Indian J Pathol Microbiol. 2003;46(3):427–8.
12. Mourad WA, al Nazer M, Tulbah A. Cytomorphologic differentiation of Hodgkin's lymphoma and Ki-1+ anaplastic large cell lymphoma in fine needle aspirates. Acta Cytol. 2003;47(5):744–8.
13. McCluggage WG, Walsh MY, Bharucha H. Anaplastic large cell malignant lymphoma with extensive eosinophilic or neutrophilic infiltration. Histopathology. 1998;32(2):110–5.
14. Vicandi B, Jimenez-Heffernan JA, Lopez-Ferrer P, Gamallo C, Viguer JM. Hodgkin's disease mimicking suppurative lymphadenitis: a fine-needle aspiration report of five cases. Diagn Cytopathol. 1999;20(5):302–6.
15. Carbone A, Gloghini A, Volpe R. Paraffin section immunohistochemistry in the diagnosis of Hodgkin's disease and anaplastic large cell (CD30+) lymphomas. Virchows Arch A Pathol Anat Histopathol. 1992;420(6):527–32.
16. Zinzani PL, Colecchia A, Festi D, Magagnoli M, Larocca A, Ascani S, et al. Ultrasound-guided core-needle biopsy is effective in the initial diagnosis of lymphoma patients. Haematologica. 1998;83(11):989–92.
17. Wotherspoon AC, et al. Diagnostic fine needle core biopsy of deep lymph nodes for the diagnosis of lymphoma in patients unfit for surgery. J Pathol. 1989;158(2):115–21.
18. Demharter J, Muller P, Wagner T, Schlimok G, Haude K, Bohndorf K. Percutaneous core-needle biopsy of enlarged lymph nodes in the diagnosis and subclassification of malignant lymphomas. Eur Radiol. 2001;11(2):276–83.
19. Ryu YJ, Cha W, Jeong WJ, Choi SI, Ahn SH. Diagnostic role of core needle biopsy in cervical lymphadenopathy. Head Neck. 2015;37(2):229–33.
20. Seif H, Soliman R, Farouk M, Khairallah MK. Fine need aspiration cytology versus TruCut biopsy in diagnosis of lymphadenopathy. In European Society of Radiology. 2017.
21. Metzgeroth G, Schneider S, Walz C, Reiter S, Hofmann WK, Marx A, et al. Fine needle aspiration and core needle biopsy in the diagnosis of lymphadenopathy of unknown aetiology. Ann Hematol. 2012;91(9):1477–84.
22. Kim BM, Kim EK, Kim MJ, Yang WI, Park CS, Park SI. Sonographically guided core needle biopsy of cervical lymphadenopathy in patients without known malignancy. J Ultrasound Med. 2007;26(5):585–91.
23. Kraft M, Laeng H, Schmuziger N, Arnoux A, Gurtler N. Comparison of ultrasound-guided core-needle biopsy and fine-needle aspiration in the assessment of head and neck lesions. Head Neck. 2008;30(11):1457–63.
24. Crespo M, Bosch F, Villamor N, Bellosillo B, Colomer D, Rozman M, et al. ZAP-70 expression as a surrogate for immunoglobulin-variable-region mutations in chronic lymphocytic leukemia. N Engl J Med. 2003;348(18):1764–75.
25. Stetler-Stevenson, M, Davis B, Wood B, Braylan R. 2006 Bethesda International Consensus Conference on flow cytometric immunophenotyping of hematolymphoid neoplasia. Cytometry B Clin Cytom. 2007;72 Suppl 1:S3.
26. Dey P, Amir T, Al Jassar A, Al Shemmari S, Jogai S, Bhat MG, et al. Combined applications of fine needle aspiration cytology and flow cytometric immunophenotyping for diagnosis and classification of non-Hodgkin lymphoma. CytoJournal. 2006;3:24.
27. Dunphy CH, Ramos R. Combining fine-needle aspiration and flow cytometric immunophenotyping in evaluation of nodal and extranodal sites for possible lymphoma: a retrospective review. Diagn Cytopathol. 1997;16(3):200–6.
28. Young NA, Al-Saleem TI, Ehya H, Smith MR. Utilization of fine-needle aspiration cytology and flow cytometry in the diagnosis and subclassification of primary and recurrent lymphoma. Cancer. 1998;84(4):252–61.
29. Meda BA, Buss DH, Woodruff RD, Cappellari JO, Rainer RO, Powell BL, et al. Diagnosis and subclassification of primary and recurrent lymphoma. The usefulness and limitations of combined fine-needle aspiration cytomorphology and flow cytometry. Am J Clin Pathol. 2000;113(5):688–99.
30. Zeppa P, Marino G, Troncone G, Fulciniti F, De Renzo A, Picardi M, et al. Fine-needle cytology and flow cytometry immunophenotyping and subclassification of non-Hodgkin lymphoma: a critical review of 307 cases with technical suggestions. Cancer. 2004;102(1):55–65.
31. Bangerter M, Brudler O, Heinrich B, Griesshamnuer M. Fine needle aspiration cytology and flow cytometry in the diagnosis and subclassification of non-Hodgkin's lymphoma based on the World Health Organization classification. Acta Cytol. 2007;51(3):390–8.
32. Barrena S, Almeida J, Del Carmen Garcia-Macias M, Lopez A, Rasillo A, Sayagues JM, et al. Flow cytometry immunophenotyping of fine-needle aspiration specimens: utility in the diagnosis and classification of non-Hodgkin lymphomas. Histopathology. 2011;58(6):906–18.
33. Stacchini A, Carucci P, Pacchioni D, Accinelli G, Demurtas A, Aliberti S, et al. Diagnosis of deep-seated lymphomas by endoscopic ultrasound-guided fine needle aspiration combined with flow cytometry. Cytopathology. 2012;23(1):50–6.
34. Volmar KE, Singh HK, Gong JZ. The advantages and limitations of the role of core needle and fine needle aspiration biopsy of lymph nodes in the modern era: Hodgkin and non-Hodgkin lymphomas and metastatic disease. AJSP Rev Rep. 2007;12(1):10–26.
35. Cozzolino I, Rocco M, Villani G, Picardi M. Lymph node fine-needle cytology of non-Hodgkin lymphoma: diagnosis and classification by flow cytometry. Acta Cytol. 2016;60(4):302–14.

36. Craig FE, Foon KA. Flow cytometric immunophenotyping for hematologic neoplasms. Blood. 2008;111(8):3941–67.
37. Dong HY, Gorczyca W, Liu Z, Tsang P, Wu CD, Cohen P, et al. B-cell lymphomas with coexpression of CD5 and CD10. Am J Clin Pathol. 2003;119(2):218–30.
38. Jaso JM, Yin CC, Wang SA, Miranda RN, Jabcuga CE, Chen L, et al. Clinicopathologic features of CD5-positive nodal marginal zone lymphoma. Am J Clin Pathol. 2013;140(5):693–700.
39. Baseggio L, Traverse-Glehen A, Petinataud F, Callet-Bauchu E, Berger F, Ffrench M, et al. CD5 expression identifies a subset of splenic marginal zone lymphomas with higher lymphocytosis: a clinico-pathological, cytogenetic and molecular study of 24 cases. Haematologica. 2010;95(4):604–12.
40. Hunter ZR, Branagan AR, Manning R, Patterson CJ, Santos DD, Tournilhac O, et al. CD5, CD10, and CD23 expression in Waldenstrom's macroglobulinemia. Clin Lymphoma. 2005;5(4):246–9.
41. Maeshima AM, Taniguchi H, Toyoda K, Yamauchi N, Makita S, Fukuhara S, et al. Clinicopathological features of histological transformation from extranodal marginal zone B-cell lymphoma of mucosa-associated lymphoid tissue to diffuse large B-cell lymphoma: an analysis of 467 patients. Br J Haematol. 2016;174(6):923–31.
42. Jaso J, Chen L, Li S, Lin P, Chen W, Miranda RN, et al. CD5-positive mucosa-associated lymphoid tissue (MALT) lymphoma: a clinicopathologic study of 14 cases. Hum Pathol. 2012;43(9):1436–43.
43. Ho AK, Hill S, Preobrazhensky SN, Miller ME, Chen Z, Bahler DW, et al. Small B-cell neoplasms with typical mantle cell lymphoma immunophenotypes often include chronic lymphocytic leukemias. Am J Clin Pathol. 2009;131(1):27–32.
44. Nelson BP, Variakojis D, Peterson LC. Leukemic phase of B-cell lymphomas mimicking chronic lymphocytic leukemia and variants at presentation. Mod Pathol. 2002;15(11):1111–20.
45. Gong JZ, Lagoo AS, Peters D, Horvatinovich J, Benz P, Buckley PJ. Value of CD23 determination by flow cytometry in differentiating mantle cell lymphoma from chronic lymphocytic leukemia/small lymphocytic lymphoma. Am J Clin Pathol. 2001;116(6):893–7.
46. Schlette E, Fu K, Medeiros LJ. CD23 expression in mantle cell lymphoma: clinicopathologic features of 18 cases. Am J Clin Pathol. 2003;120(5):760–6.
47. Klener P, Fronkova E, Berkova A, Jaksa R, Lhotska H, Forsterova K, et al. Mantle cell lymphoma-variant Richter syndrome: detailed molecular-cytogenetic and backtracking analysis reveals slow evolution of a pre-MCL clone in parallel with CLL over several years. Int J Cancer. 2016;139(10):2252–60.
48. Hoeller S, Zhou Y, Kanagal-Shamanna R, Xu-Monette ZY, Hoehn D, Bihl M, et al. Composite mantle cell lymphoma and chronic lymphocytic leukemia/small lymphocytic lymphoma: a clinicopathologic and molecular study. Hum Pathol. 2013;44(1):110–21.
49. Gong Y, Caraway N, Gu J, Zaidi T, Fernandez R, Sun X, et al. Evaluation of interphase fluorescence in situ hybridization for the t(14;18)(q32;q21) translocation in the diagnosis of follicular lymphoma on fine-needle aspirates: a comparison with flow cytometry immunophenotyping. Cancer. 2003;99(6):385–93.
50. Eshoa C, Perkins S, Kampalath B, Shidham V, Juckett M, Chang CC. Decreased CD10 expression in grade III and in interfollicular infiltrates of follicular lymphomas. Am J Clin Pathol. 2001;115(6):862–7.
51. Schraders M, de Jong D, Kluin P, Groenen P, van Krieken H. Lack of Bcl-2 expression in follicular lymphoma may be caused by mutations in the BCL2 gene or by absence of the t(14;18) translocation. J Pathol. 2005;205(3):329–35.
52. Li S, Eshleman JR, Borowitz MJ. Lack of surface immunoglobulin light chain expression by flow cytometric immunophenotyping can help diagnose peripheral B-cell lymphoma. Am J Clin Pathol. 2002;118(2):229–34.
53. Kojima M, Sato E, Oshimi K, Murase T, Koike T, Tsunoda S, et al. Characteristics of CD5-positive splenic marginal zone lymphoma with leukemic manifestation; clinical, flow cytometry, and histopathological findings of 11 cases. J Clin Exp Hematop. 2010;50(2):107–12.
54. Ott G, Katzenberger T, Greiner A, Kalla J, Rosenwald A, Heinrich U, et al. The t(11;18)(q21;q21) chromosome translocation is a frequent and specific aberration in low-grade but not high-grade malignant non-Hodgkin's lymphomas of the mucosa-associated lymphoid tissue (MALT-) type. Cancer Res. 1997;57(18):3944–8.
55. Dierlamm J, Pittaluga S, Wlodarska I, Stul M, Thomas J, Boogaerts M, et al. Marginal zone B-cell lymphomas of different sites share similar cytogenetic and morphologic features. Blood. 1996;87(1):299–307.
56. Wotherspoon AC, Finn TM, Isaacson PG. Trisomy 3 in low-grade B-cell lymphomas of mucosa-associated lymphoid tissue. Blood. 1995;85(8):2000–4.
57. Baldini L, Fracchiolla NS, Cro LM, Trecca D, Romitti L, Polli E, et al. Frequent p53 gene involvement in splenic B-cell leukemia/lymphomas of possible marginal zone origin. Blood. 1994;84(1):270–8.
58. Insuasti-Beltran G, Gale JM, Wilson CS, Foucar K, Czuchlewski DR. Significance of MYD88 L265P mutation status in the subclassification of low-grade B-cell lymphoma/leukemia. Arch Pathol Lab Med. 2015;139(8):1035–41.
59. Liu Z, Dong HY, Gorczyca W, Tsang P, Cohen P, Stephenson CF, et al. CD5- mantle cell lymphoma. Am J Clin Pathol. 2002;118(2):216–24.
60. Hans CP, Weisenburger DD, Greiner TC, Gascoyne RD, Delabie J, Ott G, et al. Confirmation of the molecular classification of diffuse large B-cell lymphoma by immunohistochemistry using a tissue microarray. Blood. 2004;103(1):275–82.
61. Karube K, Guo Y, Suzumiya J, Sugita Y, Nomura Y, Yamamoto K, et al. CD10-MUM1+ follicular lymphoma lacks BCL2 gene translocation and shows characteristic biologic and clinical features. Blood. 2007;109(7):3076–9.
62. Soo KL, Shustik D, Yusoff LZ, Tan L, Tan SY. An algorithmic approach to the diagnosis of NK and T cell lymphomas. Pathology. 2011;43(7):673–81.
63. Charafe-Jauffret E, Bertucci F, Ramuz O, Devilard E, Gaulard P, Brousset P, et al. Characterization of Hodgkin's lymphoma-like undifferentiated carcinoma of the nasopharyngeal type as a particular UCNT subtype mimicking Hodgkin's lymphoma. Int J Oncol. 2003;23(1):97–103.
64. Gomez-Gelvez JC, Smith LB. Reed-Sternberg-like cells in non-Hodgkin lymphomas. Arch Pathol Lab Med. 2015;139(10):1205–10.
65. Bossard C, Dobay MP, Parrens M, Lamant L, Missiaglia E, Haioun C, et al. Immunohistochemistry as a valuable tool to assess CD30 expression in peripheral T-cell lymphomas: high correlation with mRNA levels. Blood. 2014;124(19):2983–6.
66. Barry TS, Jaffe ES, Sorbara L, Raffeld M, Pittaluga S. Peripheral T-cell lymphomas expressing CD30 and CD15. Am J Surg Pathol. 2003;27(12):1513–22.
67. Nicolae A, Pittaluga S, Venkataraman G, Vijnovich-Baron A, Xi L, Raffeld M, et al. Peripheral T-cell lymphomas of follicular T-helper cell derivation with Hodgkin/Reed-Sternberg cells of B-cell lineage: both EBV-positive and EBV-negative variants exist. Am J Surg Pathol. 2013;37(6):816–26.
68. Rashmi Kumari T, Rajalakshmi T. Fine needle aspiration cytology in the diagnosis of Hodgkin lymphoma: hits and misses. J Cytol. 2008;25(1):10–2.
69. Jimenez-Heffernan JA, Vicandi B, Lopez-Ferrer P, Hardisson D, Viguer JM. Value of fine needle aspiration cytology in the initial diagnosis of Hodgkin's disease. Analysis of 188 cases with an emphasis on diagnostic pitfalls. Acta Cytol. 2001;45(3):300–6.
70. Macon WR, Levy NB, Kurtin PJ, Salhany KE, Elkhalifa MY, Casey TT, et al. Hepatosplenic alphabeta T-cell lymphomas: a

report of 14 cases and comparison with hepatosplenic gammadelta T-cell lymphomas. Am J Surg Pathol. 2001;25(3):285–96.
71. Tan SY, Ooi AS, Ang MK, Koh M, Wong JC, Dykema K, et al. Nuclear expression of MATK is a novel marker of type II enteropathy-associated T-cell lymphoma. Leukemia. 2011;25(3):555–7.
72. Deleeuw RJ, Zettl A, Klinker E, Haralambieva E, Trottier M, Chari R, et al. Whole-genome analysis and HLA genotyping of enteropathy-type T-cell lymphoma reveals 2 distinct lymphoma subtypes. Gastroenterology. 2007;132(5):1902–11.
73. Kucuk C, Jiang B, Hu X, Zhang W, Chan JK, Xiao W, et al. Activating mutations of STAT5B and STAT3 in lymphomas derived from gammadelta-T or NK cells. Nat Commun. 2015;6:6025.
74. Nairismagi ML, Tan J, Lim JQ, Nagarajan S, Ng CC, Rajasegaran V, et al. JAK-STAT and G-protein-coupled receptor signaling pathways are frequently altered in epitheliotropic intestinal T-cell lymphoma. Leukemia. 2016;30(6):1311–9.
75. Laurent C, Fazilleau N, Brousset P. A novel subset of T-helper cells: follicular T-helper cells and their markers. Haematologica. 2010;95(3):356–8.
76. Marafioti T, Paterson JC, Ballabio E, Chott A, Natkunam Y, Rodriguez-Justo M, et al. The inducible T-cell co-stimulator molecule is expressed on subsets of T cells and is a new marker of lymphomas of T follicular helper cell-derivation. Haematologica. 2010;95(3):432–9.
77. Das DK, Gupta SK, Datta BN, Sharma SC. Fine needle aspiration cytodiagnosis of Hodgkin's disease and its subtypes. I. Scope and limitations. Acta Cytol. 1990;34(3):329–36.
78. Chhieng DC, Cangiarella JF, Symmans WF, Cohen JM. Fine-needle aspiration cytology of Hodgkin disease: a study of 89 cases with emphasis on false-negative cases. Cancer. 2001;93(1):52–9.
79. Moreland WS, Geisinger KR. Utility and outcomes of fine-needle aspiration biopsy in Hodgkin's disease. Diagn Cytopathol. 2002;26(5):278–82.
80. Steel BL, Schwartz MR, Ramzy I. Fine needle aspiration biopsy in the diagnosis of lymphadenopathy in 1,103 patients. Role, limitations and analysis of diagnostic pitfalls. Acta Cytol. 1995;39(1):76–81.
81. Wilsher MJ. Inflammatory melanoma: a potential diagnostic pitfall. Pathology. 2010;42(6):603–6.
82. Jabbour MN, Nassif S, Chakhachiro Z. Undifferentiated nasopharyngeal carcinoma mimicking Hodgkin lymphoma with CD30 expression. Int J Surg Pathol. 2016;24(8):715–7.
83. Strum SB, Park JK, Rappaport H. Observation of cells resembling Sternberg-Reed cells in conditions other than Hodgkin's disease. Cancer. 1970;26(1):176–90.
84. Leoncini L, Del Vecchio MT, Kraft R, Megha T, Barbini P, Cevenini G, et al. Hodgkin's disease and CD30-positive anaplastic large cell lymphomas–a continuous spectrum of malignant disorders. A quantitative morphometric and immunohistologic study. Am J Pathol. 1990;137(5):1047–57.
85. Schmidt U, Metz KA, Leder LD. T-cell-rich B-cell lymphoma and lymphocyte-predominant Hodgkin's disease: two closely related entities? Br J Haematol. 1995;90(2):398–403.
86. Oertel YC. Fine needle aspiration in Hodgkin's disease. Acta Cytol. 2002;46(3):617.
87. Fromm JR, Thomas A, Wood BL. Flow cytometry can diagnose classical Hodgkin lymphoma in lymph nodes with high sensitivity and specificity. Am J Clin Pathol. 2009;131(3):322–32.
88. Roshal M, Wood BL, Fromm JR. Flow cytometric detection of the classical Hodgkin lymphoma: clinical and research applications. Adv Hematol. 2011;2011:387034.
89. Carbone A, Gloghini A. The role of current and new discriminating markers in the immunodiagnosis of Hodgkin's disease and other phenotypically related lymphomas. Pathologica. 1996;88(3):169–74.
90. Metkar SS, Naresh KN, Redkar AA, Soman CS, Advani SH, Nadkarni JJ. Expression of Fas and Fas ligand in Hodgkin's disease. Leuk Lymphoma. 1999;33(5–6):521–30.
91. Pileri S, Sabattini E, Tazzari PL, Gherlinzoni F, Zucchini L, Bigerna B, et al. Hodgkin's disease: update of findings. Haematologica. 1991;76(3):175–82.
92. Ascani S, Zinzani PL, Gherlinzoni F, Sabattini E, Briskomatis A, de Vivo A, et al. Peripheral T-cell lymphomas. Clinico-pathologic study of 168 cases diagnosed according to the R.E.A.L. Classification. Ann Oncol. 1997;8(6):583–92.
93. Pileri SA, Poggi S, Sabattini E, De Vivo A, Falini B, Stein H. Is Hodgkin's disease a unique entity? Leuk Lymphoma. 1995;15(Suppl 1):3–6.
94. von Wasielewski R, Mengel M, Fischer R, Hansmann ML, Hubner K, Franklin J, et al. Classical Hodgkin's disease. Clinical impact of the immunophenotype. Am J Pathol. 1997;151(4):1123–30.
95. Patkar N, Mehta J, Kulkarni B, Pande R, Advani S, Borges A. Immunoprofile of Hodgkin's lymphoma in India. Indian J Cancer. 2008;45(2):59–63.
96. Tzankov A, Mehta J, Kulkarni B, Pande R, Advani S, Borges A, et al. Rare expression of T-cell markers in classical Hodgkin's lymphoma. Mod Pathol. 2005;18(12):1542–9.

Small B-Cell Lymphomas With and Without Plasmacytic Differentiation

5

Juan Camilo Gómez-Gélvez and Kedar V. Inamdar

List of Frequently Asked Questions

1. What are the major subtypes of small B-cell lymphomas? How to evaluate them?
2. What are the characteristic clinical, morphological, and immunophenotypic findings in CD5+ small B-cell lymphomas?
3. What are the characteristic clinical, morphological, and immunophenotypic findings in CD10+ small B-cell lymphomas?
4. What are the characteristic clinical, morphological, and immunophenotypic findings in CD5-negative/CD10-negative small B-cell lymphomas?
5. What are unusual morphological variants of follicular lymphoma which can mimic other lymphomas and reactive lymphoid proliferation?
6. What is the differential diagnosis of small B-cell lymphomas with plasmacytic or plasmacytoid differentiation?
7. How to distinguish small B-cell lymphomas with extensive plasmacytic differentiation from nodal involvement by a plasma cell neoplasm?
8. Which immunophenotypic markers are diagnostic or exclude a specific subtype of small B-cell lymphoma?
9. Which ancillary molecular/genetic tests are useful in the diagnosis or classification of small B-cell lymphomas?
10. Which are the most common genetic abnormalities seen in small B-cell lymphomas, and how these results can be used for differential diagnosis along with immunophenotypic data?
11. Which ancillary tests provide prognostic and/or therapeutic information for small B-cell lymphomas?
12. How to distinguish small B-cell lymphomas from reactive follicular or paracortical hyperplasias and other reactive lymphadenopathies?
13. How frequently does each subtype of small B-cell lymphoma involve the bone marrow and what are their typical patterns of involvement?
14. How to distinguish bone marrow involvement by a small B-cell lymphoma from benign lymphoid aggregates?
15. What is considered an adequate specimen for diagnosis and classification of small B-cell lymphomas?
16. What information can be conveyed to the clinician during each workup stage of small B-cell lymphomas?
17. What should be the approach to provide maximum, but defensible, information from limited specimen or workup? What is a descriptive diagnosis appropriate in such situations?
18. When is a diagnostic comment necessary and what should be discussed in the diagnostic comment of small B-cell lymphomas?
19. When is it appropriate to seek external consultation for diagnosis or classification of small B-cell lymphomas?

1. What are the major subtypes of small B-cell lymphomas? How to evaluate them?

- Small B-cell lymphomas with or without plasmacytic differentiation include all B-cell non-Hodgkin lymphomas in which the neoplastic cells constitute a clonal population of predominantly small, mature lymphocytes intermixed with a variable number of larger B-cells. Lymph-node-based small B-cell lymphomas are characterized by distortion or total effacement of the nodal architecture. They display distinct morphologic and immunophenotypic features that are essential for accurate diagnosis.
- Although evaluation of cytomorphology and architectural patterns is necessary in the diagnosis of small B-cell

J. C. Gómez-Gélvez
Department of Pathology and Laboratory Medicine, Henry Ford Health System, Detroit, MI, USA
e-mail: jgomez1@hfhs.org

K. V. Inamdar (✉)
Department of Pathology, Henry Ford Hospital, Detroit, MI, USA
e-mail: kinamda1@hfhs.org

E. Wang, A. S. Lagoo (eds.), *Practical Lymph Node and Bone Marrow Pathology*, Practical Anatomic Pathology,
https://doi.org/10.1007/978-3-030-32189-5_5

lymphomas, immunophenotypic profiling by flow cytometry and/or IHC is essential to establish a definitive diagnosis with accurate subclassification.

- Flow cytometry is useful in determination of clonality by assessment of immunoglobulin light restriction and is highly sensitive in identifying even a small percent of clonal lymphoid cells in a predominantly polyclonal background.
- IHC allows for assessment of immunoarchitecture in the context of morphology and allows for accentuation of subtle morphologic features not easily identified during morphologic examination.
- Additionally, IHC plays in important role in identifying the recently described in situ neoplasias (follicular and mantle cell) in otherwise reactive lymph nodes.
- The most widely accepted initial panel of antibodies includes CD20, CD3, CD5, CD10, BCL2, BCL6, and cyclin D1. Some of the antibodies such as BCL2, BCL6, and cyclin D1 are better evaluated by IHC rather than flow cytometry.
- After confirming the B-cell lineage of the small cell lymphoma, it is useful to follow an algorithmic approach, initially dividing small B-cell lymphomas into CD5+ and CD5-negative subgroups [1]. CD5+ small B-NHLs include predominantly CLL/SLL and MCL [2, 3]. CD5-negative small B-cell lymphomas are further classified into CD10+ and CD10-negative subgroups. Thus, most small B-cell lymphomas can be divided into three broad groups: CD5+ small B-cell lymphomas, CD10+ small B-cell lymphomas, and CD5-/CD10- small B-cell lymphomas (Table 5.1).

- This chapter will focus primarily on nodal-based entities including monoclonal B-cell lymphocytosis (MBL), chronic lymphocytic leukemia/small lymphocytic lymphoma (CLL/SLL), marginal zone lymphoma (MZL), mantle cell lymphoma (MCL), follicular lymphoma (FL), and lymphoplasmacytic lymphoma/ Waldenström macroglobulinemia (LPL/WM). The uncommon splenic diffuse red pulp small B-cell lymphoma (SDRPL) and hairy cell leukemia variant (HCLv) also belong in this group; however, these are discussed elsewhere [4]. Precursor B-cell neoplasms (B-lymphoblastic leukemia/lymphoma) as well as high-grade B-cell neoplasms like Burkitt lymphoma, though composed of small B-cells, will not be considered further in this chapter.
- While the above categorization is useful, it is not flawless. For instance, CD5 expression is found in approximately 10% of nodal MZL and 7% of LPL/WM [2, 5]. Additionally, rare CLL/SLL and MCL cases can be CD5 negative. Small B-cell lymphomas with coexpression of both CD5 and CD10 are extremely rare but do occur [6]. It is important to remember that high-grade B-cell lymphomas (discussed in Chap. 7 in this book) can also express CD5 and/or CD10.
- Plasmacytic differentiation, which refers to the terminal differentiation of neoplastic B-lymphocytes into mature plasma cells, may be seen in any subtype of this group to a varying degree and frequency, but it is most commonly encountered in LPL and MZL [7]. See Questions 6 and 7 for additional information.
- The distinguishing architectural and cytological features of the main types of small B-cell lymphomas are shown in Table 5.2.

Table 5.1 Immunophenotypic groups of small B-cell lymphomas with and without plasmacytic differentiation

Immunophenotypic group	Lymphoma	Tendency to plasmacytic differentiation
CD5+	Monoclonal B-cell lymphocytosis (MBL)	–
	Chronic lymphocytic leukemia/small lymphocytic lymphoma (CLL/SLL)	–/+
	Mantle cell lymphoma (MCL)	–
CD10+	Follicular lymphoma (FL)	–/+
	Burkitt lymphoma (BL)[a]	–
	Other high-grade B-cell lymphomas[a]	–
	B-lymphoblastic leukemia/lymphoma	–
CD5-,CD10-	Marginal zone lymphoma (MZL)	++
	Lymphoplasmacytic lymphoma/ Waldenström macroglobulinemia (LPL/WM)	++
	Hairy cell leukemia[b]	–
	Splenic diffuse red pulp small B-cell lymphoma (SDRPL)	+

[a]See Question 3 for some key differences between FL and BL
[b]These entities are not considered in detail in this chapter
– usually not, –/+ occasionally, + often, ++ usually

Table 5.2 Differential diagnosis of small B-cell lymphomas by morphologic features

	Architectural pattern	Cytomorphology
CLL/ SLL	Vaguely nodular to diffuse	Small with round monotonous nuclei Occasional larger prolymphocytes and paraimmunoblasts
MCL	Diffuse/nodular/mantle zone	Small to intermediate with irregular nuclei resembling centrocytes Epithelioid macrophages and hyalinized vessels
FL	Follicular/diffuse	Small to intermediate with angulated or twisted nuclei (centrocytes), admixed with various numbers of large centroblasts
Nodal MZL	Interfollicular/perifollicular/ diffuse/nodular	Small with round nuclei and abundant clear cytoplasm (monocytoid) Occasional larger cells and plasmacytoid lymphocytes
LPL/ WM	Diffuse/vaguely nodular/often patent sinuses	Small lymphocytes, plasmacytoid lymphocytes, and plasma cells Scattered mast cells

2. What are the characteristic clinical, morphological, and immunophenotypic findings in CD5+ small B-cell lymphomas?

Three entities are considered below – MBL, CLL/SLL, and MCL. *Note*: While 20–30% cases of B-prolymphocytic leukemia (B-PLL) also can be CD5+, the disease itself, particularly one with lymph node involvement, is very rare, constituting less than 1% of all B-cell lymphomas/leukemias. The morphology of the prolymphocytes is rather characteristic, typically medium-sized lymphocytes with a round nucleus containing moderately condensed chromatin and a central prominent nucleolus. This entity is not further discussed in this chapter.

Monoclonal B-Cell Lymphocytosis (MBL)

- Definition: This entity is characterized by presence of less than 5×10^9/L clonal B-lymphocytes in peripheral blood in the absence of lymphadenopathy, organomegaly, extramedullary disease, or other evidence of lymphoma. While the diagnosis is primarily based on the absolute number of clonal B-lymphocytes in peripheral blood, MBL can also present in the lymph nodes and bone marrow.
  - Based on the immunophenotypic profile of the clonal B-cells, three subtypes of MBL are recognized: (1) CLL type, the most common subtype, accounting for 70–75% of all cases, characterized by an immunophenotype indistinguishable from CLL/SLL with expression of CD19, CD5, CD20, CD23, and surface immunoglobulin light chain restriction; (2) atypical CLL type, characterized by a similar phenotype to CLL/SLL or CLL-type MBL, however with atypical features including brighter intensities of expression for markers CD5, CD20, and surface immunoglobulin light chain restriction; (3) non-CLL type, characterized by CD19+, CD5-negative, and CD23-negative immunoprofile [8, 9].
  - CLL-type MBL is further divided into low count ($<0.5 \times 10^9$/L) and high count ($\geq 0.5 \times 10^9$/L) based on the absolute number of clonal B-lymphocytes in peripheral blood [10, 11]. Low-count MBL is biologically different from high-count MBL and CLL in terms of immunoglobulin repertoire usage and genetic abnormalities and is considered a stable nonprogressive disease without significant clinical implications. High-count MBL is biologically similar to CLL and is considered a precursor of CLL with a progression rate of approximately 1–2% per year [10–14]. Among patients with high-count MBL, the absolute number of clonal B-lymphocytes is an independent risk factor for evolution to CLL [11, 13, 14].
- Morphology: Although specific criteria for the diagnosis of tissue-based MBL have not been established, one retrospective study suggested that cases of nodal involvement by clonal B-cells with CLL/SLL-like phenotype but absent proliferation centers in patients without lymphadenopathy greater 1.5 cm on radiological survey are most likely to represent tissue-based MBL since these patients showed absence of progression and do not require treatment [15].

Chronic Lymphocytic Leukemia/Small Lymphocytic Lymphoma (CLL/SLL)

- Clinical features and epidemiology: CLL/SLL is the most common leukemia in adults in the western hemisphere accounting for approximately one-third of new leukemia cases and approximately 20% of mature B-cell neoplasms [16].
  - The annual incidence in the United States is approximately 4.7 cases per 100,000 individuals. Men are more frequently affected than women. It is more frequently diagnosed among people aged 65–74 (median age of 70) and is rarely seen before the age of 40 [17].

- The majority of CLL/SLL patients is asymptomatic and diagnosed incidentally after detection of absolute lymphocytosis during routine peripheral blood examination. Less frequently, patients may present with lymphadenopathy, hepatosplenomegaly, or systemic symptoms such as weight loss and night sweats.
- Patients can also present with cytopenias secondary to involvement of the bone marrow with suppression of hematopoiesis or as a consequence of an autoimmune process [4]. A small monoclonal paraprotein may be seen frequently in these patients [18].

- Morphology: CLL/SLL typically demonstrates complete effacement of the nodal architecture by diffuse proliferation of small, mature, and monotonous lymphocytes with round nuclei, smooth nuclear contours, condensed chromatin, and scant cytoplasm. At low magnification, alternating light and dark zones impart a vaguely nodular or even pseudo-follicular pattern due to the presence of proliferation centers.
  - The dark zones represent compact clusters of small, mature lymphocytes, whereas the light zones represent proliferation centers comprised of medium-sized prolymphocytes and paraimmunoblasts with slightly open chromatin, pale cytoplasm, and small nucleoli.
  - Variation in typical morphologic features including absence of the vague nodular pattern and cytologic atypia can be seen in some cases. Correct diagnosis in such cases is achieved by demonstration of classic CLL/SLL immunophenotype.
- Clinically relevant morphologic variants: A subset of CLL/SLL demonstrates presence of "expanded and confluent proliferation centers" defined as proliferation centers that are broader than a 20× magnification field (equivalent to an area of 0.95 mm^2 in the microscope) and an increased proliferation index (i.e., either >2.4 mitoses per proliferation center or > 40% proliferative index per proliferation center by Ki-67 stain) [19, 20].
  - These cases are associated with 17p deletion and trisomy 12, genetic markers associated with poor prognosis, and aggressive behavior [19–21]. Recognition of expanded proliferation centers is important as these cases show an aggressive clinical behavior akin to Richter transformation (CLL transformation to DLBCL) with much shorter median survival than typical CLL cases [19]. They are clinically recognized as "accelerated CLL/SLL."
- Immunophenotype: CLL/SLL demonstrates characteristic immunophenotypic features (better demonstrated by flow cytometry) that are useful to differentiate it from other small B-cell lymphomas. CLL/SLL cells show weak expression of B-cell markers CD19, CD20, and CD22 as well as dim coexpression of CD5 and CD23. They are negative for FMC7 and CD79b although the latter can show dim and partial expression in a subset of the cases. Additionally, CLL cases show monotypic dim expression of surface or cytoplasmic light chains. LEF1, a recently described marker, is considered a highly sensitive and specific marker for CLL/SLL, although it may be positive in approximately 40% of diffuse large B-cell lymphomas (DLBCL) and rare cases of small B-cell lymphomas other than CLL/SLL [22, 23]. Immunophenotypic variations can be seen in cases that still demonstrate clinical and morphologic features of typical CLL/SLL. These usually include bright expression of CD20, bright surface light chain immunoglobulin, or, rarely, lack of CD5. Such cases are referred to as "atypical CLL/SLL," a term that can also be used for cases showing variation of the classical morphologic features (see above). CD200 is a helpful marker in the differential diagnosis of CLL/SLL from MCL since it is expressed in virtually all cases of CLL/SLL (less frequently in other small B-cell lymphomas) and is typically negative in the MCL [24]. CD200 expression though has now been shown to be expressed in a significant subset of leukemic non-nodal variant of MCL [25].

Mantle Cell Lymphoma (MCL)

- Clinicopathological features: MCL accounts for approximately 3–6% of all non-Hodgkin lymphomas diagnosed in the USA with an annual incidence of 0.5 cases per 100,000 individuals. The median age at diagnosis is 68 years with a male predilection (2–3:1) [16, 26].
  - MCL is an aggressive disease with frequent relapses. Approximately 75% of patients present with advanced clinical stage (III–IV) including widespread lymphadenopathy with bone marrow, peripheral blood, and splenic involvement [26].
  - The gastrointestinal tract and Waldeyer's tonsillar ring in the nasopharynx are also frequently affected [27]. In the gastrointestinal tract, MCL shows a peculiar pattern of involvement known as lymphomatous polyposis characterized by multiple lymphoid polyps throughout the small and large bowel.
  - Other extranodal sites commonly involved include the central nervous system, skin, and lacrimal glands [27].
  - Some patients present with prominent peripheral blood involvement which may indicate the aggressive leukemic phase of nodal disease, especially in cases with blastoid morphology.
  - A leukemic, non-nodal subtype of MCL has been recently described and is now included in the 2017 WHO classification of tumors of the hematopoietic and lymphoid tissues. This variant type is characterized by indolent clinical behavior and frequent involvement of

the peripheral blood, bone marrow, and spleen (without significant lymphadenopathy) [28, 29].

Unlike classic nodal-based MCL, the leukemic non-nodal variant has hypermutated *IGH* gene variable region (*IGHV*) and lacks SOX11 expression [28, 30, 31].

Recognizing this entity is clinically important for two reasons. Firstly, it resembles CLL/SLL in morphologic and immunophenotypic aspects. The small monotonous circulating lymphocytes are similar to those of CLL/SLL. Additionally, they coexpress CD5 and CD200 and are negative for SOX11. Diagnosis relies on detection of *IGH-CCND1* rearrangement by FISH. Secondly, recognition of this entity is important to avoid overtreatment as the majority of these patients tend to follow an indolent clinical course with slow or no clinical progression [32]. However, some patients may develop secondary genetic alterations (usually inactivating *TP53* mutations) and progress to aggressive MCL [28, 30, 31].

- Morphology: MCL in its most classic form involves the lymph nodes in a diffuse, nodular, or mantle zone pattern; diffuse pattern is most common [33].
  - The neoplastic lymphocytes are small to medium-sized with irregular nuclear contours, granular and uneven chromatin, inconspicuous nucleoli, and scant cytoplasm.
  - Scattered epithelioid histiocytes and hyalinized vessels are commonly encountered and aid in differentiation from other small B-cell lymphomas.
  - Non- neoplastic plasma cells may be present; in rare cases clusters of clonal plasma cells can be found within tumor nodules or within reactive germinal centers constituting what is described as MCL with plasmacytic differentiation [34].
  - Large transformed cells such as centroblasts, immunoblasts, or paraimmunoblasts are conspicuously absent.
  - Mantle-zone pattern is characterized by expansion of the mantle zones surrounding reactive germinal centers. The mantle zones often merge leaving little interfollicular areas in between. This pattern can be difficult to distinguish from in situ mantle cell neoplasia (ISMCN) (discussed below).
  - Nodular pattern is characterized by presence of expanded and disrupted germinal centers due to the infiltration by the neoplastic mantle cells.
- Clinically relevant morphologic variants of MCL: Approximately 10% of MCL exhibit morphologic and immunophenotypic variations. The blastoid and pleomorphic morphologic variants of MCL warrant specific designation in the final diagnosis as they are associated with a highly aggressive clinical behavior compared to classic MCL.
  - In the blastoid variant, the mitotic activity is brisk (20–30 mitoses per 10 hpf), and lymphoma cells resemble lymphoblasts, thus invoking lymphoblastic lymphoma in the differential. Genetically, blastoid MCL harbors additional genetic abnormalities such as complex karyotype, *TP53*, p16^{CDKN2A}, and p18^{CDKN2C} mutations [35, 36]. Clinically, blastoid MCL behaves far more aggressively than classic MCL with much lower median overall survival (1 year) than classic MCL (4–5 years) [37–39].
  - Pleomorphic MCL resembles and can be misdiagnosed as diffuse large B-cell lymphoma. While CD5 and cyclin D1 expression can avoid this diagnostic pitfall, some cases of DLBCL can express CD5, and rare are positive for cyclin D1 [40, 41]. Furthermore, pleomorphic MCL can often be negative for cyclin D1 [42]. Recognition of pleomorphic MCL and its distinction from DLBCL is of clinical relevance as these two entities vary in their behavior as well as treatment outcomes. Clinicians are likely to opt for more intense chemotherapeutic regimens for aggressive variants of MCL than for DLBCL.
  - Morphologic variants such as monocytoid, plasmacytic, and small cell MCL may not be clinically relevant, but they pose a diagnostic challenge in routine practice, thus requiring diligent use of ancillary studies such as IHC and FISH to exclude diagnostic mimics such as MZL, LPL, CLL/SLL, and plasma cell neoplasm. In majority of cases, correlation with clinical presentation, IHC for cyclin D1 and/or FISH for t(11,14)(q13;q32), allows for accurate diagnosis.
- In situ mantle cell neoplasia: ISMCN, previously mantle cell lymphoma in situ, has been recently incorporated in the 2017 WHO classification. ISMCN constitutes a precursor lesion detected incidentally which poses very low risk of progression to overt lymphoma and requires no therapeutic intervention [4, 43, 44]. However, detection of ISMCN should prompt a thorough systemic workup to exclude the possibility of overt lymphoma at other sites [43–45]. While no additional treatment is recommended in the absence of overt lymphoma elsewhere, given the more aggressive nature of MCL, a closer follow-up is advised for ISMCN in comparison to the analogous condition of in situ follicular neoplasia ISFN [46].
  - ISMCN is characterized by presence of scattered cyclin D1-positive cells in mantle zones of reactive follicles in the background of intact nodal architecture or follicular hyperplasia. The neoplastic cells are only detected by immunostaining for cyclin D1.

Table 5.3 Differential diagnosis of in situ mantle cell neoplasia and mantle cell lymphoma with mantle zone pattern

	In situ mantle cell neoplasia	Mantle cell lymphoma with mantle cell pattern
Morphologic features	Preserved nodal architecture with morphologic features of reactive follicular hyperplasia Mantle zones exhibit normal thickness Germinal centers exhibit reactive features	Distorted nodal architecture by proliferation of follicles with expanded mantle zones Germinal centers exhibit reactive features
Immunophenotype	Cyclin D1 highlights positive cells confined in the mantle zones, mostly in inner mantle zones Germinal centers express CD10 and BCL6 and lack BCL2	Cyclin D1 highlights the full thickness of the mantle zones, which also show aberrant expression of CD5 Germinal centers express CD10 and BCL6 and lack BCL2

Table 5.4 Differential diagnosis of CLL/SLL versus MCL

	CLL/SLL	MCL
Morphology	Vaguely nodular to diffuse Small lymphocytes with round monotonous nuclei Slightly larger lymphocytes at proliferation centers	Diffuse, nodular, or mantle zone patterns Small to intermediate with irregular nuclei Epithelioid macrophages and hyalinized vessels
Immunophenotype	Positive CD20(dim) CD19 Positive CD23(bright) Aberrant loss of FMC7 and aberrant expression of CD5 Dim expression of surface Ig light chain Negative cyclin D1	Positive CD20 (bright) and CD19 Negative CD23 Positive FMC7 with aberrant expression of CD5 Expression of surface Ig light chain with normal intensity Positive cyclin D1
Genetic abnormalities	Trisomy 12 or deletions 13q14, 11q, and 17p	t(11;14); *IGH-CCND1*

  – The mantle zones are not thickened and the neoplastic cells are confined in the mantle zone, most often in the inner mantle zones, without involvement of interfollicular areas or infiltration into the germinal centers, as seen in overt MCL. ISMCN is to be distinguished from MCL with mantle zone pattern (Table 5.3) in which the mantle zones are expanded and entirely made up of cyclin D1-positive cells [44].
- Immunophenotype of MCL: MCL cells, like CLL/SLL, express pan B-cell markers CD19, CD20, CD22, and CD79a. When assessed by flow cytometry, these markers are expressed with much brighter intensity compared to CLL/SLL. However, unlike CLL/SLL, MCL cells are usually negative for CD23 and positive for CD79b and FMC7.
  – Immunohistochemical expression of cyclin D1, a highly sensitive marker for MCL, is of value in establishing a definitive diagnosis. Cyclin D1 is useful even in rare cases of CD5-negative MCL. Cyclin D1 is also expressed in approximately 30% of plasma cell myeloma, in majority of hairy cell leukemia as well as in the proliferation centers of approximately 20% of CLL/SLL cases [47–49]. While cyclin D1 overexpression in MCL is caused by *IGH-CCND1* gene fusion resulting from the characteristic translocation t(11;14)(q13;q32), in non-MCL cases, its overexpression is often attributed to other genetic alterations [50].
  – MCL cases lacking *IGH-CCND1* rearrangement and thus cyclin D1 expression by IHC (cyclin D1-negative MCL) are important to recognize because it may lead to a misdiagnosis and can impact therapeutic decision. SOX11, another specific marker for MCL, is especially useful to identify cyclin D1-negative MCL [51, 52]. Its use is strongly recommended, in order to avoid misdiagnosis, in cases of CD5+/cyclin D1-negative small B-cell lymphoma that do not entirely fit morphologic or immunophenotypic criteria for other types of small B-cell lymphoma (e.g., CD23- CLL/SLL, CD5+ MZL, or CD5+ LPL/WM).
- Differentiating MCL from CLL/SLL: The features useful in differentiating these two lymphomas with overlapping features, but clinically distinctive behaviors, are summarized in Table 5.4.

3. What are the characteristic clinical, morphological, and immunophenotypic findings in CD10+ small B-cell lymphomas?

- Here we will consider only follicular lymphoma in detail. Burkitt lymphoma (BL) is discussed in Chap. 7 with other high-grade/aggressive lymphomas and B- lymphoblastic leukemia/lymphoma is discussed in Chap. 22 with other acute leukemias. Clinical features and epidemiology of follicular lymphoma (FL): FL is the second most common non-Hodgkin lymphoma in western countries and accounts for approximately 20% of the cases. However, it is strikingly less frequent in other areas of the world [16, 53]. It commonly occurs in the sixth decade of life with a slight female preponderance. Patients usually present with asymptomatic progressive lymphadenopathy. B-symptoms are less frequent, seen in less than 30% of the patients. Bone marrow involvement is seen in up to 70% of the patients but involvement of other organs is uncommon [54]. Transformation to DLBCL over time occurs in 20–60% of cases [54, 55].

- Morphology of FL: Follicular lymphoma is characterized by effacement of nodal architecture by proliferation of densely packed, back-to-back follicles giving a classic follicular pattern. The neoplastic follicles are generally similar in size and shape with attenuated mantle zones and have ill-defined germinal centers with loss of polarity and absence of tingible body macrophages. These histologic features differentiate neoplastic follicles from reactive follicles. The neoplastic cells within the follicles are homogeneous centrocytes, centroblasts, or a mixture of both.
  - Centrocytes are small lymphocytes with irregular nuclear contours (often angulated or twisted), coarsely condensed chromatin, inconspicuous nucleoli, and scant cytoplasm. Centroblasts are large cells, 3–4 times the size of normal resting lymphocytes with rounded or slightly irregular nuclear contours, vesicular chromatin, and prominent membrane-bound nucleoli.
  - Although follicular pattern is the most common pattern seen in FL, interfollicular spread of neoplastic cells can impart either partial or a predominantly diffuse pattern. In this case, there is diffuse proliferation of centrocytes and a variable proportion of centroblasts with complete lack of follicular dendritic cell meshworks highlighted by an immunohistochemistry for CD21 and/or CD23.
- Grading of FL: The WHO recommends grading of FL into 3 grades based on the number of centroblasts in 10 representative neoplastic follicles at high-power field (high-power field of 0.159 mm^2–40 × objective, 18 mm field of view ocular) [4]. Grade 1 FL contains between 0 and 5 centroblasts; grade 2 FL shows 6–15 centroblasts, while grade 3 FL is characterized by presence of 15 or more centroblasts per high-power field.
  - Grades 1 and 2 are grouped together (as grade 1–2) due to lack of clinical differences and significant interobserver variability in grading.
  - Grade 3 FL is further divided into grade 3A when centroblasts are more than 15 per high-power field but also contain some centrocytes and grade 3B when centroblasts are present in sheets without intervening centrocytes.
- Clinical significance of grading FL: Histologic grading of FL is clinically important since grade 1–2 is usually an indolent disease that does not require aggressive chemotherapy. FL grade 3, on the other hand, bears a worse clinical outcome and benefits from aggressive chemotherapy [4]. There is still controversy on whether distinction between FL grade 3A and 3B is clinically relevant [56]. Although a diffuse pattern comprising of mixed populations of centrocytes with less than 15 centroblasts does not constitute histologic progression, the presence of more than 15 centroblasts per high power in areas lacking FDC meshworks is considered as morphologic evidence of DLBCL [4].
- Clinically relevant morphologic variants of FL: A number of morphologic variants are recognized. While they are rare, pathologists should be aware of these in order to avoid missing FL diagnosis.
  - A recently described subtype of FL confined to the inguinal region is characterized by a predominantly diffuse pattern, lack of the classic translocation t(14;18), and deletion in the terminal parts of the short arm of chromosome 1, del(1p36) [57, 58]. These patients typically present with large inguinal masses and have a low clinical stage at diagnosis. Histologically, although a predominantly diffuse pattern is encountered (mixture of predominantly centrocytes and fewer centroblasts), focal follicular areas may be present. By immunohistochemistry (IHC), the neoplastic cells in the diffuse areas show frequent coexpression CD10, BCL2, and CD23. Interestingly, BCL2 expression is quite variable in the follicular areas [57].
  - Another subtype of low-grade FL, low-grade FL with high proliferation index (LGFL-HPI), is characterized by a high proliferation index within the neoplastic germinal centers. In general, low-grade (grade 1–2) FLs are characterized by a Ki-67 proliferation rate of less than 20%, indolent behavior, and longer disease-free survival. In this subtype, proliferation rate by Ki-67 is greater than ≥30% in the neoplastic follicles [59]. *LGFL-HPI behaves more aggressively than traditional low-grade FL and similar to grade 3 FL* [59, 60]. *Recognition of this subtype is of prognostic value although not mandated by the WHO classification scheme at this time* [59].
  - Pediatric variant of FL (described elsewhere in detail) and testicular FL are important to recognize due to their distinct prognosis; however, these are less likely to be confused with small B-NHL as they usually have a high-grade (grade 3) cytomorphology.
  - In situ follicular neoplasia (ISFN): This was previously designated as follicular lymphoma in situ (FLIS). ISFN is a precursor lesion detected incidentally during evaluation of lymph nodes for other reasons other than lymphoma such as staging of carcinomas. While it poses very low risk of progression to overt lymphoma and no therapeutic intervention is necessary [4, 43, 44], its identification should prompt the clinician to initiate thorough systemic workup to exclude the possibility of overt FL at other sites [43–45]. From a clinical management

standpoint, no treatment and a "wait and watch" policy is recommended for ISFN: in the absence of overt lymphoma elsewhere. Follow-up with radiologic imaging is recommended in patients who develop B-symptoms [46]. ISFN is characterized by presence of occasional germinal centers with strong CD10 and strong BCL2 expression in an otherwise reactive lymph node with preserved nodal architecture and lymphoid follicular hyperplasia [45, 61]. On the other hand, FL exhibits effacement of nodal architecture by proliferation of densely packed, back-to-back follicles displaying the neoplastic features as described above (Table 5.5).

Table 5.5 Differential diagnosis of in situ follicular neoplasia versus follicular lymphoma

	In situ follicular neoplasia	Follicular lymphoma
Morphologic features	Preserved nodal architecture with morphologic features of reactive follicular hyperplasia Presence of mantle zones around abnormal follicles	Effaced nodal architecture by proliferation of back-to back follicles with similar size and shapes Attenuated and ill-defined mantle zones Germinal centers lack polarity and tingible bode macrophages
Immunophenotype	Germinal centers express CD10 and BCL6 There is aberrant expression of BCL2 CD10 and BCL2 are strongly coexpressed	Germinal centers express CD10 and BCL6 There is aberrant expression of BCL2 CD10 and BCL2 are typically strong but variations on intensity may be seen

– Immunophenotype of FL and other CD10+ B-cell lymphomas: The small B-cell lymphoma prototype with CD5-/CD10+ immunoprofile is FL. Importantly, some nodal high-grade B-cell lymphomas (such as Burkitt lymphoma or DLBCL germinal center subtype) are also typically CD5-/CD10+ (Table 5.6). Besides expression of common pan B-cell markers (CD19, CD20, CD22, CD79a, and PAX5), FL expresses germinal center markers CD10 and BCL6 in majority of cases. Both markers however can be downregulated in neoplastic cells that escape the germinal centers and infiltrate into the interfollicular areas [62], such as in FL with diffuse pattern and FL with marginal zone differentiation [62, 63]. CD10 is expressed in approximately 80% of low-grade FL but is less common in high-grade FL [62]. Approximately 10% of FLs are negative for BCL2 [64]. The lack of BCL2 expression in FLs is attributed to the absence of translocation t(14;18)(q32;q21), the hallmark of FL. However, some of these cases carry mutations involving the common residues of BCL2 protein recognized by the traditional anti-BCL2 antibodies [65, 66]. Additionally, three recently described germinal center markers, GCET1, HGAL, and LMO2, are useful in identifying FL with the caveat that they are also present in other germinal-center-derived B-cell lymphomas [67].

4. What are the characteristic clinical, morphological, and immunophenotypic findings in CD5-/CD10- small B-cell lymphomas?

We will discuss marginal zone lymphoma (MZL) and lymphoplasmacytic lymphoma/Waldenström macroglobulinemia (LPL/WM) in the answer below. Hairy cell leukemia is

Table 5.6 Differential diagnosis of FL versus other CD10+ B-cell lymphomas

	FL	Burkitt lymphoma	DLCBL (germinal center subtype)
Morphology	Follicular or diffuse pattern Mixture of cells with centrocytes and centroblasts	Diffuse pattern with complete effacement of the nodal architecture Intermediate-sized lymphocytes with round monotonous nuclei and clumped chromatin Increase in apoptosis or mitosis	Diffuse pattern with complete effacement of the nodal architecture Diffuse proliferation of large lymphocytes with irregular nuclei and vesicular chromatin May show increased mitosis or apoptosis
Immunophenotype	Expression of common B-cell markers Coexpression of CD10 and BCL6 Aberrant expression of BCL2	Expression of common B-cell markers Positive CD10 and BCL6 Negative BCL2	Expression of common B-cell markers Positive CD10 Variable expression of BCL6 and BCL2 Negative MUM1
Genetic abnormalities	t(14;18) *IGH-BCL2*	*MYC* rearrangements	Complex genetic abnormalities *MYC* and t(14;18) *IGH-BCL2* rearrangement are present in a subset of cases

discussed in Chap. 27, while B-prolymphocytic leukemia (B-PLL), which can be either CD5+ or CD5-/CD10-, has been discussed in Question 2 above.

Marginal Zone Lymphoma (MZL)

The term MZL encompasses three closely related yet distinct lymphoma subtypes: nodal, splenic, and extranodal marginal zone lymphoma of mucosa-associated lymphoid tissue (MALT lymphoma).

- Clinical features and epidemiology of MZL: Taken together, MZL constitutes approximately 1% of all lymphoid neoplasms in the USA [16]. MALT lymphomas are relatively common and represent 5–8% of all non-Hodgkin lymphomas, while nodal and splenic subtypes are less common and represent less than 1% of all non-Hodgkin lymphomas [68]. MZL typically occurs in adults with a median age of 69 years for nodal MZL and 66 years for extranodal MZL lymphoma (including both MALT and splenic MZL) [69].
  - MALT lymphomas have been related to acquisition of mucosa-associated lymphoid tissue in organs that do not normally contain it and develop as a result of autoimmunity or chronic infection at specific sites such as the stomach (*Helicobacter Pylori*), duodenum (*Campylobacter jejuni*), skin (*Borrelia burgdorferi*), and ocular adnexa (*Chlamydia psittaci*). Depending on the site of involvement, patients with MALT lymphoma usually present with localized disease [68].
  - Patients with splenic MZL by definition present with splenomegaly and frequently show bone marrow, peripheral blood, and liver involvement [70].
  - Nodal MZL, which will be the focus of this chapter, is slightly more common in men. Extranodal MZL shows equal gender distribution but disparities are seen depending on site of involvement [69]. Patients with nodal MZL typically present with generalized lymphadenopathy. As a general rule, nodal MZL is diagnosed after exclusion of MALT and splenic MZL secondarily involving the lymph node. Involvement of bone marrow and peripheral blood can occur but is rare in nodal MZL [71].
  - Monoclonal paraprotein can be found in approximately 15% of the patients [70].
- Morphology of MZL: Nodal MZL shares cytomorphologic features of splenic MZL or MALT lymphoma, but exclusively involves lymph nodes without evidence of extranodal or splenic disease. The nodal architecture is effaced by neoplastic cells in one or more of the five reported patterns of lymph node infiltration by NMZL [72, 73].
  - Perifollicular pattern – neoplastic cells are seen in expanded marginal zones surrounding follicles with reactive or atrophic germinal centers.
  - Nodular pattern – characterized by presence of neoplastic nodules with absent or atrophic germinal centers [73]. The presence of residual follicles imparts a nodular or vaguely nodular appearance at low magnification.
  - Diffuse pattern – the nodal architecture is totally effaced by a polymorphous infiltrate with prominent follicular colonization [74].
  - Inverse follicular pattern – characterized by presence of darker cells in the center of follicles and paler monocytoid cells in the interfollicular areas.
  - Interfollicular pattern – characterized by proliferation of neoplastic cells in between attenuated and hyperplastic follicles.
  - Most frequently the neoplastic cells proliferate in a marginal zone-like pattern surrounding reactive follicles that expand into the interfollicular areas. A combination of any or all of these patterns can be found in a single lymph node.
  - Follicular colonization characterized by infiltration of reactive germinal centers by tumor cells leading to their expansion is seen in some cases, however not as frequent a feature in NMZL as in MALT lymphoma. The neoplastic cells are mixed populations of centrocyte-like (clumped chromatin, irregular nuclei, and scant cytoplasm) and monocytoid (condensed chromatin, round nuclei, abundant pale cytoplasm with well-delineated cell borders) marginal zone B-cells and a variable number of plasma cells. Large transformed B-cells, resembling centroblasts, are also typically seen scattered among small- and intermediate-sized cells. Plasmacytic differentiation is common and at times can be exuberant causing difficulty in distinction from LPL or nodal plasmacytoma.
- Immunophenotype of MZL: See below, comparison of phenotype of MZL and LPL.

Lymphoplasmacytic Lymphoma/Waldenström Macroglobulinemia (LPL/WM)

- Clinical features and epidemiology: LPL/WM typically presents in adults with a median age of 70 years at diagnosis and with a slight male predilection [75]. This entity represents less than 1% of all lymphoid neoplasms with approximately 1000–1500 new cases diagnosed each year in the USA [16, 76]. The majority of the patients present with bone marrow involvement meeting criteria for WM, which is defined as the combination of bone marrow involvement by LPL and an IgM monoclonal paraprotein of any level. Some patients may also present with involve-

ment of peripheral blood, lymph nodes, or extranodal organs including the liver, spleen, lung, gastrointestinal tract, skin, and soft tissues among others [77, 78].
  - Clinical manifestations are related to circulating paraprotein and include autoimmune disorders, cryoglobulinemia, cold agglutinin disease, and most commonly, hyperviscosity syndrome. Development of cytopenias is attributed to bone marrow involvement [79–81]. Peripheral neuropathy can be caused by several mechanisms and is commonly seen in patients with LPL/WM [82, 83].
  - Primary AL amyloidosis, while uncommon in patients with LPL/WM, is important to recognize since it may lead to dysfunction of vital organs (e.g., amyloid cardiomyopathy) [84]. The monoclonal protein is most frequently IgM but other isotypes (mainly IgG or IgA), or even complete absence of a paraprotein, may rarely be seen [85].
  - Bing-Neel syndrome, a rare complication of WM, is characterized by central nervous system involvement by LPL/WM. It usually presents as a feature of relapsing disease, although it may also occur at initial presentation [86].
- Morphological findings in LPL/WM: LPL is characterized by proliferation of three cell types, small lymphocytes with scant cytoplasm, plasmacytoid lymphocytes displaying slightly more abundant basophilic cytoplasm, and variable numbers of plasma cells. Lymph nodes are involved in some cases but bone marrow involvement is characteristic.
  - In the lymph node, the neoplastic cells exhibit a diffuse to vaguely nodular proliferation with widely patent sinuses. The neoplastic cells comprise of monotonous lymphocytes, plasmacytoid lymphocytes, and plasma cells in the regions between sinuses. Large transformed B-cells are not increased. Increased mast cells, Dutcher bodies (PAS-positive intranuclear pseudoinclusions), and hemosiderin deposits are other features that can be seen as part of the infiltrate, and their presence serves as a useful clue in the diagnosis of LPL.
  - Plasmacytic differentiation is a hallmark of the disease, and plasma cell component in some cases may be quite prominent accounting for majority of the neoplastic infiltrate, thus mimicking a plasmacytoma.

5. What are unusual morphological variants of follicular lymphoma which can mimic other lymphomas and reactive lymphoid proliferation?

Some morphological variants of follicular lymphoma mimic other lymphomas or benign lymphoid hyperplasia.

- The “floral variant” of FL is characterized by follicles having a flower-like appearance on sections, rather than the smooth round or oval outlines of neoplastic follicles in usual FL. Two related histologic subtypes are recognized: (a) the macrogerminal center pattern in which the mantle zone lymphocytes invaginate into the neoplastic follicles causing a compartmentalization or lobulation of the latter imparting a flower-like or cloud-like appearance [87] and (b) the microgerminal center pattern characterized by an exuberant infiltration of neoplastic follicles by the mantle zone cells [88]. The former pattern mimics progressive transformation of the germinal centers, whereas the microgerminal pattern resembles nodular lymphocyte predominant Hodgkin lymphoma (NLPHL). Identification of neoplastic follicles with aberrant expression of BCL2 is key in recognizing the floral variant of FL.
- Marginal zone differentiation is seen in approximately 8% of FLs in which the neoplastic follicles are surrounded by monocytoid cells with abundant clear cytoplasm, small cleaved nuclei, clumped chromatin, and inconspicuous nucleoli. The diagnosis rests on demonstration of germinal center phenotype with expression of CD10 and BCL6 in the perifollicular monocytoid component in addition to the typical CD10+, BCL2+, and BCL6+ immunoprofile of the neoplastic follicles.
  - FL with marginal zone differentiation can pose a diagnostic challenge in its distinction from nodal marginal zone lymphoma (NMZL), particularly when the latter shows prominent follicular colonization. This is particularly an issue when FL with marginal zone differentiation lacks CD10 or BCL6 expression by IHC or t(14;18) by cytogenetic analysis. In such cases, additional GC markers such as HGAL and LMO2 can aid in establishing a GC phenotype in the neoplastic follicles as well as in the perifollicular monocytoid component [89].
  - Recognition of FL with marginal zone differentiation is clinically important because it is clinically more aggressive than conventional FL with an inferior disease-free and overall survival [90, 91].
- Plasmacytic differentiation, which is commonly encountered in other small B-cell lymphomas (see below, Question 6), is relatively rare in FL, affecting only 3% cases [92, 93]. Plasma cells are found inside follicles within the germinal centers as well as in the interfollicular areas. The neoplastic follicles demonstrate otherwise typical morphologic and immunophenotypic features of FL. The plasma cells are highlighted by CD138, MUM1/IRF4, or CD79a and demonstrate light chain restriction identical to the FL lymphoid cells.
  - Like marginal zone differentiation, plasmacytic differentiation often poses diagnostic challenges in its distinction from MZL with plasmacytic differentiation, LPL, or plasma cell neoplasm.
  - Its recognition may be clinically important due to propensity for higher stage at presentation and a higher likelihood of leukemic dissemination [94].

6. What is the differential diagnosis of small B-cell lymphomas with plasmacytic or plasmacytoid differentiation?

The main types of small B-cell lymphomas which frequently show plasmacytic or plasmacytoid differentiation are MZL and LPL/WM. Plasmacytic differentiation in other small B-cell lymphomas is infrequent or rare, seen with decreasing frequency in CLL/SLL, FL, and MCL. In addition, primary plasma cell neoplasm involving a lymph node (Question 7), reactive plasmacytosis in a lymph node, and lymph node simultaneously involved by a small B-cell lymphoma and a separate clonal plasma cell neoplasm (discussed in Chap. 16) also have overlapping morphologic and immunophenotypic findings. Differentiation from reactive lymphoid hyperplasia with plasmacytosis is discussed in Question 12.

- MZL and LPL/WM: The distinction between these two entities can be challenging due to marked overlap in immunophenotypic profile, especially when MZL exhibits plasmacytic differentiation.
  - Both MZL and LPL express pan B-cell markers and are negative for germinal center markers CD10 and BCL6. CD43, a T-cell marker, is aberrantly expressed in approximately 50% of nodal MZL cases but is also seen in a small proportion of LPL/WM cases [95, 96].
  - A particularly useful feature in the recognition of MZL is the presence of markedly expanded and disrupted follicular dendritic cell meshworks highlighted by CD21 or CD23 stain.
  - The plasmacytic component in MZL with plasmacytic differentiation or in LPL/WM is highlighted by plasma cell markers such as CD79a or CD138. By flow cytometry, the plasma cells are CD19+ and CD56 negative. Plasma cell phenotype can distinguish LPL/WM or MZL with plasmacytic differentiation from plasma cell neoplasms which typically show loss of CD19 and aberrant expression of CD56 [97].
  - In cases where morphologic and immunophenotypic features do not allow a clear-cut separation between LPL and MZL, testing for *MYD88* L265P mutation proves to be of immense value. The presence of *MYD88* L256P mutation in a small B-cell NHL with plasmacytic differentiation is consistent with LPL, whereas lack of this mutation makes LPL less likely (Table 5.7).
- Small lymphocytic lymphoma/chronic lymphocytic leukemia (SLL/CLL): Chronic lymphocytic leukemia/small lymphocytic lymphoma (CLL/SLL): Although a monoclonal IgM paraprotein can be detected frequently, second only to LPL [98], very few cases of SLL show morphologically identifiable plasmacytic differentiation [99].
- Follicular lymphoma (FL): Plasmacytic differentiation is uncommon in FL, affecting only 3% cases [92, 93].
- Mantle cell lymphoma (MCL): Non-neoplastic plasma cells may be present in variable numbers but only rarely clusters of clonal plasma cells are found within nodules of neoplastic mantle cells or within residual reactive germinal centers. These cases are described in the literature as MCL with plasmacytic differentiation [34].

Table 5.7 Differential diagnosis of MZL versus LPL/WM versus plasma cell neoplasms

	MZL	LPL/WM	Plasma cell neoplasm
Morphology	Nodular or diffuse architecture Lymphocytes are small with monocytoid features Occasional larger cells Plasmacytoid lymphocytes and plasma cells may be present at varying proportions	Diffuse or vaguely nodular architecture Patent sinuses Mixture of small lymphocytes, plasmacytoid lymphocytes, and plasma cells	Diffuse proliferation of plasma cells with effacement of the nodal architecture Predominantly plasma cells Lymphocytoid plasma cells may be present at varying proportions
Immunophenotype	B-lymphocytes Positive for CD19, CD20, CD22, CD79a, CD79b, and PAX5 Aberrant expression of CD43 in ~50% of cases Expanded follicular dendritic cell meshworks highlighted by CD21 or CD23 Plasma cells Positive for CD45, CD19, CD79a, CD38, CD138 Negative for CD56, cyclin D1	B-lymphocytes Positive for CD19, CD20, CD22, CD79a, CD79b, and PAX5 Plasma cells Positive for CD45, CD19, CD79a, CD38, CD138 Negative for CD56, cyclin D1	B-lymphocytes No significant number of B-cells; not clonal, if present Plasma cells Positive for CD79a, CD38, CD138 Aberrant loss of CD45 and CD19 Subset of cases show aberrant expression of CD56, CD20, CD117 or cyclin D1
Genetic abnormalities	*MYD88* L265P may be seen in few cases (exact percentage varies in the literature 0–20%)	*MYD88* L265P in more than 90% of cases	Absent *MYD88* mutations

See also Chap. 16 for cases in which lymph node shows involvement by two separate clonal processes – a small B-cell lymphoma and a plasma cell neoplasm

7. How to distinguish small B-cell lymphomas with extensive plasmacytic differentiation from nodal involvement by a plasma cell neoplasm?

- This is a clinically important distinction because the clinical approaches and therapeutic regimens are different. Plasma cell neoplasms, like small B-NHLs, can present with partial or complete effacement of the nodal architecture by diffuse proliferation of atypical plasma cells. Nuclear pseudo-inclusions known as Dutcher bodies can be seen in both plasma cell neoplasms and small B-cell lymphomas with plasmacytic differentiation. Although the latter frequently display at least a small proportion of B-cells, in some cases the plasmacytic differentiation can be so extensive that it may completely obscure the B-cell lymphocytic component.
- Immunophenotypic analysis of plasma cells plays an essential role in this differential diagnosis.
  - Plasma cells in B-NHLs are CD45+, CD19+, CD56-, and cyclin D1- (except for MCL and HCL) [97] and lack the typical immunophenotypic aberrations seen in most plasma cell neoplasms such as loss of CD19 and gain of CD56.
  - Plasma cells in a plasma cell neoplasm are often CD45-, CD19-, CD56+/−, and cyclin D1−/+ [100, 101].
- In some cases, despite extensive ancillary studies, correlation with presenting clinical features is required to reach a final diagnosis. Lytic bone lesions, hypercalcemia, or evidence of target organ damage as well as the identification of a non-IgM monoclonal paraprotein generally support a diagnosis of plasma cell neoplasm over a mature B-cell lymphoma.

8. Which immunophenotypic markers are diagnostic or exclude a specific subtype of small B-cell lymphoma?

- Flow cytometry and IHC as described in the previous section are extremely useful in the diagnosis of these small B-NHLs. Flow cytometric immunoprofiles of certain small B-NHLs with characteristic marker intensities or expression of specific markers by IHC allow specific diagnoses in this category.
- For example, demonstration of the classic CLL/SLL immunophenotype (CD19+, weak CD20+, FMC7-, CD5+, CD23+, CD200+, and weak surface light chain immunoglobulin expression by flow cytometry) is very useful to distinguish CLL/SLL from other B-cell lymphomas.
  - One must however not solely rely on immunoprofile and must incorporate clinical data in final diagnosis as CLL-type MBL has an immunoprofile identical to CLL/SLL.
- Strong and diffuse expression of cyclin D1 by IHC in a CD5+ small-to-medium B-NHL is diagnostic of MCL.
- Expression of CD10 (by IHC or flow cytometry) when accompanied by expression of germinal center marker BCL6 is consistent with follicle center cell derivation and in an appropriate morphologic context would be diagnostic of FL.

9. Which ancillary molecular/genetic tests are useful in the diagnosis or classification of small B-cell lymphomas?

- In routine practice, immunophenotyping alone (by flow cytometry and/or IHC) is adequate in establishing a correct diagnosis. Molecular genetic methods are used where immunophenotypic analysis is either not possible due to the nature of specimen or the immunophenotype is not definitive or does not follow the expression patterns in correlating with clinical findings or morphology.
  - Molecular methods are commonly applied in the diagnosis of lymphomas for two main reasons – to determine clonality and to detect lymphoma-specific chromosomal abnormalities, translocations in particular (see also Chap. 2 for general discussion of these tests).
  - Clonality assessment in B-NHLs is done using polymerase chain reaction (PCR) for detection of clonal immunoglobulin gene rearrangements. Sensitivity of PCR in CLL/SLL is more than 95%, whereas in other small B-NHLs, it varies between 50% and 70%. Notably, clonal B-cell populations can be found in reactive lymphoid hyperplasias secondary to bacterial or viral antigenic stimulation such as in *H. pylori* gastritis, HCV hepatitis, *EBV* infections, or autoimmune disorders such as Hashimoto's thyroiditis or Sjögren's syndrome [102–105] and immunodeficiency states as in posttransplant setting or in acquired immunodeficiency syndrome (AIDS) [106, 107].
  - Conversely, in some cases of small B-cell lymphomas (especially those undergoing somatic hypermutation), a clonal *IGH* gene rearrangement may not be detected due to mutations in the primer binding sites (false negative) and often requires additional *IGK* gene rearrangement analysis for a clonal population to be detected [108].
  - Assessment of lymphoma-specific chromosomal translocations can be achieved by a variety of techniques including PCR, FISH (fluorescence in situ hybridization), and conventional cytogenetics. Conventional cytogenetics is considered a "gold standard" in the diagnosis of lymphomas due to its ability to detect genome-wide abnormalities. This methodol-

ogy is however not routinely applied in daily practice due to logistic issues involving requirement of fresh tissue for culture and skilled labor thus making it labor intensive and expensive. Additionally, indolent small B-cell lymphomas may fail to grow in culture and thus not yield diagnostic information. In contrast, FISH is relatively easy to perform, does not require fresh tissue, and has a much shorter turnaround time compared with chromosomal analysis. FISH however allows for detection of only specific genetic abnormalities instead of genome-wide aberrations.

10. Which are the most common genetic abnormalities seen in small B-cell lymphomas and how these results can be used for differential diagnosis along with immunophenotypic data? (Table 5.8)

- Chromosomal aberrations: Seen in up to 80% of CLL/SLL patients and carry prognostic significance, the most common being del13q14 (55% of cases), del11q (18%), trisomy 12(16%), and del17p (7%) [109].
- The most common chromosomal abnormalities seen in nodal MZL are trisomies 3, 7, 12, and 18 [110]. Translocation (11;18) (q21;q21) and deletions in 7q31 are more common in MALT lymphoma and splenic MZL respectively and not as much in nodal MZL [111].
- Approximately 85% of FL harbor the translocation t(14;18) (q32;q21) resulting in *IGH-BCL2* fusion responsible for dysregulated expression of BCL2 in neoplastic follicles [112].
- Translocation t(11;14) (q13;q32) resulting in *IGH-CCND1* fusion is the most common cytogenetic alteration in MCL and is responsible for the overexpression of cyclin D1.
- The recent advent of next-generation sequencing (NGS) technologies has produced a wealth of data on the molecular landscape of small B-cell lymphomas, although the majority of these alterations are non-specific and not routinely used for diagnostic purposes. A notable exception is the *MYD88* L265P mutation used to confirm a suspected LPL/WM. Provided typical clinical and pathologic features are present, the mutation is detected in more than 90% of such cases [113].
  - In practice, *MYD88* L265P mutational analysis is most useful in small B-NHLs with plasmacytic differentiation in which LPL is suspected, but clinical presentation and morphologic and immunophenotypic features are non-specific. A positive result increases the likelihood of LPL but absence of the mutation does not rule out LPL.
  - This mutation is particularly useful in the differential between LPL/WM and MZL with significant plasmacytic differentiation, since it is not usually detected in the latter [114].
  - *MYD88* L265P has not been reported in plasma cell neoplasms and can also be used in this differential [113, 114].
  - Nonetheless, it must be kept in mind that this mutation is not specific for LPL/WM and can be found in other B-cell lymphomas including primary DLBCL of the central nervous system (CNS) (>70% of cases), primary DLCBL of the testis (approximately 70% of cases), primary cutaneous DLBCL, leg type (approximately 60% of cases), DLCBL, and activated B-cell subtype (approximately 30% of cases), as well as in

Table 5.8 Immunophenotypes and common genetic alterations seen in small B-cell lymphomas

	Typical immunophenotypic profiles	Common genetic alteration
CLL/SLL	Positive for CD20(dim), CD22(dim), CD19, and CD23(bright) Aberrant loss of FMC7 and aberrant expression of CD5 Expression of surface Ig light chain is typically dim Negative for cyclin D1	Deletions 13q14, 11q, and 17p Trisomy 12 *NOTCH1* mutations (10%)
MCL	Positive for CD19, CD20, CD22, CD79a, CD79b, and PAX5 Strong aberrant expression of cyclin D1+ Negative for CD23 Majority of cases are positive for SOX11, which is especially useful in cyclin D1-negative cases	t(11;14); *IGH-CCND1* *ATM* mutations (40–50%) *TP53* mutations (15–20%)
FL	Positive for CD19, CD20, CD22, CD79a, and PAX5 Expression of germinal center markers CD10(bright) and BCL6 Aberrant expression of BCL2 on neoplastic germinal centers	t(14;18); *IGH-BCL2* *CREEBBP* mutations (50%) *EZH2* mutations (10–20%) *EP300* mutations (10–15%)
Nodal MZL	Positive for CD19, CD2, CD22, CD79a, CD79b, and PAX5 Aberrant expression of CD43 in ~50% of cases Expanded follicular dendritic meshworks highlighted by CD21 or CD23	Trisomies 3, 7, 12, and 18 *KMT2D* mutations (34%) *PTPRD* mutations (20%) *NOTCH2* mutations (20%)
LPL/WM	B-cells: Positive for CD19, CD20, CD22, CD79a, CD79b, and PAX5 Plasma cells: Positive for CD45, CD138(bright), CD38(bright), and CD19 Negative for CD56 and cyclin D1	Deletion 6q *MYD88* L265P (>90%) *CXCR4* mutations (~25%)

few cases of CLL/SLL and MZL [114–118]. Lastly, *MYD88* L265P has also been reported in more than 50% of IgM monoclonal gammopathy of undetermined significance (IgM MGUS) which is currently considered a precursor of LPL/WM [119].

11. Which ancillary tests provide prognostic and/or therapeutic information for small B-cell lymphomas?

The prognosis varies widely, not only among the various small B-cell lymphomas, but also within the same type of lymphoma. For example, some patients with CLL/SLL may not require therapy and benefit from "watch and wait" strategies, while others behave more aggressively. Even within MCL, the majority are generally considered to require more intensified cytarabine-based chemotherapeutic regimens [120]; the lymphoma may have subtypes with less aggressive behavior.

- CLL/SLL is divided into prognostic subgroups based on expression of CD38, zeta-associated protein (ZAP)-70, and CD49d, mutational status of immunoglobulin heavy-chain variable region (IgVH), and cytogenetic abnormalities determined by interphase FISH [109, 121–125].
  - Approximately 40% of CLL have unmutated immunoglobulin genes, while in 60% the immunoglobulin genes undergo somatic hypermutations. CLL patients with mutated *IGHV* tend to have better prognosis with significantly higher rate of survival beyond 20 years compared to those with unmutated *IGHV* who clinically behave more aggressively with a shorter median survival (8–9 years) [121, 126].
  - Expression of CD38, ZAP-70, or CD49d in CLL is typically determined by flow cytometry. CD38 expression by more than 30% of leukemic cells is associated with an aggressive clinical course and adverse prognosis [123]. ZAP-70 gene expression in CLL cells correlates with the unmutated CLL group [127]. While published studies have validated the prognostic value of ZAP-70 detected by flow cytometry and IHC as well as RT-PCR [128–130], assessment of ZAP-70 (by flow cytometry or IHC) is fraught with technical issues. Nevertheless, ZAP-70 expression in CLL correlates with *IGHV* mutational status and serves as a useful surrogate to *IGHV* mutational status [109, 131–133]. Furthermore, ZAP-70 by itself may have prognostic value, independent of *IGHV* mutational status, higher expression of ZAP-70 being associated with rapid progression of disease.
  - Cytogenetic analysis by interphase FISH is of value in the prognostication of CLL/SLL. There are four genetic abnormalities of prognostic relevance in CLL/SLL: (1) del 13q involving *miR15a, miR16-1,* and *LEU2* gene, (2) del 11q involving the ataxia telangiectasia mutated (*ATM*) gene, (3) trisomy 12, and (4) del 17p involving *TP53*.

    Isolated deletion of 13q14, the most common cytogenetic abnormality, is associated with favorable prognosis, while deletion in 17p and 11q confers poor prognosis due to resistance to conventional therapy and rapid disease progression [109].

    Aberrations in *TP53* are perhaps the only genetic alteration with therapeutic impact in patients with CLL/SLL. These aberrations can present as 17p deletions associated with *TP53* mutations (seen in 5–10% of patients with CLL/SLL) or only mutations in *TP53* without 17p deletions (seen in few cases; 3–6% of patients with CLL/SLL) [109, 134–136]. Besides portending an inferior prognosis, aberrations in *TP53* predict refractoriness to standard fludarabine-containing regimens. Therefore, analysis for *TP53* aberrations is currently recommended in CLL/SLL patients before initiation of therapy [134–137]. Additionally, these patients have shown major benefit from treatment with the newly approved agents targeting the B-cell receptor signaling pathway such as ibrutinib (BTK inhibitor) and idelalisib (phosphatidylinositol 3-kinase delta inhibitor) [134, 137]. Aberrancies in *TP53* have also been identified in the majority of other small B-cell lymphomas and are associated with adverse prognosis; however, there is currently no sufficient data on its therapeutic significance in these entities [134].
- Mantle cell lymphoma (MCL): Ki-67 proliferation index measured by Ki-67 immunostaining is the single most important and independent prognostic factor in MCL and has been incorporated with other clinical parameters in the Mantle Cell Lymphoma International Prognostication Index (MIPI) score to predict prognosis and guide risk-adapted treatment decisions [138, 139].
  - Ki-67 proliferation index of >30% is associated with adverse prognosis in MCL, while cases with a proliferation of index <10% tend to have better outcome [138–140].
  - More recently, SOX11 has been recognized as a useful diagnostic and prognostic marker in MCL. Like cyclin D1, SOX11 is a specific marker for classic MCL and is useful in its distinction for other small B-NHLs. It is however of greater value in MCLs that lack cyclin D1 expression [141]. SOX11 expression is associated with a more aggressive clinical course. Lack of SOX11 expression correlates with a non-nodal, leukemic form of MCL that shows predominantly hypermutated *IGHV* and indolent clinical course [28].

- *TP53* plays an important role in the pathogenesis of MCL and is mutated in approximately one-third of MCL cases [142, 143]. MCLs with *TP53* abnormalities tend to have blastoid cytomorphology [144], high proliferation index, and aggressive behavior [145]. Thus, assessment of *TP53* mutation status is of prognostic value in MCL.

- Marginal zone lymphoma (MZL): While reliable prognostic markers are not described in nodal and splenic MZL, in MALT-type MZL (MALT lymphomas), particularly in gastric MALT lymphomas, the presence or absence of *Helicobacter pylori* has therapeutic significance as *H. pylori*-positive gastric MALT lymphomas respond favorably to antibiotic therapy leading to prolonged remission [146]. Thus, all cases of gastric MALT lymphomas should be investigated for *H. pylori* by IHC.
  - Additionally, t(11;18) (q21;q21), commonly associated with pulmonary and gastric MALT lymphoma, carries prognostic and therapeutic significance in the latter. Translocation(11;18)(q21;q21)-positive gastric MALT lymphomas do not respond to *H. pylori* eradication therapy, present with higher stage of disease and a clinically aggressive course with a higher risk for relapse [147, 148]. Thus, cytogenetic analysis by FISH to assess for t(11;18)(q21;q21) should be considered in the workup of gastric MALT lymphoma.
- Lymphoplasmacytic lymphoma/Waldenström macroglobulinemia (LPL/WM): Cytogenetic analysis for del(6q) and molecular analysis for *MYD88* L265P and *CXCR4* mutations are of prognostic and therapeutic relevance. Presence of del(6q) is associated with adverse prognosis. LPL cases with *MYD88* L265P mutation carry an adverse prognosis and show resistance to treatment by ibrutinib. *CXCR4* mutations (including WHIM-like and frameshift mutations) are present in 27% of LPL/WM patients [149]. *MYD88*L265P-mutated/*CXCR4* wild-type LPL patients show much better response to ibrutinib than *MYD88* L265P-mutated/*CXCR4*-mutated or *MYD88* wild-type/*CXCR* wild-type patients [150, 151]. No specific IHC or flow cytometric markers are currently considered to have definitive prognostic or therapeutic value in this lymphoma.

12. How to distinguish small B-cell lymphomas from reactive follicular hyperplasia or paracortical hyperplasias and other reactive lymphadenopathies?

Please see Chap. 19 for a general discussion of reactive lymphoid conditions causing lymph node enlargement. Here we emphasize the common morphological findings that overlap with small B-cell lymphomas and may create diagnostic dilemmas. In addition, we present a diagnostic approach to correctly identify the cases of common small B-cell lymphomas, such as FL and CLL/SLL, which have nonclassic morphological or immunophenotypic features mimicking other lymphomas.

- Reactive follicular hyperplasia (RFH): This is the most common histologic pattern observed in majority of benign lymphadenopathies. In RFH nodal architecture is preserved unlike in lymphomas where it is often effaced. Follicles in RFH have characteristic morphologic features that help distinguish them from their neoplastic counterparts of FL (Table 5.9). While the morphological findings on H&E-stained excisional biopsies mentioned in Table 5.9 are sufficiently characteristic to distinguish RFH from FL, these findings may be ambiguous and ancillary tests are required to rule out lymphoma in the following situations:
  - Markedly expanded germinal centers with elongated or serpiginous shapes as well as confluent germinal centers may be seen in florid reactive follicular hyperplasia.
  - Sometimes, the reactive follicles may become massively expanded by marked infiltration of naïve B-lymphocytes from mantle zones and paracortical T-lymphocytes into the germinal centers, a process known as progressive transformation of germinal centers (PTGC) [152]. This reactive expansion can mimic

Table 5.9 Differential diagnosis of reactive follicular hyperplasia versus follicular lymphoma

	Reactive follicular hyperplasia	Follicular lymphoma
Morphologic features	Preserved nodal architecture with proliferation of follicles with different sizes and shapes Well-demarcated mantle zones Germinal centers exhibit polarity and tingible body macrophages Patent sinusoids	Effaced nodal architecture by proliferation of back-to-back follicles with similar size and shapes Attenuated and ill-defined mantle zones Germinal centers lack polarity and tingible bode macrophages Collapsed sinuses
Immunophenotype	Germinal centers express CD10 and BCL6 Germinal centers are negative for BCL2 High proliferative index with polarity highlighted by Ki-67 stain	Germinal centers express CD10 and BCL6 Neoplastic germinal centers show aberrant expression of BCL2 In cases negative for BCL2, lack of polarity highlighted by Ki-67 may help

the nodular or vaguely nodular architectural pattern seen in some of the small B-cell lymphomas.
- IHC staining for CD10, BCL6, CD21, and/or CD23 is useful to demonstrate the follicle center phenotype of the cells and the follicular architecture. A negative BCL2 stain is generally associated with a reactive germinal center, but some high-grade FL can be negative for BCL2. Ki-67 staining may be helpful to show the "zonation" in reactive germinal centers.
- In rare difficult cases, it may be necessary to demonstrate absence of a clonal B-cell population by flow cytometry or *IGH/K* gene rearrangement to establish the correct diagnosis. This is particularly important in small biopsies in which other morphologic features that support a neoplastic proliferation over a reactive lymphoid hyperplasia, such as complete effacement of the nodal architecture with collapsed sinuses and extension of the atypical infiltrate into the perinodal adipose and soft tissues, cannot be evaluated adequately.

  Conversely, both primary follicles, which contain few if any BCL6+ B-cells, as well as regressed germinal centers containing many follicular helper T-cells may have BCL2 positivity and should not be misinterpreted as FL.
- BCL2-positive staining in follicle centers containing B-cells may also occur due to "follicular colonization" by any one of the other four small B-cell lymphomas (MZL, MCL, SLL, or LPL).
- The presence of reactive lymphoid follicles does NOT exclude the diagnosis of small B-cell lymphoma, as these can be present in variable numbers in MZL (in particular MALT lymphomas), MCL (in early cases with mantle zone pattern but also in some nodular and diffuse pattern), CLL/SLL (with an interfollicular pattern), and even some cases of FL (early or partial involvement of a node).

- Reactive paracortical hyperplasia of lymph nodes is characterized by distortion of the nodal architecture due to expanded superficial cortex and/or interfollicular areas. A polymorphous infiltrate including small T-lymphocytes, histiocytes, and immunoblasts is typically seen along with residual follicles imparting a moth-eaten pattern. Although morphologically the small T-lymphocytes could potentially mimic a small B-cell lymphoma, differential diagnosis is usually less of an issue since a predominant T-cell population can easily be demonstrated immunohistochemically.
  - In nodular lymphocyte predominant Hodgkin lymphoma, these paracortical areas may contain a high proportion of B-cells. However, clonal B-cell population is not demonstrated.
- Reactive mantle zone hyperplasia and plasmacytosis: In Castleman disease the nodal architecture is partially distorted by reactive follicles with regressed germinal centers surrounded by concentric layers of small B-lymphocytes in mantle zones (known as onion skinning). When a reactive plasma cell component is sparse, the mantle zone hyperplasia may raise concerns for early involvement by MCL, but a negative stain for cyclin D and SOX11 may rule it out. On the other hand, the more typical interfollicular infiltrate of plasma cells, which can be quite numerous in some cases, may raise concern for a plasma cell neoplasm or B-cell lymphoma with plasmacytic differentiation, such as nodal MZL. The plasma cells and B-lymphocytes in Castleman disease however are polytypic without immunophenotypic aberrancies.

13. How frequently does each subtype of small B-cell lymphoma involve the bone marrow and what are their typical patterns of involvement? (Table 5.10)

Bone marrow (BM) involvement by lymphomas is comprehensively covered in Chap. 27.

- Follicular lymphoma is the most common NHL to involve the BM. It characteristically shows a paratrabecular pattern of involvement in which the lymphoma cells are in close contact with bony trabeculae in a linear fashion without any intervening adipocytes.
- This pattern however is not entirely specific for FL. It can be seen in other B-NHLs except in CLL/SLL. Nevertheless, when the pattern is exclusively paratrabecular, 9 out of 10 cases are FL [153]. An exclusive paratrabecular pattern can sometimes be seen in MCL. It is noteworthy that an obvious follicular pattern and germinal centers are infrequently, if ever, encountered in FL involving BM. Chronic inflammatory conditions (such as rheumatoid arthritis) are more likely to show lymphoid follicles with active germinal centers than FL. Germinal centers can also be seen in reactive lymphoid aggregates, MCL and MZL cases. CLL/SLL involves the BM in nodular, interstitial, mixed, and diffuse patterns [154]. Paratrabecular infiltrates of lymphoma cells generally exclude CLL/SLL. Proliferation centers, a characteristic feature of CLL/SLL in the lymph nodes, can be present especially when BM involvement is diffuse and can aid in the diagnosis.
- Monoclonal B-cell lymphocytosis (MBL) with a CLL phenotype (CLL-type MBL) involving the BM is indistinguishable from CLL/SLL by morphology and immunophenotyping. The upper limit of bone marrow involvement which separates MBL from CLL/SLL has

Table 5.10 Bone marrow involvement by small B-cell lymphomas

	Frequency	Morphologic pattern	Useful ancillary tests
CLL/SLL	85%	Nodular, interstitial, diffuse, or mixed	Classic immunophenotype: CD19+, weak CD20+, FMC7-, CD5+, CD23+, CD200+, and weak surface light chain Trisomy 12 or deletions 13q14, 11q, and 17p
FL	40–70%	Paratrabecular	Expression of common B-cell markers Coexpression of CD10 and BCL6 Aberrant expression of BCL2 on germinal centers t(14;18) *IGH-BCL2*
MCL	50–80%	Nodular, interstitial, diffuse, or mixed Paratrabecular	Expression of common B-cell markers Aberrant expression of CD5 and cyclin D1 t(11;14) *IGH-CCND1*
MZL	30–40% in nodal MZL 70–100% in splenic MZL Rare in MALT lymphomas	Nodular, interstitial, or mixed Sinusoidal pattern in splenic MZL	Small B-lymphocytes express common B-cell markers Negative for CD5 and CD10 If present, plasma cells express CD45, CD19, and CD138; and lack expression of CD56 and cyclin D1 No distinct genetic abnormalities
LPL/WM	100% (by definition LPL/WM involves bone marrow)	Interstitial, diffuse, or mixed	Small B-lymphocytes express common B-cell markers Negative for CD5 and CD10 Plasma cells express CD45, CD19, and CD138; and lack expression of CD56 and cyclin D1 *MYD88* L265P in more than 90% of cases

Refs. [153–156]

not been clearly defined [157] unlike the clonal B-cell threshold of 5.0×10^9/L defined for peripheral blood [9].

- MCL involves bone marrow in various patterns similar to CLL/SLL, but MCL can also involve the BM in a paratrabecular distribution which can cause confusion with FL. Immunophenotypic analysis with cyclin D1 or genetic analysis for t(11;14) (q13;q32) can usually resolve this diagnostic pitfall.
- MZLs of different types can involve the BM in a variety of patterns including non-paratrabecular, nodular infiltrates that may contain reactive germinal centers. SMZL, MALT lymphoma, and NMZL in the BM have overlapping features in terms of the extent and pattern of involvement.
  - A mixed pattern of infiltration is the most frequent pattern seen in 83% of cases of SMZL and MALT lymphoma and 50% of cases of NMZL [158], and nodular pattern and interstitial pattern are commonly observed in all MZL types.
  - Sinusoidal pattern of infiltration is commonly associated with SMZL, and while considered fairly specific for this entity, this pattern has been found in other MZLs as well as other B-NHLs including rare cases of FL, MCL, CLL/SLL, and HCL [159]. Regardless of its non-specificity, it is almost always seen and often prominent in SMZL compared to other MZLs and thus increases the likelihood of SMZL.
  - Well-formed germinal centers are found in SMZL but not in NMZL or MALT lymphoma, and presence of follicular dendritic cells (FDCs) identified by CD21 or CD23 immunostaining within lymphoma aggregates in the BM may be helpful in suggesting the diagnosis of SMZL. Although FDCs are less common in other small B-cell lymphomas within the BM, they can be observed in FL in the BM, particularly in cases where follicles are formed [158].
- LPL/WM: A B-cell non-Hodgkin lymphoma in the BM when accompanied by a clinical syndrome of Waldenström's macroglobulinemia is by definition lymphoplasmacytic lymphoma. Importantly, the diagnosis of Waldenström's macroglobulinemia requires identification of a clonal B-cell lymphoplasmacytic infiltrate in the BM.
  - The infiltrates usually show a mixed pattern of interstitial and focal non-paratrabecular involvement by small lymphocytes, plasmacytoid lymphocytes, and plasma cells.
  - Increased mast cells is a common finding in these cases and serves as a useful diagnostic clue [154].
  - Intranuclear inclusions (Dutcher bodies) or cytoplasmic inclusions (Russell bodies) in plasma cells are typically present in LPL.
  - None of the features described are disease-defining features for LPL and do not differentiate LPL from MZL.

14. How to distinguish bone marrow involvement by a small B-cell lymphoma from benign lymphoid aggregates?

The features in distinguishing between benign lymphoid aggregates and lymphomas in general involving the BM are addressed in Chap. 27. The following points are worth noting:

- Benign lymphoid aggregates are commonly encountered in old age, autoimmune disorders [160], inflammatory conditions, post-chemotherapy marrow specimens, as well as certain myeloproliferative neoplasms [161].

- Benign lymphoid aggregates are usually few in number and small in size, show perivascular distribution (non-paratrabecular location), and display non-infiltrative edges [162]. They are comprised of a mixture of predominantly small lymphocytes and a smaller proportion of large cells and plasma cells. Cytologic atypia (open chromatin, irregular nuclear contours, prominent nucleoli, or karyorrhexis) is absent [162]. Reactive germinal centers with tingible body macrophages may be present.
- Immunohistochemically, reactive lymphoid aggregates often show predominance of T-cells, mixed populations of B- and T-cells, or central cores of T-cells surrounded by a rim of B-cells.
- In contrast, malignant lymphoid aggregates are large in size, have ill-defined margins with extensions of lymphocytes into surrounding interstitium, and usually show juxtatrabecular or paratrabecular localization, and the lymphoid cells show cytologic atypia.
- Immunohistochemically, neoplastic lymphoid aggregates are composed of predominantly B-cells or central cores of B-cells surrounded by T-cells. In addition, individual lymphoma subtypes exhibit 5 main infiltration patterns that could be highlighted by IHC – diffuse, paratrabecular, interstitial, nodular, and mixed [153, 163]. While these patterns suggest a lymphoma diagnosis, they are not specific by themselves.

15. What is considered an adequate specimen for diagnosis and classification of small B-cell lymphomas?

- Diagnosis of small B-cell lymphomas relies heavily on morphologic and immunophenotypic features in addition to cytomorphology of lymphoma cells. Architectural pattern assessment is possible in larger specimen such as incisional or excisional lymph node biopsies. The European Society of Medical Oncology (ESMO), the WHO system for lymphoma classification, the British Committee for Standards in Haematology, and the National Comprehensive Cancer Network (NCCN) recommend excisional biopsy for lymphoma diagnosis and subtyping.
  - The current NCCN clinical practice guidelines in oncology specifically state that FNA or core needle biopsy are insufficient in the diagnosis of FL, DLBCL, MCL, and MZL, and furthermore, FNAs are not ideal specimens for grading of FL (National Comprehensive Cancer Network. NCCN clinical practice guidelines in oncology for non-Hodgkin's lymphomas. http://www.nccn.org/professionals/physician_gls/pdf/nhl.pdf).
- Excisional biopsy offers several advantages over core needle biopsy for lymphoma diagnosis. Since architectural context is available in an excisional biopsy, a pathologist is more likely to use specific antibody panels and thus lesser number of markers to reach a final diagnosis. A study at the lymph node registry found that when encountered with a core needle biopsy for evaluation, pathologists tend to use more immunomarkers and are more likely to provide an inconclusive diagnosis requiring surgical excision or additional core needle biopsies [164].
- Additionally, due to limitations of architectural assessment, core needle biopsies are less effective in identifying all components in lymphomas that tend to have complex histologic patterns including transformation and composite lymphoma [164].
- Nonetheless, core needle biopsy is likely the choice when the enlarged lymph nodes are deep-seated, next to or encasing a vital structure, or when patients are a surgical risk or critically ill to undergo excisional biopsy.
- Core needle biopsy should be reserved for these situations when an excisional biopsy is contraindicated and must be supplemented by the full repertoire of ancillary testing to reach an accurate diagnosis. See Chap. 4 for guidelines to handle diagnostic dilemmas inherent to small biopsies. In general, when core needle biopsies show morphologically atypical lymphocytes, but lack evidence of clonality or an overtly aberrant immunophenotype, it might be prudent to provide a descriptive diagnosis and recommend excision biopsy for further evaluation.
- Core needle biopsy and fine needle aspiration, even when accompanied by flow cytometric and genetic ancillary studies, demonstrate an inferior diagnostic yield compared to excisional biopsy, and in many cases, the latter is still required for definitive diagnosis [164, 165]. Therefore, an excision biopsy is preferred as clinically feasible.
- It is worth noting that a definitive diagnosis for some small B-cell lymphomas can also be achieved from bone marrow biopsy provided sufficient diagnostic criteria are met and bone marrow specimen is adequate for analysis. This is possible in entities displaying characteristic immunophenotype such as CLL/SLL (CD19+, weak, CD20+, FMC7-, CD5+, CD23+, CD200+, and weak surface light chain immunoglobulin), or MCL (strong and diffuse expression of cyclin D1) [166, 167].

16. What information can be conveyed to the clinician during each workup stage of small B-cell lymphomas?

The following information can be conveyed to the clinician as various parts of the diagnostic workup are completed:

- Based on immediate assessment of a touch imprint or cytology smear, it may be possible to communicate that a large cell lymphoma or high-grade lymphoma is NOT present. If monotypic B-cells are detected by flow cytometry and constitute a majority of the total lymphoid cells analyzed, it is possible to communicate to the clinician that this is likely a small B-cell lymphoma.
- Presence of one of the characteristic immunophenotype (CD5+/CD23+ or CD5+/CD23-, or CD10+) usually, but not invariably, indicates the presence of a specific type of small B-cell lymphoma. However, given the possibility of atypical immunophenotypes occurring in each of the small B-cell lymphomas described in this chapter, it is prudent to wait communicating the type of lymphoma until the morphology and IHC staining results (where necessary) are completed.
- If the type of small B-cell lymphoma cannot be accurately determined due to insufficient tissue, the clinician should be alerted as soon as possible that a small B-cell lymphoma is present, but additional tissue is required for complete workup.
- In addition to the specific diagnosis, information regarding morphologic attributes of clinical relevance (e.g., evidence of histologic transformation to DLBCL, morphologic variants), prognostic markers, and cytogenetic and/or molecular features should be reported if available.
- If the results from cytogenetic and molecular studies have a bearing on the final diagnosis, it is appropriate to discuss these results with the clinician to ask if they want to have an interim diagnosis stating the type of lymphoma or a final diagnosis integrating all ancillary test results.

17. What should be the approach to provide maximum, but defensible, information from limited specimen or workup? What is a descriptive diagnosis appropriate in such situations?

- The small B-cell lymphoma cells generally are well suited for flow cytometry that provides dependable information about presence of clonal B-cells. With multiparameter flow cytometry, additional immunophenotypic information can be obtained even from cells obtained by fine needle aspiration. If only a cytology smear and immunophenotype of the clonal population is available, it is appropriate to inform the clinician that a CD5+ or CD10+ or CD5-/CD10- small B-cell lymphoma is detected and to give a differential diagnosis of possible entities.
- If a core needle biopsy is also available and key IHC stains such as cyclin D1, BCL6, and Ki-67 can be performed, then it is appropriate to provide the type of small B-cell lymphoma. However, the limitations of the examination, such as inability to exclude prognostically relevant morphological variants or focal presence of a more aggressive process, should be clearly stated.
- When flow cytometry is not performed, because lymphoma was not suspected before FNA, and if an adequate core biopsy also is not obtained, it may be appropriate to request another biopsy with samples for flow cytometry and histologic evaluation. With an adequate tissue biopsy, it may be possible to establish clonality of the B-cells and/or obtain sufficiently detailed immunophenotype and molecular genetic profiles based on IHC and paraffin FISH, respectively, to allow a definitive diagnosis in conjunction with available histology and cytomorphology.
- If all diagnostic and/or prognostic tests cannot be performed due to limitations of resources or patient preference despite the availability of ample tissue, then it is appropriate to provide a descriptive diagnosis based on morphology alone. This should be followed by a reasonable list of possible types of lymphomas (and reactive mimics) and suggest a minimal workup which may provide at least some guidance to the clinician for appropriate management.
- One must also bear in mind that rendering a definitive lymphoma diagnosis with subclassification is only prudent when morphologic and immunophenotypic features provide reasonable confidence to issue such as diagnosis. In cases with limitations of tissue and variations in morphology and immunophenotype, a conservative diagnosis may be wise in order to prevent diagnostic errors, avoids subjecting the patient to unnecessary or overtreatment and prompt a clinician to opt for additional biopsy to get a definitive diagnosis.

18. When is a diagnostic comment necessary and what should be discussed in the diagnostic comment of small B-cell lymphomas?

A diagnostic comment may be necessary in the pathology report for various reasons.

- As discussed before, a definite diagnosis can be challenging when the submitted material is limited or the biopsy size is small. A comment in these situations can clarify the diagnostic difficulties and emphasize the need for additional tissue for a definitive lymphoma diagnosis and subclassification.
- When cases demonstrate morphologic and/or immunophenotypic variations from a "classic" pattern, a definite

subclassification can be challenging. For example, histologically low-grade FLs with an entirely diffuse pattern, FLs that lack CD10 or BCL2 expression, CLL/SLL with expanded proliferation centers, and MCLs that lack cyclin D1 expression often pose diagnostic challenges.

- When the biopsy is fragmented, morphologic clues are lacking, and immunophenotypic analysis is incomplete due to tissue exhaustion, a definitive diagnosis of lymphoma is precluded. A comment is warranted in such cases detailing the pathologic features (or lack thereof) and emphasizing the need for another biopsy for definitive diagnosis.
- Lymphomas can have complex histologic patterns in the same lymph node and a core needle biopsy or fragmented biopsy may not entirely represent the variations. A diagnostic comment is often warranted describing limitations posed by the unusual morphologic or immunophenotypic features in the absence of an architectural context for a definitive subclassification of lymphoma.
- When a definitive diagnosis and subclassification can be rendered, a comment may be issued to discuss information of prognostic or therapeutic relevance obtained from morphology and ancillary studies. The discussion may include information on whether there is evidence of histologic transformation to DLBCL, any variant morphologic patterns of clinical relevance, any immunophenotypic aberrations, specific immunomarkers, and cytogenetic or molecular markers of prognostic significance. For example, in CLL/SLL, discussion in comment should address the prognostic significance of expanded proliferation centers.
  - In FL, morphologic variations (ISFN, floral variant, pediatric FL, low-grade FL with high proliferation rate, diffuse FL variant with 1p36 deletion), FLs at specific sites such as the duodenum and testis, or immunophenotypic variations (lack of CD10 or BCL2 or aberrant CD5 coexpression) need a comment on their diagnostic and/or prognostic significance.
  - In FL, information on overall grade, presence of any grade 3 or diffuse large B-cell component, and whether pattern is follicular, follicular and diffuse, or entirely diffuse is essential as a part of the final diagnostic report. The number of follicles in a core needle biopsy may not reach the threshold thus precluding optimal and accurate grading in FL. In such cases, the inability to accurately grade FL in a core needle biopsy due to insufficient amount of follicles should be discussed in a comment. A need for excisional biopsy for accurate grading may be emphasized. In spite of limitations, it is not unreasonable however to comment on the overall appearance of the lymphoma (low versus high grade), any areas with centroblast clusters, or diffuse areas of large cells which may raise suspicion for transformation. Such information should be communicated to the clinician to prompt another biopsy to rule out a grade 3 FL or diffuse large B-cell component.
- In MCL, a comment is warranted to discuss the prognostic impact of any morphologic (blastoid, pleomorphic variants, ISMCN) or immunophenotypic (cyclin D1-negative) variations.
- A definitive diagnosis is not always possible when the differential involves MZL versus LPL or plasma cell neoplasm versus a small B-cell lymphoma with extensive plasmacytic differentiation, especially in core needle biopsy specimens. In these situations, depending upon the extent of ancillary workup, it may be reasonable to issue a diagnosis of "low-grade B-cell lymphoma with plasmacytic differentiation" without a definitive subtype. A comment is then necessary to discuss the differential diagnoses, the limitations in further distinction between the diagnostic entities, and the need for a larger, preferably excisional biopsy. The pathologist may also wish to recommend laboratory workup such as serum viscosity, bone marrow examination, serum protein electrophoresis, and immunofixation as well as molecular studies for *MYD88* L265P mutation to further differentiate between the entities.
- A comment is generally warranted in cases where a definitive diagnosis is not possible and includes descriptive terms such as "low-grade NHL" or noncommittal language such as "suggestive of," "favor," "compatible with," and "suspicious for." In these situations, the pathologist should attempt to clarify reasons behind his/her reluctance to commit to a definitive diagnosis, whether it is the lack of an architectural context, morphologic or immunophenotypic variations, or scant tissue leading to an incomplete workup.

19. When is it appropriate to seek external consultation for diagnosis or classification of small B-cell lymphomas?

Our understanding of different lymphoma types is in a constant flux with changing terminologies, introduction of new provisional entities, and novel immunophenotypic and genetic features that refine specific lymphoma categories. In general, small B-NHLs in this category do not pose a significant diagnostic challenge in routine practice especially with the use of comprehensive immunophenotyping and genetic testing in the current WHO classification scheme.

Nevertheless, the following general points for expertise consultation are worth noting:

- Lack or perceived lack of content-specific expertise and/or technical capabilities: some pathology groups routinely obtain second opinion on all lymphoma cases due to lack of a subspecialty expertise in hematopathology. Also, some practices may not have resources for comprehensive immunophenotyping and cutting-edge cytogenetic and molecular studies.
- Diagnostic challenges due to causes as below:
  - Scant tissue and morphologic and immunophenotypic variations which may influence treatment
  - Cases with inconclusive findings where the differential diagnoses involve entities with significantly different clinical behavior, prognosis, and treatment options
  - Cases of limited tissue material from critically ill patients who may not tolerate larger biopsies and require prompt therapy

Case Presentations

Case 1

Learning Objectives

1. To become familiar with the histologic features of chronic lymphocytic leukemia/small lymphocytic lymphoma, particularly the one with expanded proliferation centers
2. To become familiar with the immunophenotypic features of chronic lymphocytic leukemia/small lymphocytic lymphoma including flow cytometric and immunohistochemical findings
3. To generate differential diagnosis

Case History

A 62-year-old male complaining of fatigue, night sweats, and unintentional weight loss. Radiologic studies demonstrate diffuse lymphadenopathy. An axillary lymph node is excised.

Histologic Findings (Fig. 5.1a–c)

- Effacement of the nodal architecture with expanded and coalescent proliferation centers which are broader than a 20× objective field (**a**, **b**).
- Proliferation centers are comprised of prolymphocytes and paraimmunoblasts (**c**).

Differential Diagnosis

- Reactive lymphoid hyperplasia
- Chronic lymphocytic leukemia/small lymphocytic lymphoma
- Mantle cell lymphoma
- Nodal marginal zone lymphoma
- Follicular lymphoma

IHC and Other Ancillary Studies (Fig. 5.1d–f)

- Positive for PAX5 (**d**).
- Positive for aberrant CD5 (**e**).
- Ki-67 demonstrates an increased proliferation index >40% (**f**).
- Negative for cyclin D1 (data not shown).

Flow Cytometric Analysis (Fig. 5.2a–f)

- Monoclonal B-cell population with aberrant CD5 and CD23.
- CD10 is negative.

Final Diagnosis

Chronic lymphocytic leukemia/small lymphocytic lymphoma with expanded proliferation centers

Take-Home Messages

1. Typical immunophenotypic profile of chronic lymphocytic leukemia/small lymphocytic lymphoma is monoclonal B-cell population with CD5 and CD23 and negative for CD10 and cyclin D1.
2. CLL/SLL with expanded proliferation centers is characterized by expanded and confluent proliferation centers broader than a 20× magnification field and an increased proliferation index (either >2.4 mitoses per proliferation center or Ki-67 >40% per proliferation center).
3. Distinction of chronic lymphocytic leukemia/small lymphocytic lymphoma with expanded proliferation centers is clinically relevant since these features are associated with a more aggressive clinical behavior compared with the usual type of CLL/SLL.

Case 2

Learning Objectives

1. To become familiar with the histologic features of mantle cell lymphoma, particularly blastoid morphologic variant
2. To become familiar with the immunophenotypic features of mantle cell lymphoma
3. To generate differential diagnosis

Case History

An 85-year-old male patient presenting with diffuse lymphadenopathy fatigue and unintentional weight loss. A 1.5-cm subcutaneous mass identified on the left thigh on physical examination was excised

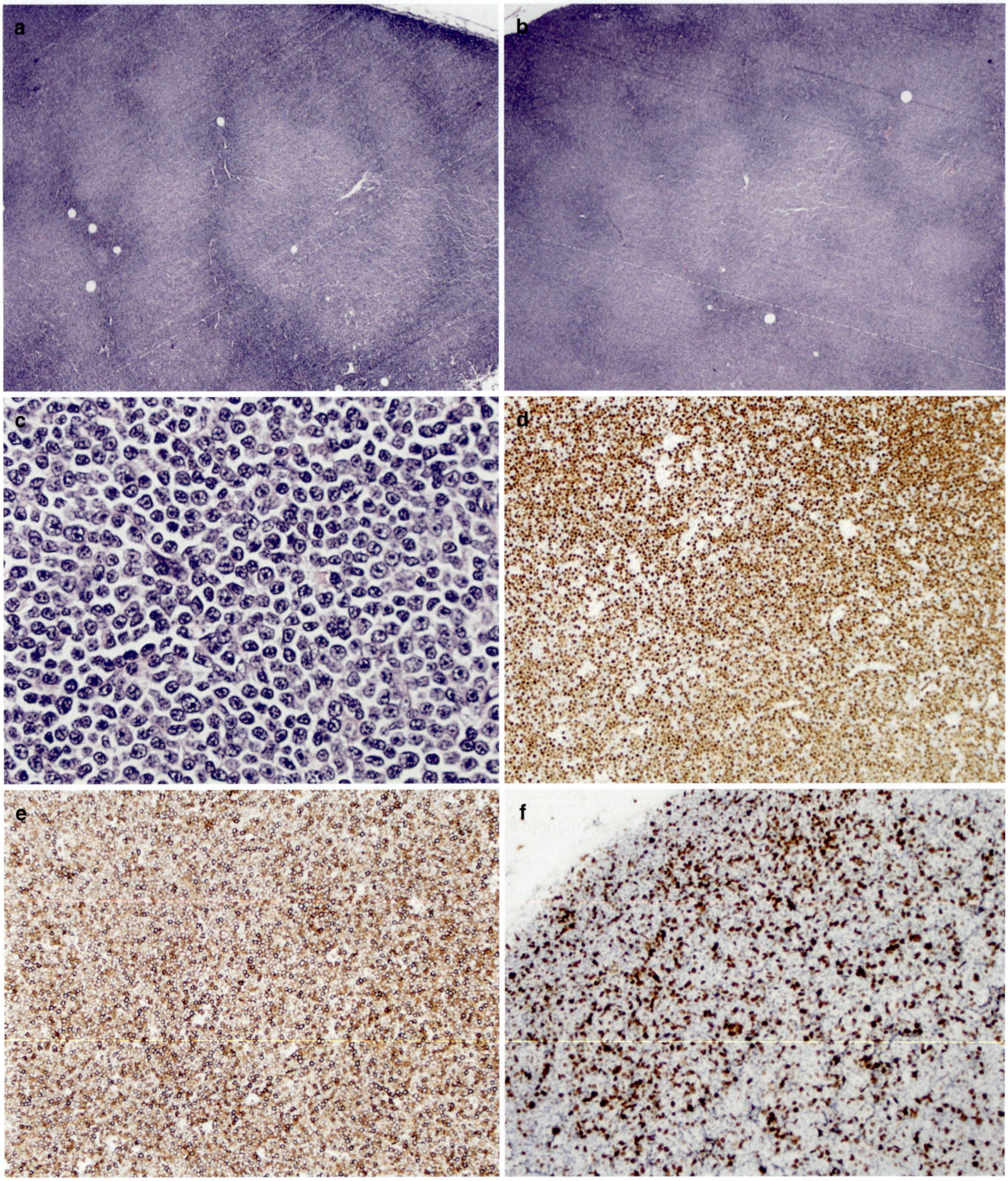

Fig. 5.1 (Case #1). Small lymphocytic lymphoma with expanded proliferation centers. (**a**, **b**) Lymph node biopsy shows effacement of the nodal architecture with nodular lymphoid proliferation. The lymphoid nodules appear paler than surrounding lymphocytes, corresponding to expanded and coalescent proliferation centers. H&E stain, 200×. (**c**) A high magnification demonstrates the pale nodules are comprised of large lymphocytes with morphology consistent with prolymphocyte and paraimmunoblasts. H&E stain, 400×. (**d**) The majority of lymphocytes are positive for PAX5. 100×. (**e**) These lymphocytes coexpress CD5. CD5 stain, 100×. (**f**) Ki-67 stain shows increase in proliferative index in expanded nodules. 100×

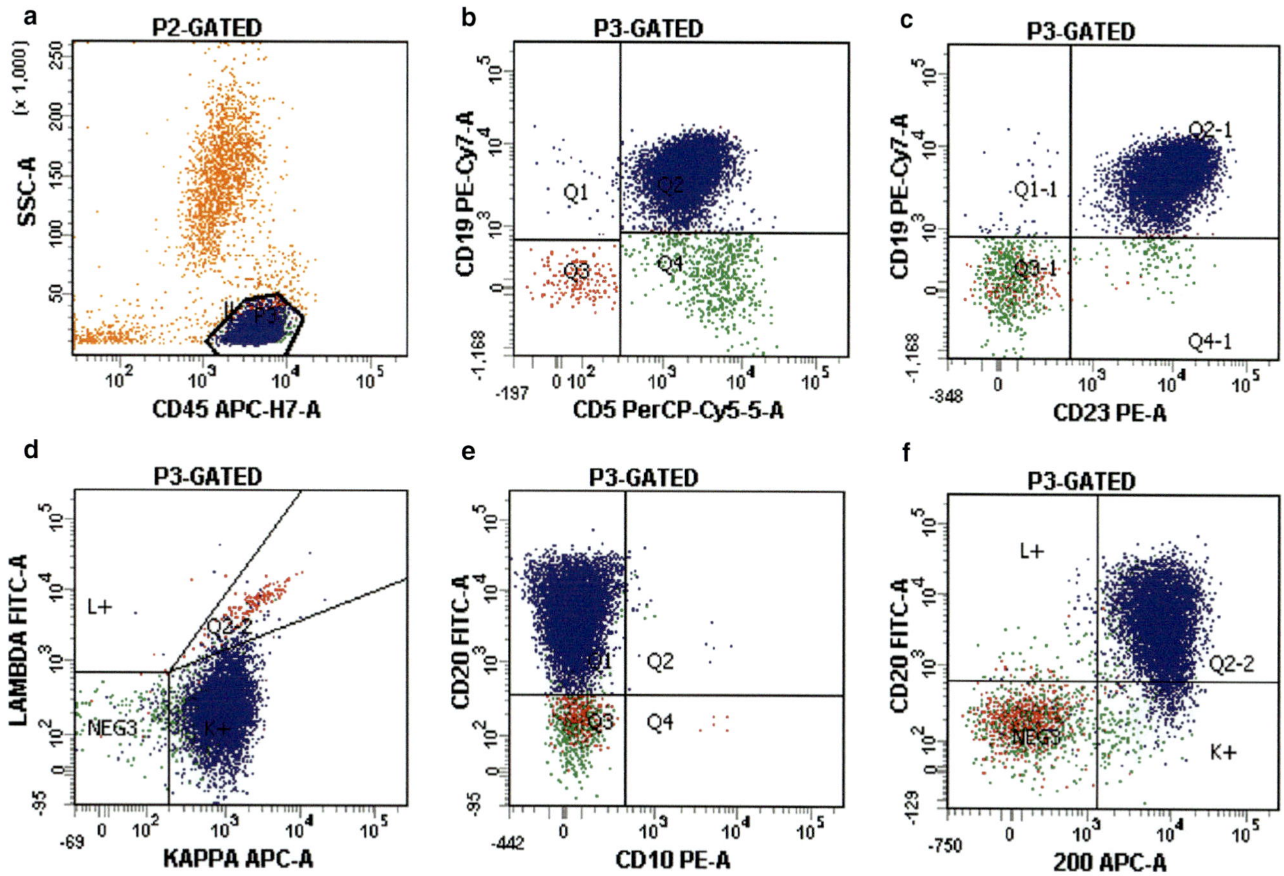

Fig. 5.2 (Case #1). Detection of small lymphocytic lymphoma by flow cytometry. (**a**) CD45 versus side scatter plot showing increased mature lymphocytes (blue population). (**b**) coexpression of CD19 and CD5 in the lymphoid population. Cells with isolated CD5 corresponding to T-cells are highlighted by green color. (**c**) B-cells (CD19+) express CD23. (**d**) The B-cell population is restricted to immunoglobulin kappa light chain. (**e**) This B-cell population expresses CD20 (heterogeneous), but is negative for CD10. (**f**) The B-cell population expresses bright CD200

Histologic Findings (Fig. 5.3a, b)

- Diffuse proliferation of large neoplastic cells displaying fine chromatin, inconspicuous nucleoli, scant cytoplasm, and increased mitotic activity (**a**, **b**)

Differential Diagnosis

- Mantle cell lymphoma, blastoid variant
- Diffuse large B-cell lymphoma
- Lymphoblastic lymphoma
- Burkitt lymphoma

IHC and Other Ancillary Studies (Fig. 5.3c–h)

- Positive for CD20 (**c**).
- Negative for CD3 (**d**).
- Positive for aberrant CD5 (**e**).
- The neoplastic cells are diffusely and strongly positive for cyclin D1 (**f**).
- Ki-67 demonstrates a high proliferation index (**g**).
- In peripheral blood, the neoplastic cells mimic lymphoblasts with very irregular nuclear contours (**h**).

Final Diagnosis

Mantle cell lymphoma, blastoid variant

Take-Home Messages

1. Mantle cell lymphoma with blastoid morphology is comprised of medium-sized lymphocytes with brisk mitotic activity and lymphoblastoid morphology including scant cytoplasm, rounded nuclei, fine chromatin, and inconspicuous nucleoli.
2. Mantle cell lymphoma with blastoid morphology shows similar immunophenotypic features as classic mantle cell lymphoma including strong and diffuse expression of cyclin D1.
3. The blastoid variant of mantle cell lymphoma warrant specific designation in the final diagnosis as this entity is associated to a highly aggressive clinical behavior compared to classic mantle cell lymphoma.

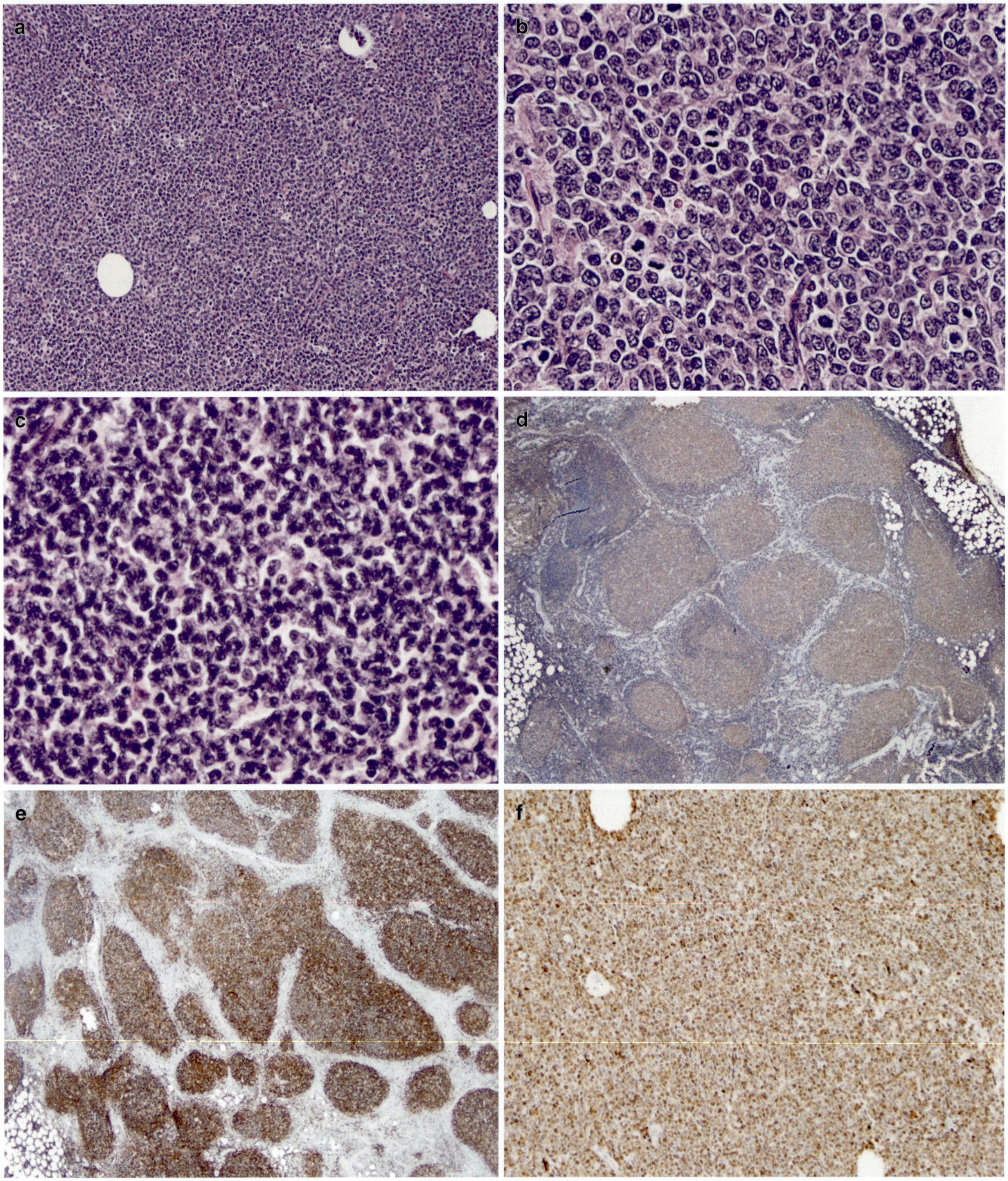

Fig. 5.3 (Case #2). Mantle cell lymphoma, blastoid variant. (**a**) Lymph node biopsy shows effacement of nodal architecture by diffuse proliferation of lymphoid cells. H&E stain, 100×. (**b**) A high magnification demonstrates the medium-sized lymphoid cells with slightly irregular nuclear contours, fine chromatin, inconspicuous nucleoli, scant cytoplasm, and increased mitotic activity. H&E stain, 400×. The majority of lymphoid cells are positive for CD20 (**c**, 100×) and negative for CD3 (**d**, 100×) and show aberrant expression of CD5 (**e**, 100×). (**f**) The lymphoid cells are diffusely and strongly positive for cyclin D1. 100×. (**g**) Ki-67 stain demonstrates a high proliferation index. 100×. (**h**) Peripheral blood smear shows circulating abnormal lymphocytes with morphologic features resembling lymphoblasts. Wright Giemsa stain, 600×

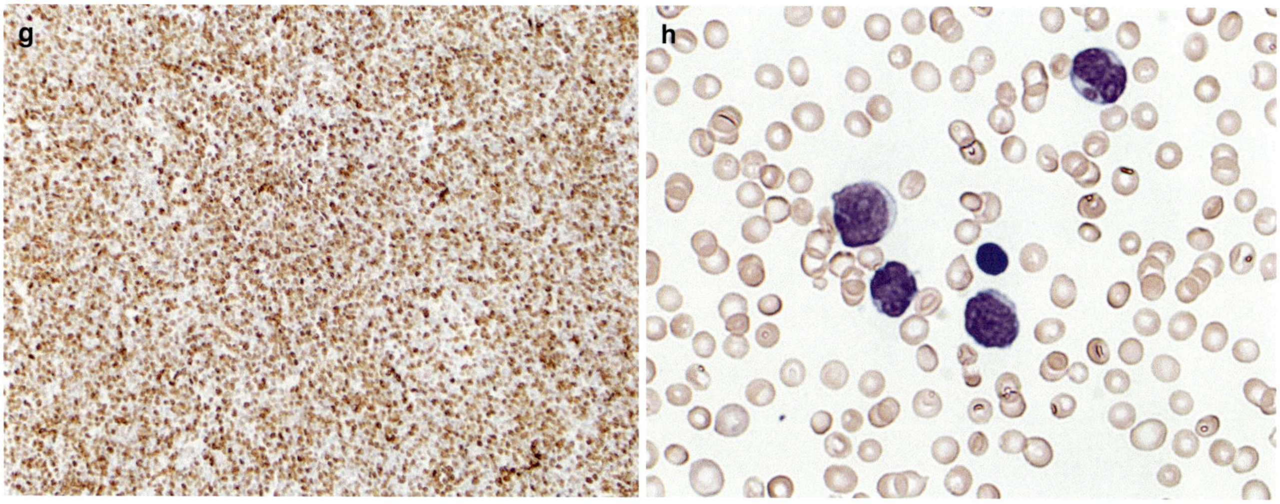

Fig. 5.3 (continued)

Case 3

Learning Objectives

1. To become familiar with the histologic features of low-grade follicular lymphoma, particularly the one with high proliferative index within neoplastic follicles
2. To become familiar with the immunophenotypic features of low-grade follicular lymphoma
3. To generate differential diagnosis

Case History

A 49-year-old male patient presenting with anemia, night sweats, and diffuse lymphadenopathy. Excisional lymph node biopsy was performed.

Histologic Findings (Fig. 5.4a, b)

- Effaced nodal architecture showing back-to-back proliferation of neoplastic follicles (**a**).
- Loss of polarity and absence of tingible body macrophages with neoplastic follicles (**a**).
- The neoplastic lymphocytes within the follicles show small round nuclei instead of the typical centrocyte/centroblast morphology (**b**). There are less than 15 centroblasts per high-power field.

Differential Diagnosis

- Follicular lymphoma
- Reactive follicular hyperplasia
- Chronic lymphocytic leukemia/small lymphocytic lymphoma
- Nodal marginal zone lymphoma
- Mantle cell lymphoma
- Nodular lymphocyte predominant Hodgkin lymphoma
- Otherwise typical low-grade follicular lymphoma (without a high proliferation index)

IHC and Other Ancillary Studies (Fig. 5.4c–h)

- Neoplastic follicles express CD20 (**c**), CD10 (**d**), BCL6 (**e**), and aberrant BCL2 (**f**).
- Ki-67 demonstrates a proliferation index >30% in the neoplastic follicles which is key for identification of this subtype of follicular lymphoma (**g**, **h**).

Final Diagnosis

Follicular lymphoma, low grade (grade 1–2), with high proliferation index

Take-Home Messages

1. Follicular lymphoma is characterized by proliferation of densely packed, back-to-back follicles giving a classic follicular pattern.
2. Neoplastic follicles exhibit similar size and shape, attenuated mantle zones, and germinal centers with loss of polarity and absence of tingible body macrophages.
3. Histologic grading of follicular lymphoma is based on identification and quantification of centroblasts.
4. Low-grade follicular lymphoma with high proliferation index contains less than 15 centroblasts per high-power field (morphologically low grade) but demonstrates a high proliferation index within the neoplastic germinal centers.
5. Identification of low-grade follicular lymphoma with high proliferation index is clinically relevant since this diagnosis portrays a more aggressive clinical behavior.

Case 4

Learning Objectives

1. To become familiar with the histologic features of follicular lymphoma, floral variant

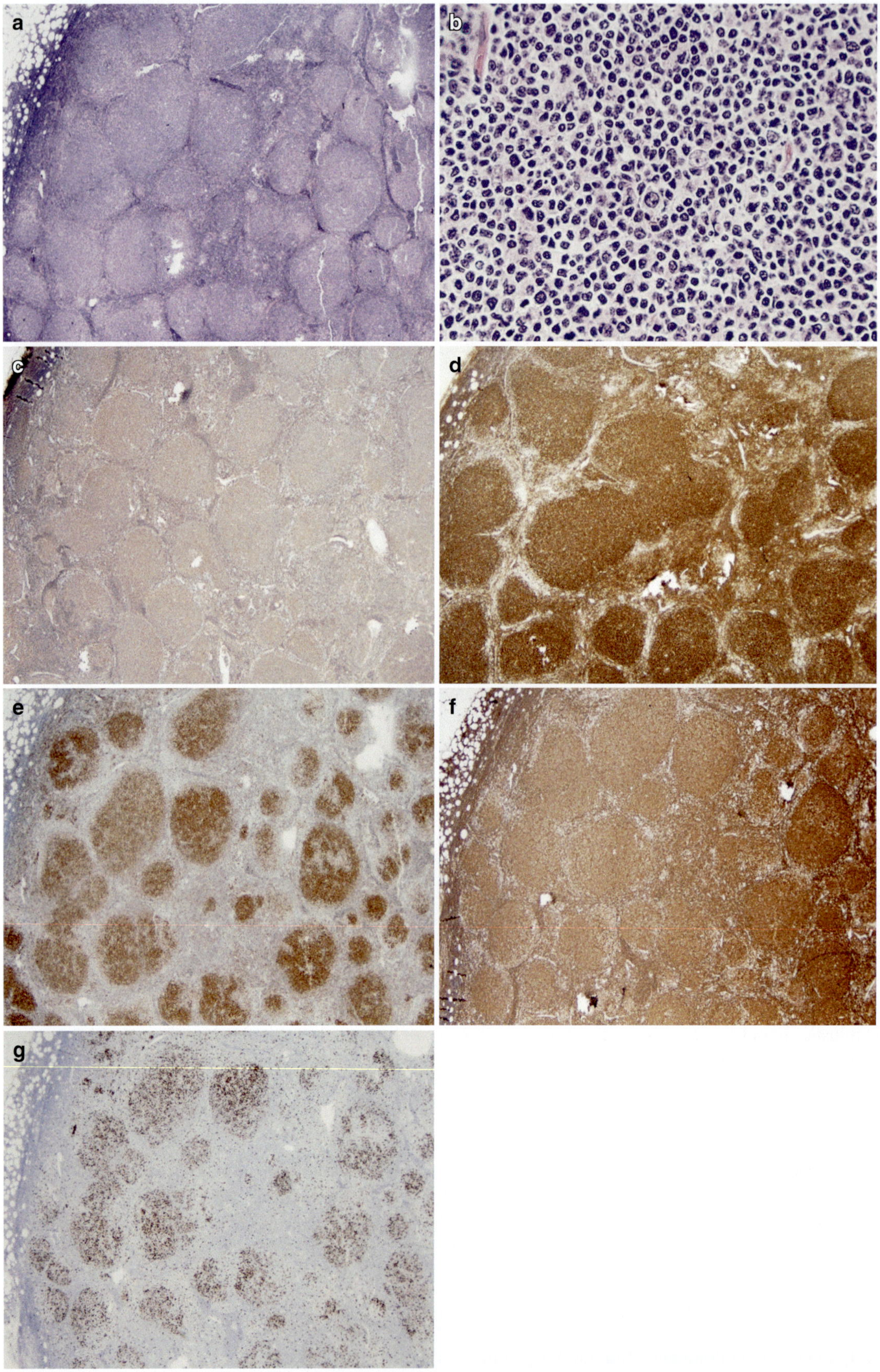

Fig. 5.4 (Case #3). Follicular lymphoma with a high proliferative index. (**a**) Lymph node biopsy shows nodal architecture effaced by a back-to-back proliferation of lymphoid follicles. H&E stain, 20×. (**b**) The lymphoid cells within the follicles are small in size with slightly irregular nuclei and moderate amount of clear cytoplasm. H&E stain, 400×. Cells in lymphoid follicles express CD20 (**c**, 20×), CD10 (**d**, 20×), BCL6 (**e**, 20×), and BCL2 (strong) (**f**, 20×). (**g**) Ki-67 stain demonstrates a proliferation index >30% in the neoplastic follicles. 20×

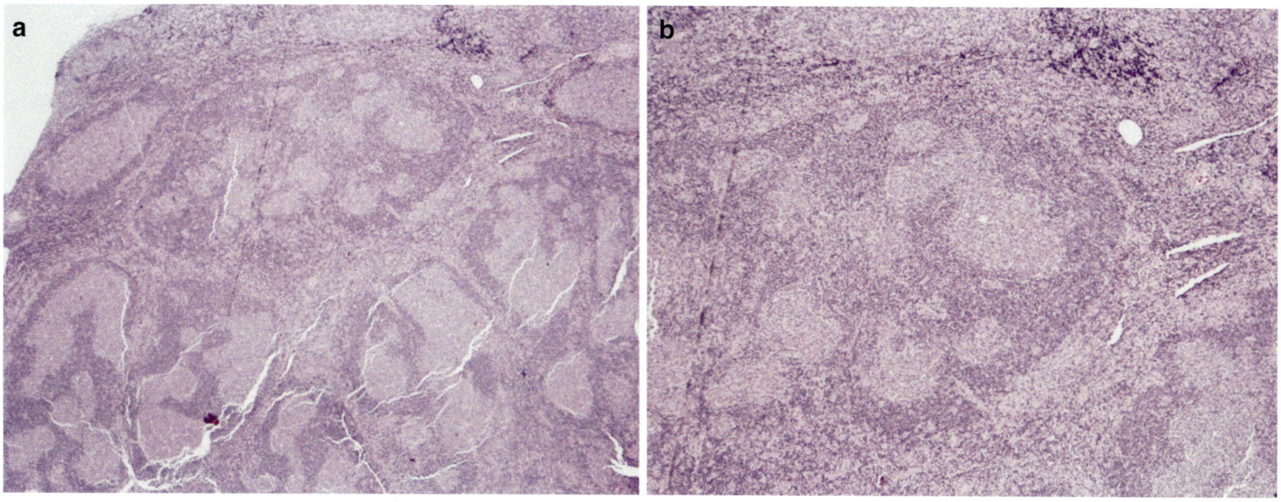

Fig. 5.5 (Case #4). Follicular lymphoma, floral morphologic variant. (**a**, **b**) The lymph node biopsy shows nodal architecture effaced or largely altered by proliferation of lymphoid follicles. In contrast to typical follicular lymphoma, the germinal centers in this lymph node biopsy are well defined with mantle zone, but demonstrate no polarity or tingible body macrophages. Follicle centers impart a flowerlike or cloud-like morphology. H&E stain, 20× and 40×, respectively

2. To become familiar with the immunophenotypic features of follicular lymphoma floral variant
3. To generate differential diagnosis

Case History

A 58-year-old male patient with diffuse lymphadenopathy identified on physical examination during routine check-up. Excisional lymph node biopsy was performed.

Histologic Findings (Fig. 5.5a, b)

- The germinal centers show neoplastic features and are surrounded by robust mantle zones that invaginate into the follicles imparting a flowerlike or cloud-like morphology (**a**, **b**).

Differential Diagnosis

- Follicular lymphoma
- Reactive follicular hyperplasia
- Mantle cell lymphoma (mantle zone pattern)

IHC and Other Ancillary Studies

- Same immunohistochemical features as otherwise typical follicular lymphoma.
- Mantle zones are negative for cyclin D1.

Final Diagnosis

Follicular lymphoma, low grade (grade 1–2), floral variant

Take-Home Messages

1. Floral variant of follicular lymphoma demonstrates similar immunophenotypic features to otherwise typical low-grade follicular lymphoma.
2. Identification of floral variant of follicular lymphoma is relevant for differential diagnosis although it bears no clinical significance.

Case 5

Learning Objectives

1. To become familiar with the histologic features of nodal marginal zone lymphoma
2. To become familiar with the immunophenotypic features of nodal marginal zone lymphoma
3. To generate differential diagnosis

Case History

A 71-year-old female patient presenting with bilateral axillary lymphadenopathy and recurrent pleural effusions. Excisional axillary lymph node biopsy was performed.

Histologic Findings (Fig. 5.6a, b)

- Nodal architecture is effaced by a diffuse to vaguely nodular polymorphous infiltrate (**a**).
- Neoplastic cells range from small to intermediate and occasionally large size (**b**).

Differential Diagnosis

- Nodal marginal zone lymphoma
- Reactive lymphoid hyperplasia
- Chronic lymphocytic leukemia/small lymphocytic lymphoma
- Mantle cell lymphoma
- Lymphoplasmacytic lymphoma
- Follicular lymphoma
- Peripheral T-cell lymphoma

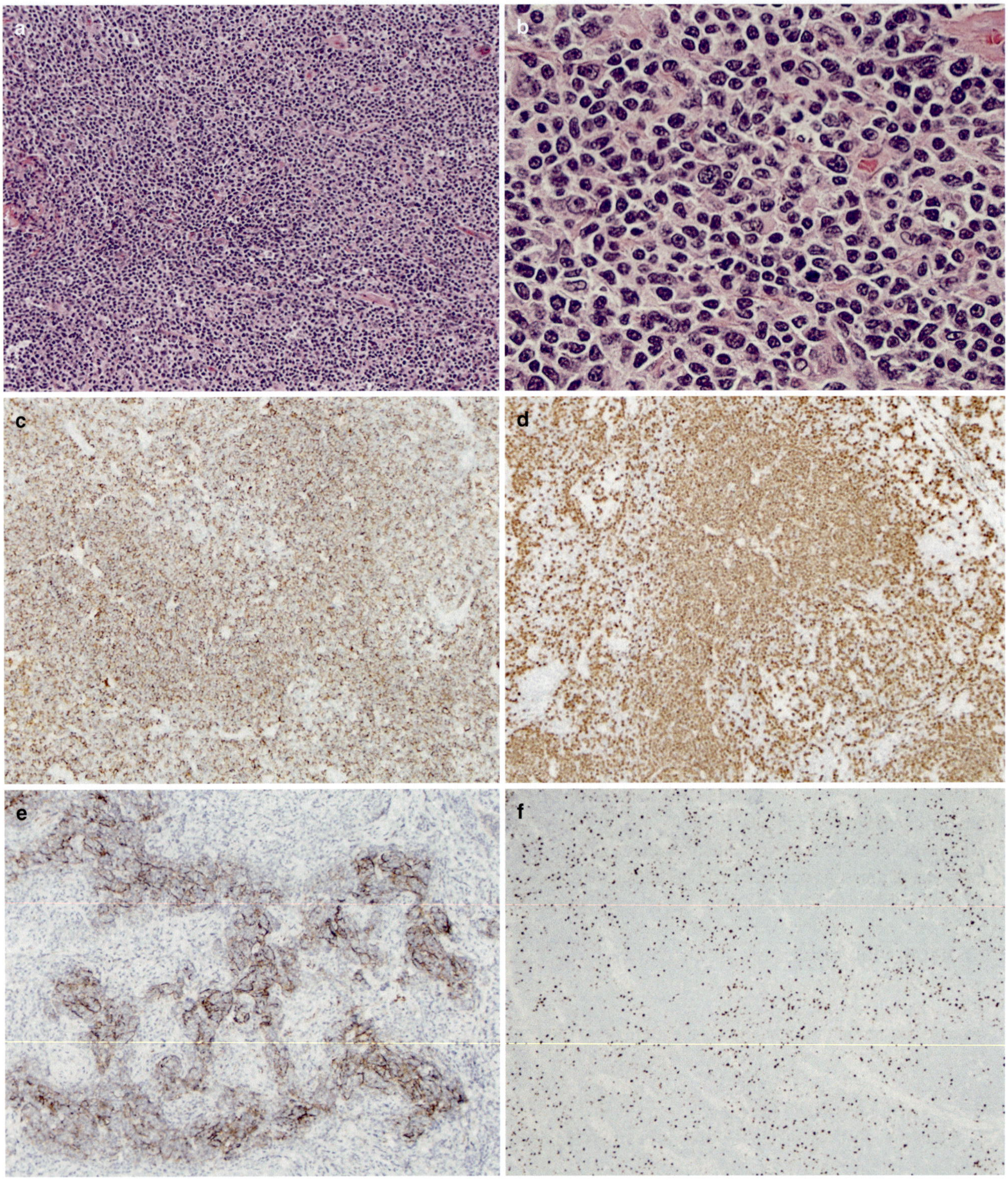

Fig. 5.6 (Case #5). Nodal marginal zone lymphoma. (**a**) This lymph node biopsy shows nodal architecture effaced by a diffuse to vaguely nodular polymorphous infiltrate. H&E stain, 100×. (**b**) A high magnification shows small to intermediate lymphocytes with irregular nuclear contours and moderate amount of cytoplasm. A few plasmacytoid cells and occasional large cells are present. H&E stain, 400×. The majority of lymphocytes express CD20 (**c**, 100×) and PAX5 (**d**, 100×). (**e**) The markedly expanded and disrupted follicular dendritic meshworks are highlighted by CD21 stain. 100×. (**f**) Ki-67 stain demonstrates a low proliferation index. Note the positive cells are distributed in peripheries of the lymphoid nodules (marginal zone pattern). 20×

IHC and Other Ancillary Studies (Fig. 5.6c–f)

- The neoplastic lymphocytes express CD20 (**c**) and PAX5 (**d**).
- The markedly expanded and disrupted follicular dendritic cell meshworks are highlighted by CD21 stain (**e**).
- Ki-67 demonstrates a low proliferation index (**f**).

Final Diagnosis

Nodal marginal zone lymphoma

Take-Home Messages

1. Nodal marginal zone lymphoma is diagnosed when the disease is exclusively nodal based without evidence of extranodal or splenic disease.
2. The nodal architecture is effaced by neoplastic cells in one or more of the five reported patterns of infiltration.
3. Nodal marginal zone lymphoma lacks a specific immunophenotypic profile and is usually positive for B-cell markers such as CD19, CD20, CD22, CD79a, and PAX5.
4. Identification of markedly expanded follicular dendritic cell meshworks with CD21 or CD23 is a useful diagnostic tool.

Case 6

Learning Objectives

1. To become familiar with the histologic features of lymphoplasmacytic lymphoma/Waldenström macroglobulinemia involving lymph node
2. To become familiar with the histologic features of lymphoplasmacytic lymphoma/Waldenström macroglobulinemia in bone marrow
3. To become familiar with the immunophenotypic features of lymphoplasmacytic lymphoma/Waldenström macroglobulinemia
4. To generate differential diagnosis

Case History

A 48-year-old female patient complaining of intermittent numbness on lower extremities. Workup studies revealed anemia, thrombocytopenia, IgM kappa monoclonal protein of 1.8 gr/dL, and mild abdominal and iguana lymphadenopathy. Excisional inguinal lymph node biopsy was performed, followed by staging bone marrow examination.

Histologic Findings (Fig. 5.7a–d)

- Nodal architecture is effaced by a diffuse to vaguely nodular polymorphous infiltrate with preserved patent sinuses (**a**)
- The polymorphous neoplastic infiltrate is comprised of small lymphocytes, plasmacytoid lymphocytes, and plasma cells (**b**)
- Bone marrow aspirate smear (**c**) and biopsy (**d**) show increased small mature lymphoma and plasmacytoid cells with interstitial infiltrating pattern.

Differential Diagnosis

- Lymphoplasmacytic lymphoma
- Nodal marginal zone lymphoma
- Plasma cell neoplasms
- Chronic lymphocytic leukemia/small lymphocytic lymphoma
- Mantle cell lymphoma

IHC and Other Ancillary Studies (Fig. 5.7e–f)

- Lymphoplasmacytic lymphoma/Waldenström macroglobulinemia lacks a specific immunophenotypic profile.
- Neoplastic lymphocytes demonstrate B-cell markers such as CD19, CD20 (e), CD22, CD79a, CD79b, and PAX5.
- Plasma cells typically demonstrate expression of CD45, CD138 (f), and CD19, while negative for CD56 and cyclin D1.

Final Diagnosis

Lymphoplasmacytic lymphoma/Waldenström macroglobulinemia

Take-Home Messages

1. Lymphoplasmacytic lymphoma/Waldenström macroglobulinemia is comprised by a polymorphous cellular infiltrate including small lymphocytes with scant cytoplasm, lymphocytes with plasmacytoid features, and plasma cells.
2. Lymphoplasmacytic lymphoma/Waldenström macroglobulinemia lacks specific morphologic and immunophenotypic features which makes differential diagnosis with other small B-cell lymphomas with plasmacytic differentiation difficult.
3. Presence of the *MYD88* L265P mutation is a useful diagnostic tool for lymphoplasmacytic lymphoma/Waldenström macroglobulinemia.

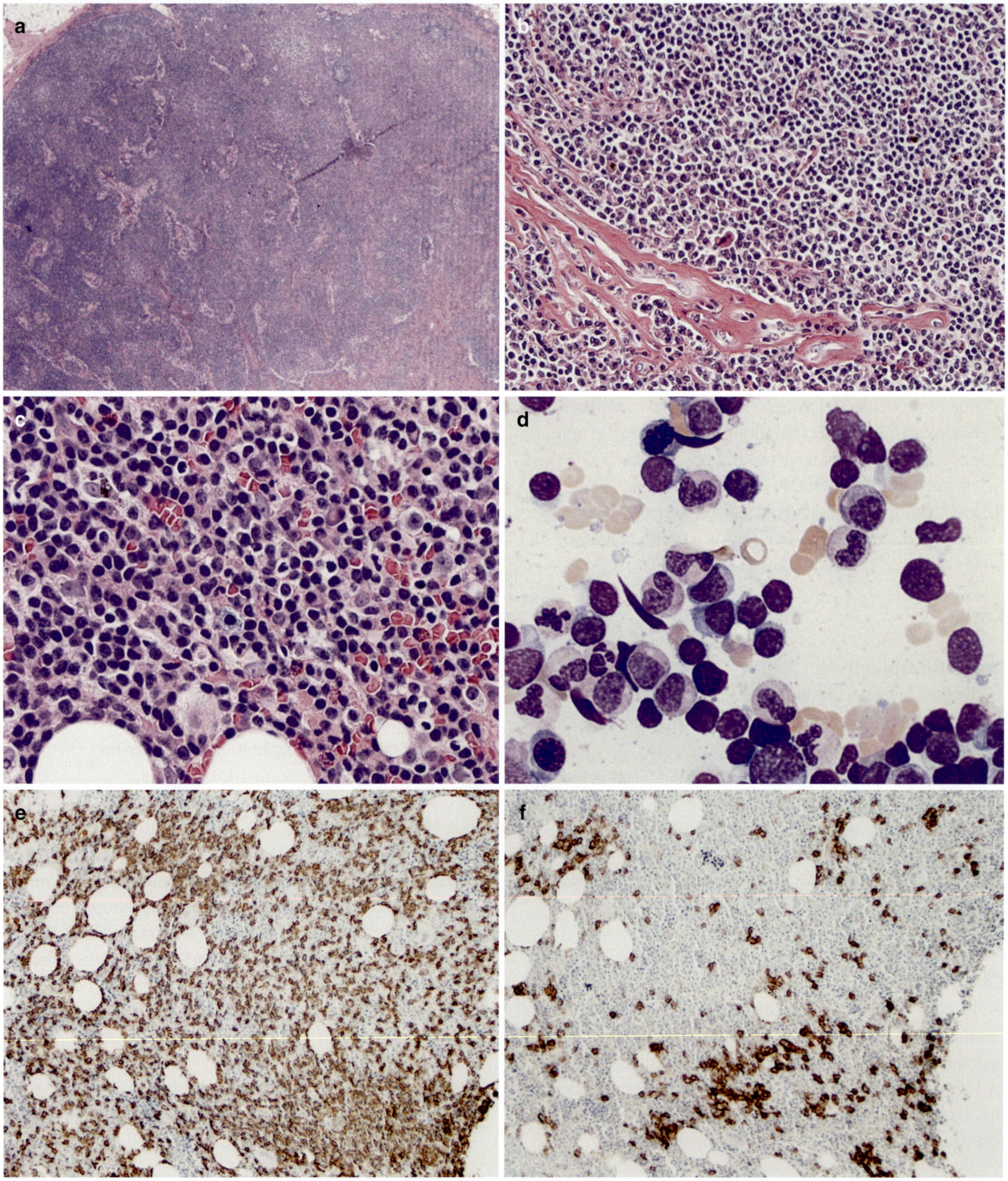

Fig. 5.7 (Case #6). Lymphoplasmacytic lymphoma. (**a**) Lymph node biopsy shows nodal architecture partially effaced by a diffuse to vaguely nodular lymphoid proliferation with patent sinuses. H&E stain, 20×. (**b**) A higher magnification demonstrates a polymorphous lymphoid population comprised of small lymphocytes, plasmacytoid lymphocytes, and plasma cells. H&E stain, 200×. (**c**) Bone marrow aspirate smear shows increase in small lymphocytes and plasmacytoid lymphocytes/plasma cells in the background of hematopoiesis. Wright-Giemsa stain, 600×. (**d**) Bone marrow biopsy demonstrates infiltration of small mature lymphocytes with scattered plasmacytoid cells or plasma cells. H&E stain, 400×. (**e**) CD20 stain highlights an increase in B-cells with interstitial distribution. 100×. (**f**) CD138 stain highlights the plasma cells that appear increased and form small clusters. 100×

References

1. Wang HY, Zu Y. Diagnostic algorithm of common mature B-cell lymphomas by immunohistochemistry. Arch Pathol Lab Med. 2017;141(9):1236–46.
2. Jaso JM, Yin CC, Wang SA, Miranda RN, Jabcuga CE, Chen L, et al. Clinicopathologic features of CD5-positive nodal marginal zone lymphoma. Am J Clin Pathol. 2013;140(5):693–700.
3. Gimeno E, Salido M, Sole F, Florensa L, Granada I, Domingo A, et al. CD5 negative and CD5 positive splenic marginal B-cell lymphomas have differential cytogenetic patterns. Leuk Res. 2005;29(8):981–2.
4. Swerdlow S, Campo E, Harris N, Jaffe E, Pileri S, Stein H, et al. WHO classification of tumours of haematopoietic and lymhoid tissues. Revised 4th ed. Lyon: IARC; 2017.
5. Hunter ZR, Branagan AR, Manning R, Patterson CJ, Santos DD, Tournilhac O, et al. CD5, CD10, and CD23 expression in Waldenstrom's macroglobulinemia. Clin Lymphoma. 2005;5(4):246–9.
6. Dong HY, Gorczyca W, Liu Z, Tsang P, Wu CD, Cohen P, et al. B-cell lymphomas with coexpression of CD5 and CD10. Am J Clin Pathol. 2003;119(2):218–30.
7. Molina TJ, Lin P, Swerdlow SH, Cook JR. Marginal zone lymphomas with plasmacytic differentiation and related disorders. Am J Clin Pathol. 2011;136(2):211–25.
8. Marti GE, Rawstron AC, Ghia P, Hillmen P, Houlston RS, Kay N, et al. Diagnostic criteria for monoclonal B-cell lymphocytosis. Br J Haematol. 2005;130(3):325–32.
9. Hallek M, Cheson BD, Catovsky D, Caligaris-Cappio F, Dighiero G, Dohner H, et al. Guidelines for the diagnosis and treatment of chronic lymphocytic leukemia: a report from the International Workshop on Chronic Lymphocytic Leukemia updating the National Cancer Institute-Working Group 1996 guidelines. Blood. 2008;111(12):5446–56.
10. Rawstron AC, Shanafelt T, Lanasa MC, Landgren O, Hanson C, Orfao A, et al. Different biology and clinical outcome according to the absolute numbers of clonal B-cells in monoclonal B-cell lymphocytosis (MBL). Cytometry B Clin Cytom. 2010;78(Suppl 1):S19–23.
11. Kostopoulos IV, Paterakis G, Papadimitriou K, Pavlidis D, Tsitsilonis OE, Papadhimitriou SI. Immunophenotypic analysis reveals heterogeneity and common biologic aspects in monoclonal B-cell lymphocytosis. Genes Chromosomes Cancer. 2015;54(4):210–21.
12. Fazi C, Scarfo L, Pecciarini L, Cottini F, Dagklis A, Janus A, et al. General population low-count CLL-like MBL persists over time without clinical progression, although carrying the same cytogenetic abnormalities of CLL. Blood. 2011;118(25):6618–25.
13. Rawstron AC, Bennett FL, O'Connor SJ, Kwok M, Fenton JA, Plummer M, et al. Monoclonal B-cell lymphocytosis and chronic lymphocytic leukemia. N Engl J Med. 2008;359(6):575–83.
14. Shanafelt TD, Kay NE, Rabe KG, Call TG, Zent CS, Maddocks K, et al. Brief report: natural history of individuals with clinically recognized monoclonal B-cell lymphocytosis compared with patients with Rai 0 chronic lymphocytic leukemia. J Clin Oncol. 2009;27(24):3959–63.
15. Gibson SE, Swerdlow SH, Ferry JA, Surti U, Dal Cin P, Harris NL, et al. Reassessment of small lymphocytic lymphoma in the era of monoclonal B-cell lymphocytosis. Haematologica. 2011;96(8):1144–52.
16. Morton LM, Wang SS, Devesa SS, Hartge P, Weisenburger DD, Linet MS. Lymphoma incidence patterns by WHO subtype in the United States, 1992-2001. Blood. 2006;107(1):265–76.
17. Noone AM, Howlader N, Krapcho M, Miller D, Brest A, Yu M, et al. SEER cancer statistics review, 1975–2015. Bethesda: National Cancer Institute; 2018.
18. Deegan MJ, Abraham JP, Sawdyk M, Van Slyck EJ. High incidence of monoclonal proteins in the serum and urine of chronic lymphocytic leukemia patients. Blood. 1984;64(6):1207–11.
19. Gine E, Martinez A, Villamor N, Lopez-Guillermo A, Camos M, Martinez D, et al. Expanded and highly active proliferation centers identify a histological subtype of chronic lymphocytic leukemia ("accelerated" chronic lymphocytic leukemia) with aggressive clinical behavior. Haematologica. 2010;95(9):1526–33.
20. Ciccone M, Agostinelli C, Rigolin GM, Piccaluga PP, Cavazzini F, Righi S, et al. Proliferation centers in chronic lymphocytic leukemia: correlation with cytogenetic and clinicobiological features in consecutive patients analyzed on tissue microarrays. Leukemia. 2012;26(3):499–508.
21. Falchi L, Keating MJ, Marom EM, Truong MT, Schlette EJ, Sargent RL, et al. Correlation between FDG/PET, histology, characteristics, and survival in 332 patients with chronic lymphoid leukemia. Blood. 2014;123(18):2783–90.
22. Menter T, Trivedi P, Ahmad R, Flora R, Dirnhofer S, Tzankov A, et al. Diagnostic utility of lymphoid enhancer binding factor 1 immunohistochemistry in small B-cell lymphomas. Am J Clin Pathol. 2017;147(3):292–300.
23. Tandon B, Peterson L, Gao J, Nelson B, Ma S, Rosen S, et al. Nuclear overexpression of lymphoid-enhancer-binding factor 1 identifies chronic lymphocytic leukemia/small lymphocytic lymphoma in small B-cell lymphomas. Mod Pathol. 2011;24(11):1433–43.
24. Palumbo GA, Parrinello N, Fargione G, Cardillo K, Chiarenza A, Berretta S, et al. CD200 expression may help in differential diagnosis between mantle cell lymphoma and B-cell chronic lymphocytic leukemia. Leuk Res. 2009;33(9):1212–6.
25. Espinet B, Ferrer A, Bellosillo B, Nonell L, Salar A, Fernandez-Rodriguez C, et al. Distinction between asymptomatic monoclonal B-cell lymphocytosis with cyclin D1 overexpression and mantle cell lymphoma: from molecular profiling to flow cytometry. Clin Cancer Res. 2014;20(4):1007–19.
26. Zhou Y, Wang H, Fang W, Romaguer JE, Zhang Y, Delasalle KB, et al. Incidence trends of mantle cell lymphoma in the United States between 1992 and 2004. Cancer. 2008;113(4):791–8.
27. Samaha H, Dumontet C, Ketterer N, Moullet I, Thieblemont C, Bouafia F, et al. Mantle cell lymphoma: a retrospective study of 121 cases. Leukemia. 1998;12(8):1281–7.
28. Fernandez V, Salamero O, Espinet B, Sole F, Royo C, Navarro A, et al. Genomic and gene expression profiling defines indolent forms of mantle cell lymphoma. Cancer Res. 2010;70(4):1408–18.
29. Orchard J, Garand R, Davis Z, Babbage G, Sahota S, Matutes E, et al. A subset of t(11;14) lymphoma with mantle cell features displays mutated IgVH genes and includes patients with good prognosis, nonnodal disease. Blood. 2003;101(12):4975–81.
30. Bea S, Valdes-Mas R, Navarro A, Salaverria I, Martin-Garcia D, Jares P, et al. Landscape of somatic mutations and clonal evolution in mantle cell lymphoma. Proc Natl Acad Sci U S A. 2013;110(45):18250–5.
31. Jares P, Colomer D, Campo E. Molecular pathogenesis of mantle cell lymphoma. J Clin Invest. 2012;122(10):3416–23.
32. Ondrejka SL, Lai R, Smith SD, Hsi ED. Indolent mantle cell leukemia: a clinicopathological variant characterized by isolated lymphocytosis, interstitial bone marrow involvement, kappa light chain restriction, and good prognosis. Haematologica. 2011;96(8):1121–7.
33. Majlis A, Pugh WC, Rodriguez MA, Benedict WF, Cabanillas F. Mantle cell lymphoma: correlation of clinical outcome and biologic features with three histologic variants. J Clin Oncol. 1997;15(4):1664–71.
34. Young KH, Chan WC, Fu K, Iqbal J, Sanger WG, Ratashak A, et al. Mantle cell lymphoma with plasma cell differentiation. Am J Surg Pathol. 2006;30(8):954–61.

35. Pinyol M, Hernandez L, Cazorla M, Balbin M, Jares P, Fernandez PL, et al. Deletions and loss of expression of p16INK4a and p21Waf1 genes are associated with aggressive variants of mantle cell lymphomas. Blood. 1997;89(1):272–80.
36. Ott G, Kalla J, Hanke A, Muller JG, Rosenwald A, Katzenberger T, et al. The cytomorphological spectrum of mantle cell lymphoma is reflected by distinct biological features. Leuk Lymphoma. 1998;32(1–2):55–63.
37. Bea S, Ribas M, Hernandez JM, Bosch F, Pinyol M, Hernandez L, et al. Increased number of chromosomal imbalances and high-level DNA amplifications in mantle cell lymphoma are associated with blastoid variants. Blood. 1999;93(12):4365–74.
38. Bosch F, Lopez-Guillermo A, Campo E, Ribera JM, Conde E, Piris MA, et al. Mantle cell lymphoma: presenting features, response to therapy, and prognostic factors. Cancer. 1998;82(3):567–75.
39. Herrero-Vicent C, Machado I, Illueca C, Avaria A, Salazar C, Hernandez A, et al. Diagnostic and therapeutic update of mantle cell lymphoma (MCL): analysis of seven cases treated in a centre in one year. Ecancermedicalscience. 2016;10:627.
40. Yamaguchi M, Seto M, Okamoto M, Ichinohasama R, Nakamura N, Yoshino T, et al. De novo CD5+ diffuse large B-cell lymphoma: a clinicopathologic study of 109 patients. Blood. 2002;99(3):815–21.
41. Al-Kawaaz M, Mathew S, Liu Y, Gomez ML, Chaviano F, Knowles DM, et al. Cyclin D1-positive diffuse large B-cell lymphoma with IGH-CCND1 translocation and BCL6 rearrangement. a report of two cases Am J Clin Pathol. 2015;143(2):288–99.
42. Chuang WY, Chang H, Chang GJ, Wang TH, Chang YS, Wang TH, et al. Pleomorphic mantle cell lymphoma morphologically mimicking diffuse large B cell lymphoma: common cyclin D1 negativity and a simple immunohistochemical algorithm to avoid the diagnostic pitfall. Histopathology. 2017;70(6):986–99.
43. Bermudez G, Gonzalez de Villambrosia S, Martinez-Lopez A, Batlle A, Revert-Arce JB, Cereceda Company L, et al. Incidental and isolated follicular lymphoma in situ and mantle cell lymphoma in situ lack clinical significance. Am J Surg Pathol. 2016;40(7):943–9.
44. Carvajal-Cuenca A, Sua LF, Silva NM, Pittaluga S, Royo C, Song JY, et al. In situ mantle cell lymphoma: clinical implications of an incidental finding with indolent clinical behavior. Haematologica. 2012;97(2):270–8.
45. Jegalian AG, Eberle FC, Pack SD, Mirvis M, Raffeld M, Pittaluga S, et al. Follicular lymphoma in situ: clinical implications and comparisons with partial involvement by follicular lymphoma. Blood. 2011;118(11):2976–84.
46. Carbone A, Santoro A. How I treat: diagnosing and managing "in situ" lymphoma. Blood. 2011;117(15):3954–60.
47. Gradowski JF, Sargent RL, Craig FE, Cieply K, Fuhrer K, Sherer C, et al. Chronic lymphocytic leukemia/small lymphocytic lymphoma with cyclin D1 positive proliferation centers do not have CCND1 translocations or gains and lack SOX11 expression. Am J Clin Pathol. 2012;138(1):132–9.
48. Sherman MJ, Hanson CA, Hoyer JD. An assessment of the usefulness of immunohistochemical stains in the diagnosis of hairy cell leukemia. Am J Clin Pathol. 2011;136(3):390–9.
49. Teixeira Mendes LS, Peters N, Attygalle AD, Wotherspoon A. Cyclin D1 overexpression in proliferation centres of small lymphocytic lymphoma/chronic lymphocytic leukaemia. J Clin Pathol. 2017;70(10):899–902.
50. Hoechtlen-Vollmar W, Menzel G, Bartl R, Lamerz R, Wick M, Seidel D. Amplification of cyclin D1 gene in multiple myeloma: clinical and prognostic relevance. Br J Haematol. 2000;109(1):30–8.
51. Chen YH, Gao J, Fan G, Peterson LC. Nuclear expression of sox11 is highly associated with mantle cell lymphoma but is independent of t(11;14)(q13;q32) in non-mantle cell B-cell neoplasms. Mod Pathol. 2010;23(1):105–12.
52. Narurkar R, Alkayem M, Liu D. SOX11 is a biomarker for cyclin D1-negative mantle cell lymphoma. Biomark Res. 2016;4:6.
53. Muller AM, Ihorst G, Mertelsmann R, Engelhardt M. Epidemiology of non-Hodgkin's lymphoma (NHL): trends, geographic distribution, and etiology. Ann Hematol. 2005;84(1):1–12.
54. Freedman A. Follicular lymphoma: 2018 update on diagnosis and management. Am J Hematol. 2018;93(2):296–305.
55. Montoto S, Davies AJ, Matthews J, Calaminici M, Norton AJ, Amess J, et al. Risk and clinical implications of transformation of follicular lymphoma to diffuse large B-cell lymphoma. J Clin Oncol. 2007;25(17):2426–33.
56. Hans CP, Weisenburger DD, Vose JM, Hock LM, Lynch JC, Aoun P, et al. A significant diffuse component predicts for inferior survival in grade 3 follicular lymphoma, but cytologic subtypes do not predict survival. Blood. 2003;101(6):2363–7.
57. Katzenberger T, Kalla J, Leich E, Stocklein H, Hartmann E, Barnickel S, et al. A distinctive subtype of t(14;18)-negative nodal follicular non-Hodgkin lymphoma characterized by a predominantly diffuse growth pattern and deletions in the chromosomal region 1p36. Blood. 2009;113(5):1053–61.
58. Siddiqi IN, Friedman J, Barry-Holson KQ, Ma C, Thodima V, Kang I, et al. Characterization of a variant of t(14;18) negative nodal diffuse follicular lymphoma with CD23 expression, 1p36/TNFRSF14 abnormalities, and STAT6 mutations. Mod Pathol. 2016;29(6):570–81.
59. Wang SA, Wang L, Hochberg EP, Muzikansky A, Harris NL, Hasserjian RP. Low histologic grade follicular lymphoma with high proliferation index: morphologic and clinical features. Am J Surg Pathol. 2005;29(11):1490–6.
60. Koster A, Tromp HA, Raemaekers JM, Borm GF, Hebeda K, Mackenzie MA, et al. The prognostic significance of the intrafollicular tumor cell proliferative rate in follicular lymphoma. Haematologica. 2007;92(2):184–90.
61. Cong P, Raffeld M, Teruya-Feldstein J, Sorbara L, Pittaluga S, Jaffe ES. In situ localization of follicular lymphoma: description and analysis by laser capture microdissection. Blood. 2002;99(9):3376–82.
62. Eshoa C, Perkins S, Kampalath B, Shidham V, Juckett M, Chang CC. Decreased CD10 expression in grade III and in interfollicular infiltrates of follicular lymphomas. Am J Clin Pathol. 2001;115(6):862–7.
63. Yegappan S, Schnitzer B, Hsi ED. Follicular lymphoma with marginal zone differentiation: microdissection demonstrates the t(14;18) in both the follicular and marginal zone components. Mod Pathol. 2001;14(3):191–6.
64. Lai R, Arber DA, Chang KL, Wilson CS, Weiss LM. Frequency of bcl-2 expression in non-Hodgkin's lymphoma: a study of 778 cases with comparison of marginal zone lymphoma and monocytoid B-cell hyperplasia. Mod Pathol. 1998;11(9):864–9.
65. Pezzella F, Tse AG, Cordell JL, Pulford KA, Gatter KC, Mason DY. Expression of the bcl-2 oncogene protein is not specific for the 14;18 chromosomal translocation. Am J Pathol. 1990;137(2):225–32.
66. Schraders M, de Jong D, Kluin P, Groenen P, van Krieken H. Lack of Bcl-2 expression in follicular lymphoma may be caused by mutations in the BCL2 gene or by absence of the t(14;18) translocation. J Pathol. 2005;205(3):329–35.
67. Menter T, Gasser A, Juskevicius D, Dirnhofer S, Tzankov A. Diagnostic utility of the germinal center-associated markers GCET1, HGAL, and LMO2 in hematolymphoid neoplasms. Appl Immunohistochem Mol Morphol. 2015;23(7):491–8.
68. Ferreri AJ, Zucca E. Marginal-zone lymphoma. Crit Rev Oncol Hematol. 2007;63(3):245–56.
69. Khalil MO, Morton LM, Devesa SS, Check DP, Curtis RE, Weisenburger DD, et al. Incidence of marginal zone lymphoma in the United States, 2001-2009 with a focus on primary anatomic site. Br J Haematol. 2014;165(1):67–77.

70. Chacon JI, Mollejo M, Munoz E, Algara P, Mateo M, Lopez L, et al. Splenic marginal zone lymphoma: clinical characteristics and prognostic factors in a series of 60 patients. Blood. 2002;100(5):1648–54.
71. Berger F, Felman P, Thieblemont C, Pradier T, Baseggio L, Bryon PA, et al. Non-MALT marginal zone B-cell lymphomas: a description of clinical presentation and outcome in 124 patients. Blood. 2000;95(6):1950–6.
72. Traverse-Glehen A, Bertoni F, Thieblemont C, Zucca E, Coiffier B, Berger F, et al. Nodal marginal zone B-cell lymphoma: a diagnostic and therapeutic dilemma. Oncology (Williston Park). 2012;26(1):92-9, 103-4.
73. Campo E, Miquel R, Krenacs L, Sorbara L, Raffeld M, Jaffe ES. Primary nodal marginal zone lymphomas of splenic and MALT type. Am J Surg Pathol. 1999;23(1):59–68.
74. Mollejo M, Camacho FI, Algara P, Ruiz-Ballesteros E, Garcia JF, Piris MA. Nodal and splenic marginal zone B cell lymphomas. Hematol Oncol. 2005;23(3–4):108–18.
75. Castillo JJ, Olszewski AJ, Kanan S, Meid K, Hunter ZR, Treon SP. Overall survival and competing risks of death in patients with Waldenström macroglobulinaemia: an analysis of the Surveillance, Epidemiology and End Results database. Br J Haematol. 2015;169(1):81–9.
76. Sekhar J, Sanfilippo K, Zhang Q, Trinkaus K, Vij R, Morgensztern D. Waldenstrom macroglobulinemia: a surveillance, epidemiology, and end results database review from 1988 to 2005. Leuk Lymphoma. 2012;53(8):1625–6.
77. Banwait R, Aljawai Y, Cappuccio J, McDiarmid S, Morgan EA, Leblebjian H, et al. Extramedullary Waldenstrom macroglobulinemia. Am J Hematol. 2015;90(2):100–4.
78. Lin P, Bueso-Ramos C, Wilson CS, Mansoor A, Medeiros LJ. Waldenstrom macroglobulinemia involving extramedullary sites: morphologic and immunophenotypic findings in 44 patients. Am J Surg Pathol. 2003;27(8):1104–13.
79. Cesana C, Barbarano L, Miqueleiz S, Lucchesini C, Ricci F, Varettoni M, et al. Clinical characteristics and outcome of immunoglobulin M-related disorders. Clin Lymphoma. 2005;5(4):261–4.
80. Dimopoulos MA, Gertz MA, Kastritis E, Garcia-Sanz R, Kimby EK, Leblond V, et al. Update on treatment recommendations from the Fourth International Workshop on Waldenstrom's Macroglobulinemia. J Clin Oncol. 2009;27(1):120–6.
81. Merlini G, Baldini L, Broglia C, Comelli M, Goldaniga M, Palladini G, et al. Prognostic factors in symptomatic Waldenstrom's macroglobulinemia. Semin Oncol. 2003;30(2):211–5.
82. Nobile-Orazio E, Marmiroli P, Baldini L, Spagnol G, Barbieri S, Moggio M, et al. Peripheral neuropathy in macroglobulinemia: incidence and antigen-specificity of M proteins. Neurology. 1987;37(9):1506–14.
83. Silberman J, Lonial S. Review of peripheral neuropathy in plasma cell disorders. Hematol Oncol. 2008;26(2):55–65.
84. Gertz MA, Kyle RA, Noel P. Primary systemic amyloidosis: a rare complication of immunoglobulin M monoclonal gammopathies and Waldenstrom's macroglobulinemia. J Clin Oncol. 1993;11(5):914–20.
85. Cao X, Medeiros LJ, Xia Y, Wang X, Thomas SK, Loghavi S, et al. Clinicopathologic features and outcomes of lymphoplasmacytic lymphoma patients with monoclonal IgG or IgA paraprotein expression. Leuk Lymphoma. 2016;57(5):1104–13.
86. Minnema MC, Kimby E, D'Sa S, Fornecker LM, Poulain S, Snijders TJ, et al. Guideline for the diagnosis, treatment and response criteria for Bing-Neel syndrome. Haematologica. 2017;102(1):43–51.
87. Policepatil SM, Go RS, Zeng GG. Floral variant of follicular lymphoma. Am J Hematol. 2011;86(6):503.
88. Kojima M, Yamanaka S, Yoshida T, Shimizu K, Murayama K, Ohno Y, et al. Histological variety of floral variant of follicular lymphoma. APMIS. 2006;114(9):626–32.
89. Younes SF, Beck AH, Lossos IS, Levy R, Warnke RA, Natkunam Y. Immunoarchitectural patterns in follicular lymphoma: efficacy of HGAL and LMO2 in the detection of the interfollicular and diffuse components. Am J Surg Pathol. 2010;34(9):1266–76.
90. Nathwani BN, Anderson JR, Armitage JO, Cavalli F, Diebold J, Drachenberg MR, et al. Clinical significance of follicular lymphoma with monocytoid B cells. Non-Hodgkin's Lymphoma Classification Project. Hum Pathol. 1999;30(3):263–8.
91. Muller-Hermelink HK, Zettl A, Pfeifer W, Ott G. Pathology of lymphoma progression. Histopathology. 2001;38(4):285–306.
92. Keith TA, Cousar JB, Glick AD, Vogler LB, Collins RD. Plasmacytic differentiation in follicular center cell (FCC) lymphomas. Am J Clin Pathol. 1985;84(3):283–90.
93. Matsuda I, Shimizu Y, Okamoto T, Hirota S. Follicular lymphoma mimicking marginal zone lymphoma in lymph node: a case report. Int J Clin Exp Pathol. 2014;7(10):7076–81.
94. Vago JF, Hurtubise PE, Redden-Borowski MM, Martelo OJ, Swerdlow SH. Follicular center-cell lymphoma with plasmacytic differentiation, monoclonal paraprotein, and peripheral blood involvement. Recapitulation of normal B-cell development. Am J Surg Pathol. 1985;9(10):764–70.
95. Lai R, Weiss LM, Chang KL, Arber DA. Frequency of CD43 expression in non-Hodgkin lymphoma. A survey of 742 cases and further characterization of rare CD43+ follicular lymphomas. Am J Clin Pathol. 1999;111(4):488–94.
96. van den Brand M, van Krieken JH. Recognizing nodal marginal zone lymphoma: recent advances and pitfalls. A systematic review. Haematologica. 2013;98(7):1003–13.
97. Seegmiller AC, Xu Y, McKenna RW, Karandikar NJ. Immunophenotypic differentiation between neoplastic plasma cells in mature B-cell lymphoma vs plasma cell myeloma. Am J Clin Pathol. 2007;127(2):176–81.
98. Lin P, Hao S, Handy BC, Bueso-Ramos CE, Medeiros LJ. Lymphoid neoplasms associated with IgM paraprotein: a study of 382 patients. Am J Clin Pathol. 2005;123(2):200–5.
99. Evans HL, Polski JM, Deshpande V, Dunphy CH. CD5+ true SLL/CLL with plasmacytic differentiation and an unusual 1p36 translocation: case report and review of the literature. Leuk Lymphoma. 2000;39(5–6):625–32.
100. Lin P, Molina TJ, Cook JR, Swerdlow SH. Lymphoplasmacytic lymphoma and other non-marginal zone lymphomas with plasmacytic differentiation. Am J Clin Pathol. 2011;136(2):195–210.
101. Rosado FG, Morice WG, He R, Howard MT, Timm M, McPhail ED. Immunophenotypic features by multiparameter flow cytometry can help distinguish low grade B-cell lymphomas with plasmacytic differentiation from plasma cell proliferative disorders with an unrelated clonal B-cell process. Br J Haematol. 2015;169(3):368–76.
102. Cozzolino I, Vigliar E, Sosa Fernandez LV, Selleri C, Pepe S, Vitale M, et al. Non lymphomatous clonal B-cell populations in enlarged lymph nodes in acquired immunodeficiency syndrome. Infez Med. 2012;20(Suppl 2):35–42.
103. Jordan RC, Masaki Y, Takeshita S, Speight PM, Sugai S. High prevalence of B-cell monoclonality in labial gland biopsies of Japanese Sjogren's syndrome patients. Int J Hematol. 1996;64(1):47–52.
104. Kussick SJ, Kalnoski M, Braziel RM, Wood BL. Prominent clonal B-cell populations identified by flow cytometry in histologically reactive lymphoid proliferations. Am J Clin Pathol. 2004;121(4):464–72.
105. Matsubayashi S, Tamai H, Morita T, Fukata S, Matsuzuka F, Suzuki T, et al. Hashimoto's thyroiditis manifesting monoclonal lymphocytic infiltration. Clin Exp Immunol. 1990;79(2):170–4.
106. Locker J, Nalesnik M. Molecular genetic analysis of lymphoid tumors arising after organ transplantation. Am J Pathol. 1989;135(6):977–87.

107. Pelicci PG, Knowles DM, Arlin ZA, Wieczorek R, Luciw P, Dina D, et al. Multiple monoclonal B cell expansions and c-myc oncogene rearrangements in acquired immune deficiency syndrome-related lymphoproliferative disorders. Implications for lymphomagenesis. J Exp Med. 1986;164(6):2049–60.
108. Lu C, He Q, Zhu W, Fu C, Zhou J, Tao Y, et al. The value of detecting immunoglobulin gene rearrangements in the diagnosis of B-cell lymphoma. Oncotarget. 2017;8(44):77009–19.
109. Dohner H, Stilgenbauer S, Benner A, Leupolt E, Krober A, Bullinger L, et al. Genomic aberrations and survival in chronic lymphocytic leukemia. N Engl J Med. 2000;343(26):1910–6.
110. Arcaini L, Lucioni M, Boveri E, Paulli M. Nodal marginal zone lymphoma: current knowledge and future directions of an heterogeneous disease. Eur J Haematol. 2009;83(3):165–74.
111. Ayyappan S, William BM. Marginal zone lymphoma: clinicopathologic variations and approaches to therapy. Curr Oncol Rep. 2018;20(4):33.
112. Leich E, Salaverria I, Bea S, Zettl A, Wright G, Moreno V, et al. Follicular lymphomas with and without translocation t(14;18) differ in gene expression profiles and genetic alterations. Blood. 2009;114(4):826–34.
113. Treon SP, Xu L, Yang G, Zhou Y, Liu X, Cao Y, et al. MYD88 L265P somatic mutation in Waldenstrom's macroglobulinemia. N Engl J Med. 2012;367(9):826–33.
114. Gachard N, Parrens M, Soubeyran I, Petit B, Marfak A, Rizzo D, et al. IGHV gene features and MYD88 L265P mutation separate the three marginal zone lymphoma entities and Waldenstrom macroglobulinemia/lymphoplasmacytic lymphomas. Leukemia. 2013;27(1):183–9.
115. Ngo VN, Young RM, Schmitz R, Jhavar S, Xiao W, Lim KH, et al. Oncogenically active MYD88 mutations in human lymphoma. Nature. 2011;470(7332):115–9.
116. Nakamura T, Tateishi K, Niwa T, Matsushita Y, Tamura K, Kinoshita M, et al. Recurrent mutations of CD79B and MYD88 are the hallmark of primary central nervous system lymphomas. Neuropathol Appl Neurobiol. 2016;42(3):279–90.
117. Kraan W, Horlings HM, van Keimpema M, Schilder-Tol EJ, Oud ME, Scheepstra C, et al. High prevalence of oncogenic MYD88 and CD79B mutations in diffuse large B-cell lymphomas presenting at immune-privileged sites. Blood Cancer J. 2013;3:e139.
118. Pham-Ledard A, Beylot-Barry M, Barbe C, Leduc M, Petrella T, Vergier B, et al. High frequency and clinical prognostic value of MYD88 L265P mutation in primary cutaneous diffuse large B-cell lymphoma, leg-type. JAMA Dermatol. 2014;150(11):1173–9.
119. Landgren O, Tageja N. MYD88 and beyond: novel opportunities for diagnosis, prognosis and treatment in Waldenstrom's Macroglobulinemia. Leukemia. 2014;28(9):1799–803.
120. Cheah CY, Seymour JF, Wang ML. Mantle cell lymphoma. J Clin Oncol. 2016;34(11):1256–69.
121. Damle RN, Wasil T, Fais F, Ghiotto F, Valetto A, Allen SL, et al. Ig V gene mutation status and CD38 expression as novel prognostic indicators in chronic lymphocytic leukemia. Blood. 1999;94(6):1840–7.
122. Durig J, Naschar M, Schmucker U, Renzing-Kohler K, Holter T, Huttmann A, et al. CD38 expression is an important prognostic marker in chronic lymphocytic leukaemia. Leukemia. 2002;16(1):30–5.
123. Ibrahim S, Keating M, Do KA, O'Brien S, Huh YO, Jilani I, et al. CD38 expression as an important prognostic factor in B-cell chronic lymphocytic leukemia. Blood. 2001;98(1):181–6.
124. Jelinek DF, Tschumper RC, Geyer SM, Bone ND, Dewald GW, Hanson CA, et al. Analysis of clonal B-cell CD38 and immunoglobulin variable region sequence status in relation to clinical outcome for B-chronic lymphocytic leukaemia. Br J Haematol. 2001;115(4):854–61.
125. Bulian P, Shanafelt TD, Fegan C, Zucchetto A, Cro L, Nuckel H, et al. CD49d is the strongest flow cytometry-based predictor of overall survival in chronic lymphocytic leukemia. J Clin Oncol. 2014;32(9):897–904.
126. Hamblin TJ, Davis Z, Gardiner A, Oscier DG, Stevenson FK. Unmutated Ig V(H) genes are associated with a more aggressive form of chronic lymphocytic leukemia. Blood. 1999;94(6):1848–54.
127. Rosenwald A, Alizadeh AA, Widhopf G, Simon R, Davis RE, Yu X, et al. Relation of gene expression phenotype to immunoglobulin mutation genotype in B cell chronic lymphocytic leukemia. J Exp Med. 2001;194(11):1639–47.
128. Durig J, Nuckel H, Cremer M, Fuhrer A, Halfmeyer K, Fandrey J, et al. ZAP-70 expression is a prognostic factor in chronic lymphocytic leukemia. Leukemia. 2003;17(12):2426–34.
129. Bakke AC, Purtzer Z, Leis J, Huang J. A robust ratio metric method for analysis of Zap-70 expression in chronic lymphocytic leukemia (CLL). Cytometry B Clin Cytom. 2006;70(4):227–34.
130. Gibbs G, Bromidge T, Howe D, Hopkins J, Johnson S. Comparison of flow cytometric methods for the measurement of ZAP-70 expression in a routine diagnostic laboratory. Clin Lab Haematol. 2005;27(4):258–66.
131. Chen YH, Peterson LC, Dittmann D, Evens A, Rosen S, Khoong A, et al. Comparative analysis of flow cytometric techniques in assessment of ZAP-70 expression in relation to IgVH mutational status in chronic lymphocytic leukemia. Am J Clin Pathol. 2007;127(2):182–91.
132. Dal-Bo M, Del Giudice I, Bomben R, Capello D, Bertoni F, Forconi F, et al. B-cell receptor, clinical course and prognosis in chronic lymphocytic leukaemia: the growing saga of the IGHV3 subgroup gene usage. Br J Haematol. 2011;153(1):3–14.
133. Crespo M, Bosch F, Villamor N, Bellosillo B, Colomer D, Rozman M, et al. ZAP-70 expression as a surrogate for immunoglobulin-variable-region mutations in chronic lymphocytic leukemia. N Engl J Med. 2003;348(18):1764–75.
134. Rosenquist R, Rosenwald A, Du MQ, Gaidano G, Groenen P, Wotherspoon A, et al. Clinical impact of recurrently mutated genes on lymphoma diagnostics: state-of-the-art and beyond. Haematologica. 2016;101(9):1002–9.
135. Malcikova J, Smardova J, Rocnova L, Tichy B, Kuglik P, Vranova V, et al. Monoallelic and biallelic inactivation of TP53 gene in chronic lymphocytic leukemia: selection, impact on survival, and response to DNA damage. Blood. 2009;114(26):5307–14.
136. Zenz T, Eichhorst B, Busch R, Denzel T, Habe S, Winkler D, et al. TP53 mutation and survival in chronic lymphocytic leukemia. J Clin Oncol. 2010;28(29):4473–9.
137. Stilgenbauer S, Furman RR, Zent CS. Management of chronic lymphocytic leukemia. Am Soc Clin Oncol Educ Book. 2015: 164–75.
138. Hoster E, Dreyling M, Klapper W, Gisselbrecht C, van Hoof A, Kluin-Nelemans HC, et al. A new prognostic index (MIPI) for patients with advanced-stage mantle cell lymphoma. Blood. 2008;111(2):558–65.
139. Geisler CH, Kolstad A, Laurell A, Raty R, Jerkeman M, Eriksson M, et al. The Mantle Cell Lymphoma International Prognostic Index (MIPI) is superior to the International Prognostic Index (IPI) in predicting survival following intensive first-line immunochemotherapy and autologous stem cell transplantation (ASCT). Blood. 2010;115(8):1530–3.
140. Determann O, Hoster E, Ott G, Wolfram Bernd H, Loddenkemper C, Leo Hansmann M, et al. Ki-67 predicts outcome in advanced-stage mantle cell lymphoma patients treated with anti-CD20 immunochemotherapy: results from randomized trials of the European MCL Network and the German Low Grade Lymphoma Study Group. Blood. 2008;111(4):2385–7.

141. Mozos A, Royo C, Hartmann E, De Jong D, Baro C, Valera A, et al. SOX11 expression is highly specific for mantle cell lymphoma and identifies the cyclin D1-negative subtype. Haematologica. 2009;94(11):1555–62.
142. Halldorsdottir AM, Lundin A, Murray F, Mansouri L, Knuutila S, Sundstrom C, et al. Impact of TP53 mutation and 17p deletion in mantle cell lymphoma. Leukemia. 2011;25(12):1904–8.
143. Zhang J, Jima D, Moffitt AB, Liu Q, Czader M, Hsi ED, et al. The genomic landscape of mantle cell lymphoma is related to the epigenetically determined chromatin state of normal B cells. Blood. 2014;123(19):2988–96.
144. Bernard M, Gressin R, Lefrere F, Drenou B, Branger B, Caulet-Maugendre S, et al. Blastic variant of mantle cell lymphoma: a rare but highly aggressive subtype. Leukemia. 2001;15(11):1785–91.
145. Louie DC, Offit K, Jaslow R, Parsa NZ, Murty VV, Schluger A, et al. p53 overexpression as a marker of poor prognosis in mantle cell lymphomas with t(11;14)(q13;q32). Blood. 1995;86(8):2892–9.
146. Wotherspoon AC, Doglioni C, Diss TC, Pan L, Moschini A, de Boni M, et al. Regression of primary low-grade B-cell gastric lymphoma of mucosa-associated lymphoid tissue type after eradication of Helicobacter pylori. Lancet. 1993;342(8871):575–7.
147. Liu H, Ye H, Ruskone-Fourmestraux A, De Jong D, Pileri S, Thiede C, et al. T(11;18) is a marker for all stage gastric MALT lymphomas that will not respond to H. pylori eradication. Gastroenterology. 2002;122(5):1286–94.
148. Ye H, Liu H, Raderer M, Chott A, Ruskone-Fourmestraux A, Wotherspoon A, et al. High incidence of t(11;18)(q21;q21) in Helicobacter pylori-negative gastric MALT lymphoma. Blood. 2003;101(7):2547–50.
149. Hunter ZR, Xu L, Yang G, Zhou Y, Liu X, Cao Y, et al. The genomic landscape of Waldenstrom macroglobulinemia is characterized by highly recurring MYD88 and WHIM-like CXCR4 mutations, and small somatic deletions associated with B-cell lymphomagenesis. Blood. 2014;123(11):1637–46.
150. Treon SP, Cao Y, Xu L, Yang G, Liu X, Hunter ZR. Somatic mutations in MYD88 and CXCR4 are determinants of clinical presentation and overall survival in Waldenstrom macroglobulinemia. Blood. 2014;123(18):2791–6.
151. Treon SP, Tripsas CK, Meid K, Warren D, Varma G, Green R, et al. Ibrutinib in previously treated Waldenstrom's macroglobulinemia. N Engl J Med. 2015;372(15):1430–40.
152. Chang CC, Osipov V, Wheaton S, Tripp S, Perkins SL. Follicular hyperplasia, follicular lysis, and progressive transformation of germinal centers. A sequential spectrum of morphologic evolution in lymphoid hyperplasia. Am J Clin Pathol. 2003;120(3):322–6.
153. Arber DA, George TI. Bone marrow biopsy involvement by non-Hodgkin's lymphoma: frequency of lymphoma types, patterns, blood involvement, and discordance with other sites in 450 specimens. Am J Surg Pathol. 2005;29(12):1549–57.
154. Zhang QY, Foucar K. Bone marrow involvement by Hodgkin and non-Hodgkin lymphomas. Hematol Oncol Clin North Am. 2009;23(4):873–902.
155. Viswanatha D, Foucar K. Hodgkin and non-Hodgkin lymphoma involving bone marrow. Semin Diagn Pathol. 2003;20(3):196–210.
156. Schmidt B, Kremer M, Gotze K, John K, Peschel C, Hofler H, et al. Bone marrow involvement in follicular lymphoma: comparison of histology and flow cytometry as staging procedures. Leuk Lymphoma. 2006;47(9):1857–62.
157. Strati P, Shanafelt TD. Monoclonal B-cell lymphocytosis and early-stage chronic lymphocytic leukemia: diagnosis, natural history, and risk stratification. Blood. 2015;126(4):454–62.
158. Inamdar KV, Medeiros LJ, Jorgensen JL, Amin HM, Schlette EJ. Bone marrow involvement by marginal zone B-cell lymphomas of different types. Am J Clin Pathol. 2008;129(5):714–22.
159. Kent SA, Variakojis D, Peterson LC. Comparative study of marginal zone lymphoma involving bone marrow. Am J Clin Pathol. 2002;117(5):698–708.
160. Engels K, Oeschger S, Hansmann ML, Hillebrand M, Kriener S. Bone marrow trephines containing lymphoid aggregates from patients with rheumatoid and other autoimmune disorders frequently show clonal B-cell infiltrates. Hum Pathol. 2007;38(9):1402–11.
161. Franco V, Florena AM, Aragona F, Campesi G. Immunohistochemical evaluation of bone marrow lymphoid nodules in chronic myeloproliferative disorders. Virchows Arch A Pathol Anat Histopathol. 1991;419(4):261–6.
162. Johnston A, Brynes RK, Naemi K, Reisian N, Bhansali D, Zhao X, et al. Differentiating benign from malignant bone marrow B-cell lymphoid aggregates: a statistical analysis of distinguishing features. Arch Pathol Lab Med. 2015;139(2):233–40.
163. Sovani V, Harvey C, Haynes AP, McMillan AK, Clark DM, O'Connor SR. Bone marrow trephine biopsy involvement by lymphoma: review of histopathological features in 511 specimens and correlation with diagnostic biopsy, aspirate and peripheral blood findings. J Clin Pathol. 2014;67(5):389–95.
164. Johl A, Lengfelder E, Hiddemann W, Klapper W. Core needle biopsies and surgical excision biopsies in the diagnosis of lymphoma-experience at the Lymph Node Registry Kiel. Ann Hematol. 2016;95(8):1281–6.
165. Frederiksen JK, Sharma M, Casulo C, Burack WR. Systematic review of the effectiveness of fine-needle aspiration and/or core needle biopsy for subclassifying lymphoma. Arch Pathol Lab Med. 2015;139(2):245–51.
166. Zhang QY, Chabot-Richards D, Evans M, Spengel K, Andrews J, Kang H, et al. A retrospective study to assess the relative value of peripheral blood, bone marrow aspirate and biopsy morphology, immunohistochemical stains, and flow cytometric analysis in the diagnosis of chronic B cell lymphoproliferative neoplasms. Int J Lab Hematol. 2015;37(3):390–402.
167. Gujral S, Polampalli SN, Badrinath Y, Kumar A, Subramanian PG, Nair R, et al. Immunophenotyping of mature B-cell non Hodgkin lymphoma involving bone marrow and peripheral blood: critical analysis and insights gained at a tertiary care cancer hospital. Leuk Lymphoma. 2009;50(8):1290–300.

6 Large B-Cell Lymphoma

Zenggang Pan

List of Frequently Asked Questions

1. How is diffuse large B-cell lymphoma (DLBCL) classified?
2. What are the major subtypes of DLBCL?
3. What are the typical clinical features of DLBCL?
4. What are the common morphologic features of DLBCL?
5. What are the unusual morphologic variants of DLBCL?
6. What are the major genetic changes in DLBCL?
7. What are the important poor prognostic factors in DLBCL?
8. What are the major differential diagnoses of DLBCL?
9. What is the initial workup for the cases with morphologic features of DLBCL?
10. What is the further workup after initial studies of the potential DLBCL cases?
11. What are the major pitfalls and recommendations in the workup of DLBCL with immunohistochemical stains?
12. What are the major clinicopathologic features of T-cell/histiocyte-rich large B-cell lymphoma (THRLBCL)?
13. How is THRLBCL distinguished from conventional DLBCL?
14. How is THRLBCL distinguished from nodular lymphocyte predominant Hodgkin lymphoma (NLPHL)?
15. What are the major clinicopathologic features of primary central nervous system DLBCL (PCNS DLBCL)?
16. What are the major clinicopathologic features of primary mediastinal (thymic) large B-cell lymphoma (PMLBCL)?
17. What is the initial workup for the cases with morphologic features of PMLBCL?
18. How is PMLBCL distinguished from mediastinal classic Hodgkin lymphoma (CHL)?
19. How is PMLBCL distinguished from conventional DLBCL?
20. What are the other differential diagnoses of PMLBCL?
21. What are the major clinicopathologic features of intravascular large B-cell lymphoma (IVLBCL)?
22. What are the major clinicopathologic features of primary cutaneous DLBCL, leg type (PCDLBCL-LT)?
23. What are the major clinicopathologic features of lymphomatoid granulomatosis (LyG)?
24. How is LyG distinguished from extranodal NK-/T-cell lymphoma, nasal type?
25. How is LyG distinguished from granulomatosis with polyangiitis (GPA), formerly known as Wegener granulomatosis?
26. What are the major clinical features of ALK+ large B-cell lymphoma (ALK+ LBCL)?
27. What are the typical morphologic and immunophenotypic features of ALK+ LBCL?
28. What are the common and uncommon chromosomal rearrangements in ALK+ LBCL?
29. How is ALK+ LBCL distinguished from ALK+ anaplastic large cell lymphoma?
30. What are the major differential diagnoses of a high-grade neoplasm in the lymph node with predominant sinus infiltrative pattern?
31. What are the major clinicopathologic features of plasmablastic lymphoma (PBL)?
32. How is PBL distinguished from solid variant of primary effusion lymphoma (PEL)?
33. How is PBL distinguished from plasmablastic plasmacytoma?
34. What are the major clinicopathologic features of extracavitary PEL?
35. What are the major clinicopathologic features of conventional PEL?
36. What is the initial workup for the cases with plasmablastic morphologic features?
37. What is the definition of *EBV*+ DLBCL, NOS?

Z. Pan (✉)
Department of Pathology, Yale University School of Medicine, New Haven, CT, USA
e-mail: zenggang.pan@yale.edu

E. Wang, A. S. Lagoo (eds.), *Practical Lymph Node and Bone Marrow Pathology*, Practical Anatomic Pathology,
https://doi.org/10.1007/978-3-030-32189-5_6

38. What are the major clinicopathologic features of *EBV*+ DLBCL, NOS?
39. How is *EBV*+ DLBCL, NOS, distinguished from mucocutaneous ulcer (MCU)?
40. What is the definition of "high-grade B-cell lymphoma (HGBL) with *MYC* and *BCL2* and/or *BCL6* rearrangement?"
41. What are the major clinicopathologic features of "high-grade B-cell lymphoma with *MYC* and *BCL2* and/or *BCL6* rearrangement?"
42. How is "HGBL with *MYC* and *BCL2* and/or *BCL6* rearrangement" distinguished from Burkitt lymphoma?

1. How is diffuse large B-cell lymphoma (DLBCL) classified?

DLBCL is heterogeneous with variable clinical presentations, morphologic features, immunophenotype, genetic changes, and outcomes. Thus, classification of DLBCL takes account of all these aspects. A large proportion of DLBCLs cannot fit into any specific subtype and therefore is classified as "DLBCL, not otherwise specified (NOS)." [1–8]

2. What are the major subtypes of DLBCL?

DLBCL shows diverse morphologic features and is divided into three major morphologic variants, centroblastic, immunoblastic, and anaplastic. In addition, several minor morphologic variants have rarely been reported. By cell of origin, two major subtypes of DLBCL have been identified based on gene expression profiling and immunohistochemical staining, germinal center B-cell-like (GCB) and activated B-cell-like (ABC), representing ~50% and ~40% of DLBCL, respectively. The ABC-DLBCL is associated with inferior progression-free survival (PFS), event-free survival, and overall survival (OS), in contrast to the GCB subtype. Several specific types of DLBCLs are also defined based on clinicopathological features. Finally, three categories of large B-cell lymphomas with borderline features are also clinically important.

Classification of DLBCLs

DLBCL, NOS

- Morphologic variants
  - Centroblastic
  - Immunoblastic
  - Anaplastic
  - Other rare variants
- Molecular subtypes
  - Germinal center B-cell-like (GCB)
  - Activated B-cell type (ABC)

Specific types of DLBCLs

- T-cell/histiocyte-rich LBCL
- Primary DLBCL of the central nervous system
- Primary cutaneous DLBCL, leg type
- *EBV*+ DLBCL, NOS
- Primary mediastinal (thymic) LBCL
- Intravascular LBCL
- DLBCL associated with chronic inflammation
- Lymphomatoid granulomatosis
- ALK+ LBCL
- Plasmablastic lymphoma
- HHV8-positive DLBCL
- Primary effusion lymphoma
- LBCL with *IRF4* rearrangement (provisional entity)

Borderline types of DLBCLs (See also Chap. 7 for detailed discussion of high grade B-cell lymphomas).

- High-grade B-cell lymphoma with *MYC* and *BCL2* and/or *BCL6* rearrangement
- High-grade B-cell lymphoma, NOS
- B-cell lymphoma, unclassifiable, with features intermediate between DLBCL and classic Hodgkin lymphoma [2, 8, 9]

3. What are the typical clinical features of DLBCL?

- Mostly affects the old patients with a median age of 64 years and a slight male predominance, with a male to female ratio of 1.2:1.
- Majority of cases involve the lymph nodes primarily, but ~30% are diagnosed in extranodal sites.
- Clinical presentations: Rapidly growing lymph nodes or masses in the extranodal sites. Nearly 50% of patients show advanced disease at diagnosis (stage III to IV). Approximately 1/3 of patients present with B symptoms. Bone marrow involvement is not common, detected in <20% of cases.
- Prognosis: Although DLBCL is aggressive, it is potentially curable, and >50% of DLBCLs can be cured with R-CHOP.

4. What are the common morphologic features of DLBCL?

DLBCL reveals a diffuse infiltration in the tissue by medium to large tumor cells. In the lymph nodes, the architecture is completely or partially effaced, and rare cases may show an interfollicular or sinusoidal infiltrative pattern. Frequent apoptotic cells and mitotic figures are present, and areas of coagulative necrosis are commonly noted. Occasional cases may display a "starry sky" appearance, which resemble Burkitt lymphoma at low magnification.

Cytologically, DLBCLs show centroblastic, immunoblastic, and/or cells with intermediate features. Centroblasts are large in size and have a high N/C ratio with a thin rim of amphophilic or basophilic cytoplasm. The nuclei are round and have vesicular chromatin with several small nucleoli adjacent to the nuclear membrane. In contrast to centroblasts, immunoblasts are larger and have variable amounts of cytoplasm. The nuclei of immunoblasts are large and round with vesicular chromatin. A prominent, centrally located, eosinophilic nucleolus is present in most cells. Classification of DLBCL based on cytology is optional. Lymphomas with >90% immunoblasts are considered as the immunoblastic variant, which is associated with more aggressive clinical behaviors and an inferior survival. The DLBCLs with <90% immunoblasts and mixed centroblasts are considered as the centroblastic variant, which is the most common morphologic subtype.

Rare DLBCLs (~3.4%) demonstrate anaplastic cytology, with large to gigantic, bizarre nuclei. These cases show a high frequency of *TP53* mutations and genetic abnormalities of *MYC*, *BCL2*, and *BCL6*. The patients usually have an aggressive clinical course with a poor overall survival [10–12].

5. What are the unusual morphologic variants of DLBCL?

In rare cases, the DLBCL cells show a cohesive growth, closely resembling a carcinoma. There are also cases with a predominantly sinusoidal infiltration, mimicking metastatic carcinoma and anaplastic large cell lymphoma. Exceptionally, DLBCL may show spindle cell morphology with abundant mixed inflammatory cells, which can be confused with inflammatory myofibroblastic tumor and other spindle cell lesions [13–15].

6. What are the major genetic changes in DLBCL?

DLBCLs are positive for clonal rearrangements of immunoglobulin heavy chain (*IGH*) and/or light chains (*IGK* and *IGL*), whereas there is no rearrangement of T-cell receptor genes (*TCR*). Approximately 20% of DLBCLs have t(14;18)(q32;q21) translocation, involving *IGH-BCL2* rearrangement. *BCL6* rearrangement is detected in ~ 30% of cases, and *MYC* rearrangement is found in ~10%. Gene mutations have been commonly detected in DLBCLs. Particularly, *EZH2*, *SGK1*, *GNA13*, *SOCS1*, *STAT6*, and *TNFRSF14* are more frequently mutated in GCB-DLBCLs, while mutations of *ETV6*, *MYD88*, *PIM1*, and *TBL1XR1* are more common in ABC-DLBCLs [7].

7. What are the important poor prognostic factors in DLBCL?

Clinically, a high International Prognostic Index (IPI) is one of the most important factors associated with unfavorable prognosis. Based on the gene expression profiling and immunohistochemical staining, the DLBCL of ABC subtype has a worse prognosis than the GCB subtype. The ABC-DLBCL typically has no or decreased expression of germinal center B-cell markers, including CD10, GCET1, BCL6, GCET2/HGAL, and LMO2. DLBCLs with immunoblastic morphology are clinically more aggressive than the ones with centroblastic cytology. Other poor prognostic indicators include double expression of MYC and BCL2, CD5 expression, lack of CD30 expression, CD43 expression, *BCL2* gene rearrangement, *MYC* gene rearrangement, *TP53* mutation, and lack of *BCL6* gene rearrangement or mutation [2, 8, 9, 16].

8. What are the major differential diagnoses of DLBCL?

DLBCL has to be separated from reactive conditions with abundant reactive immunoblasts, Burkitt lymphoma, blastoid mantle cell lymphoma, and non-hematopoietic malignancies. The major differential diagnoses of DLBCL are summarized in Table 6.1.

Table 6.1 Differential diagnosis of DLBCL

Entities	Caveats	Features against DLBCL and workup
Reactive immunoblastosis	Associated with multiple underlying causes, including infection (particularly *EBV*), medication, autoimmune, and nonspecific reactions to adjacent non-hematologic malignancy Variable number of large immunoblasts in the paracortex and even sinuses, which may form loose clusters	Nodal architecture at least partially preserved Polymorphous paracortical lymphoid proliferation with a spectrum of cytology, from small lymphocytes, larger transformed cells, immunoblasts, and plasmacytoid cells to plasma cells Not significant atypia of immunoblasts Mostly positive for CD30, MUM1, BOB1, and OCT2; CD20, CD45, and PAX5 variably expressed Rule out *EBV* infection and other etiology Lack of clonal *IGH* rearrangement
Burkitt lymphoma (BL)	DLBCL may show a "starry-sky" appearance with medium-sized cells and abundant mitoses and apoptotic cells DLBCL can be negative for BCL2 while expressing BCL6 and CD10	Clinical presentations in BL: jaw bone of kids in endemic BL and ileocecal region in sporadic BL Typical cytology of BL: medium size, round nuclei, several small peripheral nucleoli, and scant basophilic cytoplasm (with vacuoles on smear) Simple karyotype with *MYC* translocation
Blastoid mantle cell lymphoma (MCL)	Blastoid MCL has medium to large lymphoma cells and a high proliferation index Blastoid MCL may express CD10 and BCL6 but not CD5 Rare DLBCLs may show variable cyclin D1 expression in a subset of lymphoma cells	Albeit large size, tumor cells in blastoid MCL generally have small or inconspicuous nucleoli Diffuse and strong expression of cyclin D1 and SOX11 Recommend cyclin D1 stain in the initial workup of DLBCL
Plasmablastic or anaplastic plasma cell neoplasm (PCN)	Plasmablastic or anaplastic PCN may show immunoblastic or pleomorphic cytology with no obvious plasmablastic or plasmacytic cytology PCN can express CD20 and/or CD45 diffusely	Solid sheets of tumor cells with minimal reactive inflammatory cells Diffuse positivity for CD138 Recommend CD138 and at least two pan-B-cell markers in the initial workup of DLBCL
Non-hematopoietic malignancies	Metastatic non-hematopoietic tumors in the lymph node may mimic lymphoma morphologically, including carcinoma, melanoma, seminoma, and other soft tissue sarcoma Metastatic tumor may show paracortical and/or sinusoidal infiltrative pattern Metastatic tumor cells may be dyscohesive or even obscured by lymphocytes, i.e., lymphoepithelioma-like nasopharyngeal carcinoma	Clinical history of nonlymphoid malignancy Careful morphologic examination and search for hints indicative for nonlymphoid neoplasm For a high-grade neoplasm, recommend multiple lineage markers in the initial workup (cytokeratin, S100, and OCT3/4), in addition to lymphoid markers

9. What is the initial workup for the cases with morphologic features of DLBCL?

For a high-grade neoplasm suspicious for DLBCL, it is recommended to include the following immunohistochemical stains:

- CD45: To confirm the nature of hematopoietic neoplasm. If CD45 negative, may consider CD43.
- CD3: To rule out a T-cell or NK neoplasm. However, rare cases of DLBCL may aberrantly express CD3.
- CD20: DLBCL is diffusely and strongly positive for CD20, although rare cases can be negative, including the ones after rituximab therapy. CD20 is occasionally expressed in plasma cell neoplasms, particularly the cases with t(11;14). In addition, T-cell lymphomas may rarely show aberrant CD20 expression.
- Additional B-cell markers, including CD19, CD79a, PAX5, BOB1, and OCT2. Incorporation of at least one of these B-cell markers is necessary to confirm the B-cell lineage of a high-grade lymphoma and to rule out aberrant expression of B-cell markers in a T-cell lymphoma.
- MIB1 (Ki-67): To determine the proliferation index and therefore the high-grade nature of the lymphoma. Furthermore, a very high proliferation fraction may raise a suspicion for a double-hit lymphoma (now high-grade B-cell lymphoma with rearrangements of *BCL2* and *MYC* and/or *BCL6*), Burkitt lymphoma, and lymphoblastic lymphoma, in conjunction with morphology.
- Cyclin D1: Blastoid MCL closely mimics DLBCL. A diffuse and strong expression of cyclin D1 should point to the diagnosis of MCL. Conversely, rare cases of DLBCL may have a variable expression of cyclin D1 in

a subset of tumor cells, which is not associated *CCND1* rearrangement.

- CD138: It is recommended that CD138 be applied to the initial workup of a high-grade B-cell neoplasm. Plasmablastic lymphoma and plasmablastic/anaplastic plasma cell neoplasm may show variable cytologic features, including immunoblastic, anaplastic, and plasmablastic. Moreover, the tumor cells may occasionally have a diffuse expression of CD20, which may lead to misinterpretation to DLBCL.

10. What is the further workup after initial studies of possible DLBCL cases?

- CD10/BCL6/MUM1: For classification of DLBCL into GCB or ABC subtype based on the Hans algorithm.
- BCL2 and MYC: Dual expression of MYC and BCL2 in DLBCL is predictive of a poor survival [17, 18].
- CD30: Expression of CD30 in DLBCL is associated with a favorable prognosis and may serve as an alternative therapeutic target.
- CD34/TdT: It is necessary to rule out lymphoblastic lymphoma in certain cases with suspicious morphologic features and a very high proliferation index.
- CD5: CD5-positive DLBCL is associated with a poorer overall survival rate than the CD5-negative case.
- EBER-ISH: Qualified *EBV*+ cases should be further classified as "*EBV*+ DLBCL."
- FISH studies for rearrangements of *MYC*, *BCL2*, and *BCL6* are performed in many institutions after the diagnosis of DLBCL.

11. What are the major pitfalls and recommendations in the workup of DLBCL with immunohistochemical stains?

- CD3 is expressed in rare cases of DLBCL. In addition, expression of CD2, CD7, and CD8 is detected in approximately 2.7%, 4.0%, and 1.3% cases of DLBCL, respectively.
- PAX5 is positive in most cases of Merkel cell carcinoma and neuroendocrine tumor of the lung, although the expression is usually heterogeneous. Thus, PAX5 shouldn't be used as the sole B-cell marker in the initial workup of a high-grade neoplasm.
- Cyclin D1 is recommended in the initial workup of DLBCL to rule out blastoid MCL.
- CD138 is recommended in the initial workup of DLBCL to rule out plasmablastic lymphoma and plasma cell neoplasm with CD20 expression.
- Cytokeratin may be positive in rare cases of DLBCL, but the expression is usually weak and variable. Therefore, for a high-grade neoplasm with focal and variable expression of cytokeratin, additional cytokeratins should be stained.
- P63 is commonly used as a maker for squamous cell carcinoma. However, it is also positive in 42.5% of DLBCLs, and the expression is associated with a favorable prognosis [19–25]

12. What are the major clinicopathologic features of T-cell/histiocyte-rich large B-cell lymphoma (THRLBCL)?

THRLBCL is a morphologic variant of DLBCL with scattered large lymphoma cells in a background of abundant reactive CD8+/TIA-1+ T lymphocytes and histiocytes. It mostly arises in the lymph nodes and rarely extranodal sites. The patients are mostly old with a median age of 57 years and a male predominance (male to female ratio of 2.7:1). Approximately 2/3 of patients present at high clinical stages of III to IV, and up to 60% cases have bone marrow involvement at the time of diagnosis.

Morphologically, the lymph node architecture is completely effaced with a diffuse infiltration of a polymorphous cellular population. Presence of nodular proliferation or NLPHL component essentially excludes the diagnosis of THRLBCL. The large lymphoma cells are dispersed singly, without forming clusters or sheets. They display a spectrum of morphologic features, including centroblastic, immunoblastic, cytology between centroblast and immunoblast, LP cell, Reed-Sternberg cell, and pleomorphic large cell cytology. There are typically abundant small lymphocytes in the background, mostly reactive T lymphocytes, with no or mild cytologic atypia. In addition, scattered and/or small clusters of histiocytes are present. Other inflammatory cells, including eosinophils and plasma cells, are commonly noted.

The scattered large lymphoma cells express pan-B-cell markers (CD19, CD20, and CD79a) but not CD15, CD30, or CD138. No *EBV* infection is detected in the tumor cells. The background is composed of mixed CD3+/CD8+ T-cells and variable numbers of CD68+/CD163+ histiocytes. There are no PD1+ T-cell rosettes around the large tumor cells. In addition, residual follicular dendritic cell meshworks are essentially absent [26–28].

13. How is T-cell/histiocyte-rich large B-cell lymphoma (THRLBCL) distinguished from conventional DLBCL?

Although THRLBCL represents a distinct clinicopathologic variant of DLBCL, it has to be separated from conventional DLBCL. THRLBCL usually shows a diffuse proliferation with only scattered large tumor cells, which account for

<10% of all cells in the tissue. Therefore, presence of solid clusters or sheets of tumor cells essentially rules out the diagnosis of THRLBCL and would lead to conventional DLBCL. However, it is not uncommon to identify focal areas of conventional DLBCL during the course of THRLBCL progression.

14. How is THRLBCL distinguished from nodular lymphocyte predominant Hodgkin lymphoma (NLPHL)?

The separation of THRLBCL from typical NLPHL is usually straightforward. However, there are cases of NLPHL with prominent diffuse growth and inconspicuous nodules, which places a great diagnostic challenge. In general, NLPHL occurs in younger patients with early stage disease. Morphologically, NLPHL shows a nodular proliferation at least focally, which can be highlighted by CD21 and/or CD23 immunostaining. Rare cases of NLPHL may have a pure diffuse growth without follicular dendritic cell meshworks; it is not certain whether they should be classified as a variant of NLPHL or B-cell lymphoma with features intermediate between NLPHL and THRLBCL. The large lymphoma cells in NLPHL display LP (or L&H) cytology, and some cells may show immunoblastic or RS-like morphology. Furthermore, the small lymphocytes in the diffuse areas of NLPHL are mostly T-cells with no expression of TIA-1, and the lymphocytes surrounding the tumor cells are positive for CD57 and PD1 [29].

15. What are the major clinicopathologic features of primary central nervous system DLBCL (PCNS DLBCL)?

PCNS DLBCL is an extranodal NHL, involving the brain parenchyma, leptomeninges, eyes, and spinal cord, which does not include systemic lymphomas spreading to the CNS. It is usually confined to the CNS, without evidence of systemic disease. PCNS DLBCL accounts for ~1.7% of all lymphomas and ~2.2% of all primary brain tumors in the United States with an incidence of 0.39–0.55/100,000 per year and ~1500 new cases annually. PCNS DLBCL may occur in immunocompetent patients and immunosuppressed patients (particularly AIDS patients). The PCNS DLBCL in immunocompetent patients accounts for 67.7% with a medium age of 63 years and an M/F ratio of 5:4. Approximately 32.3% cases affect HIV+ patients with a medium age of 37 years and an M/F ratio of 11:1. By clinical imaging studies, PCNS DLBCL usually presents as an intracranial mass lesion, mostly single in immunocompetent patients and often multiple in HIV+ patients. Steroids often cause rapid but temporary tumor lysis, making radiological and pathologic diagnosis difficult.

Morphologically, PCNS DLBCL reveals a diffuse infiltration of large cells with a characteristic angiocentric pattern, forming cuffs within and around the blood vessels. There are frequent mitoses, apoptotic cells, and areas of necrosis. Lymphoma cells express pan-B-cell markers (CD20, CD79a, and PAX5), and most cases (75–96%) are of ABC subtype. *EBV* infection is commonly detected in the cases from HIV+ patients but rarely from immunocompetent patients.

16. What are the major clinicopathologic features of primary mediastinal (thymic) large B-cell lymphoma (PMLBCL)?

PMLBCL accounts for ~2.4% of NHLs and typically affects young adults (median age, 37 years) with a female predominance (female to male ratio, 2: 1). The patient usually presents with a bulky anterior mediastinal mass, which causes symptoms of superior vena cava obstruction and dyspnea. PMLBCL may invade the adjacent organs, including the pleura, lung, pericardium, and chest wall. Rare cases initially occur at the extra-mediastinal sites with similar morphology and gene profiling to the primary mediastinal cases. Approximately 2/3 of patients are diagnosed at early clinical stage of I or II, and only 2% cases have bone marrow involvement. The serum LDH is elevated in most cases (76%), whereas serum β2-microglobulin is not increased likely due to lack of expression of HLA class I molecules in the tumor.

Morphologically, PMLBCL shows a diffuse infiltrate of tumor cells in a background of delicate fibrosis. The lymphoma cells are large in size with variable cytologic features, including centroblastic, immunoblastic, anaplastic or pleomorphic, unclassifiable, and RS-like cytology. Rare cells may have spindle cytology. The cytoplasm is usually abundant and clear staining. Characteristically, the background contains delicate fibrosis surrounding individual or small groups of lymphoma cells, so called compartmentalized fibrosis.

PMLBL is positive for pan-B-cell markers, CD20, CD79a, and PAX5. Most cases do not express surface or cytoplasmic light chains. BCL6, CD23, and CD30 are expressed in the majority of cases, whereas CD10 is only detected in a small proportion of cases. Several immunohistochemical markers are preferentially expressed in PMLBCL over conventional DLBCL, including MAL, CD200, TNFAIP2, and PD-L2. *EBV* infection is not detected [30–34].

17. What is the initial workup for the cases with morphologic features of PMLBCL?

For the mediastinal biopsy with clinical and morphologic features highly suggestive for PMLBCL, a selective initial study panel may include:

- CD3, CD20, CD45, and PAX5: These are basic immunohistochemical markers for lymphoid neoplasms.
- CD15 and CD30: PMLBCL is mostly positive for CD30 but negative for CD15. A positive CD15 should raise the possibility of classic Hodgkin lymphoma.
- CD10 and BCL6: BCL6 is positive in most cases of PMLBCL, whereas CD10 is detected in a small proportion of cases.
- CD23: A positive CD23 immunostain is also suggestive for PMLBCL.
- EBER-ISH: PMLBCL is negative for *EBV* infection, and a positive EBER-ISH essentially excludes this entity.
- Ki-67: Used to assess the proliferative index.
- MAL: MAL is very specific for PMLBCL, although it is not commonly used in many institutions.

18. How is PMLBCL distinguished from mediastinal classic Hodgkin lymphoma (CHL)?

Mediastinal CHL is nearly always the nodular sclerosis variant (NS), which may closely resemble PMLBCL with similar clinical presentations and morphology. CHL-NS also contains large tumor cells with abundant clear cytoplasm and fibrosis, although CHL-NS usually does not have the delicate fibrosis as noted in PMLBL. The detailed differential diagnosis is summarized in Table 6.2.

Rare cases of mediastinal high-grade B-cell lymphoma have significant overlapping clinical, morphological, and immunophenotypic features between CHL and PMLBCL, which has been designated as "gray zone lymphoma."

Table 6.2 Differential diagnosis between PMLBCL and CHL-NS

	PMLBCL	CHL-NS
BOB.1	+	Mostly –
CD15	–	+, 80%
CD20	+	–/+
CD30	+, 86%	+, diffuse, strong
CD79a	+	–/+
Cyclin E	–	+, 79%
MAL	+	–
OCT2	+	Mostly –
PAX5	+, strong	+, weak
PU.1	+	–
EBER-ISH	–	–/+, 20–30%

Table 6.3 Differential diagnosis between PMLBCL and DLBCL

	PMLBCL	DLBCL
Age (years)	37	65
Gender	Male < female	Male ≥ female
Stage III/IV	1/3	1/2
CD30	86%	Mostly negative
CD200/OX2	94%	7%
REL	31/48 (65%)	28/160 (18%)
TRAF1	48/78 (62%)	20/173 (12%)
REL+/TRAF1+	24/45 (53%)	3/156 (2%)
TNFAIP2	27/31 (87%)	2/45 (4%)

Actually, PMLBCL has a similar gene expression profile to that in CHL.

19. How is PMLBCL distinguished from conventional DLBCL?

Although PMLBCL commonly shows compartmentalized fibrosis, there are cases with diffuse and solid infiltration of lymphoma cells, which are reminiscent of conventional DLBCL. The major differential diagnosis of these two entities is summarized in Table 6.3.

20. What are the other differential diagnoses of PMLBCL?

Other differential diagnosis of PMLBCL includes anaplastic large cell lymphoma (ALCL), mediastinal seminoma, and thymic carcinoma. Particularly, mediastinal seminoma is cytologically similar to PMLBL, with abundant clear cytoplasm. However, mediastinal seminoma exclusively occurs in male, and the tumor cells have a central, "inclusion-like" nucleolus. In addition, the tumor cells are positive for OCT3/4, PLAP, SALL4, and CD117 with no expression of CD45 or B-cell markers.

21. What are the major clinicopathologic features of intravascular large B-cell lymphoma (IVLBCL)?

IVLBCL is a unique and aggressive extranodal lymphoma with proliferation of tumor cells in small vessels, particularly capillaries. IVLBCL is very rare with a frequency < 1/1,000,000. It mostly affects old patients with a median age of 67 years and no gender predilection. Most (>90%) patients present with advanced clinical stages (III or IV) and high IPI.

The clinical presentations are largely dependent upon the variants of IVLBL:

- Classic variant: Typically in Western countries with frequent CNS and skin involvement.
- Asian variant: Often associated with hemophagocytic syndrome, fever, hepatosplenomegaly, thrombocytopenia, and bone marrow involvement. Does not commonly involve the CNS and skin.
- Cutaneous variant: A subtype of classic variant, with only skin involvement; almost exclusively in females, with a mean age of 59 years and normal platelet and leukocyte counts.

The large lymphoma cells are predominantly or exclusively in the small blood vessels, with centroblastic, immunoblastic, or unclassifiable cytology. Frequent mitotic figures may be noted. Occasionally, the lymphoma cells palisade along vascular wall, mimicking angiosarcoma, and they can be deceptively cohesive, resembling carcinoma. In areas with fibrin thrombi in the vessels, hemorrhage and necrosis can be noted. Hemophagocytosis is commonly present in the Asian variant.

IVLBCL is positive for CD45 and pan-B-cell markers. A small subset of cases may express CD5 and CD10. The lack of expression of CD29 (β1-integrin) and CD54 (ICAM-1) may explain the intravascular nature of this lymphoma, since both molecules are important for transvascular lymphocyte migration. No *EBV* or HTLV-1 infection is detected [35–40].

22. What are the major clinicopathologic features of primary cutaneous DLBCL, leg type (PCDLBCL-LT)?

PCDLBCL-LT involves old patients with a median age of ~78 years and female predominance. Clinically, the tumor usually presents as rapidly growing subcutaneous mass lesions within the lower extremities. However, approximately 20% cases affect the locations other than the legs. In contrast to other DLBCL, PCDLBCL-LT is associated with more aggressive clinical behaviors and unfavorable prognosis.

PCDLBCL-LT shows a diffuse infiltration of solid or confluent sheets of tumor cells in the dermis and frequently extends into the subcutaneous adipose tissue with no epidermotropism. The lymphoma cells are monotonous and possess centroblastic and/or immunoblastic cytology with frequent mitoses and apoptotic cells. Reactive lymphocytes and follicular dendritic cells are typically scant in the tumor.

The lymphoma cells are positive for pan-B-cell markers, CD20, CD79a, and PAX5. Particularly, BCL2, MUM1, and FOXP1 are strongly positive in most cases. BCL6 is commonly positive, whereas CD10 is typically negative. Therefore, PCDLBCL-LT is mostly classified as the "activated B-cell" subtype based on the Hans algorithm. The proliferation index is generally high with >75% in most cases [41, 42].

23. What are the major clinicopathologic features of lymphomatoid granulomatosis (LyG)?

LyG occurs in immunocompetent individuals, and some cases may affect patients with underlying primary or secondary immunodeficiencies, including Wiskott-Aldrich syndrome, HIV infection, and iatrogenic immunosuppression. Patients are mostly in their fourth and sixth decade of life and have a male predominance with a male to female ratio of 2:1.

Almost all patients present with pulmonary symptoms, including cough, dyspnea, and chest pain. Clinical image studies frequently show bilateral pulmonary nodules of variable sizes with occasional cavitary lesions. Extrapulmonary organs are also commonly involved, particularly the CNS, skin, liver, and kidneys.

Morphologically, LyG displays a characteristic angiocentric infiltration with angioinvasion and angiodestruction. Areas of coagulative necrosis are commonly seen around the destructed vessels. The lymphoma cells are variable in number with a polymorphous background, containing mixed reactive lymphocytes, histiocytes, and plasma cells. Granulomas, multinucleated giant cells, and neutrophilic abscesses are usually absent. The neoplastic cells are mostly large in size with a spectrum of morphologic features, including immunoblastic and HRS-like cytology.

LyG is further graded based on the number of large cells, which are readily highlighted by CD20. Grade 1 LyG contains scattered large cells in a polymorphous background, and occasional cases may show focal necrosis. By EBER-ISH, the *EBV*-positive cells are <5 cells/HPF. Grade 2 lesion has frequent large cells with necrosis commonly, whereas in grade 3, the tumor cells are more numerous and form small clusters or aggregates in a background with reactive cells. A diagnosis of DLBCL should be made when the lymphoma cells form solid sheets with no polymorphic background.

The tumor cells in LyG are positive for B-cell markers, including CD20, CD79a, and PAX5. CD30 is positive in a subset of cases. They are also positive for EBER-ISH, LMP-1, EBNA-2, and ZEBRA, indicating a type III latency pattern. The background lymphocytes are mostly T-cells with a predominance of CD4+ lymphocytes [43, 44].

24. How is LyG distinguished from extranodal NK-/T-cell lymphoma, nasal type?

Extranodal NK-/T-cell lymphoma, nasal type, may initially occur in the lung and show angiocentric invasion, geographic necrosis, and *EBV* infection, which closely resembles LyG. The major differential diagnosis of these two lymphomas is summarized in Table 6.4.

Table 6.4 Comparison between LyG and extranodal NK-/T-cell lymphoma, nasal type

	Lymphomatoid granulomatosis	Extranodal NK-/T-cell lymphoma, nasal type
Angioinvasion and angiodestruction	Present	Present
Coagulative necrosis	Present	Present
B-cell markers	Positive	Negative
CD3-IHC	Negative	Positive
CD56	Negative	Positive
Cytotoxic markers	Negative	Positive
EBER-ISH	Positive	Positive
IGH PCR	Clonal	Polyclonal
TRG PCR	Polyclonal	Germline

Table 6.5 Comparison between LyG and GPA

	Lymphomatoid granulomatosis	Granulomatosis with polyangiitis
Extrapulmonary involvement	Present, including the brain, skin, and liver	Present, typically the kidney
C-ANCA	Negative	Positive
Geographic necrosis	Present	Present
Palisading granulomas	No	Present
Necrosis with neutrophils and microabscesses	No	Present
Angioinvasion	Present	Present
Capillaritis	No	Present
Atypical lymphoid cells	Present	No
CD20	Positive in variable numbers of large cells	Positive in small reactive lymphocytes
EBER-ISH	Positive	Negative
IGH PCR	Clonal	Polyclonal

25. How is LyG distinguished from granulomatosis with polyangiitis (GPA), formerly known as Wegener granulomatosis?

GPA shares some clinicopathologic features with LyG, including involvement of the lung and kidney, angioinvasion, and presence of geographic necrosis (Table 6.5).

26. What are the major clinical features of ALK+ large B-cell lymphoma (ALK+ LBCL)?

ALK+ LBCL is a rare subtype of DLBCL with characteristic *ALK* rearrangements, and it mostly occurs in the lymph nodes of young and middle-aged, immunocompetent patients. The medium age is 35 years with a male to female ratio of 3.5:1. The 5-year overall survival is ~34% and the median survival is 1.8 years. In patients with stage III/IV disease, the 5-year survival is only 8%. Moreover, patients <35 years have a significantly better survival than those ≥35 years [13, 24, 45–53].

27. What are the typical morphologic and immunophenotypic features of ALK+ LBCL?

ALK+ LBCL typically shows a diffuse infiltration in the lymph node. Some cases have focal or even purely sinusoidal infiltrative pattern. The lymphoma cells are large in size with plasmablastic and/or immunoblastic cytology. Anaplastic or pleomorphic morphology is present focally in rare cases.

ALK staining shows the characteristic cytoplasmic granular pattern in the vast majority of cases, and very few cases have nuclear positivity in addition to cytoplasmic or membranous staining. Most cases are positive for CD45, whereas pan-B-cell markers (CD20, CD79a, and PAX5) are negative. However, BOB1 and OCT2 are very sensitive for ALK+ LBCL. Most cases express plasma cell markers, such as CD138, EMA, and MUM1 with either kappa or lambda light chain restriction. IgA is detected in ~80% cases, and ~50% cases aberrantly express CD4. No *EBV* or HHV8 infection has been detected in any reported cases [13].

28. What are the common and uncommon chromosomal rearrangements in ALK+ LBCL?

With conventional cytogenetic and FISH assays, *ALK* rearrangements have been detected in 94% cases of ALK+ LBCL. The most translocation is t(2;17)(p23;q23), as noted in 72% cases, which results in a *CLTC-ALK* fusion gene and gives a cytoplasmic granular or dotted pattern in lymphoma cells. Other partner genes include *NPM1*, *SEC31A*, *SQSTM1*, *RANBP2*, and *IGL* [13].

29. How is ALK+ LBCL distinguished from ALK+ anaplastic large cell lymphoma?

ALK+ LBCL significantly overlaps ALK+ ALCL: Both lymphomas commonly occur in young patients and frequently show a characteristic sinusoidal infiltration in the lymph nodes. Cytologically, ALK+ LBCL displays plasmablastic and/or immunoblastic features, whereas ALK+ ALCL shows anaplastic morphology with characteristic "hallmark cells." Particularly, ALK+ LBCL has a cytoplasmic granular ALK expression pattern, in contrast to the nuclear and cytoplasmic pattern in most cases of ALK+ ALCL (Table 6.6) [13].

Table 6.6 Comparison between ALK+ ALCL and ALK+ LBCL

	ALK+ ALCL	ALK+ LBCL
Incidence	Not uncommon	Extremely rare
Gender (M/F)	1.7/1	3.5/1
Age (years)	34	38
5-year overall survival	70%	25%
Growth pattern	Sinusoidal or sheets	Sinusoidal or sheets
Cytology	Mostly anaplastic, "hallmark" cells	Plasmablastic, immunoblastic
ALK	Cytoplasmic and nuclear	Cytoplasmic granular pattern
CD45	+	+
CD3	Mostly negative	–
CD4	40%	53%
CD20/CD79a/PAX5	–	Mostly negative
BOB1/OCT2	–	Mostly positive
CD30	100%	Mostly negative
CD138	–	Positive
EMA	Mostly positive	Mostly positive
Cytotoxic markers	Mostly positive	–
EBER-ISH	–	–
IGH PCR	Polyclonal	Monoclonal
TRG PCR	Monoclonal	Polyclonal
ALK rearrangement	Mostly t(2;5)(p23;35) with *NPM/ALK* rearrangement	Mostly t(2;17)(p23;q23) with *CLTC/ALK* rearrangement

30. What are the major differential diagnoses of a high-grade neoplasm in the lymph node with predominant sinus infiltrative pattern?

In addition to ALK+ LBCL and ALK+ ALCL, other metastatic tumors may show a prominent sinusoidal infiltrative pattern in the lymph node, and they should be considered in the initial workup:

- Melanoma: The tumor cells may show a variety of cytology in the sinuses of lymph node. In general, they have more cytologic atypia than the sinus histiocytes. Immunostains with melanocytic markers are necessary in cases with subtle morphologic changes.
- Carcinoma: Undifferentiated nasopharyngeal carcinoma, papillary carcinoma, and other metastatic carcinoma may initially show a sinus pattern in the lymph node.
- Seminomatous tumor: The tumor cells are large in size and have abundant clear cytoplasm. The nuclei are large with an "inclusion-like" nucleolus.
- Rare case of rhabdomyosarcoma may show a sinusoidal infiltrative pattern in the lymph nodes, and the tumor cells may express ALK but not CD30.

31. What are the major clinicopathologic features of plasmablastic lymphoma (PBL)?

- Typically arises in the oral cavity of HIV-positive patients, and approximately 34% of cases initially occur in the extraoral sites
- Morphology: Diffuse infiltration of large plasmablastic and/or immunoblastic cells
- Usually negative for CD20 and PAX5, but CD79a often positive
- Positive for plasma cell markers, CD138, EMA, and MUM1
- Mostly positive for BOB1 and OCT2
- Positive for *EBV* infection in >70% of cases, but negative for KSHV/HHV8 [54–56].

32. How is PBL distinguished from solid variant of primary effusion lymphoma (solid PEL)?

Both PBL and solid PEL typically occur in HIV+ patients with plasmablastic and/or immunoblastic morphology and *EBV* infection. The major difference is the presence of HHV8 infection in solid PEL. In addition, most cases of solid PEL express CD45 and CD30, whereas CD138 can be negative in ~30% cases. Particularly, the light chain expression is undetectable in ~50% cases of solid PEL by immunohistochemical and/or in situ hybridization assays. Furthermore, up to 29% of solid PEL aberrantly express CD3 with variable intensity [57–63].

33. How is PBL distinguished from plasmablastic plasmacytoma?

The separation of *EBV*+ PBL from plasmablastic plasmacytoma is straightforward, but it is very challenging to differentiate *EBV*-negative PBL from plasmablastic plasmacytoma without sufficient clinical information. Detection of CD56 and/or cyclin D1 expression would lean toward plasmacytoma. However, currently there are no solid diagnostic criteria to separate these two neoplasms, particularly in the extraoral locations. Therefore, a descriptive diagnosis of "plasmablastic neoplasm" can be made to the problematic cases with a comment suggesting correlation with further clinical and laboratory studies.

34. What are the major clinicopathologic features of extra-cavitary primary effusion lymphoma (PEL)?

Extra-cavitary PEL (or "solid PEL") has been observed in the lymph nodes and extranodal sites without lymphomatous effusions during the course of disease. Otherwise, extracavitary PEL is similar to classic PEL based on the clinical features (HIV+ male), morphology (immunoblastic, plasmablastic, or anaplastic), immunophenotype (CD45+, CD20-, CD79a-, CD30+, CD138+, and EMA+), presence of *EBV* infection, and clonal *IGH* rearrangements. Up to 29% cases of solid PEL have aberrant CD3 expression, which may mislead to a diagnosis of T-cell lymphoma, particularly anaplastic large cell lymphoma in combination with the anaplastic morphology and expression of CD30 and EMA [57].

35. What are the major clinicopathologic features of conventional PEL?

- A rare and unique lymphoma, nearly exclusively in HIV+ male
- Presents as lymphomatous effusions in the body cavities without solid tumor formation
- Cytology: plasmablastic, immunoblastic, and/or anaplastic
- Negative for pan-B-cell markers (CD20, CD79a, and PAX5)
- Positive for CD45, CD30, and plasma cell markers (CD138, MUM1, and EMA)
- Occasional cases with aberrant expression of CD3
- All cases positive for HHV8 infection and most cases positive for *EBV* infection [59, 61, 64].

36. What is the initial workup for the cases with plasmablastic morphology?

The malignant tumors with plasmablastic morphology include hematopoietic neoplasms (plasma cell neoplasm, ALK+ LBCL, PEL and its solid variant, and DLBCL) and non-hematopoietic tumors (melanoma, seminomatous tumor, and poorly differentiated carcinoma or sarcoma). Therefore, an initial immunohistochemical panel may include, but not limited to, the following (Table 6.7):

Table 6.7 Initial workup for neoplasms with plasmablastic cytology

Antibody	Differential diagnosis	Pitfall/comment
CK AE1/3	Poorly differentiated carcinoma	Can be positive in rare sarcomas Lymphoma may rarely express CKs May consider other cytokeratins
CD45	Hematologic neoplasm	May consider CD3 and CD20 as well
CD43	Hematologic neoplasm	More sensitive than CD45, positive in both lymphoid and myeloid neoplasms
S100	Melanoma or neuroendocrine tumor	May need synaptophysin or chromogranin A
BOB1, OCT2	Poorly differentiated B-cell and plasmacytic neoplasms	Very sensitive and specific for both B-cell and plasmacytic differentiation, especially the ones negative for conventional B-cell markers, including PEL, ALK+ LBCL, and PBL
PAX5	B-cell lymphoma	Positive in most Merkel cell carcinoma and neuroendocrine tumor of the lung; usually heterogeneous staining, weak to moderate
OCT3/4	Seminoma	Also positive for CD117 and PLAP
CD138	Plasma cell neoplasm	Also positive in carcinomas
CD30	ALCL or PTCL lymphoma with aberrant CD30+	Also positive in some B-cell lymphomas and embryonal carcinoma

37. What is the definition of *EBV*+ DLBCL, NOS?

"*EBV*+ DLBCL, NOS" is an *EBV*-related lymphoma with exclusion of other specific types of *EBV*+ B-cell neoplasms, including lymphomatoid granulomatosis, plasmablastic lymphoma, DLBCL associated with chronic inflammation, and *EBV*-positive mucocutaneous ulcer. It was previously designated as "*EBV*+ DLBCL of the elderly" since it usually occurs in patients >50 years of age. However, recently data indicated that it can present in younger patients, and the restriction to elderly patients has been eliminated [8].

38. What are the major clinicopathologic features of *EBV*+ DLBCL, NOS?

EBV+ DLBCL, NOS, accounts for <5% of DLBCLs in Western patients, with no documented predisposing immunodeficiency. It mostly occurs in patients >50 years of age with a male predominance. However, there are sporadic cases diagnosed in younger patients.

EBV+ DLBCL, NOS, often involves the lymph nodes, particularly in younger patients. The extranodal sites can be involved, especially the lungs and gastrointestinal tract. The clinical presentations are variable, with >50% of the patients having a high or high-intermediate International Prognostic Index (IPI) score. The *EBV* DNA is detected in the blood of most patients.

Morphologically, there is a diffuse infiltration of monotonous large tumor cells, similar to that in *EBV*-negative DLBCL. Cases often consist of a variable number of neoplastic cells, including immunoblastic cells, large pleomorphic cells, and Hodgkin/Reed-Sternberg-like cells. Some cases contain abundant reactive lymphocytes and histiocytes in the background, as typically seen in young patients. Characteristic geographic necrosis and angioinvasion are commonly noted. The lymphoma cells are mostly positive for MUM1 but negative for CD10 and BCL6, representing the activated B-cell subtype. CD30 is frequently expressed. By EBER-ISH, the tumor cells have evidence of *EBV* infection [65–67].

39. How is *EBV*+ DLBCL, NOS, distinguished from mucocutaneous ulcer (MCU)?

MCU is *EBV*-related and occurs in patients with immunosuppression due to aging or iatrogenic causes (medication or organ transplant). MCU mostly arises in the skin and mucosa with an indolent clinical course. Many cases regress spontaneously, particularly after discontinuation of immunosuppressive medication.

Morphologically, MCU is different from *EBV*+ DLBCL, NOS, despite some overlapping features. MCU lesion is limited with surface ulceration in the skin or mucosa. It is usually well-demarcated with a band of reactive small lymphocytes in the periphery, which are mostly CD8+ T-cells. Within the lesion, there are a variable number of large atypical cells, including immunoblastic and HRS-like cells, which are positive for CD20 and frequently CD30 and MUM1. By EBER-ISH, *EBV* is detected in many large atypical cells, as well as some small lymphocytes and larger transformed cells. In contrast, *EBV*+ DLBCL, NOS, is clinically and histologically more aggressive, with an extensive infiltration of lymphoma cells and a diffuse positivity of *EBV* limited to the large cells. Discontinuation of immunosuppressant will not result in disease regression [68, 69].

40. What is the definition of "high-grade B-cell lymphoma, with *MYC* and *BCL2* and/or *BCL6* rearrangement?" (See also Chap. 7)

"High-grade B-cell lymphoma (HGBL) with *MYC* and *BCL2* and/or *BCL6* rearrangement" is a specific type of aggressive B-cell lymphoma, which is different to "DLBCL, NOS" and Burkitt lymphoma. It includes the HGBLs with *MYC* rearrangement in combination with *BCL2* and/or *BCL6* rearrangement, which are also known as "double-hit lymphomas" or "triple-hit lymphomas." Rare cases of follicular lymphoma and B-lymphoblastic leukemia/lymphoma harbor similar genetic alterations, and they are not included in this category. In addition, this classification is applicable to the de novo cases only, and the cases transformed from low-grade lymphomas should be diagnosed descriptively, e.g., "HGBL with *MYC* and *BCL2* rearrangements, transformed from follicular lymphoma." [70, 71].

41. What are the major clinicopathologic features of "HGBL with *MYC* and *BCL2* and/or *BCL6* rearrangement?" (See also Chap. 7)

HGBL with *MYC* and *BCL2* and/or *BCL6* rearrangement mostly occurs in elderly patients at their sixth to seventh decade with a slight male predominance. Most patients present with advanced diseases with involvement of multiple sites. The morphology of "HGBL with *MYC* and *BCL2* and/or *BCL6* rearrangement" is very similar to DLBCL, NOS. In general, the tumor shows a diffuse infiltration of large cells with increased mitotic figures and apoptotic cells. However, there are occasional cases with a low number of mitotic figures and a low Ki-67 proliferation rate.

Approximately 50% of cases show morphologic features mimicking that of Burkitt lymphoma (BL) or have features intermediate between DLBCL and BL. In these cases, the lymphoma cells show a diffuse infiltration with a frequent starry-sky pattern at low-power magnification. The cells are medium to large in size, and nuclei are uniform or variable in sizes, which are typically more irregular than those in BL.

These lymphomas are positive for pan-B-cell markers and express BCL6 and CD10 in most cases, whereas MUM1 is typically negative. In contrast to BL, cases of HGBL with *MYC* and *BCL2* and/or *BCL6* rearrangement express BCL2, with a strong and diffuse cytoplasmic staining pattern. MYC can be detected in most cases by immunohistochemical staining, particularly in cases with *MYC* rearrangement. However, MYC protein expression is not always correlated with gene rearrangement. The proliferation index is greater than 80% in most cases, and occasional cases may have a low rate of <30% [70, 71].

42. How is "HGBL, with *MYC* and *BCL2* and/or *BCL6* rearrangement" distinguished from Burkitt lymphoma? (See also Chap. 7)

Some cases of "HGBL with *MYC* and *BCL2* and/or *BCL6* rearrangement" may resemble Burkitt lymphoma. However, they can be separated based on the morphology, immunophenotype, and genetic changes (Table 6.8).

Table 6.8 Comparison between "HGBL with *MYC* and *BCL2* and/or *BCL6* rearrangement" and Burkitt lymphoma

	HGBL with *MYC* and *BCL2* and/or *BCL6* rearrangement	Burkitt lymphoma
Starry-sky pattern	Present in a subset of cases	Nearly always present
Nuclei	Medium to large, variably sized	Medium size, round, several peripherally located nucleoli
Cytoplasm	Variable in amounts; may be moderate to abundant	Scant, deeply basophilic, cytoplasmic vacuoles
BCL6, CD10	Mostly positive	Often positive
BCL2	Diffusely and strongly positive mostly	Mostly negative; weakly positive in a small subset of cases
Ki-67	Mostly 80–95%, occasionally low	Typically >90%
Karyotype	Mostly complex	Mostly simple
MYC partner gene	40% non-*IG*	Always *IG*, mostly *IGH*, less commonly *IGK* and *IGL*

Case Presentations

Case 1

Learning Objectives

1. To recognize the typical morphologic features of DLBCL
2. To generate the differential diagnosis based on morphologic features
3. To know the initial and further workup of cases suspicious for DLBCL

Case History

A 65-year-old female was found to have several enlarged right axillary lymph nodes, with the largest one measuring 2.8 cm. A large axillary lymph node was excised.

Histologic Findings

- The lymph node architecture is effaced by a diffuse infiltration of tumor cells (Fig. 6.1a).
- Lymphoma cells are large in size and have round nuclei with vesicular chromatin and one to several small nucleoli.

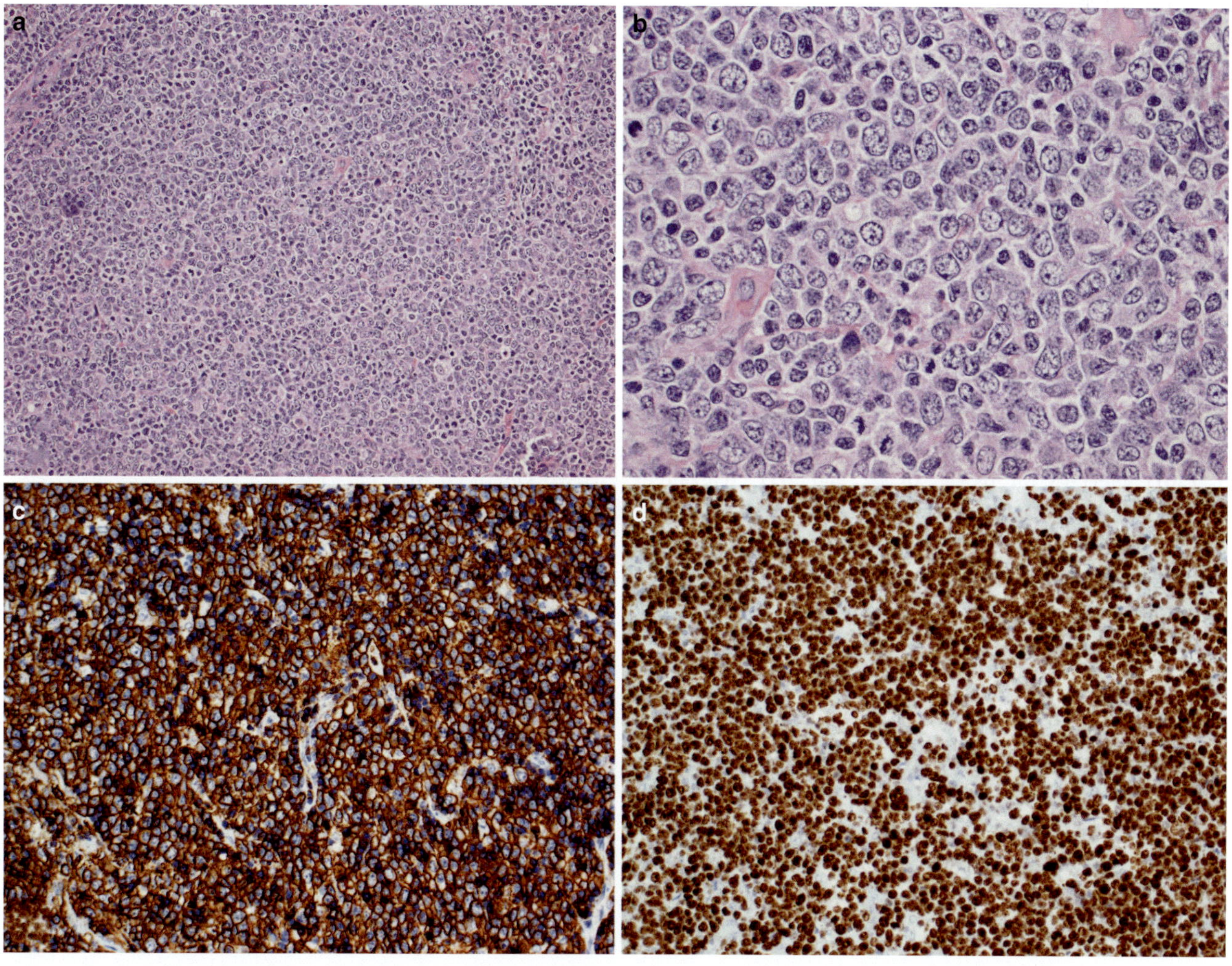

Fig. 6.1 Diffuse large B-cell lymphoma. There is a diffuse infiltration (**a**) by large lymphoma cells with round nuclei, vesicular chromatin, and one to several small nucleoli (**b**). The lymphoma cells are positive for CD20 (**c**) with a high proliferation index >90% by Ki-67 immunostaining (**d**)

The cytoplasm is moderate to abundant and pale staining (Fig. 6.1b).

Differential Diagnosis

- High-grade lymphoma, particularly diffuse large B-cell lymphoma (DLBCL)
- Other hematopoietic neoplasms, including high-grade T-cell lymphoma, lymphoblastic lymphoma, blastoid mantle cell lymphoma, and myeloid sarcoma.
- Metastatic tumor, including carcinoma, germ cell tumors, and melanoma

Initial Workup

- Positive for CD45, CD20 (Fig. 6.1c), and Ki-67 (Fig. 6.1d; >90%)
- Negative for CD3, CK AE1/AE3, and S100

Further Workup and Other Ancillary Studies

- Positive for BCL2, BCL6, CD10, and PAX5
- Negative for CD34, CD138, cyclin D1, MUM1, MYC, TdT, and EBER-ISH
- By FISH assays, positive for *BCL2* rearrangement, but negative for *BCL6* or *MYC* rearrangement

Final Diagnosis

Diffuse large B-cell lymphoma, germinal center B-cell (GCB) subtype

Take-Home Messages

1. DLBCL typically reveals a diffuse growth of large tumor cells.
2. An initial panel should include several lineage markers, including B-cell, T-cell, and other non-hematopoietic markers depending upon morphologic suspicion.
3. After establishing the diagnosis of DLBCL, additional studies are necessary for subclassification, including CD10, BCL6, MUM1, and EBER-ISH.
4. FISH analyses for *BCL2*, *BCL6*, and *MYC* rearrangements are required to rule out "high-grade B-cell lymphoma, with *MYC* and *BCL2* and/or *BCL6* rearrangement." [1–7, 70, 71]

Case 2

Learning Objectives

1. To recognize the blastoid cytology
2. To know the differential diagnosis of high-grade B-cell neoplasms with blastoid cytology
3. To know the important workup to reach an accurate diagnosis

Case History

A 63-year-old male presented with dysphagia for 3 weeks. A CT scan showed circumferential thickening of the distal esophagus extending into the stomach. A biopsy was performed on the gastric side.

Histologic Findings

- There is a diffuse infiltration of monotonous cells in the gastric mucosa. Scattered tingible-body macrophages are noted (Fig. 6.2a).
- The tumor cells are medium sized and have a high N/C ratio with scant cytoplasm. The nuclei are irregular with fine chromatin and inconspicuous nucleolus. Frequent apoptotic cells are present (Fig. 6.2b).

Differential Diagnosis

- Burkitt lymphoma
- Diffuse large B-cell lymphoma
- Lymphoblastic lymphoma, B-cell or T-cell
- Mantle cell lymphoma with blastoid cytology
- Poorly differentiated non-hematopoietic neoplasm

Ancillary Studies

- Positive for CD45, CD20, PAX5, CD10 (Fig. 6.2c), BCL2, cyclin D1 (Fig. 6.2d), and Ki-67 (>90%)
- Negative for CD3, CD5 (Fig. 6.2e), CD34, CD138, CK AE1/AE3, MPO, and TdT
- FISH study positive for *CCND1* rearrangement

Final Diagnosis

Mantle cell lymphoma with blastoid cytology

Take-Home Messages

1. Blastoid mantle cell lymphoma closely resembles DLBCL, Burkitt lymphoma, and lymphoblastic lymphoma morphologically.
2. Cyclin D1 should be frequently considered in the initial workup of DLBCL [72–76].

Case 3

Learning Objectives

1. To recognize the immunoblastic and/or plasmablastic cytology
2. To review the major differential diagnosis of malignant neoplasms with immunoblastic and/or plasmablastic cytology
3. To know the workup of malignant neoplasms with immunoblastic and/or plasmablastic cytology

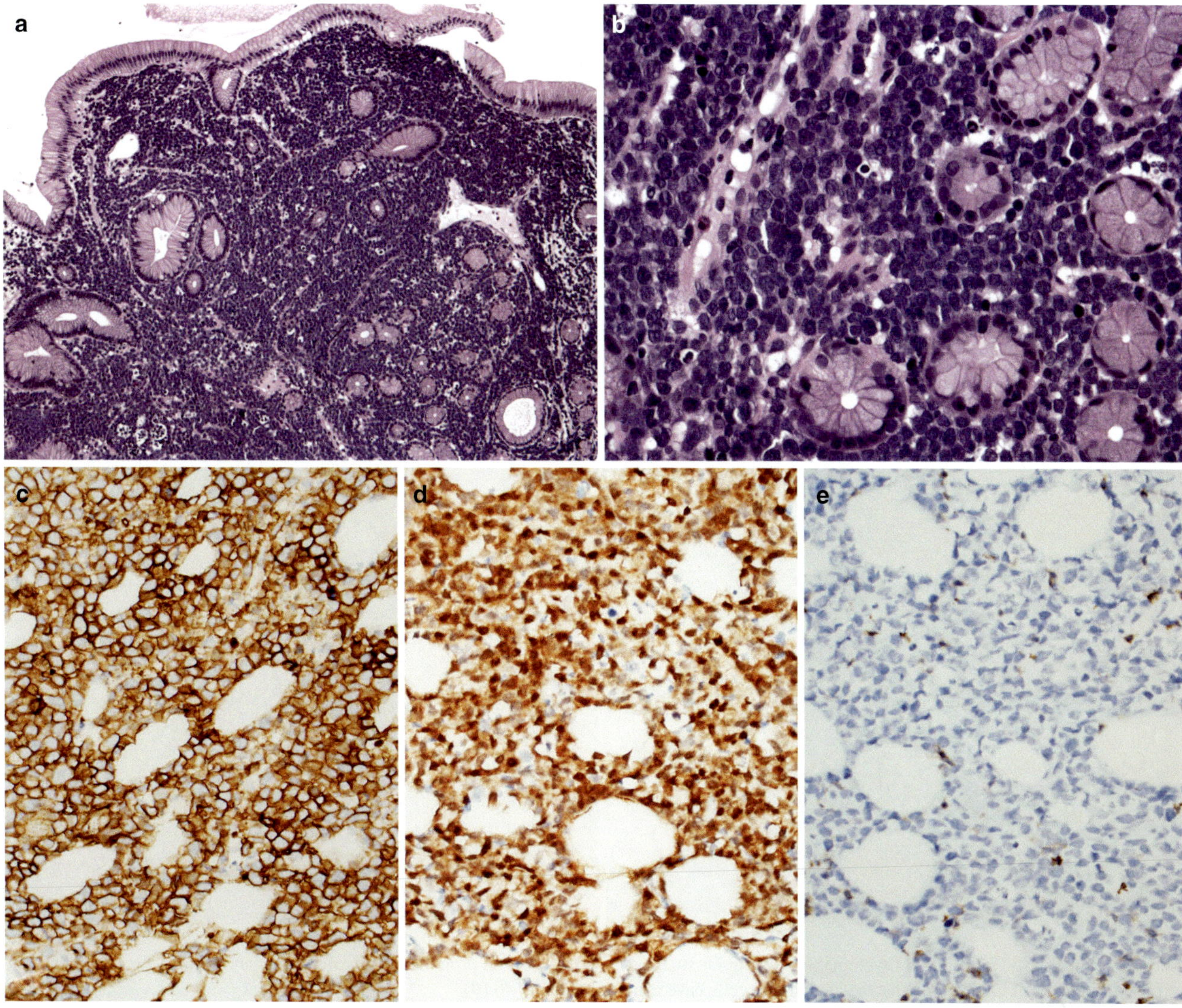

Fig. 6.2 Blastoid mantle cell lymphoma resembling DLBCL. (**a**), diffuse infiltration of monotonous lymphoma cells in the gastric mucosa. (**b**), the lymphoma cells are medium sized and have a high N/C ratio with scant cytoplasm. The nuclei are irregular with fine chromatin and inconspicuous nucleolus. Tumor cells are positive for CD10 (**c**) and cyclin D1 (**d**), but lack expression of CD5 (**e**)

Case History

A 72-year-old male was found to have a 3.7 cm peri-sacral mass. An incisional biopsy was performed.

Histologic Findings

- The biopsy displays a diffuse proliferation of tumor cells with frequent tingible-body macrophages and minimal reactive inflammatory cells (Fig. 6.3a).
- The tumor cells are large in size and have abundant amphophilic cytoplasm. The nuclei are round with vesicular chromatin and a central prominent nucleolus. There are frequent apoptotic cells and mitotic figures (Fig. 6.3b).

Differential Diagnosis

- Diffuse large B-cell lymphoma
- Plasmablastic neoplasm, including plasmablastic lymphoma and plasmacytoma
- Poorly differentiated carcinoma
- Other high-grade neoplasms, including melanoma and sarcoma

Initial Workup

- Positive for CD20 (Fig. 6.3c) and CD138 (Fig. 6.3d)
- Negative for CK AE1/3, S100, CD3, and CD45

Further Studies

- Positive for BOB1, OCT2, kappa, and Ki-67 (>90%)
- Negative for lambda, PAX5, cyclin D1, and EBER-ISH
- Subsequent clinical and laboratory studies revealed multiple lytic bone lesions, extensive bone marrow

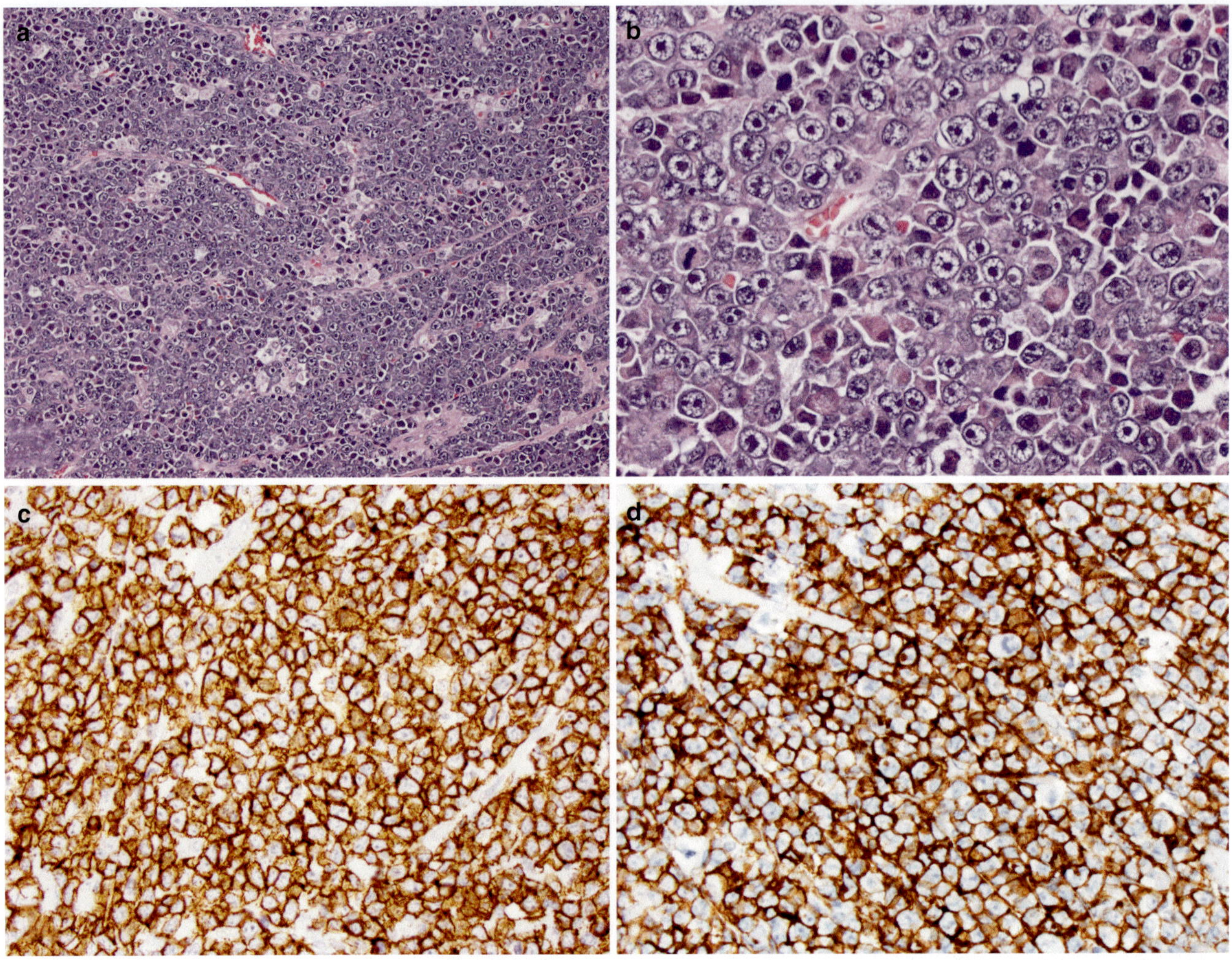

Fig. 6.3 Plasmablastic plasma cell myeloma resembling DLBCL. (**a**), a diffuse infiltration of tumor cells. (**b**), the large tumor cells have abundant amphophilic cytoplasm and round nuclei with vesicular chromatin and a central prominent nucleolus. They are positive for both CD20 (**c**) and CD138 (**d**)

involvement, and serum IgG paraprotein with kappa light chain restriction

Final Diagnosis

Plasma cell myeloma with plasmablastic morphology

Take-Home Messages

1. Plasma cell myeloma occasionally shows plasmablastic and/or immunoblastic cytology.
2. CD20 is expressed in a small proportion of plasma cell neoplasms.
3. CD138 should be frequently incorporated in the initial workup of DLBCL, even in cases with CD20 expression [13, 55, 57, 63, 77–88].

Case 4

Learning Objectives

1. To be aware of aberrant expression of markers in DLBCL
2. To know the important studies for lymphoid neoplasms to avoid misinterpretation

Case History

A 47-year-old female had GI symptoms and was found to have a large ileal mass. Multiple small biopsies were obtained from the terminal ileum.

Histologic Findings

- The ileal mucosa shows a diffuse intramucosal involvement (Fig. 6.4a).

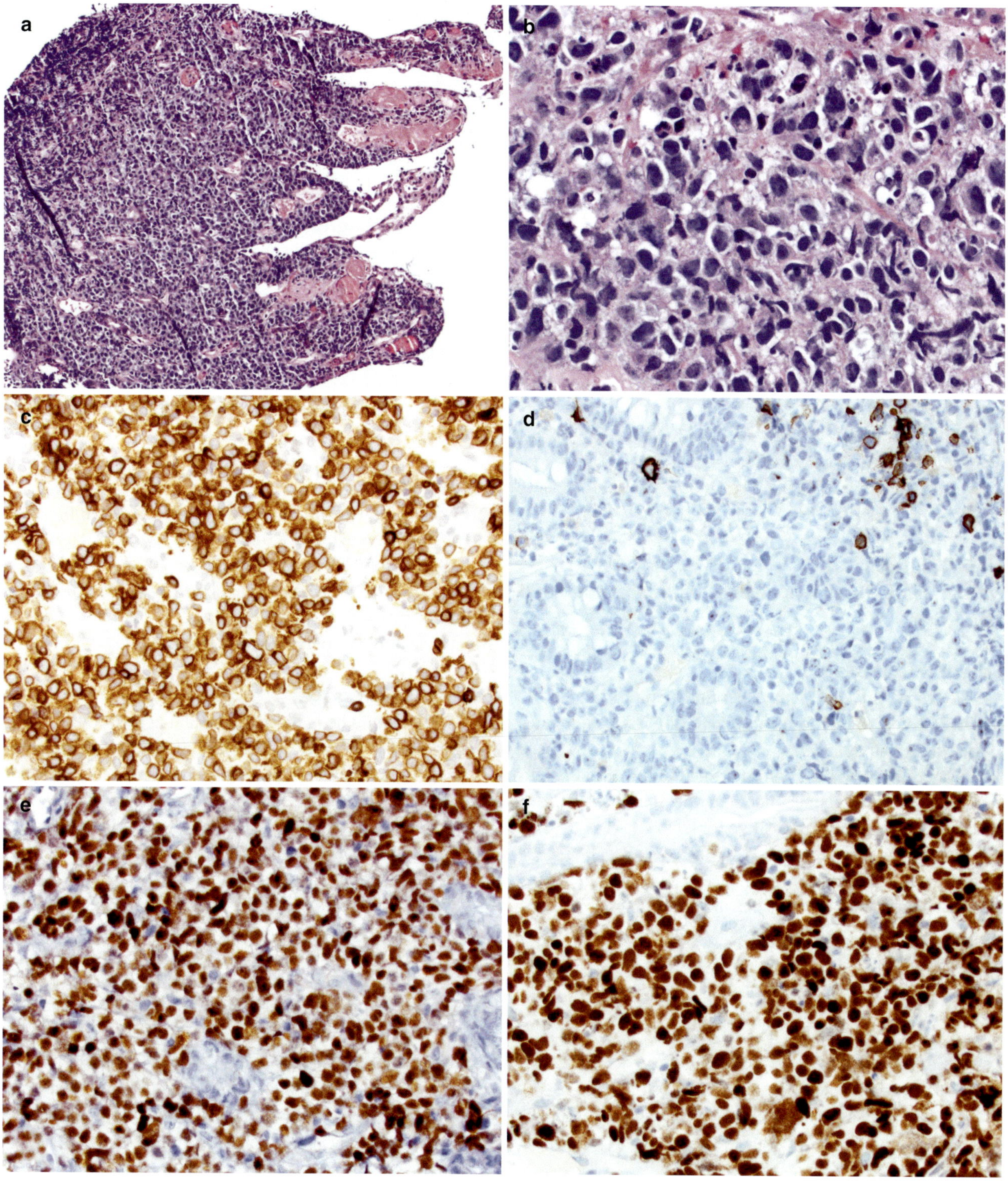

Fig. 6.4 Diffuse large B-cell lymphoma with aberrant CD3 expression. (**a**), diffuse intramucosal infiltration of lymphoma cells. (**b**), the large tumor cells have round or irregular nuclei with vesicular chromatin and prominent nucleoli. Lymphoma cells are positive for CD3 (**c**) but negative for CD20 (**d**). Additional studies show that the tumor cells express PAX5 (**e**) and OCT2 (**f**)

- The tumor cells are large in size and have round or irregular nuclei with vesicular chromatin and prominent nucleoli. There are frequent apoptotic bodies (Fig. 6.4b).

Differential Diagnosis

- Diffuse large B-cell lymphoma
- High-grade T-cell neoplasm, including peripheral T-cell lymphoma and anaplastic large cell lymphoma
- Poorly differentiated carcinoma or sarcoma

Initial Workup

- Positive for CD45 and CD3 (Fig. 6.4c)
- Negative for CD20 (Fig. 6.4d), CK AE1/AE3, S100, and CD138

Further Workup

- Positive for PAX5 (Fig. 6.4e), BOB1, OCT2 (Fig. 6.4f), MUM1, and Ki-67 (>90%)
- Negative for BCL6, CD4, CD5, CD7, CD8, CD10, CD30, CD56, and EBER-ISH

Final Diagnosis

Diffuse large B-cell lymphoma, with aberrant CD3 expression

Take-Home Messages

1. Rare cases of DLBCL may aberrantly express CD3.
2. DLBCL may rarely lose expression of CD20, even without rituximab treatment.
3. Besides CD20, at least one additional B-cell marker (usually PAX5) is recommended in the initial workup of DLBCL, even in cases positive for CD3.
4. PAX5 should NOT be used as the sole B-cell lineage marker in the initial workup since it can be expressed in non-hematopoietic neoplasms, including small cell carcinoma of the lung and Merkel cell carcinoma [63, 89–96].

Case 5

Learning Objectives

1. To recognize the morphologic mimicries of DLBCL
2. To utilize necessary studies in the initial workup of DLBCL

Case History

A 22-year-old male had increased left extremity weakness and pain. CT scans showed a T6 epidural mass. An incisional biopsy was performed.

Histologic Findings

- The biopsy reveals a diffuse infiltrate of lymphoid cells in the soft tissue (Fig. 6.5a).
- The tumor cells are medium sized and have a high N/C ratio. The nuclei are round to irregular with fine chromatin and small nucleoli. There are brisk mitotic figures (Fig. 6.5b).

Differential Diagnosis

- Hematopoietic neoplasms, including DLBCL, blastoid mantle cell lymphoma, and lymphoblastic lymphoma
- Other small round blue cell soft tissue sarcoma

Initial Workup

- Positive for CD45 and CD20 (Fig. 6.5c)
- Negative for CK AE1/3, CD3, CD30, CD138, and S100

Further Workup

- Positive for CD10, PAX5 (Fig. 6.5d), TdT (Fig. 6.5e), CD99 (Fig. 6.5f), and Ki-67 (>95%)
- Negative for CD34 and cyclin D1

Final Diagnosis

B-cell lymphoblastic lymphoma (LBL)

Take-Home Messages

1. B-LBL should be in the differential diagnosis of DLBCL, particularly in cases with blastoid cytology (medium-sized tumor cells, high N/C ratio, round or irregular nuclei, fine chromatin, and brisk mitoses).
2. Frequently incorporate CD34 and TdT in the initial workup of DLBCL, particularly in cases with blastoid cytology.
3. TdT may be expressed in rare cases of DLBCL, usually with a heterogeneous intensity.

Case 6

Learning Objectives

1. To understand the major histomorphologic features of T-cell/histiocyte-rich large B-cell lymphoma (THRLBCL)
2. To distinguish THRLBCL from its mimicries

Case History

A 33-year-old female presented with abdominal pain due to umbilical hernia, and image studies revealed a periportal lymph node of 3.9 cm, which was excised.

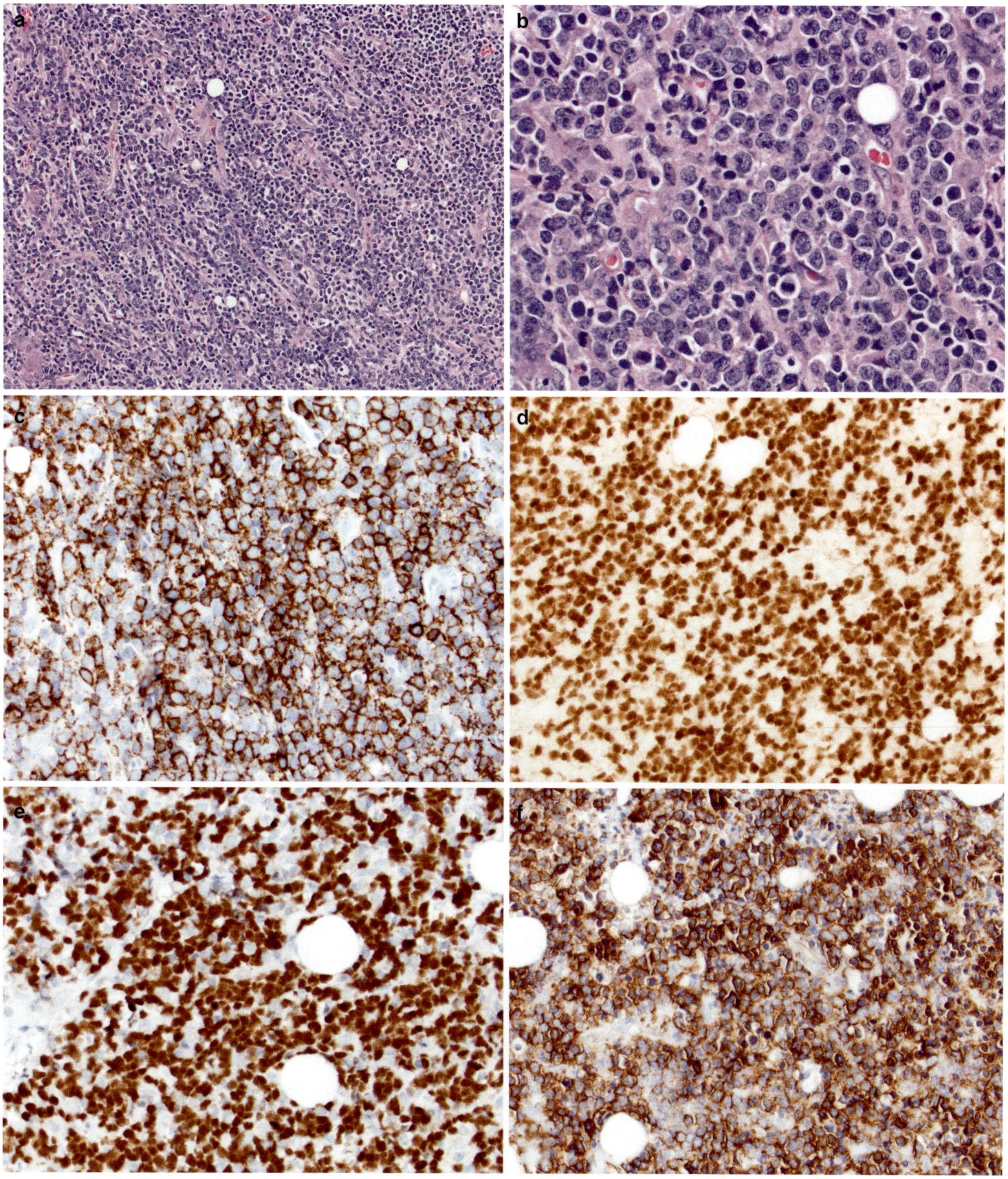

Fig. 6.5 B-cell lymphoblastic lymphoma resembling DLBCL. (**a**), diffuse infiltrate in the soft tissue by lymphoid cells. (**b**), the lymphoma cells are medium sized and have a high N/C ratio with round to irregular nuclei, fine chromatin, and small nucleoli. The tumor cells express CD20 (**c**), PAX5 (**d**), TdT (**e**), and CD99 (**f**)

Histologic Findings

- The lymph node architecture is effaced by a diffuse infiltration with no follicular or nodular pattern (Fig. 6.6a).
- There are scattered large atypical cells, with variable cytologic features, resembling centroblasts, immunoblasts, LP cells, and Reed-Sternberg cells. The background contains abundant reactive small lymphocytes and scattered and/or small clusters of histiocytes (Fig. 6.6b).

Differential Diagnosis

- T-cell/histiocyte-rich large B-cell lymphoma (THRLBCL)
- Nodular lymphocyte predominant Hodgkin lymphoma (NLPHL)
- Conventional DLBCL
- Classic Hodgkin lymphoma

Ancillary Studies

- The scattered large atypical cells are strongly positive for CD20 (Fig. 6.6c) and PAX5 without forming clusters or aggregates. They are negative for CD15, CD30, and EBER-ISH.
- Abundant reactive T-cells and histiocytes are highlighted by CD3 (Fig. 6.6d) and CD68 (Fig. 6.6e), respectively.
- CD23 shows no residual or expanded follicular dendritic meshworks.

Final Diagnosis

T-cell/histiocyte-rich large B-cell lymphoma (THRLBCL)

Take-Home Messages

1. In THRLBCL, the tumor cells are dispersed and account for <10% of all cells in the tissue. The significant increase

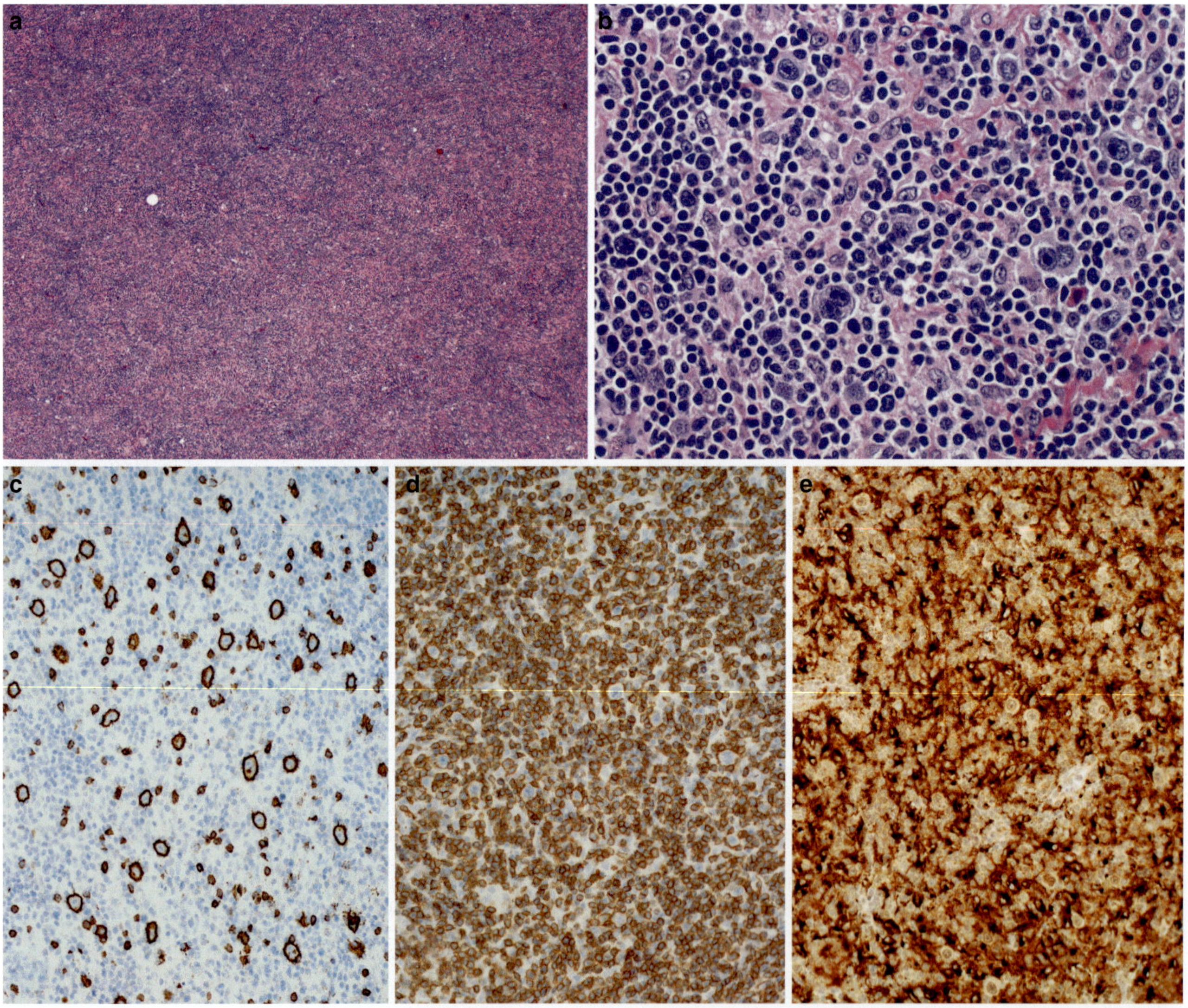

Fig. 6.6 T-cell/histiocyte-rich large B-cell lymphoma. (**a**), the lymph node shows a diffuse infiltration. (**b**), scattered large atypical cells in a background of abundant reactive lymphocytes and histiocytes. The scattered large cells are strongly positive for CD20 (**c**) and the background contains abundant reactive small T-cells (**d**; CD3) and histiocytes (**e**; CD68)

in large lymphoma cells (>10%) or formation of focal solid sheets of tumor cells would lean toward a diagnosis of conventional DLBCL.
2. NLPHL can be separated from THRLBCL with at least focally expanded follicular dendritic meshworks and/or presence of rosettes of follicular T-helper cells around the large lymphoma cells.
3. THRLBCL is typically negative for CD15, CD30, and *EBV* infection, in contrast to classic Hodgkin lymphoma [26–28].

Case 7

Learning Objectives

1. To know the major morphologic features of lymphomatoid granulomatosis (LyG)
2. To differentiate LyG from "granulomatosis with polyangiitis (GPA)" and "NK-/T-cell lymphoma, nasal type"

Case History

A 71-year-old female presented with persistent cough, chest pain, fever, and weight loss. Clinical images studies revealed multiple mass lesions in the bilateral lungs. An open biopsy was performed from the left upper lobe.

Histologic Findings

- The mass lesion from the left upper lobe shows a diffuse infiltration of atypical cells with focal coagulative necrosis (Fig. 6.7a).
- There are abundant large atypical cells (Fig. 6.7b) in a background of reactive inflammatory cells and focal angioinvasion (Fig. 6.7c).

Differential Diagnosis

- Lymphomatoid granulomatosis (LyG)
- NK-/T-cell lymphoma, nasal type
- Granulomatosis with polyangiitis (GPA)
- Poorly differentiated carcinoma

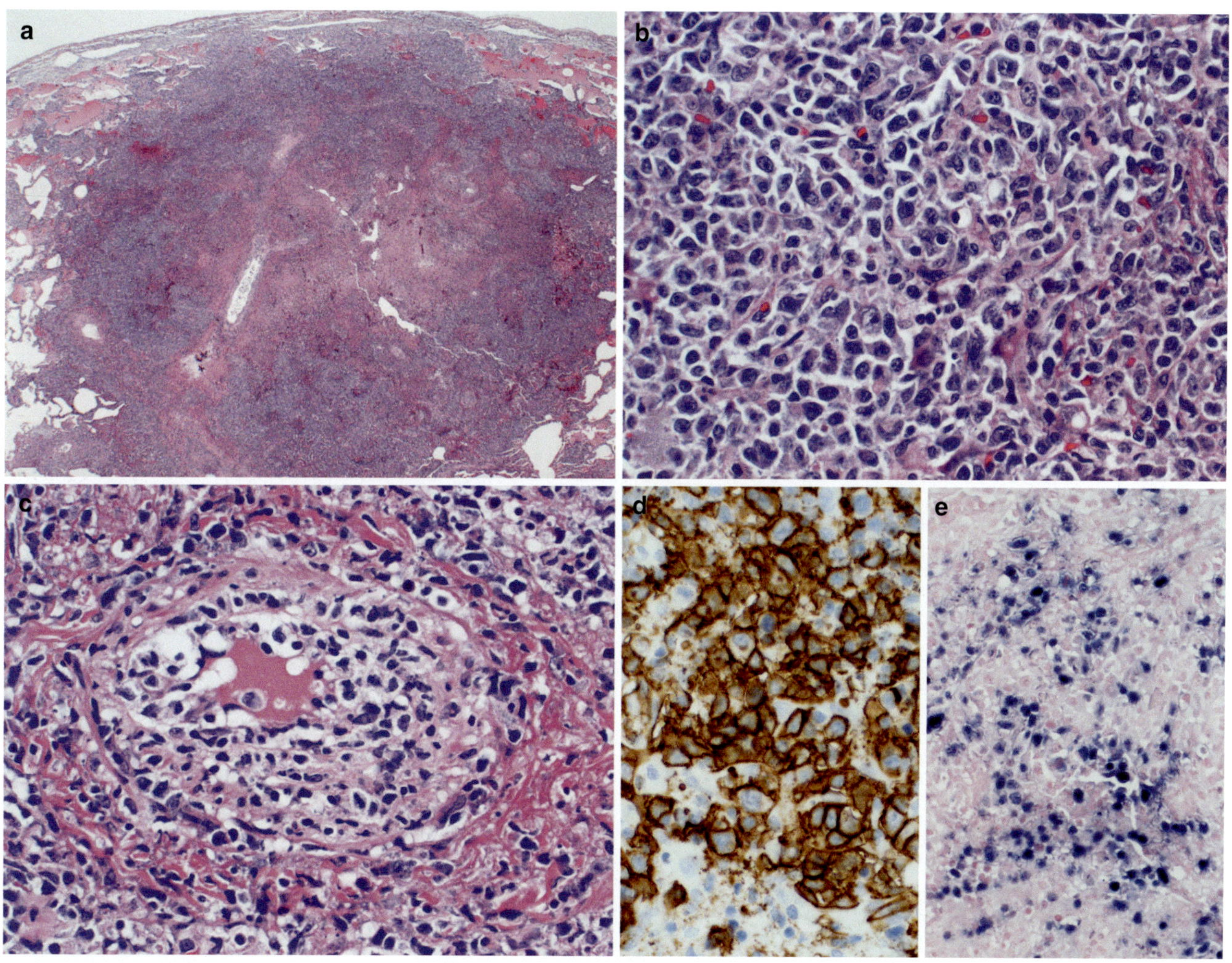

Fig. 6.7 Lymphomatoid granulomatosis. (**a**), a nodular infiltration in the lung with focal coagulative necrosis. (**b**), abundant large atypical cells in a background of reactive inflammatory cells and focal angioinvasion (**c**). The large cells are positive for CD20 (**d**) with *EBV* infection (**e**)

Ancillary Studies

- The large cells are positive for CD45, CD20 (Fig. 6.7d), PAX5, BCL6, MUM1, and EBER-ISH (Fig. 6.7e)
- Negative for CD3, CD10, CD30, and CD138

Final Diagnosis

Lymphomatoid granulomatosis (LyG)

Take-Home Messages

1. Typical morphologic features of LyG: presence of large tumor cells, scattered or in sheets with *EBV* infection, angioinvasion and angiodestruction, and coagulative necrosis.
2. NK-/T-cell lymphoma, nasal type, overlaps LyG with angioinvasion, coagulative necrosis, and *EBV* infection. However, NK-/T-cell lymphoma is positive for CD3, CD56, and cytotoxic markers.
3. GPA shares some features with LyG, including angioinvasion and presence of geographic necrosis. However, in GPA there are microabscesses and palisading granulomas with no atypical lymphocytes or *EBV* infection. Instead, the serum is positive for C-ANCA [43, 44].

Case 8

Learning Objective

1. To recognize the major clinicopathologic features of intravascular large B-cell lymphoma (IVLBCL)

Case History

A 65-year-old female presented with changes of mental status, fatigue, and renal failure. Further clinical studies revealed anemia and multiple nonspecific white matter lesions and meningeal enhancement. She also had scattered painful indurated erythematous skin eruptions, particularly on the bilateral legs. A skin punch biopsy was performed from her left lower leg.

Histologic Findings

- The skin shows unremarkable epidermis and dermis except groups of large atypical cells in some small vessels (Fig. 6.8a)
- The atypical cells in the vessels possess round nuclei, prominent nucleoli, and small to moderate amount of cytoplasm (Fig. 6.8b)

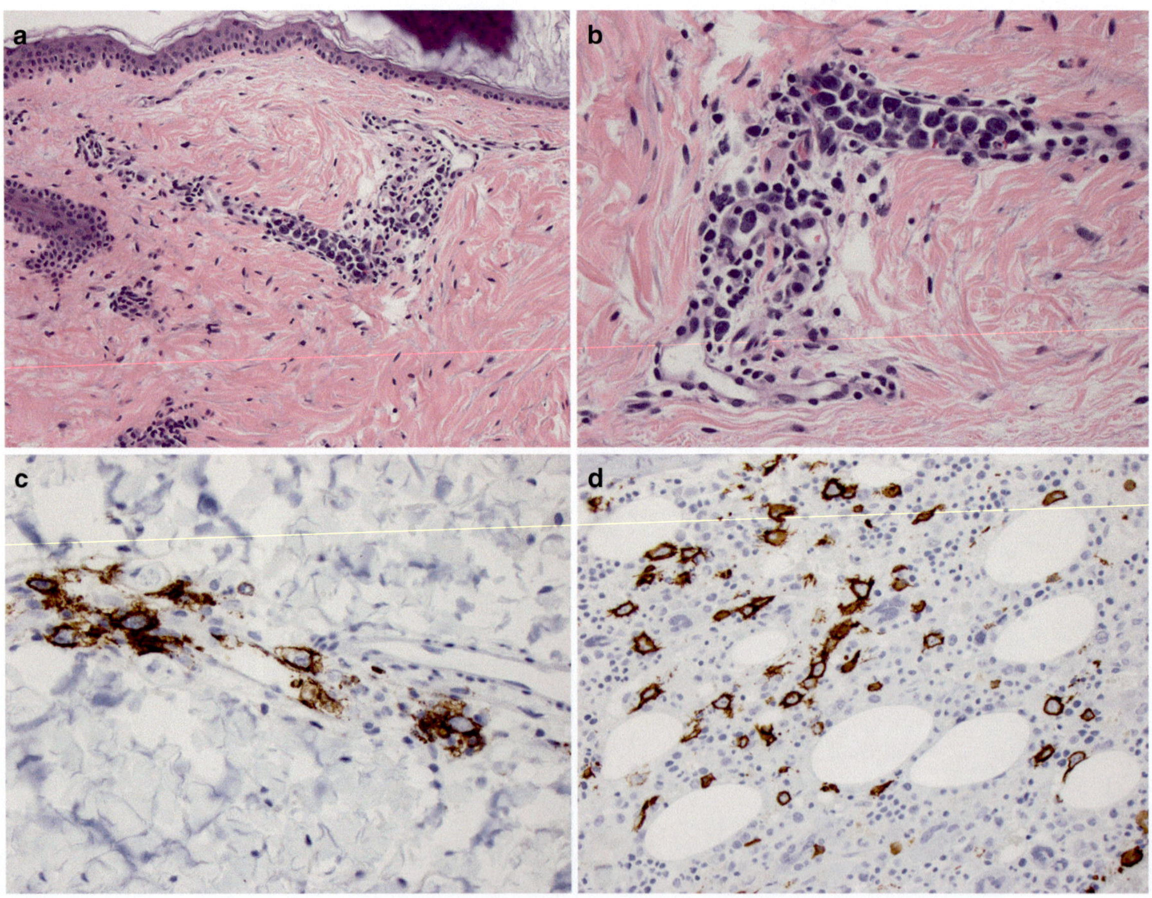

Fig. 6.8 Intravascular large B-cell lymphoma. (**a**), a skin biopsy contains large atypical cells in small vessels within the dermis. (**b**), the intravascular atypical cells have round nuclei and prominent nucleoli, and they are positive for CD20 (**c**). Scattered and focal sinusoidal lymphoma cells are also noted in the bone marrow, as highlighted by CD20 (**d**)

Differential Diagnosis

- Intravascular large B-cell lymphoma (IVLBCL)
- Other hematopoietic neoplasms, including anaplastic large cell lymphoma and acute myeloid leukemia

Ancillary Studies

- Positive for CD45, CD20 (Fig. 6.8c), and PAX5
- Negative for CD3 and CD30
- A subsequent bone marrow biopsy reveals scattered and sinusoidal lymphoma cells, which are highlighted by CD20 (Fig. 6.8d)

Final Diagnosis

Intravascular large B-cell lymphoma (IVLBCL)

Take-Home Message

1. IVLBCL is usually a systemic B-cell lymphoma with involvement in the small blood vessels [35–40].

Case 9

Learning Objectives

1. To know the important clinicopathologic features of primary mediastinal large B-cell lymphoma (PMLBCL)
2. To be familiar with the ancillary studies to reach an accurate diagnosis of PMLBCL
3. To distinguish PMLBCL from its mimicries

Case History

A 27-year-old male presented with superior vena cava syndrome, and subsequent image studies showed a 15 cm anterior mediastinal mass. An incisional biopsy was performed.

Histologic Findings

- The biopsy shows a diffuse infiltration of tumor cells with marked background fibrosis (Fig. 6.9a).
- The tumor cells are large in size and have round or irregular nuclei, vesicular chromatin, and prominent nucleoli. The cytoplasm is abundant and clear staining. Characteristically, there are delicate fibrotic bundles surrounding small groups of or individual cells (Fig. 6.9b).

Differential Diagnosis

- Primary mediastinal large B-cell lymphoma (PMLBCL)
- Classic Hodgkin lymphoma, nodular sclerosis variant (CHL-NS)
- Germ cell tumor

Ancillary Studies

- Positive for CD45, CD20, PAX5, CD30, CD23, and BCL6
- Negative for CD3, CD10, CD15, and EBER-ISH

Final Diagnosis

Primary mediastinal large B-cell lymphoma (PMLBCL)

Take-Home Messages

1. PMLBCL typically affects young patients with a bulky anterior mediastinal mass. The lymphoma cells often show abundant clear cytoplasm in a background with delicate fibrosis. CD23 and CD30 are commonly expressed.
2. CHL-NS overlaps PMLBCL in many clinicopathologic features. However, CHL-NS is typically positive for CD15 with weak expression of PAX5, whereas CD20 and CD45 are usually negative [30–34].

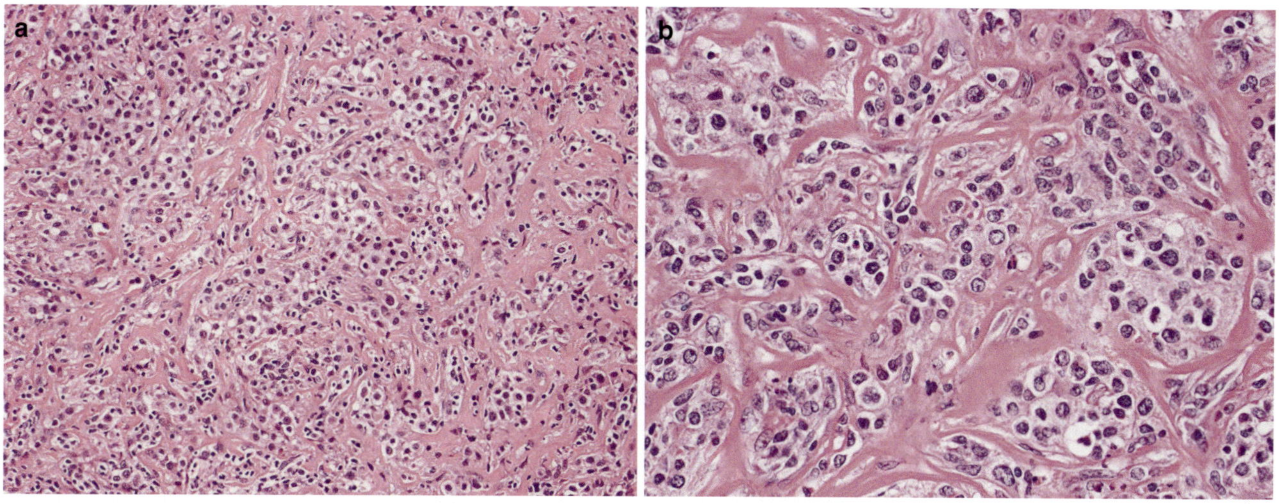

Fig. 6.9 Primary mediastinal large B-cell lymphoma. (**a**), the excisional biopsy from a large mediastinal mass shows a diffuse infiltration of tumor cells with marked background fibrosis. (**b**), the large tumor cells have round or irregular nuclei, vesicular chromatin, and prominent nucleoli. The cytoplasm is abundant and clear staining. In the background, there are characteristic, delicate fibrotic bundles surrounding small groups of or individual lymphoma cells

Case 10

Learning Objectives

1. To learn the clinicopathologic characteristic of ALK-positive large B-cell lymphoma (ALK+ LBCL)
2. To distinguish ALK+ LBCL from its mimicries
3. To know the necessary workups to diagnose ALK+ LBCL

Case History

A 32-year-old male presented with fatigue, weight loss, and night sweats for several weeks. Physical examinations revealed multiple enlarged cervical lymph nodes. Subsequent clinical image studies showed systemic lymphadenopathy, particularly in the cervical region with the largest one measuring up to 3.1 cm. A large cervical lymph node was excised.

Histologic Findings

- The cervical lymph node has a diffuse infiltration of tumor cells (Fig. 6.10a).
- The tumor cells are large in size with a spectrum of cytologic features, including plasmacytic and plasmablastic cells (Fig. 6.10b).

Differential Diagnosis

- Plasmablastic lymphoma
- Plasma cell neoplasm with plasmablastic cytology

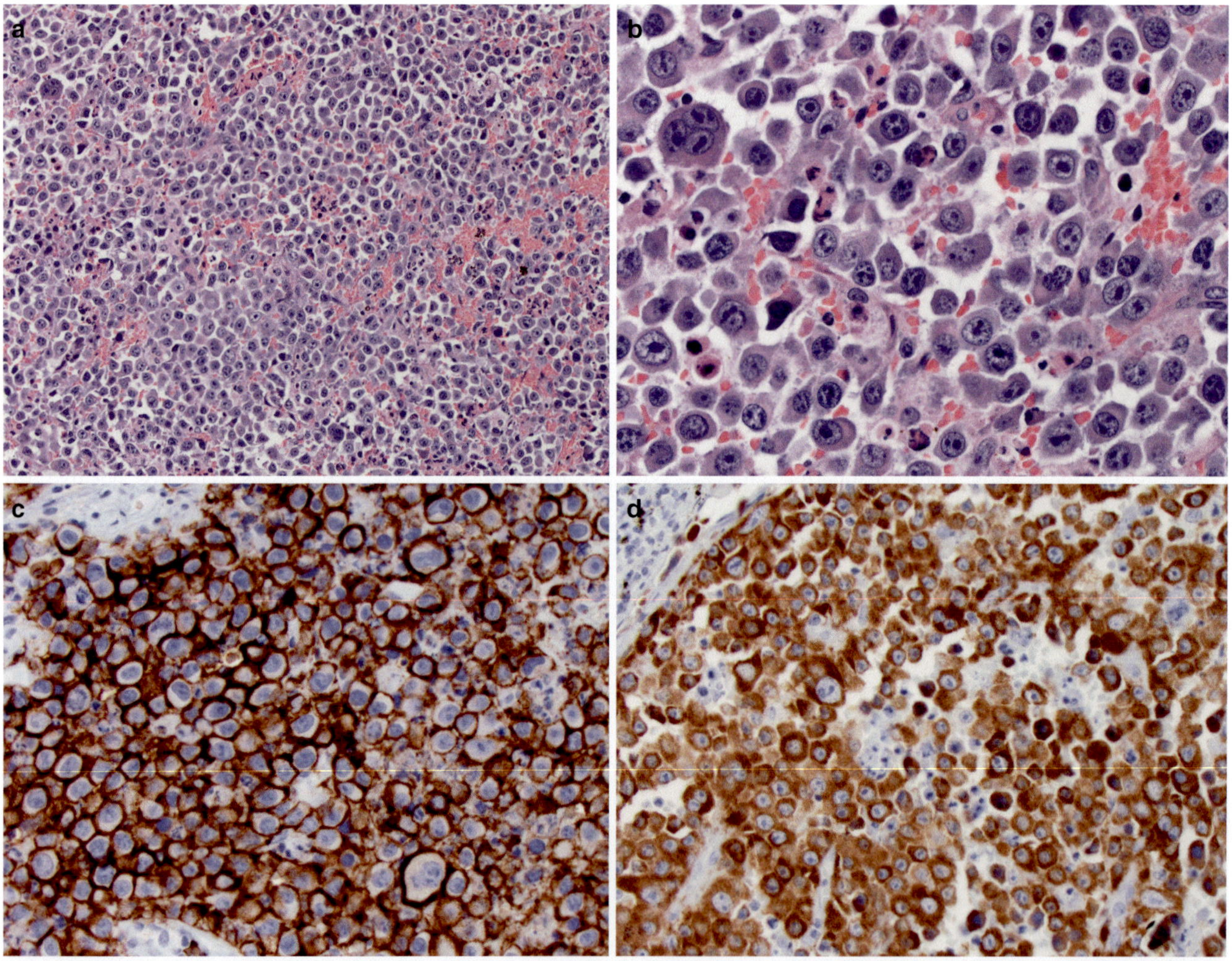

Fig. 6.10 ALK-positive large B-cell lymphoma. (**a**), the lymph node shows a diffuse infiltration of tumor cells, which are large in size with a spectrum of cytologic features, including plasmacytic and plasmablastic cells (**b**). The lymphoma cells are positive for CD138 (**c**), ALK (**d**)

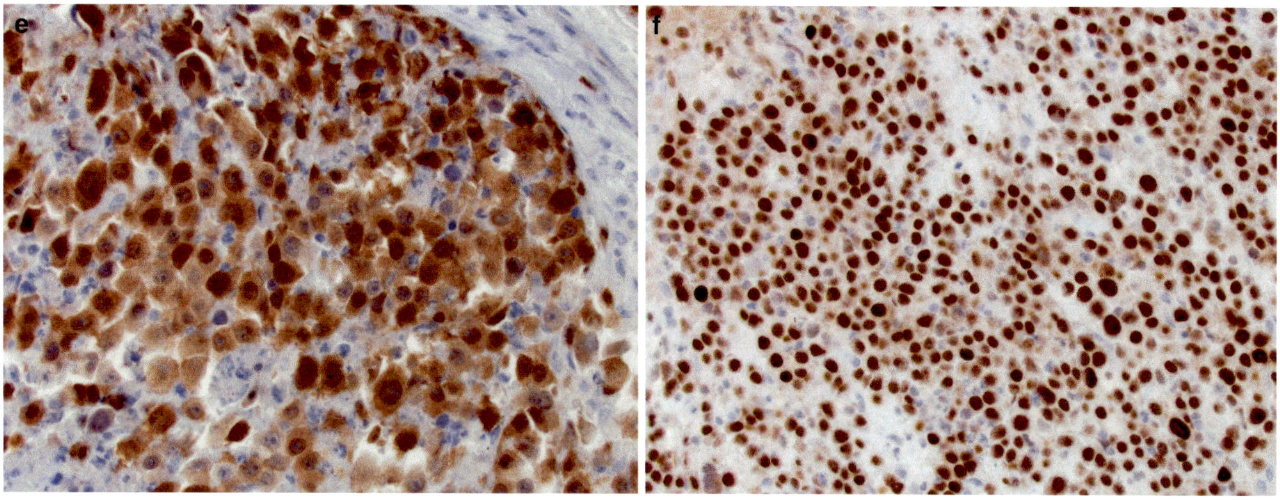

Fig. 6.10 (continued) BOB1 (**e**), and OCT2 (**f**)

- ALK-positive large B-cell lymphoma (ALK+ LBCL)
- Other high-grade neoplasms, including melanoma and poorly differentiated carcinoma

Initial Workup
- Positive for CD45, CD138 (Fig. 6.10c), and MUM1
- Negative for CD3, CD20, CD30, CK AE1/AE3, and S100

Further Workup
- Positive for ALK (Fig. 6.10d), BOB1 (Fig. 6.10e), OCT2 (Fig. 6.10f), CD4, and IgA with kappa light chain restriction
- Negative for PAX5, CD2, CD5, CD7, CD8, lambda, and EBER-ISH
- Positive for *ALK* rearrangement by FISH assay

Final Diagnosis
ALK-positive large B-cell lymphoma (ALK+ LBCL)

Take-Home Messages
1. ALK+ LBCL has to be separated from ALK+ anaplastic large cell lymphoma; ALK+ LBCL is negative for CD30 and T-cell markers except CD4. In addition, ALK+ LBCL expresses BOB1 and OCT2, and ALK stain shows a characteristic cytoplasmic dotted staining pattern.
2. ALK+ LBCL may have plasmablastic, immunoblastic, and/or anaplastic cytology, which may be reminiscent of DLBCL and plasmablastic neoplasm.
3. ALK may be considered in plasmablastic neoplasms with the following features:
   - Immunocompetent young patients
   - Involvement of extramedullary sites, especially lymph nodes
   - Presence of sinusoidal infiltration in the lymph node
   - Co-expression of CD45 but not routine B-cell markers (CD20 and PAX5) [13, 24, 45–53]

Case 11

Learning Objectives
1. To recognize the typical clinicopathologic features of plasmablastic lymphoma (PBL)
2. To distinguish PBL from plasmablastic plasma cell neoplasm and extra-cavitary primary effusion lymphoma

Case History
A 34-year-old male had a long history of HIV infection. Recently he presented with a 3.4 cm ulcerated mass in the oral cavity. An incisional biopsy was performed.

Histologic Findings
- The oral biopsy displays an extensive infiltration by nested and diffuse tumor cells in the submucosa (Fig. 6.11a).
- The tumor cells are large in size and have moderate to abundant amphophilic cytoplasm. The nuclei are round with vesicular chromatin and a central prominent nucleolus. Frequent apoptotic cells and mitotic figures are noted (Fig. 6.11b).

Differential Diagnosis
- Hematopoietic neoplasm, including DLBCL, PBL, and plasmacytoma
- Poorly differentiated carcinoma
- Mucosal melanoma

Initial Workup
- Positive for CD138 (Fig. 6.11c)
- Negative for CD45, CD3, CD20, CK AE1/AE3, and S100

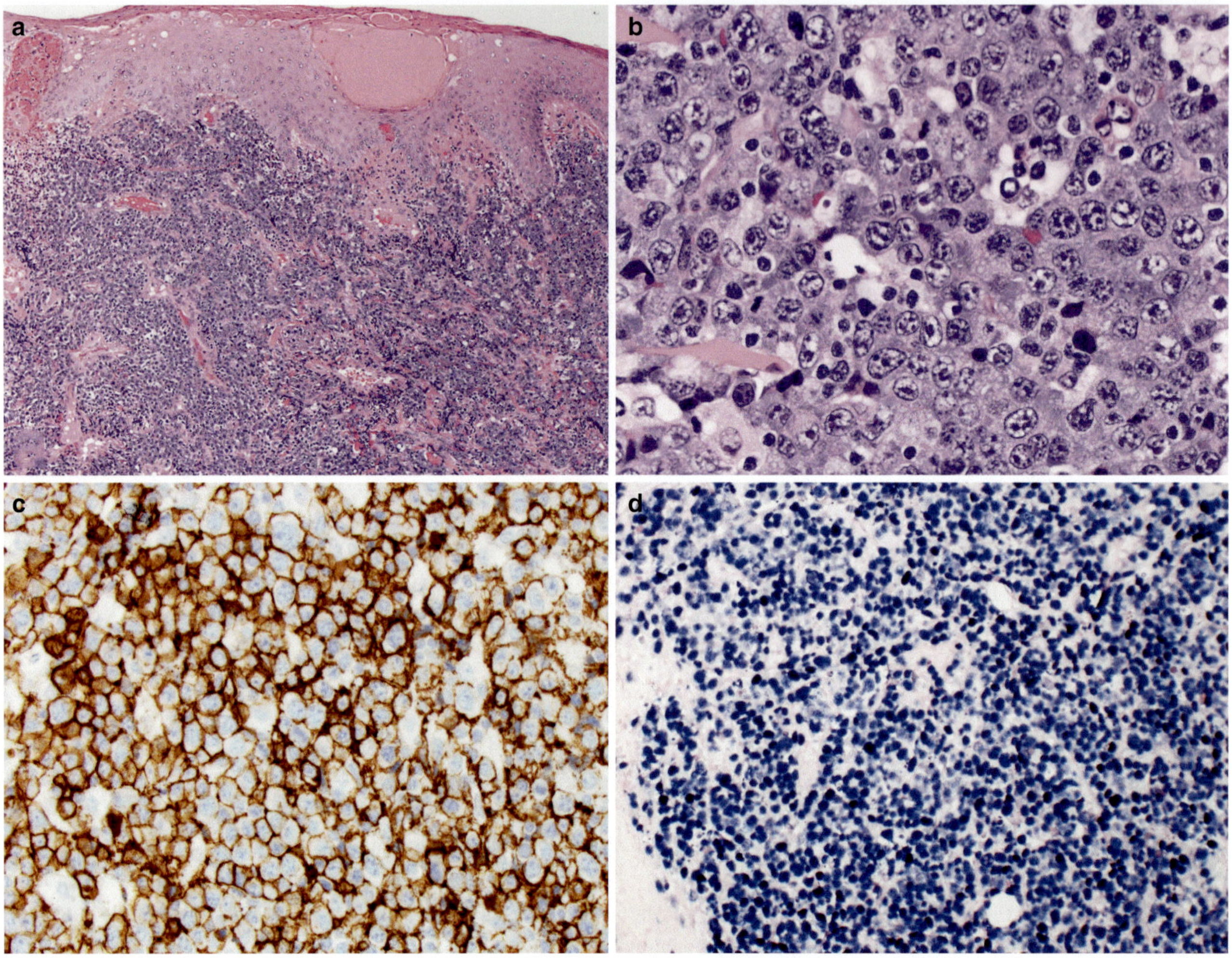

Fig. 6.11 Plasmablastic lymphoma. (**a**), the oral biopsy from an AIDS male displays a diffuse infiltration of tumor cells in the submucosa. (**b**), the large tumor cells have moderate to abundant amphophilic cytoplasm and round nuclei with vesicular chromatin and a central prominent nucleolus. There are frequent apoptotic cells and mitotic figures. The tumor cells are positive for CD138 (**c**) with *EBV* infection (**d**)

Further Workup

- Positive for lambda, BOB1, OCT2, and EBER-ISH (Fig. 6.11d)
- Negative for kappa and HHV8

Final Diagnosis

Plasmablastic lymphoma (PBL)

Take-Home Messages

1. PBL commonly arises in the oral cavity of AIDS patient.
2. PBL can be separated from plasmablastic plasma cell neoplasm with positive *EBV* infection.
3. PBL shares many clinicopathologic features with extracavitary primary effusion lymphoma. However, HHV8 is negative in PBL [78, 83, 97–100].

Case 12

Learning Objectives

1. To know the typical clinical features of primary effusion lymphoma (PEL)
2. To recognize the cytologic features of PEL
3. To learn the major immunophenotype of PEL

Case History

A 39-year-old male had uncontrolled HIV infection for 6 years. He recently presented to the emergency room with shortness of breath, and clinical examinations revealed abundant bilateral pleural effusions, which were sent for cytology evaluation.

Histologic Findings

- The pleural effusion smears (Wright-Giemsa stained) show abundant large atypical cells with plasmablastic features. They have round or irregular nuclei with prominent nucleoli (Fig. 6.12a). The cytoplasm is moderate to abundant and basophilic.

Differential Diagnosis

- Primary effusion lymphoma
- Other high-grade hematopoietic neoplasms, including DLBCL and anaplastic large cell lymphoma
- Poorly differentiated carcinoma or sarcoma

Initial Workup

- Positive for CD45 (Fig. 6.12b), CD3 (weak and subset), CD138, HHV8 (Fig. 6.12c), and EBER-ISH
- Negative for CD20, PAX5, and CK AE1/AE3

Further Studies

- Positive for CD30, BOB1, and OCT2
- Negative for other T-cell markers, including CD2, CD4, CD5, CD7, and CD8
- Negative for kappa or lambda by immunohistochemical staining and in situ hybridization

Final Diagnosis

Primary effusion lymphoma (PEL)

Take-Home Messages

1. PEL occurs in the body cavities of AIDS patients.
2. Mostly positive for CD45, CD30, and *EBV* infection. CD138 and light chains are mostly detectable but are negative in a small proportion of cases.
3. CD20 and PAX5 are negative, whereas BOB1 and OCT2 are expressed in the majority of cases.
4. HHV8 positivity is diagnostic for PEL, even in cases with CD3 expression [54, 61, 101, 102].

Case 13

Learning Objectives

1. To be aware of the rare type of extra-cavitary primary effusion lymphoma (PEL)
2. To know the immunophenotype of extra-cavitary PEL
3. To distinguish extra-cavitary PEL from plasmablastic lymphoma and other entities

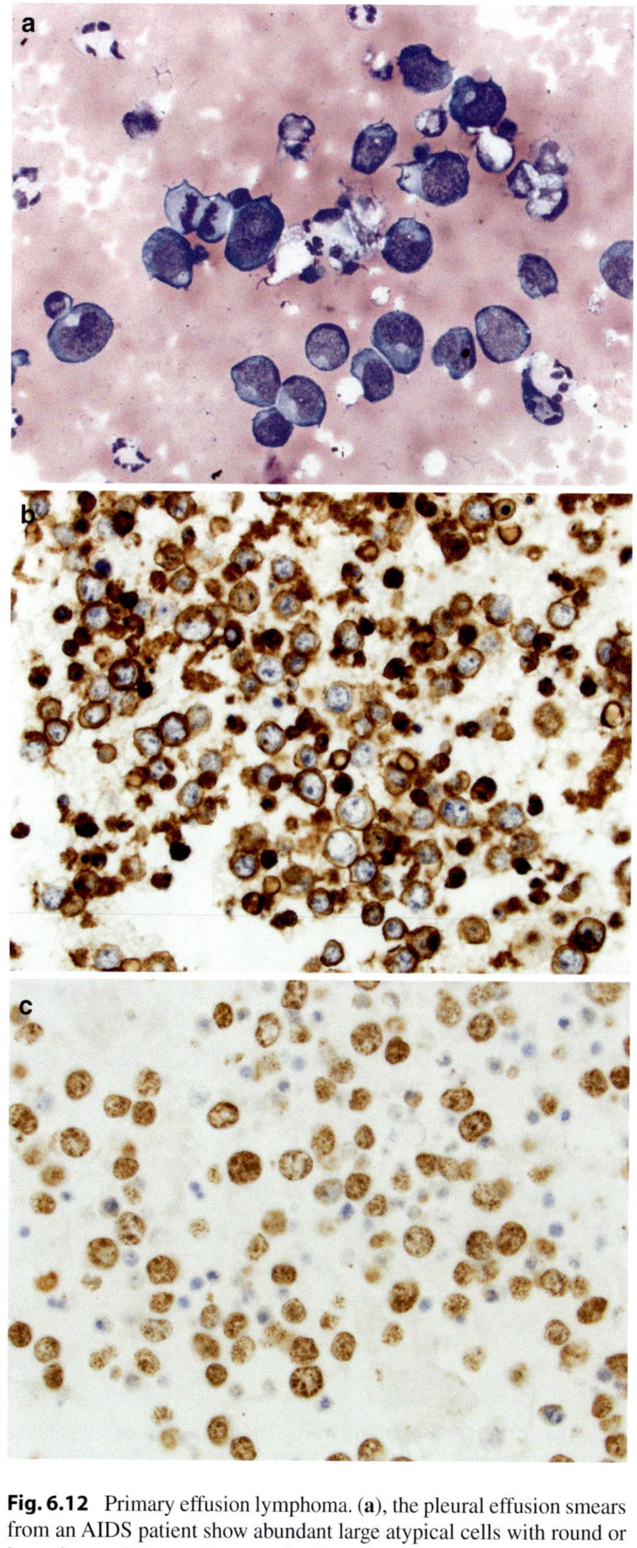

Fig. 6.12 Primary effusion lymphoma. (**a**), the pleural effusion smears from an AIDS patient show abundant large atypical cells with round or irregular nuclei, prominent nucleoli, and moderate to abundant basophilic cytoplasm. The atypical cells express CD45 (**b**) and HHV8 (**c**)

Case History

A 39-year-old HIV+ male presented with diarrhea and abdominal pain. Colonoscopy showed several mass lesions in the transverse colon and descending colon. Multiple biopsies were performed from the masses and revealed similar morphologic features.

Histologic Findings

- The colon has a prominent intramucosal infiltrate by sheets of tumor cells (Fig. 6.13a).
- The tumor cells are large in size and have round nuclei with vesicular chromatin and prominent nucleoli. There are brisk mitotic figures and apoptotic bodies (Fig. 6.13b).

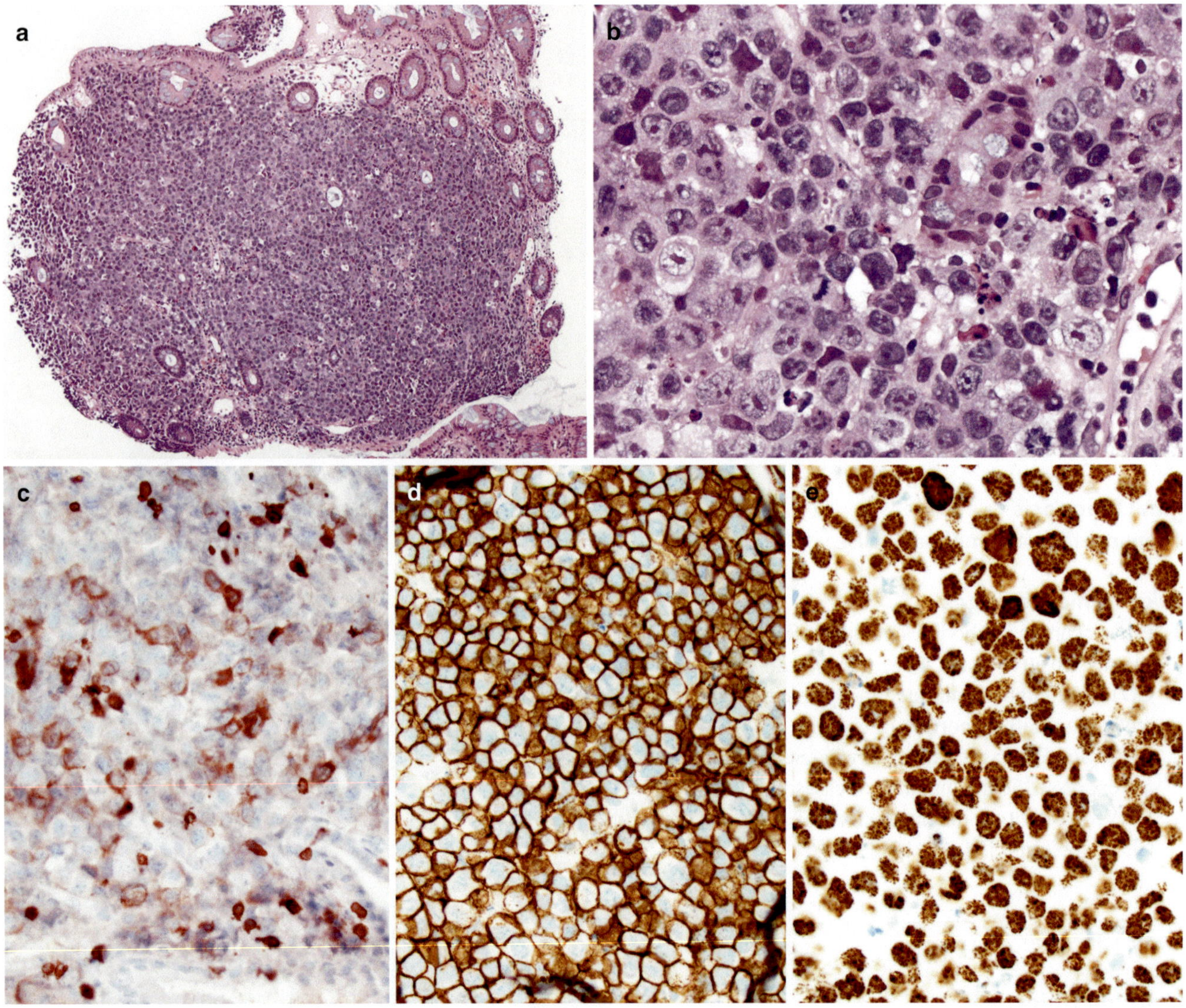

Fig. 6.13 Extra-cavitary primary effusion lymphoma. (**a**), the colon biopsy from an HIV+ male shows sheets of tumor cells in the mucosa. (**b**), the large tumor cells have round nuclei with vesicular chromatin and prominent nucleoli. They are positive for CD3 (**c**), CD138 (**d**), and HHV8 (**e**).

Differential Diagnosis

- Diffuse large B-cell lymphoma
- Plasmablastic lymphoma
- Anaplastic large cell lymphoma or other high-grade T-cell lymphoma
- Poorly differentiated carcinoma

Initial Workup

- Positive for CD3 (subset and variable; Fig. 6.13c), CD30, and CD138 (Fig. 6.13d)
- Negative for CD45, CD20, CK AE1/AE3, and S100

Further Workup and Other Ancillary Studies

- Positive for BOB1, OCT2, HHV8 (Fig. 6.13e), and EBER-ISH (Fig. 6.13f)
- Negative for CD2, CD79a, and PAX5

Final Diagnosis

Extra-cavitary primary effusion lymphoma (PEL)

Take-Home Messages

1. Extra-cavitary PEL is very rare and not associated with effusions in the body cavities.
2. The cytology and immunophenotype are otherwise similar to classic PEL [54, 57, 58, 60, 103, 104].

Case 14

Learning Objectives

1. To understand the definition of "high-grade B-cell lymphoma (HGBL) with *MYC* and *BCL2* and/or *BCL6* rearrangement"
2. To know the differential diagnosis of "HGBL with *MYC* and *BCL2* and/or *BCL6* rearrangement"
3. To be aware of the necessary studies to diagnose "HGBL with *MYC* and *BCL2* and/or *BCL6* rearrangement"

Case History

A 78-year-old male had several enlarged inguinal lymphomas, with the largest one 3.1 cm.

Histologic Findings

- The lymph node reveals entire architectural effacement by a diffuse infiltration of tumor cells (Fig. 6.14a).
- The tumor cells are large in size and have a small to moderate amount of cytoplasm. The nuclei are round to irregular with vesicular chromatin and prominent nucleoli (Fig. 6.14b).

Differential Diagnosis

- Diffuse large B-cell lymphoma, NOS
- Other hematopoietic neoplasms, including Burkitt lymphoma, blastoid mantle cell lymphoma, and high-grade T-cell lymphoma
- Metastatic poorly differentiated carcinoma or sarcoma

Initial Workup

- Positive for CD45, CD20, and PAX5
- Negative for CD3, CK AE1/AE3, and S100

Further Workup and Other Ancillary Studies

- Positive for BCL2 (Fig. 6.14c), MUM1, MYC (Fig. 6.14d), and Ki-67 (>90%)
- Negative for CD10, BCL6, CD34, cyclin D1, CD138, TdT, and EBER-ISH
- FISH studies positive for *BCL2* and *MYC* rearrangements, but negative for *BCL6* rearrangement (Fig. 6.14e and Fig. 6.14f)

Final Diagnosis

High-grade B-cell lymphoma with *MYC* and *BCL2* and/or *BCL6* rearrangement

Take-Home Messages

1. It is necessary to perform FISH studies for *BCL2*, *BCL6*, and *MYC* rearrangements in high-grade B-cell lymphomas after ruling out other specific entities.
2. BCL2, BCL6, or MYC protein expression does not always reflect the gene rearrangement status, and therefore FISH studies are required for the diagnosis of this entity [70, 105, 106].

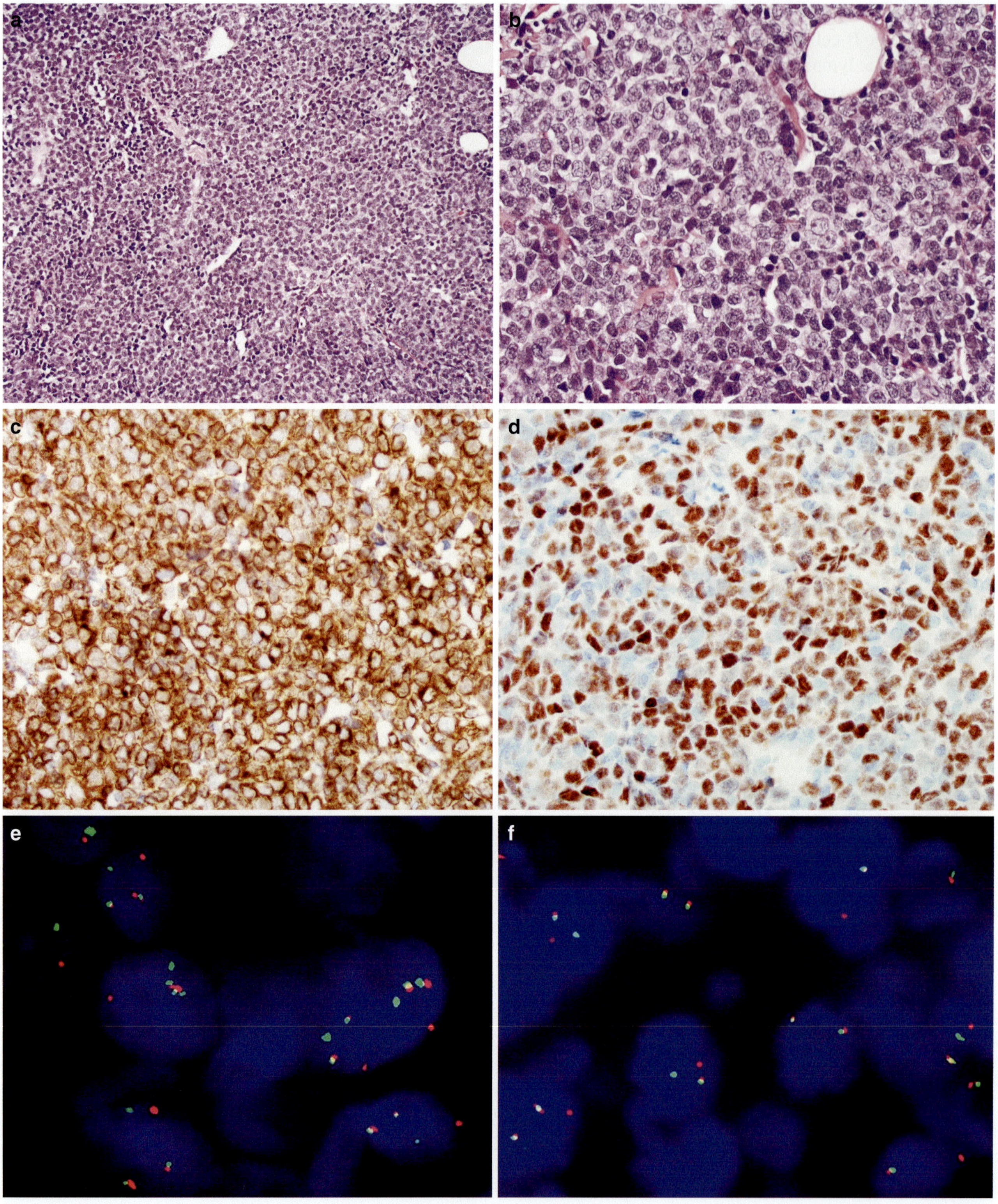

Fig. 6.14 High-grade B-cell lymphoma with *MYC* and *BCL2* and/or *BCL6* rearrangement. (**a**), the lymph node architecture is effaced by a diffuse infiltration of tumor cells, which are large in size and have round to irregular nuclei with vesicular chromatin and prominent nucleoli (**b**). The lymphoma cells are positive for BCL2 (**c**) and MYC (**d**). FISH studies detect *BCL2* and *MYC* rearrangements (**e** and **f**). (Images courtesy of Dr. Shaoying Li from the MD Anderson Cancer Center, Houston, TX)

References

1. Anonymous. A clinical evaluation of the International Lymphoma Study Group classification of non-Hodgkin's lymphoma. The Non-Hodgkin's Lymphoma Classification Project. Blood. 1997;89:3909–18.
2. Alizadeh AA, Eisen MB, Davis RE, Ma C, Lossos IS, Rosenwald A, et al. Distinct types of diffuse large B-cell lymphoma identified by gene expression profiling. Nature. 2000;403:503–11.
3. Armitage JO, Weisenburger DD. New approach to classifying non-Hodgkin's lymphomas: clinical features of the major histologic subtypes. Non-Hodgkin's Lymphoma Classification Project. J Clin Oncol. 1998;16:2780–95.
4. Dobashi A. Molecular pathogenesis of diffuse large B-cell lymphoma. J Clin Exp Hematop. 2016;56:71–8.
5. Leonard JP, Kolibaba KS, Reeves JA, Tulpule A, Flinn IW, Kolevska T, et al. Randomized phase II study of R-CHOP with or without bortezomib in previously untreated patients with non-germinal center B-cell-like diffuse large B-cell lymphoma. J Clin Oncol. 2017;35:3538–46.
6. Miyazaki K. Treatment of diffuse large B-cell lymphoma. J Clin Exp Hematop. 2016;56:79–88.
7. Reddy A, Zhang J, Davis NS, Moffitt AB, Love CL, Waldrop A, et al. Genetic and functional drivers of diffuse large B cell lymphoma. Cell. 2017;171:481,494.e15.
8. Swerdlow SH, Campo E, Pileri SA, Harris NL, Stein H, Siebert R, et al. The 2016 revision of the World Health Organization classification of lymphoid neoplasms. Blood. 2016;127:2375–90.
9. Hans CP, Weisenburger DD, Greiner TC, Gascoyne RD, Delabie J, Ott G, et al. Confirmation of the molecular classification of diffuse large B-cell lymphoma by immunohistochemistry using a tissue microarray. Blood. 2004;103:275–82.
10. Li M, Liu Y, Wang Y, Chen G, Chen Q, Xiao H, et al. Anaplastic variant of diffuse large B-cell lymphoma displays intricate genetic alterations and distinct biological features. Am J Surg Pathol. 2017;41:1322–32.
11. Ott G, Ziepert M, Klapper W, Horn H, Szczepanowski M, Bernd HW, et al. Immunoblastic morphology but not the immunohistochemical GCB/nonGCB classifier predicts outcome in diffuse large B-cell lymphoma in the RICOVER-60 trial of the DSHNHL. Blood. 2010;116:4916–25.
12. Camara DA, Stefanoff CG, Pires AR, Soares F, Biasoli I, Zalcberg I, et al. Immunoblastic morphology in diffuse large B-cell lymphoma is associated with a nongerminal center immunophenotypic profile. Leuk Lymphoma. 2007;48:892–6.
13. Pan Z, Hu S, Li M, Zhou Y, Kim YS, Reddy V, et al. ALK-positive large B-cell lymphoma: a clinicopathologic study of 26 cases with review of additional 108 cases in the literature. Am J Surg Pathol. 2017;41:25–38.
14. Carbone A, Gloghini A, Libra M, Gasparotto D, Navolanic PM, Spina M, et al. A spindle cell variant of diffuse large B-cell lymphoma possesses genotypic and phenotypic markers characteristic of a germinal center B-cell origin. Mod Pathol. 2006;19:299–306.
15. Kimura Y, Arakawa F, Kiyasu J, Miyoshi H, Yoshida M, Ichikawa A, et al. A spindle cell variant of diffuse large B-cell lymphoma is characterized by T-cell/myofibrohistio-rich stromal alterations: analysis of 10 cases and a review of the literature. Eur J Haematol. 2012;89:302–10.
16. Xu-Monette ZY, Dabaja BS, Wang X, Tu M, Manyam GC, Tzankov A, et al. Clinical features, tumor biology, and prognosis associated with MYC rearrangement and Myc overexpression in diffuse large B-cell lymphoma patients treated with rituximab-CHOP. Mod Pathol. 2015;28:1555–73.
17. Sohani AR, Abramson JS. MYC/BCL2 double-expression vs. cell-of-origin classification in diffuse large B-cell lymphoma: do we need to know both? Leuk Lymphoma. 2016;57:509–11.
18. Staiger AM, Ziepert M, Horn H, Scott DW, Barth TFE, Bernd HW, et al. Clinical impact of the cell-of-origin classification and the MYC/ BCL2 dual expresser status in diffuse large B-cell lymphoma treated within prospective clinical trials of the German High-Grade Non-Hodgkin's Lymphoma Study Group. J Clin Oncol. 2017;35:2515–26.
19. Suzuki Y, Yoshida T, Wang G, Aoki T, Katayama T, Miyamoto S, et al. Incidence and clinical significance of aberrant T-cell marker expression on diffuse large B-cell lymphoma cells. Acta Haematol. 2013;130:230–7.
20. Pan Z, Chen YY, Wu X, Trisal V, Wilczynski SP, Weiss LM, et al. Merkel cell carcinoma of lymph node with unknown primary has a significantly lower association with Merkel cell polyomavirus than its cutaneous counterpart. Mod Pathol. 2014;27:1182–92.
21. Song J, Li M, Tretiakova M, Salgia R, Cagle PT, Husain AN. Expression patterns of PAX5, c-met, and paxillin in neuroendocrine tumors of the lung. Arch Pathol Lab Med. 2010;134:1702–5.
22. Adams H, Schmid P, Dirnhofer S, Tzankov A. Cytokeratin expression in hematological neoplasms: a tissue microarray study on 866 lymphoma and leukemia cases. Pathol Res Pract. 2008;204:569–73.
23. Donner LR, Mott FE, Tafur I. Cytokeratin-positive, CD45-negative primary centroblastic lymphoma of the adrenal gland: a potential for a diagnostic pitfall. Arch Pathol Lab Med. 2001;125:1104–6.
24. Reichard KK, McKenna RW, Kroft SH. ALK-positive diffuse large B-cell lymphoma: report of four cases and review of the literature. Mod Pathol. 2007;20:310–9.
25. Xu-Monette ZY, Zhang S, Li X, Manyam GC, Wang XX, Xia Y, et al. p63 expression confers significantly better survival outcomes in high-risk diffuse large B-cell lymphoma and demonstrates p53-like and p53-independent tumor suppressor function. Aging (Albany NY). 2016;8:345–65.
26. Pittaluga S, Jaffe ES. T-cell/histiocyte-rich large B-cell lymphoma. Haematologica. 2010;95:352–6.
27. Kommalapati A, Tella SH, Go RS, Nowakowski GS, Goyal G. T cell/histiocyte-rich large B cell lymphoma: incidence, demographic disparities, and long-term outcomes. Br J Haematol. 2019;185(1):140–2.
28. El Weshi A, Akhtar S, Mourad WA, Ajarim D, Abdelsalm M, Khafaga Y, et al. T-cell/histiocyte-rich B-cell lymphoma: clinical presentation, management and prognostic factors: report on 61 patients and review of literature. Leuk Lymphoma. 2007;48:1764–73.
29. Boudova L, Torlakovic E, Delabie J, Reimer P, Pfistner B, Wiedenmann S, et al. Nodular lymphocyte-predominant Hodgkin lymphoma with nodules resembling T-cell/histiocyte-rich B-cell lymphoma: differential diagnosis between nodular lymphocyte-predominant Hodgkin lymphoma and T-cell/histiocyte-rich B-cell lymphoma. Blood. 2003;102:3753–8.
30. Abou-Elella AA, Weisenburger DD, Vose JM, Kollath JP, Lynch JC, Bast MA, et al. Primary mediastinal large B-cell lymphoma: a clinicopathologic study of 43 patients from the Nebraska Lymphoma Study Group. J Clin Oncol. 1999;17:784–90.
31. Dorfman DM, Shahsafaei A, Alonso MA. Utility of CD200 immunostaining in the diagnosis of primary mediastinal large B cell lymphoma: comparison with MAL, CD23, and other markers. Mod Pathol. 2012;25:1637–43.
32. Steidl C, Gascoyne RD. The molecular pathogenesis of primary mediastinal large B-cell lymphoma. Blood. 2011;118:2659–69.
33. Zinzani PL, Martelli M, Bendandi M, De Renzo A, Zaccaria A, Pavone E, et al. Primary mediastinal large B-cell lymphoma with sclerosis: a clinical study of 89 patients treated with MACOP-B chemotherapy and radiation therapy. Haematologica. 2001;86:187–91.
34. Zinzani PL, Martelli M, Magagnoli M, Pescarmona E, et al. Treatment and clinical management of primary mediastinal large B-cell lymphoma with sclerosis: MACOP-B regimen and mediastinal radiotherapy monitored by (67)Gallium scan in 50 patients. Blood. 1999;94:3289–93.

35. Hall JM, Meyers N, Andrews J. Hemophagocytosis-related (Asian variant) intravascular large B-cell lymphoma in a hispanic patient: a case report highlighting a micronodular pattern in the spleen. Am J Clin Pathol. 2016;145:727–35.
36. Nakashima MO, Roy DB, Nagamine M, Roullet MR, Gabriel CA, Sood SL, et al. Intravascular large B-cell lymphoma: a mimicker of many maladies and a difficult and often delayed diagnosis. J Clin Oncol. 2011;29:e138–40.
37. Orwat DE, Batalis NI. Intravascular large B-cell lymphoma. Arch Pathol Lab Med. 2012;136:333–8.
38. Ponzoni M, Campo E, Nakamura S. Intravascular large B-cell lymphoma: a chameleon with multiple faces and many masks. Blood. 2018;132:1561–7.
39. Ponzoni M, Ferreri AJ, Campo E, Facchetti F, Mazzucchelli L, Yoshino T, et al. Definition, diagnosis, and management of intravascular large B-cell lymphoma: proposals and perspectives from an international consensus meeting. J Clin Oncol. 2007;25:3168–73.
40. Saab J, Nassif S, Boulos F. Asian-type intravascular large B-cell lymphoma of the spleen and bone marrow with Hodgkin-like morphology and immunophenotype. Br J Haematol. 2013;163:294.
41. Hristov AC. Primary cutaneous diffuse large B-cell lymphoma, leg type: diagnostic considerations. Arch Pathol Lab Med. 2012;136:876–81.
42. Pham-Ledard A, Prochazkova-Carlotti M, Andrique L, Cappellen D, Vergier B, Martinez F, et al. Multiple genetic alterations in primary cutaneous large B-cell lymphoma, leg type support a common lymphomagenesis with activated B-cell-like diffuse large B-cell lymphoma. Mod Pathol. 2014;27:402–11.
43. Katzenstein AL, Doxtader E, Narendra S. Lymphomatoid granulomatosis: insights gained over 4 decades. Am J Surg Pathol. 2010;34:e35–48.
44. Song JY, Pittaluga S, Dunleavy K, Grant N, White T, Jiang L, et al. Lymphomatoid granulomatosis – a single institute experience: pathologic findings and clinical correlations. Am J Surg Pathol. 2015;39:141–56.
45. Beltran B, Castillo J, Salas R, Quinones P, Morales D, Hurtado F, et al. ALK-positive diffuse large B-cell lymphoma: report of four cases and review of the literature. J Hematol Oncol. 2009;2:11,8722-2-11.
46. De Paepe P, Baens M, van Krieken H, Verhasselt B, Stul M, Simons A, et al. ALK activation by the CLTC-ALK fusion is a recurrent event in large B-cell lymphoma. Blood. 2003;102:2638–41.
47. Delsol G, Lamant L, Mariame B, Pulford K, Dastugue N, Brousset P, et al. A new subtype of large B-cell lymphoma expressing the ALK kinase and lacking the 2; 5 translocation. Blood. 1997;89:1483–90.
48. Gascoyne RD, Lamant L, Martin-Subero JI, Lestou VS, et al. ALK-positive diffuse large B-cell lymphoma is associated with Clathrin-ALK rearrangements: report of 6 cases. Blood. 2003;102:2568–73.
49. Isimbaldi G, Bandiera L, d'Amore ES, Conter V, Milani M, Mussolin L, et al. ALK-positive plasmablastic B-cell lymphoma with the clathrin-ALK gene rearrangement. Pediatr Blood Cancer. 2006;46:390–1.
50. Lee HW, Kim K, Kim W, Ko YH. ALK-positive diffuse large B-cell lymphoma: report of three cases. Hematol Oncol. 2008;26:108–13.
51. Lee SE, Kang SY, Takeuchi K, Ko YH. Identification of RANBP2-ALK fusion in ALK positive diffuse large B-cell lymphoma. Hematol Oncol. 2014;32:221–4.
52. Takeuchi K, Soda M, Togashi Y, Ota Y, Sekiguchi Y, Hatano S, et al. Identification of a novel fusion, SQSTM1-ALK, in ALK-positive large B-cell lymphoma. Haematologica. 2011;96:464–7.
53. Van Roosbroeck K, Cools J, Dierickx D, Thomas J, Vandenberghe P, Stul M, et al. ALK-positive large B-cell lymphomas with cryptic SEC31A-ALK and NPM1-ALK fusions. Haematologica. 2010;95:509–13.
54. Carbone A, Gloghini A. HHV-8-associated lymphoma: state-of-the-art review. Acta Haematol. 2007;117:129–31.
55. Sarode SC, Sarode GS, Patil A. Plasmablastic lymphoma of the oral cavity: a review. Oral Oncol. 2010;46:146–53.
56. Tavora F, Gonzalez-Cuyar LF, Sun CC, Burke A, Zhao XF. Extra-oral plasmablastic lymphoma: report of a case and review of literature. Hum Pathol. 2006;37:1233–6.
57. Pan ZG, Zhang QY, Lu ZB, Quinto T, Rozenvald IB, Liu LT, et al. Extracavitary KSHV-associated large B-Cell lymphoma: a distinct entity or a subtype of primary effusion lymphoma? Study of 9 cases and review of an additional 43 cases. Am J Surg Pathol. 2012;36:1129–40.
58. Boulanger E, Meignin V, Afonso PV, Duprez R, Oksenhendler E, Agbalika F, et al. Extracavitary tumor after primary effusion lymphoma: relapse or second distinct lymphoma? Haematologica. 2007;92:1275–6.
59. Carbone A, Gloghini AKSHV. HHV8-associated lymphomas. Br J Haematol. 2008;140:13–24.
60. Carbone A, Gloghini A, Vaccher E, Cerri M, Gaidano G, Dalla-Favera R, et al. Kaposi's sarcoma-associated herpesvirus/human herpesvirus type 8-positive solid lymphomas: a tissue-based variant of primary effusion lymphoma. J Mol Diagn. 2005;7:17–27.
61. Nador RG, Cesarman E, Chadburn A, Dawson DB, Ansari MQ, Sald J, et al. Primary effusion lymphoma: a distinct clinicopathologic entity associated with the Kaposi's sarcoma-associated herpes virus. Blood. 1996;88:645–56.
62. Simonelli C, Spina M, Cinelli R, Talamini R, Tedeschi R, Gloghini A, et al. Clinical features and outcome of primary effusion lymphoma in HIV-infected patients: a single-institution study. J Clin Oncol. 2003;21:3948–54.
63. Yin L, Xu J, Li M, Reddy V, Zhou Q, Liu H, et al. Oct2 and Bob1 are sensitive and specific markers in lineage determination of B-cell lymphomas with no expression of conventional B-cell markers. Histopathology. 2016;69(5):775–83.
64. Cesarman E, Mesri EA. Kaposi sarcoma-associated herpesvirus and other viruses in human lymphomagenesis. Curr Top Microbiol Immunol. 2007;312:263–87.
65. Castillo JJ, Beltran BE, Miranda RN, Young KH, Chavez JC, Sotomayor EM. EBV-positive diffuse large B-cell lymphoma of the elderly: 2016 update on diagnosis, risk-stratification, and management. Am J Hematol. 2016;91:529–37.
66. Montes-Moreno S, Odqvist L, Diaz-Perez JA, Lopez AB, de Villambrosia SG, Mazorra F, et al. EBV-positive diffuse large B-cell lymphoma of the elderly is an aggressive post-germinal center B-cell neoplasm characterized by prominent nuclear factor-kB activation. Mod Pathol. 2012;25:968–82.
67. Ok CY, Papathomas TG, Medeiros LJ, Young KH. EBV-positive diffuse large B-cell lymphoma of the elderly. Blood. 2013;122:328–40.
68. Dojcinov SD, Venkataraman G, Raffeld M, Pittaluga S, Jaffe ES. EBV positive mucocutaneous ulcer – a study of 26 cases associated with various sources of immunosuppression. Am J Surg Pathol. 2010;34:405–17.
69. Gratzinger D, Jaffe ES. Mucocutaneous ulcer: a mimic of EBV + diffuse large B cell lymphoma in the immunodeficiency setting. Leuk Lymphoma. 2016;57:1982–3.
70. Huang W, Medeiros LJ, Lin P, Wang W, Tang G, Khoury J, et al. MYC/BCL2/BCL6 triple hit lymphoma: a study of 40 patients with a comparison to MYC/BCL2 and MYC/BCL6 double hit lymphomas. Mod Pathol. 2018;31:1470–8.
71. Scott DW, King RL, Staiger AM, Ben-Neriah S, Jiang A, Horn H, et al. High-grade B-cell lymphoma with MYC and BCL2 and/or BCL6 rearrangements with diffuse large B-cell lymphoma morphology. Blood. 2018;131:2060–4.
72. Hao S, Sanger W, Onciu M, Lai R, Schlette EJ, Medeiros LJ. Mantle cell lymphoma with 8q24 chromosomal abnormalities: a report of 5 cases with blastoid features. Mod Pathol. 2002;15:1266–72.

73. Zhou DM, Chen G, Zheng XW, Zhu WF, Chen BZ. Clinicopathologic features of 112 cases with mantle cell lymphoma. Cancer Biol Med. 2015;12:46–52.
74. Zeng W, Fu K, Quintanilla-Fend L, Lim M, Ondrejka S, Hsi ED. Cyclin D1-negative blastoid mantle cell lymphoma identified by SOX11 expression. Am J Surg Pathol. 2012;36:214–9.
75. Vose JM. Mantle cell lymphoma: 2017 update on diagnosis, risk-stratification, and clinical management. Am J Hematol. 2017;92:806–13.
76. Hoster E, Rosenwald A, Berger F, Bernd HW, Loddenkemper C, Barth TF, et al. Prognostic value of Ki-67 index, cytology, and growth pattern in mantle-cell lymphoma: results from randomized trials of the European mantle cell lymphoma network. J Clin Oncol. 2016;34:1386–94.
77. Colomo L, Loong F, Rives S, Pittaluga S, Martinez A, Lopez-Guillermo A, et al. Diffuse large B-cell lymphomas with plasmablastic differentiation represent a heterogeneous group of disease entities. Am J Surg Pathol. 2004;28:736–47.
78. Delecluse HJ, Anagnostopoulos I, Dallenbach F, Hummel M, Marafioti T, Schneider U, et al. Plasmablastic lymphomas of the oral cavity: a new entity associated with the human immunodeficiency virus infection. Blood. 1997;89:1413–20.
79. Deloose ST, Smit LA, Pals FT, Kersten MJ, van Noesel CJ, Pals ST. High incidence of Kaposi sarcoma-associated herpesvirus infection in HIV-related solid immunoblastic/plasmablastic diffuse large B-cell lymphoma. Leukemia. 2005;19:851–5.
80. Flaitz CM, Nichols CM, Walling DM, Hicks MJ. Plasmablastic lymphoma: an HIV-associated entity with primary oral manifestations. Oral Oncol. 2002;38:96–102.
81. Greipp PR, Leong T, Bennett JM, Gaillard JP, Klein B, Stewart JA, et al. Plasmablastic morphology – an independent prognostic factor with clinical and laboratory correlates: Eastern Cooperative Oncology Group (ECOG) myeloma trial E9486 report by the ECOG Myeloma Laboratory Group. Blood. 1998;91:2501–7.
82. Greipp PR, Raymond NM, Kyle RA, O'Fallon WM. Multiple myeloma: significance of plasmablastic subtype in morphological classification. Blood. 1985;65:305–10.
83. Hsi ED, Lorsbach RB, Fend F, Dogan A. Plasmablastic lymphoma and related disorders. Am J Clin Pathol. 2011;136:183–94.
84. Montes-Moreno S, Montalban C, Piris MA. Large B-cell lymphomas with plasmablastic differentiation: a biological and therapeutic challenge. Leuk Lymphoma. 2012;53:185–94.
85. Rafaniello Raviele P, Pruneri G, Maiorano E. Plasmablastic lymphoma: a review. Oral Dis. 2009;15:38–45.
86. Sasaki S, Hashimoto K, Nakatsuka S, Hasegawa M, Nakano T, Nagata S, et al. Plasmablastic extramedullary plasmacytoma associated with Epstein-Barr virus arising in an immunocompetent patient with multiple myeloma. Intern Med. 2011;50:2615–20.
87. Teruya-Feldstein J. Diffuse large B-cell lymphomas with plasmablastic differentiation. Curr Oncol Rep. 2005;7:357–63.
88. Vega F, Chang CC, Medeiros LJ, Udden MM, Cho-Vega JH, Lau CC, et al. Plasmablastic lymphomas and plasmablastic plasma cell myelomas have nearly identical immunophenotypic profiles. Mod Pathol. 2005;18:806–15.
89. Ismail A, Mallick JA, Qin D, Hussaini MO. Sentinel case of Richter transformation from chronic lymphocytic leukaemia/small lymphocytic lymphoma to CD3+ diffuse large B-cell lymphoma. J Clin Pathol. 2017;70(7):575–8.
90. Kaleem Z, White G, Zutter MM. Aberrant expression of T-cell-associated antigens on B-cell non-Hodgkin lymphomas. Am J Clin Pathol. 2001;115:396–403.
91. Lee M, Cha HJ, Yoon DH, Suh C, Huh J. EBV-positive diffuse large B-cell lymphoma of the elderly with aberrant expression of CD3 and TIA-1. Blood Res. 2013;48:156–60.
92. Luo X, Kuklani R, Bains A. Dual CD3 and CD4 positive plasma cell neoplasm with indistinct morphology: a diagnostic pitfall. Pathology. 2016;48:378–80.
93. Mishra P, Kakri S, Gujral S. Plasmablastic transformation of plasma cell myeloma with heterotropic expression of CD3 and CD4: a case report. Acta Clin Belg. 2017;72(4):250–253.
94. Oliveira JL, Grogg KL, Macon WR, Dogan A, Feldman AL. Clinicopathologic features of B-cell lineage neoplasms with aberrant expression of CD3: a study of 21 cases. Am J Surg Pathol. 2012;36:1364–70.
95. Wallentine JC, Perkins SL, Tripp SR, Bruggman RD, Bayerl MG. Diffuse large B-cell lymphoma with coexpression of CD3 in a pediatric patient: a case report, review of the literature, and tissue microarray study. J Pediatr Hematol Oncol. 2009;31:124–7.
96. Wang J, Chen C, Lau S, Raghavan RI, Rowsell EH, Said J, Weiss LM, Huang Q. CD3-positive large B-cell lymphoma. Am J Surg Pathol. 2009;33:505–12.
97. Bogusz AM, Seegmiller AC, Garcia R, Shang P, Ashfaq R, Chen W. Plasmablastic lymphomas with MYC/IgH rearrangement: report of three cases and review of the literature. Am J Clin Pathol. 2009;132:597–605.
98. Chetty R, Hlatswayo N, Muc R, Sabaratnam R, Gatter K. Plasmablastic lymphoma in HIV+ patients: an expanding spectrum. Histopathology. 2003;42:605–9.
99. Dong HY, Scadden DT, de Leval L, Tang Z, Isaacson PG, Harris NL. Plasmablastic lymphoma in HIV-positive patients: an aggressive Epstein-Barr virus-associated extramedullary plasmacytic neoplasm. Am J Surg Pathol. 2005;29:1633–41.
100. Morscio J, Dierickx D, Nijs J, Verhoef G, Bittoun E, Vanoeteren X, et al. Clinicopathologic comparison of plasmablastic lymphoma in HIV-positive, immunocompetent, and posttransplant patients: single-center series of 25 cases and meta-analysis of 277 reported cases. Am J Surg Pathol. 2014;38:875–86.
101. Cesarman E, Nador RG, Aozasa K, Delsol G, Said JW, Knowles DM. Kaposi's sarcoma-associated herpesvirus in non-AIDS related lymphomas occurring in body cavities. Am J Pathol. 1996;149:53–7.
102. Walts AE, Shintaku IP, Said JW. Diagnosis of malignant lymphoma in effusions from patients with AIDS by gene rearrangement. Am J Clin Pathol. 1990;94:170–5.
103. Mylona E, Baraboutis IG, Georgiou O, Rondogianni D, Lekakis LJ, Papastamopoulos V, Apostolidis I, Skoutelis AT. Solid variant of primary effusion lymphoma in successfully treated HIV infection: a case report. Int J STD AIDS. 2008;19:570–2.
104. Zhang H, Yang XY, Hong T, Feldman T, Bhattacharyya PK. Kaposi sarcoma-associated herpesvirus (human herpesvirus type 8)-associated extracavitary lymphoma: report of a case in an HIV-positive patient with simultaneous Kaposi sarcoma and a review of the literature. Acta Haematol. 2010;123:237–41.
105. Jaffe ES, Pittaluga S. Aggressive B-cell lymphomas: a review of new and old entities in the WHO classification. Hematology Am Soc Hematol Educ Program. 2011;2011:506–14.
106. Wang XJ, L Jeffrey M, Bueso-Ramos CE, Tang G, Wang S, Oki Y, et al. P53 expression correlates with poorer survival and augments the negative prognostic effect of MYC rearrangement, expression or concurrent MYC/BCL2 expression in diffuse large B-cell lymphoma. Mod Pathol. 2017;30:194–203.

High-Grade B-Cell Lymphoma

7

Xiaoqiong Wang and Qin Huang

List of Frequently Asked Questions

1. What are "aggressive" B-cell lymphomas and what are "high-grade B-cell lymphomas?"
2. How are the major types of aggressive (high-grade) B-cell lymphomas defined?
3. What are the clinical features of the major types of aggressive (high-grade) B-cell lymphomas?
4. What are the morphological features of the major types of aggressive (high-grade) B-cell lymphomas?
5. What is the immunophenotype in each of the major types of aggressive (high-grade) B-cell lymphomas?
6. What are the characteristic cytogenetic and molecular genetic findings in the major types of aggressive (high-grade) B-cell lymphomas?
7. Why is the status of *MYC* a central defining characteristic of most aggressive/high-grade lymphomas?
8. What are the morphological mimics of aggressive (high-grade) B-cell lymphomas and how are they differentiated?
9. Which findings are suggestive of the diagnosis, which are definitively diagnostic, and which rule out the diagnosis of specific types of aggressive/high-grade B-cell lymphomas?
10. What is the prognostic and therapeutic significance of identification of these subtypes of aggressive/high-grade B-cell lymphomas?

X. Wang
Robert J. Tomisch Pathology and Laboratory Medicine Institute, Cleveland Clinic, Cleveland, OH, USA
e-mail: wangx9@ccf.org

Q. Huang (✉)
Pathology and Laboratory Medicine, Cedars-Sinai Medical Center, Los Angeles, CA, USA
e-mail: qin.huang@cshs.org

1. What are "aggressive" B-cell lymphomas and what are "high-grade B-cell lymphomas"?

- Historically, in previous lymphoma classifications, B-cell lymphomas were divided into two groups: low-grade (indolent) lymphomas and high-grade (aggressive) lymphomas according to their morphology [1]. These classifications aimed to predict clinical behavior and guide appropriate treatment.
  - Morphologically, high-grade or aggressive B-cell lymphomas were defined as lymphomas composed of either large, abnormal lymphoid cells or small- to medium-size lymphoid cells with blastoid nuclear features.
  - This schema included diverse entities such as diffuse large B-cell lymphoma and its subtypes such as centroblastic B-cell lymphoma, immunoblastic B-cell lymphoma, large cell anaplastic B-cell lymphoma, plasmablastic lymphoma, Burkitt lymphoma, B-lymphoblastic leukemia/lymphoma (B-ALL), and other rare types of B-cell lymphomas (Table 7.1).
  - It was also recognized that low-grade B-cell lymphomas can undergo transformation to clinically aggressive, "high-grade" lymphomas.
- As our understanding of these diseases evolved, these entities are now further delineated. Thus the new category of high-grade B-cell lymphoma (HGBL) introduced in the 2017 WHO classification now specifically refers to a heterogeneous but select group of mature but aggressive B-cell lymphomas that are biologically and clinically distinct. Lymphomas in this category are now separated from diffuse large B-cell lymphoma (DLBCL), NOS, as well as from Burkitt lymphoma [2].
  - This new category of HGBL essentially replaces the provisional category in the prior, 2008 WHO classification, called "B-cell lymphoma, unclassifiable, with features intermediate between diffuse large B-cell lymphoma and Burkitt lymphoma (DLBCL-BL)." It also incorporates

E. Wang, A. S. Lagoo (eds.), *Practical Lymph Node and Bone Marrow Pathology*, Practical Anatomic Pathology,
https://doi.org/10.1007/978-3-030-32189-5_7

other B-cell lymphomas with blastoid morphology provided they do not fulfill diagnostic criteria for other entities listed in the 2017 WHO classification such as precursor B lymphoblastic lymphoma/leukemia or blastoid mantle cell lymphoma (Fig. 7.1) [2, 3].

– Two entities are defined under this new category and they are distinguished by morphology and the presence or absence of specific gene rearrangements: (1) high-grade B-cell lymphoma with *MYC* and *BCL2* and/or *BCL6* rearrangement (HGBL-DH) and (2) high-grade B-cell lymphoma, not otherwise specified (HGBL, NOS).

1. HGBL-DH encompasses all B-cell lymphomas (except rare transformed follicular lymphomas and B-lymphoblastic leukemia/lymphomas) that simultaneously carry gene rearrangements of *MYC* with additional *BCL2* and/or *BCL6* (double hit or triple hit).

   Provided there is a double- or triple-hit cytogenetic abnormality, the lymphoma cells may have typical DLBCL morphology, or have features intermediate between DLBL and BL (DLBL-BL), or show blastoid morphology (but blastoid variants of mantle cell lymphoma or B-lymphoblastic leukemia/lymphoma are excluded).
2. HGBL, NOS, refers to all lymphomas with DLBCL-BL and blastoid morphologies (but not those with typical DLBCL morphology) which do not carry a "double- or triple-hit" cytogenetic abnormality and do not represent BL, B-ALL, or blastoid mantle cell lymphoma.

- Two clinically aggressive lymphomas which have overlapping features with the "high grade B-cell lymphomas" defined in the 2017 WHO calcifications deserve special attention. These are:
  – Burkitt lymphoma (BL), as one of the top differential of HGBL, is a highly aggressive but curable mature B-cell lymphoma that mainly occurs in children and young adults as an extranodal mass or acute leukemia

Table 7.1 "Aggressive B-cell Lymphomas" in the WHO 2017 classification

B-lymphoblastic leukemia/lymphoma
Burkitt lymphoma
Burkitt-like lymphoma with 11q aberration
High-grade B-cell lymphoma
High-grade B-cell lymphoma with *MYC* and *BCL2* and/or *BCL6* rearrangements
High-grade B-cell lymphoma, not otherwise specified
Variants and subtypes of diffuse large B-cell lymphoma (DLBCL)
DLBCL, not otherwise specified
Germinal center B-cell type
Activated B-cell type
T-cell/histiocyte-rich large B-cell lymphoma
Primary DLBCL of the central nervous system
Primary cutaneous DLBCL, leg type
EBV+ DLBCL, not otherwise specified
DLBCL associated with chronic inflammation
Lymphomatoid granulomatosis
Primary mediastinal large B-cell lymphoma
Intravascular large B-cell lymphoma
ALK+ large B-cell lymphoma
Plasmablastic lymphoma
Primary effusion lymphoma
HHV8-positive DLBCL, not otherwise specified

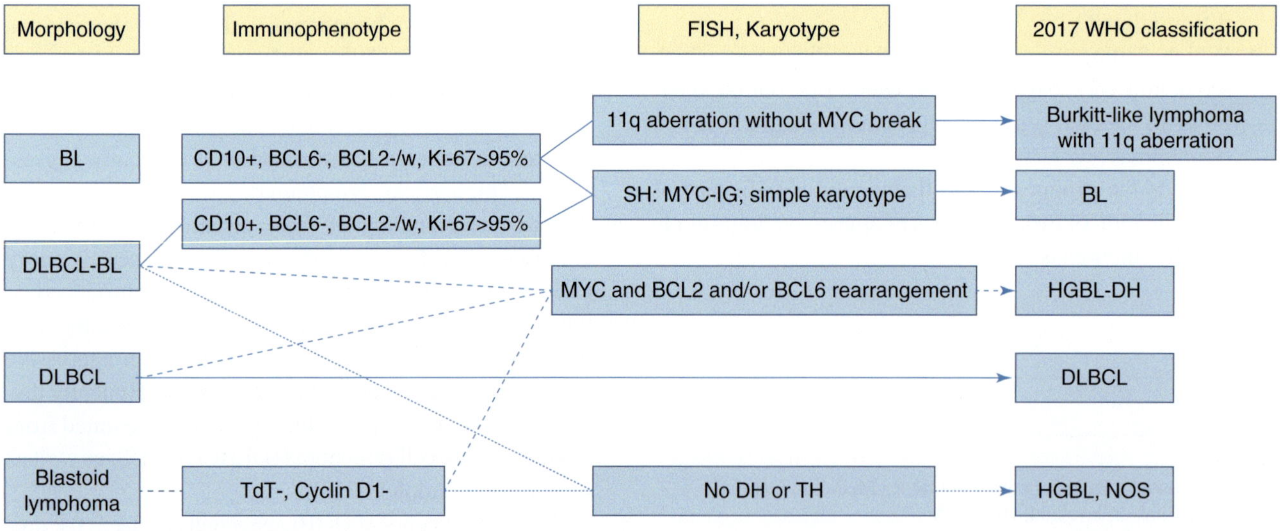

Fig. 7.1 Diagnostic algorithm for differential diagnosis of high-grade B-cell lymphomas. The combinations of morphology, immunophenotype, and molecular analysis are necessary to approach the correct diagnosis. FISH fluorescence in situ hybridization, BL Burkitt lymphoma, DLBCL-BL B-cell lymphoma with features intermediate between diffuse large B-cell lymphoma and Burkitt lymphoma, DLBCL diffuse large B-cell lymphoma, blastoid lymphoma, either blastoid variant of mantle cell lymphoma without expression of cyclin D1 or B-lymphoblastic leukemia/lymphoma without expression of TdT, SH single hit, DH double hit, TH triple hit, HGBL-DH high-grade B-cell lymphoma with *MYC* and *BCL2* and/or *BCL6* rearrangement, HGBL, NOS high-grade B-cell lymphoma, not otherwise specified

(so-called ALL-L3). It has a characteristic oncogenic translocation involving *MYC-IG* and a simple karyotype.
 - Burkitt-like lymphoma with 11q aberration is a new provisional entity in the 2017 WHO classification. Rare cases have been reported that have typical BL morphology and gene expression profile but lack *MYC* aberration by FISH and karyotype [3–5]. Subsequent studies have identified that at least a subset of these cases without detectable *MYC* translocation have chromosome 11q aberration and more complex cytogenetics [6–8].

2. How are the major types of aggressive (high-grade) B-cell lymphomas defined?

Below we describe the defining features of four categories: (1) high-grade B-cell lymphoma with *MYC* and *BCL2* and/or *BCL6* rearrangement (HGBL-DH); (2) high-grade B-cell lymphoma, not otherwise specified (HGBL, NOS); (3) Burkitt lymphoma (BL); and (4) Burkitt-like lymphoma with 11q aberration.

1. High-grade B-cell lymphoma with *MYC* and *BCL2* and/or *BCL6* rearrangements (HGBL-DH): These are de novo, aggressive, mature B-cell lymphomas that have a *MYC* gene (chromosome 8q24) rearrangement and a rearrangement at *BCL2* gene (chromosome 18q21) and/or *BCL6* gene (chromosome 3q27) [2].
   - It is also called as double-hit (DH)/triple-hit (TH) lymphoma, and the term only refers to the lymphomas with gene rearrangements of *BCL2* and/or *BCL6* in addition to *MYC* that are commonly detected by FISH, chromosomal karyotype, or molecular analysis.
   - Lymphomas with pre-existing or coexisting indolent lymphomas should be diagnosed as such, for example, large B-cell lymphoma with *MYC* and *BCL2* rearrangements, transformed from follicular lymphoma [2].
   - Excluded from this category:
     - Excisional biopsy-proven follicular lymphoma with DH, including FL grade 3B, should still be diagnosed as FL with a comment on the presence of DH [2]. Many studies indicated that *MYC* breakpoint in these FL is a secondary event and is acquired during the course of the disease transformation [9, 10].
     - Similarly, occasional B-lymphoblastic leukemia/lymphoma with DH, mostly transformed from an antecedent or synchronous FL, should be classified as B-lymphoblastic leukemia/lymphoma [10–13].
     - Lymphomas with double expression of MYC and BCL2 proteins ("double expressors") without DH/TH, mutation/copy number increase/amplification without DH/TH, two gene rearrangements other than *MYC* (e.g., *BCL2* and *BCL6*), or other gene rearrangements with *MYC* (e.g., *CCND1*) are not included in this category [2].
2. High-grade B-cell lymphoma, not otherwise specified (HGBL, NOS)

This is the other heterogeneous but specific category that is under HGBL. By definition these lymphomas lack *MYC* and *BCL2* and/or *BCL6* rearrangements and do not fulfill the category of DLBCL, NOS, or Burkitt lymphoma [2].

   - This category also includes some cases that resemble BL with a *MYC* translocation and gain or amplification of *BCL2* or *BCL6* or, conversely, with *BCL2* or *BCL6* translocation and gain or amplification of *MYC* [14].
   - HGBL, NOS, are actually very rare and should only be diagnosed as such when it is truly impossible to classify a case as DLBCL or BL.
     - Cases with morphology of DLBCL that have a *MYC* rearrangement, either in combination or not with gain/amplification *BCL2* or *BCL6*, should be diagnosed as DLBCL with a comment of *MYC* rearrangement [2].
     - Pediatric DLBCL-BL is recommended to be classified as BL or DLBCL instead of HGBL. Because HGBL does not occur in pediatric patients, most of pediatric DLBCL-BL have molecular BL or intermediate profile and show an excellent prognosis [15].
3. Burkitt lymphoma (BL) is a highly aggressive but curable mature B-cell lymphoma that primarily presents as an extranodal mass or an acute leukemia (ALL-L3 in French-American-British classification) in children and young adults.
   - It was first described by Dennis Burkitt in 1958 as a rapidly enlarging jaw mass in children in the malarial belt of equatorial Africa and Papua, New Guinea. Since then, enormous achievements have been made including delineation of three clinical variants, discovery of Epstein-Barr virus (*EBV*) and its effects in BL, unravelling the oncogenic role of *MYC* translocation, profiling molecular signature of BL, and introduction of novel and curable chemotherapy [4, 16–22].
   - It is derived from germinal center B-cells and composed of a diffuse infiltrate of monomorphic, medium-sized B-cells with clumped chromatin, multiple nucleoli, basophilic cytoplasm, and high mitotic rate.

- There are three clinical variants of BL: endemic, sporadic, and immunodeficiency-associated [2]. *MYC* translocation (chromosome 8q24) is a consistent feature but *EBV* infection varies among the clinical variants.

4. Burkitt-like lymphoma with 11q aberration: It is a new entity in the 2017 WHO classification which is indistinguishable from BL by morphology, immunophenotype, and genetic profile but has 11q aberration and undetectable of *MYC* breakpoint or *MYC/IGH* fusion [2, 16].

3. What are the clinical features of the major types of aggressive (high-grade) B-cell lymphomas?

1. HGBL-DH and HGBL, NOS: Most published literature describes these two entities together. These lymphomas predominantly affect elderly patients with a median age of 60–70 years and slightly male predominance [2, 9, 23–27]. Patients mainly have advanced disease (Ann Arbor stage III or VI disease) with more than one extranodal sites, most frequently involving the bone marrow and CNS, and elevated LDH and high international prognostic index (IPI).
2. Burkitt lymphoma: Often presents as a rapidly growing tumor in children and young adults. Because of the short doubling time of the tumor, pediatric patients typically present with symptoms of only a few weeks. There are three clinical variants of BL: endemic, sporadic, and immunodeficiency-associated [2]. Clinical symptoms may vary by the site of involvement.
   - Sites of involvement: Extranodal sites are usually involved, with some variations of preferred sites among the three clinical variants. Bone marrow and lymph node involvement are less commonly seen.
     – Serious medical emergencies may happen, including bowel obstruction and perforation, spinal cord compression, and post-chemotherapy acute tumor lysis syndrome.
   - Staging: Pediatric cases are staged according to the St. Jude system which was established in 1980 [28]. A revised international pediatric non-Hodgkin's lymphoma staging system has been recently proposed [29]. Adult cases are staged according to the traditional Ann Abor system and the updated Lugano classification [30]. Advanced-stage disease is 2–3 times more common than localized-stage disease in both age groups [31–33].
   - Clinical variants of BL: Variants differ from each other mainly in geographical distribution and clinical presentation, but subtle in morphology, and biological and molecular features (Table 7.2) [2, 14, 15, 34–36].

Table 7.2 Clinicopathological features of three clinical variants of Burkitt lymphoma

	Epidemiology	Clinical features	Morphology	*EBV* positivity	MYC breakpoint	IGH breakpoint
Endemic BL	Malaria belt of equatorial Africa and Papua, New Guinea	Young children with a peak age of 4–7 years; extranodal sites, mostly face >>bone marrow	Predominantly classic: diffuse infiltrate of monotonous medium-sized cells with multiple small nucleoli and basophilic squared-off cytoplasm	>95%	Predominantly: class III: far 5′ (>100 kb) MYC	Predominantly VDJ region
Sporadic BL	Throughout the world	Bimodal age: peak in children of 5–15 years and young adult of 30 years; extranodal sites, mostly intra-abdominal structures >bone marrow, lymph node	Predominantly classic	20–30%	Predominantly: class I: first exon and intron of *MYC* or class II: immediately 5′ *MYC*	Predominantly switch region
Immunodeficiency-associated BL	Immunodeficient patients, mostly HIV-infected patients	Bimodal age: early stage of AIDS with a peak in 10–19 years; extranodal sites, mostly intra-abdominal structures > bone marrow, lymph node	Predominantly classic, some may show slightly increased cell pleomorphism or plasmacytoid differentiation	25–40%	Predominantly: class I: first exon and intron of *MYC*	Predominantly switch region

- Endemic Burkitt lymphoma was the first described variant that occurs in the malaria belt of equatorial Africa and Papua New Guinea [17]. It mainly affects young children with a peak incidence in 4–7 years and 2:1 male-to-female ratio [2]. *EBV* is present in >95% cases and translocation primarily involves far upstream of the *MYC* and VDJ region of IGH [15, 35–37]. Endemic BL presents in extranodal sites, mostly jaws and other facial bones (e.g., orbit). Other less common sites may include distal ileum, cecum, omentum, ovaries, kidneys, and breasts. Involvement of bone marrow or peripheral blood is rare.
- Sporadic Burkitt lymphoma occurs throughout the world. It commonly afflicts bimodal age: children with a peak age between 5 and 15 years and young adult with a median age of 30 years [2]. Recent studies also suggested trimodal age distribution with an extra geriatric peak in 70 years [38, 39]. The male-to-female ratio is 2–3:1. *EBV* is present in 20–30% of cases, and most translocations involve nearby or within *MYC* and switch region of IGH, which are different from endemic BL [15, 35, 36]. Sporadic BL mostly present with abdominal masses with ileocecum as the most frequent involved region. The ovary, kidneys, and breasts are less common sites. Involvement of the jaw, other facial structures, Waldeyer ring, and mediastinum is rare. Lymph node involvement is rarely seen and is more common in adults than in children. Sporadic patients in endemic regions may lack *EBV* infection and present with different clinical and molecular features from endemic BL patients.
- Immunodeficiency-associated Burkitt lymphoma occurs primarily in HIV-infected patients and accounts for one third of AIDS-related lymphomas [40]. Patients usually present in the early stage of AIDS with younger age between 10 and 19 years and relatively high CD4+ T-cell accounts, and the increased risk of BL with HIV infection persists over time, especially in patients without highly active antiretroviral therapy (HAART) [2, 41]. *EBV* is detected in 25–40% of cases, and the breakpoint of *MYC* and *IGH* is similar to sporadic BL [15, 35, 36].

- This variant may also occasionally occur in other immunodeficient diseases, including congenital disorders such as Duncan's disease or iatrogenic immunosuppressed states [42]. Extranodal involvement especially the gastrointestinal tract remains frequent, but bone marrow and nodal involvement are more common than endemic BL [43].

3. Burkitt-like lymphoma with 11q aberration: Based on a few reported cases, the disease mainly occurs in children and young adults with an age range of 6–76 years and male predominance [7, 44–46]. Lymph node and tonsil involvement are common, whereas bone marrow and CNS involvement are unlikely.

4. What are the morphological features of the major types of aggressive (high-grade) B-cell lymphomas?

1. HGBL-DH: Morphologically, HGBL-DH is variable and includes cases that appear similar to DLBCL, BL, DLBL-BL, and blastoid lymphomas either like blastoid variant of mantle cell lymphoma or B-lymphoblastic leukemia/lymphoma. Double-hit status should be investigated in these cases by FISH, chromosomal karyotype, or other molecular analysis because these entities require different therapeutic approaches and have distinctive prognosis.
   - Many HGBL-DH cases may be morphologically reminiscent of DLBCL, NOS, which is the most common subtype of non-Hodgkin's lymphoma [2, 9, 26, 47–49]. Approximately 2–12% DLBCLs (most studies ≤6%) are proved to be double-hit lymphomas. These lymphomas usually show diffuse infiltrate of large-/medium-sized cell with variable nuclei size and shape, moderate amount of cytoplasm, and relatively few admixed small lymphocytes (Fig. 7.2). Mitotic and apoptotics are variable among the cases, and starry-sky macrophage may be seen.
   - Some cases have morphological features intermediate between DLBCL and BL or morphologically resemble BL but have atypical clinical presentation, immunophenotype, and genetic findings [9, 24, 26, 47, 49]. These cases were previously defined as a provisional entity as DLBCL-BL in the 2008 WHO classification. In fact, about 32–78% of them are indeed double-hit lymphomas.
     - The lymphoma cells may vary from monomorphic to more pleomorphic among the cases. Compared to BL, the cytoplasm is less basophilic and lacks vacuoles. Starry-sky macrophages are usually present with many mitotic and apoptotic bodies.
   - Rare cases of HGBL-DH may have a blastoid morphology with fine chromatin, inconspicuous nucleoli, and scant cytoplasm [2, 50, 51]. Morphologically, they resemble B-lymphoblastic leukemia/lymphoma and blastoid variant of mantle cell lymphoma, but they do not express characteristic TdT or cyclin D1/SOX11.
2. HGBL, NOS: Most cases are intermediate between BL and DLBCL. They either morphologically mimic BL but

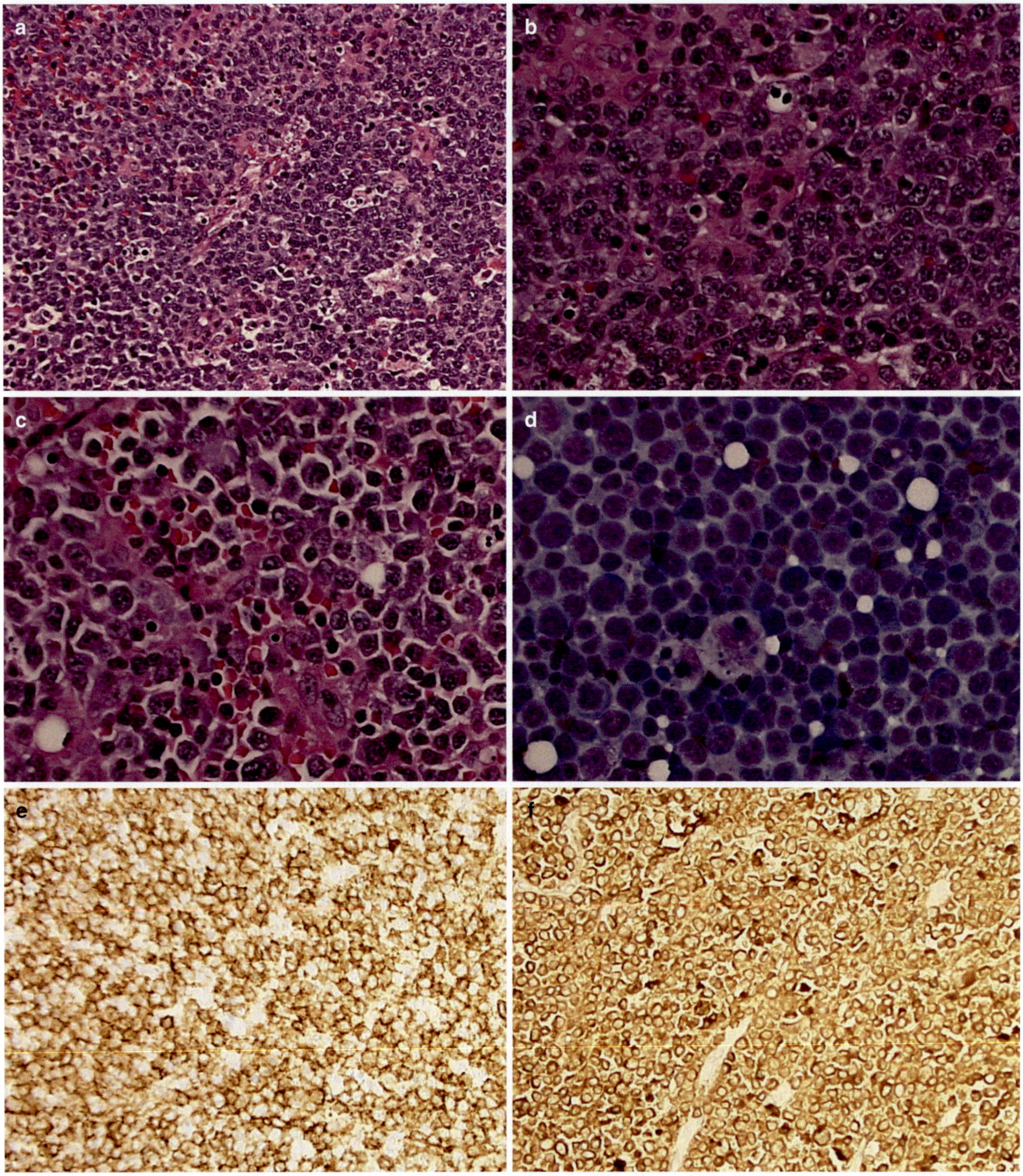

Fig. 7.2 High-grade B-cell lymphoma with *MYC* and *BCL2*. (**a**) Diffuse infiltrating pattern of medium-/large-sized cells (H&E, ×100). (**b**) The cells show variable nuclei and amount of cytoplasm (H&E, ×200). (**c**) Mitotic and apoptosis are present (H&E, ×400). (**d**) Imprint morphology of the lymphoma cells with variation of size and nuclear shape (×400). (**e**) Positive for CD10 (IHC, ×200). (**f**) Positive for CD20 (IHC, ×200)

with atypical clinical features, immunophenotype, and/or molecular findings or vice versa. Rare mature B-cell lymphoma with a blastoid cytomorphology but lacking TdT, cyclin D1, and DH/TH is also included in this category.

3. Burkitt lymphoma: The classical morphological feature of BL is observed in endemic BL, most sporadic BL (especially in children), and many cases of immunodeficiency-related BL [2].
   - Under low magnification, there is a diffuse infiltrate of monomorphous medium-sized cells with scattered pale tingible body macrophage (Fig. 7.3).
     - Follicular pattern has been reported in rare cases possibly representing colonization of residual germinal center [52, 53].
   - The cells usually appear cohesive with squared-off retracted cytoplasm caused by formalin fixing artifact. The nuclei are uniform, round with a size approximately the nuclei of a histiocyte. The chromatin is finely clumped with multiple small basophilic, paracentric nucleoli. The cytoplasm is moderate in amount and deeply basophilic. Cytoplasmic lipid vacuoles due to dysregulated lipid metabolism are usually seen in imprint preparations or fine needle aspiration of BL, which are characteristic but not specific [54–56]. The lymphoma cells have extremely high rate of mitosis and apoptosis with nearby macrophage engulfing cellular debris, imparting a starry-sky pattern.
   - Tumor-infiltrating T-cells in BL are usually very limited, which is consistent with lack of host immune response.
   - Atypical morphology: Apart from morphological alterations caused by specimen quality and tissue processing problems, BL with atypical morphology, such as some degree of variation in cell size and nuclear shape, has been observed. Atypical BL is more commonly presented in adults, in HIV-associated variant, and in lymph node [2, 16]. These cases are biologically and clinically indistinguishable from BL and have typical BL immunophenotype and molecular features, including >95% Ki-67, negative or weak BCL2, and presence of *MYC* translocation [2, 57].
     - In HIV-associated BL, besides slightly increased cellular pleomorphism, the tumor cells may show plasmacytoid differentiation with single central nucleoli and eccentric cytoplasm [58].
   - Occasionally, typical BL cases are associated with marked granulomatous reaction which may suggest usual immune response to *EBV* infection [59, 60]. Most of these cases have localized disease and are associated with good prognosis.
4. Burkitt-like lymphoma with 11q aberration: Morphologically, it is indistinguishable from BL and has diffuse infiltrate of monotonous medium-sized cells with fine chromatin and multiple small basophilic nucleoli and scattered tingible body macrophages.

5. What is the immunophenotype in each of the major types of aggressive (high-grade) B-cell lymphomas?

1. HGBL-DH: The tumor cells express mature B-cell markers (CD19, CD20, CD79a, PAX5) and lack immature marker (TdT) [2, 50]. Some cases may lose surface immunoglobulin expression which may contribute to translocations involving IG locus [61]. None of the IHCs (e.g., high Ki-67, high MYC, GC phenotype) may be used as a surrogate marker for preselecting cases for DH/TH rearrangement tests [26].
   - Most HGBL-DH cases have germinal cell (GC) B-cell phenotype with expression of CD10 and BCL6 (75–90%). However, small proportions of HGBL-DH, mostly with *MYC/BCL6* DH, may have non-GC phenotype with IRF4/MUM1 expression [25, 48].
   - Most, but not all, cases show double expression of BCL2 and MYC protein.
     - Notably, the majority of double expressers are *not* double-hit lymphomas, and their cell of origin tends to be non-GC/activated B-cell (ABC) subtype of DLBCL.
     - BCL2 expression is positive in a majority of cases which correlate well with *BCL2* rearrangement in HGBL with *MYC* and *BCL2* rearrangements, but may be negative in HGBL with *MYC* and *BCL6* rearrangements. MYC staining is variable and not reliable enough to be used for preselecting cases for DH/TH status. Ki-67 also has variable positivity and may be deceptively low in cases that morphologically resemble DLBCL.
2. HGBL, NOS: The immunophenotype is not well documented in the limited studies.
   - All cases are mature B-cell lymphoma with expression of CD20 [2]. MYC expression is variable and partially related to the presence of *MYC* translocations and its partners.
   - Most cases have BCL6 expression, but CD10, BCL2, and Ki-67 are variable. IRF4/MUM1 is typically absent.
3. Burkitt lymphoma (BL): The normal counterpart of the tumor cells is mature B-cells from the germinal center (GC). Accordingly, the tumor cells typically express B-cell markers (CD19, CD20, CD22, PAX5, and CD79a), membrane IgM with light chain restriction, and germinal center markers (CD10 and BCL6 but not BCL2).
   - Characteristically, almost all BLs have high expression of MYC and nearly 100% Ki-67 [2].
     - Cases with <95% Ki-67 should be carefully evaluated to exclude other diagnosis unless this could be explained by a histotechnologic problem.
   - CD38, CD43, TCL1 (T-cell leukemia-1, oncogene overexpressed in some T-cell lymphomas, and B-cell lymphomas), and adipophilin (staining for cytoplas-

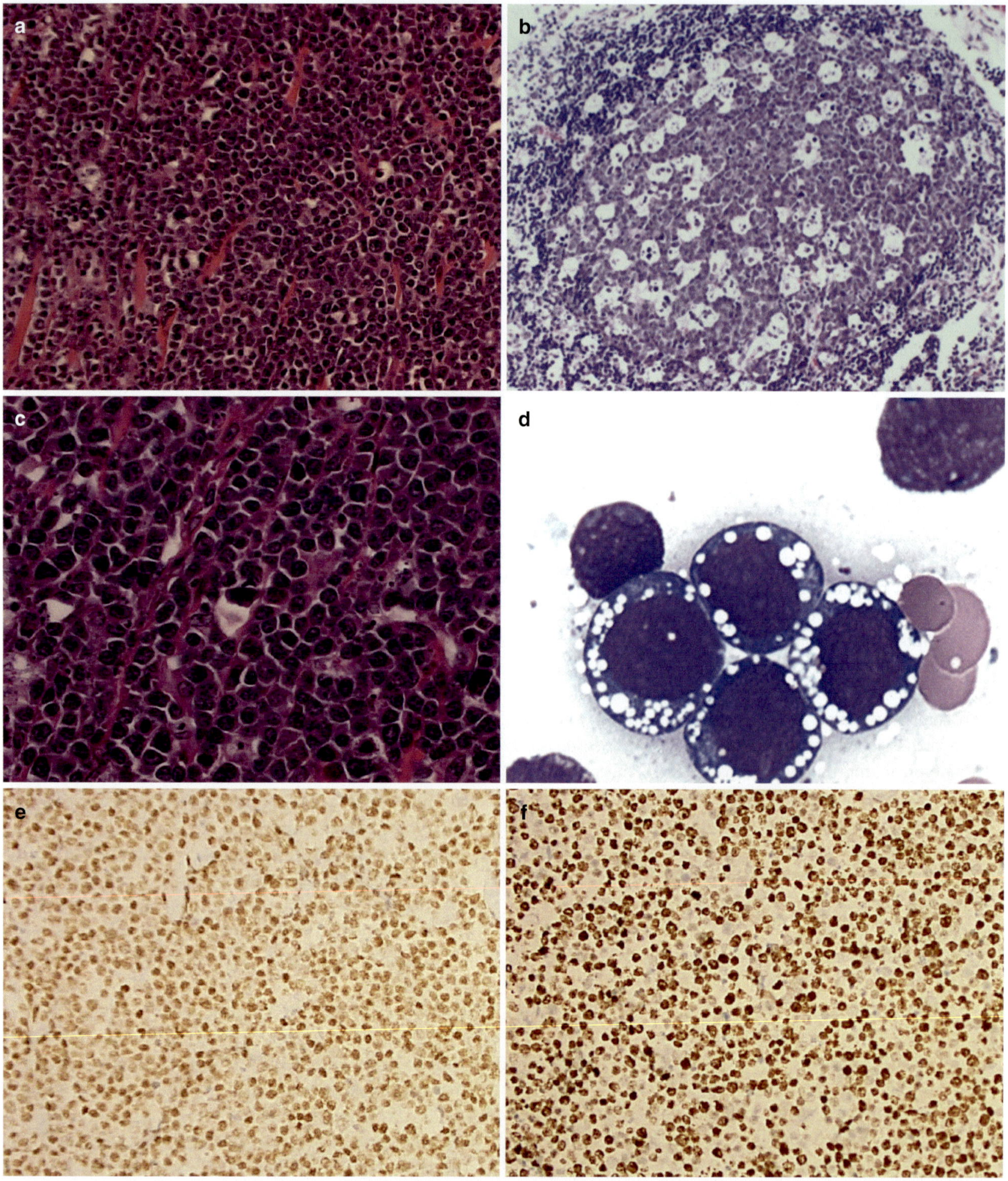

Fig. 7.3 Burkitt lymphoma. (**a**) Diffuse infiltrate of monomorphous medium-sized cell with admixed macrophages (H&E, ×200). (**b**) Colonization of residual germinal center (H&E, ×200). (**c**) Medium-sized cells with round or oval nuclei, clumped chromatin, small nucleoli, and basophilic and squared-off cytoplasm (H&E, ×400). (**d**) Imprint morphology of lymphoma cells with moderate basophilic cytoplasm and lipid vacuoles (×1000). (**e**) Strong expression of MYC protein (IHC, ×200). (**f**) Nearly 100% Ki-67 (IHC ×200)

mic lipid vesicles) are also frequently positive [62]. The cells are usually negative for CD5, CD23, cyclin D1, TdT, CD138, and MUM1/IRF4. A subset of the cases may be positive for MUM1/IRF4 which may suggest a late GC phenotype [63].

- Cases associated with *EBV* infection will show a type I latent *EBV* infection pattern with positive EBER and negative LMP1.
- Aberrant immunophenotype, such as CD5 expression, lack of CD10, or weak/focal positive of BCL2, may be seen in older patients with sporadic BL [2, 4, 64]. However, strong BCL2 positivity should raise the possibility of high-grade B-cell lymphoma with *MYC* and *BCL2* and/or *BCL6* rearrangements.
- Blasts of pediatric Burkitt leukemia show mature B-cell immunophenotype as typical BL. However, a few of these cases may have an immunophenotype of precursor B-cells with expression of TdT and CD34 and absence of CD20 and surface immunoglobulin [65].

4. Burkitt-like lymphoma with 11q aberrations: The tumor cells resemble BL by immunohistochemical staining.
   - They express pan B-cell markers (CD19, CD20, PAX5, and CD9a), germinal center markers (CD10 and BCL6), MYC (weaker than BL), and nearly 100% Ki-67. The cells are usually negative for CD5, BCL2, MUM1, cyclin D1, TdT, and *EBV*.
   - Recent flow cytometric data from these cases indicate subtle differences from typical BL: expression of CD16/CD56, lower frequency of CD45low, and CD38high [66].

6. What are the characteristic cytogenetic and molecular genetic findings in the major types of aggressive (high-grade) B-cell lymphomas?

1. HGBL-DH:
   - Approximately 65% of the cases have *MYC/IG* translocation, whereas in the rest of the cases, *MYC* is juxtaposed to a non-IG partner, most commonly 9p13 (gene unknown) and 3q27 (*BCL6*) [2, 47, 67]. Similar to *MYC/IG* light chain translocation, the breaks in *MYC* in *MYC*/non-IG translocation occur mostly in 3′/telomeric of *MYC* (Fig. 7.4).
   - About 60–70% of HGBL-DH have *MYC/BCL2* rearrangements (Fig. 7.5), whereas 15–30% of the cases have *MYC/BCL6* rearrangement and 10% have three rearrangements [2, 68]. The strong preference for *BCL2* involvement in DH lymphomas suggests complementary role for *MYC* and *BCL2* [9].
     - Cases with a combination of a chromosomal rearrangement and mutation, gain, or amplification of other genes, for example, *MYC* rearrangement and amplification of *BCL2*, are not sufficient to classify a case as HGBL-DH [2].

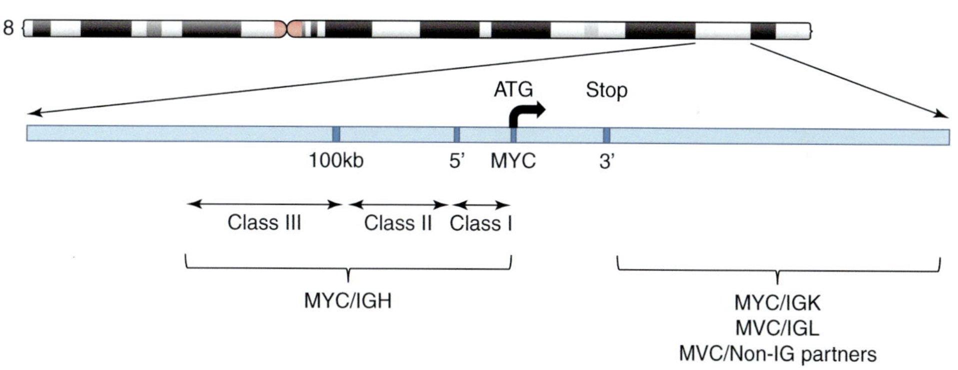

Fig. 7.4 The MYC locus at chromosome 8q24. Various *MYC* breakpoint regions with their partners

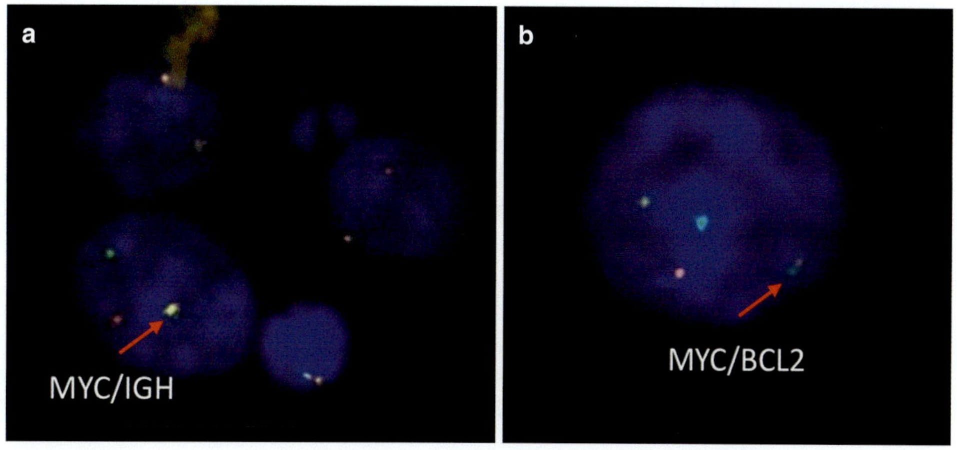

Fig. 7.5 FISH analysis of double rearrangements of *MYC* and *BCL2* genes: (**a**) *MYC/IGH* fusion signal (*yellow*) in addition to isolated green and red signals on chromosome 8 and 14, respectively. (**b**) *BCL2/IGH* fusion signal (*yellow*) in addition to isolated red and green signals on chromosome 14 and 18, respectively

- Most cases have complex karyotype and other molecular changes, such as *ID3*, *TP53*, *CREBBP/EP300*, and *MYD88* mutations [2, 47, 62–64].

2. HGBL, NOS: Cases with DH/TH should be excluded.
   - About one third of the cases have a *MYC* rearrangement with or without increased copy number or amplification of *BCL2*. Vice versa, cases with a *BCL2* rearrangement and increased copy number or amplification of *MYC* are also detected [2, 24, 65, 69].
3. Burkitt lymphoma: The characteristic *MYC/IG* translocation of BL juxtapose *MYC* gene (chromosome 8q24) to one of the three immunoglobulin genes: Ig heavy chain (IGH, chromosome 14q32), κ light chain (IGK, chromosome 2p12), or λ light chain (IGL, chromosome 22q11).
   - The translocation t(8;14)(q24;q32) is prototypic and present in 75–80% of the cases, and the other two variants t(8;22)(q24;q11) and t(2;8)(p12;q24) are less common [2, 16, 54].
   - The translocation results in constitutive expression of MYC. As a transcription factor, overexpression of MYC can induce expression of many genes which are involved in apoptosis, proliferation, metabolism, and angiogenesis.
   - The position of the *MYC* breakpoint differs according to the IG partner (Fig. 7.4). In the cases of *MYC/IGH* with t(8;14), the breakpoint mainly occurs within the centromeric (5′) part of *MYC*.
     - There is some heterogeneity of t(8;14) breakpoints among three clinical variants [2, 16, 70]. Endemic BL predominantly breaks at far upstream (>100 kb) to 5' *MYC* and J region of IGH, whereas sporadic and HIV-associated BL mostly breaks nearby or within *MYC* and one of the switch regions of IGH. In contrast, in t(2;8) and t(8;22), the *MYC* breakpoints are dispersed from 3′ to 2 Mb telomeric of *MYC*.
   - Fluorescence in situ hybridization (FISH) assays are commonly applied to detect these translocations. In regard to variable distribution of the breakpoints, various *MYC* break-apart probes and *MYC/IGH* fusion probes are available to increase the sensitivity.
   - A few studies have reported that rare cases of phenotypically typical BL expressing MYC protein lack detectable *MYC* translocation [3–5, 71–73].
     - Most of these cases are true negative of *MYC* rearrangement that harbor 11q aberration and activate other alternative pathways to overexpress MYC.
     - Subsets of these cases are false negative because technically all methods currently used to diagnose genetics aberration (cytogenetics, FISH, and PCR) may miss some cryptic or variant *MYC* translocations.
   - BL usually has a simple karyotype with fewer than two additional chromosomal aberrations. The most common secondary abnormalities are gains of chromosome 1q, 7, 9q, and 12 and losses of 6q, 13q32–34, and 17p [2, 16, 74].
   - Molecular studies with genome sequencing also confirmed the infrequency of chromosomal imbalance. These studies also revealed a unique molecular profile of BL with relatively few mutations. The recurrent mutations identified include *TCF3*, *ID3*, *PIK3R1*, *CCND3*, *TP53*, *GNA13*, and *SMARCA4* [14, 34].
4. Burkitt-like lymphoma with 11q aberrations: While there are similarities in the overall genetic profile with that of BL, this disease has unique aberration of chromosome 11q instead of *MYC* rearrangement.
   - The 11q alteration includes interstitial gains at 11q23.2–q23.3 and/or telomeric losses at 11q24.1-qter. These abnormalities potentially affect genes such as *PAFAH1B at 11q23.3* (constant overexpression) and *FLI1* (downregulated) and *ETS1* (recurrently mutated) at 11q24 [16].
   - Recent studies also found alternative genetic changes that may result in equivalent molecular effects, such as inverted duplication of 11q and uniparental disomy at 11q24. These chromosome abnormalities can usually be detected by conventional karyotype and/or FISH but are best identified by CGH and SNP array.
   - Compared to BL, Burkitt-like lymphoma with 11q aberration has more complex chromosome alterations with the most frequent additional aberration of 6q24. However, 18q21 [7, 44]. *ID3*, which leads to *PI3K* activation in BL, is not mutated in this disease.

7. Why is the status of MYC a central defining characteristic of most aggressive/high-grade lymphomas?

- In normal lymph nodes, *MYC* is essential in germinal center formation and is transiently expressed during the initial expansion of naive B-cells when they are exposed to antigens and at stages immediately preceding the light zone to dark zone transition [75].
- Overexpression of *MYC* has many roles in lymphomagenesis including promoting cell proliferation, increasing apoptosis, and suppressing human leukocyte antigen (HLA) class I antigen expression to evade host immunity [66, 76, 77].
- The constant detection of *MYC* translocation in BL implies its primary driver effect in the lymphomagenesis of BL.
  - However, *MYC* alone may not be sufficient to cause BL. It cooperates with many other mechanisms, such as *EBV* infection, and dysregulated *ARF-P53*, *TCF-ID3*, and *BCR-NF-KB* pathway [78–80].

- Recent studies suggest that BL may be related to polymicrobial factors. *EBV*, one member of the human herpesviruses (HHV), is the first infectious factor that was found to be important in the pathogenesis of BL [81]. *EBV* infection can be persistent within B-cells in the latent state (mostly latency pattern I in BL) and transform and drive clonal expansion of B-cells. *EBV* is present in >95% of the endemic BL but is variably detected in 20–30% of sporadic BL and in 25–40% of immunodeficiency-associated BL. There are two contrasting theories about the timing of *EBV* infection and *MYC* translocation [82–87]. The variation of *EBV* positivity among three clinical variants and among different countries makes it difficult to reconcile if *EBV* infection or vice versa *MYC* translocation is a prerequisite for BL.
- Microbial factors other than *EBV*, e.g., malaria, human immunodeficiency virus (HIV), HHV5, HHV8, arbovirus, and schistosomiasis, were reported to have roles in the pathogenesis of BL [88–93]. The precise mechanisms of these infectious factors have yet to be established.

8. What are the morphological mimics of aggressive (high-grade) B-cell lymphomas and how are they differentiated?

- Non-hematopoietic neoplasms with a "small blue cell" morphology such as poorly differentiated neuroendocrine tumors, neuroblastoma, and Ewing sarcoma can potentially mimic BL, while poorly differentiated carcinomas, melanomas, dendritic cell sarcomas, etc. can mimic large cell lymphomas. These tumors can be easily differentiated from aggressive B-cell lymphomas by their histology and immunophenotype.
- The main differential diagnosis includes the other subtypes of aggressive/high-grade lymphomas, various subtypes of DLBCL, lymphoblastic leukemia/lymphoma (LBL), blastoid mantle cell lymphoma, and myeloid sarcoma (Table 7.3).
- HGBL-DH can be morphologically and immunophenotypically indistinguishable from DLBCL, NOS and the presence or absence of DH/TH is essential for accurate diagnosis. It may be prudent to perform the appropriate

Table 7.3 Differential diagnosis of BL

	Architecture	Cytology	Immunophenotype	Molecular genetics
BL	Diffuse and starry-sky pattern	Medium-sized monotonous cells with multiple small nucleoli and basophilic squared-off cytoplasm	CD19+, CD20+, CD10+, BCL6+, MYC+, CD5−, BCL2−, cyclin D1−, TdT− Ki-67~100% EBER + (variable among clinical variants)	*MYC* rearrangement Simple cytogenetics
Burkitt-like lymphoma with 11q aberration	Similar to Burkitt lymphoma	Similar to Burkitt lymphoma	CD19+, CD20+, CD10+, BCL6+, MYC+; CD5−, BCL2−, cyclin D1−, TdT− Ki-67~100% EBER – (based on limited reports)	11q aberration, no *MYC* rearrangement Complex cytogenetics
DLBCL subtypes and variants	Diffuse, +/− follicular pattern	Large-/medium-sized centroblastic, immunoblastic cells	CD19+, CD20+, CD10+/−, BCL6+/−, MUM1+/−, BCL2+/−, MYC−/+,CD5−/+,cyclinD1−,TdT− Ki-67 <90% EBER−/+	No DH, isolated *MYC* rearrangement in 10% Complex cytogenetics
HGBL-DH	Diffuse, +/− follicular pattern	DLBCL, intermediate BL-DLBCL, blastoid cells	CD19+, CD20+, CD10+/−, BCL6+/−, MUM1+/−, BCL2+/−, MYC+/−, cyclin D1−, TdT− Ki-67 <90% EBER −/+	DH or TH Complex cytogenetics
HGBL, NOS	Diffuse, +/− follicular pattern	DLBCL, intermediate BL-DLBCL, blastoid cells	CD19+, CD20+, CD10+/−, BCL6+/−, MUM1+/−, BCL2+/−, MYC−/+, cyclin D1−, TdT− Ki-67 <90% EBER−/+	No DH, may have isolated *MYC*, *BCL2*, or *BCL6* rearrangement Complex cytogenetics
Blastoid MCL	Mantle zone, nodular or diffuse	Medium-sized cells with immature fine chromatin and inconspicuous nucleoli	CD19+, CD20+, CD10−, BCL6−, BCL2+, CD5+, cyclin D1+, TdT− Ki-67 <90% EBER−	t(11.14)
B-lymphoblastic leukemia/lymphoma	Diffuse, or paracortical/sinusoidal if involves lymph nodes	Medium-sized cells with immature fine chromatin and inconspicuous nucleoli	CD19+, CD20+/−, CD10+, cyclin D1−, TdT+, CD34+ Ki-67 <90% EBER−	No DH (rare cases may have *BCL2* and *MYC* rearrangement)

FISH assay in all cases of DLBCL with a GC-B-cell like phenotype, especially if the Ki-67 proliferation fraction is high.

- Compared to HGBL-DH, BL mostly occurs in children, young adult, or patients with HIV and consists of monotonous medium-sized cells with high mitotic rate and starry-sky macrophages. BL cells usually have strong expression of MYC but lack BCL2 and harbor *MYC/IG* translocation, simple cytogenetics, and molecular BL profile.
- The principle mimics of BL include Burkitt-like lymphoma with 11q aberration, HGBL, NOS, blastoid variant of mantle cell lymphoma, and B-lymphoblastic leukemia/lymphoma (Table 7.3).
  - Burkitt-like lymphoma with 11q aberration is morphologically undistinguishable from Burkitt lymphoma. However, instead of *MYC* translocation, it has 11q aberration that can be detected by conventional karyotype and/or FISH or more sensitive methods, such as array comparative genomic hybridization (CGH) or single nucleotide polymorphism (SNP) array [2, 16].
  - The remaining entities are distinguished from BL by the combined analysis of clinical, morphologic, immunophenotypic, and molecular features.
- LBL often shows leukemic pattern of infiltration with paracortical, sinusoidal involvement. It expresses immature lymphocyte markers, such as TdT and CD34, and lacks surface immunoglobulin. Rare cases of B-LBL, mostly transformed from follicular lymphoma, may have a double hit, but they should not be classified as HGBL-DH [2].
- Blastoid variant mantle cell lymphoma may show mantle zone, nodular, or diffuse pattern with expression of cyclin D1/SOX11. Rare cases may undergo aggressive transformation and acquire secondary *MYC* rearrangement, but without DH/TH, these cases should not be diagnosed as HGBL-DH [94].
- Myeloid sarcoma can involve the lymph node in a sinusoidal pattern or show diffuse infiltration of blastoid cells with fine chromatin and granular cytoplasm and admixed immature eosinophils. Immunostains for granulocytic markers, including CD33, lysosome, myeloperoxidase, CD15, and CD68, are very helpful for differential diagnosis.

9. Which findings are suggestive of the diagnosis, which are definitively diagnostic, and which rule out the diagnosis of specific types of aggressive/high-grade B-cell lymphomas?

- Findings suggestive of an aggressive lymphoma:
  - Cytomorphology: Large cells, blastic or blastoid morphology of lymphoma cells, high number of mitoses, high number of apoptotic cells, tingible body macrophages, and cytoplasmic vacuoles.
  - Histology: Diffuse growth pattern with medium to large cells, starry-sky pattern, areas of necrosis
  - IHC: High proliferation index with Ki-67 staining, positive staining for MYC with or without *EBV*, GCB phenotype in a diffuse pattern lymphoma, especially if BCL2 staining is positive
- Findings diagnostic of aggressive/high-grade lymphomas:
  - The presence appropriate cytogenetic abnormality or combination of abnormalities with the corresponding morphology of lymphoma cells is required for definitive diagnosis. For example, detection of translocations involving *MYC* with either *BCL2* or *BCL6* by conventional karyotype, FISH, and other molecular methods is required for the diagnosis of HGBL-DH. See questions 4 and 8 above for defining features of the four main categories of aggressive lymphomas.
- Caution:
  - Translocation of *MYC* is characteristic but not specific of BL. *MYC* rearrangement can also be detected in some de novo and transformed lymphomas, including mantle cell lymphoma, follicular lymphoma, DLBCL, plasmablastic lymphoma, plasma cell myeloma, and the new category in the 2017 WHO classification of high-grade B-cell lymphoma [21]. Some of these *MYC* translocations detected by break-apart probes are actually *MYC* juxtaposed to non-IG loci, which preclude the diagnosis of BL.
  - The 11q aberration is not specific for the new entity of Burkitt-like lymphoma with 11q aberration. It has also been detected in BL or high-grade B-cell lymphoma, not otherwise specified (HGBL, NOS), DLBCL, and even large B-cell lymphoma with *IRF4* rearrangement [7, 44, 95].
- Findings that rule out the diagnosis of specific types of high-grade or aggressive lymphoma (see also exclusionary criteria in question 2):
  - Morphology: Typical diffuse large B-cell lymphoma morphology rules out a diagnosis of HGBL, NOS irrespective of proliferation fraction and/or double or triple "expressor" phenotype (diagnosis of HGBL-HD is possible with DLBCL morphology if appropriate cytogenetic abnormalities are present).
  - Earlier biopsy-proven diagnoses of follicular lymphoma, mantle cell lymphoma, or lymphoblastic lymphoma rule out a subsequent diagnosis of HGBL-DH even when a *MYC* translocation is acquired as a secondary transformation event.

10. What is the prognostic and therapeutic significance of identification of these subtypes of aggressive/high-grade B-cell lymphomas?

- HGBL-DH often has a significantly poorer prognosis compared with DLBCL [2, 96].

- With R-CHOP or comparable chemotherapies, complete response rate remains very low and overall survival time is short with a median of 4.5–18.5 months. Several factors, including extent of the disease, the tumor morphology, and *MYC* partner, have prognostic impact [2, 97].

- HGBL, NOS, has a slightly better prognosis than HGBL-DH. However, in general, HGBL, NOS, has a poor outcome, especially in cases with rearrangement/amplification of *MYC* [2, 24, 69]. More clinical data are required to better stratify the prognosis of this disease.
- Burkitt lymphoma is a highly aggressive but potentially curable neoplasm.
  - High-intensity, short-duration chemotherapy with CNS chemoprophylaxis has achieved high percentage of survival rate for this highly proliferative neoplasm [2, 16, 98, 99].
    - Acute tumor lysis syndrome may develop as massive tumor death after intense chemotherapy. The chemotherapy may be compromised by the limited availability of medical resources in underdeveloped counties and increased risk of opportunistic infection in immunodeficiency-associated BL.
    - Surgical resection may be helpful especially for patients presenting with ileocecal involvement but irradiation therapy does not improve the prognosis.
  - Several adverse prognostic factors are reported: advanced stage, unresected tumor >10 cm, bone marrow and CNS involvement, and high serum LDH [2]. In these cases, relapse is often seen within 1 year after diagnosis.
- Burkitt-like lymphoma with 11q aberrations:
  - Burkitt lymphoma-directed chemotherapy has better effects in this disease than R-CHOP.
  - Patients who are treated with BL regimens have relapse-free outcome similar to BL patients. The 5-year overall survival is 80% with a plateau after initial non-relapse mortality [45].

Case Presentations

Case 1

Learning Objectives

1. To become familiar with morphologic presentation, immunohistochemical features, flow cytometric findings, and cytogenetic/molecular profile of high-grade B-cell lymphoma
2. To become familiar with the differentials and essential work-ups for high-grade B-cell lymphoma

Case History

A 67-year-old male with no significant past medical history presented with left leg discomfort. He underwent chest/abdomen CT and lumbar spine MRI and was found to have 11 cm retroperitoneal soft tissue masses encasing multiple organs and structures. A CT-guided needle biopsy was performed.

Histologic Findings

- The biopsy showed diffuse infiltrate of pleomorphic large cells. The atypical cells have large irregular nuclei, multiple nucleoli, and moderate amount of cytoplasm. Numerous mitoses are seen.

Differential Diagnosis (Fig. 7.6)

- High-grade B-cell lymphoma
- Diffuse large B-cell lymphoma
- Mantle cell lymphoma, blastoid variant
- Follicular lymphoma, transformed to DLBCL
- Lymphoblastic leukemia/lymphoma
- Burkitt lymphoma

IHC Findings

- The large atypical cells are positive for PAX5, BCL6, BCL2 (100%, strong), and MYC (40%, variable intensity) and negative for MUM1.
- A CD21 stain is negative.
- A Ki-67 stain is positive in approximately 90% of large cell nuclei.

Flow Cytometric Findings

Sixty-seven percent monoclonal B-cell population with CD10 and lambda surface immunoglobin light chain restriction

Cytogenetic Analysis

- FISH: *MYC* rearrangement in 85% of the total interphase nuclei
- *MYC/IGH* in 1% of the total interphase nuclei
- *BCL6* rearrangement in 90% of the total interphase nuclei
- *BCL2* rearrangement in 95% of the total interphase nuclei

Final Diagnosis

High-grade B-cell lymphoma with *MYC, BCL2,* and *BCL6* rearrangements

Take-Home Messages

1. HGBL refers to a heterogeneous group of aggressive mature B-cell lymphomas that do not meet the criteria for DLBCL or Burkitt lymphoma.
2. HGBL with *MYC* and *BCL2* and/or *BCL6* translocations is highly aggressive and responds poorly to standard

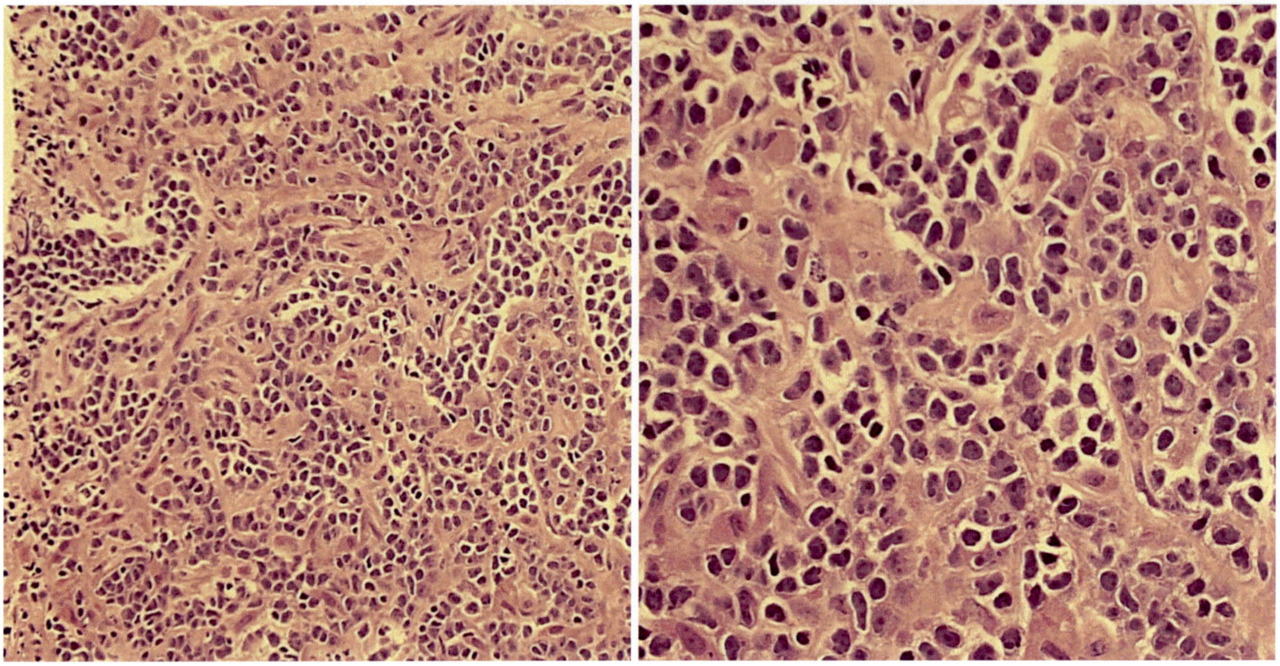

Fig. 7.6 Retroperitoneal mass, CT-guided core needle biopsy (H&E, left pane 10×, right pane 40×)

DCBCL therapy (R-CHOP). So it is mandatory to do cytogenetic tests to differentiate it from other aggressive B-cell lymphomas.

3. The 2017 WHO classification recommends exclusion of the following lymphomas from this category:
   - Follicular lymphoma with *MYC* and *BCL2* rearrangement.
   - Follicular lymphoma with lymphoblastic transformation.
   - Lymphomas with double expression of MYC and BCL2 proteins ("double expressors") without DH/TH, mutation/copy number increase/amplification without DH/TH, two gene rearrangements other than *MYC* (e.g., *BCL2* and *BCL6*), or other gene rearrangements with *MYC* (e.g., *CCND1*) are not included in this category.

Case 2

Learning Objectives

1. To learn the clinical presentation, morphologic findings, immunohistochemical features, flow cytometric, and cytogenetic/molecular profile of Burkitt lymphoma
2. To become familiar with the differentials and essential work-ups for the differentials of Burkitt lymphoma

Case History

A 14-year-old male with no significant past medical history presented with a non-tender but rapidly increasing left neck mass. CT showed a 4.5 × 3 × 3 cm left neck mass, favoring an enlarged lymph node. A biopsy was performed to rule out neoplasm versus infection (e.g., *EBV*, mumps).

Histologic Findings

- The nodal architecture is largely effaced by a diffuse proliferation of monotonous intermediate-sized cells with prominent starry-sky macrophages.
- The atypical cells have moderate basophilic cytoplasm and irregular nuclei with clumped chromatin and multiple small nucleoli.

Differential Diagnosis (Fig. 7.7)

- Burkitt lymphoma
- Burkitt-like lymphoma with 11q aberration
- Lymphoblastic leukemia/lymphoma
- Mantle cell lymphoma, blastoid variant
- Diffuse large B-cell lymphoma
- High-grade B-cell lymphoma

IHC Findings

- The proliferation consists of CD20-positive cells that coexpress CD10 and BCL6.
- MYC is expressed in at least 60–70% of cells. The atypical cells are negative for BCL2.
- A CD21 stain shows rare residual follicular dendritic cell meshwork.
- A Ki-67 stain is positive in greater than 95% of tumor nuclei.
- An EBER in situ hybridization stain is negative.

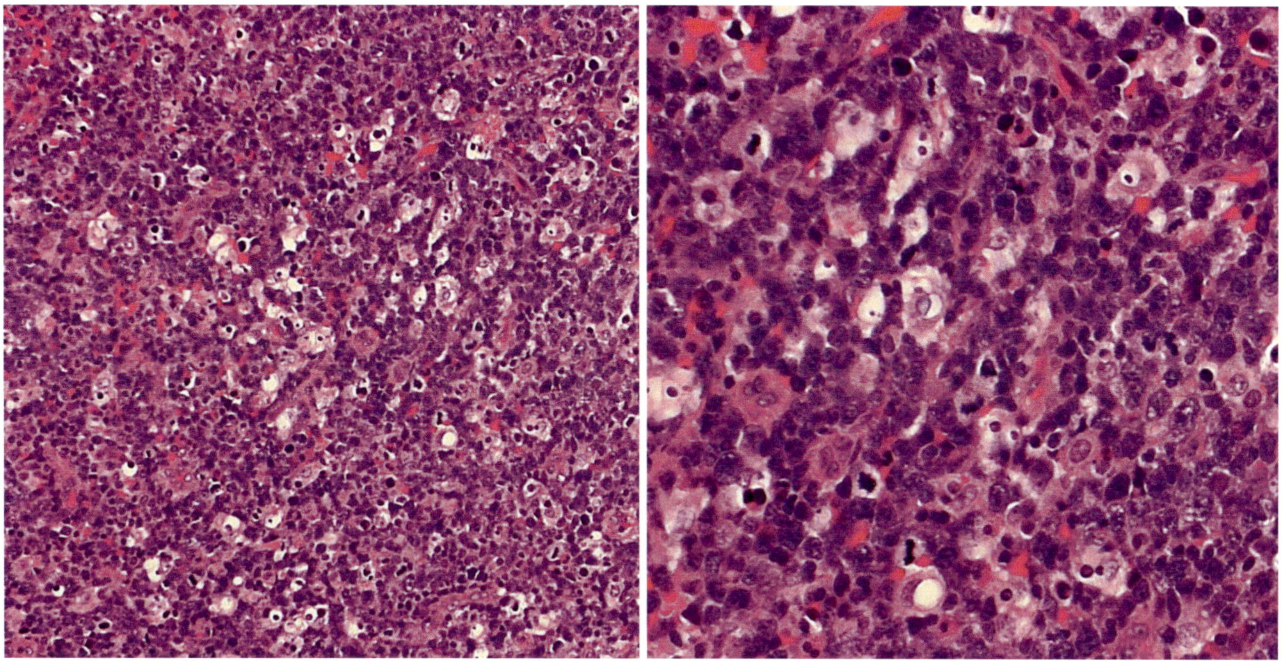

Fig. 7.7 Rapidly enlarging, non-tender neck mass in a 14-year-old patient, biopsy (H&E, left pane 10×, right pane 40×)

Flow Cytometric Findings

Thirty-two percent monoclonal B-cell population with CD10, kappa surface immunoglobin light chain restriction

Cytogenetic Analysis

- Karyotype: 46, XY, t(8;14)(q24.1;q32) [12]/46, XY [8].
- FISH: *MYC* (8q24) translocation in 94% of the total interphase nuclei

Final Diagnosis

Burkitt lymphoma

Take-Home Messages

1. Burkitt lymphoma has three clinicopathological variants: endemic, sporadic, and immunodeficiency-associated. It accounts for 30–50% of childhood lymphomas, and most presented with extranodal involvement.
2. BL exhibits monotonous intermediate-sized cells with clumped chromatin, multiple nucleoli, and moderate basophilic cytoplasm. The cells show high mitotic rate with starry-sky macrophages.
3. BL is germinal center derivation and expresses B-cell markers but is negative for BCL2. It harbors characteristic *MYC* translocation with *IGH*, or kappa/lambda gene loci.
4. A subset of MYC-negative Burkitt lymphoma cases having 11q aberrations are now regarded as a new provisional entity in the 2017 WHO classification.

References

1. Lennert K, Feller AC. Histopathology of non-Hodgkin's lymphomas. 2nd ed. Berlin: Springer; 1992. p. 115–64.
2. Swerdlow SH, Campo E, Harris NL, Jaffe ES, Pileri SA, Stein H, et al. WHO classification of tumours of haematopoietic and lymphoid tissues. Revised 4th ed. IARC: Lyon; 2017. p. 330–44.
3. Haralambieva E, Boerma EJ, van Imhoff GW, Rosati S, Schuuring E, Muller-Hermelink HK, et al. Clinical, immunophenotypic, and genetic analysis of adult lymphomas with morphologic features of Burkitt lymphoma. Am J Surg Pathol. 2005;29(8):1086–94.
4. Hummel M, Bentink S, Berger H, Klapper W, Wessendorf S, Barth TF, et al. A biologic definition of Burkitt's lymphoma from transcriptional and genomic profiling. N Engl J Med. 2006;354(23):2419–30.
5. Boerma EG, Siebert R, Kluin PM, Baudis M. Translocations involving 8q24 in Burkitt lymphoma and other malignant lymphomas: a historical review of cytogenetics in the light of todays knowledge. Leukemia. 2009;23(2):225–34.
6. Pienkowska-Grela B, Rymkiewicz G, Grygalewicz B, Woroniecka R, Krawczyk P, Czyz-Domanska K, et al. Partial trisomy 11, dup(11)(q23q13), as a defect characterizing lymphomas with Burkitt pathomorphology without MYC gene rearrangement. Med Oncol. 2011;28(4):1589–95.

7. Salaverria I, Martin-Guerrero I, Wagener R, Kreuz M, Kohler CW, Richter J, et al. A recurrent 11q aberration pattern characterizes a subset of MYC-negative high-grade B-cell lymphomas resembling Burkitt lymphoma. Blood. 2014;123(8):1187–98.
8. Ferreiro JF, Morscio J, Dierickx D, Marcelis L, Verhoef G, Vandenberghe P, et al. Post-transplant molecularly defined Burkitt lymphomas are frequently MYC-negative and characterized by the 11q-gain/loss pattern. Haematologica. 2015;100(7):e275–9.
9. Aukema SM, Siebert R, Schuuring E, van Imhoff GW, Kluin-Nelemans HC, Boerma EJ, et al. Double-hit B-cell lymphomas. Blood. 2011;117(8):2319–31.
10. De Jong D, Voetdijk BM, Beverstock GC, van Ommen GJ, Willemze R, Kluin PM. Activation of the c-myc oncogene in a precursor-B-cell blast crisis of follicular lymphoma, presenting as composite lymphoma. N Engl J Med. 1988;318(21):1373–8.
11. Geyer JT, Subramaniyam S, Jiang Y, Elemento O, Ferry JA, de Leval L, et al. Lymphoblastic transformation of follicular lymphoma: a clinicopathologic and molecular analysis of 7 patients. Hum Pathol. 2015;46(2):260–71.
12. Kobrin C, Cha SC, Qin H, Raffeld M, Fend F, Quintanilla-Martinez L, et al. Molecular analysis of light-chain switch and acute lymphoblastic leukemia transformation in two follicular lymphomas: implications for lymphomagenesis. Leuk Lymphoma. 2006;47(8):1523–34.
13. Young KH, Xie Q, Zhou G, Eickhoff JC, Sanger WG, Aoun P, et al. Transformation of follicular lymphoma to precursor B-cell lymphoblastic lymphoma with c-myc gene rearrangement as a critical event. Am J Clin Pathol. 2008;129(1):157–66.
14. Schmitz R, Young RM, Ceribelli M, Jhavar S, Xiao W, Zhang M, et al. Burkitt lymphoma pathogenesis and therapeutic targets from structural and functional genomics. Nature. 2012;490(7418):116–20.
15. Boxer LM, Dang CV. Translocations involving c-myc and c-myc function. Oncogene. 2001;20(40):5595–610.
16. Jaffe ES, Arber DA, Campo E, Harris NL, Quintanilla-Martinez L. Hematopathology. 2nd ed. Philadelphia: Elsevier; 2017.
17. Burkitt D. A sarcoma involving the jaws in African children. Br J Surg. 1958;46(197):218–23.
18. Burkitt D. Burkitt's lymphoma outside the known endemic areas of Africa and New Guinea. Int J Cancer. 1967;2(6):562–5.
19. Facer CA, Playfair JH. Malaria, Epstein-Barr virus, and the genesis of lymphomas. Adv Cancer Res. 1989;53:33–72.
20. Manolov G, Manolova Y, Klein G, Levan A, Kieler J. Chromosome #14 markers in two Epstein-Barr virus (EBV)-transformed lymphoblastoid cell lines of normal origin differ from the Burkitt lymphoma (BL)-associated 14q+ marker. Cancer Genet Cytogenet. 1981;4(2):179–84.
21. Magrath IT. Treatment of Burkitt lymphoma in children and adults: lessons from Africa. Curr Hematol Malig Rep. 2006;1(4):230–40.
22. Klapper W, Szczepanowski M, Burkhardt B, Berger H, Rosolowski M, Bentink S, et al. Molecular profiling of pediatric mature B-cell lymphoma treated in population-based prospective clinical trials. Blood. 2008;112(4):1374–81.
23. Lindsley RC, LaCasce AS. Biology of double-hit B-cell lymphomas. Curr Opin Hematol. 2012;19(4):299–304.
24. Perry AM, Crockett D, Dave BJ, Althof P, Winkler L, Smith LM, et al. B-cell lymphoma, unclassifiable, with features intermediate between diffuse large B-cell lymphoma and Burkitt lymphoma: study of 39 cases. Br J Haematol. 2013;162(1):40–9.
25. Pillai RK, Sathanoori M, Van Oss SB, Swerdlow SH. Double-hit B-cell lymphomas with BCL6 and MYC translocations are aggressive, frequently extranodal lymphomas distinct from BCL2 double-hit B-cell lymphomas. Am J Surg Pathol. 2013;37(3):323–32.
26. Swerdlow SH. Diagnosis of 'double hit' diffuse large B-cell lymphoma and B-cell lymphoma, unclassifiable, with features intermediate between DLBCL and Burkitt lymphoma: when and how, FISH versus IHC. Hematology Am Soc Hematol Educ Program. 2014;2014(1):90–9.
27. Wang W, Hu S, Lu X, Young KH, Medeiros LJ. Triple-hit B-cell lymphoma with MYC, BCL2, and BCL6 translocations/rearrangements: clinicopathologic features of 11 cases. Am J Surg Pathol. 2015;39(8):1132–9.
28. Murphy SB. Classification, staging and end results of treatment of childhood non-Hodgkin's lymphomas: dissimilarities from lymphomas in adults. Semin Oncol. 1980;7(3):332–9.
29. Rosolen A, Perkins SL, Pinkerton CR, Guillerman RP, Sandlund JT, Patte C, et al. Revised international pediatric non-Hodgkin lymphoma staging system. J Clin Oncol. 2015;33(18):2112–8.
30. Cheson BD, Fisher RI, Barrington SF, Cavalli F, Schwartz LH, Zucca E, et al. Recommendations for initial evaluation, staging, and response assessment of Hodgkin and non-Hodgkin lymphoma: the Lugano classification. J Clin Oncol. 2014;32(27):3059–68.
31. Oosten LEM, Chamuleau MED, Thielen FW, de Wreede LC, Siemes C, Doorduijn JK, et al. Treatment of sporadic Burkitt lymphoma in adults, a retrospective comparison of four treatment regimens. Ann Hematol. 2018;97(2):255–66.
32. Hoelzer D, Walewski J, Döhner H, Viardot A, Hiddemann W, Spiekermann K, et al. Improved outcome of adult Burkitt lymphoma/leukemia with rituximab and chemotherapy: report of a large prospective multicenter trial. Blood. 2014;124(26):3870–9.
33. Barnes JA, LaCasce AS, Feng Y, Toomey CE, Neuberg D, Michaelson JS, et al. Evaluation of the addition of rituximab to CODOX-M/IVAC for Burkitt's lymphoma: a retrospective analysis. Ann Oncol. 2011;22(8):1859–64.
34. Dave SS, Fu K, Wright GW, Lam LT, Kluin P, Boerma EJ, et al. Molecular diagnosis of Burkitt's lymphoma. N Engl J Med. 2006;354(23):2431–42.
35. Hecht JL, Aster JC. Molecular biology of Burkitt's lymphoma. J Clin Oncol. 2000;18(21):3707–21.
36. Neri A, Barriga F, Knowles DM, Magrath IT, Dalla-Favera R. Different regions of the immunoglobulin heavy-chain locus are involved in chromosomal translocations in distinct pathogenetic forms of Burkitt lymphoma. Proc Natl Acad Sci U S A. 1988;85(8):2748–52.
37. Magrath IT. African Burkitt's lymphoma. History, biology, clinical features, and treatment. Am J Pediatr Hematol Oncol. 1991;13(2):222–46.
38. Mbulaiteye SM, Anderson WF, Ferlay J, Bhatia K, Chang C, Rosenberg PS, et al. Pediatric, elderly, and emerging adult-onset peaks in Burkitt's lymphoma incidence diagnosed in four continents, excluding Africa. Am J Hematol. 2012;87(6):573–8.
39. Mbulaiteye SM, Anderson WF, Bhatia K, Rosenberg PS, Linet MS, Devesa SS. Trimodal age-specific incidence patterns for Burkitt lymphoma in the United States, 1973–2005. Int J Cancer. 2010;126(7):1732–9.
40. Levine AM. Acquired immunodeficiency syndrome-related lymphoma. Blood. 1992;80(1):8–20.
41. Lim ST, Karim R, Nathwani BN, Tulpule A, Espina B, Levine AM. AIDS-related Burkitt's lymphoma versus diffuse large-cell lymphoma in the pre-highly active antiretroviral therapy (HAART) and HAART eras: significant differences in survival with standard chemotherapy. J Clin Oncol. 2005;23(19):4430–8.
42. Kaplan MA, Ferry JA, Harris NL, Jacobson JO. Clonal analysis of posttransplant lymphoproliferative disorders, using both episomal Epstein-Barr virus and immunoglobulin genes as markers. Am J Clin Pathol. 1994;101(5):590–6.
43. Roithmann S, Toledano M, Tourani JM, Raphael M, Gentilini M, Gastaut JA, et al. HIV-associated non-Hodgkin's lymphomas: clinical characteristics and outcome. The experience of the French registry of HIV-associated tumors. Ann Oncol. 1991;2(4):289–95.
44. Grygalewicz B, Woroniecka R, Rymkiewicz G, Rygier J, Borkowska K, Kotyl A, et al. The 11q-gain/loss aberration occurs recurrently in

MYC-negative Burkitt-like lymphoma with 11q aberration, as well as MYC-positive Burkitt lymphoma and MYC-positive high-grade B-cell lymphoma, NOS. Am J Clin Pathol. 2018;149(1):17–28.
45. Rymkiewicz G, Grygalewicz B, Chechlinska M, Blachnio K, Bystydzienski Z, Romejko-Jarosinska J, et al. A comprehensive flow-cytometry-based immunophenotypic characterization of Burkitt-like lymphoma with 11q aberration. Mod Pathol. 2018;31(5):732–43.
46. Ferreiro JF, Morscio J, Dierickx D, Marcelis L, Verhoef G, Vandenberghe P, et al. Post-transplant molecularly defined Burkitt lymphomas are frequently MYC-negative and characterized by the 11q-gain/loss pattern. Haematologica. 2015;100(7):e275–e9.
47. Aukema SM, Kreuz M, Kohler CW, Rosolowski M, Hasenclever D, Hummel M, et al. Biological characterization of adult MYC-translocation-positive mature B-cell lymphomas other than molecular Burkitt lymphoma. Haematologica. 2014;99(4):726–35.
48. Li S, Desai P, Lin P, Yin CC, Tang G, Wang XJ, et al. MYC/BCL6 double-hit lymphoma (DHL): a tumour associated with an aggressive clinical course and poor prognosis. Histopathology. 2016;68(7):1090–8.
49. Snuderl M, Kolman OK, Chen YB, Hsu JJ, Ackerman AM, Dal Cin P, et al. B-cell lymphomas with concurrent IGH-BCL2 and MYC rearrangements are aggressive neoplasms with clinical and pathologic features distinct from Burkitt lymphoma and diffuse large B-cell lymphoma. Am J Surg Pathol. 2010;34(3):327–40.
50. Kanagal-Shamanna R, Medeiros LJ, Lu G, Wang SA, Manning JT, Lin P, et al. High-grade B-cell lymphoma, unclassifiable, with blastoid features: an unusual morphological subgroup associated frequently with BCL2 and/or MYC gene rearrangements and a poor prognosis. Histopathology. 2012;61(5):945–54.
51. Vaidyanathan G, Ngamphaiboon N, Hernandez-Ilizaliturri FJ. Clinical spectrum and prognosis of follicular lymphoma with blastoid transformation: case series and a review of the literature. Ann Hematol. 2011;90(8):955–62.
52. Mann RB, Jaffe ES, Braylan RC, Nanba K, Frank MM, Ziegler JL, et al. Non-endemic Burkitts's lymphoma. A B-cell tumor related to germinal centers. N Engl J Med. 1976;295(13):685–91.
53. Pavlova Z, Parker JW, Taylor CR, Levine AM, Feinstein DI, Lukes RJ. Small noncleaved follicular center cell lymphoma: Burkitt's and non-Burkitt's variants in the US. II. Pathologic and immunologic features. Cancer. 1987;59(11):1892–902.
54. Koo CH, Rappaport H, Sheibani K, Pangalis GA, Nathwani BN, Winberg CD. Imprint cytology of non-Hodgkin's lymphomas based on a study of 212 immunologically characterized cases: correlation of touch imprints with tissue sections. Hum Pathol. 1989;20(12 Suppl 1):1–137.
55. Bhatt AP, Jacobs SR, Freemerman AJ, Makowski L, Rathmell JC, Dittmer DP, et al. Dysregulation of fatty acid synthesis and glycolysis in non-Hodgkin lymphoma. Proc Natl Acad Sci. 2012;109(29):11818.
56. Stastny JF, Almeida MM, Wakely PE Jr, Kornstein MJ, Frable WJ. Fine-needle aspiration biopsy and imprint cytology of small non-cleaved cell (Burkitt's) lymphoma. Diagn Cytopathol. 1995;12(3):201–7.
57. Braziel RM, Arber DA, Slovak ML, Gulley ML, Spier C, Kjeldsberg C, et al. The Burkitt-like lymphomas: a Southwest Oncology Group study delineating phenotypic, genotypic, and clinical features. Blood. 2001;97(12):3713–20.
58. Carbone A, Gloghini A, Gaidano G, Cilia AM, Bassi P, Polito P, et al. AIDS-related Burkitt's lymphoma. Morphologic and immunophenotypic study of biopsy specimens. Am J Clin Pathol. 1995;103(5):561–7.
59. Haralambieva E, Rosati S, van Noesel C, Boers E, van Marwijk Kooy M, Schuuring E, et al. Florid granulomatous reaction in Epstein-Barr virus-positive nonendemic Burkitt lymphomas: report of four cases. Am J Surg Pathol. 2004;28(3):379–83.
60. Hollingsworth HC, Longo DL, Jaffe ES. Small noncleaved cell lymphoma associated with florid epithelioid granulomatous response. A clinicopathologic study of seven patients. Am J Surg Pathol. 1993;17(1):51–9.
61. Kramer MH, Raghoebier S, Beverstock GC, de Jong D, Kluin PM, Kluin-Nelemans JC. De novo acute B-cell leukemia with translocation t(14;18): an entity with a poor prognosis. Leukemia. 1991;5(6):473–8.
62. Gebauer N, Bernard V, Feller AC, Merz H. ID3 mutations are recurrent events in double-hit B-cell lymphomas. Anticancer Res. 2013;33(11):4771–8.
63. Gebauer N, Bernard V, Gebauer W, Thorns C, Feller AC, Merz H. TP53 mutations are frequent events in double-hit B-cell lymphomas with MYC and BCL2 but not MYC and BCL6 translocations. Leuk Lymphoma. 2015;56(1):179–85.
64. Gebauer N, Bernard V, Thorns C, Feller AC, Merz H. Oncogenic MYD88 mutations are rare events in double-hit B-cell lymphomas. Acta Haematol. 2015;133(1):113–5.
65. Li S, Seegmiller AC, Lin P, Wang XJ, Miranda RN, Bhagavathi S, et al. B-cell lymphomas with concurrent MYC and BCL2 abnormalities other than translocations behave similarly to MYC/BCL2 double-hit lymphomas. Mod Pathol. 2015;28(2):208–17.
66. Andersson ML, Stam NJ, Klein G, Ploegh HL, Masucci MG. Aberrant expression of HLA class-I antigens in Burkitt lymphoma cells. Int J Cancer. 1991;47(4):544–50.
67. Pedersen MO, Gang AO, Poulsen TS, Knudsen H, Lauritzen AF, Nielsen SL, et al. MYC translocation partner gene determines survival of patients with large B-cell lymphoma with MYC- or double-hit MYC/BCL2 translocations. Eur J Haematol. 2014;92(1):42–8.
68. Hsi ED. Hematopathology. 3rd ed. Philadelphia, PA: Elsevier/Saunders; 2018. xiv, 744 p. p.
69. Lin P, Dickason TJ, Fayad LE, Lennon PA, Hu P, Garcia M, et al. Prognostic value of MYC rearrangement in cases of B-cell lymphoma, unclassifiable, with features intermediate between diffuse large B-cell lymphoma and Burkitt lymphoma. Cancer. 2012;118(6):1566–73.
70. Guikema JE, de Boer C, Haralambieva E, Smit LA, van Noesel CJ, Schuuring E, et al. IGH switch breakpoints in Burkitt lymphoma: exclusive involvement of noncanonical class switch recombination. Genes Chromosomes Cancer. 2006;45(9):808–19.
71. May PC, Foot N, Dunn R, Geoghegan H, Neat MJ. Detection of cryptic and variant IGH-MYC rearrangements in high-grade non-Hodgkin's lymphoma by fluorescence in situ hybridization: implications for cytogenetic testing. Cancer Genet Cytogenet. 2010;198(1):71–5.
72. Leucci E, Cocco M, Onnis A, De Falco G, van Cleef P, Bellan C, et al. MYC translocation-negative classical Burkitt lymphoma cases: an alternative pathogenetic mechanism involving miRNA deregulation. J Pathol. 2008;216(4):440–50.
73. Haralambieva E, Schuuring E, Rosati S, van Noesel C, Jansen P, Appel I, et al. Interphase fluorescence in situ hybridization for detection of 8q24/MYC breakpoints on routine histologic sections: validation in Burkitt lymphomas from three geographic regions. Genes Chromosomes Cancer. 2004;40(1):10–8.
74. Aukema SM, Theil L, Rohde M, Bauer B, Bradtke J, Burkhardt B, et al. Sequential karyotyping in Burkitt lymphoma reveals a linear clonal evolution with increase in karyotype complexity and a high frequency of recurrent secondary aberrations. Br J Haematol. 2015;170(6):814–25.
75. Dominguez-Sola D, Victora GD, Ying CY, Phan RT, Saito M, Nussenzweig MC, et al. c-MYC is required for germinal center selection and cyclic re-entry. Nat Immunol. 2012;13(11):1083–91.
76. Kelly GL, Rickinson AB. Burkitt lymphoma: revisiting the pathogenesis of a virus-associated malignancy. Hematology Am Soc Hematol Educ Program. 2007:277–84.

77. Bissonnette RP, Echeverri F, Mahboubi A, Green DR. Apoptotic cell death induced by c-myc is inhibited by bcl-2. Nature. 1992;359(6395):552–4.
78. Bouska A, Bi C, Lone W, Zhang W, Kedwaii A, Heavican T, et al. Adult high-grade B-cell lymphoma with Burkitt lymphoma signature: genomic features and potential therapeutic targets. Blood. 2017;130(16):1819–31.
79. De Souza MT, Vera-Lozada G, Othman M, Marques-Salles TJ, Pinto LW, da Rocha MM, et al. Molecular and cytogenetic studies in a child with Burkitt lymphoma and ataxia-telangiectasia syndrome harboring MYC overexpression and partial trisomy 8. Ann Lab Med. 2018;38(1):63–6.
80. Dittmer DP. Not like a wrecking ball: EBV fine-tunes MYC lymphomagenesis. Blood. 2014;123(4):460–1.
81. Epstein MA, Achong BG, Barr YM. Virus particles in cultured lymphoblasts from Burkitt's lymphoma. Lancet. 1964;1(7335):702–3.
82. Raab-Traub N, Flynn K. The structure of the termini of the Epstein-Barr virus as a marker of clonal cellular proliferation. Cell. 1986;47(6):883–9.
83. Brown NA, Liu CR, Wang YF, Garcia CR. B-cell lymphoproliferation and lymphomagenesis are associated with clonotypic intracellular terminal regions of the Epstein-Barr virus. J Virol. 1988;62(3):962–9.
84. Gutierrez MI, Bhatia K, Cherney B, Capello D, Gaidano G, Magrath I. Intraclonal molecular heterogeneity suggests a hierarchy of pathogenetic events in Burkitt's lymphoma. Ann Oncol. 1997;8(10):987–94.
85. Young LS, Murray PG. Epstein-Barr virus and oncogenesis: from latent genes to tumours. Oncogene. 2003;22(33):5108–21.
86. Seitz V, Butzhammer P, Hirsch B, Hecht J, Gutgemann I, Ehlers A, et al. Deep sequencing of MYC DNA-binding sites in Burkitt lymphoma. PLoS One. 2011;6(11):e26837.
87. Gutierrez MI, Bhatia K, Barriga F, Diez B, Muriel FS, de Andreas ML, et al. Molecular epidemiology of Burkitt's lymphoma from South America: differences in breakpoint location and Epstein-Barr virus association from tumors in other world regions. Blood. 1992;79(12):3261–6.
88. Wilmore JR, Asito AS, Wei C, Piriou E, Sumba PO, Sanz I, et al. AID expression in peripheral blood of children living in a malaria holoendemic region is associated with changes in B cell subsets and Epstein-Barr virus. Int J Cancer. 2015;136(6):1371–80.
89. Robbiani DF, Deroubaix S, Feldhahn N, Oliveira TY, Callen E, Wang Q, et al. Plasmodium infection promotes genomic instability and AID-dependent B cell lymphoma. Cell. 2015;162(4):727–37.
90. Molyneux EM, Rochford R, Griffin B, Newton R, Jackson G, Menon G, et al. Burkitt's lymphoma. Lancet. 2012;379(9822):1234–44.
91. Mannucci S, Luzzi A, Carugi A, Gozzetti A, Lazzi S, Malagnino V, et al. EBV reactivation and chromosomal polysomies: Euphorbia tirucalli as a possible cofactor in endemic Burkitt lymphoma. Adv Hematol. 2012;2012:149780.
92. van den Bosch C. A role for RNA viruses in the pathogenesis of Burkitt's lymphoma: the need for reappraisal. Adv Hematol. 2012;2012:494758.
93. van den Bosch CA. Is endemic Burkitt's lymphoma an alliance between three infections and a tumour promoter? Lancet Oncol. 2004;5(12):738–46.
94. Reddy K, Ansari-Lari M, Dipasquale B. Blastic mantle cell lymphoma with a Burkitt translocation. Leuk Lymphoma. 2008;49(4):740–50.
95. Havelange V, Ameye G, Théate I, Callet-Bauchu E, Lippert E, Luquet I, et al. The peculiar 11q-gain/loss aberration reported in a subset of MYC-negative high-grade B-cell lymphomas can also occur in a MYC-rearranged lymphoma. Cancer Genet. 2016;209(3):117–8.
96. Zelenetz AD, Gordon LI, Abramson JS, Advani R, Andreadis CB, Bartlett NL, et al. NCCN Clinical Practice Guidelines in Oncology: B-cell lymphomas. 3.2018 ed: National comprehensive cancer network; 2018.
97. Moore EM, Aggarwal N, Surti U, Swerdlow SH. Further exploration of the complexities of large B-cell lymphomas with MYC abnormalities and the importance of a blastoid morphology. Am J Surg Pathol. 2017;41(9):1155–66.
98. Sullivan MP, Ramirez I. Curability of Burkitt's lymphoma with high-dose cyclophosphamide-high-dose methotrexate therapy and intrathecal chemoprophylaxis. J Clin Oncol. 1985;3(5):627–36.
99. Patte C, Auperin A, Michon J, Behrendt H, Leverger G, Frappaz D, et al. The Societe Francaise d'Oncologie Pediatrique LMB89 protocol: highly effective multiagent chemotherapy tailored to the tumor burden and initial response in 561 unselected children with B-cell lymphomas and L3 leukemia. Blood. 2001;97(11):3370–9.

Major Subtypes of Mature T- and NK-Cell Neoplasms

8

Lina Irshaid and Mina L. Xu

List of Frequently Asked Questions

1. What are the major subtypes mature T- and NK-cell neoplasms
2. What is the most important clinical information to collect for this category?
3. What are the typical morphological findings in lymph node and extranodal sites involved by various subtypes of T- and NK-cell neoplasms?
4. What are the mimics and what is the clinical relevance of misinterpretation between the true diagnosis and mimics with reference to mistreatment and/or wrong prognosis?
5. Which morphological findings in the peripheral blood/BM/lymph node biopsy are reliably diagnostic? Which ones suggest the diagnosis? Which is (are) unreliable for diagnosis? Which findings rule out the diagnosis?
6. What is the minimal and optimal ancillary workup for diagnosis and subclassification mature T- and NK-cell neoplasms?
7. Which ancillary test results are diagnostic, suggestive of diagnosis, unreliable for diagnosis, or rule out the diagnosis?
8. What is the workup to provide prognostic and therapeutic target information? (Corollary – what treatments are available for this entity?)
9. Which subtypes of mature T- and NK-cell neoplasms are clinically relevant and which are morphologically defined but have unproven/minimal clinical relevance?
10. What is an adequate specimen for this condition?
11. What information can be conveyed to the clinician during each stage of the workup?
12. What should be the approach to provide maximum, but defensible, information from limited specimen or workup? When is a descriptive diagnosis appropriate in such situations?
13. When is a diagnostic comment necessary and what should be discussed in the diagnostic comment for mature T- and NK-cell neoplasms?
14. When is it appropriate to seek external consultation for mature T- and NK-cell neoplasms?

1. What are the major subtypes mature T- and NK-cell neoplasms?

- Nodal T-cell lymphomas
  - Peripheral T-cell lymphoma, not otherwise specified
  - Angioimmunoblastic T-cell lymphoma
  - Anaplastic large cell lymphoma, ALK-positive
  - Anaplastic large cell lymphoma, ALK-negative
- Extranodal T- and NK-cell neoplasms
  - Breast implant-associated anaplastic large cell lymphoma
  - NK-/T-cell lymphoma, nasal type
  - Hepatosplenic T-cell lymphoma
  - Subcutaneous panniculitis-like T-cell lymphoma
- T-cell neoplasms with frequent leukemic presentation
  - Adult T-cell leukemia/lymphoma
  - T-cell large granular lymphocytic leukemia
  - T-cell prolymphocytic leukemia
- Cutaneous T-cell lymphomas
  - Mycosis fungoides
  - Primary cutaneous CD30-positive T-cell lymphoproliferative disorders
- Intestinal T-cell lymphomas
  - Enteropathy-associated T-cell lymphoma
  - Monomorphic epitheliotropic intestinal T-cell lymphoma

Cutaneous T-cell lymphomas and T-cell lymphomas of the gastrointestinal tract will be discussed in more detail in Chapter 12.

L. Irshaid · M. L. Xu (✉)
Departments of Pathology and Laboratory Medicine, Yale University School of Medicine, New Haven, CT, USA
e-mail: lina.irshaid@yale.edu; mina.xu@yale.edu

E. Wang, A. S. Lagoo (eds.), *Practical Lymph Node and Bone Marrow Pathology*, Practical Anatomic Pathology,
https://doi.org/10.1007/978-3-030-32189-5_8

2. What is the most important clinical information to collect for this category?

The most relevant clinical information to collect for each case includes [1–3]:

- Patient age and gender
- History of neoplasm(s)
- B-symptoms
- Degree of adenopathy and speed of progression
- Extranodal involvement including the skin, bone marrow, liver, spleen, and/or lungs
- Immune suppression
- Infectious and autoimmune workup
- Breast implant surgery and date
- Travel history
- Geographic region and racial characteristics
- Peripheral blood workup including peripheral blood counts, autoimmune serology, and calcium and lactate dehydrogenase levels
- Bone scan for assessment of lytic bone lesions

3. What are the typical morphological findings in lymph node and extranodal sites involved by various subtypes of T- and NK-cell neoplasms?

In contrast to the B-cell lymphomas, cell morphology in diverse T- / NK-cell lymphomas may overlap and cell size is not a reliable guide to aggressiveness of disease. Nevertheless, following T- / NK-cell lymphomas have relatively characteristic morphological findings:

- Angioimmunoblastic T-cell lymphoma (AITL): Partial to complete effacement of lymph node architecture by small- to medium-sized lymphocytes in a background of prominent, arborizing high endothelial venules (HEVs), extra-follicular proliferation of follicular dendritic cells (FDCs), and a polymorphous infiltrate of reactive lymphocytes, plasma cells, and histiocytes are typical morphologic features of AITL [1, 2, 4] (see Fig. 8.1a and Table 8.1).
- Anaplastic large cell lymphoma (ALCL): A neoplastic proliferation of a spectrum of small to large cells with

Table 8.1 Differential diagnosis for angioimmunoblastic T-cell lymphoma

Lymphoma subtype	Lymph node architecture	Cytology	IHC	Molecular	Clinical features
AITL	Expanded dendritic meshworks with partial to total nodal effacement; arborization of high endothelial venules and polymorphic inflammatory background	Small- to intermediate-sized lymphocytes with pale cytoplasm	Positive for CD4, CD10, BCL6, PD1, CXCL13 (TFH phenotype) with scattered *EBV*+ B-cells	Frequent mutations in *TET2*, *IDH2*, *DNMT3A*, *RHOA*	Often with generalized lymphadenopathy, hepatosplenomegaly, polyclonal hypergammaglobulinemia, B symptoms
Follicular TCL	Predominantly follicular growth pattern	Intermediate-sized monotonous lymphocytes with pale cytoplasm	In addition to AITL markers, can also have prominent RS-like cells	20% show t(5;9)(q33;q22), *ITK-SYK* fusion	Similar to AITL; a subset with localized disease and no B symptoms
Nodal PTCL TFH	Predominantly diffuse growth pattern; a subset are T-zone in distribution	Small- to intermediate-sized cells with atypia	Has at least 2–3 of the TFH phenotype listed for AITL	Can show similar mutations as AITL: *TET2*, *DNMT3A*, *RHOA*	Similar to AITL
TCHRLBCL	Typically diffuse growth pattern	Single scattered large cells with numerous surrounding small T-cells	Large CD20-positive B-cells that are *EBV* negative	TCR in germline configuration. BCR should be clonal if enough neoplastic cells present	B symptoms, occasionally with hepatosplenomegaly; usually presents at advanced stage
Infectious mononucleosis lymphadenitis	Intact follicles with expanded paracortex	Numerous large immunoblasts in paracortex with normal/ hyperplastic germinal centers	Immunoblasts often CD30+ *EBV*+	TCR in germline configuration	Fatigue, fever, lymphadenopathy, splenomegaly, sore throat

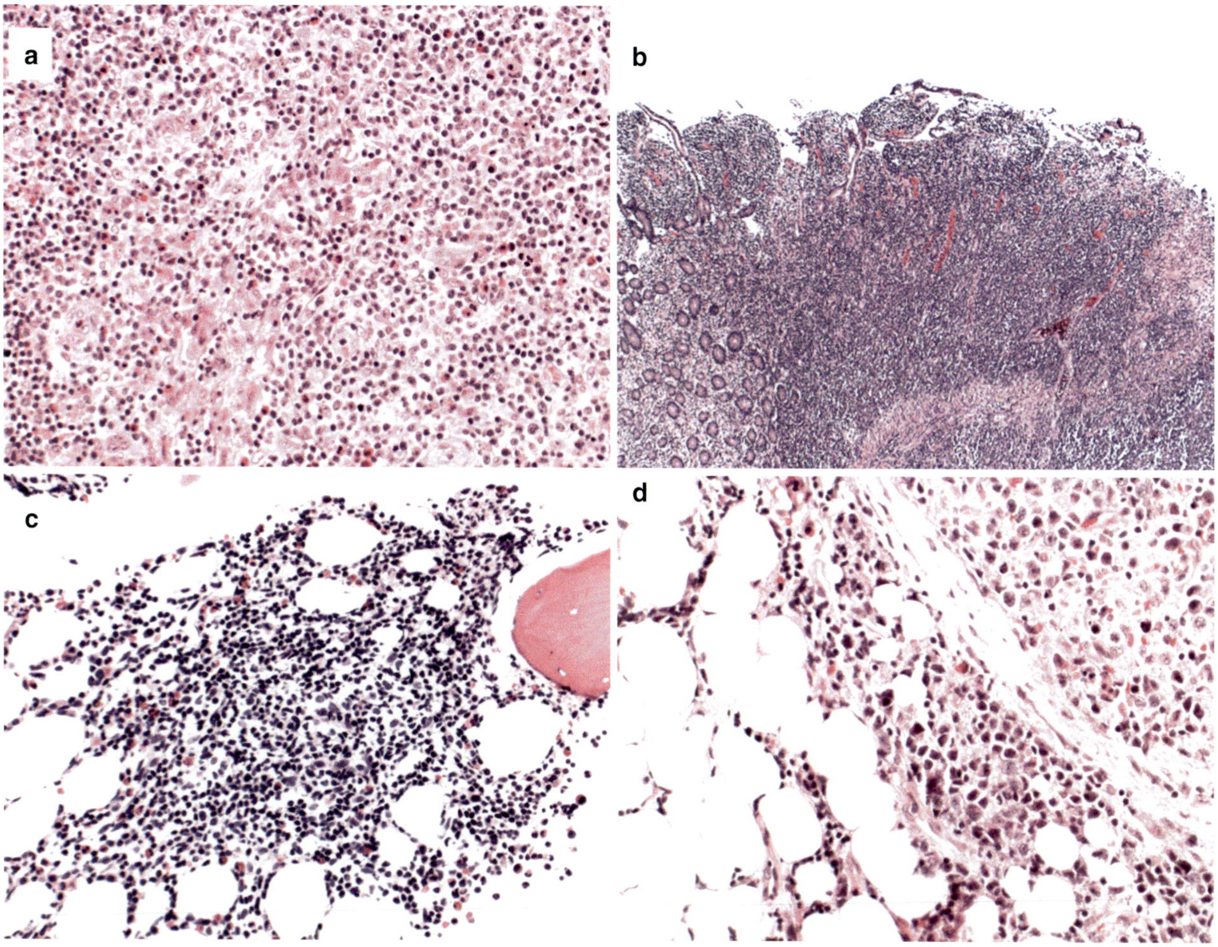

Fig. 8.1 (**a**) Morphologic features of angioimmunoblastic T-cell lymphoma, (**b**) enteropathy-associated T-cell lymphoma, (**c**) marrow involvement by angioimmunoblastic T-cell lymphoma, and (**d**) marrow clot section involvement by ALK-negative anaplastic large cell lymphoma

irregular nuclei, in the presence of hallmark cells characterized as large cells with eccentric, horseshoe-shaped nuclei, distinct nucleoli, prominent eosinophilic Golgi region, and abundant cytoplasm are findings typical of ALCL. Sinusoidal involvement is common. ALK-positive and ALK-negative ALCL are morphologically indistinguishable [1, 2, 5] (see Fig. 8.1d).

- Adult T-cell leukemia/lymphoma (ATLL): The distinctive "flower cells" on peripheral blood smear, characterized as medium- to large-sized lymphocytes with polylobulated nuclei, coarse chromatin, and agranular basophilic cytoplasm, make the diagnosis of ATLL more likely. Lymph nodes in ATLL exhibit varied morphology and require further studies to render a diagnosis [1, 3, 6] (see Table 8.2).
- NK-/T-cell lymphoma, nasal type: This lymphoma typically demonstrates an angiocentric and angiodestructive growth pattern and is commonly associated with high mitotic activity, necrosis, and ulceration. The neoplastic cells are small to medium in size, with infrequent large forms. Nasal-type NK-/T-cell lymphoma preferentially involves the lymph node paracortex and/or medulla with relative sparing of the cortex [1, 2, 7] (see Fig. 8.2).
- Hepatosplenic T-cell lymphoma (HSTL): This lymphoma is characterized by an infiltrate of small- to intermediate-sized T-cells with clumped chromatin and inconspicuous nucleoli, most often limited to the sinusoids of the liver, spleen, and bone marrow [1, 2, 8].
- Subcutaneous panniculitis-like T-cell lymphoma (SPTCL): As the name suggests, SPTCL primarily involves the subcutaneous adipose tissue and spares the overlying epidermis and dermis. SPTCL is composed of neoplastic cells that infiltrate the lobules, spare the septa, and often surround individual adipocytes and disrupt their membrane. While there is a range in cell size across tumors, it is often uniform within an individual tumor. Fat necrosis and an inflammatory reaction involving histiocytes and multinucleated giant cells are common findings [1, 2, 9].
- T-cell large granular lymphocytic leukemia (T-LGLL): Typical morphologic features of T-LGLL on peripheral blood smear are an increase in cells with round to indented nuclei, inconspicuous nucleoli, clumped chromatin, and

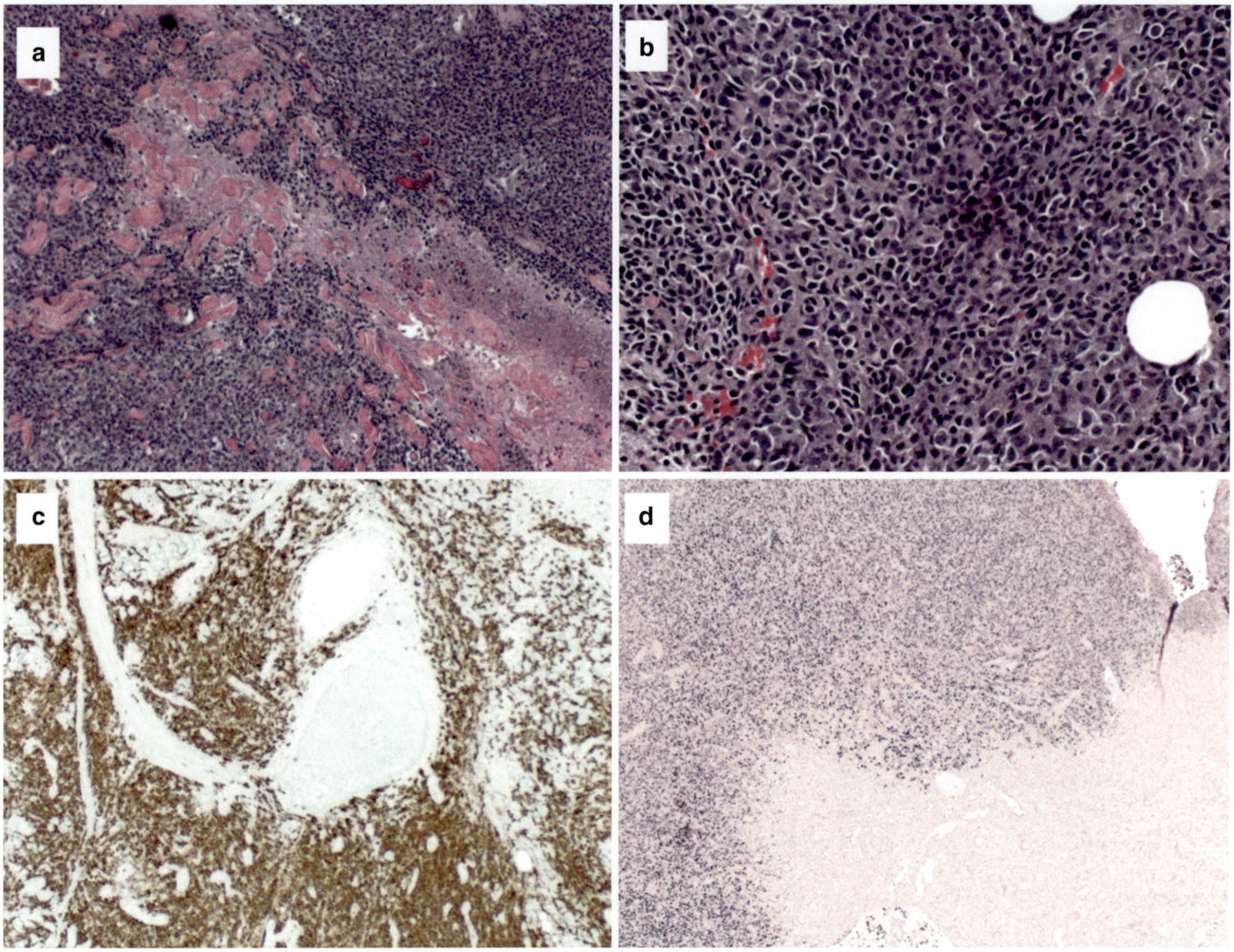

Fig. 8.2 (**a**, **b**) H&E of NK/T-cell lymphoma, nasal type, shows a dense lymphoid infiltrate adjacent to necrosis. (**c**) The tumor is CD3 positive by immunostain and exhibits strong uniform expression of (**d**) *EBV* by in situ hybridization (EBER)

cytoplasm containing azurophilic granules. T-LGLL is commonly associated with neutropenia and may be associated with pure red cell aplasia. Involvement of the spleen and bone marrow is commonly seen [1, 3].

- T-cell prolymphocytic leukemia (T-PLL): This lymphoma demonstrates a variety of morphologies. Most commonly, the neoplastic cells exhibit classic features of prolymphocytes, with small- to intermediate-sized cells, round to irregular nuclear borders, condensed chromatin, a single prominent nucleolus, and basophilic cytoplasm. Less commonly, small cell and cerebriform variants of T-PLL are encountered, characterized by small cells with absent nucleoli and cells with cerebriform nuclei, respectively [1, 3, 10].
- Mycosis fungoides (MF)/Sézary syndrome (SS): Mycosis fungoides is a primary cutaneous T-cell lymphoma characterized by a lichenoid-like infiltrate of neoplastic cells at the dermal-epidermal junction with invasion of the epidermis in the absence of significant edema. The characteristic cell in MF is an intermediate-sized cell with irregular "cerebriform" nuclear borders and clumped chromatin. Involvement of peripheral blood by these malignant lymphocytes at presentation is a defining feature of Sézary syndrome [1, 3].
- Enteropathy-associated T-cell lymphoma (EATL): EATL is characterized by small intestinal mucosal to transmural infiltration of pleomorphic intermediate- to large-sized lymphocytes with round to angulated nuclei, distinct nucleoli, and moderate pale cytoplasm, in a mixed inflammatory background. Occasionally, the neoplastic cells are anaplastic. EATL commonly occurs in the setting of celiac disease and small intestinal mucosa distant from the lymphoma often demonstrates enteropathy-associated changes including villous blunting and increased intraepithelial lymphocytes [1, 2, 11] (see Fig. 8.1b).
- Monomorphic epitheliotropic intestinal T-cell lymphoma (MEITL): In contrast to EATL, MEITL is characterized by transmural infiltration of monomorphic small- to medium-sized lymphocytes with round nuclei, indistinct

Table 8.2 Differential diagnosis for predominantly leukemic T-cell neoplasms

Neoplastic subtype	Cytology	Flow phenotype	Molecular/cytogenetics	Clinical features
T-PLL	Cells with irregular nuclei and often distinct to prominent nucleoli; size ranges from small to intermediate	CD3+ with CD4+ CD8+ (25% of cases) being helpful for diagnosis, TCL1+ CD52+	Inversion of chromosome 14 is frequent: inv(14)(q11q32), t(14;14)(q11;q32), t(X;14)(q28;q11); recurrent alterations in genes of JAK/STAT pathway	Typically aggressive at onset with hepatosplenomegaly and lymphadenopathy as well as skin involvement (~20%)
Sézary	Typically small- to intermediate-sized cells with cerebriform nuclei	CD3+ CD4+ with ratio of CD4:CD8 >10 and loss of CD7 or CD26	No recurrent chromosomal translocations known; gain-of-function mutations in genes affecting TCR signaling recently found	Erythroderma, lymphadenopathy, often associated with pruritus, alopecia
ATLL	Variable, commonly intermediate-sized cells with markedly irregular nuclei "flower cells" and condensed chromatin	CD3+ CD4+ CD25+ CCR4+ FOXP3(subset)+ in some cases	Tumor cells demonstrate monoclonal integration of HTLV-1 (not a routine clinical test)	Heterogeneous, ranging from chronic to acute and lymphomatous; often associated with cutaneous lesions
T-LGL	Large lymphocytes with abundant cytoplasm and azurophilic granules; in bone marrow, shows interstitial/ intrasinusoidal infiltrates	CD3+ CD8+ CD57+ CD2+ and usually alpha beta TCR positive, TIA+ granzyme B+ granzyme M+	Approximately 30% show *STAT3* SH2 domain mutations. Rare *STAT5B* SH2 domain mutations have also been seen (a subset of the latter have been associated with more aggressive disease)	Majority are indolent and associated with neutropenia with or without anemia
HSTCL	Intermediate-sized lymphocytes with pale cytoplasm; tumor involves cords and sinuses of splenic red pulp; usually seen in marrow and liver in intrasinusoidal distribution	CD3+ gamma delta TCR+ CD56+/- CD4- CD8-/+ CD5- TIA1+ granzymeM+granzymeB-	Isochromosome 7q is usually found; missense mutations in *STAT5B* and rarely *STAT3* seen in ~40% of cases	Hepatosplenomegaly, thrombocytopenia, and systemic symptoms

nucleoli, and scant cytoplasm with minimal background inflammation. Adjacent small intestinal mucosa often demonstrates marked intraepithelial lymphocytosis. In contrast to EATL, MEITL is often not associated with celiac disease [1, 2, 11].

4. What are the mimics and what is the clinical relevance of misinterpretation between the true diagnosis and mimics with reference to mistreatment and/or wrong prognosis?

Several benign and malignant conditions can mimic T- and NK-cell lymphomas.

- Reactive lymph nodes as in the case of *EBV* lymphadenitis (infectious mononucleosis) can mimic lymphoma with lymph node architectural distortion and effacement by atypical interfollicular immunoblasts and small- to intermediate-sized lymphocytes. Likewise, Kikuchi-Fujimoto disease, particularly in the proliferative phase, can mimic T- and NK-cell lymphomas with a proliferation of immunoblasts and predominance of CD8-positive T-cells [12]. These reactive conditions usually present a self-limited clinical course with spontaneous resolution and typically harbor an excellent prognosis.
- On the malignant spectrum, several hematopoietic and solid cancers can mimic T- and NK-cell lymphomas. Classic Hodgkin lymphoma rich in large, CD30-positive Reed-Sternberg cells with a scant inflammatory background may easily mimic a large cell T-cell lymphoma, such as anaplastic large cell lymphoma. On the other hand, the lymphocyte-rich subtype of classic Hodgkin lymphoma can mimic the follicular variant of peripheral T-cell lymphoma. In these cases, PAX5 immunostain (which is typically positive in Hodgkin lymphomas and negative in T-cell lymphomas) may be helpful in distinguishing the two, along with absence of monoclonal T-cell receptor gene rearrangements and/or aberrant T-cell immunophenotype. T-cell/histiocyte-rich large B-cell lymphoma and diffuse large B-cell lymphoma that are poor in B-cells and rich in polymorphic, reactive T-cells demonstrating a diffuse growth pattern with effacement of lymph node architecture may also mimic T-cell lymphoma. In these cases, immunostains to highlight the neoplastic cells as B-cells in the absence of monoclonal T-cell receptor gene rearrangements are clues to the diagnosis. Finally, carcinomas metastatic to lymph nodes may mimic T-cell lymphomas with sinus involvement, such as anaplastic large cell lymphoma, and are a pitfall particularly in CD30-positive carcinomas,

such as embryonal carcinoma. A high index of suspicion and generous use of multiple immunostains to confirm or refute these differentials diagnoses is key to making the correct interpretation [5, 13].

- Caution should be exercised when diagnosing T- and NK-cell lymphomas and the clinical history should be a fundamental component of the evaluation, particularly in children and young adults. A high index of suspicion of the abovementioned mimics should be maintained and evidence of aberrant T-cell immunophenotype and/or monoclonal T-cell receptor gene rearrangements should be sought in the right clinical, morphologic, and immunophenotypic picture to confirm a diagnosis of T-cell lymphoma. It is useful to note that clonality analysis may be deceptive in some reactive mimics, particularly in the setting of *EBV* infection.

5. Which morphological findings in the peripheral blood/BM/lymph node biopsy are reliably diagnostic? Which ones suggest the diagnosis? Which is (are) unreliable for diagnosis? Which findings rule out the diagnosis?

- In the peripheral blood, patients with Sézary syndrome, T-PLL, or T-LGLL show a range of cytologic features, but all exhibit nuclear atypia. The finding of abnormal cytologic features in any of these predominantly blood-based lymphomas in the appropriate clinical and flow immunophenotypic context is reliably diagnostic. For T-PLL, the cytogenetic finding of inversion chromosome 14 or t(14;14) is further supportive of the diagnosis. In T-LGLL, *STAT3* mutations have been found in about a third of cases and may also aid in challenging cases.
- The predominantly nodal or extranodal lymphomas may be difficult to evaluate on staging bone marrow biopsies. Of the subtypes discussed in detail above (see answer to Question #3), AITL and HSTL most commonly show marrow involvement. In the case of HSTL, the finding of abnormal sinusoidal infiltration (supported by stains for CD3, TCR gamma/delta, and TIA1 and/or concurrent flow) is relatively reliable, as well as the finding of isochromosome 7q, in the correct clinical setting of hepatosplenomegaly. In AITL, marrow involvement typically presents as paratrabecular lymphohistiocytic aggregates with an abnormal T-cell infiltrate. Immunostains for T-follicular helper cell phenotype can be useful to further confirm the diagnosis (see Fig. 8.1c).
- In general, the finding of necrosis, increased interfollicular T-cells, or partial lymph node architectural distortion is not reliable as these can be seen in neoplastic lymph nodes or lymph nodes involved by other processes (infection, inflammation, or immune dysfunction).
- Special note should be made that the finding of a positive T-cell receptor (*TCR*) gene rearrangement is not a reliable indicator of malignancy without the correct morphologic findings. Due to varying sensitivities and specificities of the *TCR* gene rearrangement, patients with underlying autoimmune disorders or other diseases may exhibit restricted TCR repertoire and, hence, can lead to false-positive results [14, 15]. On the other hand, due to technical issues, alterations in DNA during processing or the failure of PCR primers to properly anneal with target sequences, certain clonal populations may not be detectable using current methods [16].

6. What is the minimal and optimal ancillary workup for diagnosis and subclassification of mature T- and NK-cell neoplasms?

- The diagnostic workup for T- and NK-cell lymphomas is diverse, owing to a variety of factors including the heterogeneity of clinical presentations, morphologic findings, and the availability of ancillary workup at the diagnostic medical center. Recently a tiered diagnostic panel including morphologic, immunophenotypic, and molecular characterization has been proposed, with confirmed high diagnostic consensus [17]. At Tier 0, the diagnostic workup includes basic clinical and demographic information as well as simple H&E morphologic examination. Next, Tier 1 includes a panel of immunohistochemical studies (CD3, CD5, CD10, CD20, CD21, CD30, CD45, and PAX5), to aid in distinguishing T- and NK-cell lymphomas from B-cell lymphomas, Hodgkin lymphoma, and reactive processes. Subsequently, a Tier 2 diagnostic panel (CD2, CD4, CD7, CD8, CD23, CD56, PD1, ALK, TIA1, TCRB, TCRG, EBER) can help in confirming and subclassifying the T-cell lymphoma. Use of gene rearrangement studies can be helpful as a third tier/Tier 2b, but was not shown to add significantly to achieving consensus on a majority of cases. WHO diagnosis and subclassification of T- and NK-cell lymphomas was made in 16.5%, 37.1%, 82.8%, and 85.9% of cases receiving Tier 0, 1, 2, and 2b diagnostic workups, respectively. It is important to note that not all cases can be subclassified, with major reasons being incompletely defined boundaries between certain entities and/or lack of tissue for complete diagnostic workup.
- Over the past few years, a variety of therapeutic agents have been approved to target T-cell lymphomas, some of which are subtype specific, supporting the use of diagnostic panels to increase accurate diagnoses and subclassification and help guide targeted therapy (see answer to Question #8).

7. Which ancillary test results are diagnostic, suggestive of diagnosis, unreliable for diagnosis, or rule out the diagnosis?

- Expression of T-cell markers with coexpression or absence of both CD4 and CD8 and/or loss of one or more pan T-cell antigens in the appropriate clinical and flow immunophenotypic context is suggestive of T-cell lymphoma. CD7 is lost more frequently compared to CD2 and CD5 in AITL, ALK-negative ALCL, and PTCL-NOS, whereas CD3 is lost more frequently in ALK-positive ALCL and CD5 is most often absent in extranodal T-/NK-cell lymphoma, EATL and HSTCL [17]. In this setting, strong and uniform CD30 positivity suggests a diagnosis of ALCL, although CD30-expressing AITL and PTCL-NOS need to be excluded. T-follicular helper cell (TFH) immunophenotype with expression of CD10, BCL6, CXCL13, CXCR5, and/or PD1, particularly in the setting of scattered *EBV* positivity in B-cells, is most suggestive of AITL, although other T-cell lymphomas such as PTCL-NOS need to be excluded [17]. In the most recent revision to the WHO *Classification of Tumors of Haematopoietic and Lymphoid Tissues*, T-cell lymphomas with TFH phenotype but without classic features of AITL are classified under the same umbrella as AITL [1]. These can be considered as nodal peripheral T-cell lymphoma with TFH phenotype (see Fig. 8.3). NK-cell phenotype (TIA, granzyme-B, perforin) in the setting of *EBV* positivity suggests extranodal T-/NK-cell lymphoma. HTLV-1 positivity in the correct clinical and pathologic setting suggests ATLL.

- Novel molecular studies can also be used to further classify or confirm a diagnosis. Chromosomal translocations involving the *ALK* gene at 2p23 confirms ALK-positive ALCL (this is largely replaced by ALK immunostain). Likewise, translocation of the *DUSP22* gene at 6p25.3 or *TP63* gene at 3q28, in the appropriate setting, confirms ALK-negative ALCL [1, 2, 18, 19] (see Fig. 8.4). *TET2*, *IDH2*, *DNMT3A*, and *RHOA* mutations support the diagnosis of AITL [1, 2, 4]. Similarly, *SETD2*, *INO80*, *ARID1B*, and/or *STAT5B* mutation can support HSTCL [1, 2, 8]. *STAT3* mutations, although only present in a third of cases, aid in the diagnosis of challenging T-LGL cases [1, 3].

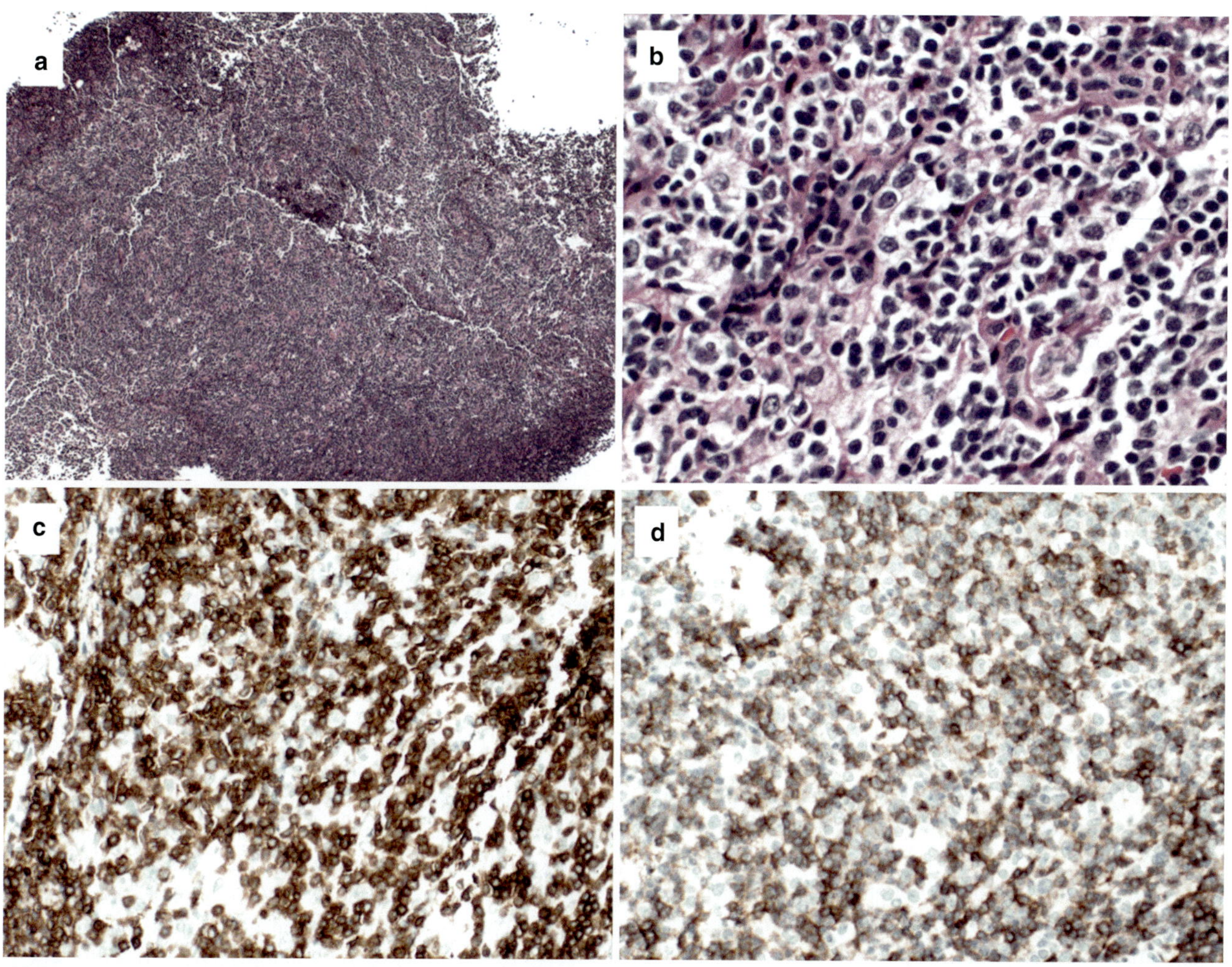

Fig. 8.3 (**a**, **b**) H&E of an enlarged inguinal lymph node showing architectural effacement by numerous atypical intermediate-sized lymphocytes with irregular nuclei and variably dispersed chromatin. (**c**) These are CD3-positive T-cells that coexpress (**d**) PD1. This neoplasm also expressed BCL6, CD4, and CXCL13. It did not have typical architectural morphologic features or presence of *EBV* positive large B cells typically seen in angioimmunoblastic T-cell lymphoma. Hence, it was classified as nodal peripheral T-cell lymphoma with TFH phenotype

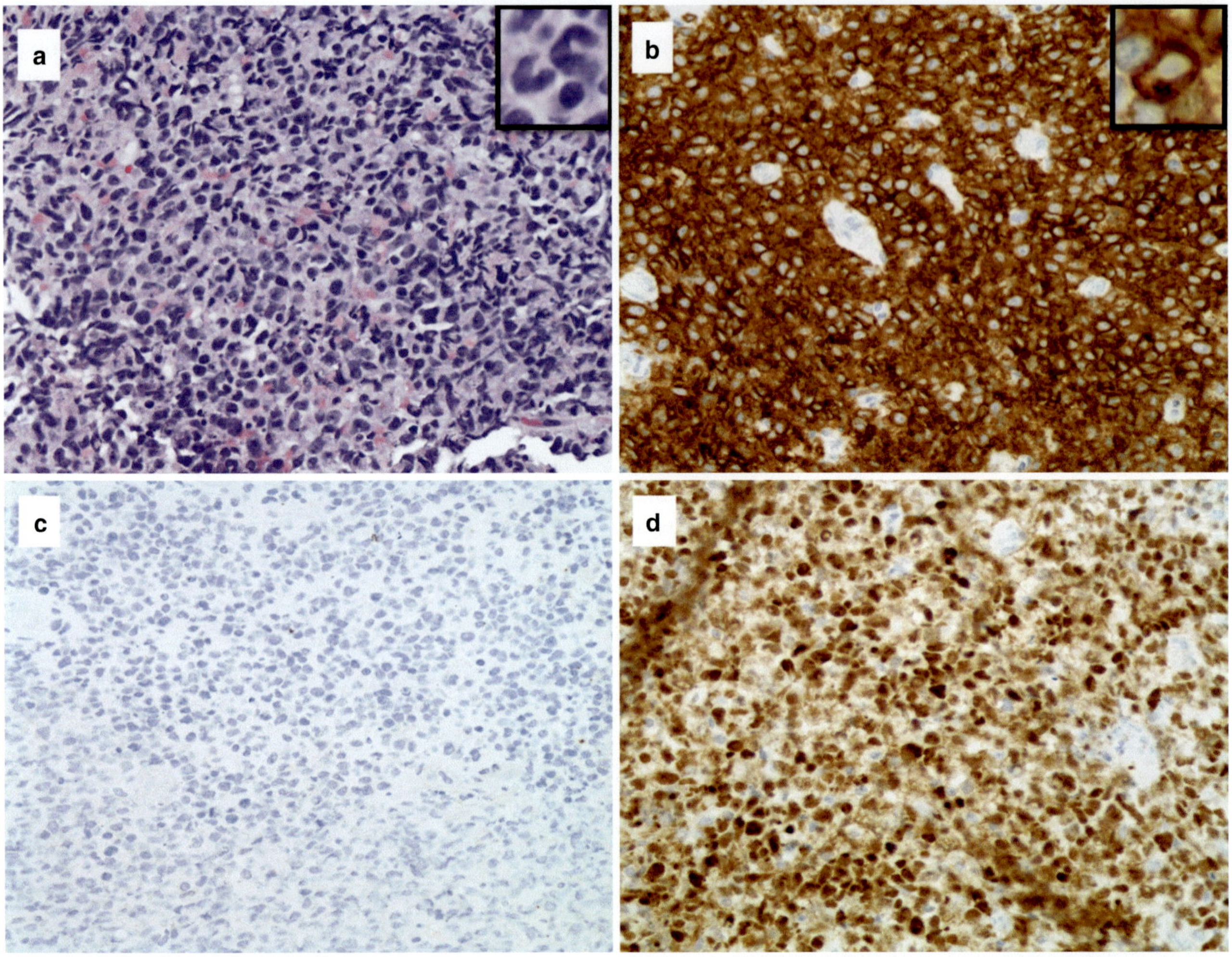

Fig. 8.4 (**a**) H&E of anaplastic large cell lymphoma (ALCL) growing in sheets composed of atypical cells with irregular ovoid nuclei, open chromatin, large nucleoli, and a moderate amount of eosinophilic cytoplasm with indistinct cells borders. Hallmark cells characterized by eccentric, horseshoe-shaped nuclei are seen (*inset*). Scattered mitotic figures are also seen. (**b**) CD30 is strongly expressed in the tumor cells, in a membrane and Golgi pattern (*inset*). (**c**) ALK is negative. (**d**) p63 is expressed strongly and diffusely; p63 immunostain may be used in ALK-negative ALCL as a screening tool for *TP63* gene rearrangement before further confirmatory FISH testing. *TP63* gene rearrangement is associated with a poor prognosis

- As previously discussed, monoclonal T-cell receptor gene rearrangement is an unreliable indicator of malignancy without the correct morphologic findings and may be seen in patients with reactive or inflammatory conditions including autoimmune disorders [14, 15]. On the other hand, due to technical issues, alterations in DNA during processing or the failure of PCR primers to properly anneal with target sequences, certain clonal populations may not be detectable using current methods [16].
- The presence of a B-cell clone does not automatically rule out the diagnosis of T-cell lymphoma. Secondary B-cell clones may be present in a variety of T-cell lymphomas and are associated with *EBV* positivity [20].

8. What is the workup to provide prognostic and therapeutic target information? (Corollary – what treatments are available for this entity?)

- Clinically, the International Prognostic Index (IPI) is a tool established to help predict the prognosis of patients with aggressive non-Hodgkin lymphomas. The IPI takes into account the patient's age, performance status, LDH level, stage of disease, and extranodal involvement. Pathologically, subtyping T-cell lymphomas also provides critical prognostic information. Of the most common subtypes of T- and NK-cell lymphomas, ALK-positive ALCL exhibits the best 5-year overall survival (70%), followed by ALK-negative ALCL (49%), PTCL-NOS, AITL and all NKTCL (32%), and ATLL (14%) [21].

- Prognostic information can also be provided based on individual marker expression in these lymphomas. For example, CD4 expression in PTCL-NOS has been associated with a favorable prognosis [17] and CD30 expression in PTCL-NOS has been associated with a dismal prognosis [22]. Likewise, recent studies demonstrated that distinct genetic alterations in ALK-negative ALCL lead to significantly different clinical outcomes. ALK-negative ALCL harboring *DUSP22* (6p25.3) gene rearrangement demonstrates a 5-year overall survival of 90%, compared to 17% in ALK-negative ALCL with *TP63* (3q28) gene rearrangement and 42% in triple-negative ALCL [18]. P63 immunostain may be used in ALK-negative ALCL as a screening tool for *TP63* gene rearrangement before confirmatory FISH testing [19]. Of the less common subtypes of T- and NK-cell lymphomas, primary cutaneous T-cell lymphoma has the most favorable 5-year overall survival (90%), followed by subcutaneous panniculitis-like TCL (64%), nasal NKTCL (42%), enteropathy-associated TCL (20%), extranasal NKTCL and aggressive or unclassifiable NK-cell leukemia/lymphoma (9%), and hepatosplenic TCL (7%) [21].
- Treatment regimens for T- and NK-cell lymphomas have generally resulted from clinical trials for patients with aggressive non-Hodgkin lymphomas, 10% of which are T-cell lymphomas. While there is no generally accepted first-line treatment, the vast majority of patients receive anthracycline-based multi-agent chemotherapy or a CHOP-like regimen with or without radiation therapy, with the goal being long-term remission or cure. In cases of *EBV*-positive lymphoma arising in the setting of immunosuppression, reducing the degree of immunosuppression may also be useful. Lately, the efficacy of l-asparaginase in NKTCL, nasal type has been established [23]. In more aggressive T- and NK-cell lymphomas, including high-risk ALK-positive ALCL, ALK-negative ALCL, PTCL-NOS, and AITL, consolidation in first remission with autologous stem cell transplant may be considered in the appropriate clinical context. Relapsed and/or refractory disease is managed with second-line systemic therapy followed by autologous or allogeneic stem cell transplant. Second-line targeted therapeutic options include alemtuzumab (anti-CD52), daratumumab (anti-CD38), brentuximab (anti-CD30), daclizumab (anti-CD25), mogamulizumab (anti-CCR4), and crizotinib (ALK inhibitor). Other second-line treatment options include pralatrexate, romidepsin, belinostat, bendamustine, and gemcitabine [24, 25].

9. Which subtypes of mature T- and NK-cell neoplasms are clinically relevant and which are morphologically defined but have unproven/ minimal clinical relevance?

- The major subgroups of nodal and extranodal T- and NK-cell lymphomas are pathologically, prognostically, and therapeutically distinct, as discussed in Question 8. However, under the umbrella of nodal lymphomas of T-follicular helper cell origin with AITL, follicular T-cell lymphoma and nodal peripheral T-cell lymphoma with T-follicular helper phenotype are histopathologically distinct entities without proven clinical significance.
- Of the T- and NK-cell leukemias, T-PLL, T-LGL, ATLL, aggressive NK-cell leukemia (ANKL), and Sézary syndrome (SS) are clinically distinct diagnoses with unique prognostic features and therapeutic targets. On the other hand, chronic lymphoproliferative disorder of NK-cells (CLPD-NKs), characterized by persistently increased peripheral blood NK-cells without an identifiable cause, is a disorder that is often difficult to distinguish as neoplastic versus reactive. Furthermore, the clinical course is often indolent and no therapy is typically required [1].
- In the gastrointestinal tract, EATL and MEITL are morphologically and epidemiologically distinct entities, with EATL associated with celiac disease. Otherwise, EATL and MEITL are similar in terms of complications, treatment, and overall prognosis [1, 11].

10. What is an adequate specimen for this condition?

- Excisional lymph node or soft tissue samples are, by far, the optimal specimens for workup of suspected T-cell lymphoma.
- Core needle biopsies can be cautiously used to triage cases. It is only rare cases in which core needle samples or very small excisional biopsy samples will suffice in making a WHO subclassified diagnosis within the mature T- and NK-cell neoplasm category. For example, if sheets of large cells with hallmark morphology, strong and uniform CD30 positivity, CD3 positivity, and ALK positivity can be demonstrated, even relatively small samples can be adequate for diagnosis. However, if a core needle biopsy demonstrates no morphologic or immunophenotypic abnormality, but clinical features remain suspicious, a larger sample is warranted.
- In the majority of cases, fine needle aspiration or other cytology-only specimens are not sufficient. In some special cases, such as breast implant-associated anaplastic large cell lymphomas, the bulk of the tumor may not be in solid tissue but, instead, be found in cytology specimens.

11. What information can be conveyed to the clinician during each stage of the workup?

- The first layer of information, depending on the specimen type, may be regarding adequacy. Particularly if the patient is in a critical condition, it is very important for the clinician to know whether or not to schedule a re-biopsy or excisional biopsy when core needle is insufficient for diagnosis. At this juncture, if full subclassification is not necessary to deliver life-saving therapies, it would be helpful for the clinician to understand how valuable additional tissue can be for his or her decision making. Alternatively, if the pathologist determines that adequacy has been achieved and is proceeding carefully with ancillary studies, the clinician can be comfortable starting high-dose steroids at this point to stabilize the patient. Otherwise, steroid use can contribute to cytomorphologic artifacts in subsequent biopsies.
- Subsequent to or concurrent with the discussion on adequacy, a conversation about the current status of the patient should be pursued. Hence, additional clinical information should be conveyed to the pathologist as workup proceeds. The pathologist may direct further laboratory testing, depending on the information available. In our experience, checking LDH, HIV, HTLV-1 (if ATLL is suspected), and peripheral blood smear (if T-PLL or T-LGL is suspected) are relatively low-cost, high-yield laboratory tests in the appropriate clinical context.
- Note should be made that flow cytometric interpretations often result prior to the tissue diagnosis. These interpretations, while they can be discussed with the clinician as soon as possible, must be couched with the appropriate caveat. For example, a flow finding of atypical CD4+ CD8+ "double-positive" T-cells is often seen in nodular lymphocyte-predominant Hodgkin lymphoma and should not lead the clinician to jump to the conclusion of a peripheral T-cell lymphoma or T-ALL [26]. Conversely, small B-cell clones can be found incidentally in some T-cell lymphomas.
- As the immunohistochemical studies are being completed, the pathologist may decide to pursue molecular studies such as T-cell gene rearrangement. Since the extraction of DNA and other preparatory work may account for significant delay to diagnosis, and since the specificity of T-cell gene rearrangement is not 100%, it is not always necessary to wait for the molecular results in order to issue a morphologic diagnosis.

12. What should be the approach to provide maximum, but defensible information, from limited specimen or workup? When is a descriptive diagnosis appropriate in such situations?

- In situations where the initial diagnostic specimen is limited (such as small core needle biopsy without supportive flow data), it is reasonable to render a diagnosis of "atypical lymphoid proliferation" with the addition of "suspicious for T-cell lymphoma" if morphologic and immunohistochemical studies are supportive of it. Depending on the clinical context, the clinician should be contacted in order to strongly recommend an adequate tissue biopsy such as lymph node excision.
- It may be tempting to rely on molecular evidence of T-cell clonality in these limited tissue biopsies, but this is a major pitfall given occasionally suboptimal positive predictive value of T-cell gene rearrangement studies.
- A descriptive diagnosis is entirely appropriate when T-cell lymphoma is suspected clinically and/or pathologically but only a fine needle aspiration (FNA) has been obtained. In this setting, even with the addition of flow markers of aberrancy (loss of pan T-cell antigens such as CD7/CD2/CD5), it is dangerous to issue a definitive diagnosis of malignancy without supporting morphologic evidence obtained by biopsy.
- Certain exceptions exist, primarily for neoplasms that do not generally exhibit solid tumor proliferations such as T-PLL, T-LGL, and ATLL. For predominantly blood-based infiltrations, if the diagnosis has been rendered on peripheral blood specimen (along with clinical, flow, and molecular correlations), an FNA of additional sites of involvement can be cytologically compared to the prior in order to give a more summative interpretation.

13. When is a diagnostic comment necessary and what should be discussed in the diagnostic comment for mature T- and NK-cell neoplasms?

- Diagnostic comments are most useful in biopsies where the morphology and immunophenotype are not typical "textbook" cases. This is where the pathologist can explain why a definitive diagnosis requires additional correlation. For example, in a case of overt T-cell lymphoma that has TFH phenotype but no significant proliferation of high endothelial venules, or large *EBV*-positive B-cells, a comment would be useful to explain why the pathologist is rendering a diagnosis of nodal peripheral T-cell lymphoma with TFH phenotype rather than angioimmunoblastic T-cell lymphoma. Another example would be the diagnosis of peripheral T-cell lymphoma, not otherwise specified, when the tumor exhibits significant CD30 expression. It would be helpful to clinicians or subsequent pathologists viewing the case to understand that anaplastic large cell lymphoma had been a consideration, but that the staining quality and morphologic features did not suit the latter diagnosis.

- In addition, cases where tissue adequacy is questionable, or clinical information is limited, a comment should be made to qualify the histopathologic interpretation. Often, patients with an ultimate diagnosis of peripheral T-cell lymphoma have had previous biopsy attempts. If comparisons were made with prior available biopsies, a comment that summarizes the findings can also be very useful in achieving a comprehensive picture of the patient's disease.

14. When is it appropriate to seek external consultation for mature T- and NK-cell neoplasms?

- In a large study employing 131 T-cell lymphoma cases that were ultimately reviewed at a referral center with expert hematopathologists, 24% of cases were discordant with high variability among the T-cell lymphoma subtypes. In particular, 44% of the discordant cases could have resulted in a different clinical management decision [26]. This study revealed that some previously diagnosed benign lymphoid infiltrates and classic Hodgkin lymphoma were reclassified as T-cell lymphomas. The use of less commonly available immunohistochemical studies, such as CXCL13 and PD1, resulted in further subclassification. However, in many cases, the diagnosis was altered based on already performed ancillary testing [27]. Hence, it may be prudent to have a low threshold of referring cases suspicious for T-cell lymphoma to a center where they are more commonly diagnosed.
- A subsequent study in France that reviewed concordance rates among all lymphomas found similar results and highlighted the particular challenge of T-cell lymphoma diagnoses. In a total of 31,910 patients, concordance between referral and expert review was relatively high for diffuse large B-cell lymphomas (83.8%) and classic Hodgkin lymphoma (93.3%), whereas AITL was only 68.7%; PTCL, NOS was at 63.8%; and ALK-negative ALCL was quite low at 47.2% [28]. A separate, international cooperative study also discovered a discordance rate of 13.1% cases when initial biopsies were centrally reviewed, with 4.6% of cases misclassified and found to be disorders other than T-cell lymphomas. In 13 cases initially diagnosed as ALK-negative ALCL, 6 were later diagnosed as B-cell lymphomas [29]. Part of the reason for these discrepancies may be the general lack of reliable markers and objective criteria. However, as seen in the 2014 study mentioned above, concordance was quite adequate among hematopathologists at NCCN centers that are exposed to a higher volume of T-cell lymphoma cases. In addition, as the WHO classification includes more consideration for the results obtained by less widely available antibodies and molecular studies, seeking external consultation may be more routine for these rare tumors.

Case Presentations

Case 1

Learning Objectives

1. To become familiar with the typical clinical and histologic features of the neoplasm
2. To generate a differential diagnosis
3. To become familiar with the typical immunohistochemical and molecular features of the neoplasm

Case History

A 65-year-old male presented with fever, arthralgias, fatigue, night sweats, weight loss, and a generalized maculopapular rash. Physical examination revealed generalized lymphadenopathy. Laboratory workup was significant for pancytopenia with hypereosinophilia and polyclonal hypergammaglobulinemia.

Histologic Features (Fig. 8.1a)

- Effacement of lymph node architecture by small- to medium-sized lymphocytes with pale cytoplasm
- Prominent arborizing high endothelial venules
- Extra-follicular proliferation of follicular dendritic cells
- Polymorphous inflammatory background

Differential Diagnosis

- Reactive hyperplasia
- Drug reaction
- T-cell/histiocyte-rich large B-cell lymphoma
- PTCL-NOS
- Classic Hodgkin lymphoma

Immunohistochemistry and Other Ancillary Studies

- Positive for CD4, CD10, BCL6, PD1, and CXCL13 with scattered *EBV*+ B-cells
- Expanded follicular dendritic meshworks highlighted with CD23

- Negative for CD7, CD8, and CD20
- Often normal CD4/CD8 ratio by flow (due to abundant background reactive T-cells); occasional cases demonstrate CD10+ T-cells by flow
- T-cell receptor rearrangement detected

Final Diagnosis

Angioimmunoblastic T-cell lymphoma

Case 2

Learning Objectives

1. To become familiar with the typical clinical and histologic features of the neoplasm
2. To generate a differential diagnosis
3. To become familiar with the typical immunohistochemical and molecular features of the neoplasm

Case History

A 45-year-old female with a history of celiac disease presented with sudden onset severe abdominal pain. An x-ray showed air under the diaphragm. Emergency laparotomy revealed a transmural defect in the jejunum with enlarged mesenteric lymph nodes. The jejunum and proximal ileum were resected.

Histologic Features (Fig. 8.1b)

- Transmural infiltration of intestinal wall by intermediate- to large-sized lymphocytes with round to angulated nuclei, distinct nucleoli, and moderate pale cytoplasm
- Mucosal ulceration
- Background polymorphic inflammatory infiltrate
- Pathologic celiac disease-related changes in small intestinal mucosa distant from the lymphoma

Differential Diagnosis

- Monomorphic epitheliotropic intestinal T-cell lymphoma
- Peripheral T-cell lymphoma, not otherwise specified
- Anaplastic large cell lymphoma
- Diffuse large B-cell lymphoma

Immunohistochemistry and Other Ancillary Studies

- Positive for CD3, CD7, CD103, TIA, and granzyme B
- Negative for CD4, CD5, CD8, CD56, TCR-G, and *EBV*
- Overexpression of p53

Final Diagnosis

Enteropathy-associated T-cell lymphoma

Case 3

Learning Objectives

1. To become familiar with the typical clinical and histologic features of the neoplasm
2. To generate a differential diagnosis
3. To become familiar with the typical immunohistochemical and molecular features of the neoplasm

Case History

A 58-year-old female from Colombia presented with fatigue, shortness of breath, and epistaxis. CT scan revealed a lesion in her left nasal cavity with surrounding edema. A biopsy was performed.

Histologic Features (Fig. 8.2)

- Small- to medium-sized cells with a diffuse, angiocentric, and angiodestructive growth pattern
- High mitotic activity, necrosis, and ulceration

Differential Diagnosis

- Peripheral T-cell lymphoma – not otherwise specified
- Diffuse large B-cell lymphoma
- Inflammatory conditions including Wegner granulomatosis

Immunohistochemistry and Other Ancillary Studies

- Positive for CD2, cytoplasmic CD3, CD56, TIA, granzyme B, and *EBV*
- Negative for CD4, CD5, and CD8

Final Diagnosis

NK-/T-cell lymphoma, nasal type

Case 4

Learning Objectives

1. To become familiar with the typical clinical and histologic features of the neoplasm
2. To generate a differential diagnosis
3. To become familiar with the typical immunohistochemical and molecular features of the neoplasm

Case History

A 40-year-old female presented with fatigue, fever, night sweats, and generalized lymphadenopathy. Laboratory workup revealed leukocytosis and elevated lactate dehydrogenase. An axillary lymph node biopsy was performed.

Histologic Features (Fig. 8.3)

- Effacement of lymph node architecture by intermediate-sized lymphocytes with pleomorphic cytology and abundant pale cytoplasm
- Absence of prominent vascular proliferation, expanded follicular dendritic cell meshworks, and polymorphic inflammatory background

Differential Diagnosis

- Peripheral T-cell lymphoma, not otherwise specified
- Angioimmunoblastic T-cell lymphoma
- Follicular peripheral T-cell lymphoma

Immunohistochemistry and Other Ancillary Studies

- Positive for CD3, CD4, PD1, CXCL13, and BCL6
- Negative for CD10, CD30, CD34, and TdT
- Negative for *EBV* RNA by FISH

Final Diagnosis

Peripheral T-cell lymphoma with T-follicular helper phenotype

Case 5

Learning Objectives

1. To become familiar with the typical clinical and histologic features of the neoplasm
2. To generate a differential diagnosis
3. To become familiar with the typical immunohistochemical and molecular features of the neoplasm

Case History

A 60-year-old male presented with abdominal pain, fever, night sweats, and cervical lymphadenopathy. CT scan revealed hepatomegaly. Biopsy of the largest cervical lymph node was performed.

Histologic Features (Fig. 8.4)

- Effacement of lymph node architecture by predominantly large cells with areas of necrosis.
- Hallmark cells with eccentric horseshoe-shaped nuclei and a prominent eosinophilic Golgi region and abundant cytoplasm.
- Neoplastic cells grow cohesively and typically involve lymph node sinusoids.

Differential Diagnosis

- ALK-positive ALCL
- PTLC-NOS
- Classic Hodgkin lymphoma
- Metastatic carcinoma

Immunohistochemistry and Other Ancillary Studies

- Positive for CD3, CD30 (membrane and Golgi pattern), and granzyme B
- Negative for CD20, CD4, CD8, CD34, TDT, CD56, EMA, *EBV*, and ALK
- Positive for p63 followed by confirmatory FISH testing revealing TP63 gene rearrangement

Final Diagnosis

ALK-negative anaplastic large cell lymphoma with TP63 gene rearrangement

Case 6

Learning Objectives

1. To become familiar with the typical clinical and cytologic features of the neoplasm
2. To generate a differential diagnosis
3. To become familiar with the typical flow cytometry features of the neoplasm

Case History

A 45-year-old female from Japan presented with a scaly skin rash, back pain, and generalized lymphadenopathy. Laboratory workup revealed leukocytosis, hypercalcemia, and HTLV-1 positivity by serology.

Cytologic Features

- Intermediate-sized cells with markedly irregular nuclei "flower cells," condensed chromatin, and agranular basophilic cytoplasm on peripheral blood smear

Differential Diagnosis

- HTLV-1-positive reactive lymphadenitis
- Mycosis fungoides/Sézary syndrome
- T-lymphoblastic leukemia/lymphoma
- Diffuse large B-cell lymphoma

Flow Immunophenotype and Other Ancillary Studies

- Positive for CD2, CD3, CD4, CD5, CD25, CD45, CCR4, and FOXP3
- Negative for CD7, CD8, CD1a, CD10, and PD1
- Monoclonal TCR gene rearrangement

Final Diagnosis

Adult T-cell leukemia/lymphoma, HTLV-1-positive

Author Disclosures Neither LI nor MLX have conflicts of interest.

References

1. Swerdlow SH, Campo E, Harris N, Jaffe E, Pileri S, Stein H, et al. WHO classification of tumours of haematopoietic and lymphoid tissues. In: World Health Organization classification of tumours. Lyon, France: IARC. p. 2017.
2. Hsi ED. Peripheral T-cell lymphomas. In: Hematopathology. 3rd ed. Elsevier; 2018. p. 306–39.
3. Hsi ED. Mature T-cell and natural killer–cell leukemias. In: Hematopathology. 3rd ed. Philadelphia: Elsevier; 2018. p. 414–28.
4. Bal M, Gujral S, Gandhi J, Shet T, Epari S, Subramanian PG. Angioimmunoblastic T-cell lymphoma: a critical analysis of clinical, morphologic and immunophenotypic features. Indian J Pathol Microbiol. 2010;53(4):640–5.
5. Kinney MC, Higgins RA, Medina EA. Anaplastic large cell lymphoma: twenty-five years of discovery. Arch Pathol Lab Med. 2011;135(1):19–43.
6. Qayyum S, Choi JK. Adult T-cell leukemia/lymphoma. Arch Pathol Lab Med. 2014;138(2):282–6.
7. Gill H, Liang RHS, Tse E. Extranodal natural-killer/T-cell lymphoma, nasal type. Adv Hematol. 2010;2010:627401.
8. Yang S, Wang E. Hepatosplenic T-cell lymphoma: a clinicopathologic review with an emphasis on diagnostic differentiation from other T-cell/natural killer–cell neoplasms. Arch Pathol Lab Med. 2015;139(9):1173–80.
9. Parveen Z, Thompson K. Subcutaneous panniculitis-like T-cell lymphoma: redefinition of diagnostic criteria in the recent World Health Organization-European Organization for Research and Treatment of Cancer classification for cutaneous lymphomas. Arch Pathol Lab Med. 2009;133(2):303–8.
10. Chen X, Cherian S. Immunophenotypic characterization of T-cell prolymphocytic leukemia. Am J Clin Pathol. 2013;140(5, 1):727–35.
11. Arps DP, Smith LB. Classic versus type II enteropathy-associated T-cell lymphoma: diagnostic considerations. Arch Pathol Lab Med. 2013;137(9):1227–31.
12. Attygalle AD, Cabeçadas J, Gaulard P, Jaffe ES, de Jong D, Ko YH, et al. Peripheral T-cell and NK-cell lymphomas and their mimics; taking a step forward - report on the lymphoma workshop of the XVIth meeting of the European Association for Haematopathology and the Society for Hematopathology. Histopathology. 2014;64(2):171–99.
13. Moroch J, Copie-Bergman C, de Leval L, Plonquet A, Martin-Garcia N, Delfau-Larue MH, et al. Follicular peripheral T-cell lymphoma expands the spectrum of classical Hodgkin lymphoma mimics. Am J Surg Pathol. 2012;36(11):1636–46.
14. Wang CY, Yu PF, He XB, Fang YX, Cheng WY, Jing ZZ. αβ T-cell receptor bias in disease and therapy (review). Int J Oncol. 2016;48(6):2247–56.
15. Fitzgerald JE, Ricalton NS, Meyer AC, West SG, Kaplan H, Behrendt C, et al. Analysis of clonal CD8+ T cell expansions in normal individuals and patients with rheumatoid arthritis. J Immunol. 1995;154(7):3538–47.
16. Raess PW, Bagg A. The role of molecular pathology in the diagnosis of cutaneous lymphomas. Pathol Res Int. 2012;2012:913523.
17. Hsi ED, Said J, Macon WR, Rodig SJ, Ondrejka SL, Gascoyne RD, et al. Diagnostic accuracy of a defined immunophenotypic and molecular genetic approach for peripheral T/NK-cell lymphomas: a North American PTCL Study Group Project. Am J Surg Pathol. 2014;38(6):768–75.
18. Parrilla Castellar ER, Jaffe ES, Said JW, Swerdlow SH, Ketterling RP, Knudson RA, et al. ALK-negative anaplastic large cell lymphoma is a genetically heterogeneous disease with widely disparate clinical outcomes. Blood. 2014;124(9):1473–80.
19. Wang X, Boddicker RL, Dasari S, Sidhu JS, Kadin ME, Macon WR, et al. Expression of p63 protein in anaplastic large cell lymphoma: implications for genetic subtyping. Hum Pathol. 2017;64:19–27.
20. Zaki MA, Wada N, Kohara M, Ikeda J, Hori Y, Fujita S, et al. Presence of B-cell clones in T-cell lymphoma. Eur J Haematol. 2011;86(5):412–9.
21. Vose J, Armitage J, Weisenburger D. International T-cell lymphoma project. International peripheral T-cell and natural killer/T-cell lymphoma study: pathology findings and clinical outcomes. J Clin Oncol. 2008;26(25):4124–30.
22. Savage KJ, Harris NL, Vose JM, Ullrich F, Jaffe ES, Connors JM, et al. ALK- anaplastic large cell lymphoma is clinically and immunophenotypically different from both ALK+ ALCL and peripheral T-cell lymphoma not otherwise specified: report from the International Peripheral T-cell Lymphoma Project. Blood. 2008;111:5496–504.
23. Yong W. Clinical study of l-asparaginase in the treatment of extranodal NK/T-cell lymphoma, nasal type. Hematol Oncol. 2016;34(2):61–8.
24. Moskowitz AJ, Lunning MA, Horwitz SM. How I treat the peripheral T-cell lymphomas. Blood. 2014;123(17):2636–44.
25. d'Amore F, Gaulard P, Trümper L, Corradini P, Kim WS, Specht L, et al. ESMO Guidelines Committee. Peripheral T-cell lymphomas: ESMO Clinical Practice Guidelines for diagnosis, treatment and follow-up. Ann Oncol. 2015;26(Suppl 5):v108–15.
26. Rahemtullah A, Reichard KK, Preffer FI, Harris NL, Hasserjian RP. A double-positive CD4+ CD8+ T-cell population is commonly found in Nodular Lymphocyte Predominant Hodgkin Lymphoma. Am J Clin Pathol. 2006;126:805–14.
27. Herrera AF, Crosby-Thompson A, Friedberg JW. Comparison of referring and final pathology for patients with T-cell lymphoma in the National Comprehensive Cancer Network. Cancer. 2014;120(13):1993–9.
28. Laurent C, Baron M, Amara N, Haioun C, Dandoit M, Maynadié M, et al. Impact of expert pathologic review of lymphoma diagnosis: study of patients from the French Lymphopath Network. J Clin Oncol. 2017;35(18):2008–17.
29. Bellei M, Sabattini E, Pesce EA, Ko YH, Kim WS, Cabrera ME, et al. Pitfalls and major issues in the histologic diagnosis of peripheral T-cell lymphomas: results of the central review of 573 cases from the T-cell Project, an international cooperative study. Hematol Oncol. 2017;35:630–6.

Hodgkin Lymphomas

9

Jinming Song and Shiyong Li

List of Frequently Asked Questions

1. What are the major subtypes of Hodgkin lymphoma?
2. What are the major clinicopathological features of Hodgkin lymphoma?
3. What are the typical morphological findings in Hodgkin lymphoma?
4. What are the most typical immunophenotypes of classic Hodgkin lymphoma?
5. How to distinguish CD30 and CD15 staining in classic Hodgkin cells from those in non-Hodgkin cells?
6. How to further classify classic Hodgkin lymphoma into subtypes?
7. How to distinguish nodular lymphocyte-predominant Hodgkin lymphoma (NLPHL) from classic Hodgkin lymphoma (cHL)?
8. What are the mimics of Hodgkin lymphoma and what are the clinical consequences of misinterpretation between Hodgkin lymphomas and their mimics?
9. How to distinguish nodular lymphocyte-predominant Hodgkin lymphoma (NLPHL) from progressive transformation of germinal centers (PTGC)?
10. How to distinguish nodular lymphocyte-predominant Hodgkin lymphoma (NLPHL) from T-cell/histiocyte-rich large B-cell lymphoma (THRLBCL)
11. How to distinguish nodular lymphocyte-predominant Hodgkin lymphoma (NLPHL) from follicular lymphoma (FL)?
12. How to distinguish classic Hodgkin lymphoma (cHL) from T-cell/histiocyte-rich large B-cell lymphoma (THRLBCL)?
13. How to distinguish nodular sclerosis classic Hodgkin lymphoma (NSCHL) from primary mediastinal (thymic) large B-cell lymphoma (PMLBCL)?
14. How to distinguish classic Hodgkin lymphoma (cHL) from B-cell lymphoma, unclassifiable, with features intermediate between diffuse large B-cell lymphoma and classic Hodgkin lymphoma (gray zone lymphoma, GZL)?
15. How to distinguish cHL from *EBV*+ diffuse large B-cell lymphoma NOS (*EBV*+ DLBCL)?
16. How to distinguish classic Hodgkin lymphoma (cHL) from peripheral T-cell lymphoma (PTCL NOS)?
17. How to distinguish classic Hodgkin lymphoma from anaplastic large cell lymphoma (ALCL)?
18. How to distinguish lymphocyte-rich classic Hodgkin lymphoma (LRCHL) from mantle cell lymphoma (MCL)?
19. How to distinguish lymphocyte-rich classic Hodgkin lymphoma (LRCHL) from follicular lymphoma?
20. How to distinguish lymphocyte-depleted classic Hodgkin lymphoma (LDCHL) from histiocytic sarcoma?
21. For peripheral blood and bone marrow biopsies, what morphological findings are diagnostic and what findings are suspicious for classic Hodgkin lymphoma?
22. What is the minimal and optimal ancillary workup for the diagnosis of Hodgkin lymphomas?
23. What information provides prognostic and therapeutic target information for Hodgkin lymphomas?
24. What are adequate specimens for the diagnosis of Hodgkin lymphomas?
25. What information can be conveyed to the clinician during each stage of the workup?
26. When are comments necessary and what should be discussed in the comments for Hodgkin lymphoma?
27. When is it appropriate to seek external consultation for Hodgkin lymphomas?

J. Song (✉)
Department of Hematopathology and Laboratory Medicine, Moffitt Cancer Center, Tampa, FL, USA
e-mail: Jinming.Song@Moffitt.org

S. Li
Hematopathology, Pathology and Laboratory Medicine, Emory University School of Medicine, Atlanta, GA, USA
e-mail: sli2@emory.edu

E. Wang, A. S. Lagoo (eds.), *Practical Lymph Node and Bone Marrow Pathology*, Practical Anatomic Pathology,
https://doi.org/10.1007/978-3-030-32189-5_9

1. What are the major subtypes of Hodgkin lymphoma?

Hodgkin lymphomas (HLs) are mature B-cell malignancies characterized by a minor population of large neoplastic cells in a background of reactive inflammatory cells. Based on the cytomorphology and immunophenotypic profile of the neoplastic cells and the background reactive inflammatory cells, HLs are categorized as nodular lymphocyte-predominant Hodgkin lymphoma (NLPHL) and classic Hodgkin lymphoma (cHL). Classic Hodgkin lymphomas (cHLs) are further divided into four subtypes: nodular sclerosis (NSCHL), lymphocyte-rich (LRCHL), mixed cellularity (MCCHL), and lymphocyte-depleted classic Hodgkin lymphoma (LDCHL). cHLs comprise approximately 90% of all HL cases with nodular sclerosis classic Hodgkin lymphoma being the most common subtype (about 70% of cHLs), while nodular lymphocyte-predominant Hodgkin lymphoma accounts for the remaining cases [1–5].

- Nodular lymphocyte-predominant Hodgkin lymphoma (NLPHL)
- Classic Hodgkin lymphoma (cHL)
  - Nodular sclerosis classic Hodgkin lymphoma (NSCHL)
  - Lymphocyte-rich classic Hodgkin lymphoma (LRCHL)
  - Mixed cellularity classic Hodgkin lymphoma (MCCHL)
  - Lymphocyte-depleted classic Hodgkin lymphoma (LDCHL)

2. What are the major clinicopathological features of Hodgkin lymphoma?

- Hodgkin lymphomas are lymphoid neoplasms that usually affect lymph nodes and cause lymphadenopathy or masses.
- Classic Hodgkin lymphomas (cHLs) preferentially involve cervical lymph nodes and mediastinum (especially NSCHL), while NLPHL preferentially involves peripheral lymph nodes.
- Splenic involvement is more common in MCCHL. Bone marrow involvement is much less common.
- The patients can present with B symptoms, including fever, drenching night sweats, and weight loss [1]. Most of the Hodgkin lymphomas have male predominance except for NSCHL.
- *EBV* infection is more likely to be associated with classic Hodgkin lymphoma, especially MCCHL and LDCHL, but rarely with NLPHL [1, 6–10].
- In some patients, LDCHL is associated with HIV infection [11] and has more adverse risk factors than other subtypes of cHLs [12].

The clinicopathological features of Hodgkin lymphomas are summarized in Table 9.1 [1].

3. What are the typical morphological findings in Hodgkin lymphoma?

The typical morphological findings of Hodgkin lymphoma are summarized in Table 9.2 [1]. Morphological assessment for HLs involves the identification of the large neoplastic cells and the background inflammatory cells.

- Nodular lymphocyte-predominant Hodgkin lymphoma (NLPHL)
  - The neoplastic cells in NLPHL are derived from germinal center B cells with intact clonal immunoglobulin gene rearrangements.
  - They are characterized by a nodular or at least partial nodular pattern. The nodules contain a minor population of individual large neoplastic cells surrounded by a predominant small B lymphocytic proliferation with background follicular dendritic meshworks (Table 9.2).
  - The large neoplastic cells show a lobulated nucleus and prominent but not inclusion-like nucleoli (popcorn, lymphocytic-histiocytic, or lymphocyte-predominant (LP) cells). Mononuclear variant resembling Hodgkin cells may occasionally be seen.

Table 9.1 Clinicopathological features of Hodgkin lymphomas

	NLPHL	NSCHL	LRCHL	MCCHL	LDCHL
Socioeconomic status	No association	High	Unknown	Low	Low
Gender predominance	Male	Female	Male	Male	Male
Age	Young adults	Young adults	Young adults	Children or elderly	Children or elderly
HIV infection	Rare	Rare	Unknown	Common	Common
EBV infection	Rare	Rare	Unknown	Common	Common
Anatomic sites	Peripheral and mesenteric lymph nodes	Mediastinal, cervical, and axial lymph nodes	Variable	Systemic with frequent bone marrow involvement	Systemic with frequent bone marrow involvement

Table 9.2 Histomorphologic features of Hodgkin lymphoma [1]

		NLPHL	NSCHL	LRCHL	MCCHL	LDCHL
Neoplastic cell	Classical LP cell	Frequent	Rare	Rare	Rare	Rare
	Classical RS/H cell	Rare	Rare	Frequent	Frequent	Frequent
	Lacunar cell variant	Rare	Frequent	Rare	Rare	Rare
	Mummified cell variant	Rare	Frequent	Rare	Variable	Variable
Histological pattern	Thickened capsule	Rare	Frequent	Rare	Rare	Rare
	Collagen fibrosis	Rare	Frequent	Rare	Rare	Rare
	Nodular pattern	Frequent	Frequent	Frequent	Rare	Rare
	Diffuse pattern	Rare	Rare	Rare	Frequent	Frequent
Background inflammatory cell	Small lymphocytes	Frequent	Frequent	Frequent	Variable	Rare
	Neutrophils/eosinophils	Rare	Frequent	Rare	Variable	Variable
	Histiocytes	Rare	Rare	Rare	Variable	Frequent
	Plasma cells	Rare	Variable	Rare	Variable	Frequent

  - The LP cells are ringed by PD1+/CD57+ T follicular helper cells in almost all the cases, while the reactive small lymphocytes in the nodules are mainly B cells.
  - Progression of NLPHL to diffuse large B-cell lymphoma is reported in approximately 3–5% of the cases [1, 13–15]. NLPHL can occur with diffuse large B-cell lymphoma concurrently or sequentially.
- Classic Hodgkin lymphoma (cHL)
  - The neoplastic cells in cHLs are also derived from germinal center B cells with crippled but clonal immunoglobulin gene rearrangements that somehow escaped the normal apoptotic process.
  - cHLs typically show scattered large atypical cells in the background of reactive inflammatory cells, including small lymphocytes, eosinophils, neutrophils, histiocytes, and plasma cells. The neoplastic cells are characterized by large cell size, abundant slightly basophilic cytoplasm, and a single nucleus (Hodgkin or H cell) or multiple nuclei (Reed-Sternberg or RS cell) with inclusion-like eosinophilic nucleoli.
  - Variants of RS/H cells include lacunar cells and mummified cells. Lacunar cells have smaller nuclei, less prominent nucleoli, and more abundant cytoplasm due to cytoplasmic membrane retraction. They are typically seen in NSCHL subtype.
  - Mummified cells have condensed cytoplasm and pyknotic hyperchromatic nuclei that can be seen in any of the subtypes. The neoplastic cells in cHLs account for less than 10% of the cellular infiltrate and generally do not form cohesive sheets or large aggregates except in the syncytial variant of NSCHL.
  - RS cells are not required for patients with cHLs diagnosed at another site [16].

4. What are the most typical immunophenotypes of classic Hodgkin lymphoma?

- cHL cells are transformed B cells that have lost the expression of B-cell markers.
- CD30 is positive in nearly all the cases, while CD15 is positive in subset of the cases or a minority of the cells [1, 17–19].
- CD20 is positive in 30–40% of the cases and is usually weak and in a minority of the cells [20, 21]. PAX5 is usually weaker than background reactive B cells [22]. Either OCT2 or BOB1 might be expressed in cHL but not both positive at the same time. CD79a is usually negative [23].
- Rare cases of cHL, especially NSCHL, can show aberrant expression of T-cell antigens, especially CD2 or CD4 [24, 25], and are reported to be associated with poorer prognosis [26]. Therefore, the most typical immunophenotype of cHL is as follows: CD45−, CD30+, CD15+/−, CD20 negative or weak+, PAX5 weak+, MUM1 strong +, EBER in situ hybridization for *EBV*+, CD79a−, OCT2−/+, BOB1−/+, EMA−.
- Diagnosis of classic Hodgkin lymphoma needs both positive and negative markers for a definitive diagnosis.

5. How to distinguish CD30 and CD15 staining in classic Hodgkin cells from those in non-Hodgkin cells?

- CD30 is the most sensitive marker for classic Hodgkin lymphoma. CD30 should be included in the initial workup of any lymphoma to detect potential or rare H or RS cells. However, CD30 is a non-specific marker and can also be positive in reactive immunoblasts of the lymph nodes, in other B-cell lymphomas, as well as in T-cell lymphomas.

- CD15 positivity will help to confirm the diagnosis of cHL when positive with CD30. However, CD15 can also stain granulocytes or neutrophils in the background.
- It is important to tell the difference between real Hodgkin cell staining from non-Hodgkin cell staining. The typical Hodgkin CD30 and CD15 stains should be membrane staining of mostly large atypical cells with Golgi zone accentuation, while the staining of non-Hodgkin cells might show a spectrum of size and most cells do not show Golgi zone staining. CD15 staining of neutrophils usually shows small cells.

6. How to further classify classic Hodgkin lymphoma into subtypes?

- cHL is further subclassified into nodular sclerosis classic Hodgkin lymphoma (NSCHL), lymphocyte-rich classic Hodgkin lymphoma (LRCHL), mixed cellularity classic Hodgkin lymphoma (MCCHL), and lymphocyte-depleted classic Hodgkin lymphoma (LDCHL), depending on the degree of fibrosis and the number of background reactive lymphocytes.
- The histological pattern and composition of background inflammatory cells vary among the different subtypes of cHLs. For example, band-like collagen fibrosis is characteristic of NSCHL, but is absent in other subtypes. Eosinophilic microabscesses and necrosis are also frequently seen within the nodules of NSCHL, but are uncommon in other subtypes. In contrast, histiocytes are more common in LDCHL than in other subtypes of classic Hodgkin lymphomas (Table 9.2).
- If there is at least one broad band-like fibrosis surrounding the atypical lymphoid nodules, it is most likely to be NSCHL. The cytoplasm of H/RS cells frequently shows retraction of the cell membranes, and H/RS cells are called lacunar cells. When H/RS cells form prominent aggregates, the term syncytial variant can be used.
- If the fibrosis is minor and the background lymphocytes are rich and forming nodules, it is most likely LRCHL [27].
- If there are no lymphocyte nodules and the background consists of mixture of eosinophils, neutrophils, histiocytes, and plasma cells, it is likely to be MCCHL.
- If there are few lymphocytes and no band-like fibrosis but numerous H/RS cells, it should be called LDCHL [28].
- In some needle core biopsies with limited tissue, precise subclassification is not always feasible.

7. How to distinguish nodular lymphocyte-predominant Hodgkin lymphoma (NLPHL) from classic Hodgkin lymphoma (cHL)?

- Both NLPHL and classic Hodgkin lymphoma, especially lymphocyte-rich classic Hodgkin lymphoma (LRCHL), can show nodules of lymphocytes with scattered large atypical cells, making it necessary to keep them in the differentials of each other. NLPHL usually shows popcorn cells in B-cell nodules, while cHL shows H or RS cells in an inflammatory background including lymphocytes, eosinophils, neutrophils, and plasma cells.
- NLPHL and cHL also differ in that the neoplastic cells in NLPHL are positive for most of the B-cell markers, while H or RS cells lose most of the B-cell markers. NLPHL shows scattered popcorn cells that are usually CD20 strong +, CD30−, CD45+, CD79a+, CD15−, OCT2+, Bob1+ [29–34], while LRCHL shows H or RS cells that are usually CD20− or weak+, CD30+ with mostly Golgi zone staining, CD45−, CD15 subset+, CD79a−, OCT2−, and Bob.1− or positive but not both at the same time.
- CD21 can also show follicular dendritic meshwork and CD3/CD57/PD1 [35] rosette formation around popcorn cells in NLPHL, but not in cHLs. CD4/CD8 double positive T cell in the background is frequent in NLPHL [36, 37].
- EBER in situ hybridization for *EBV* might be positive in cHLs, but is usually negative in NLPHL.

8. What are the mimics of Hodgkin lymphoma and what are the clinical consequences of misinterpretation between Hodgkin lymphomas and their mimics?

- Hodgkin lymphomas have an excellent prognosis with 80–95% cure rate. Standard treatment for cHLs is chemotherapy with ABVD (doxorubicin, bleomycin, vinblastine, dacarbazine) and involved field radiation. Replacement of bleomycin with anti-CD30 antibody (brentuximab vedotin) has become the new frontline therapy for cHL with less pulmonary toxicity [38].
- Patients with low-stage or non-bulky NLPHL require no treatment or only require site radiation therapy. Those with high-stage or bulky disease are treated with ABVD or CHOP (cyclophosphamide, doxorubicin, vincristine, and prednisone) plus rituximab. Care should be taken to differentiate HLs from non-Hodgkin lymphoma mimics that usually have a poor prognosis and require a different or more aggressive therapy.
- The main mimics of Hodgkin lymphomas are listed in Table 9.3.

Table 9.3 Hodgkin lymphomas and their main morphologic mimics

Hodgkin lymphomas	Morphologic mimics
NLPHL	Progressive transformation of germinal center (PTGC) LRCHL T-cell/histiocyte-rich large B-cell lymphoma (THRLBCL) Follicular lymphoma (FL)
NSCHL	Primary mediastinal large B-cell lymphoma (PMLBCL) B-cell lymphoma, unclassifiable, with features intermediate between diffuse large B-cell lymphoma and classic Hodgkin lymphoma (gray zone lymphoma, GZL) Anaplastic large cell lymphoma (ALCL) T-cell/histiocyte-rich large B-cell lymphoma (THRLBCL)
LRCHL	NLPHL Mantle cell lymphoma (MCL) Marginal zone B-cell lymphoma (MZL) Follicular lymphoma (FL)
MCCHL	T-cell/histiocyte-rich large B-cell lymphoma (THRLBCL) Peripheral T-cell lymphoma, not otherwise specified (PTCL NOS) Angioimmunoblastic T-cell lymphoma (AITCL)
LDCHL	NSCHL syncytial variant Anaplastic large cell lymphoma (ALCL) Diffuse large B-cell lymphoma (DLBCL) *EBV*+ diffuse large B-cell lymphoma NOS (*EBV*+ DLBCL) Histiocytic sarcoma Carcinoma Melanoma

9. How to distinguish nodular lymphocyte-predominant Hodgkin lymphoma (NLPHL) from progressive transformation of germinal centers (PTGC)?

- Both NLPHL and PTGC, a benign process, can show nodular structures. PTGC can occur prior to or co-occur with NLPHL. However, NLPHL shows large atypical popcorn cells in B-cell nodules that were ringed by rosette of PD1+ or CD57+ T follicular helper cells, while PTGC shows germinal centers with no popcorn cells and only occasional centroblasts.

10. How to distinguish nodular lymphocyte-predominant Hodgkin lymphoma (NLPHL) from T-cell/histiocyte-rich large B-cell lymphoma (THRLBCL)?

- Both NLPHL and THRLBCL show numerous lymphocytes with scattered large atypical B cells, which are positive for CD20, CD45, OCT2, and BOB1, so can be confused with each other in some cases.
- NLPHL usually presents as a local disease, while THRLBCL usually presents as a more aggressive or systemic disease.
- NLPHL shows popcorn cells in B-cell nodules that are ringed by CD3/CD57/PD1+ T cells, while THRLBCL shows large atypical lymphocytes in mostly T cell and histiocyte background without obvious nodular formation.
- Demonstration of at least one follicular dendritic meshwork by CD21 is sufficient to exclude THRLBCL.
- Predominance of CD8+ and TIA+ T cells favors THRLBCL.
- There is close relationship between NLPHL and THRLBCL in that NLPHL may progress into or contain areas indistinguishable from THRLBCL. In some small biopsies, differentiation between them may be impossible.

11. How to distinguish nodular lymphocyte-predominant Hodgkin lymphoma (NLPHL) from follicular lymphoma (FL)?

- In rare cases, NLPHL might be confused with FL when nodules of lymphocytes are seen with scattered large atypical cells in the centers. Both show lack of normal germinal center architecture (polarization and tingible body macrophages). The large atypical lymphocytes in both entities are positive for CD45, CD20, and other B-cell markers.
- The germinal centers in FL are usually more recognizable than those in NLPHL. The large cells in FL are centroblasts, while the large cells in NLPHL are popcorn cells. The germinal centers of FL also show clefted small atypical lymphocytes (centrocytes) that are positive for CD10, BCL6, and BCL2, while the B-cell nodules in NLPHL will be negative for CD10.
- FISH study might show diagnostic t(14;18) (*IGH/BCL2*) translocation in FL.

12. How to distinguish classic Hodgkin lymphoma (cHL) from T-cell/histiocyte-rich large B-cell lymphoma (THRLBCL)?

- Classic Hodgkin lymphoma, especially mixed cellularity classic Hodgkin lymphoma (MCCHL), can show scattered large atypical cells in the background of numerous inflammatory cells (small reactive lymphocytes, eosinophils, and plasma cells) and should be distinguished from THRLBCL [39, 40].
- Unsurprisingly, the H or RS cells in cHL should be CD30+ with Golgi zone staining, CD15+/−, CD45−,

CD20−/weak+, PAX5 weak+, Mum-1+, OCT2−, and BOB1− or not positive at the same time, while the large atypical lymphocytes in THRLBCL should be CD30− or small subset + without Golgi zone staining, CD15−, CD45+, CD20 strong +, PAX5 strong +, OCT2+, and BOB1+.
- cHL could be *EBV*+, while THRLBCL is usually *EBV*−. According to the WHO classification, large B-cell lymphoma with *EBV*+ and T-cell-rich background should be classified as *EBV*+ DLBCL instead of THRLBCL.

13. How to distinguish nodular sclerosis classic Hodgkin lymphoma (NSCHL) from primary mediastinal (thymic) large B-cell lymphoma (PMLBCL)?

- Both of these two entities commonly present as mediastinal masses and have a female preference [41–43]. Both entities can show large CD30+ atypical cells or Hodgkin/Reed-Sternberg-like cells in the background of fibrosis [44, 45]; therefore, they deserve to be differentiated from each other.
- The atypical cells in PMLBCL are usually medium-sized to large with abundant pale cytoplasm and relatively round or ovoid nuclei, while NSCHL will show typical Hodgkin or Reed-Sternberg cells. PMLBCL usually shows compartmentalization alveolar fibrosis [41, 46–49], while NSCHL usually shows broad band-like fibrosis.
- The Hodgkin or Reed-Sternberg cells in cHL are usually CD30+ with Golgi zone staining, CD15+/−, CD20−/weak+, PAX5 weak+, BOB1−, and OCT2− or not positive at the same time, CD45−, and CD23−, while the large atypical cells in PMLBCL are usually weak and homogenous CD30+ [49, 50], CD15− or + in minority of the cells, CD20 strong+, PAX5 strong+, OCT2+, and BOB1+, CD23+ [51–54], and CD45+ [41, 54–56].
- NSCHL could be positive for EBER ISH (*EBV*), while PMLBCL is usually negative for *EBV* [41].

14. How to distinguish classic Hodgkin lymphoma (cHL) from B-cell lymphoma, unclassifiable, with features intermediate between diffuse large B-cell lymphoma and classic Hodgkin lymphoma (gray zone lymphoma, GZL)?

- Both cHL (especially NSCHL) and diffuse large B-cell lymphoma (DLBCL) especially PMLBCL can present with mediastinal mass [1, 45, 57]. Sometimes, the lymphoma cells exhibit atypical morphology or immunophenotype that is difficult to distinguish between cHL and DLBCL/PMLBCL [45] and is therefore called gray zone lymphoma. GZL generally has more aggressive clinical course and poorer outcome than either cHL or PMLBCL [1, 58]; therefore, it is important to distinguish them in diagnosis.
- cHL typically shows scattered Hodgkin or Reed-Sternberg cells that are CD30+ with frequent Golgi zone staining, CD15+ with Golgi zone staining or −, CD20− or weak+, PAX5 weak+, Bob.1−, and Oct.2− or not both positive at the same time, CD45−, while PMLBCL typically shows large atypical lymphocytes that are CD20+, PAX5 strong +, OCT2+, and BOB1+, CD15−, and CD45+.
- In GZL, the morphology might appear like cHL, but the large atypical cells are CD20 strong+, PAX5 not weak, CD79a+, or show Bob.1 and Oct.2 staining at the same time. CD45 usually shows diffuse staining of all the cells and most of the time is hard to unambiguously define.
- In other cases of GZL, the morphology might appear like PMLBCL, but the large atypical cells show weaker than typical CD20 and PAX5 staining and ambiguous BOB1 and OCT2 staining. CD30 is usually positive and CD15 may be expressed. In these cases, it is very difficult to unequivocally call it cHL or PMLBCL/DLBCL. A diagnosis of B-cell lymphoma, unclassifiable, with features intermediate between Hodgkin lymphoma and diffuse large B-cell lymphoma (gray zone lymphoma) is justified.
- Composite cHL and DLBCL/PMLBL in the same specimen are not strictly called GZL [1, 59, 60].

15. How to distinguish cHL from *EBV*+ diffuse large B-cell lymphoma NOS (*EBV*+ DLBCL)?

- Both cHL and *EBV*+ DLBCL can show *EBV*+ and CD30+ large atypical lymphocytes, including Hodgkin or RS-like cells. CD15 sometimes might be positive in *EBV*+ DLBCL too [61–63]. They should therefore be distinguished from each other.
- CD30 stain of cHL usually shows more typical Golgi zone staining in scattered large cells, while *EBV*+ DLBCL usually shows less typical Golgi zone staining.
- cHLs are usually CD45−, CD20 negative or weak+, PAX5 weak+, CD79a−, OCT2−, and BOB1− or not positive at the same time, while *EBV*+ DLBCL is usually CD45+, CD20+, PAX5+, CD79a+, OCT2+, and BOB1+.
- Cases that show sparse CD45+, CD20+, *EBV*+, large neoplastic cells, even though with Hodgkin-like morphology, should be considered *EBV*+ DLBCL, instead of classic Hodgkin lymphoma or THRLBCL [63, 64].

16. How to distinguish classic Hodgkin lymphoma (cHL) from peripheral T-cell lymphoma (PTCL)?

- cHL can show diffuse (MCCHL) lymphocyte infiltrate as PTCL NOS. PTCL NOS can also have large atypical *EBV*+ Hodgkin or Reed-Sternberg-like cells that are CD30+ [65, 66], and rarely CD15+, which is associated with adverse prognosis [67, 68]. PTCL can rarely be *EBV*-positive in standby B-cell immunoblasts [69–71]. Therefore, these two entities should be distinguished from each other in some situations.
- Typically, the Hodgkin or Reed-Sternberg cells in cHL should be CD30+ with Golgi zone staining, CD15+/−, CD45−, PAX5 weak+, and negative for CD3 and other T-cell markers, while PTCL NOS should be CD30+ without less typical Golgi zone staining or CD30−, CD15−, CD45+, and positive for one or more of the T-cell markers (CD2, CD3, CD4 or CD8, CD5, CD7).
- Rare cases of cHL, especially NSCHL, can show aberrant expression of T-cell antigens, especially CD2 or CD4. So a combination of positive and negative markers should be considered during the differentials.
- Abnormal T cells with pan T-cell antigen loss or alteration could be detected by flow cytometry in majority of PTCL, while reactive T cells in microenvironment of cHL often show no aberrant changes.

17. How to distinguish classic Hodgkin lymphoma from anaplastic large cell lymphoma (ALCL)?

- cHL, especially LDCHL or NSCHL syncytial variants, can show clusters or sheets of large atypical cells without many lymphocytes, morphologically similar to ALCL [72–74]. The large atypical cells in both entities are also positive for CD30 with potentially Golgi zone staining [1, 18, 74] and occasional CD15 expression [75], making it necessary to keep them in the differentials of each other. Rare cases of cHL can show aberrant expression of CD2 or CD4 [24], which are positive in ALCL.
- Typically, the large atypical cells in ALCL have abundant cytoplasm and eccentric pleomorphic horseshoe-shaped or kidney-shaped nuclei, often with an eosinophilic region near the nucleus (hallmark cells) [75].
- The Hodgkin or Reed-Sternberg cells in cHL should be CD15+/−, CD20− or weak+, PAX5 weak+, Mum-1+, and negative for the T-cell markers (CD3, CD2, CD4, CD5, CD7) and EMA, while the ALCL cells should be CD15− and positive for one or more of the T-cell markers (usually CD4, CD2, CD5), EMA, and/or ALK1.
- ALK+ ALCL will also show t(2;5)(*NPM1/ALK*) or variant translocations by FISH study. The small T cells in ALCL are also neoplastic and might have irregular nuclei [75].
- cHL could be *EBV*+, while ALCL is usually negative.

18. How to distinguish lymphocyte-rich classic Hodgkin lymphoma (LRCHL) from mantle cell lymphoma (MCL)?

- Both LRCHL and MCL can present as nodules of small mature lymphocytes. MCL with blastoid transformation could also show some large atypical lymphocytes. Therefore, it might be necessary to distinguish these two entities in rare instances.
- cHL should show Hodgkin or RS cells in clusters in expanded mantle zone. These clusters of Hodgkin cells are highlighted by pertinent immunohistochemical stains.
- cHLs are CD30+ with Golgi zone staining, CD15+/−, CD45−, CD20−/weak+, PAX5 weak+, BCL1−, MUM1+, OCT2−, and BOB1−, and SOX11−, while the mantle lymphoma cells should be CD30−, CD15−, CD45+, CD20 strong +, PAX5 strong +, BCL1+, SOX11+, OCT2+, and BOB1+.
- FISH study will show t(11;14) (*CCND1/IGH*) translocation in MCL.

19. How to distinguish lymphocyte-rich classic Hodgkin lymphoma (LRCHL) from follicular lymphoma?

- Both LRCHL and FL can present as nodules of small mature lymphocytes. High-grade FL could also show some large atypical lymphocytes. Therefore, it might be necessary to distinguish these two entities in rare instances.
- Typically, FL should show lymphoid follicles with germinal centers that can be demonstrated by CD21 immunostain. The lymphoma cells in FL should be CD30−, CD15−, CD45+, CD20+, PAX5 strong +, CD10+, BCL2+, BCL6+, OCT2+, and BOB1+, while the Hodgkin or Reed-Sternberg cells in cHL should be CD30+ with Golgi zone staining, CD15+/−, CD45−, CD20−/weak+, PAX5 weak+, CD10−, BCL2−, BCL6−, MUM1+, OCT2−, and BOB1− or not both positive at the same time.
- FISH study will likely show t(14;18) (*BCL2/IGH*) translocation in FL.

20. How to distinguish lymphocyte-depleted classic Hodgkin lymphoma (LDCHL) from histiocytic sarcoma?

- LDCHL usually shows clusters or sheets of large atypical cells without many lymphocytes, morphologically could resemble histiocytic sarcoma. Histiocytic sarcoma can rarely show weak expression of CD15 too [76].
- The Hodgkin or RS cells in LDCHL should be CD30+ with Golgi zone staining, PAX5 weak+, Mum-1+, and negative for histiocytic markers (lysozyme, CD4, CD64, CD68, CD163), while histiocytic sarcoma cells should be CD30−, CD45+, and positive for one or more of the above histiocytic markers.
- cHL could be *EBV*+, while histiocytic sarcoma will be negative.

21. For peripheral blood and bone marrow biopsies, what morphological findings are diagnostic and what findings are suspicious for classic Hodgkin lymphoma?

- Peripheral blood may show mild leukocytosis with left shift at the time of HL diagnosis. Mild eosinophilia may also be present. Circulating neoplastic cells are never seen in the peripheral blood. These findings are non-specific.
- Bone marrow involvement by cHLs occurs in less than 5% of the cases. Bone marrow aspirate smear usually shows left-shifted myelopoiesis. Neoplastic cells are rarely seen unless there is an extensive bone marrow involvement, particularly in LDCHL. These cells, if present, should be distinguished from the immature megakaryocytes that do not display inclusion-like nucleoli. Immunostain for CD61 will confirm the megakaryocytes, while CD30 positivity will favor cHL.
- The core biopsy of involved bone marrow usually shows lymphohistiocytic aggregates that contain scattered large atypical cells with monolobated or multilobated nuclei and prominent nucleoli. Classic RS/H cells are difficult to find, and immunohistochemical stains are essential to confirm the diagnosis and distinguish cHL from its morphologic mimics involving bone marrow. In the absence of typical H or RS cells, the presence of lymphohistiocytic aggregates is highly suspicious for cHL. Deeper sections sometimes might be helpful to reveal H or RS cells.

22. What is the minimal and optimal ancillary workup for the diagnosis of Hodgkin lymphomas?

- Immunohistochemistry with a panel of antibodies is the main ancillary tool for the diagnosis and classification/subclassification of HLs. A minimal panel of antibodies should include CD45, CD30, CD15, CD3, PAX5, CD20, CD45, and EBER ISH. CD57, CD79a, BOB1, OCT2, MUM1, BCL6, and PD1 should be added to the minimal panel in difficult cases for differential diagnosis.
- Flow cytometry is not helpful in the follow-up of classic Hodgkin lymphomas, but should be included in the initial workup for NLPHL or cHL, to exclude non-Hodgkin lymphomas or a composite HL. The increased CD4:CD8 ratio in the sample may be suggestive of, but is unreliable for, diagnosis or to exclude the diagnosis of classic HLs. An increase in CD4/CD8-double negative cells may suggest the diagnosis of NLPHL, but again is non-diagnostic.
- B-cell gene rearrangement and cytogenetic studies are usually not helpful to the diagnosis of Hodgkin lymphoma due to small number and the fragility of the large atypical lymphocytes. Molecular testing for immunoglobulin heavy/K (IgH/IgK) light chain and T-cell receptor gamma (*TCR*) gene rearrangements is of very limited utility in establishing or excluding the diagnosis of HLs. Monoclonal *IGH/IGK* gene rearrangements may be seen in a small subset of HLs. However, it may occasionally be needed to distinguish HL from its morphologic mimics.

23. What information provides prognostic and therapeutic target information for Hodgkin lymphomas?

- Strong CD30 expression provides an ideal target for anti-CD30 (brentuximab vedotin or Adcetris) treatment in patients with cHLs [77, 78]. More recently, it has reported to be useful when used in combination with chemotherapy adriamycin or doxorubicin, vinblastine, and dacarbazine (AVD) as a frontline treatment for adult patients with stage III or IV cHL [79, 80].
- Expression of CD20 is known to be associated with a worse prognosis in cHLs [81].
- *EBV* positivity is also associated with worse prognosis in cHL patients older than 60 years, but not in patients younger than 15 years [82].

- Immunostains for PD1/PDL1 are also helpful for immune check point inhibitor/immunomodulatory therapy with anti-PD1/PDL1 antibodies in cHLs [83, 84]. Anti-PD1 nivolumab (Opdivo) was approved by FDA in 2016 to treat relapsed/refractory HLs.
- In advanced cHL, increased expression of CD163 and c-Met is reported to have significant association with adverse prognostic parameters and poor response to treatment [85].

24. What are adequate specimens for the diagnosis of Hodgkin lymphomas?

- Excisional biopsy is the recommended specimen for the diagnosis of HLs. Core needle biopsy may contain too few large neoplastic cells to be diagnostic. Fine needle aspiration alone is insufficient for diagnosis of HL except when in combination with immunohistochemistry on cell block that happens to have typical H or RS cells.

25. What information can be conveyed to the clinician during each stage of the workup?

- Frozen section is not recommended for the workup of HLs. If performed for other reasons, such as staging for metastatic melanoma or carcinoma, and an HL is suspected on frozen section, the pathologist should inform the surgeon whether sufficient tissue is obtained for further morphological examination and ancillary studies. A touch imprint may be prepared at the time of frozen section. Fresh tissue can be triaged for ancillary studies, such as flow cytometric immunophenotyping, to differentiate HL from its morphological mimics of non-Hodgkin lymphomas, and to exclude a composite lymphoma.
- When hematoxylin-eosin-stained slides become available, the pathologist may discuss the preliminary diagnostic impression with the clinician and inform the clinician that additional studies are needed to confirm or exclude the diagnosis of HLs.
- The final diagnosis of HLs requires integration of histomorphology and other ancillary study results, particularly immunohistochemistry.

26. When are comments necessary and what should be discussed in the comments for Hodgkin lymphoma?

- With a definitive diagnosis, a diagnostic comment may just include the immunohistochemical profile of the neoplastic cells to support the diagnosis. When the diagnosis is inconclusive due to various limitations, such as small sample size or ambiguous immunohistochemical results, it is imperative to comment on the limitation of the biopsy, the degree of confidence, the atypical findings, the potential differential diagnoses, and the recommendation for additional tissue or external expert consultation.

27. When is it appropriate to seek external consultation for Hodgkin lymphomas?

- In academic centers with more than one hematopathologist, intradepartmental consultation should be obtained first. When a consensus diagnosis cannot be reached, the primary hematopathologists should seek an external consultation, especially when low confidence in diagnosis is encountered.

Case Presentations

Case 1 (Fig. 9.1)

Learning Objectives

1. To become familiar with the histologic morphologic features of NLPHL
2. To become familiar with the immunohistochemical features of the NLPHL
3. To become familiar with the differential diagnosis of NLPHL

Case History

A 40-year-old male presented with cervical lymphadenopathy.

Histologic Findings

- Nodular atypical lymphoid infiltrate with scattered popcorn cells

Differential Diagnosis

- NLPHL
- Progressive transformation of germinal center (PTGC)
- Lymphocyte-rich classic Hodgkin lymphoma (LRCHL)
- T-cell/histiocyte-rich large B-cell lymphoma (THRLBCL)
- Follicular lymphoma (FL)
- Diffuse large B-cell lymphoma (DLBCL)

IHC Studies

- CD20+, Oct2+, popcorn cells surrounded by PD1 T-cell rosettes.
- CD21 demonstrate expanded follicular dendritic meshworks.

Additional IHC Studies

- PAX5+ (strong), CD79a+, BOB1+, CD30−, CD15−, EBER for *EBV*−

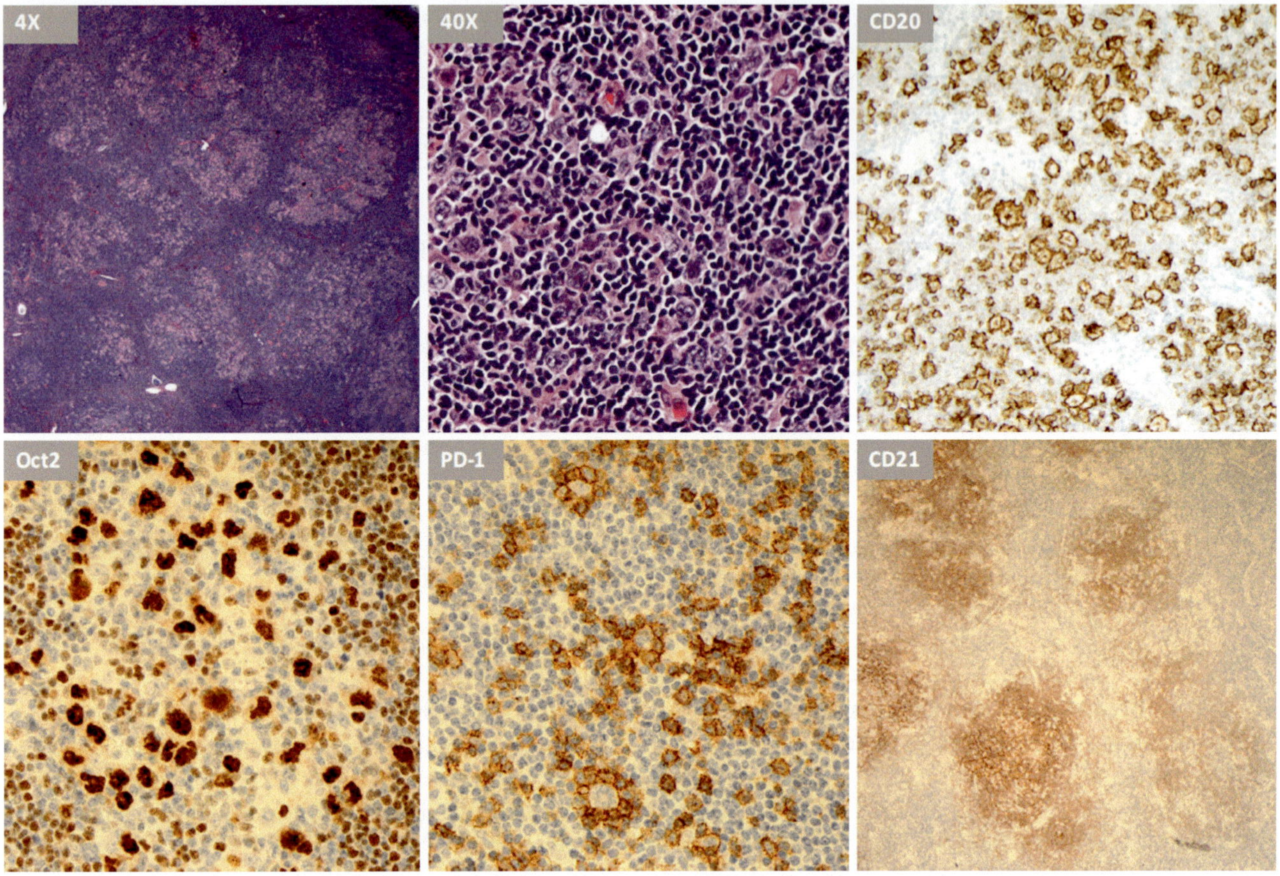

Fig. 9.1 Case 1, nodular lymphocyte-predominant Hodgkin lymphoma (NLPHL). Nodular lymphoid infiltrate (40×) with a minor population of large neoplastic cells (40×) with popcorn cells or lymphocyte-predominant (LP) cells, which are positive for CD20 and Oct2 and ringed by PD1 positive T-helper cells. CD21 shows the presence of follicular dendritic meshworks

Final Diagnosis

Nodular lymphocyte-predominant classic Hodgkin lymphoma (NLPHL)

Take-Home Messages

1. NLPHL shows CD20+ popcorn cells in expanded follicular nodules and surrounded by CD57+/PD1 follicular helper T cells.
2. Popcorn cells often retain B-cell antigens, including CD19, CD20, CD79a, and leukocyte common antigen CD45.
3. Popcorn cells are usually negative for CD30 and CD15, which is in contrast to cHL.

Case 2 (Fig. 9.2)

Learning Objectives

1. To become familiar with the histologic morphologic features of NSCHL
2. To become familiar with the immunohistochemical features of the NSCHL
3. To become familiar with the differential diagnosis of NSCHL

Case History

A 30-year-old female presented with a mediastinal mass.

Histologic Findings

- Nodular atypical lymphoid infiltrate surrounded by broad band fibrosis
- Hodgkin, RS, or lacunar cells in the background of small reactive lymphocytes, histiocytes, plasma cells, and rare plasma cells

Differential Diagnosis

- NSCHL
- PMLBCL
- ALCL
- Gray zone lymphoma

IHC Studies

- CD30+, CD15+, CD20−, PAX5 weak+

Additional IHC Studies

- CD45−, Mum-1+, Oct2−, BOB1−, EBER for *EBV*−

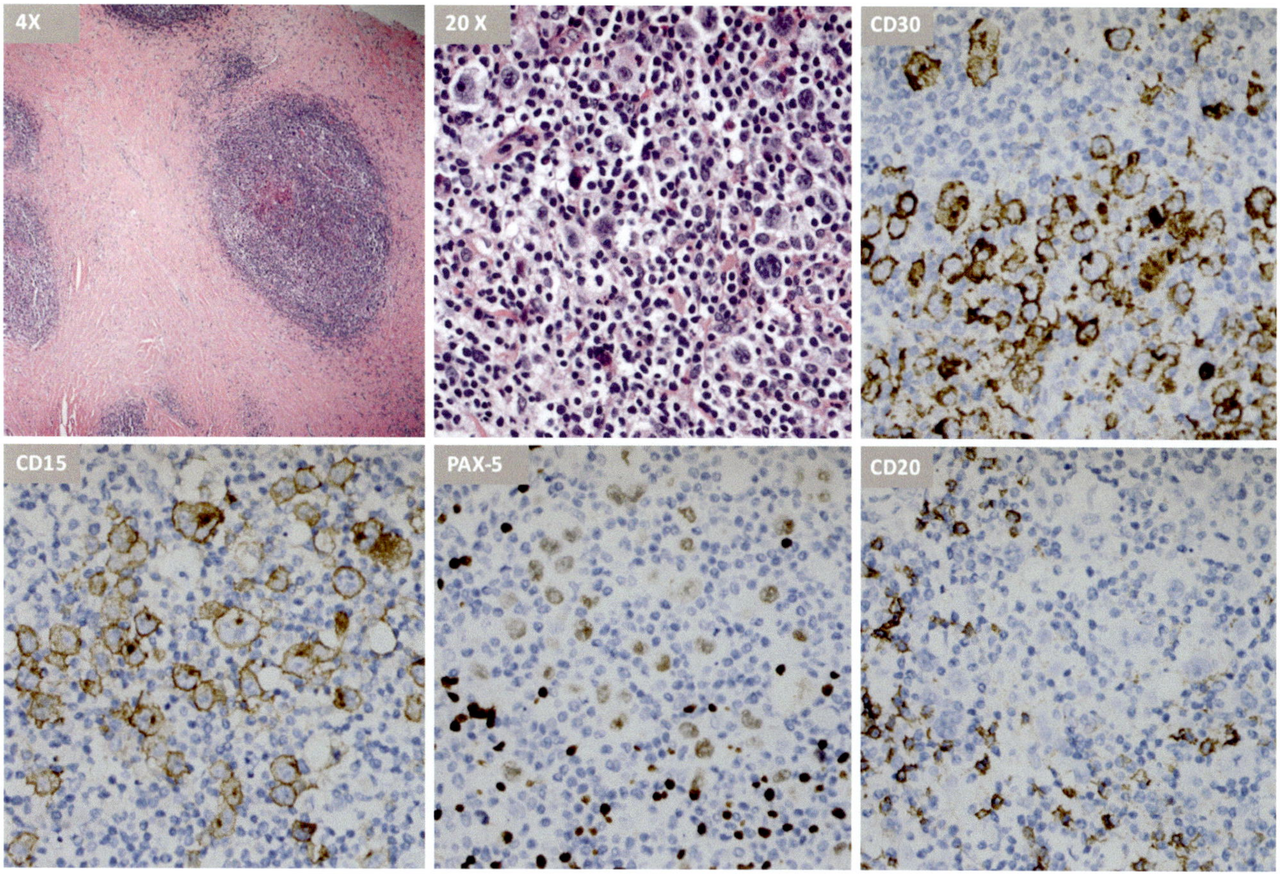

Fig. 9.2 Case 2, nodular sclerosis classic Hodgkin lymphoma (NSCHL). Nodular lymphoid infiltrate (40×) with broad band fibrosis. The nodular infiltrate consists of Hodgkin, Reed-Sternberg, or Lacunar RS cells. The background of reactive inflammatory cells includes eosinophils, small lymphocytes, neutrophils, histiocytes, and plasma cells (40×). The H or RS cells are positive for CD30, CD15, weak positive for PAX5 and negative for CD20

Final Diagnosis

Nodular sclerosis classic Hodgkin lymphoma (NSCHL)

Take-Home Messages

1. NSCHL show broad band fibrosis.
2. RS cells or variants in cHL have their B-cell program down-regulated, thus demonstrating negative staining for majority of B-cell antigens.
3. Typical cHLs are CD30+, CD15+, PAX5 weak+, CD20−, CD45−, Mum-1+, *EBV*+/−, OCT2−, BOB1−.

Case 3 (Fig. 9.3)

Learning Objectives

1. To become familiar with the histologic morphologic features of LRCHL
2. To become familiar with the immunohistochemical features of the LRCHL
3. To become familiar with the differential diagnosis of LRCHL

Case History

A 37-year-old male presented with left axillary lymphadenopathy.

Histologic Findings

- Nodular lymphoid proliferation with apparently reactive follicles and expanded perifollicular or interfollicular areas; no significant fibrosis is identified around the lymphoid nodules.
- Hodgkin or RS cells in the background of small lymphocytes and histiocytes.

Differential Diagnosis

- LRCHL
- NLPHL
- FL
- Castleman lymphadenopathy

IHC Studies

- CD30+, CD20−, PAX5 weak+, *EBV*-LMP1+

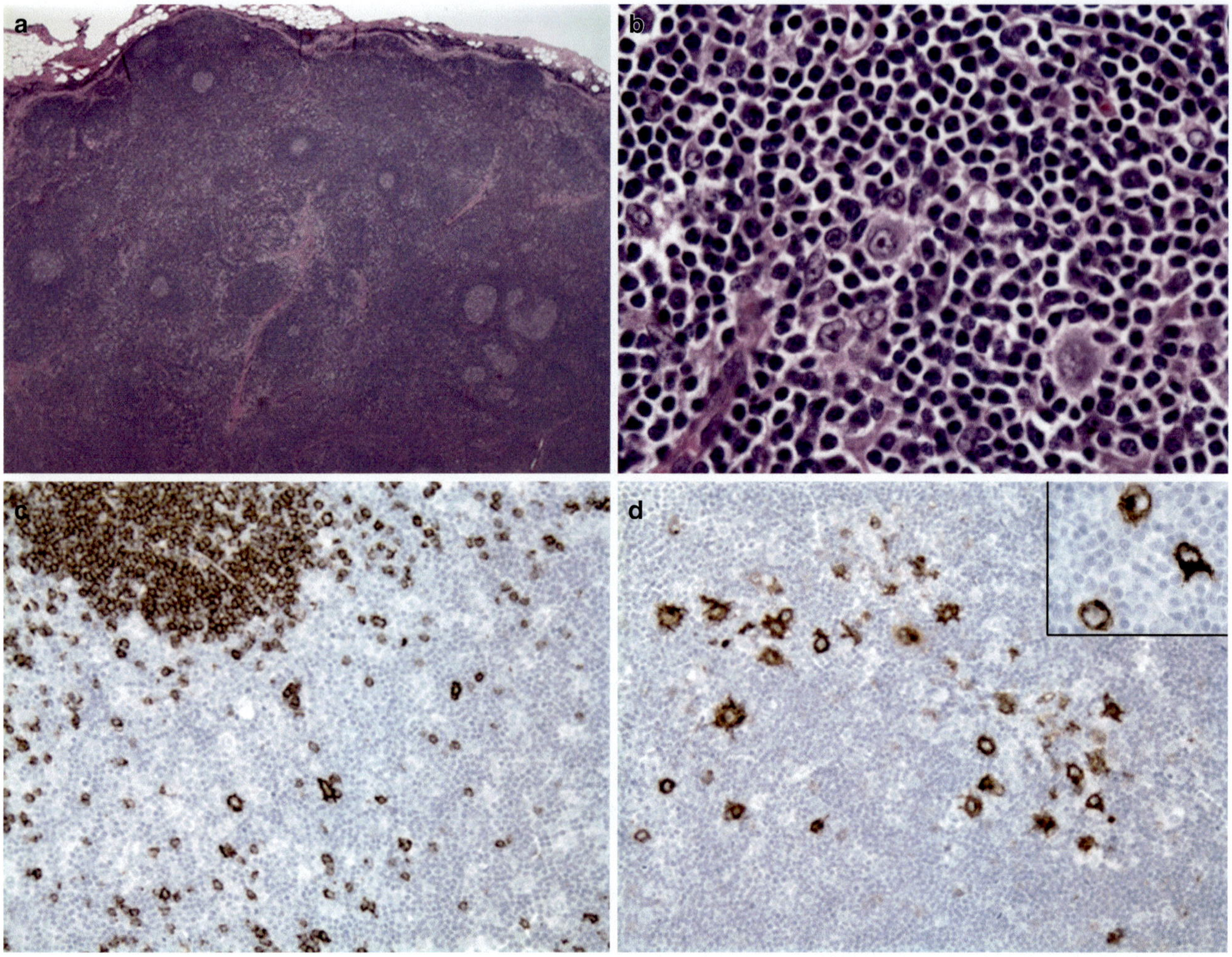

Fig. 9.3 Case 3, lymphocyte-rich classic Hodgkin lymphoma (LRCHL). (**a**) Section of lymph node biopsy shows largely preserved nodal architecture with apparently reactive lymphoid follicles and slight expansion of perifollicular/interfollicular areas. H&E stain, ×40. (**b**) High magnification shows scattered large atypical cells with prominent nucleoli in the background of many small lymphocytes in interfollicular area. H&E stain, 40×. (**c**) CD20 stain highlights aggregates of B cells, but the large atypical cells are negative for the stain. 20×. (**d**) The large atypical cells are positive for CD30, 20×. Inset shows three large cells positive for *EBV* latent membrane protein, 40×

Additional IHC Studies

- CD45−, CD15+, Mum-1+, OCT2−, BOB1−

Final Diagnosis

Lymphocyte-rich classic Hodgkin lymphoma (LRCHL)

Take-Home Messages

1. LRCHL show nodular lymphoid proliferation with RS or Hodgkin cells in expanded mantle zone, which could be highlighted by immunohistochemistry.
2. RS cells or variants in cHL have their B-cell program down-regulated, thus demonstrating negative staining for majority of B-cell antigens.
3. Typical cHLs are CD30+, CD15+, PAX5 weak+, CD20−, CD45−, Mum-1+, *EBV*+/−, OCT2−,BOB1−.

Case 4 (Fig. 9.4)

Learning Objectives

1. To become familiar with the histologic morphologic features of MCCHL
2. To become familiar with the immunohistochemical features of the MCCHL
3. To become familiar with the differential diagnosis of MCCHL

Case History

A 38-year-old male presented with right axillary lymphadenopathy.

Histologic Findings

- Diffuse atypical lymphoid infiltrate with mixed inflammatory background and scattered Hodgkin and RS cells

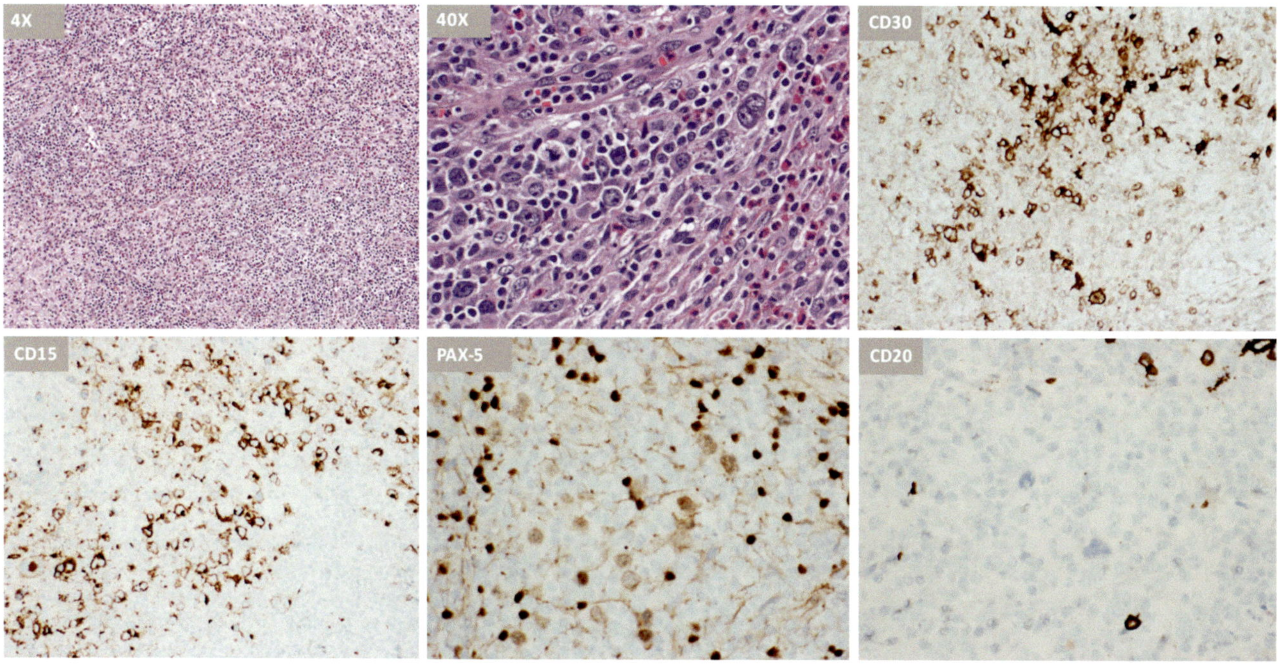

Fig. 9.4 Case 4, mixed cellularity classic Hodgkin lymphoma (MCCHL). The background shows mixed inflammatory cells without obvious nodular formation (40×). Large H or RS cells are seen (40×) and are positive for CD30, CD15, weak positive for PAX5, and negative for CD20

Differential Diagnosis

- T-cell/histiocyte-rich large B-cell lymphoma (T/HRLBCL)
- Peripheral T-cell lymphoma (PTCL), not otherwise specified

IHC Studies

- CD30+, CD15+, PAX5 weak+, CD20−

Additional IHC Studies

- Mum-1+, CD45−, OCT2−, BOB1−, EBER for *EBV*+

Final Diagnosis

Mixed cellularity classic Hodgkin lymphoma (MCCHL)

Take-Home Message

1. MCCHL shows CD30+, CD15+/−, PAX5 weak+, Mum-1+, CD20−, CD45−, Hodgkin or RS cells in the background of mixed inflammatory background, including significant eosinophils.

Case 5 (Fig. 9.5)

Learning Objectives

1. To become familiar with the histologic morphologic features of LDCHL
2. To become familiar with the immunohistochemical features of the LDCHL
3. To become familiar with the differential diagnosis of LDCHL

Case History

A 51-year-old male presented with a retroperitoneal mass.

Histologic Findings

- Enlarged lymph node with nodal architecture effaced by diffuse proliferation of large atypical cells with pleomorphic nuclei in a background of fibrosis and devoid of lymphoid cells.
- Hodgkin and RS are abundant with sarcomatoid morphology.

Differential Diagnosis

- LDCHL
- ALCL
- Sarcoma, including histiocytic sarcoma or other dendritic cell sarcoma

IHC Studies

- CD30+, CD15+, CD20−, PAX5 weak+

Additional IHC Studies

- CD45−, Mum-1+, Oct2−, Bob1−, CD163−, lysozyme−, CD21−, EBER for *EBV*+

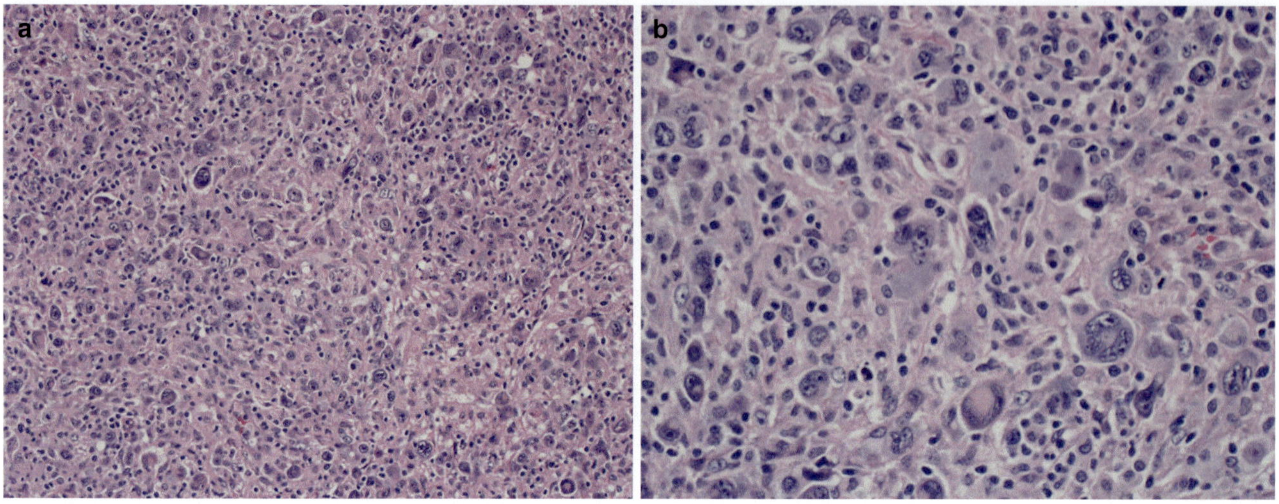

Fig. 9.5 Case 5, lymphocyte-depleted classic Hodgkin lymphoma (LDCHL). (**a**) Section of lymph node biopsy shows nodal architecture effaced by proliferation of large cells with pleomorphic nuclei admixed with other inflammatory cells. H&E stain, 10×. (**b**) A high magnification demonstrates many large cells with pleomorphic nuclei including a few with multinucleation and wreath-like nuclei. The background cells consist of small lymphocytes and histiocytes, though lymphocytes are apparently fewer than other subtypes of cHL. H&E stain, 40×

Final Diagnosis

Lymphocyte-depleted classic Hodgkin lymphoma (LDCHL)

Take-Home Messages

1. LDCHL shows pleomorphic morphology resembling sarcoma.
2. RS cells or variants in cHL have their B-cell program down-regulated, thus demonstrating negative staining for majority of B-cell antigens.
3. Typical cHLs are CD30+, CD15+, PAX5 weak+, CD20−, CD45−, Mum-1+, *EBV*+/−, OCT2−, BOB1−.

Case 6 (Fig. 9.6)

Learning Objectives

1. To become familiar with the histologic morphologic features of PTGC
2. To become familiar with the immunohistochemical features of the PTGC
3. To become familiar with its differentiation from NLPHL

Case History

A 32-year-old male presented with cervical lymphadenopathy.

Histologic Findings

- Mostly maintained lymph node architecture
- Occasional expanded lymphoid follicles with mantle cell invasion but without obvious large atypical cells

Differential Diagnosis

- Nodular lymphocyte-predominant Hodgkin lymphoma (NLPHL)
- T-cell/histiocyte-rich large B-cell lymphoma (THRLBCL)
- Follicular lymphoma (FL)

IHC Studies

- CD20+ and OCT2 show no obvious large atypical lymphocytes.

Additional IHC Studies

- CD30 and CD15 show no large atypical cells.

Final Diagnosis

Progressive transformation of germinal centers (PTGC)

Take-Home Messages

1. PTGC shows overall maintained lymph node architecture, expanded lymphoid follicles with mantle cell invagination into germinal centers, but no obvious large atypical B cells by morphology or by IHC, in comparison to NLPHL.
2. Often demonstrates coexisting reactive hyperplasic follicles.
3. Often demonstrates patent sinuses.

Case 7 (Fig. 9.7)

Learning Objectives

1. To become familiar with the histologic morphologic features of THRLBCL

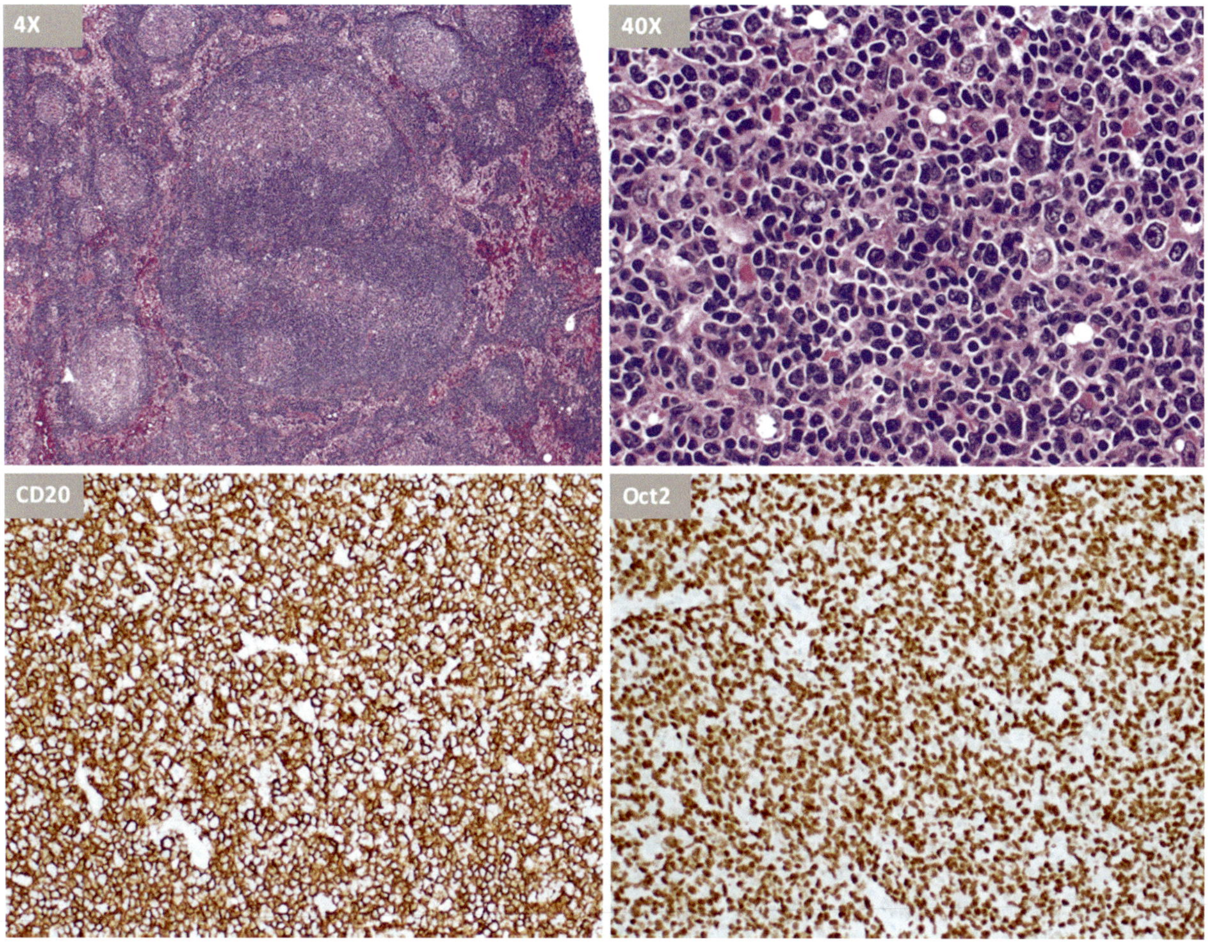

Fig. 9.6 Case 6, progressive transformation of germinal centers (PTGC). Large expanded lymphoid follicles are seen in the background of follicular hyperplasia (40×). No large atypical lymphocytes are present except for occasional immunoblasts (40×). CD20 and OCT2 only show small reactive B cells and no large atypical B cells, as seen in NLPHL

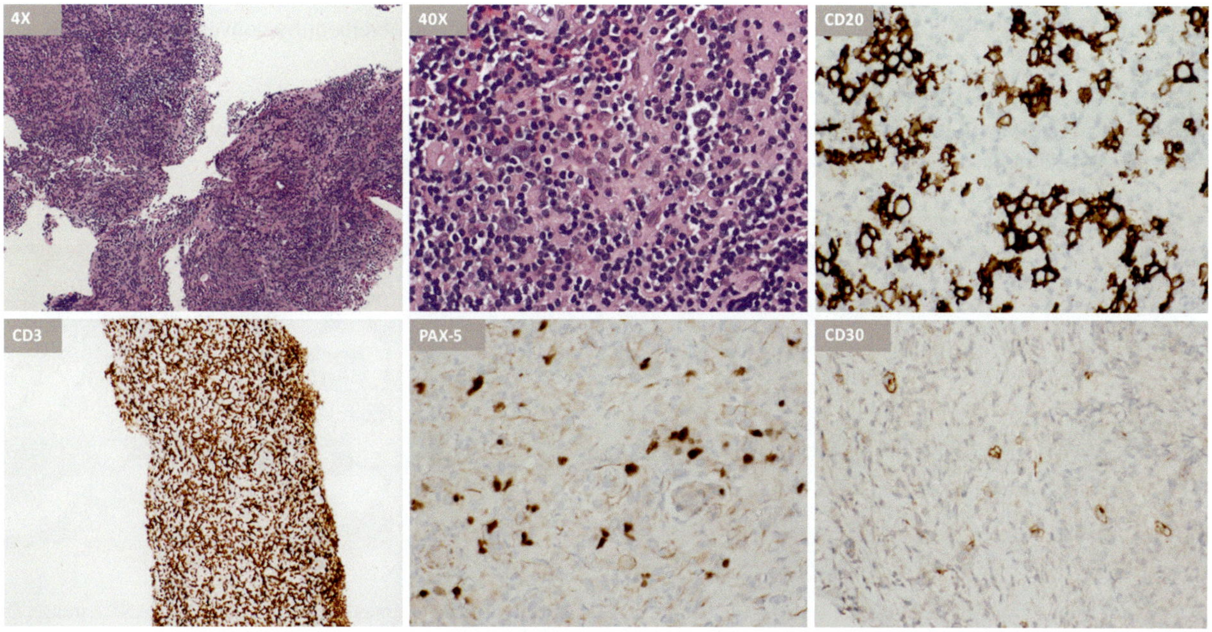

Fig. 9.7 Case 7, T-cell/histiocyte-rich large B-cell lymphoma (THRLBCL). Diffuse lymphoid infiltrate (4×) with scattered large atypical cells including some Hodgkin-like cells (40×) that are strong positive for CD20, PAX5 occasionally positive for CD30. CD3 shows numerous T cells in the background

2. To become familiar with the immunohistochemical features of the THRLBCL
3. To become familiar with its differentiation from Hodgkin lymphoma

Case History

A 50-year-old male presented with fever, malaise, splenomegaly, hepatomegaly, and right inguinal lymphadenopathy.

Histologic Findings

- Diffuse atypical lymphoid infiltrate with scattered large atypical cells

Differential Diagnosis

- MCCHL
- LRCHL
- PTGC
- PTCL

IHC Studies

- CD20 strong +, PAX5 strong+, occasional CD30+ large typical lymphocytes.
- CD3 shows mostly T cell in the background.

Additional IHC Studies

- OCT2+, BOB1+, CD30−, CD15−, CD45+, EBER for *EBV*−.
- CD21 demonstrate no obvious follicular dendritic meshworks.

Final Diagnosis

T-cell/histiocyte-rich large B-cell lymphoma (THRLBCL)

Take-Home Messages

1. THRLBCL shows a few CD20+, PAX5+, OCT2+, BOB1+ large atypical B cells in the background of diffuse T-cell or histiocytic infiltrate without follicular dendritic meshworks.
2. NLPHL, particularly diffuse T-cell-rich variant, show similar large atypical B cells ringed by CD57+/PD1 T cells in the background of B-cell nodules with at least one follicular dendritic meshwork.
3. MCCHL or LRCHL shows CD30+, CD15+/−, PAX5 weak+, CD20−, CD45−, OCT2−, BOB1− H or RS cells in the background of lymphocytes.
4. Those cases with similar morphologic features but *EBV* infection in large cells are best classified as *EBV*-positive DLBCL per the recent WHO classification, rather than THRLBCL.

Case 8 (Fig. 9.8)

Learning Objectives

1. To become familiar with the histologic morphologic features of PMLBCL
2. To become familiar with the immunohistochemical features of the PMLBCL
3. To become familiar with its differentiation from classic Hodgkin lymphoma

Case History

A 35-year-old female presented with large mediastinal mass.

Histologic Findings

- Diffuse large atypical lymphocytes in the background of fine fibrosis

Differential Diagnosis

- cHL
- GZL
- Mediastinal involvement by conventional DLBCL

IHC Studies

- CD20+ (strong), CD30 occasionally +
- CD79a+, CD45+, CD15−

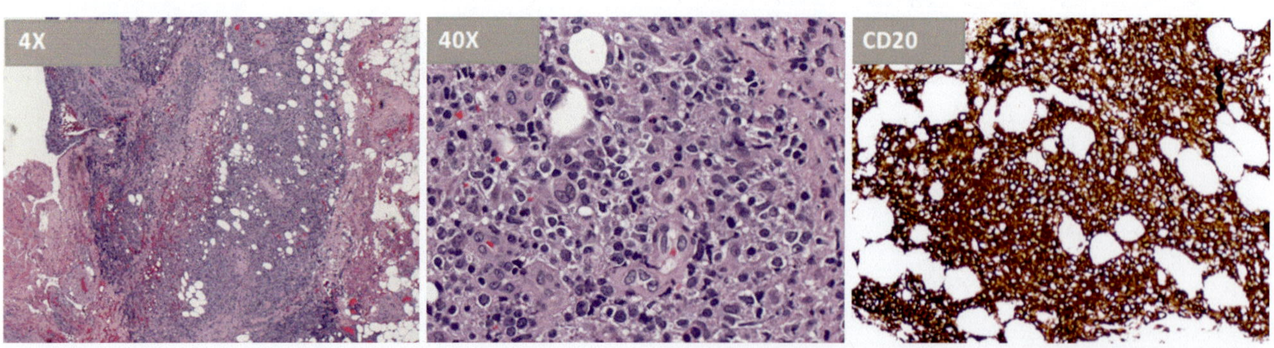

Fig. 9.8 Case 8, primary mediastinal (thymic) large B-cell lymphoma (PMLBCL). Sheets of large atypical lymphocytes in the background of compartmentalization alveolar fine fibrosis (4× and 40×). The large atypical lymphocytes are positive for CD20, and PAX5 (strong), Oct2, and CD23, and occasionally positive for CD30 (not shown)

Additional IHC Studies

- PAX5 strong +, CD30 occasionally+, CD23 subset+, EBER for *EBV*−

Final Diagnosis

Primary mediastinal (thymic) large B-cell lymphoma (PMLBCL)

Take-Home Messages

1. PMLBCL shows medium-sized to large atypical cells that are partially CD30+, but also strongly positive for CD20, CD45, PAX5, OCT2, and BOB1, which are usually negative or only weak positive in cHL.
2. The diagnosis of primary mediastinal (thymic) large B-cell lymphoma can be established only after ruling extrathoracic involvement of the disease.

Case 9 (Fig. 9.9)

Learning Objectives

1. To become familiar with the histologic morphologic features of gray zone lymphoma
2. To become familiar with the immunohistochemical features of gray zone lymphoma
3. To become familiar with its differentiation from classic Hodgkin lymphoma

Case History

A 30-year-old male presented with a large anterior mediastinal mass.

Histologic Findings

- Diffuse infiltrate of Hodgkin or RS cells or like cells (40×)

Differential Diagnosis

- Nodular sclerosis classic Hodgkin lymphoma (NSCHL)
- Primary mediastinal large B-cell lymphoma (PMLBCL)
- Anaplastic large cell lymphoma (ALCL)
- T-cell/histiocyte-rich large B-cell lymphoma (T/HRLBCL)

IHC Studies

- CD30+, CD20 strong+, OCT2 strong+, CD45 strong+

Additional IHC Studies

- CD15−, PAX5 weak+, EBER for *EBV*−

Final Diagnosis

B-cell lymphoma, unclassifiable, with features intermediate between diffuse large B-cell lymphoma and classic Hodgkin lymphoma (gray zone lymphoma)

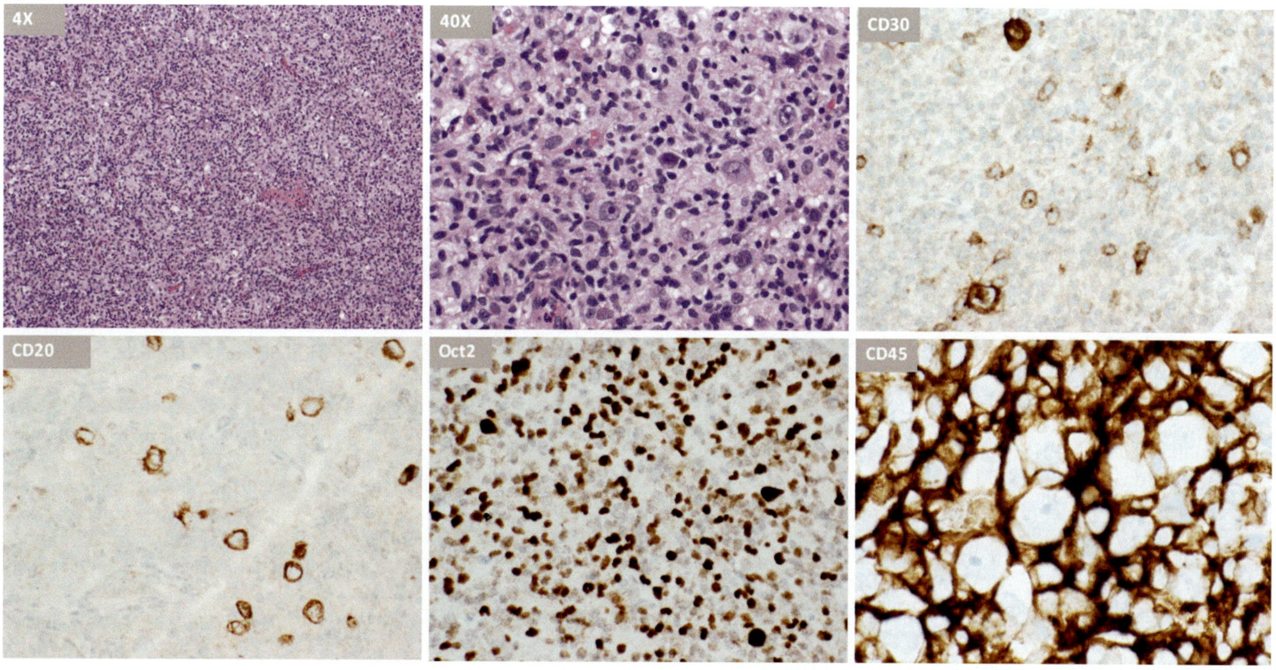

Fig. 9.9 Case 9, gray zone lymphoma (GZL). Numerous large atypical lymphocytes, including some Hodgkin or Hodgkin-like cells in an inflammatory background (4× and 40×). The large atypical cells are positive for CD30, but also show strong positivity for CD20, OCT2, CD45, as well as Bob1 (not shown)

Take-Home Messages

1. Gray zone lymphoma shows classic Hodgkin lymphoma-like morphology but with strong CD20 or OCT2/CD79a/BOB1 or CD45 expression (DLBCL phenotype) or, otherwise, demonstrates diffuse large B-cell lymphoma-like morphology but with weak CD20 and other B-cell markers (phenotype resembling cHL).
2. While most cases of gray zone lymphoma occur in anterior mediastinum, rare cases are reported in other anatomic sites.

References

1. Swerdlow SH, Campo E, Harris NL, Jaffe ES, Pileri S, Stein H, et al. WHO classification of tumours of haematopoietic and lymphoid tissues. 4th ed: World Health Organization Classification of Tumours; 2017: WHO International Agency for Research on Cancer (IARC). 585.
2. Connors JM. State-of-the-art therapeutics: Hodgkin's lymphoma. J Clin Oncol. 2005;23(26):6400–8.
3. Diehl V, Engert A, Re D. New strategies for the treatment of advanced-stage Hodgkin's lymphoma. Hematol Oncol Clin North Am. 2007;21(5):897–914.
4. Board, P.P.T.E. Childhood Hodgkin Lymphoma Treatment (PDQ(R)): Health Professional Version, in PDQ Cancer Information Summaries. Bethesda, MD; 2002.
5. Laurent C, Do C, Gourraud PA, de Paiva GR, Valmary S, Brousset P. Prevalence of common non-Hodgkin lymphomas and subtypes of Hodgkin lymphoma by nodal site of involvement: a systematic retrospective review of 938 cases. Medicine (Baltimore). 2015;94(25):e987.
6. Huppmann AR, Nicolae A, Slack GW, Pittaluga S, Davies-Hill T, Ferry JA, et al. EBV may be expressed in the LP cells of nodular lymphocyte-predominant Hodgkin lymphoma (NLPHL) in both children and adults. Am J Surg Pathol. 2014;38(3):316–24.
7. Herbst H, Dallenbach F, Hummel M, Niedobitek G, Pileri S, Muller-Lantzsch N, et al. Epstein-Barr virus latent membrane protein expression in Hodgkin and Reed-Sternberg cells. Proc Natl Acad Sci U S A. 1991;88(11):4766–70.
8. Herbst H, Niedobitek G, Kneba M, Hummel M, Finn T, Anagnostopoulos I, et al. High incidence of Epstein-Barr virus genomes in Hodgkin's disease. Am J Pathol. 1990;137(1):13–8.
9. Weiss LM. Epstein-Barr virus and Hodgkin's disease. Curr Oncol Rep. 2000;2(2):199–204.
10. Weiss LM, Movahed LA, Warnke RA, Sklar J. Detection of Epstein-Barr viral genomes in Reed-Sternberg cells of Hodgkin's disease. N Engl J Med. 1989;320(8):502–6.
11. Shiels MS, Movahed LA, Warnke RA, Sklar J. Prevalence of HIV Infection among U.S. Hodgkin lymphoma cases. Cancer Epidemiol Biomark Prev. 2014;23(2):274–81.
12. Karube K, Niino D, Kimura Y, Ohshima K. Classic Hodgkin lymphoma, lymphocyte depleted type: clinicopathological analysis and prognostic comparison with other types of classic Hodgkin lymphoma. Pathol Res Pract. 2013;209(4):201–7.
13. Chittal SM, Alard C, Rossi JF, al Saati T, Le Tourneau A, Diebold J, et al. Further phenotypic evidence that nodular, lymphocyte-predominant Hodgkin's disease is a large B-cell lymphoma in evolution. Am J Surg Pathol. 1990;14(11):1024–35.
14. Hansmann ML, Stein H, Fellbaum C, Hui PK, Parwaresch MR, Lennert K. Nodular paragranuloma can transform into high-grade malignant lymphoma of B type. Hum Pathol. 1989;20(12):1169–75.
15. Miettinen M, Franssila KO, Saxen E. Hodgkin's disease, lymphocytic predominance nodular. Increased risk for subsequent non-Hodgkin's lymphomas. Cancer. 1983;51(12):2293–300.
16. Rappaport H, Berard CW, Butler JJ, Dorfman RF, Lukes RJ, Thomas LB. Report of the committee on histopathological criteria contributing to staging of Hodgkin's disease. Cancer Res. 1971;31(11):1864–5.
17. Schwarting R, Gerdes J, Durkop H, Falini B, Pileri S, Stein H. BER-H2: a new anti-Ki-1 (CD30) monoclonal antibody directed at a formol-resistant epitope. Blood. 1989;74(5):1678–89.
18. Stein H, Mason DY, Gerdes J, O'Connor N, Wainscoat J, Pallesen G, et al. The expression of the Hodgkin's disease associated antigen Ki-1 in reactive and neoplastic lymphoid tissue: evidence that Reed-Sternberg cells and histiocytic malignancies are derived from activated lymphoid cells. Blood. 1985;66(4):848–58.
19. Stein H, Gerdes J, Kirchner H, Schaadt M, Diehl V. Hodgkin and Sternberg-Reed cell antigen(s) detected by an antiserum to a cell line (L428) derived from Hodgkin's disease. Int J Cancer. 1981;28(4):425–9.
20. Schmid C, Pan L, Diss T, Isaacson PG. Expression of B-cell antigens by Hodgkin's and Reed-Sternberg cells. Am J Pathol. 1991;139(4):701–7.
21. Zukerberg LR, Collins AB, Ferry JA, Harris NL. Coexpression of CD15 and CD20 by Reed-Sternberg cells in Hodgkin's disease. Am J Pathol. 1991;139(3):475–83.
22. Foss HD, Reusch R, Demel G, Lenz G, Anagnostopoulos I, Hummel M, et al. Frequent expression of the B-cell-specific activator protein in Reed-Sternberg cells of classical Hodgkin's disease provides further evidence for its B-cell origin. Blood. 1999;94(9):3108–13.
23. Slack GW, Ferry JA, Hasserjian RP, Sohani AR, Longtine JA, Harris NL, et al. Lymphocyte depleted Hodgkin lymphoma: an evaluation with immunophenotyping and genetic analysis. Leuk Lymphoma. 2009;50(6):937–43.
24. Tzankov A, Bourgau C, Kaiser A, Zimpfer A, Maurer R, Pileri SA, et al. Rare expression of T-cell markers in classical Hodgkin's lymphoma. Mod Pathol. 2005;18(12):1542–9.
25. Tzankov A, Zimpfer A, Pehrs AC, Lugli A, Went P, Maurer R, et al. Expression of B-cell markers in classic Hodgkin lymphoma: a tissue microarray analysis of 330 cases. Mod Pathol. 2003;16(11):1141–7.
26. Venkataraman G, Song JY, Tzankov A, Dirnhofer S, Heinze G, Kohl M, et al. Aberrant T-cell antigen expression in classic Hodgkin lymphoma is associated with decreased event-free survival and overall survival. Blood. 2013;121(10):1795–804.
27. Sakai J, Tanae K, Takahashi N, Nagata K, Yoshino T, Tamaru J, et al. Lymphocyte-rich classic Hodgkin lymphoma. A case with difficulty in distinguishing from nodular lymphocyte-predominant Hodgkin lymphoma. J Clin Exp Hematop. 2015;55(1):23–8.
28. Chang KL, Weiss LM. Lymphocyte depletion Hodgkin lymphoma. In: Weiner N, et al., editors. Modern surgical pathology. 2nd ed: Science Direct; 2009.
29. Coles FB, Cartun RW, Pastuszak WT. Hodgkin's disease, lymphocyte-predominant type: immunoreactivity with B-cell antibodies. Mod Pathol. 1988;1(4):274–8.
30. Pinkus GS, Said JW. Hodgkin's disease, lymphocyte predominance type, nodular--a distinct entity? Unique staining profile for L&H variants of Reed-Sternberg cells defined by monoclonal antibodies to leukocyte common antigen, granulocyte-specific antigen, and B-cell-specific antigen. Am J Pathol. 1985;118(1):1–6.
31. Pinkus GS, Said JW. Hodgkin's disease, lymphocyte predominance type, nodular--further evidence for a B cell derivation. L & H variants of Reed-Sternberg cells express L26, a pan B cell marker. Am J Pathol. 1988;133(2):211–7.
32. Stein H, Marafioti T, Foss HD, Laumen H, Hummel M, Anagnostopoulos I, et al. Down-regulation of BOB.1/OBF.1 and Oct2 in classical Hodgkin disease but not in lymphocyte predomi-

nant Hodgkin disease correlates with immunoglobulin transcription. Blood. 2001;97(2):496–501.
33. Mottok A, Hansmann ML, Brauninger A. Activation induced cytidine deaminase expression in lymphocyte predominant Hodgkin lymphoma. J Clin Pathol. 2005;58(9):1002–4.
34. Anagnostopoulos I, Hansmann ML, Franssila K, Harris M, Harris NL, Jaffe ES, et al. European Task Force on Lymphoma project on lymphocyte predominance Hodgkin disease: histologic and immunohistologic analysis of submitted cases reveals 2 types of Hodgkin disease with a nodular growth pattern and abundant lymphocytes. Blood. 2000;96(5):1889–99.
35. Poppema S. The nature of the lymphocytes surrounding Reed-Sternberg cells in nodular lymphocyte predominance and in other types of Hodgkin's disease. Am J Pathol. 1989;135(2):351–7.
36. David JA, Huang JZ. Diagnostic utility of flow cytometry analysis of reactive T cells in nodular lymphocyte-predominant Hodgkin lymphoma. Am J Clin Pathol. 2016;145(1):107–15.
37. Rahemtullah A, Reichard KK, Preffer FI, Harris NL, Hasserjian RP. A double-positive CD4+CD8+ T-cell population is commonly found in nodular lymphocyte predominant Hodgkin lymphoma. Am J Clin Pathol. 2006;126(5):805–14.
38. Connors JM, Jurczak W, Straus DJ, Ansell SM, Kim WS, Gallamini A, et al. Brentuximab vedotin with chemotherapy for stage III or IV Hodgkin's lymphoma. N Engl J Med. 2018;378(4):331–44.
39. Achten R, Verhoef G, Vanuytsel L, De Wolf-Peeters C. T-cell/histiocyte-rich large B-cell lymphoma: a distinct clinicopathologic entity. J Clin Oncol. 2002;20(5):1269–77.
40. Ramsay AD, Smith WJ, Isaacson PG. T-cell-rich B-cell lymphoma. Am J Surg Pathol. 1988;12(6):433–43.
41. Cazals-Hatem D, Lepage E, Brice P, Ferrant A, d'Agay MF, Baumelou E, et al. Primary mediastinal large B-cell lymphoma. A clinicopathologic study of 141 cases compared with 916 nonmediastinal large B-cell lymphomas, a GELA ("Groupe d'Etude des Lymphomes de l'Adulte") study. Am J Surg Pathol. 1996;20(7):877–88.
42. Savage KJ, Al-Rajhi N, Voss N, Paltiel C, Klasa R, Gascoyne RD, et al. Favorable outcome of primary mediastinal large B-cell lymphoma in a single institution: the British Columbia experience. Ann Oncol. 2006;17(1):123–30.
43. Zinzani PL, Martelli M, Poletti V, Vitolo U, Gobbi PG, Chisesi T, et al. Practice guidelines for the management of extranodal non-Hodgkin's lymphomas of adult non-immunodeficient patients. Part I: primary lung and mediastinal lymphomas. A project of the Italian Society of Hematology, the Italian Society of Experimental Hematology and the Italian Group for Bone Marrow Transplantation. Haematologica. 2008;93(9):1364–71.
44. Paulli M, Strater J, Gianelli U, Rousset MT, Gambacorta M, Orlandi E, et al. Mediastinal B-cell lymphoma: a study of its histomorphologic spectrum based on 109 cases. Hum Pathol. 1999;30(2):178–87.
45. Traverse-Glehen A, Pittaluga S, Gaulard P, Sorbara L, Alonso MA, Raffeld M, et al. Mediastinal gray zone lymphoma: the missing link between classic Hodgkin's lymphoma and mediastinal large B-cell lymphoma. Am J Surg Pathol. 2005;29(11):1411–21.
46. Barth TF, Leithauser F, Joos S, Bentz M, Moller P. Mediastinal (thymic) large B-cell lymphoma: where do we stand? Lancet Oncol. 2002;3(4):229–34.
47. Menestrina F, Chilosi M, Bonetti F, Lestani M, Scarpa A, Novelli P, et al. Mediastinal large-cell lymphoma of B-type, with sclerosis: histopathological and immunohistochemical study of eight cases. Histopathology. 1986;10(6):589–600.
48. Moller P, Lammler B, Herrmann B, Otto HF, Moldenhauer G, Momburg F. The primary mediastinal clear cell lymphoma of B-cell type has variable defects in MHC antigen expression. Immunology. 1986;59(3):411–7.
49. Pileri SA, Gaidano G, Zinzani PL, Falini B, Gaulard P, Zucca E, et al. Primary mediastinal B-cell lymphoma: high frequency of BCL-6 mutations and consistent expression of the transcription factors OCT-2, BOB.1, and PU.1 in the absence of immunoglobulins. Am J Pathol. 2003;162(1):243–53.
50. Higgins JP, Warnke RA. CD30 expression is common in mediastinal large B-cell lymphoma. Am J Clin Pathol. 1999;112(2):241–7.
51. Copie-Bergman C, Gaulard P, Maouche-Chretien L, Briere J, Haioun C, Alonso MA, et al. The MAL gene is expressed in primary mediastinal large B-cell lymphoma. Blood. 1999;94(10):3567–75.
52. Copie-Bergman C, Plonquet A, Alonso MA, Boulland ML, Marquet J, Divine M, et al. MAL expression in lymphoid cells: further evidence for MAL as a distinct molecular marker of primary mediastinal large B-cell lymphomas. Mod Pathol. 2002;15(11):1172–80.
53. Gentry M, Bodo J, Durkin L, Hsi ED. Performance of a commercially available MAL antibody in the diagnosis of primary mediastinal large B-cell lymphoma. Am J Surg Pathol. 2017;41(2):189–94.
54. Weinberg OK, Rodig SJ, Pozdnyakova O, Ren L, Arber DA, Ohgami RS. Surface light chain expression in primary mediastinal large B-cell lymphomas by multiparameter flow cytometry. Am J Clin Pathol. 2015;144(4):635–41.
55. Kanavaros P, Gaulard P, Charlotte F, Martin N, Ducos C, Lebezu M, et al. Discordant expression of immunoglobulin and its associated molecule mb-1/CD79a is frequently found in mediastinal large B cell lymphomas. Am J Pathol. 1995;146(3):735–41.
56. Loddenkemper C, Anagnostopoulos I, Hummel M, Johrens-Leder K, Foss HD, Jundt F, et al. Differential Emu enhancer activity and expression of BOB.1/OBF.1, Oct2, PU.1, and immunoglobulin in reactive B-cell populations, B-cell non-Hodgkin lymphomas, and Hodgkin lymphomas. J Pathol. 2004;202(1):60–9.
57. Garcia JF, Mollejo M, Fraga M, Forteza J, Muniesa JA, Perez-Guillermo M, et al. Large B-cell lymphoma with Hodgkin's features. Histopathology. 2005;47(1):101–10.
58. Fanale MA, Horwitz SM, Forero-Torres A, Bartlett NL, Advani RH, Pro B, et al. Brentuximab vedotin in the front-line treatment of patients with CD30+ peripheral T-cell lymphomas: results of a phase I study. J Clin Oncol. 2014;32(28):3137–43.
59. Gonzalez CL, Medeiros LJ, Jaffe ES. Composite lymphoma. A clinicopathologic analysis of nine patients with Hodgkin's disease and B-cell non-Hodgkin's lymphoma. Am J Clin Pathol. 1991;96(1):81–9.
60. Perrone T, Frizzera G, Rosai J. Mediastinal diffuse large-cell lymphoma with sclerosis. A clinicopathologic study of 60 cases. Am J Surg Pathol. 1986;10(3):176–91.
61. Chen BJ, Chapuy B, Ouyang J, Sun HH, Roemer MG, Xu ML, et al. PD-L1 expression is characteristic of a subset of aggressive B-cell lymphomas and virus-associated malignancies. Clin Cancer Res. 2013;19(13):3462–73.
62. Dojcinov SD, Venkataraman G, Pittaluga S, Wlodarska I, Schrager JA, Raffeld M, et al. Age-related EBV-associated lymphoproliferative disorders in the Western population: a spectrum of reactive lymphoid hyperplasia and lymphoma. Blood. 2011;117(18):4726–35.
63. Nicolae A, Pittaluga S, Abdullah S, Steinberg SM, Pham TA, Davies-Hill T, et al. EBV-positive large B-cell lymphomas in young patients: a nodal lymphoma with evidence for a tolerogenic immune environment. Blood. 2015;126(7):863–72.
64. Lim MS, Beaty M, Sorbara L, Cheng RZ, Pittaluga S, Raffeld M, et al. T-cell/histiocyte-rich large B-cell lymphoma: a heterogeneous entity with derivation from germinal center B cells. Am J Surg Pathol. 2002;26(11):1458–66.
65. Bossard C, Dobay MP, Parrens M, Lamant L, Missiaglia E, Haioun C, et al. Immunohistochemistry as a valuable tool to assess CD30 expression in peripheral T-cell lymphomas: high correlation with mRNA levels. Blood. 2014;124(19):2983–6.
66. Sabattini E, Pizzi M, Tabanelli V, Baldin P, Sacchetti CS, Agostinelli C, et al. CD30 expression in peripheral T-cell lymphomas. Haematologica. 2013;98(8):e81–2.

67. Barry TS, Jaffe ES, Sorbara L, Raffeld M, Pittaluga S. Peripheral T-cell lymphomas expressing CD30 and CD15. Am J Surg Pathol. 2003;27(12):1513–22.
68. Went P, Agostinelli C, Gallamini A, Piccaluga PP, Ascani S, Sabattini E, et al. Marker expression in peripheral T-cell lymphoma: a proposed clinical-pathologic prognostic score. J Clin Oncol. 2006;24(16):2472–9.
69. Attygalle AD, Cabecadas J, Gaulard P, Jaffe ES, de Jong D, Ko YH, et al. Peripheral T-cell and NK-cell lymphomas and their mimics; taking a step forward - report on the lymphoma workshop of the XVIth meeting of the European Association for Haematopathology and the Society for Hematopathology. Histopathology. 2014;64(2):171–99.
70. Dupuis J, Emile JF, Mounier N, Gisselbrecht C, Martin-Garcia N, Petrella T, et al. Prognostic significance of Epstein-Barr virus in nodal peripheral T-cell lymphoma, unspecified: a Groupe d'Etude des Lymphomes de l'Adulte (GELA) study. Blood. 2006;108(13):4163–9.
71. Ha SY, Sung J, Ju H, Karube K, Kim SJ, Kim WS, et al. Epstein-Barr virus-positive nodal peripheral T cell lymphomas: clinicopathologic and gene expression profiling study. Pathol Res Pract. 2013;209(7):448–54.
72. Cazals-Hatem D, Andre M, Mounier N, Copin MC, Divine M, Berger F, et al. Pathologic and clinical features of 77 Hodgkin's lymphoma patients treated in a lymphoma protocol (LNH87): a GELA study. Am J Surg Pathol. 2001;25(3):297–306.
73. Mani H, Jaffe ES. Hodgkin lymphoma: an update on its biology with new insights into classification. Clin Lymphoma Myeloma. 2009;9(3):206–16.
74. Falini B, Bigerna B, Fizzotti M, Pulford K, Pileri SA, Delsol G, et al. ALK expression defines a distinct group of T/null lymphomas ("ALK lymphomas") with a wide morphological spectrum. Am J Pathol. 1998;153(3):875–86.
75. Benharroch D, Meguerian-Bedoyan Z, Lamant L, Amin C, Brugieres L, Terrier-Lacombe MJ, et al. ALK-positive lymphoma: a single disease with a broad spectrum of morphology. Blood. 1998;91(6):2076–84.
76. Pileri SA, Grogan TM, Harris NL, Banks P, Campo E, Chan JK, et al. Tumours of histiocytes and accessory dendritic cells: an immunohistochemical approach to classification from the International Lymphoma Study Group based on 61 cases. Histopathology. 2002;41(1):1–29.
77. Ramchandren R, Advani RH, Ansell SM, Bartlett NL, Chen R, Connors JM, et al. Brentuximab vedotin plus chemotherapy in North American subjects with newly diagnosed stage III or IV Hodgkin lymphoma. Clin Cancer Res. 2019;25(6):1718–26.
78. Younes A, Gopal AK, Smith SE, Ansell SM, Rosenblatt JD, Savage KJ, et al. Results of a pivotal phase II study of brentuximab vedotin for patients with relapsed or refractory Hodgkin's lymphoma. J Clin Oncol. 2012;30(18):2183–9.
79. Allen PB, Winter JN. Controversies in the approach to initial therapy of Hodgkin lymphoma. Curr Oncol Rep. 2019;21(5):39.
80. Nagai H. Recent advances in Hodgkin lymphoma: interim PET and molecular-targeted therapy. Jpn J Clin Oncol. 2015;45(2):137–45.
81. Santos MAO, Lima MM. CD20 role in pathophysiology of Hodgkin's disease. Rev Assoc Med Bras (1992). 2017;63(9):810–3.
82. Koh YW, Han JH, Yoon DH, Suh C, Huh J. Epstein-Barr virus positivity is associated with angiogenesis in, and poorer survival of, patients receiving standard treatment for classical Hodgkin's lymphoma. Hematol Oncol. 2018;36(1):182–8.
83. Ansell SM. Immunotherapy in Hodgkin lymphoma: the road ahead. Trends Immunol. 2019;40:380.
84. Ansell SM, Lesokhin AM, Borrello I, Halwani A, Scott EC, Gutierrez M, et al. PD-1 blockade with nivolumab in relapsed or refractory Hodgkin's lymphoma. N Engl J Med. 2015;372(4):311–9.
85. Bedewy M, El-Maghraby S, Bedewy A. CD163 and c-Met expression in the lymph node and the correlations between elevated levels of serum free light chain and the different clinicopathological parameters of advanced classical Hodgkin's lymphoma. Blood Res. 2013;48(2):121–7.

Posttransplant Lymphoproliferative Disorders (PTLDs)

10

Jun Wang

List of Frequently Asked Questions

1. What is PTLD?
2. What is the spectrum of PTLDs?
3. How many categories of PTLDs?
4. What is required in a diagnostic workup of PTLD?
5. What are the key histologic features of nondestructive PTLDs, and how are they distinguished from other types of PTLDs?
6. What are the expected results of common immunomarkers for nondestructive PTLDs?
7. What are the expected genetic profiles of nondestructive PTLDs?
8. What is required to diagnose nondestructive PTLDs?
9. What are the key histologic features distinguishing polymorphic PTLD (P-PTLD) from nondestructive PTLDs?
10. What is the differential diagnosis of P-PTLD?
11. What are the expected results of common immunomarkers for P-PTLDs?
12. What are the expected genetic profiles of P-PTLDs?
13. How are monomorphic PTLDs (M-PTLDs) defined?
14. What are the entities included in monomorphic B-cell PTLDs?
15. What are the expected results of common immunomarkers for monomorphic B-cell PTLDs?
16. What are the expected genetic profiles of monomorphic B-cell PTLDs?
17. What are the entities included in monomorphic T/NK-cell PTLDs?
18. What are the expected results of common immunomarkers for monomorphic T/NK-cell PTLDs?
19. What are the expected genetic profiles of monomorphic T-cell PTLDs?
20. What is classic Hodgkin lymphoma PTLD (HL-PTLD)?
21. How is the previously so-called Hodgkin lymphoma-like PTLD (HL-like PTLD) differentiated from classic HL-PTLD?
22. How is PTLD on small tissue biopsy worked up?
23. How is PTLD distinguished from rejection?

J. Wang (✉)
Pathology and Laboratory Medicine, Loma Linda University Medical Center, Loma Linda, CA, USA
e-mail: JWang@llu.edu

1. What is PTLD?

- Posttransplant lymphoproliferative disorders (PTLDs) are lymphoid or plasmacytic proliferations that develop in an immunosuppressed recipient of a solid organ, bone marrow, and/or stem cell allograft [1–6].

2. What is the spectrum of PTLDs?

- The spectrum of PTLDs ranges from usually *EBV*-driven polyclonal lymphoid/plasmacytic proliferations to *EBV*-positive or *EBV*-negative monoclonal lymphomatous or plasmacytic proliferations indistinguishable from a subset of B-cell/plasma cell or less often T/NK-cell lymphomas including classic Hodgkin lymphoma, which occur in immunocompetent individuals [1–4].

3. How many categories of PTLDs?

- The 2017 revised WHO Classification of Tumours of Haematopoietic and Lymphoid Tissues describes four categories of PTLD: nondestructive, polymorphic (P-PTLD), monomorphic (M-PTLD), and classic Hodgkin lymphoma (HL-PTLD) PTLDs (Table 10.1) [4].

E. Wang, A. S. Lagoo (eds.), *Practical Lymph Node and Bone Marrow Pathology*, Practical Anatomic Pathology,
https://doi.org/10.1007/978-3-030-32189-5_10

Table 10.1 WHO categories of posttransplant lymphoproliferative disorder (PTLD)[a]

Nondestructive PTLDs
Plasmacytic hyperplasia
Infectious mononucleosis
Florid follicular hyperplasia
Polymorphic PTLD
Monomorphic PTLDs
B-cell neoplasms
DLBCL
BL/BL-like (high grade B cell lymphoma)
Plasma cell myeloma
Plasmacytoma
Other
T-cell neoplasms
PTCL, NOS
Hepatosplenic T-cell lymphoma
Other
Classic Hodgkin lymphoma (HL) PTLD[b]

[a]2017 WHO classification and [b]its reference #3198 by Pitman and Wang et al. *AJSP* 2006;30:470–6

Table 10.2 Evaluation of pathologic specimens for the diagnosis of PTLD

Evaluation	Necessity	Usage
Histomorphology	Required	Architecture/cytology for categorization
Immunophenotype (immunohistochemistry (IHC)/flow cytometry/ chromogenic in situ hybridization (CISH)	Required*	Lineage/subset or light chain monotypic* determination, required for classification
EBER in situ hybridization	Required**	Most sensitive for *EBV*+ PTLDs, diagnosis, and prognosis; distinguishing PTLD from rejection in allograft
Molecular/cytogenetics	Variably useful	Determination of clonality and/or lineage of clonal population(s), chromosomal and/or oncogene abnormalities, may be useful for categorization
EBV clonality	Not necessarily required	May be useful for identification of minor clones

(*IHC/flow/CISH useful for PC, polymorphic, monomorphic B-cell cases)
(**if LMP-1+, EBER may not be needed)

4. What is required in a diagnostic workup of PTLD?

- Histomorphology, immunophenotype, and EBER in situ hybridization analysis are typically required for the pathologic diagnosis of PTLD.
- Molecular and cytogenetic studies are helpful for demonstrating clonality and presence of lineage population as well as categorization of PTLD (Table 10.2) [1–5].

5. What are the key histologic features of nondestructive PTLDs, and how are they distinguished from other types of PTLDs?

- A lymphoid/plasmacytic proliferation in transplant recipient, characterized by some degree of architectural preservation of the involved tissue, i.e., with preservation of the nodal sinuses or tonsillar crypts, and residual or florid reactive follicles (FFH) in some cases, but an absence of any diagnostic features of a malignant lymphoma or other known explanations and nonspecific chronic inflammatory processes [1–6].
  - Plasmacytic hyperplasia (PH) is characterized by the presence of numerous plasma cells, some small lymphocytes, and rare immunoblasts in the expanded parafollicular and interfollicular zones.
  - Infectious mononucleosis (IM)-like lesion shows paracortical/interfollicular expansion with numerous immunoblasts in a background of mixed T cells, B cells, and plasma cells.
  - Florid follicular hyperplasia (FFH) shows enlarged lesional mass with marked follicular hyperplasia with prominent reactive germinal centers.

6. What are the expected results of common immunomarkers for nondestructive PTLDs?

- The proliferations contain mixed polyclonal B cells, plasma cells, and T cells with no apparent phenotypic aberrancy.
- *EBV* is positive in many of the cells in PH and FFH, as well as in nearly all of the immunoblasts in IM PTLD [1–6].

7. What are the expected genetic profiles of nondestructive PTLDs?

- Clonally rearranged IG genes are generally not expected in nondestructive PTLDs, although small monoclonal or oligoclonal populations have been reported, with unknown significance.
- Rare simple clonal cytogenetic abnormalities have also been described in FFH [1–12].

8. What is required to diagnose nondestructive PTLDs?

- Formation of a mass lesion in lymph node, tonsil, or adenoid along with the above-described morphologic changes and/or a significant *EBV* positivity (usually more than at least 20%) is necessary to make a diagnosis of one of the nondestructive PTLDs.
- In FFH the *EBV*-positive cells are more concentrated in one or few germinal centers with occasional positive cells between the follicles by EBER in situ hybridization [1–5, 8–12].

9. What are the key histologic features distinguishing polymorphic PTLD (P-PTLD) from nondestructive PTLDs?

- Polymorphic PTLDs are defined as destructive lesions composed of a heterogeneous mixture of immunoblasts, plasma cells, and small- to medium-sized lymphoid cells that efface the nodal architecture or form destructive extranodal mass(es) and do not fulfill the criteria for any of the recognized lymphomas occurring in immunocompetent hosts [1–8].

10. What is the differential diagnosis of P-PTLD?

- Since there are no established criteria for the proportion of transformed larger cells and immunoblasts in P-PTLD, its distinction from cases of IM lesions with marked architectural distortion may be hard, as is from M-PTLDs, particularly those cases with plasmacytic differentiation [4].
- There may be a continuous spectrum between P-PTLDs and monomorphic PTLD (M-PTLD), whereas others closely resemble Hodgkin lymphoma (so-called HL-like PTLD), which are currently considered to be a form of M-PTLD [1–13].
- Although they may appear quite polymorphic morphologically, PTLDs that fulfill the criteria for T-cell/histiocyte-rich large B-cell lymphoma or *EBV*-positive diffuse large B-cell lymphoma, NOS, are best regarded as a form of M-PTLD [4].
- In addition, *EBV*+ mucocutaneous ulcer needs to be distinguished from P-PTLD [4, 14].

11. What are the expected results of common immunomarkers for P-PTLDs?

- Immunostains will show presence of many B cells with or without light chain restriction, admixed with a variable proportion of heterogeneous T cells, which sometimes can be moderate to predominant in numbers.
- CD30-positive large atypical cells including Reed-Sternberg (RS)-like cells are commonly seen, but they are usually CD20+ and CD15−.
- *EBV* positivity is detected in most P-PTLD cases by EBER in situ hybridization [1–4].

12. What are the expected genetic profiles of P-PTLDs?

- Most P-PTLDs are expected to have demonstrable clonally rearranged IG genes.
- The most sensitive method for demonstrating clonal *EBV* genomes in *EBV*+ P-PTLD is the analysis of *EBV* terminal repeat.
- Cytogenetic abnormalities are variable but not universal [1–4].

13. How are monomorphic PTLDs (M-PTLDs) defined?

- M-PTLDs are defined as posttransplant lymphoproliferations that fulfill the criteria for one of the B-cell or T/NK-cell neoplasms that are identical to those occurring in immunocompetent hosts.
- M-PTLDs can be further subcategorized as either monomorphic B-cell PTLDs or monomorphic T/NK-cell PTLDs [1–4, 13–18].

14. What are the entities included in monomorphic B-cell PTLDs?

- Monomorphic B-cell PTLDs are monoclonally transformed B-lymphocytic or plasmacytic proliferations that fulfill the morphologic and immunophenotypic and/or molecular/cytogenetic criteria for a diffuse large B-cell lymphoma (DLBCL), or less often a Burkitt lymphoma, or other types of a B-cell lymphoma or a plasma cell neoplasm including plasmacytoma-like and plasma cell myeloma-type PTLDs [1–7, 13–18].

- However, most indolent small B-cell lymphomas are not considered M-PTLD, with the exception of EVB+ extranodal marginal zone lymphoma of mucosa-associated lymphoid tissue (MALT lymphoma) in skin and subcutaneous tissue in immunosuppressed transplant recipients [4, 14].

15. What are the expected results of common immunomarkers for monomorphic B-cell PTLDs?

- Most cases express B-cell-associated antigens (CD19, CD20, CD79a, PAX5), with demonstrable monotypic Ig (~50% cases) [1–4, 13–18].
- CD30 reactivity can be seen in many cases with or without anaplastic morphology.
- DLBCL-type PTLDs can be further subclassified into GC or non-GC (most cases) type based on immunohistochemistry, and most *EBV*− DLBCL PTLDs are GC type, whereas most of the *EBV*+ DLBCL PTLDs are non-GC type [1–4, 15].
- The myelomatous or plasmacytoma-like lesions can be *EBV*+ or − and are phenotypically similar to those in immunocompetent patients [4, 13, 15–18].

16. What are the expected genetic profiles of monomorphic B-cell PTLDs?

- Clonal Ig gene rearrangement is present in virtually all cases.
- *EBV* genomes (in clonal episomal forms) are detected in the majority of cases.
- Other genetic/molecular abnormalities including *BCL6* may be seen [1–4, 13–18].

17. What are the entities included in monomorphic T/NK-cell PTLDs?

- Monomorphic T/NK-cell PTLDs include PTLDs that fulfill the criteria for any type of the T- or NK-cell lymphomas, with the most being peripheral T-cell lymphoma (PTCL), NOS, followed by hepatosplenic T-cell lymphoma, and others (T-LGL, ATL/L, nasal-type NK/T-cell lymphoma, MF/Sézary syndrome, primary S-ALCL, and C-ALCL) [1–4, 19, 20].
- The interval to lymphoma development is typically longer for T-cell PTLDs than for the B-cell cases.
- Involvement of extranodal sites (PB, BM, spleen, skin, liver, GI, and lung) is commonly present, sometimes with associated lymphadenopathy.

18. What are the expected results of common immunomarkers for monomorphic T/NK-cell PTLDs?

- Expression of pan-T-cell and sometimes NK-associated antigens including CD4 or CD8, CD30, CD16, CD56, and ALK and either $\alpha\beta$ or $\gamma\delta$ T-cell receptors is expected, depending on the specific type.
- Most cases (2/3) are *EBV*−, but about 1/3 of cases are *EBV*+ [1–4, 19, 20].

19. What are the expected genetic profiles of monomorphic T-cell PTLDs?

- Demonstrable TCR gene rearrangements are present in T-cell lymphomas.
- i(7)(q10) and + 8 found in most hepatosplenic T-cell lymphomas.
- TP53 and other oncogene mutations are also reported [1–4].

20. What is classic Hodgkin lymphoma PTLD (HL-PTLD)?

- As the rarest subcategory, HL-PTLD should be morphologically and immunophenotypically identical to that of a classic Hodgkin lymphoma that is encountered in immunocompetent hosts.
- The Reed-Sternberg (RS) cells and their variants should be CD45−, CD30+, CD15+, and PAX5+ weakly, as well as *EBV*+ with no positivity in the background bystander small lymphocytes [1–4, 21–25].

21. How is the previously so-called Hodgkin lymphoma-like PTLD (HL-like PTLD) differentiated from classic HL-PTLD?

- Although HL-like PTLD morphologically simulates classic HL-PTLD, there are important immunophenotypic and molecular genetic differences. The RS-like cells in HL-like PTLD are CD45+, CD20+, CD30+/−, but CD15-, and virtually all cases are *EBV*+ in both RS-like cells and bystander small lymphocytes [23–25]. Clonally rearranged *IG* genes are often demonstrable [22, 25].

- More studies have suggested that HL-like PTLD is in fact most often a "monomorphic" B-cell PTLD, with similar immunophenotype, genotype, and clinical behavior [23–25]. Therefore, HL-like PTLD has been recategorized as a form of DLBCL-type monomorphic B-cell PTLD since the 2008 WHO classification [2, 13, 23] and remains the same in the 2017 WHO revision [4, 23].
- Distinction between HL and HL-like PTLD is important for their clinical management as rituximab can be given to this entity [13, 23–25].

22. How is PTLD on small tissue biopsy worked up?

- Histologic evaluation is essential. A basic immunohistochemical panel including B- and T-cell markers, along with Hodgkin lymphoma markers CD30 and CD15 if applicable, as well as EBER in situ hybridization is also essentially needed.
- In patients suspicious for PTLD, biopsies and larger more representative samples from multiple sites are encouraged for PTLD workup as the types of PTLD at different sites in the same patient may be different.

23. How is PTLD distinguished from rejection?

- EBER in situ hybridization analysis is the most sensitive test for *EBV*+ PTLDs, distinguishing PTLD from rejection in allograft [1–4].

Case Presentations

Cases 1–3 Learning Objectives

1. To become familiar with the histologic features of the nondestructive PTLD and its subcategories (plasmacytic hyperplasia, infectious mononucleosis, and florid follicular hyperplasia)
2. To become familiar with the immunohistochemical features of the nondestructive PTLD
3. To generate the differential diagnosis

Case 1 (Fig. 10.1)

Case History

A 6-year-old female with a history of heart transplant at age 2 and on prednisone and tacrolimus presented with an enlarged right neck mass.

Histologic Findings

- The right neck mass showing an enlarged lymph node with markedly expanded paracortical/interfollicular zones but preservation of the nodal architecture with residual lymphoid follicles containing reactive germinal centers (Fig. 10.1a)
- The expanded paracortical/interfollicular zones containing numerous mature plasma cells and rare immunoblasts without significant nuclear atypia (Fig. 10.1b)

Differential Diagnosis

- Nondestructive PTLD, plasmacytic hyperplasia type
- Nondestructive PTLD, infectious mononucleosis type
- Plasmacytoma-type M-PTLD

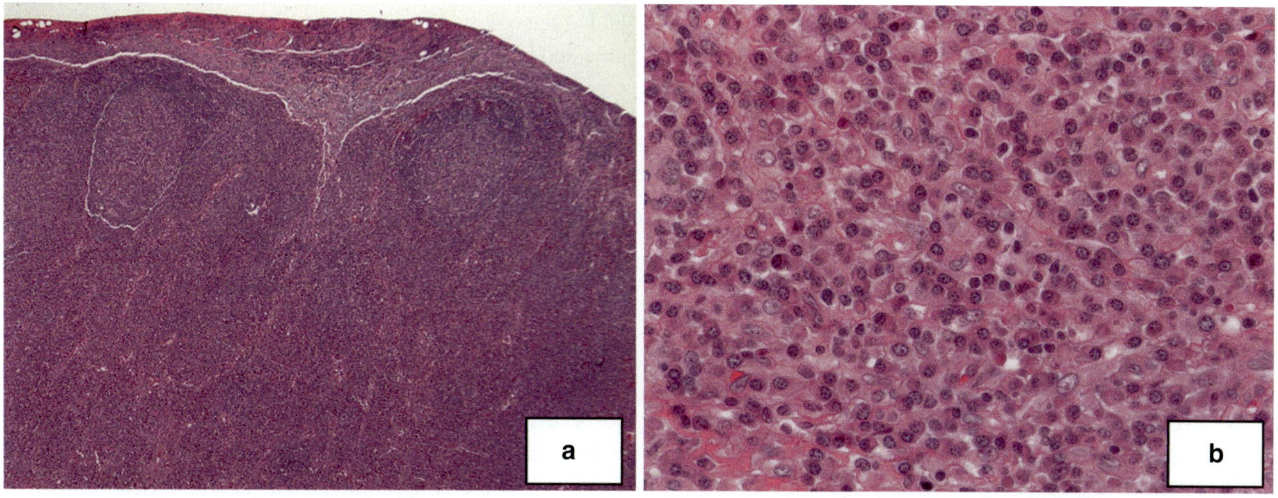

Fig. 10.1 The enlarged right neck lymph node showed markedly expanded paracortical and interfollicular zones but with preservation of the nodal architecture with residual lymphoid follicles containing reactive germinal centers (**a**). The expanded paracortical and interfollicular zones contained numerous mature plasma cells (**b**) and rare immunoblasts

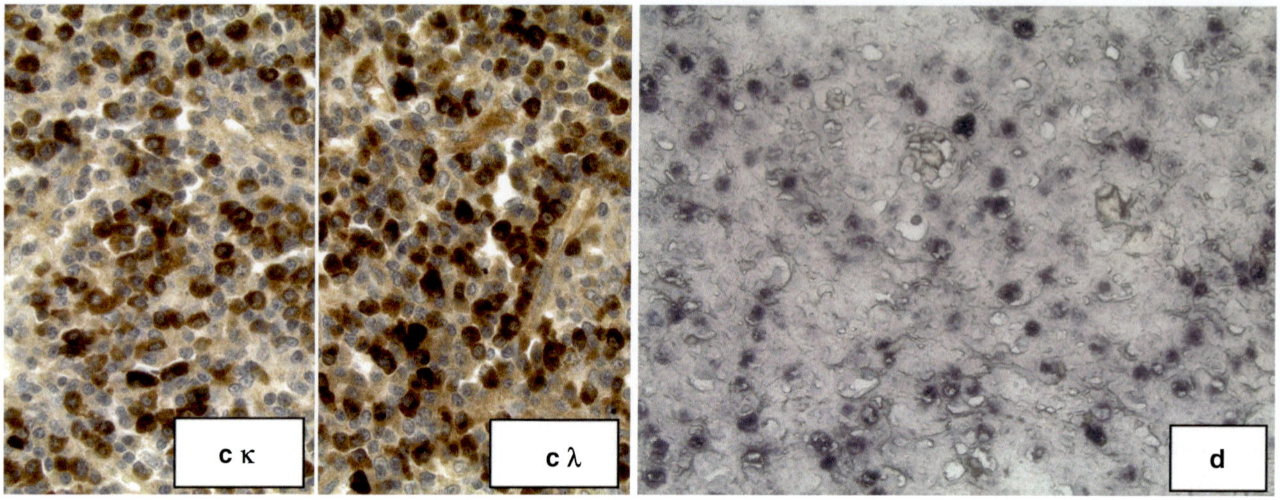

Fig. 10.1 (continued) The plasma cells were polyclonal with a kappa to lambda ratio of ~1–2:1 (**c**), and many of the cell nuclei were *EBV* positive by EBER in situ hybridization (**d**)

IHC and Other Ancillary Studies (Fig. 10.1c, d)

- Numerous CD138-positive plasma cells admixed with scattered polyclonal B cells and T cells without phenotypic aberrancy.
- The plasma cells were polyclonal with approximately a kappa to lambda ratio of ~1–2:1.
- Many of the cell nuclei showing EBER positivity.

Final Diagnosis

Nondestructive PTLD, plasmacytic hyperplasia (PH) type

Case 2 (Fig. 10.2)

Case History

A 13-year-old girl, status post heart transplant for congenital heart disease and on sirolimus and prednisone, presented with right neck lymphadenopathy.

Histologic Findings

- The biopsied left neck large lymph node showing markedly expanded paracortical/interfollicular zones but preservation of the nodal architecture with residual lymphoid follicles containing reactive germinal centers (Fig. 10.2a)
- The expanded paracortical zones containing many immunoblasts in a background of T cells and scattered plasma cells (Fig. 10.2b)

Differential Diagnosis

- Reactive viral lymphadenitis with paracortical hyperplasia
- Nondestructive PTLD, infectious mononucleosis type
- Nondestructive PTLD, plasmacytic hyperplasia type

IHC and Other Ancillary Studies (Fig. 10.2d, f)

- Numerous immunoblasts in a background of scattered polyclonal plasma cells, B cells, and many T cells without phenotypic aberrancy
- Most of the larger immunoblastic cell nuclei showing EBER positivity

Final Diagnosis

Nondestructive PTLD, infectious mononucleosis (IM) type

Case 3 (Fig. 10.3)

Case History

A 4-year-old boy with a 3-year history of small bowel, liver, and pancreatic transplantation. His *EBV* genome was detected in the blood 2 years ago, and the copies were arising recently. He had a bilateral tonsillectomy due to tonsillar hypertrophy.

Histologic Findings

- The resected bilateral tonsils showing numerous variably sized reactive follicles with large, polarized germinal centers with many mitoses. The mantle zones are attenuated (Fig. 10.3a).
- There is lack of increased numbers of plasma cells.

Differential Diagnosis

- Reactive follicular lymphoid hyperplasia
- Florid follicular hyperplasia (FFH) type PTLD

IHC and Other Ancillary Studies (Fig. 10.3b)

- The reactive lymphoid follicles stained positive for B-cell markers, and the germinal centers were BCL2 negative,

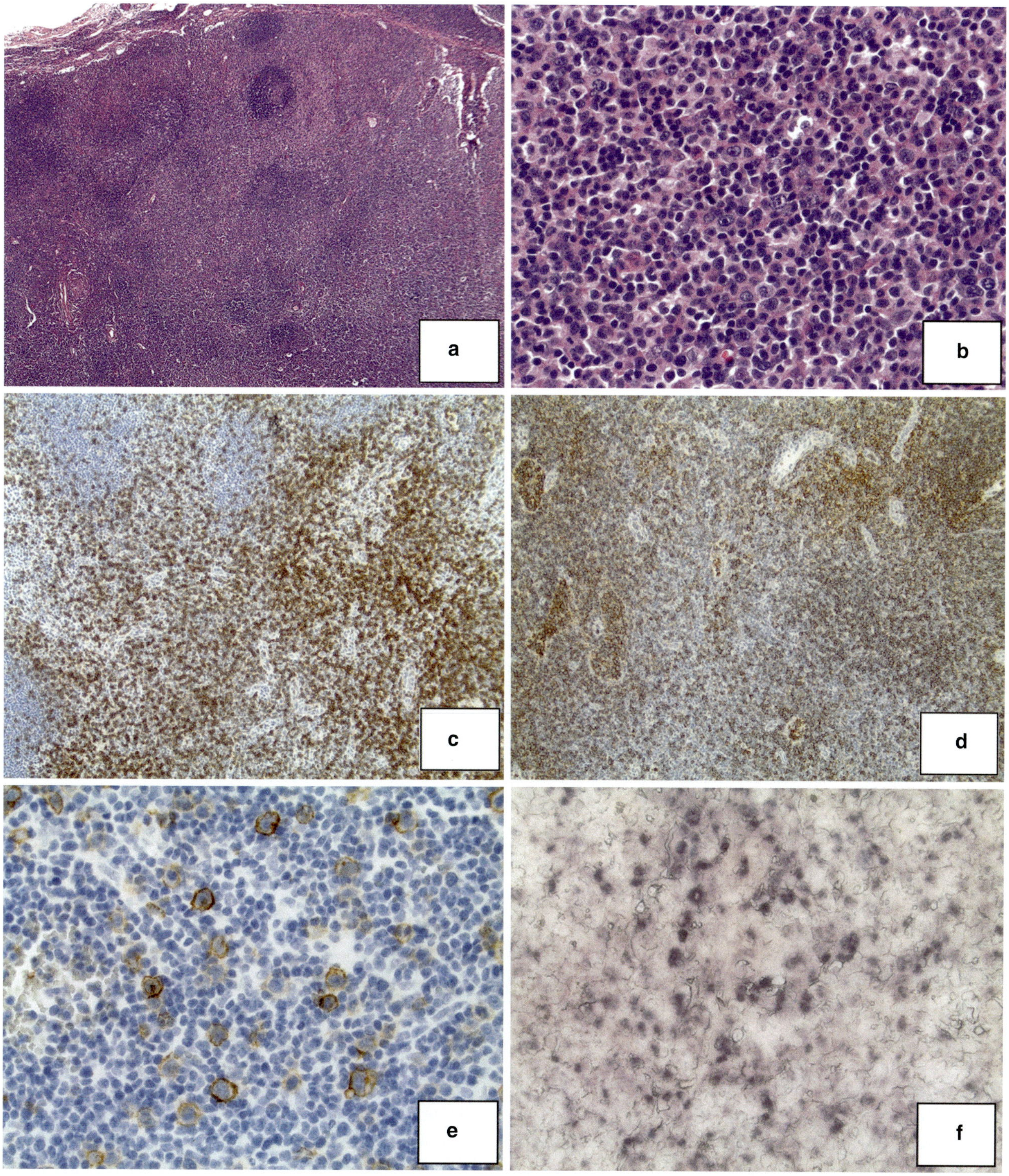

Fig. 10.2 The right neck lymph node showed markedly expansion of the paracortical/interfollicular zones but preservation of the nodal architecture with residual lymphoid follicles containing reactive germinal centers (**a**), and the expanded paracortical/interfollicular zones contained many immunoblasts in a background of lymphocytes, plasma cells, and histiocytes (**b**). The background contains scattered polyclonal plasma cells, mixed B cells and T cells without phenotypic aberrancy, as well as numerous immunoblasts (**c**–**e**). Many of the larger cell nuclei showing EBER positivity (**f**)

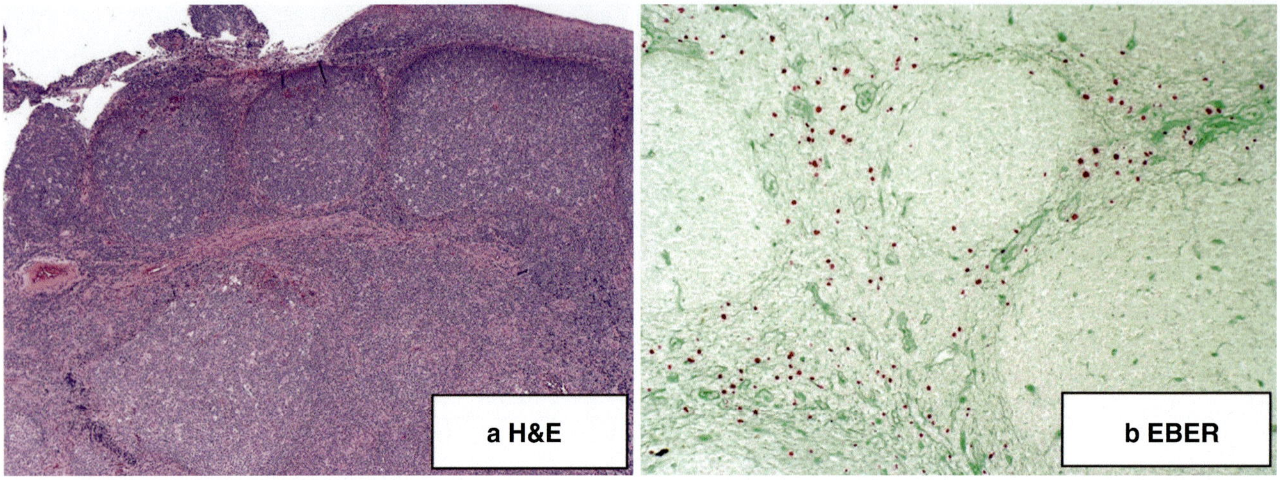

Fig. 10.3 The resected bilateral tonsils showing numerous variably sized reactive follicles with large, polarized germinal centers with many mitoses, and the mantle zones are attenuated with lack of increased numbers of plasma cells (**a**). The reactive lymphoid follicles stained positive for B-cell markers, and the germinal centers were BCL2 negative (not shown), whereas the interfollicular areas were T-cell predominance (not shown). There were increased numbers of EBER-positive cells in the interfollicular areas and sometimes numerous among one or few germinal centers (**b**)

whereas the interfollicular areas were T-cell predominance.
- There were increased numbers of EBER-positive cells in the interfollicular areas and sometimes numerous among one or few germinal centers.

Final Diagnosis

Nondestructive PTLD, florid follicular hyperplasia (FFH) type

Take-Home Messages

1. Nondestructive PTLD is a lymphoid/plasmacytic proliferation in transplant recipient in a setting of immunosuppression and is characterized by some degree of architecture preservation of the involved tissue, with preservation of the nodal sinuses or tonsillar crypts, and residual or florid reactive follicles (FFH) in some cases.
2. Plasmacytic hyperplasia-type PTLD is characterized by numerous plasma cells and rare immunoblasts, as well as detection of many *EBV* genomes by EBER in situ hybridization.
3. IM-like PTLD shows paracortical expansion and numerous immunoblasts in a background of T cells and plasma cells, as well as detection of many *EBV* genomes by EBER in situ hybridization.
4. Florid follicular hyperplasia (FFH)-type PTLD is characterized by tonsil and/or adenoid involvement with florid follicular hyperplasia. The size of the follicles varied, but they all contained large, polarized, germinal centers with many mitoses and attenuated mantle zones. These cases of FFH lacked increased numbers of plasma cells. *EBV*-positive cells are more numerous in a germinal center with occasional positive cells between the follicles.

   References [1–13]

Case 4 (Fig. 10.4)

Case History

A 57-year-old female had kidney transplant at age 40 and had been on tacrolimus and prednisone for the last few years. She now presented with left tonsillar mass.

Histologic Findings

- The resented left tonsil showing diffuse lymphoid infiltrate effacing the entire underlying tonsillar architecture (Fig. 10.4a).
- The lymphoid infiltrate is polymorphic with variably sized small, medium to large lymphoid cells with irregular nuclear contours, hyperchromatic to vesicular chromatin, occasional nucleoli, and small to moderate amount of cytoplasm. Mitotic figures and apoptotic bodies are also evident, as are some plasma cells and scattered large atypical RS-like cells (Fig. 10.4b).

Differential Diagnosis

- Nondestructive PTLD, infectious mononucleosis type with marked architectural distortion and large numbers of immunoblasts
- Monomorphic B-cell PTLD
- Classic Hodgkin lymphoma-type PTLD

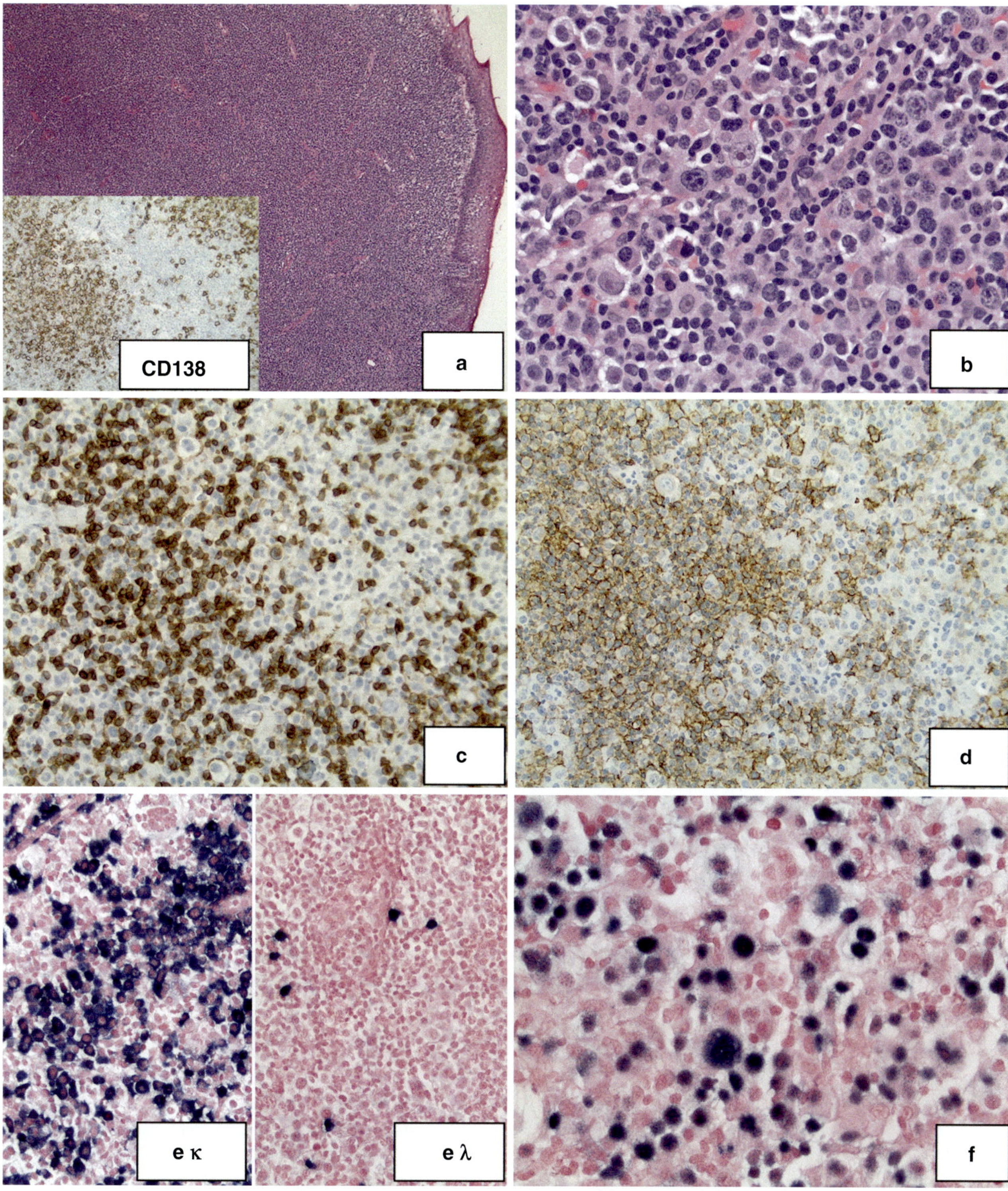

Fig. 10.4 The resected left tonsil showing a diffuse lymphoid infiltrate effacing the underlying normal tonsillar architecture (**a**). The lymphoid infiltrate is polymorphic with variably sized small, medium to large lymphoid cells with irregular nuclear contours, hyperchromatic to vesicular chromatin, occasional nucleoli, and small to moderate amount of cytoplasm. Mitotic figures and apoptotic bodies are also evident, as are rare large atypical RS-like cells (**b**). The polymorphic lymphoid infiltrate consists of mixed T cells (**c**) and B cells (**d**) and some plasma cells (**a**, *Inset*). These plasma cells and B cells were kappa light chain restricted by chromogenic in situ hybridization (**e**), and there were also many EBER-positive cells (**f**)

IHC and Other Ancillary Studies (Fig. 10.4c–f)

- The polymorphic lymphoid infiltrate consists of mixed B and T cells as well as some plasma cells (Fig 10.4a, insert).
- Most of the large lymphoid cells including rare RS-like cells were CD45, CD20, CD79a, PAX5, and/or CD30 positive but CD15 negative, with most B cells/plasma cells showing monotypic kappa light chain restriction, which was also confirmed by flow cytometry.
- There were many EBER-positive cells.
- IgH gene rearrangement was also detected by PCR.

Final Diagnosis
Polymorphic PTLD

Take-Home Messages

1. Polymorphic PTLDs are defined as destructive lesions composed of immunoblasts, plasma cells, and small- to medium-sized lymphoid cells that efface the nodal architecture or form destructive extranodal masses.
2. The polymorphic lymphoid infiltrate consists of mixed B and T cells and sometimes with T-cell predominance.
3. There may be continuous spectrum between P-PTLDs and monomorphic PTLD (M-PTLD), whereas others closely resemble Hodgkin lymphoma (so-called HL-like PTLD), which currently are better considered a form of M-PTLD [13, 21–25].
4. Although they may appear quite polymorphic morphologically, PTLDs that fulfill the criteria for T-cell/histiocyte-rich large B-cell lymphoma or *EBV*-positive diffuse large B-cell lymphoma, NOS, are best regarded as a form of M-PTLD [4].
   References [1–6, 13, 22–25]

Case 5 (Fig. 10.5)

Case History

A 56-year-old male, who had a history of right kidney transplant 4 years ago and had been on CellCept (mycophenolate mofetil) and prednisone, presented with a large left neck mass.

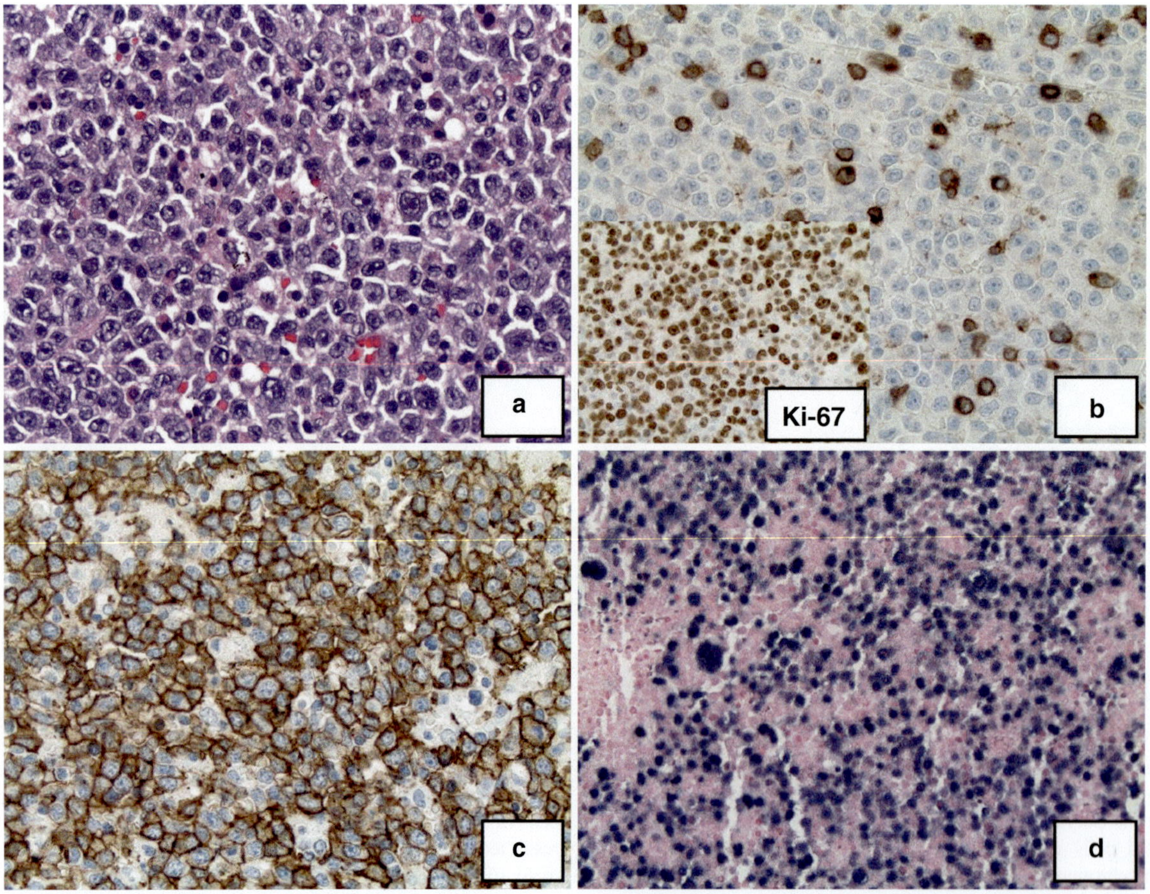

Fig. 10.5 The excised left neck mass showing complete effacement of the normal nodal architecture by diffuse lymphoid infiltrate that was relatively monomorphic with mostly medium- to large-sized lymphoid cells with round, oval, or slightly irregular nuclear contours, vesicular chromatin, prominent nucleoli, and moderate amount of cytoplasm, along with evident mitotic figures and apoptotic bodies (**a**). The lymphoid infiltrate was negative for CD3 (**b**), CD5, CD10, and BCL6, but was diffusely positive for B-cell marker CD20 (**c**), CD79a, PAX5, IRF4/MUM1, and kappa light chain (not shown). There was a high (~80–90%) Ki-67 nuclear proliferative reactivity (**b**, *inset*) with many EBER-positive cells (**d**)

Histologic Findings

- The excised left neck mass showing complete effacement of the normal nodal architecture by diffuse lymphoid infiltrate.
- The lymphoid infiltrate is relative monomorphic with mostly medium- to large-sized lymphoid cells with round, oval, or slightly irregular nuclear contours, vesicular chromatin, prominent nucleoli, and moderate amount of cytoplasm. Mitotic figures and apoptotic bodies are also evident (Fig. 10.5a).

Differential Diagnosis

- Nondestructive PTLD, infectious mononucleosis type with marked architectural distortion and large numbers of immunoblasts
- Polymorphic PTLD

IHC and Other Ancillary Studies (Fig. 10.5b–d)

- The lymphoid infiltrate consists predominantly of CD20, CD79a, CD30, IRF4/MUM1, BCL2, PAX5, and kappa light chain positive but ALK, CD3, CD10, CD15, CD5, and lambda light chain-negative B cells.
- They show a high Ki-67 nuclear proliferative reactivity (~80–90%).
- There were many EBER-positive cells.
- His peripheral blood *EBV* titer was elevated at 1,167, 300.00 copies/mL by PCR.
- FISH analyses were negative for *MYC*, *BCL6*, and *BCL2* gene rearrangements.

Final Diagnosis

Monomorphic B-cell PTLD, diffuse large B-cell lymphoma, non-germinal center (GC) immunophenotype

Take-Home Messages

1. Monomorphic B-cell PTLDs are monoclonally transformed B-lymphocytic or plasmacytic proliferations that fulfill the morphologic and immunophenotypic and/or molecular/cytogenetic criteria for a diffuse large B-cell lymphoma (DLBCL), or less often a Burkitt lymphoma, or other types of a B-cell lymphoma or a plasma cell neoplasm including plasmacytoma-like and plasma cell myeloma-type PTLDs.
2. *EBV+* cases usually have a late germinal center/post germinal center phenotype (CD10−, BCL6+/−, IRF4/MUM1+), while EVB− cases are more likely to have a germinal center phenotype (CD10+/−, BCL6+, IRF4/MUM1−, CD138−).
3. The myeloma or plasmacytoma-like lesions can be *EBV+* or − and are phenotypically similar to those in immunocompetent patients.
4. In addition, most indolent small B-cell lymphomas are not considered M-PTLD, with an exception of EVB+ extranodal marginal zone lymphoma of mucosa-associated lymphoid tissue (MALT lymphoma) in skin and subcutaneous tissue in immunosuppressed transplant recipients.
References [1–7, 13–18]

Case 6 (Fig. 10.6)

Case History

A 14-year-old boy with two times of heart transplants now presented with adenopathy.

Histologic Findings

- The biopsied left neck lymph node showing complete effacement of the normal nodal architecture by diffuse lymphoid infiltrate.
- The lymphoid infiltrate consists of mixed small-, medium- to large-sized lymphoid cells with round, oval, or slightly irregular nuclear contours, vesicular chromatin, prominent nucleoli, and moderate amount of cytoplasm. Mitotic figures and apoptotic bodies are also evident (Fig. 10.6a).

Differential Diagnosis

- Nondestructive PTLD, infectious mononucleosis type with marked architectural distortion and large numbers of immunoblasts
- Polymorphic PTLD

IHC and Other Ancillary Studies (Fig. 10.6b–f)

- The lymphoid infiltrate was predominantly positive for CD2, CD3, CD5, CD7, and CD8, but negative for CD4, CD10, and BCL6.
- There were many EBER-positive cells.
- *TCR γ chain* gene is rearranged without *IgH/K* gene rearrangements detected by PCR.

Final Diagnosis

Monomorphic T/NK-cell PTLD, peripheral T-cell lymphoma type, not otherwise specified (PTCL, NOS)

Take-Home Messages

1. Monomorphic T/NK-cell PTLDs include PTLDs that fulfill the criteria for any type of the T- or NK-cell lymphomas, with the most being PTCL, NOS, followed by hepatosplenic T-cell lymphoma, and others.
2. The interval to lymphoma development is typically longer for T-cell PTLDs than for the B-cell cases.
3. Involvement of extranodal sites (PB, BM, spleen, skin, liver, GI, and lung) is usually common, sometimes with associated lymphadenopathy.
4. Most (2/3) are *EBV−*, but about 1/3 of cases are *EBV+*
References [1–7, 13, 19, 20]

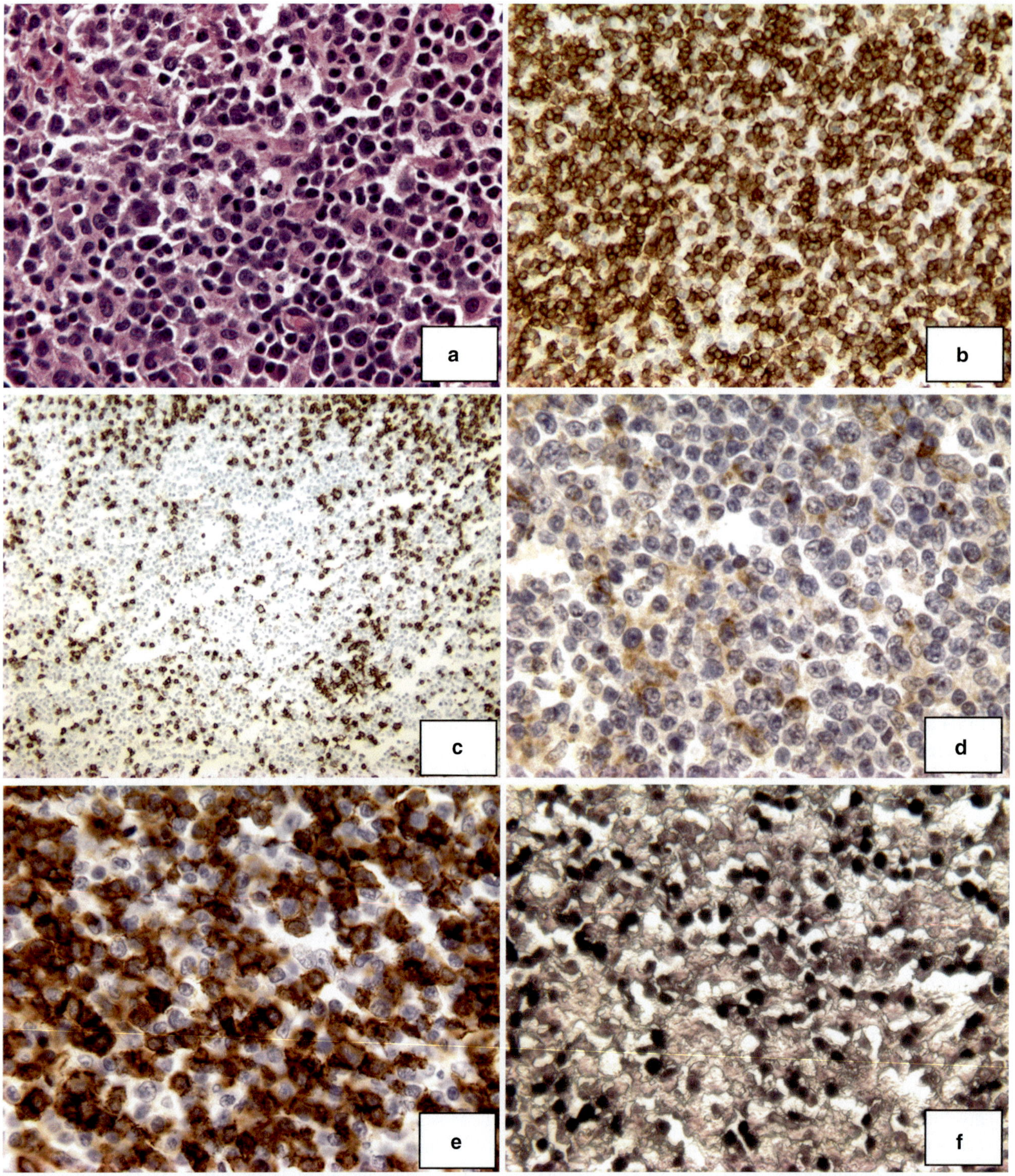

Fig. 10.6 The left neck lymph node showing complete effacement of the normal nodal architecture by diffuse lymphoid infiltrate that consisted of mixed small-, medium- to large-sized lymphoid cells with round, oval, or slightly irregular nuclear contours, vesicular chromatin, prominent nucleoli, and moderate amount of cytoplasm, along with some mitotic figures and apoptotic bodies (**a**). The lymphoid infiltrate was predominantly positive for CD3 (**b**), CD2, CD5 partial, CD7 (not shown), and CD8 (**e**), but negative for CD20 (**c**) and CD4 (**d**). Many of the neoplastic cell nuclei were positive for EBER (**f**)

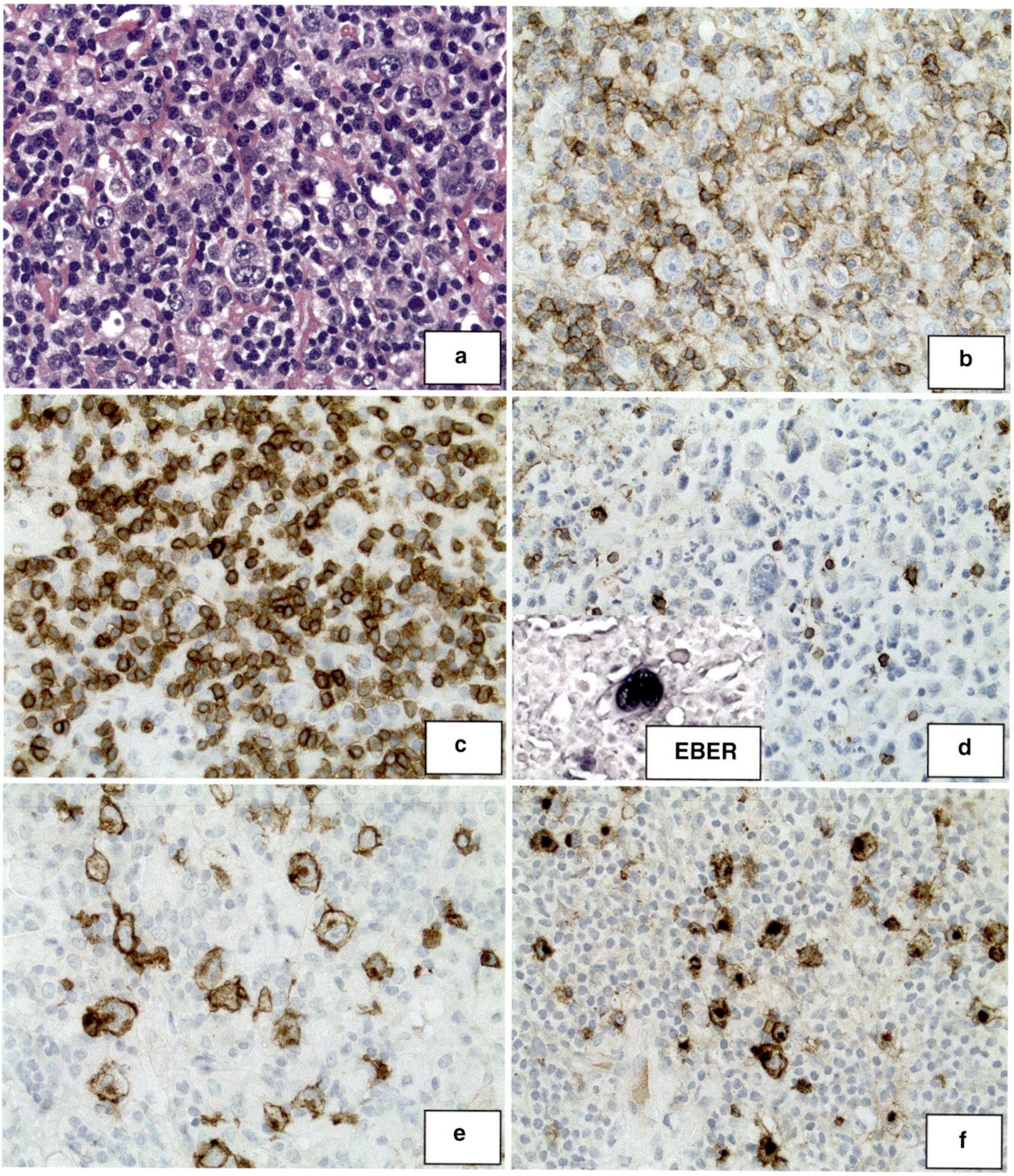

Fig. 10.7 The right neck lymph node showed a complete effacement of the normal nodal architecture by diffuse lymphohistiocytic infiltrate with some large Reed-Sternberg (RS) and their variants against an inflammatory background of small lymphocytes, some histiocytes, plasma cells, granulocytes, and occasional eosinophils (**a**). The RS cells and their variant were negative for CD45, CD3, and CD20 (**b–d**) but positive for CD30 (**e**) and CD15 (**f**), as well as for EBER (**d**, *inset*)

Case 7 (Fig. 10.7)

Case History

A 12-year-old boy with a history of cardiac transplantation at 2 months of age and had been doing well with the usual immunosuppressant treatment until recently, when he developed right cervical lymphadenopathy with weakness and weight loss.

Histologic Findings

- The right neck lymph node showing complete effacement of the normal nodal architecture by diffuse lymphohistiocytic infiltrate.
- The infiltrate consists of scattered large atypical Reed-Sternberg (RS) and their mononucleated and multinucleated variants against an inflammatory background of

small lymphocytes, some histiocytes, plasma cells, granulocytes, and occasional eosinophils (Fig. 10.7a).

Differential Diagnosis

- Nondestructive PTLD, infectious mononucleosis type with marked architectural distortion and large numbers of immunoblasts
- Polymorphic PTLD

IHC and Other Ancillary Studies (Fig. 10.7b–f)

- The RS cells and their variants were negative for CD45, CD3, and CD20 but positive for CD30, CD15, and PAX5 (weakly).
- The RS cells and their variants were also positive for *EBV* with no positivity in the background bystander small lymphocytes (Fig 10.7d, insert).

Final Diagnosis

Classic Hodgkin lymphoma-type PTLD (HL-PTLD)

Take-Home Messages

1. HL-PTLD should be morphologically and immunophenotypically identical to that of a classic Hodgkin lymphoma that is encountered in immunocompetent hosts. The Reed-Sternberg (RS) cells and their variants should be CD45−, CD30+, CD15+, and PAX5+ weakly, as well as *EBV+* with no positivity in the background bystander small lymphocytes.
2. HL-like PTLD may morphologically simulate HL-PTLD; however, there are important immunophenotypic and molecular genetic differences between them. The RS-like cells in HL-like PTLD are CD45+, CD20+, CD30+/−, but CD15-, and virtually all cases are *EBV+* in both RS-like cells and bystander small lymphocytes. Clonally rearranged IG genes are often demonstrable.
3. HL-like PTLD is in fact most often a "monomorphic" B-cell PTLD, with similar immunophenotype, genotype, and clinical behavior [13, 21–25].
4. Therefore, HL-like PTLD has been recategorized as a form of DLBCL-type monomorphic B-cell PTLD since the 2008 WHO classification and remains the same in the 2017 WHO revision. Distinction between HL and HL-like PTLD is important for their clinical management as rituximab can be given to this entity.
   References [1–7, 13, 21–25]

References

1. Harris NL, Swerdlow SH, Frizzera G, et al. Post-transplant lymphoproliferative disorders. In: Jaffe E, Harris N, Stein H, et al., editors. Pathology and genetics: tumours of haematopoietic and lymphoid tissues. World Health Organization classification of Tumuors. Lyon: IARC Press; 2001. p. 264–9.
2. Swerdlow SH, Webber SA, Chadburn A, Ferry JA. Post-transplant lymphoproliferative disorders. In: Swerdlow SH, Campo E, Harris NL, et al., editors. WHO classification of tumours of haematopoietic and lymphoid tissues. 4th ed. Lyon: IARC Press; 2008. p. 335–51.
3. Swerdlow SH, Campo E, Pileri SA, Harris NL, Stein H, Siebert R, et al. The 2016 revision of the World Health Organization (WHO) classification of lymphoid neoplasms. Blood. 2016;127(20):2375–90.
4. Swerdlow SH, Webber SA, Chadburn A, Ferry JA. Post-transplant lymphoproliferative disorders. In: Swerdlow SH, Campo E, Harris NL, et al., editors. WHO classification of Tumours of Haematopoietic and lymphoid tissues. Revised 4th ed. Lyon: IARC Press; 2017. p. p453–62.
5. Al-Mansour Z, Nelson BP, Evens AM. Post-transplant lymphoproliferative disease (PTLD): risk factors, diagnosis, and current treatment strategies. Curr Hematol Malig Rep. 2013;8(3):173–83.
6. San-Juan R, Comoli P, Caillard S, Moulin B, Hirsch HH, Meylan P, et al. Epstein-Barr virus-related post-transplant lymphoproliferative disorder in solid organ transplant recipients. Clin Microbiol Infect. 2014;20(Suppl 7):109–18.
7. Perry AM, Aoun P, Coulter DW, Sanger WG, Grant WJ, Coccia PF. Early onset, EBV(−) PTLD in pediatric liver-small bowel transplantation recipients: a spectrum of plasma cell neoplasms with favorable prognosis. Blood. 2013;121(8):1377–83.
8. Lones MA, Mishalani S, Shintaku IP, Weiss LM, Nichols WS, Said JW. Changes in tonsils and adenoids in children with posttransplant lymphoproliferative disorder: report of three cases with early involvement of Waldeyer's ring. Hum Pathol. 1995;26(5):525–30.
9. Dotti G, Fiocchi R, Motta T, et al. Primary effusion lymphoma after heart transplantation: a new entity associated with human herpes virus-8. Leukemia. 1999;13:664–70.
10. Chen W, Huang Q, Zuppan C, Rowsell EH, Cao JD, Weiss LM, Wang J. Complete absence of KSHV/HHV-8 in post-transplant lymphoproliferative disorders – an immunohistochemical and molecular study of 52 cases. Am J Clin Pathol. 2009;131:632–9.
11. Vakiani E, Nandula SV, Subramaniyam S, Keller CE, Alobeid B, Murty VV, Bhagat G. Cytogenetic analysis of B-cell posttransplant lymphoproliferations validates the World Health Organization classification and suggests inclusion of florid follicular hyperplasia as a precursor lesion. Hum Pathol. 2007;38(2):315–25.
12. Nelson BP, Wolniak KL, Evens A, Chenn A, Maddalozzo J, Proytcheva M. Early posttransplant lymphoproliferative disease: clinicopathologic features and correlation with mTOR signaling pathway activation. Am J Clin Pathol. 2012;138(4):568–78.
13. Mucha K, Foroncewicz B, Ziarkiewicz-Wroblewska B, Krawczyk M, Lerut J, Paczek L. Post-transplant lymphoproliferative disorder in view of the new WHO classification: a more rational approach to a protean disease? Nephrol Dial Transplant. 2010;25(7):2089–98.
14. Gibson SE, Swerdlow SH, Craig FE, Surti U, Cook JR, Nalesnik MA, et al. EBV-positive extranodal marginal zone lymphoma of mucosa-associated tissue in posttransplant setting: a distinct type of posttransplant lymphoproliferative disorder? Am J Surg Pathol. 2011;35(6):807–15.
15. Morscio J, Finalet Ferreiro J, Vander Borght S, Bittoun E, Gheysens O, Dierickx D, et al. Identification of distinct subgroups of EBV-positive post-transplant diffuse large B-cell lymphoma. Mod Pathol. 2017;30(3):370–81.
16. Sarkozy C, Kaltenbach S, Faurie P, Canioni D, Berger F, Traverse-Glehen A, et al. Array-CGH predicts prognosis in plasma cell post-transplantation lymphoproliferative disorders. Genes Chromosomes Cancer. 2017;56(3):221–30.
17. Trappe R, Zimmermann H, Fink S, Reinke P, Dreyling M, Pascher A, et al. Plasmacytoma-like post-transplant lymphoproliferative disorder, a rare subtype of monomorphic B-cell post-transplant lymphoproliferation, is associated with a favorable outcome

in localized as well as in advanced disease: a prospective analysis of 8 cases. Haematologica. 2011;96(7):1067–71.
18. Tcheng WY, Said J, Hall T, Al-Akash S, Malogolowkin M, Feig SA. Post-transplant multiple myeloma in a pediatric renal transplant patient. Pediatr Blood Cancer. 2006;47(2):218–23.
19. Pitman S, Rowsell EH, Cao JD, Huang Q, Wang J. Anaplastic large cell lymphoma associated with Epstein-Barr virus following cardiac transplant. Am J Surg Pathol. 2004;28(3):410–5.
20. Wang J, Pitman S, Rowsell EH, Cao JD, Huang Q. What is anaplastic large cell lymphoma? Authors' reply. Am J Surg Pathol. 2004;28(12):1664–7.
21. Adams H, Campidelli C, Dirnhofer S, Pileri SA, Tzankov A. Clinical, phenotypic and genetic similarities and disparities between post-transplant and classical Hodgkin lymphomas with respect to therapeutic targets. Expert Opin Ther Targets. 2009;13(10):1137–45.
22. Mohri T, Ikura Y, Hirakoso A, Okamoto M, Hishizawa M, Takaori-Kondo A, et al. Classical Hodgkin lymphoma type post-transplant lymphoproliferative disorder in a kidney transplant recipient: a diagnostic pitfall. Int J Hematol. 2018;108(2):218–27.
23. Ranganathan S, Webber S, Ahuja S, Jaffe R. Hodgkin-like post-transplant lymphoproliferative disorder in children: does it differ from post-transplant Hodgkin lymphoma? Pediatr Dev Pathol. 2004;7(4):348–60.
24. Pitman S, Huang Q, Zuppan C, Rowsell EH, Cao JD, Berdeja JG, Weiss LM, Wang J. Hodgkin Lymphoma-like (HD-like) Post-Transplant Lymphoproliferative Disorder (PTLD) simulates monomorphic B-cell PTLD both Clinically and Pathologically. Am J Surg Pathol. 2006;30(4):470–6.
25. Semakula B, Rittenback J, Wang J. Hodgkin lymphoma-like post-transplant lymphoproliferative disorder. Arch Pathol Lab Med. 2006;130(4):558–60.

Immunodeficiency-Associated Lymphoproliferative Disorders Other Than PTLD (in Primary Immune Deficiency, HIV, and Iatrogenic Conditions)

11

Jerald Z. Gong, Siraj M. El Jamal, and Guldeep Uppal

List of Frequently Asked Questions

1. What are the major subtypes of primary immune deficiency (PID)?
2. How is autoimmune lymphoproliferative syndrome (ALPS) different from other PIDs? What are other entities that may mimic ALPS?
3. What are the types of benign lymphoid proliferation associated with PID? What are the morphologic and phenotypic features?
4. What are the types of malignant lymphoproliferative conditions associated with PID? What are the morphologic and phenotypic features?
5. What are the diagnostic criteria for lymphoproliferative disorders associated with PIDs? What is the minimal and optimal ancillary work-up for diagnosis and subclassification of these conditions?
6. What is an adequate specimen for the diagnosis of lymphoproliferative disorders associated with PID? When is it appropriate to seek external consultation?
7. What are the benign lymphoproliferative disorders associated with human immunodeficiency virus (HIV) infection?
8. What are the morphologic stages of HIV-related benign lymphadenopathy?
9. What is the differential diagnosis of HIV-related benign lymphadenopathy?
10. What are the common types of lymphomas associated with HIV?
11. What are the common genetic abnormalities and what are the main viral and molecular driving factors in HIV-associated lymphomas?
12. What is the definition of iatrogenic immunodeficiency-associated lymphoproliferative disorder (IA-LPD)?
13. Which clinical conditions and therapies are associated with IA-LPD?
14. How common is the IA-LPD?
15. Which therapeutic agents are associated with IA-LPD?
16. What is the median interval from initiation of therapy to the diagnosis of IA-LPD?
17. What are the types of IA-LPD?

J. Z. Gong (✉) · G. Uppal
Department of Pathology, Anatomy and Cell Biology, Thomas Jefferson University, Philadelphia, PA, USA
e-mail: Jerald.Gong@jefferson.edu; Guldeep.Uppal@jefferson.edu

S. M. El Jamal
The Department of Pathology, Molecular and Cell-Based Medicine, Icahn School of Medicine at Mount Sinai, Mount Sinai Hospital, New York, NY, USA
e-mail: siraj.eljamal@mountsinai.org

1. What are the major subtypes of primary immune deficiency (PID)?

- *Common variable immune deficiency (CVID)* (see also Chap. 29).
  - The most common primary immune deficiency, with an incidence of 1 in 10,000 to 50,000.
  - It is not a single entity but rather a group of diseases with reduced serum levels of one or more of IgG, IgM, and IgA.
  - The disease first occurs in late childhood or more typically young adults and affects male and female equally.
  - The clinical presentation is broadly heterogeneous depending on the severity of the antibody deficiencies. The most common clinical manifestation is recurrent bacterial infection, which most commonly affects sinopulmonary and gastrointestinal systems. Other clinical presentation may include immune disorders, granulomatous disease, and lymphoproliferative disorders. Most cases are sporadic while only 10–25% have familiar history.

E. Wang, A. S. Lagoo (eds.), *Practical Lymph Node and Bone Marrow Pathology*, Practical Anatomic Pathology,
https://doi.org/10.1007/978-3-030-32189-5_11

- The diagnosis is established by clinical presentation, laboratory evidence of reduction in one or several immunoglobulin isotypes with or without reduced B cells, and exclusion of the other primary immune disorders.
- The etiology of the majority of cases (>90%) is unknown. Mutations in *ICOS*, *TACI*, *MSH5*, and *BAFFR* were found in a small number of CVID patients, which were thought to contribute to the diseases [1, 2].

- *Severe combined immunodeficiency (SCID)*
  - Represents a heterogeneous group of severe immune deficiency, primarily affecting cell-mediated immunity. All SCID patients have defect of T-cell immunity, and a fraction have additional defect in B-cell immunity.
  - Two major forms of SCID have been described: typical SCID and leaky SCID.
  - Typical SCID has low or absent T cells with marked compromise of both number and function of T cells.
  - Patients with typical SCID develop various symptoms from infancy including bacterial and viral respiratory infection, diarrhea and failure to thrive, lymphadenopathy, and underdeveloped thymus.
  - Patients with leaky SCID may show delayed onset of symptoms that include immune dysregulation, skin rash, granulomatous inflammation, lymphadenopathy, and hepatosplenomegaly.
  - Germline gene mutations involving lymphoid maturation and differentiation, T-cell receptor signaling, and cytokine signaling can be detected in SCID patients.
  - Diagnosis of SCID can be established by characteristic clinical presentation during infancy, numerical and/or functional T-cell defect, gene mutations, and *EBV*-associated lymphoproliferative disorders. Nearly 100% SCID patients develop *EBV*-associated lymphoproliferative disorders [3, 4].
- *Hyper IgM syndrome* (HIgM, also known as CD40 or CD40 ligand deficiency)
  - A group of rare disorders characterized by deficiency of either CD40 ligand on T cells (type 1 HIgM) or CD40 on T cells (type 3 HIgM).
  - All types of inherence including autosomal dominant, autosomal recessive, and X-linked may be seen in HIgM.
  - Impaired CD40 or CD40 ligand on T cells results in abnormal interaction of T cells with B cells and consequently impairs class switching from IgM to IgG and IgA in B cells.
  - Serum IgG and IgA levels are consistently low while IgM level is normal to high.
  - The disease onset occurs before 2 years of age and affected children usually present with neutropenia, thrombocytopenia, and recurrent opportunistic infection in respiratory and gastrointestinal tracts.
  - Patients have increased risk of *EBV*-associated large B-cell lymphoma and Hodgkin lymphoma. Some patients may develop large granular lymphocytic leukemia [5].
- *Ataxia-telangiectasia (AT)*
  - An autosomal recessive disorder primarily affecting young children. The incidence in Western countries is approximately 1 in 100,000 live births.
  - The disease is characterized by primary immunodeficiency and neurological defect with cerebellar degeneration.
  - Symptoms usually start to occur at around 1 to 4 years of age with progressive cerebellar ataxia, oculocutaneous telangiectasia, and dysarthria. Patients are highly susceptible to recurrent sinopulmonary infection and increased sensitivity of ionizing radiation.
  - Up to 20% of AT patients may develop malignancies, which are nearly all lymphoid leukemia and lymphoma.
  - AT is caused by mutations in *ATM* gene, which is a member of phosphotidyl inositol kinase (PI3K) family that functions as sensor for DNA repair.
  - Diagnosis of AT is based on family history, highly characteristic clinical presentation, and confirmation of biallelic mutations in *ATM* gene [6, 7].
- *Wiskott-Aldrich Syndrome (WAS)*
  - An X-linked primary immune disorder affecting male children. The incidence in Western countries is approximately 1 in 250,000 live male births. The onset of symptoms can be at variable ages, but thrombocytopenia is present at birth.
  - The disease is caused by mutations in *WAS* gene located at the short arm of the X chromosome, which carries important functions of actin polymerization and T-cell receptor signaling. Female carriers are asymptomatic.
  - Clinical manifestation includes frequent, recurrent infection, bleeding with thrombocytopenia and microthrombosis, severe eczema, and immune deficiency. The disease usually starts with skin rash, petechiae, and ecchymoses and progresses to recurrent bacterial, viral, and/or fungal infection, autoimmune disorders, internal bleeding, and thrombosis.
  - Hematologic malignancies develop in approximately 10–20% patients and may be lymphoid or myeloid neoplasms.
  - Diagnosis of WAS is based on family history, clinical presentation, and confirmation of either abnormal WAS protein expression or *WAS* gene mutations [8, 9].
- *X-linked lymphoproliferative disease (XLP)*
  - Also known as Duncan syndrome, XLP is an X-linked genetic disorder affecting male children. The incidence is approximately 1 to 2 in 1,000,000 male infants.

- The disease is caused by a germline mutation at *SH2D1A* gene, which encodes a protein with key role in T-cell and NK-cell signaling. Cellular immunity with suppressed NK-cell function and humoral immunity with acquired hypogammaglobulinemia are affected.
- These patients develop *EBV*-associated lymphoproliferative disorders due to impaired T-cell response to *EBV*. Symptoms of *EBV* infection appear sometime during childhood or adolescence. The gastrointestinal tract is the most common site of infection, but other extranodal and nodal site can also be affected. Most patients succumb to hepatic failure and/or hemophagocytic syndrome.
- The disease spectrum includes infectious mononucleosis-like diseases, fatal *EBV*-associated infection, and high-grade B-cell lymphomas [10, 11].

- *Autoimmune lymphoproliferative syndrome (ALPS)*
  - Also known as Canale-Smith syndrome, ALPS is an acquired genetic disorder mainly affecting lymphoid system. The disease onset occurs at a medium age of 3 years, and symptoms include unexplained lymphadenopathy and splenomegaly and multilineage cytopenia.
  - The most common presentation of ALPS is asymptomatic lymphadenopathy and/or splenomegaly in children, many patients have an incidental finding of enlarged palpable peripheral lymph nodes. A blood work may also identify multilineage cytopenia. Symptoms related with cytopenia may include fatigue, pallor, easy bruising, and infection.
  - Patients may also present with autoimmune symptoms and autoantibodies such a rheumatoid factor, ANA, as well as a positive Coombs test.
  - The disease is caused by inherited or acquired mutations in a group of genes involving programmed cell death (apoptosis), with vast majority occurring in *FAS* genes. Other genes that may be involved include *FASLG*, *CASP10*, and *CASP8*.
  - The diagnosis is established based on clinical presentation of unexplained lymphadenopathy and/or splenomegaly for greater than 6 months, increased CD4 and CD8 double-negative T cells in blood, and germline mutations of one of the aforementioned genes involving apoptotic pathways [12–14].

2. How is autoimmune lymphoproliferative syndrome (ALPS) different from other PIDs? What are other entities that may mimic ALPS?

- ALPS may be suspected when a child or young adult presents with unexplained lymphadenopathy and/or splenomegaly and cytopenia with or without symptoms. Many of the ALPS patients are initially asymptomatic in contrast to the other types of PIDs that recurrent infection is usually the initial presentation.
- The disease is characterized by the increase of CD4 and CD8 double-negative T lymphocytes in blood, bone marrow, and the lymphoid organs, which can be detected by flow cytometry and immunohistochemistry.
- ALPS can occasionally affect older adults, which are usually caused by acquisition of somatic mutations in later age. These patients may be difficult to recognize due to atypical clinical presentation and broader differential diagnosis.
- Other entities that may overlap with ALPS include Evan's syndrome, hemophagocytic lymphohistiocytosis, Castleman disease, and other benign and atypical lymphoproliferative disorders.
- The lymph node morphology from ALPS has its characteristic morphologic and phenotypic features, which is discussed in the next section [15, 16].
- An international workshop in 2010 proposed detailed diagnostic guidelines and algorithm for ALPS. A set of diagnostic criteria including major and minor criteria was listed. A definitive diagnosis requires the presence of two required criteria and one primary accessory criterion. A probable diagnosis requires the presence of two required criteria and one secondary accessory criterion [17]:
  - *Required*
    - Chronic (>6 months), nonmalignant, noninfectious lymphadenopathy or splenomegaly or both
    - Elevated CD3 + TCRab+ and CD4-CD8- double-negative T cells (≥1.5% of total lymphocytes or 2.5% of CD3+ lymphocytes) in the setting of normal or elevated lymphocyte counts
  - *Accessory*

    Primary
    - Defective lymphocyte apoptosis (in two separate assays)
    - Somatic or germline pathogenic mutation in *FAS, FASLG*, or *CASP10*

    Secondary
    - Elevated plasma sFASL levels (>200 pg/mL) or elevated serum or plasma vitamin B12 level (>1500 ng/L) or elevated plasma interleukin 18 level (>500 pg/mL)
    - Typical immunohistological findings as reviewed by an experienced hematopathologist
    - Autoimmune cytopenia (hemolytic anemia, thrombocytopenia, or neutropenia) and elevated immunoglobulin G level (polyclonal hypergammaglobulinemia)
    - Family history of a nonmalignant/noninfectious lymphoproliferation with or without autoimmunity

3. What are the types of benign lymphoid proliferation associated with the PID? What are the morphologic and phenotypic features?

- *Follicular and paracortical hyperplasia*
  - This is commonly seen in CVID and less frequently in other types of PIDs.
  - Morphologically, the lymph nodes are indistinguishable from lymphoid hyperplasia in immune-competent individuals. The lymph nodes usually show follicular hyperplasia with highly activated germinal centers. Numerous tingible body macrophages may be present in germinal centers. The paracortex is usually expanded and contains a variable number of immunoblasts. Reed-Sternberg-like cells may be present.
  - *EBV*-infected lymphocytes are invariably present in the paracortical areas and can be demonstrated by EBER in situ hybridization [18].
- *Nodular lymphoid hyperplasia of gastrointestinal tract*
  - Nodular lymphoid infiltrate of the GI tract is commonly seen in CVID.
  - The lymphoid nodules are present in the lamina propria and may extend deep into the GI wall. Reactive-appearing lymphoid follicles may or may not present. The lymphoid nodules contain a mixture of B cells and T cells.
  - *EBV*-positive cells are usually present.
  - Clonal B-cell gene rearrangement may be detected in some patients.
  - The clinical course is usually self-limited, and the detection of B-cell clonality does not indicate disease progression or lymphoma [19, 20].
- *Lymphoproliferative disorders associated with ALPS*
  - The lymph nodes show prominent follicular hyperplasia with many enlarged, often irregularly shaped follicles. Large hyperplastic germinal centers contain many increased centroblasts and tingible body macrophages. Progressive transformation of germinal center (PTGC) is frequently seen.
  - The paracortex is expanded and contains increased CD4 and CD8 double-negative T cells admixed with phenotypically normal T cells, polyclonal plasma cells, and immunoblasts. These double-negative T cells may be difficult to visualize by CD4 and CD8 immunohistochemistry due to the mixture of normal helper and suppressor T cells.
  - Flow cytometry is more accurate to detect and enumerate the percentage of the double-negative T cells. The double-negative T cells range from 51% to 78% of alpha-beta T cells according to one study [15].
  - These lesions are usually not associated with *EBV*.
  - The spleen is usually moderately to massively enlarged, which shows expansion of both white pulp and red pulp. The white pulp shows features of follicular hyperplasia with expansion of marginal zone. The red pulp shows similar features to the paracortex in the affected lymph nodes containing numerous lymphocytes, immunoblasts, and polyclonal plasma cells.
  - The peripheral blood shows variable degree of lymphocytosis. The lymphocytes are usually small mature in morphology. The double-negative T cells are invariably increased in peripheral blood (2- to 67-fold over normal value) and can be easily detected by flow cytometry. Peripheral B lymphocytes may show coexpression of CD5, but these B cells are usually polyclonal [15].
- *Lymphoid hyperplasia associated with HIgM*
  - The most characteristic feature of the lymph node morphology is hyperplastic lymphoid follicles with absent germinal centers. IgM-positive plasma cells may be increased in the paracortical and/or medullary areas.
  - These lesions are usually not associated with *EBV*.
  - In extranodal sites, such as the intestinal tract and liver, IgM-positive plasma cells may accumulate.
  - IgG-positive B cells in blood are reduced or absent and can be demonstrated by flow cytometry analysis of blood B cells [5].
- *Fatal infectious mononucleosis*
  - This is primarily seen in SCID and XLP.
  - The lymph nodes are hyperplastic containing markedly expanded T zones. There are variable numbers of immunoblasts and Hodgkin-like cells, which are forming sheets in some cases.
  - *EBV*-positive cells are usually abundant.
  - The lymphadenopathy may be extensive and fulminant in progression. Some patients have associated uncontrolled hemophagocytic syndrome which results in severe progressive pancytopenia.
  - Although this condition is benign, many patients die from fulminant *EBV* infection and bone marrow failure [21].

4. What are the types of malignant lymphoproliferative conditions associated with the PID? What are the morphologic and phenotypic features?

- *Diffuse large B-cell lymphoma (DLBCL)*
  - DLBCL is the most common lymphoma in PIDs and occurs in nearly all types of PIDs (CVID, HIgM, WAS, AT, XLP, ALPS).

- Morphologically, DLBCL in PIDs is similar to those of the immune-competent patients. Both centroblast and immunoblast morphologies can be present.
- *EBV* can be demonstrated in many, but not all, cases.
- There are insufficient data on histogenesis (germinal center vs. activated B-cell types) or MYC/BCL2 expression pattern in these lymphomas [22].

- *Hodgkin lymphoma*
  - Classic Hodgkin lymphoma (CHL) can arise from WAS and AT, and nodular lymphocyte-predominant Hodgkin lymphoma may arise from ALPS.
  - Classic Hodgkin lymphoma shows similar morphology to those from immune-competent population. The most frequent subtype is mixed cellularity followed by nodular sclerosis.
  - Most of these lesions are *EBV* positive.
  - Hodgkin-like lesions that phenotypically do not fulfill diagnostic criteria of CHL can also occur.
  - Nodular lymphocyte-predominant Hodgkin lymphoma in ALPS has similar morphologic and phenotypic features to those from immune-competent patients and is usually *EBV* negative [22, 23].
- *Lymphomatoid* granulomatosis
  - Patients with WAS have an increased incidence of lymphomatoid granulomatosis.
  - The primary sites of involvement are lung, skin, brain, and kidney.
  - The morphology and phenotype are similar to those arising from immune-competent population or other immunodeficient patients.
  - There are variable numbers of large B cells in an inflammatory background with reactive T lymphocytes, histiocytes, and granulocytes. The infiltrate is angiocentric and angiodestructive with often large areas of necrosis. The large B cells express common B-cell antigens, consistently express *EBV*, and variably express CD30. The background T lymphocytes are predominantly CD4+ with normal T-cell phenotype.
  - Clonal immunoglobulin gene rearrangement can be detected in higher-grade lesions (grades 2 and 3) [24, 25].
- *Burkitt lymphoma*
  - Burkitt lymphoma can be occasionally seen in AT, XLD, and ALPS.
  - The lymphoma shows similar morphology and phenotype to those of sporadic type and HIV-associated type.
  - Expression of *EBV* is variable from case to case.
  - Similar to that of the sporadic and HIV-associated types, confirmation of diagnosis requires evidence of rearrangement of *C-MYC* with either immunoglobulin heavy or light chains and absence of *BCL2* and *BCL6* translocations [15, 22].
- *T-cell neoplasms*
  - Peripheral T-cell lymphoma NOS, T-prolymphocytic leukemia, and T-lymphoblastic leukemia/lymphoma are increased in AT.
  - T-cell large granular lymphocytic leukemia is increased in HIgM.
  - Peripheral T-cell lymphoma NOS has been reported in ALPS.
  - These T-cell neoplasms show similar morphology and phenotype to those arising from immune-competent individuals. *EBV* expression is variable in these cases.
  - Diagnosis is based on the same criteria to those of the T-cell neoplasms in the general populations [26].

5. What are the diagnostic criteria for lymphoproliferative disorders associated with PIDs? What is the minimal and optimal ancillary work-up for diagnosis and subclassification of these conditions?

- Each entity should be worked up similarly to its corresponding disease in immune-competent individuals. The diagnostic criteria are essentially identical.
- However, EBER should be performed in all cases, and *EBV* serology is recommended in all patients.
- A thorough clinical history should be obtained for any overt or underlying immune deficiency. Severe PIDs such as SCID, WA, and AT arise at an early age, and usually the diagnoses have already been established at the time when the LPDs arise. Other more indolent PIDs, such as CVID and ALPS, primary etiologies may be inconspicuous at the time of LPDs. Careful assessment of clinical presentation, proper interaction with clinicians, and thorough assessment of biopsied specimens are essential for elucidating the underlying causes.
- In clinical practice, diagnosis of CVID is usually delayed due to its broad heterogeneity of the disease presentation. Patients presented with recurrent mild infection are often treated symptomatically without further work-up of underlying etiology.
- The presence of hypogammaglobulinemia of two or more isotypes points toward CVID. Demonstration of impaired functional antibody response confirms the diagnosis.
- Patients with ALPS usually present with asymptomatic enlargement of lymph nodes and/or the spleen, many of

which are incidental findings. These patients are often accompanied by unexplained multilineage cytopenia. The current diagnostic criteria do not require biopsy of lymph node. However, lymph node biopsy is necessary if lymphoma is suspected. The characteristic lymph node morphology and increase of CD4 and CD8 double-negative T cells in the expanded paracortex help to confirm the diagnosis of ALPS.

6. What is an adequate specimen for the diagnosis of lymphoproliferative disorders associated with PID? When is it appropriate to seek external consultation?

- Diagnosis of LPD in PIDs universally requires tissue biopsy. Excisional biopsy of an enlarged lymph node is the preferred choice, although in certain cases needle core biopsy may be sufficient to reach a diagnosis if sampled appropriately.
- Clinical tests include *EBV* serology, and quantitative *EBV* DNA tests are necessary in addition to the standard work-up on biopsied tissue samples.
- In certain conditions, such as CVID and ALPS, additional tests such as serum gamma globulin quantitation and flow cytometry analysis of blood and tissue are readily available on site or at major reference laboratories and are very useful for initial screening to rule out/rule in these diseases.
- Genetic testing for constitutional or acquired mutations at genomic level is only offered by several specialty pediatric genomic laboratories in the country. The genomic analysis on the constitutional mutations can be performed on blood samples, while for acquired mutations, testing additional tissue sample may be necessary.

7. What are the benign lymphoproliferative disorders associated with human immunodeficiency virus (HIV) infection?

- *HIV-related benign lymphadenopathy (HIV-BNL)*
  - Persistent generalized lymphadenopathy is one of the most common findings in HIV patients. The lymphadenopathy is often accompanied by systemic symptoms such as fever, fatigue, night sweat, and weight loss. The frequency of HIV-BNL has considerably declined as the disease is now effectively controlled by combination antiretroviral therapy (cART).
  - The lymphadenopathy consists of progressive conditions spanning through a series of four morphological patterns (stages): florid follicular hyperplasia, mixed follicular hyperplasia and follicular involution, follicular involution, and lymphocyte depletion. These stages advance in synergy with the decreasing CD4 count, degree of viremia, and the HIV disease progression in the untreated HIV+ individuals.
  - Nearly all biopsied lymph nodes from living individuals have the morphology of florid follicular hyperplasia and mixed follicular hyperplasia. The follicular involution and lymphocyte depletion are only seen in terminal stages of HIV infection that are exceedingly rare in the post-cART era [27–29].
- *Benign lymphoepithelial cyst (BLC)*
  - These lesions affect salivary glands, most commonly parotid gland, and accounts for 25% of salivary glands enlargements in HIV patients. Besides HIV patients, the condition often occurs in patients with autoimmune disorders such as Sjögren syndrome and other autoimmune sialadenitis. Bilateral salivary glands are usually affected, which often lead to lymphadenopathy in the regional lymph nodes.
  - The lesions are composed of epithelium-lined cysts in a background of lymphoid follicular hyperplasia. The prolonged lymphocytic proliferation results in epithelial metaplasia and duct calcification that in turn results in duct obstruction and cyst formation.
  - Histologically, there are multiple nodules consisting of hyperplastic lymphoid tissue that are surrounded by multiple cysts. The lymphoid tissue shows features of HIV lymphadenopathy with large hyperplastic follicles and highly proliferative germinal centers. The cysts are lined by columnar, cuboidal, or squamous epithelium and are filled with clear or pink amorphous material.
  - Surgical excision is typically performed on these patients for symptomatic relief and to rule out lymphoma [30, 31].
- *Multicentric Castleman disease (MCD)*
  - HIV patients have an increased risk of developing MCD.
  - Evidence of HHV8 infection can be found in nearly all MCD in these patients; otherwise, the lesions are similar in morphology and phenotype to MCD in immune-competent population.
  - HHV8+ Kaposi sarcoma is often in concurrence with MCD. In fact, most patients would have developed Kaposi sarcoma prior to the Castleman disease.
  - Most MCD cases are of the plasma cell variant or mixed variant types. The histological features of MCD

are similar to those from non-HIV patients; however, a more prominent follicular hyperplasia and hyalinization as well as greater numbers of interfollicular plasma cells may be seen.
- The risk of developing lymphoma in HIV patients who have MCD increases 15-fold as compared to those who have no MCD [32, 33].

8. What are the morphologic stages of HIV-related benign lymphadenopathy?

- *Florid follicular hyperplasia (FFH)*
  - Florid follicular hyperplasia is the first stage of HIV-BNL and is the most common lymph node finding in HIV patients.
  - The lymph nodes are usually moderately enlarged and are characterized by numerous hyperplastic lymphoid follicles with geographical shapes. Bizarre-shaped follicles such as "dumbbell-like" and other irregularly shaped follicles are commonly seen. The germinal centers are massively enlarged and are highly proliferative with numerous, often sheets, of centroblasts and abundant tingible body macrophages. Mantle zones are attenuated or absent, resulting in "naked" germinal centers.
  - Accompanying the hyperplastic follicles, clusters of monocytoid B cells are nearly always present. These clusters may be located next (abut) to the follicles, next to sinusoids, or isolated in the T zones.
  - Follicle lysis, once considered as a specific feature of HIV lymphadenopathy and later was found in other hyperplastic lymph nodes, consists of "bleeding" inside the follicles and invasion of the lymphoid follicles by small lymphocytes with effacement of the mantle zones [34–36].
- *Mixed follicular hyperplasia and follicular involution (MFHFI)*
  - When the disease progresses, some of the hyperplastic follicles regress with involuted germinal centers. The interfollicular areas are expanded more than what is seen in FFH.
  - The involuted follicles at this phase consist of less than 50% of all follicles [34–36].
- *Follicular involution (FI)*
  - At this phase, most follicles are regressed and small in size. Remnants of germinal centers are composed largely of hyalinized follicular dendritic cells with prominent hyalinized blood vessels. The interfollicular areas are further expanded between the small regressed follicles, but the cellular components are reduced.
  - Histiocytes and plasma cells preside over lymphocytes.
  - Follicular dendritic cells are markedly decreased [34–36].
- *Lymphocyte depletion (LD)*
  - This morphology represents the late stage of HIV lymphadenopathy and is usually not observed in living individuals. Much of the data were collected from autopsy cases.
  - Lymph nodes from this type are usually small in size and show absence of germinal centers and scant lymphoid elements in interfollicular areas. The lymph node parenchyma is composed of connective tissue stromal cells, medullary cords, and sinusoids.
  - Follicular dendritic cells (FDC) are virtually absent.
  - CD4-positive T cells are markedly decreased to absent, reflecting progression to the late stage of the disease.
  - The progression of morphological features from the initial follicular hyperplasia to the late stages of follicular involution and lymphocytic depletion correlates the destruction of FDC meshwork leading to loss of the normal lymphoid follicles. During clinical latency of the disease, the FDC meshwork serves as a barrier to keep the viral particles contained in the lymphoid tissue, which correlates with low viral counts in the blood. As the disease progresses and FDC meshwork degenerates, the capacity to containing the virus decreases and the blood viral count consequently rises [34–36].

9. What is the differential diagnosis of HIV-related benign lymphadenopathy?

- When typical HIV-BNL morphology is seen in a lymph node biopsy, a potential HIV infection should be suspected and further clinical investigation such as HIV serology and viral DNA test should be suggested.
- However, none of the morphologic features in HIV-BNL are unique to HIV infection, and many other diseases may share similar morphology.
- Nonspecific follicular hyperplasia is a very common finding in lymph node biopsy that may or may not have a known etiology at the time of biopsy. Follicular hyperplasia is a response of lymph node to regional antigen stimulation that can be caused by infection, autoimmune disorders, hypersensitivity, among others. When assessing such cases, a thorough review of clinical history should be performed in order to elucidate possible causes [37].
- Acute *EBV* infection (infectious mononucleosis) can occasionally mimic early stages of HIV-related lymph-

adenopathy when follicular hyperplasia is prominent. However, acute *EBV* infection typically has variously expanded paracortical zone with increased immunoblasts.

- Atypical mycobacterial infection may show regressed follicles and lymphocyte-depleted morphology with increased background fibrosis that leads to a morphological picture similar to the late stages of HIV-BL of follicular involution and lymphocytic depletion.
- Hyaline vascular Castleman disease has regressed, hyalineized germinal centers that mimic follicular involution in the late stage of HIV lymphadenopathy. However, increased vasculature is usually absent in HIV cases.
- Classic Hodgkin lymphoma, especially lymphocyte-depleted type, may resemble lymphocyte-depleted stage of HIV lymphadenopathy. Careful morphologic assessment and review of relevant immunohistochemical stains can readily differentiate between them. One should be aware that a lymphoma like CHL may develop in a lymph node previously affected by the HIV-related benign lymphadenopathy.

10. What are the common types of lymphomas associated with HIV?

- *Diffuse large B-cell lymphoma, NOS*
  - DLBCL in HIV patients is more likely to present with high-stage disease and extranodal site involvement. Some unusual sites such as the anorectal, orbit, and heart are more likely seen at the presentation in HIV DLBCL, although the CNS and gastrointestinal tract are the most common extranodal sites of involvement.
  - The histopathologic features of DLBCL in HIV patients are similar to those of the DLBCL in immune-competent population. Both centroblast and immunoblast types may be present although immunoblast type is more common in HIV DLBCL.
  - Phenotypically, germinal center-type DLBCL (GC-DLBCL) is about twice as common as activated B-cell type DLBCL (ABC-DLBCL). Patients with GC-DLBCL usually have moderate CD4 counts in mildly immunodeficient state, while those with ABC-DLBCL are more likely to have low CD4 counts with more severe immunodeficient state.
  - Similar to DLBCL in the general population, ABC-DLBCL has unfavorable outcomes as compared to GC-DLBCL [38].
- *Primary central nervous system lymphomas (PCNSL)*
  - PCNSL is the most common extranodal lymphoma in HIV patients, comprising approximately 20% of all AIDS-related lymphomas.
  - Most patients who develop PCNSL are young homosexual male who have low CD4 counts. These patients often have concurrent other AIDS-defining illnesses with various degrees of systemic symptoms, which may mask the neurologic symptoms caused by the lymphoma. Surgical biopsy is invariably necessary to differentiate between lymphoma and infection.
  - Histologically, the lymphoma may diffusely replace brain tissue or focally infiltrate perivascular space. When present at only perivascular location, the diagnosis may be difficult due to small sample size, necrosis, and sparsity of involved blood vessels. The diagnosis can be confirmed by the presence of large B cells surrounding and infiltrating the blood vessel walls.
  - Nearly all HIV-related CNS lymphomas are *EBV* positive [39].
- *HIV-related Burkitt lymphoma (HIV-BL)*
  - HIV-BL accounts for 15% of HIV-associated lymphoma and involves lymph node as well as extranodal sites.
  - HIV-BL shows the similar histologic features to the sporadic type with proliferation of monomorphic, intermediate-sized lymphoma cells. In some cases, the lymphoma cells may show plasmablastic morphology. The rapid proliferation of the tumor cells results in numerous mitosis and increased tingible body macrophages exhibiting the characteristic histomorphologic “starry-sky” pattern.
  - Similar to sporadic BL, the tumor cells express B-cell markers and germinal center markers CD10 and BCL6 and are consistently negative for BCL2.
  - Translocations of *MYC* are the molecular hallmark of Burkitt lymphoma, with t(8;14) being the most common.
  - Approximately 50% of the cases are *EBV* positive [40, 41].
- *Plasmablastic lymphoma*
  - Plasmablastic lymphoma occurs primarily in HIV patients but can also occur in other immunosuppressive conditions such as posttransplantation, iatrogenic medication, and aging.
  - The lymphoma nearly always arises from extranodal sites, most commonly from the oral cavity followed by the gastrointestinal tract, skin, bone, nasal cavity, CNS, liver, and lung.
  - The tumor cells are large in size with immature morphology and varying degrees of plasmacytic differen-

tiation with prominent nucleoli and basophilic cytoplasm. Mitotic figures are common and tingible body macrophages may be present.
  - Plasmablastic lymphoma expresses CD138, CD38, and MUM1/IRF4 and is negative or weakly positive for CD20, PAX5, and CD45. CD56 is typically negative, and if positive, a differential diagnosis of plasma cell neoplasm should be considered. The proliferation index is usually greater than 90%.
  - The vast majority of plasmablastic lymphomas are positive for *EBV*.
  - Approximately 50% cases harbor *MYC* translocation [42].
- *Primary effusion lymphoma (PEL)*
  - PEL is a *human herpesvirus* 8 (HHV8)-driven lymphoma seen almost exclusively in HIV patients and to a lesser extent in individuals in other types of immunodeficiencies.
  - The classic cases develop in body cavities with no solid tumor component.
  - The lymphoma cells are very large in size but show highly variable morphology ranging from immunoblastic, plasmablastic to large bizarre anaplastic morphology.
  - The lymphoma expresses a limited set of antigens including CD138 and MUM1/IRF4 but is negative in nearly all pan-B-cell and pan-T-cell antigens.
  - All cases are positive for *EBV* in addition to HHV-8.
  - The prognosis is dismal with an overall survival of <6 months.
  - A solid variant (extracavitary) with similar morphological and immunophenotypic features to cavitary PEL was also described. These lesions are solid masses involving extranodal sites other than body cavities. Patients with extracavitary lesions have relatively higher CD4 counts and have slightly better prognosis than the cavitary type [43, 44].
- *Classic Hodgkin lymphoma (CHL)*
  - CHL is not considered an AIDS-defining entity. The incidence of CHL in HIV patients is not increased as compared to the incidence in the general population.
  - However, CHL in HIV individuals may often have atypical clinical features with more aggressive clinical behavior and unfavorable subtypes. Although the nodular sclerosis type is still the most common subtype, the frequency of mixed cellularity type and lymphocyte-depleted type are higher than those from immune-competent populations.
  - cART treatment also alters the frequencies of subtypes. In the pre-cART era, most cases of HIV CHL were mixed cellularity subtype, whereas after the introduction of cART therapy, a paradoxical increase in the incidence of nodular sclerosis subtype is observed.
  - Patients of mixed cellularity subtype usually present with an advanced disease and bone marrow involvement, whereas patients of nodular sclerosis subtype are more likely to present with a limited disease confined to the mediastinum.
  - Lymphocyte-depleted CHL was considered more frequent in HIV patients, and many of the cases are *EBV* positive. However, the "depletion" of the background lymphocytes is often a result of reduced CD4 T cells in the late stage of HIV infection, which may provide a "lymphocyte-depleted" appearance.
  - The Hodgkin and Reed-Sternberg cells in HIV CHL have similar phenotype to those from the immune-competent individuals; however, evidence of *EBV* expression is present in nearly all HIV CHL [45, 46].
- *Polymorphic B-cell lymphoproliferative disorders (PTLD-like)*
  - Rare cases of polymorphic PTLD-like lesions were reported in HIV patients. These lesions have similar morphologic, phenotypic, and genotypic features to the polymorphic PTLD seen in patients who receive solid organ transplantation.
  - The affected lymph nodes or extranodal masses show effacement of architecture with a polymorphous infiltrate containing scattered large lymphocytes admixed with inflammatory cells in the background.
  - B-cell clonality as well as *EBV* infection can be demonstrated in some, but not all, cases.
  - In contrast to the bona fide HIV-associated lymphomas, these polymorphic infiltrates often show more limited disease distribution and lack of consistent genetic alterations.
  - Due to the small number of reported cases, the clinical behavior and outcome are unknown [47].

11. What are the common genetic abnormalities and what are the main viral and molecular driving factors in HIV-associated lymphomas?

- The most common genetic alterations in conventional NHL are also present in HIV-associated lymphomas. Translocations such as *MYC*, *BCL6*, and mutations of *TP53* play similar roles in HIV-associated lymphomas. *TP53* mutations are seen in increased frequencies in multiple types of HIV-associated lymphomas.

- Evidence of *EBV* infection can be demonstrated in all HIV-associated lymphoma types ranging from 40% to nearly 100%. Increased serum cytokines such as IL6 and IL10 are observed in *EBV*-positive cases suggesting an association of cytokine network dysregulation with *EBV*-associated lymphomas [48].
- *MYC* rearrangement is present in 100% Burkitt lymphoma, nearly all plasmablastic lymphoma, and a small percentage of DLBCL in HIV patients. The *MYC* breakpoints in Burkitt lymphoma are similar in HIV and sporadic types and are usually within first intron, first exon or 5′ of first exon. The breakpoints in immunoglobulin heavy chain gene in t(8;14) typically involve switch regions. These patterns are different from endemic type. Approximately 25% of HIV-associated DLBCL also harbors *MYC* rearrangement. *MYC*-rearranged cases tend to have higher proliferation rate, but it is unclear whether *MYC* rearrangement portends unfavorable clinical outcome [41, 49, 50].
- *BCL6* rearrangement can be detected in 20% of systematic HIV-associated DLBCL and 40% of HIV-associated CNS lymphomas. *BCL6* translocation partners with immunoglobulin heavy chain gene in most cases and with various other genes in the remaining cases. Except for rare cases of double-hit lymphoma, *BCL6* and *MYC* translocations are mutually exclusive indicating different pathogenic mechanisms between lymphomas with these two translocations [51].
- *TP53* mutations can be detected in 40% of HIV-DLBCL and 60% of HIV-BL.
  - *TP53* is a tumor suppressor gene and is typically inactivated by loss of heterozygosity with a missense or nonsense mutation.
  - Mutations of *TP53* are detected across all tumor types, but high-grade lymphomas associated with HIV appear to have relatively higher frequency of mutations.
  - Most mutations accumulate between exon 5 to exon 9 and are missense or nonsense mutations. Most mutated cases also show loss of heterozygosity resulting in inactivation of the gene by loss of function of both alleles.
  - Other cases show intact second allele, and in these cases *TP53* may be inactivated through alternative mechanisms [51].
- Similar to lymphoproliferative processes in other immune deficiency conditions, *EBV* expression is a consistent finding in HIV-associated lymphomas.
  - *EBV* can be found in nearly all classic Hodgkin lymphoma and CNS lymphoma, 60–70% plasmablastic lymphoma, approximately 50% Burkitt lymphoma, and approximately 40% systemic DLBCL in HIV patients.
  - Nearly all HIV+ individuals are seropositive for *EBV*, and many have evidence of *EBV* reactivation.
  - Clonal *EBV* genomes were found in HIV-BL and HIV-CHL, which suggest that *EBV* infection is an early event.
  - The pathogenesis of *EBV* in HIV-associated lymphoma was considered similar to that of lymphomas in congenital and iatrogenic immune deficiencies. It was hypothesized that the compromised immunity in HIV infection was prone to *EBV* reactivation and polyclonal expansion of the *EBV*-infected B cells.
  - The proliferation of *EBV*-infected lymphocytes was unstable and susceptible to genetic alterations such *MYC* translocation and mutations in oncogenes and tumor suppressor genes, which resulted in malignant transformation to lymphoma [49, 52].

12. What is the definition of iatrogenic immunodeficiency-associated lymphoproliferative disorder (IA-LPD)?

- Iatrogenic immunodeficiency-associated lymphoproliferative disorder (IA-LPD) comprises of reactive and neoplastic lymphoid proliferations that arise in patients treated with immunosuppressive and immunomodulatory drugs for autoimmune disorders and conditions other than posttransplant setting.
- Some drugs used to treat autoimmune diseases are also used in posttransplant setting (i.e., tacrolimus, mycophenolate), and it is unclear whether these agents play a direct causative role.
- This is further complicated by the fact that many autoimmune disorders have inherent risk in developing lymphoma.
- *EBV*-associated mucocutaneous ulcer is a newly described entity that can be seen after immunotherapy or can be associated with age-related immune senescence [53].

13. Which clinical conditions and therapies are associated with IA-LPD?

- Based on the underlying diseases, IA-LPDs can be grouped into two categories based on the offending agents:
  1. LPDs associated with therapy of autoimmune/chronic inflammatory disorders
  2. LPDs associated with therapy of hematologic malignancies
- The common diseases in the former category are rheumatoid arthritis, inflammatory bowel disease, psoriasis and psoriatic arthritis, systemic lupus erythematosus, and ankylosing spondylitis.

- In the setting of hematologic malignancies, IA-LPDs are more commonly reported in certain leukemias and lymphomas including chronic lymphocytic leukemia/small lymphocytic lymphoma and plasma cell myeloma, although rare cases have been reported in a wide variety of neoplastic hematologic disorders [53].

14. How common is the IA-LPD?

- While the association of various chemotherapeutic agents and immune modulators with lymphoproliferative disorders is well established, the exact frequency of IA-LPD is not known. There are various small series and case reports in the literature which are indicative of rarity of these diseases. It appears that the prevalence of IA-LPD is on the rise due to the increasing use of immunomodulatory agents in many autoimmune and rheumatologic conditions.
- Several factors affect the frequencies of these disorders including underlying diseases and their severity and the types of immunosuppressive therapy. Many of the reported patients used multiple immune suppressive agents, which prevented clear understanding of the role of each individual agent.

  However, it is generally believed that the incidence of LPDs increases 8–10 folds in patients treated with multiple immunosuppressive agents as compared to those treated with single agent [54, 55]. A large meta-analysis of 18 studies of patients with inflammatory bowel disease reported a significantly increased risk of lymphoma among patients taking thiopurines [56].
- The absolute risk was highest in patients older than 50 years of age [56].

15. Which therapeutic agents are associated with IA-LPD?

- The major classes of drugs associated with IA-LPDs are antimetabolites, methotrexate, purine analogues (fludarabine), and immunomodulators (Table 11.1).
- In the broad class of antineoplastic drugs, secondary LPDs are most common in CLL/SLL patients treated with fludarabine and cyclophosphamide.
- Other chemotherapeutic agents that may result in secondary LPDs include alemtuzumab, chlorambucil, cyclosporine, bendamustine, bortezomib, doxorubicin, melphalan (used in conditioning for autologous stem cell transplant), and vincristine (Table 11.1). Many of these agents are used in combination which precludes understanding of the precise role of individual drug in association of secondary LPDs [57].

16. What is the median interval from initiation of therapy to the diagnosis of IA-LPD?

- The time interval from initiation of therapy to diagnosis of LPD varies considerably ranging from 6 weeks to 24 years, with the median intervals from 24 months to 55 months [57, 58].
- IA-LPDs arising after treatment of autoimmune and other chronic inflammatory disorders have a shorter median

Table 11.1 List of common immune modulators and biologic agents that are associated with IA-LPD

Name	Class	Mechanism	Common indications
Methotrexate	Antimetabolite	Inhibition of DHFR	Leukemia, lymphoma, autoimmune disorders
Azathioprine	Antimetabolite	Inhibits nuclei acid synthesis	Renal transplant, RA, UC, CD, lupus nephritis
6-Mercaptopurine	Antimetabolite	Inhibits nuclei acid synthesis	ALL, CD
Infliximab	Cytokine inhibitor	TNF-α inhibitor	UC, CD, psoriatic arthritis
Adalimumab	Cytokine inhibitor	TNF-α inhibitor	RA, AS, UC, CD, psoriatic arthritis
Etanercept	Cytokine inhibitor	TNF-α inhibitor	RA, psoriasis, AS
Anakinra	Cytokine inhibitor	IL-1Ra inhibitor	RA
Tocilizumab	Cytokine inhibitor	IL-6R inhibitor	RA, juvenile idiopathic arthritis
Abatacept	Selective co-stimulation modulator	Blocks binding of the CD80/CD86 in APC to CD28 on T cells	RA, juvenile idiopathic arthritis
Tofacitinib	JAK-STAT pathway inhibitor	Inhibits JAK1, JAK3	RA, IBD, psoriasis

DHFR dihydrofolate reductase, *RA* rheumatoid arthritis, *UC* ulcerative colitis, *CD* Crohn's disease, *ALL* acute lymphoblastic leukemia, *AS* ankylosing spondylitis, *IBD* inflammatory bowel disease, *APC* antigen-presenting cell interval (24 months) as compared to those arising after chemotherapy for malignancies (55 months). However, more data with large multi-institutional studies are necessary to confirm these observations.

17. What are the types of IA-LPD?

- Lymphoproliferative disorders in the setting of prior therapy can present as overt lymphomas and polymorphic lymphoid proliferations. In general, polymorphic LPDs are less common than lymphomas (10% vs 90%).
  - The polymorphic LPDs can be nodal (atypical follicular hyperplasia, atypical paracortical T-cell hyperplasia, aberrant T-cell phenotypes, and abnormal extrafollicular proliferation of B cells) or extranodal.
  - The iatrogenic lymphomas are dominated by diffuse large B-cell lymphoma and classic Hodgkin lymphoma. Other less commonly reported lymphomas include Burkitt lymphoma, lymphoplasmacytic lymphoma, follicular lymphoma, peripheral T-cell lymphoma, and marginal zone lymphoma [58, 59].
- *Polymorphic lymphoid proliferation associated with iatrogenic immune suppression (IA-PLP)*
  - IA-PLP encompasses a wide spectrum of morphological changes that include atypical follicular hyperplasia, paracortical hyperplasia, atypical lymphohistiocytic proliferation, and lymphoid proliferation with Hodgkin-like cells.
  - *EBV*-positive cases may show areas of geographic necrosis.
  - The infiltrating lymphocytes exhibit a spectrum of differentiation (small lymphocytes, centroblasts, immunoblasts, and plasma cells). Some cases show florid follicular hyperplasia or polymorphous paracortical hyperplasia with prominent vascular proliferation. However, many of these lymphoid proliferations do not fulfill the diagnostic criteria for either reactive lesions or neoplastic proliferations.
  - Clonal immunoglobulin heavy chain (*IGH*) gene rearrangement may be detected, but the clonal peaks are usually small and are accompanied by a polyclonal background.
  - Most of these lesions regress following discontinuation of the offending drugs [60, 61].
- *Dasatinib-associated reactive follicular hyperplasia*
  - Patients treated with dasatinib have been reported to develop florid reactive follicular hyperplasia that regresses after discontinuation of the drug. The patients often present with solitary or regional lymphadenopathy.
  - This entity shows distinctive morphological features. The lymph nodes can be markedly enlarged but nodal architecture is preserved. The follicles are hyperplastic with features akin to progressive transformation of germinal centers (PTGC). However, unlike typical PTGC, the displaced mantle zone forms a cuff around capillaries. This feature is reminiscent of Castleman's disease, but other features of Castleman's disease are absent [62, 63].
- *Diffuse large B-cell lymphoma, NOS (DLBCL)*
  - DLBCL is the most common LPD in patients treated with methotrexate (MTX). Up to 40% cases show an extranodal presentation.
  - A few cases of cutaneous DLBCL have been reported after prolonged MTX administration. A case of MTX-associated LPD was reported at the injection site of MTX [64].
  - These cases show sheets of large centroblast or immunoblast lymphocytes and express a B-cell phenotype with CD20, CD79a, PAX5, BOB1, and OCT2.
  - *EBV* has been reported in up to 79% cases.
  - CD30 is more frequently expressed; otherwise, the morphology and phenotype are identical to the DLBCL in immune-competent population [58, 65, 66].
- *Classic Hodgkin lymphoma associated with iatrogenic immune suppression (IA-CHL)*
  - Diagnosis of CHL in iatrogenic clinical setting is challenging as *EBV*+ polymorphic LPD often contains Hodgkin-like cells. For accurate diagnosis, the lesions should have unequivocal morphologic and phenotypic features of CHL.
  - The histologic morphology is similar to those arising from immune-competent population with large single or multinucleated HRS cells in a background of lymphocytes, plasma cells, eosinophils, and histiocytes.
  - Up to 80% cases express EBER. The HRS cells lack a complete B-cell phenotype with frequent but not universal expression of CD15. If the large cells express strong B-cell markers, a diagnosis of T-cell/histiocyte-rich B-cell lymphoma should be entertained.
  - In terms of microenvironment, IA-CHL shows a predominance of CD163+ histiocytes with a M2 phenotype. Increased number of M2 histiocytes were reportedly associated with a worse prognosis in non-immunodeficiency-associated CHL. Prognostic significance of this finding in CHL in iatrogenic setting is unknown.
  - Subtyping of IA-CHL arising after therapy is usually difficult, although it appears that mixed cellularity is more frequent than nodular sclerosis subtype. This is the opposite of CHL in immune-competent population.
  - IA-CHL requires treatment with combination chemotherapy. Regression of CHL after cessation the offending drugs was reported only in rare cases [67].
- *EBV-positive mucocutaneous ulcer (EBV-MCU)*

  - *EBV*-MCU is a recently recognized B-cell lymphoproliferative disorder and was initially reported by Dojcinov, et al. in 2010 [68].
  - The disease presents as ulcerated lesions in gingiva or other mucocutaneous locations and is associated with immunosuppressive therapy (56%), age-related immune senescence (40%), as well as primary immune deficiencies (4%).
  - Iatrogenic medications that may increase risk of developing *EBV*-MCI are methotrexate, azathioprine, cyclosporine, mycophenolate, and tacrolimus.
  - Histologically, these lesions show polymorphic infiltrate with scattered atypical large B cells in a background of abundant T cells. The B cells may show HRS cell-like morphology and are usually positive for CD30 and EBER [68, 69].
- *Extranodal marginal zone lymphoma (ENMZL) and small B-cell lymphoma with plasmacytic differentiation*
  - In 2011, Gibson et al. described four cases of *EBV*+ marginal zone lymphoma arising after organ transplant [70]. Subsequently, similar cases arising after iatrogenic therapy were reported.
  - These lesions are nearly always positive for *EBV*, which suggests underlying immunodeficiency when expressed in mature B-cell neoplasms. ENMZL has been reported in patients with rheumatoid arthritis after treated with immunosuppressives such as methotrexate.
  - These cases frequently involve the skin and subcutaneous tissue [71].
- *EBV+ B-cell lymphoproliferative disorders of the central nervous system*
  - These lesions range from polymorphic *EBV*+ lymphoid proliferations to *EBV*+ diffuse large B-cell lymphoma and were reported after mycophenolate therapy for various autoimmune disorders.
  - They can regress with mycophenolate withdrawal with or without additional therapy.
  - Almost all the cases occur when mycophenolate is administrated alone without calcineurin inhibitors. It appears that calcineurin inhibitors have a protective effect [72, 73].
- *Peripheral T-cell lymphomas*
  - Hepatosplenic T-cell lymphoma (HSTCL), extranodal NK−/T-cell lymphoma, and breast implant-associated anaplastic large cell lymphoma (BIA-ALCL) may arise after immunosuppressive/immunomodulator therapy.
  - Up to 20% cases of HSTCL are reported in young patients treated with immunosuppressive/immunomodulator therapy for inflammatory bowel disease. Rare cases have also been reported in rheumatoid arthritis and sarcoidosis after treatment with thiopurines and TNF-α inhibitors. An FDA study reported 25 cases of iatrogenic HSTCL, of which 24 had undergone treatment with TNF-α inhibitor followed by a second immunomodulator (azathioprine, 6-mercaptopurine, or methotrexate) [74].

Case Presentations

Case 1

Learning Objectives

1. To become familiar with the clinical presentation and pathologic diagnosis of nodular lymphoid hyperplasia of gastrointestinal (GI) tract in patient with common variable immunodeficiency syndrome.
2. To become familiar with the application of laboratory evaluations to diagnose common variable immunodeficiency syndrome and associated nodular lymphoid hyperplasia of the gastrointestinal tract.
3. To be familiar with other types of benign and neoplastic lymphoid proliferations associated with primary immunodeficiency.

Case History

A 31-year-old female with history of recurrent respiratory infection presented with chronic diarrhea. Upper and lower gastrointestinal endoscopy demonstrated multiple polypoid lesions in the stomach, duodenum, ileum, and large intestine resembling what could be seen in familial adenomatous polyposis.

Histologic Findings

- H&E sections of upper and lower GI endoscopic biopsies demonstrated nodular lymphoid proliferation in the lamina propria (Figs. 11.1 and 11.2).
- In the small intestine, villous atrophy was noted, resembling the features seen in celiac disease. Some lymphoid nodules contained germinal centers.
- Immunohistochemical analysis performed on section of colonic biopsy showed mixed B cells and T cells within lymphoid nodules with B cells in the center surrounded by T cells.

Differential Diagnosis

- Nodular lymphoid hyperplasia of the gastrointestinal tract
- Follicular lymphoma of the gastrointestinal tract
- Mantle cell lymphoma of the GI tract
- Familiar adenomatous polyposis with lymphoid aggregates
- Nodular lymphoid hyperplasia of the GI tract associated with primary immunodeficiency

Ancillary Studies

- EBER ISH was positive in rare cells.
- *IGH* and *TCR* gene rearrangement analyses were negative for clonal rearrangement of the genes.

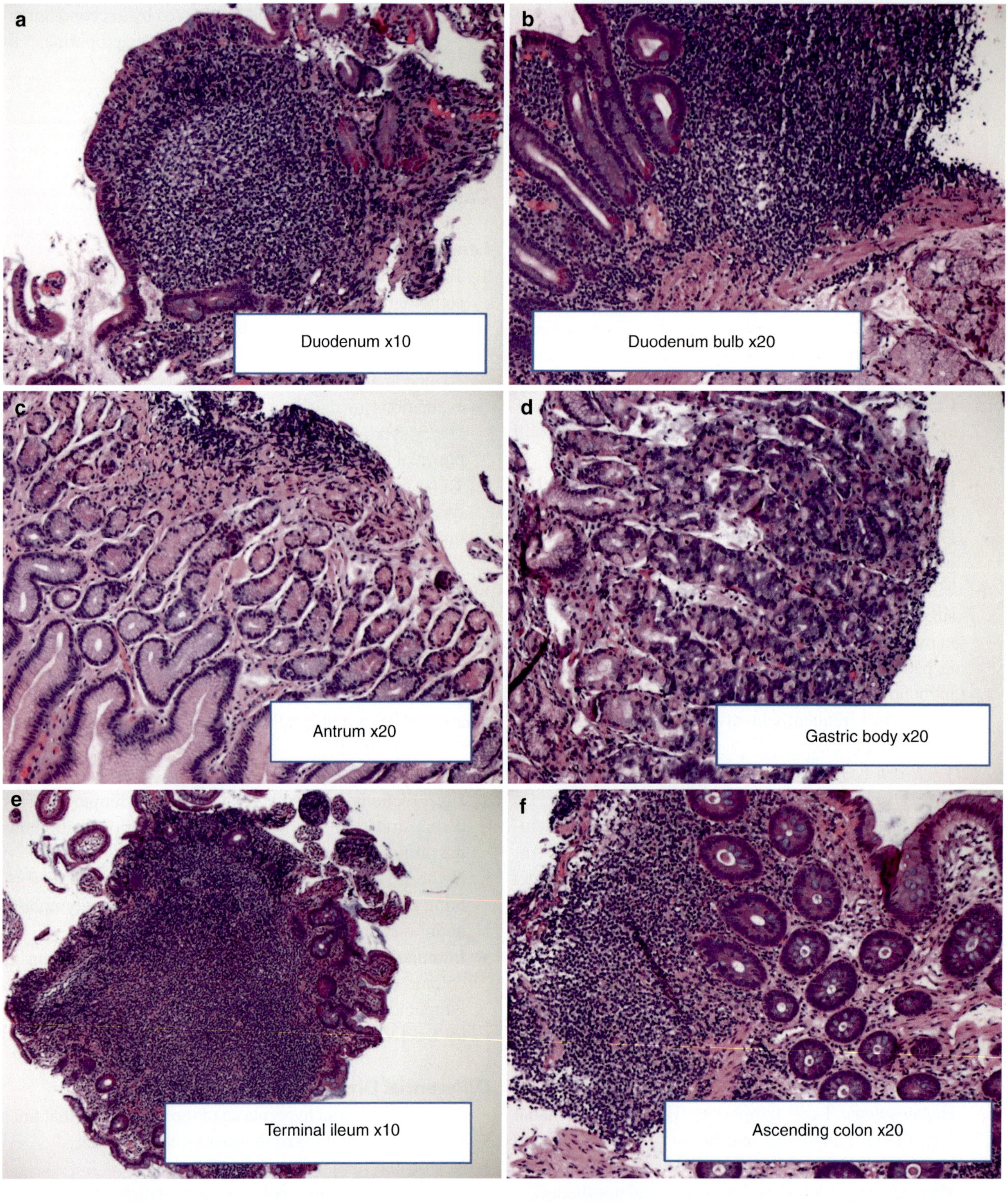

Fig. 11.1 Nodular lymphoid hyperplasia of the gastrointestinal tract associated with common variable immunodeficiency (Case 1). H&E sections of upper and lower GI endoscopic biopsies demonstrate nodular lymphoid proliferation in the lamina propria in duodenum (**a**, **b**), stomach (**c**, **d**), ileum (**e**), and ascending colon (**f**). Note villous atrophy in the small intestinal mucosa (**a**, **b**) and germinal center in lymphoid nodules (**a**)

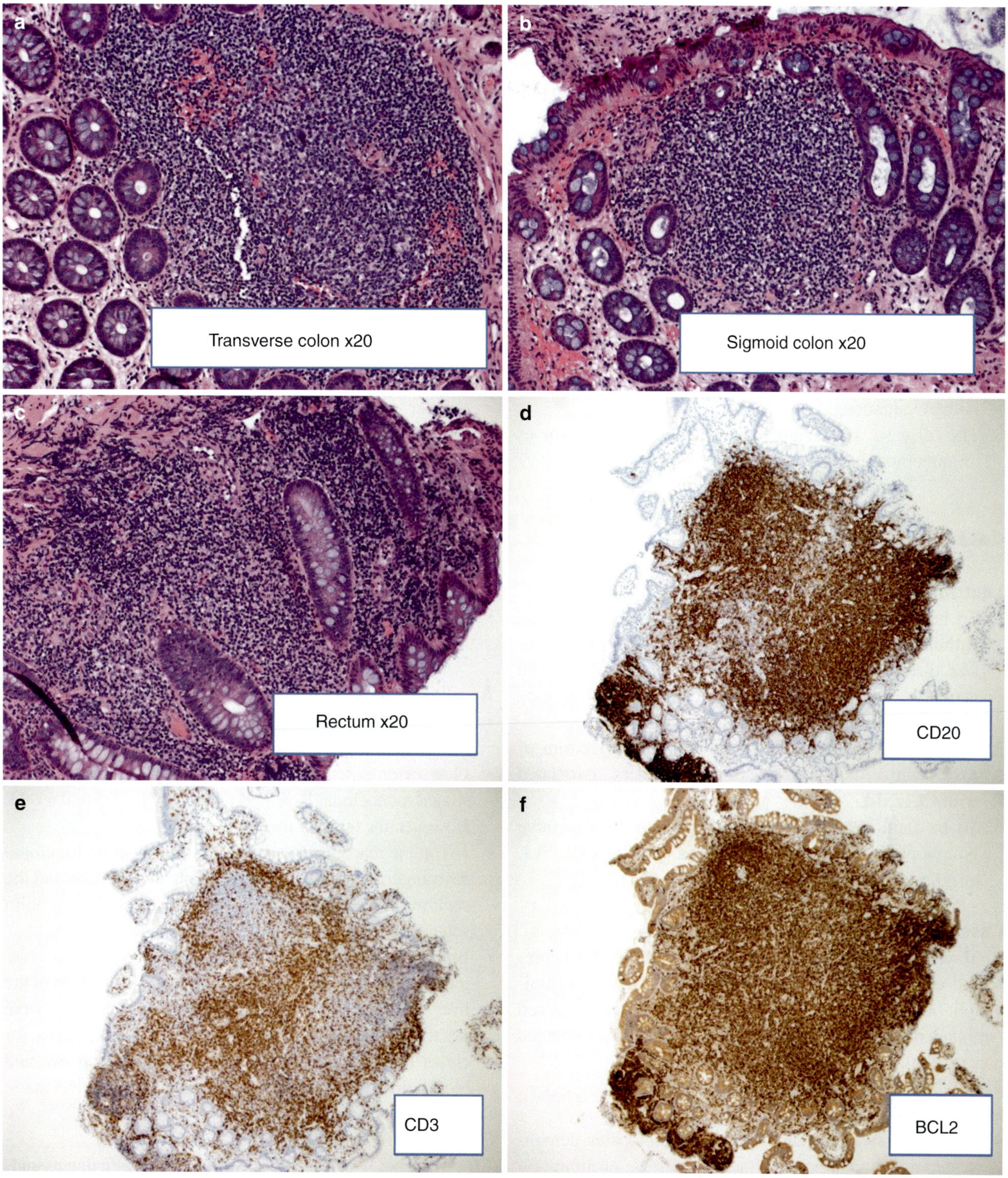

Fig. 11.2 Nodular lymphoid hyperplasia of the gastrointestinal tract associated with common variable immunodeficiency (Case 1). H&E sections of lower GI endoscopic biopsies demonstrate nodular lymphoid proliferation in the lamina propria in the transverse colon (**a**), sigmoid colon (**b**), and rectum (**c**). Immunohistochemical analysis performed on section of colonic biopsy showed mixed B cells (**d**) and T cells (**e**) within lymphoid nodules with B cells in the center surrounded by T cells. Image (**f**) is BCL2 stain that is positive in mantle zone and surrounding T cells, highlighting a small reactive germinal center at upper center (negative for the stain)

- Laboratory evaluations demonstrated serum immunoglobulin levels as follows: IgG = 600 mg/dl, IgA = 34 mg/dl, and IgM = 36 mg/dl.
- Anti-HIV 1 and 2 antibodies were not detected. Stool culture was negative for any pathogenic microorganisms.

Final Diagnosis

Nodular lymphoid hyperplasia of the gastrointestinal tract associated with common variable immunodeficiency

Take-Home Messages

1. Nodular lymphoid hyperplasia of the gastrointestinal tract can be seen in patient with common variable immunodeficiency.
2. The diagnosis relies on histologic examination and laboratory evaluations.
3. The disease is benign, and the treatment involves immunomodulators.

Case 2

Learning Objectives

1. To become familiar with the clinical presentation and pathologic diagnosis of *EBV*-positive lymphoproliferative disorder associated with another hematolymphoid neoplasm, in particular chronic lymphocytic leukemia/small lymphocytic lymphoma (CLL/SLL)
2. To become familiar with the morphologic spectrum of *EBV*-positive lymphoproliferative disorders associated with CLL/SLL
3. To be familiar with the pathogenesis of *EBV*-positive lymphoproliferative disorder associated with CLL/SLL or other indolent B-cell lymphoma/leukemia.

Case History

A 62-year-old male with remote history of CLL/SLL presented with fever, fatigue, and weight loss. Physical examination and radiologic evaluation revealed generalized lymphadenopathy and liver mass. Laboratory data showed pancytopenia.

Histologic Findings

- H&E sections of inguinal lymph node biopsies demonstrated nodal architecture effaced by diffuse proliferation of small- to medium-sized lymphocytes. Vague nodular areas consistent with proliferation centers were noted (Fig. 11.3a, b).
- Immunohistochemical analysis showed that the majority of lymphoid cells were positive for CD20 and negative for CD3 (Fig. 11.3c, d). The latter stain exhibited scattered positive cells consistent with reactive T cells.
- The majority of lymphoid cells were positive for CD5 and CD23 (Fig. 11.3e, f), suggesting that B cells coexpressed these two antigens.
- H&E section of liver biopsy showed mixed inflammatory cell infiltrate including small lymphocytes, plasma cells, histiocytes, and eosinophils with scattered large lymphoid cells (Fig. 11.4a).
- Immunohistochemical analysis showed the findings as below: the large cells were positive for CD30 (Fig. 11.4b) and CD15 (partial) (Fig. 11.4c) and negative for CD45 (Fig. 11.4d). CD68 stain highlighted many histiocytic cells in the background (Fig. 11.4e).

Differential Diagnosis

- Richter transformation of CLL, DLBCL type
- Richter transformation of CLL, classic Hodgkin lymphoma type
- Iatrogenic immunodeficiency-associated B-cell lymphoproliferative disorder, *EBV*-positive DLBCL type
- Iatrogenic immunodeficiency-associated B-cell lymphoproliferative disorder, *EBV*-positive cHL type
- Iatrogenic immunodeficiency-associated B-cell lymphoproliferative disorder, *EBV*-positive cHL-like
- Iatrogenic immunodeficiency-associated B-cell lymphoproliferative disorder, *EBV*-positive polymorphic type

Ancillary Studies

- EBER ISH revealed scattered positive lymphoid cells, most being large (Fig. 11.4f).
- Flow cytometric analysis of lymph node biopsy demonstrated monoclonal B-cell population with CD5 and CD23. However, the tests on liver mass biopsy were negative.
- *IGH* gene rearrangement analysis was positive for clonal rearrangement of the gene on lymph node section and the section of liver mass. The amplicon size and breakpoint sequences were different between the two biopsies.
- Bone marrow biopsy showed the lymphomatous involvement with morphologic features similar to those seen in the liver biopsy (Fig. 11.5). Flow cytometric analyses were negative. *IGH* gene rearrangement analysis was positive for clonal rearrangement of the gene with amplicon size and breakpoint sequences identical to that seen in the liver mass.

Final Diagnosis

***EBV*-positive B-cell lymphoproliferative disorder associated with iatrogenic immunodeficiency related to CLL therapy or CLL itself.**

Take-Home Messages

1. Patients with CLL and corresponding therapy could develop B-cell lymphoproliferative disorders.
2. This category of LPD could demonstrate a spectrum of histologic features.

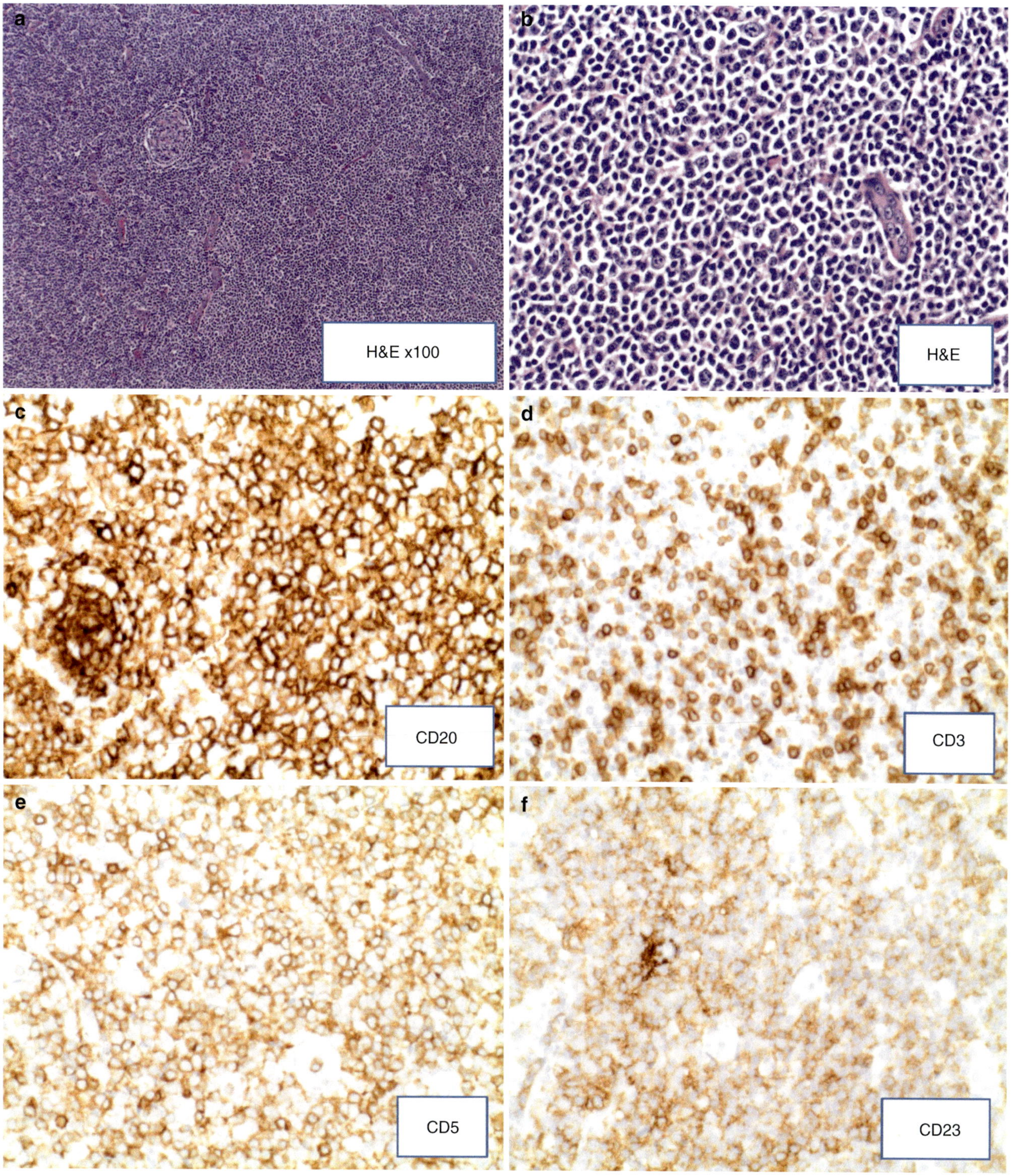

Fig. 11.3 Small lymphocytic lymphoma (Case 2). H&E section of inguinal lymph node biopsies demonstrates nodal architecture effaced by diffuse proliferation of small- to medium-sized lymphocytes (**a**, **b**). Note the size and morphology of lymphoid cells that are consistent with history of CLL/SLL. (**c**) CD20 stain. Note the weak staining in the majority of lymphoid cells. (**d**) CD3 stain. Note the scattered positive cells consistent with reactive T cells. The majority of lymphoid cells are positive for CD5 (**e**) and CD23 (**f**), suggesting coexpression of these two antigens in B cells

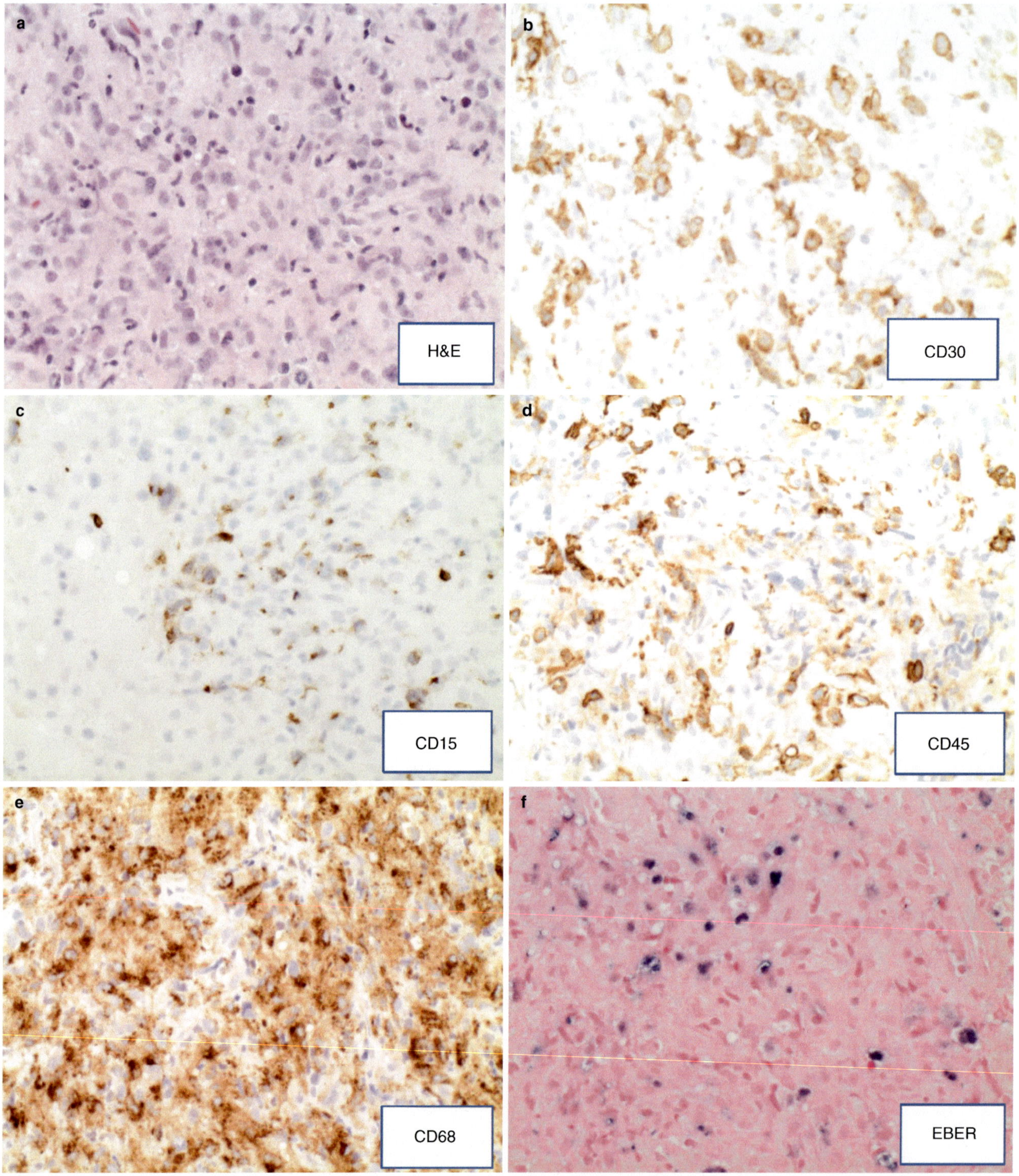

Fig. 11.4 Iatrogenic immunodeficiency-related B-cell lymphoproliferative disorder associated with CLL/SLL (Case 2). (**a**) H&E section of liver biopsy showed mixed inflammatory cell infiltrate with scattered large lymphoid cells. The large cells are positive for CD30 (**b**) and CD15 (**c**) and negative for CD45 (**d**). (**e**) CD68 stain. Note many positive cells consistent with histiocytes in the background. (**f**) EBER ISH is positive in scattered large cells

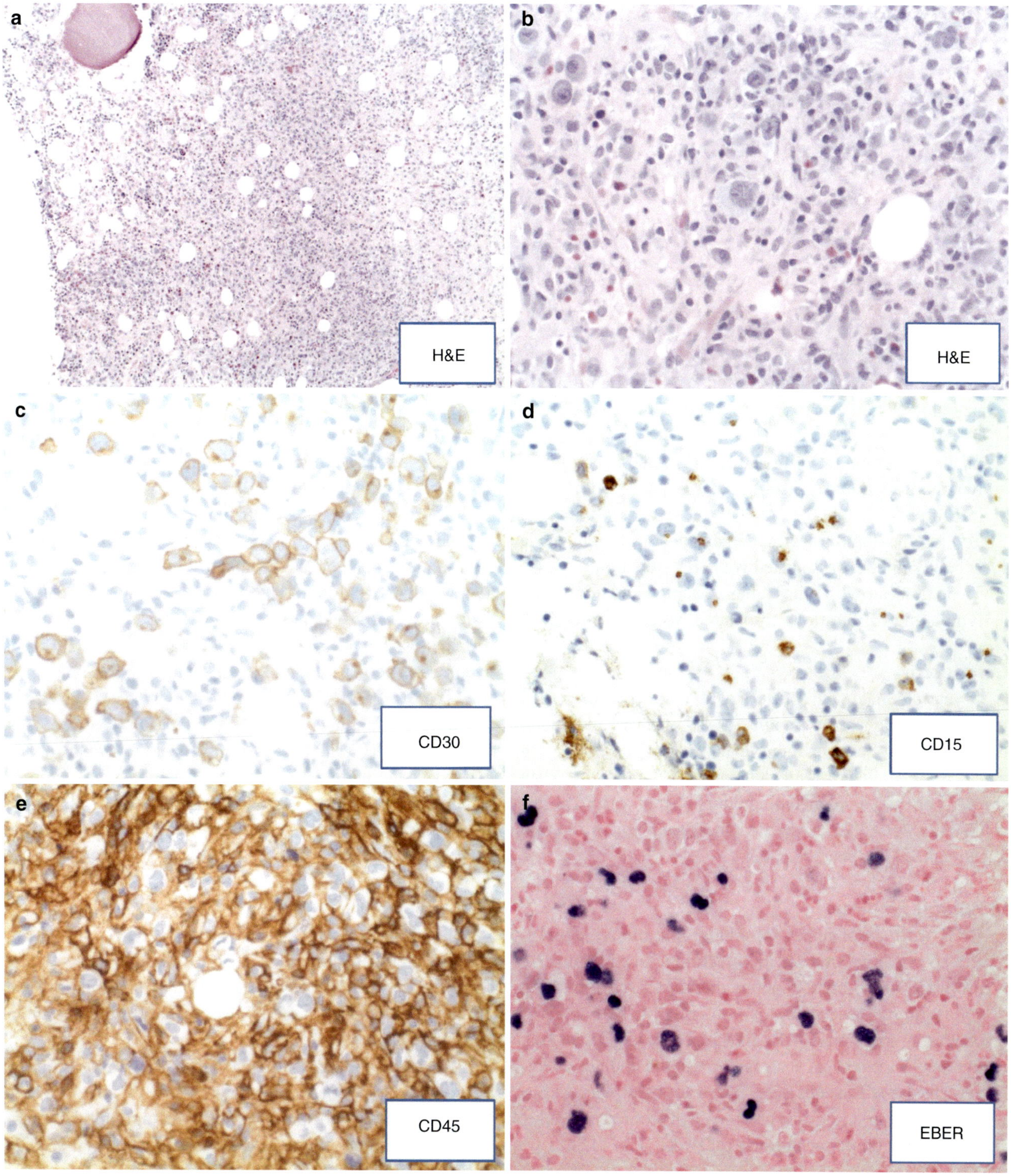

Fig. 11.5 Iatrogenic immunodeficiency-related B-cell lymphoproliferative disorder associated with CLL/SLL (Case 2). (**a**) H&E section of bone marrow biopsy shows extensive lymphomatous involvement. (**b**) A high magnification image shows scattered large lymphoid cells in a background of mixed inflammatory cell infiltrate with fibrosis. The large cells are positive for CD30 (**c**), partial weak for CD15 (**d**), and negative for CD45 (**e**). (**f**) EBER ISH is positive in scattered large cells

3. Iatrogenic immunodeficiency is the underlying pathogenesis, and the cases are often positive for *EBV*.
4. The vast majority of the cases have been demonstrated the clonal rearrangement of B-cell receptor genes that are unrelated to those seen in primary CLL.
5. Similar to posttransplant lymphoproliferative disorders (PTLD), iatrogenic immunodeficiency-associated B-cell lymphoproliferative disorders demonstrate variable clinical outcome, depending upon the histologic classification.

Case 3

Learning Objectives

1. To become familiar with the clinical presentation and pathologic diagnosis of HIV-associated lymphoproliferative disorder
2. To become familiar with the morphologic spectrum of lymphoproliferative disorders associated with HIV infection
3. To become familiar with the diagnosis of high-grade B-cell lymphoma associated with HIV infection
4. To be familiar with other types of benign and neoplastic lymphoid proliferations associated with HIV infection

Case History

A 39-year-old male with a history of HIV infection presented with fever, fatigue, and weight loss as well as abdominal pain. Physical examination and radiologic evaluation revealed generalized lymphadenopathy. Laboratory data showed pancytopenia, including lymphopenia with CD4 cell count of 258/μl. CT scan revealed intestinal mass, in addition to generalized lymphadenopathy.

Histologic Findings

- H&E sections of upper GI endoscopic biopsy demonstrated intestinal mucosa architecture effaced by diffuse proliferation of homogeneous medium-sized lymphoid cells with increased apoptosis and tingible body macrophages, giving a starry-sky-like appearance (Fig. 11.6a).
- Immunohistochemical analysis showed the findings as follows: the lymphoid cells were positive for CD20 (Fig. 11.6b) and CD10 (Fig. 11.6c) and had very high proliferation index (Fig. 11.6d); they were negative for BCL2 (Fig. 11.6e).

Differential Diagnosis

- Burkitt lymphoma
- Burkitt lymphoma associated with HIV infection
- High-grade B-cell lymphoma with *MYC* and *BCL2* and/or *BCL6* rearrangements
- High-grade B-cell lymphoma, NOS

Ancillary Studies

- EBER ISH was positive in >90% of the total abnormal lymphoid cells (Fig. 11.6f).
- Flow cytometric analysis detected a monoclonal B-cell population with bright CD45 and CD10 and bright surface light chain restriction. The events were medium-sized to large based on forward scatter features.
- FISH analysis demonstrated isolated *IGH/MYC* fusion without rearrangement of either *BCL2* or *BCL6* gene.

Final Diagnosis

Burkitt lymphoma associated with HIV infection

Take-Home Messages

1. Patients with HIV infection could develop B-cell lymphoproliferative disorders.
2. This category of lymphoproliferative disorder could demonstrate a spectrum of histologic features, as seen in PTLD, including Burkitt lymphoma.
3. Immunodeficiency is the underlying pathogenesis, and more than one third of Burkitt lymphoma in HIV patients are positive for *EBV*.
4. Diagnosis of Burkitt lymphoma associated with HIV infection relied on histologic examination, immunophenotypic profiling, and cytogenetic studies, as does the Burkitt lymphoma without HIV infection.
5. Similar to PTLD, B-cell lymphoproliferative disorders associated with HIV infection demonstrate variable clinical outcome, depending upon the histologic classification.

Case 4

Learning Objectives

1. To become familiar with the clinical presentation and pathologic diagnosis of HIV-associated benign lymphoid hyperplasia
2. To become familiar with the morphologic spectrum of lymphoid hyperplasia associated with HIV infection
3. To be familiar with other types of benign and neoplastic lymphoid proliferations associated with HIV infection

Case History

A 34-year-old male with a history of HIV infection presented with bilateral enlargement of parotid glands associated with submandibular lymphadenopathy. Physical examination and radiologic evaluation revealed enlarged

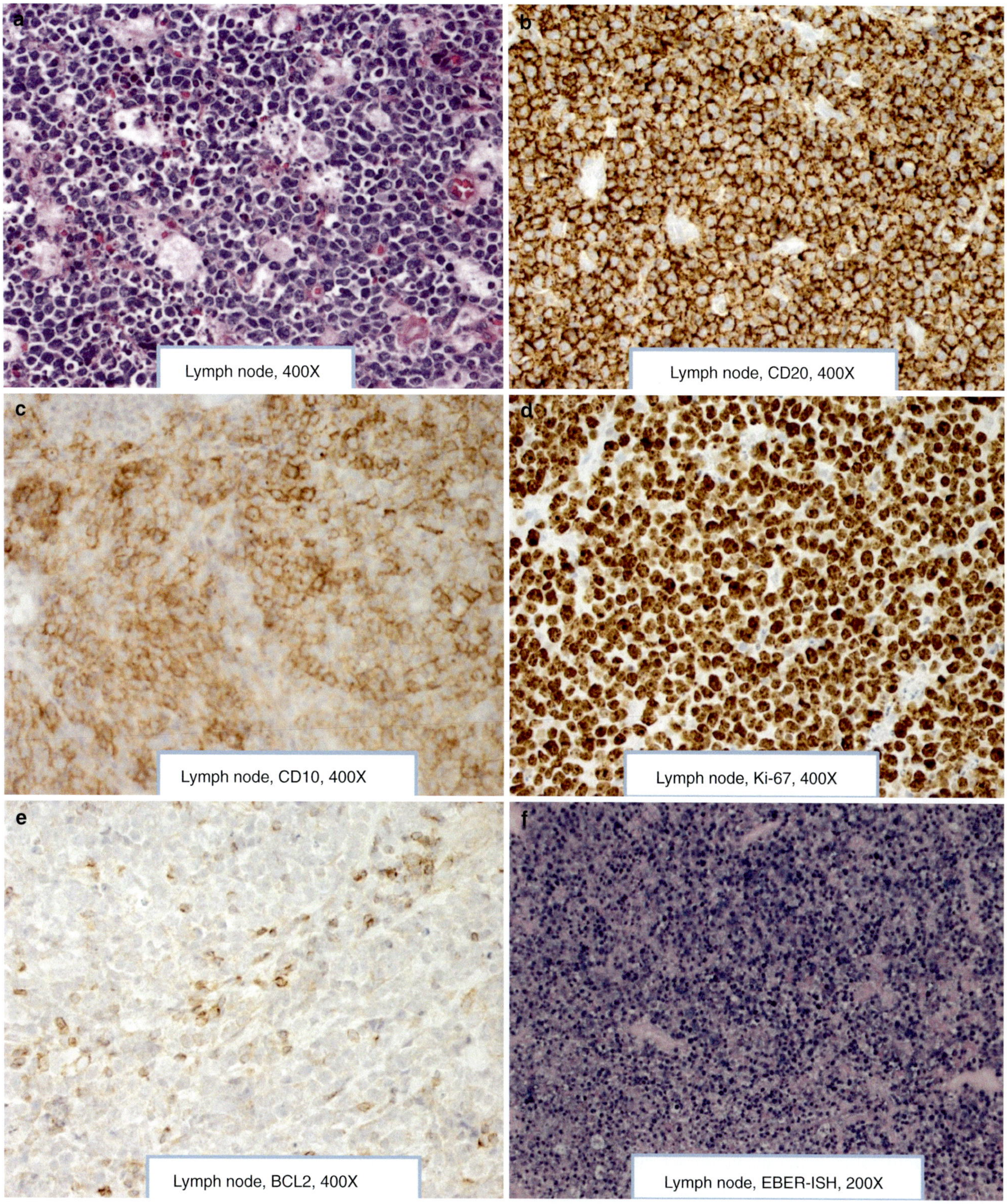

Fig. 11.6 Burkitt lymphoma associated with HIV infection (Case 3). (**a**) H&E section of upper GI endoscopic biopsy demonstrates diffuse proliferation of homogeneous medium-sized lymphoid cells with increased apoptosis and tingible body macrophages. Note the starry-sky pattern of the neoplastic proliferation. The lymphoid cells are positive for CD20 (**b**) and CD10 (**c**) and had very high proliferation index (**d**); they are essentially negative for BCL2 (**e**). (**f**) EBER ISH is positive in the majority of lymphoid cells

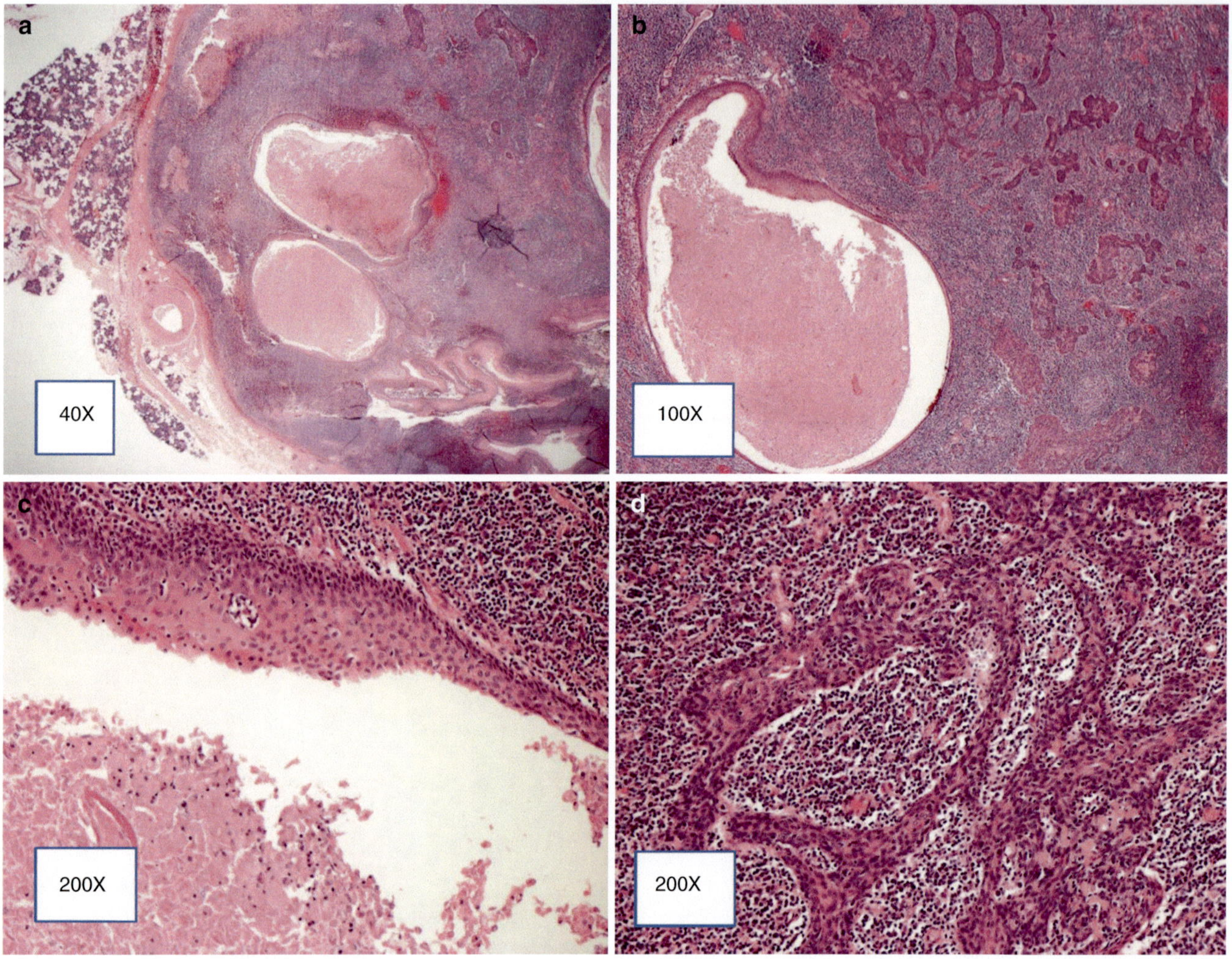

Fig. 11.7 Benign lymphoepithelial cyst associated with HIV infection (Case 4). (**a**, **b**) H&E sections of excisional biopsies demonstrate lymphoid proliferation with squamous epithelium-lined cysts. Note tissue of salivary glands in the left of image a and lymphoid follicles with germinal centers in the lower right in image **b**. Cystic content contained desquamous epithelial cells (**c**). Epithelial islets were present in the background of lymphoid hyperplasia (**d**)

bilateral parotid glands and regional lymphadenopathy. Laboratory data showed lymphopenia with CD4 cell count of 169/μl.

Histologic Findings

- Fine-needle aspiration collected clear to pink fluid with scattered lymphoid cells.
- H&E sections of excisional biopsies demonstrated lymphoid proliferation with squamous epithelium-lined cysts (Fig. 11.7a, b). A few lymphoid follicles with germinal centers were seen.
- Cystic content contained desquamous epithelial cells (Fig. 11.7c).
- Epithelial islets were present in the background of lymphoid hyperplasia (Fig. 11.7d).

Differential Diagnosis

- Epithelial inclusion cyst
- Benign lymphoepithelial cyst (BLC) associated with HIV infection
- Autoimmune sialadenitis
- Extranodal marginal zone lymphoma of mucosa-associated lymphoid tissue (MALT lymphoma)

Ancillary Studies

- Immunohistochemical analysis demonstrated lymphoid follicular hyperplasia and interfollicular hyperplasia (data not shown).
- Flow cytometric analysis showed polytypic B-cell population and unremarkable T-cell population except for an inverted CD4:CD8 ratio.

- *IGH/K* gene rearrangement analysis detected no clonal rearrangement of the genes

Final Diagnosis

Benign lymphoepithelial cyst associated with HIV infection

Take-Home Messages

1. Patients with HIV infection could develop enlargement of bilateral parotid glands that is often confirmed to be benign lymphoepithelial cyst.
2. The diagnosis relies on morphologic examination, flow cytometric analysis, and molecular diagnostic tests as well as clinical correlation.
3. Surgical excision carries diagnostic and therapeutic implications.

Case 5

Learning Objectives

1. To become familiar with the clinical presentation and pathologic diagnosis of *EBV*-positive lymphoproliferative disorder associated with treatment for underlying autoimmune diseases
2. To become familiar with the morphologic spectrum of *EBV*-positive lymphoproliferative disorders associated with iatrogenic immunodeficiency other than organ transplant
3. To be familiar with the clinical outcome of *EBV*-positive lymphoproliferative disorder associated with iatrogenic immunodeficiency other than organ transplant.

Case History

A 22-year-old female patient with a history of Sjögren's syndrome, systemic lupus erythematosus (SLE), and transverse myelitis developed cervical and axillary lymphadenopathy. Pertinent drug history included mycophenolate mofetil and prednisone. She also received pulse high-dose steroids for SLE flare. Excisional biopsy of axillary lymph node was performed for a diagnosis.

Histologic Findings

- Nodal architecture was effaced by heterogeneous lymphoid proliferation. There was a vague nodularity, but otherwise a diffuse process (Fig. 11.8a) with scattered large cells that were mostly consistent with immunoblast-like cells; rare large cells resembled Hodgkin cell variants; however, classic Reed-Sternberg cells or "popcorn" cells were not identified (Fig. 11.8b).
- Background cells included mixture of lymphocytes, plasma cells, and some histiocytes without apparent neutrophils or eosinophils.
- Summary of immunohistochemical stains: the large cells were positive for CD30 (Fig. 11.8c), CD20 (variably) (Fig. 11.8d), CD45 (variably) (Fig. 11.8e), PAX5 (strong), and MUM1, but negative for CD15.
- EBER ISH was positive in scattered small lymphocytes and some large cells (Fig. 11.8f).

Differential Diagnosis

- Iatrogenic immunodeficiency-associated B-cell lymphoproliferative disorder, *EBV*-positive DLBCL type
- Iatrogenic immunodeficiency-associated B-cell lymphoproliferative disorder, *EBV*-positive CHL type
- Iatrogenic immunodeficiency-associated B-cell lymphoproliferative disorder, *EBV*-positive CHL-like
- Iatrogenic immunodeficiency-associated B-cell lymphoproliferative disorder, *EBV*-positive polymorphic type
- Infectious mononucleosis lymphadenopathy

Ancillary Studies

- Flow cytometric analysis of lymph node biopsy demonstrated polytypic B-cell population and unremarkable T-cell population.
- *IGH* gene rearrangement analyses were positive for clonal rearrangement.
- Laboratory evaluation demonstrated a high copy number of *EBV* genome in the blood sample.

Final Diagnosis

***EBV*-positive B-cell lymphoproliferative disorder, polymorphic variant, associated with iatrogenic immunodeficiency related to the treatment for underlying autoimmune diseases**

Take-Home Messages

1. Patients with autoimmune disorder such as Sjögren's syndrome and SLE could develop B-cell lymphoproliferative disorders due to immunosuppressive therapy.
2. This category of LPD could demonstrate a spectrum of histologic features, as seen in PTLD.
3. Iatrogenic immunodeficiency is the underlying pathogenesis, and the cases are often positive for *EBV*.
4. The vast majority of the cases have clonal rearrangement of B-cell receptor genes.
5. Similar to PTLD, iatrogenic immunodeficiency-associated B-cell lymphoproliferative disorders demonstrate variable clinical outcome, depending upon the histologic classification.

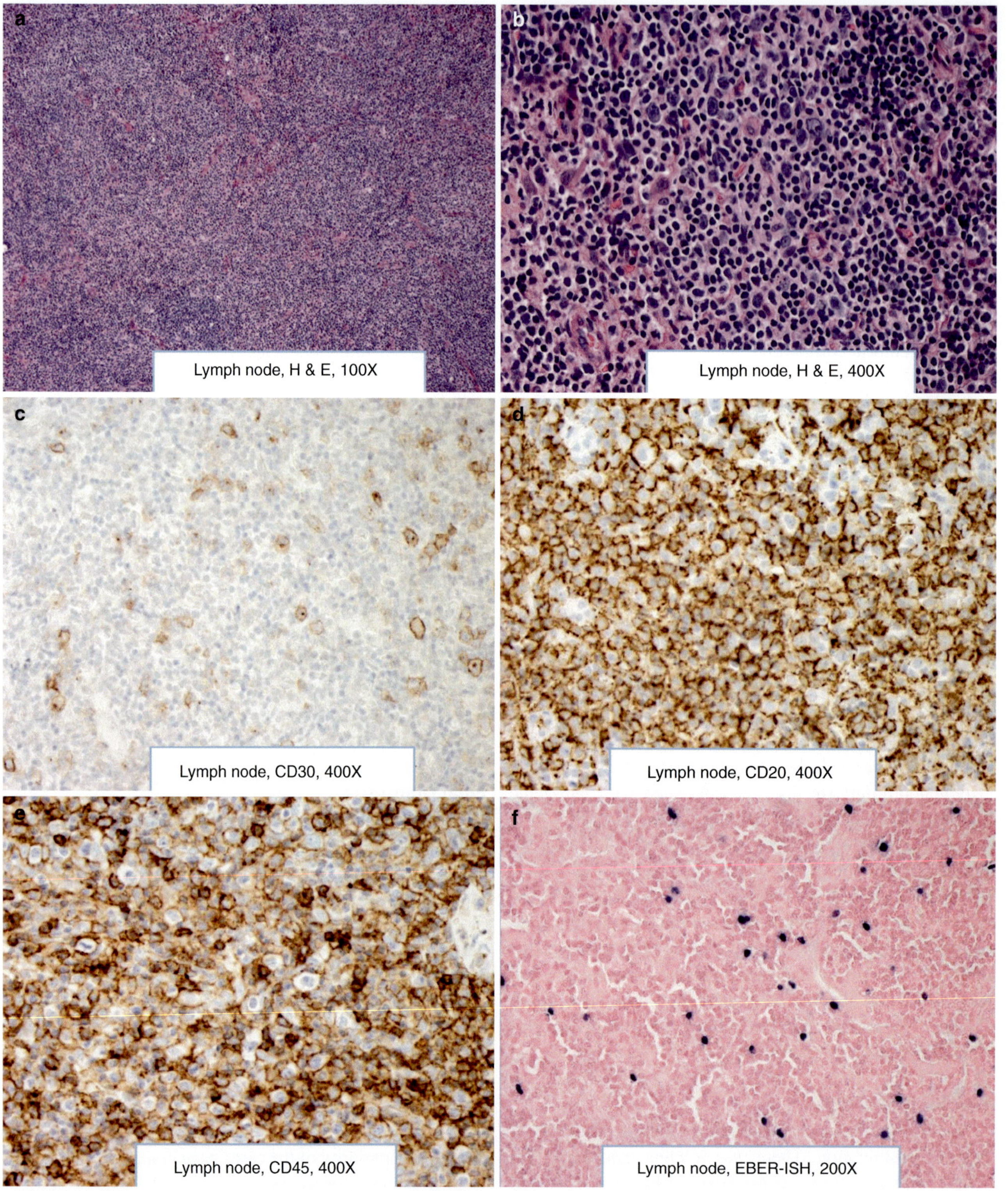

Fig. 11.8 B-cell lymphoproliferative disorder associated with iatrogenic immunodeficiency related to immunosuppressive therapy for autoimmune diseases (Case 5). (**a**) Section of axillary lymph node biopsy shows nodal architecture effaced by heterogeneous lymphoid proliferation. Note a vague nodular appearance. High magnification demonstrates scattered large cells admixed with otherwise heterogeneous lymphoid cells (**b**). The large cells are positive for CD30 (**c**), CD20 (**d**), and CD45 (**e**). Note many small and intermediate lymphoid cells are positive for CD20 and CD45 with weak staining, in addition to some positive large cells. (**f**) EBER ISH is positive in scattered cells including small cells and some large cells

References

1. Yong PF, Tarzi M, Chua I, Grimbacher B, Chee R. Common variable immunodeficiency: an update on etiology and management. Immunol Allergy Clin North Am. 2008;28:367–86.
2. Park MA, Li JT, Hagan JB, Maddox DE, Abraham RS. Common variable immunodeficiency: a new look at an old disease. Lancet. 2008;372:489–502.
3. Kalman L, Lindegren ML, Kobrynski L, Vogt R, Hannon H, Howard JT, et al. Mutations in genes required for T-cell development: IL7R, CD45, IL2RG, JAK3, RAG1, RAG2, ARTEMIS, and ADA and severe combined immunodeficiency: HuGE review. Genet Med. 2004;6:16–26.
4. Schuetz C, Huck K, Gudowius S, Megahed M, Feyen O, Hubner B, et al. An immunodeficiency disease with RAG mutations and granulomas. N Engl J Med. 2008;358:2030–8.
5. Qamar N, Fuleihan RL. The hyper IgM syndromes. Clin Rev Allergy Immunol. 2014;46:120–30.
6. Taylor AM, Harnden DG, Arlett CF, Harcourt SA, Lehmann AR, Stevens S, et al. Ataxia telangiectasia: a human mutation with abnormal radiation sensitivity. Nature. 1975;258:427–9.
7. Savitsky K, Sfez S, Tagle DA, Ziv Y, Sartiel A, Collins FS, Shiloh Y, et al. The complete sequence of the coding region of the ATM gene reveals similarity to cell cycle regulators in different species. Hum Mol Genet. 1995;4:2025–32.
8. Derry JMJ, Ochs HD, Francke U. Pillars Article: Isolation of a Novel Gene Mutated in Wiskott-Aldrich Syndrome. Cell. 1994;78:635–44. J Immunol. 2018;200:3671–80
9. Featherstone C. How does one gene cause Wiskott-Aldrich syndrome? Lancet. 1996;348:950.
10. Rezaei N, Mahmoudi E, Aghamohammadi A, Das R, Nichols KE. X-linked lymphoproliferative syndrome: a genetic condition typified by the triad of infection, immunodeficiency and lymphoma. Br J Haematol. 2011;152:13–30.
11. Booth C, Gilmour KC, Veys P, Gennery AR, Slatter MA, Chapel H, et al. X-linked lymphoproliferative disease due to SAP/SH2D1A deficiency: a multicenter study on the manifestations, management and outcome of the disease. Blood. 2011;117:53–62.
12. Sneller MC, Wang J, Dale JK, Strober W, Middelton LA, Choi Y, et al. Clinical, immunologic, and genetic features of an autoimmune lymphoproliferative syndrome associated with abnormal lymphocyte apoptosis. Blood. 1997;89:1341–8.
13. Shah S, Wu E, Rao VK, Tarrant TK. Autoimmune lymphoproliferative syndrome: an update and review of the literature. Curr Allergy Asthma Rep. 2014;14:462.
14. Price S, Shaw PA, Seitz A, Joshi G, Davis J, Niemela JE, et al. Natural history of autoimmune lymphoproliferative syndrome associated with FAS gene mutations. Blood. 2014;123:1989–99.
15. Lim MS, Straus SE, Dale JK, Fleisher TA, Stetler-Stevenson M, Strober W, et al. Pathological findings in human autoimmune lymphoproliferative syndrome. Am J Pathol. 1998;153:1541–50.
16. Bleesing JJ, Brown MR, Straus SE, Dale JK, Siegel RM, Johnson M, et al. Immunophenotypic profiles in families with autoimmune lymphoproliferative syndrome. Blood. 2001;98:2466–73.
17. Oliveira JB, Bleesing JJ, Dianzani U, Fleisher TA, Jaffe ES, Lenardo MJ, et al. Revised diagnostic criteria and classification for the autoimmune lymphoproliferative syndrome (ALPS): report from the 2009 NIH International Workshop. Blood. 2010;116:e35–40.
18. Sander CA, Medeiros LJ, Weiss LM, Yano T, Sneller MC, Jaffe ES. Lymphoproliferative lesions in patients with common variable immunodeficiency syndrome. Am J Surg Pathol. 1992;16:1170–82.
19. Caballero FM, Brown WR, Kohler PF, Hayward AR. B cell numbers and responses in patients with common variable immunodeficiency and nodular lymphoid hyperplasia of the bowel. J Clin Lab Immunol. 1984;13:59–63.
20. Washington K, Stenzel TT, Buckley RH, Gottfried MR. Gastrointestinal pathology in patients with common variable immunodeficiency and X-linked agammaglobulinemia. Am J Surg Pathol. 1996;20:1240–52.
21. Hugle B, Astigarraga I, Henter JI, Porwit-MacDonald A, Meindl A, Schuster V. Simultaneous manifestation of fulminant infectious mononucleosis with haemophagocytic syndrome and B-cell lymphoma in X-linked lymphoproliferative disease. Eur J Pediatr. 2007;166:589–93.
22. Tran H, Nourse J, Hall S, Green M, Griffiths L, Gandhi MK. Immunodeficiency-associated lymphomas. Blood Rev. 2008;22:261–81.
23. Tinguely M, Vonlanthen R, Muller E, Dommann-Scherrer CC, Schneider J, Laissue JA, et al. Hodgkin's disease-like lymphoproliferative disorders in patients with different underlying immunodeficiency states. Mod Pathol. 1998;11:307–12.
24. Cotelingam JD, Witebsky FG, Hsu SM, Blaese RM, Jaffe ES. Malignant lymphoma in patients with the Wiskott-Aldrich syndrome. Cancer Investig. 1985;3:515–22.
25. Ilowite NT, Fligner CL, Ochs HD, Brichacek B, Harada S, Haas JE, et al. Pulmonary angiitis with atypical lymphoreticular infiltrates in Wiskott-Aldrich syndrome: possible relationship of lymphomatoid granulomatosis and EBV infection. Clin Immunol Immunopathol. 1986;41:479–84.
26. Taylor AM, Metcalfe JA, Thick J, Mak YF. Leukemia and lymphoma in ataxia telangiectasia. Blood. 1996;87:423–38.
27. Miller B, Stansfield SK, Zack MM, Curran JW, Kaplan JE, Schonberger LB, et al. The syndrome of unexplained generalized lymphadenopathy in young men in New York City. Is it related to the acquired immune deficiency syndrome? JAMA. 1984;251:242–6.
28. Mathur-Wagh U, Enlow RW, Spigland I, Winchester RJ, Sacks HS, Rorat E, et al. Longitudinal study of persistent generalised lymphadenopathy in homosexual men: relation to acquired immunodeficiency syndrome. Lancet. 1984;1:1033–8.
29. O'Murchadha MT, Wolf BC, Neiman RS. The histologic features of hyperplastic lymphadenopathy in AIDS-related complex are nonspecific. Am J Surg Pathol. 1987;11:94–9.
30. Finfer MD, Schinella RA, Rothstein SG, Persky MS. Cystic parotid lesions in patients at risk for the acquired immunodeficiency syndrome. Arch Otolaryngol Head Neck Surg. 1988;114:1290–4.
31. Terry JH, Loree TR, Thomas MD, Marti JR. Major salivary gland lymphoepithelial lesions and the acquired immunodeficiency syndrome. Am J Surg. 1991;162:324–9.
32. Oksenhendler E, Duarte M, Soulier J, Cacoub P, Welker Y, Cadranel J, et al. Multicentric Castleman's disease in HIV infection: a clinical and pathological study of 20 patients. AIDS. 1996;10:61–7.
33. Katchanov J, Zimmermann U, Branding G, Arasteh K, Muller M. HIV-associated multicentric Castleman's disease after initiation of antiretroviral therapy: experience of a European Centre. Infection. 2014;42:791–3.
34. Pileri S, Rivano MT, Raise E, Gualandi G, Gobbi M, Martuzzi M, et al. The value of lymph node biopsy in patients with the acquired immunodeficiency syndrome (AIDS) and the AIDS-related complex (ARC): a morphological and immunohistochemical study of 90 cases. Histopathology. 1986;10:1107–29.
35. Biberfeld P, Ost A, Porwit A, Sandstedt B, Pallesen G, Bottiger B, et al. Histopathology and immunohistology of HTLV-III/LAV related lymphadenopathy and AIDS. Acta Pathol Microbiol Immunol Scand A. 1987;95:47–65.
36. Chadburn A, Metroka C, Mouradian J. Progressive lymph node histology and its prognostic value in patients with acquired immunodeficiency syndrome and AIDS-related complex. Hum Pathol. 1989;20:579–87.

37. Weiss LM, O'Malley D. Benign lymphadenopathies. Mod Pathol. 2013;26:S88–96.
38. Raphael MM, Audouin J, Lamine M, Delecluse HJ, Vuillaume M, Lenoir GM, et al. Immunophenotypic and genotypic analysis of acquired immunodeficiency syndrome-related non-Hodgkin's lymphomas. Correlation with histologic features in 36 cases. French Study Group of Pathology for HIV-Associated Tumors. Am J Clin Pathol. 1994;101:773–82.
39. Kasamon YL, Ambinder RF. AIDS-related primary central nervous system lymphoma. Hematol Oncol Clin North Am. 2005;19:665–87.
40. Raphael M, Gentilhomme O, Tulliez M, Byron PA, Diebold J. Histopathologic features of high-grade non-Hodgkin's lymphomas in acquired immunodeficiency syndrome. The French Study Group of Pathology for Human Immunodeficiency Virus-Associated Tumors. Arch Pathol Lab Med. 1991;115:15–20.
41. Davi F, Delecluse HJ, Guiet P, Gabarre J, Fayon A, Gentilhomme O, et al. Burkitt-like lymphomas in AIDS patients: characterization within a series of 103 human immunodeficiency virus-associated non-Hodgkin's lymphomas. Burkitt's Lymphoma Study Group. J Clin Oncol. 1998;16:3788–95.
42. Bibas M, Castillo JJ. Current knowledge on HIV-associated plasmablastic lymphoma. Mediterr J Hematol Infect Dis. 2014;6:e2014064.
43. Nador RG, Cesarman E, Chadburn A, Dawson DB, Ansari MQ, Sald J, et al. Primary effusion lymphoma: a distinct clinicopathologic entity associated with the Kaposi's sarcoma-associated herpes virus. Blood. 1996;88:645–56.
44. Guillet S, Gerard L, Meignin V, Agbalika F, Cuccini W, Denis B, et al. Classic and extracavitary primary effusion lymphoma in 51 HIV-infected patients from a single institution. Am J Hematol. 2016;91:233–7.
45. Tirelli U, Errante D, Dolcetti R, Gloghini A, Serraino D, Vaccher E, et al. Hodgkin's disease and human immunodeficiency virus infection: clinicopathologic and virologic features of 114 patients from the Italian Cooperative Group on AIDS and Tumors. J Clin Oncol. 1995;13:1758–67.
46. Clifford GM, Rickenbach M, Lise M, Dal Maso L, Battegay M, Bohlius J, et al. Hodgkin lymphoma in the Swiss HIV Cohort Study. Blood. 2009;113:5737–42.
47. Nador RG, Chadburn A, Gundappa G, Cesarman E, Said JW, Knowles DM. Human immunodeficiency virus (HIV)-associated polymorphic lymphoproliferative disorders. Am J Surg Pathol. 2003;27:293–302.
48. Bellan C, De Falco G, Lazzi S, Leoncini L. Pathologic aspects of AIDS malignancies. Oncogene. 2003;22:6639–45.
49. Pelicci PG, Knowles DM 2nd, Magrath I, Dalla-Favera R. Chromosomal breakpoints and structural alterations of the c-myc locus differ in endemic and sporadic forms of Burkitt lymphoma. Proc Natl Acad Sci U S A. 1986;83:2984–8.
50. Liapis K, Clear A, Owen A, Coutinho R, Greaves P, Lee AM, et al. The microenvironment of AIDS-related diffuse large B-cell lymphoma provides insight into the pathophysiology and indicates possible therapeutic strategies. Blood. 2013;122:424–33.
51. Ballerini P, Gaidano G, Gong JZ, Tassi V, Saglio G, Knowles DM, et al. Multiple genetic lesions in acquired immunodeficiency syndrome-related non-Hodgkin's lymphoma. Blood. 1993;81:166–76.
52. Okano M, Gross TG. A review of Epstein-Barr virus infection in patients with immunodeficiency disorders. Am J Med Sci. 2000;319:392–6.
53. Gaulard P, Swerdlow SH, Harris NL, Sundstrom C, Jaffe ES. Other iatrogenic immunodeficiency-associated lymphoproliferative disorders. WHO classification of tumours of haematopoietic and lymphoid tissues. 2016:462–4.
54. Kinlen L. Cancer epidemiology and prevention. 2nd ed. New York: Oxford University Press; 1996. p. 532–45.
55. Farrell RJ, Ang Y, Kileen P, O'Briain DS, Kelleher D, Keeling PW, et al. Increased incidence of non-Hodgkin's lymphoma in inflammatory bowel disease patients on immunosuppressive therapy but overall risk is low. Gut. 2000;47:514–9.
56. Kotlyar DS, Lewis JD, Beaugerie L, Tierney A, Brensinger CM, Gisbert JP, et al. Risk of lymphoma in patients with inflammatory bowel disease treated with azathioprine and 6-mercaptopurine: a meta-analysis. Clin Gastroenterol Hepatol. 2015;13:847–58.e4; quiz e48–50
57. Pina-Oviedo S, Miranda RN, Medeiros LJ. Cancer therapy-associated lymphoproliferative disorders: an under-recognized type of immunodeficiency-associated lymphoproliferative disorder. Am J Surg Pathol. 2018;42:116–29.
58. Hasserjian RP, Chen S, Perkins SL, de Leval L, Kinney MC, Barry TS, et al. Immunomodulator agent-related lymphoproliferative disorders. Mod Pathol. 2009;22:1532–40.
59. Bernatsky S, Clarke AE, Suissa S. Hematologic malignant neoplasms after drug exposure in rheumatoid arthritis. Arch Intern Med. 2008;168:378–81.
60. Salloum E, Cooper DL, Howe G, Lacy J, Tallini G, Crouch J, et al. Spontaneous regression of lymphoproliferative disorders in patients treated with methotrexate for rheumatoid arthritis and other rheumatic diseases. J Clin Oncol. 1996;14:1943–9.
61. Abruzzo LV, Rosales CM, Medeiros LJ, Vega F, Luthra R, Manning JT, et al. Epstein-Barr virus-positive B-cell lymphoproliferative disorders arising in immunodeficient patients previously treated with fludarabine for low-grade B-cell neoplasms. Am J Surg Pathol. 2002;26:630–6.
62. Mustjoki S, Ekblom M, Arstila TP, Dybedal I, Epling-Burnette PK, Guilhot F, et al. Clonal expansion of T/NK-cells during tyrosine kinase inhibitor dasatinib therapy. Leukemia. 2009;23:1398–405.
63. Ozawa MG, Ewalt MD, Gratzinger D. Dasatinib-related follicular hyperplasia: an underrecognized entity with characteristic morphology. Am J Surg Pathol. 2015;39:1363–9.
64. Giard C, Avenel-Audran M, Croue A, Verret JL, Martin L. Primary cutaneous Epstein-Barr virus-associated B-cell lymphoma arising at the site of subcutaneous injections of methotrexate. J Clin Oncol. 2010;28:e717–8.
65. Hoshida Y, Xu JX, Fujita S, Nakamichi I, Ikeda J, Tomita Y, et al. Lymphoproliferative disorders in rheumatoid arthritis: clinicopathological analysis of 76 cases in relation to methotrexate medication. J Rheumatol. 2007;34:322–31.
66. Bhamidipati PK, Jabbour E, Konoplev S, Estrov Z, Cortes J, Daver N. Epstein-Barr virus-induced CD30-positive diffuse large B-cell lymphoma in a patient with mixed-phenotypic leukemia treated with clofarabine. Clin Lymphoma Myeloma Leuk. 2013;13:342–6.
67. Loo EY, Medeiros LJ, Aladily TN, Hoehn D, Kanagal-Shamanna R, Young KH, et al. Classical Hodgkin lymphoma arising in the setting of iatrogenic immunodeficiency: a clinicopathologic study of 10 cases. Am J Surg Pathol. 2013;37:1290–7.
68. Dojcinov SD, Venkataraman G, Raffeld M, Pittaluga S, Jaffe ES. EBV positive mucocutaneous ulcer–a study of 26 cases associated with various sources of immunosuppression. Am J Surg Pathol. 2010;34:405–17.
69. Roberts TK, Chen X, Liao JJ. Diagnostic and therapeutic challenges of EBV-positive mucocutaneous ulcer: a case report and systematic review of the literature. Exp Hematol Oncol. 2015;5:13. https://doi.org/10.1186/s40164-016-0042-5.
70. Gibson SE, Swerdlow SH, Craig FE, Surti U, Cook JR, Nalesnik MA, et al. EBV-positive extranodal marginal zone lymphoma of mucosa-associated lymphoid tissue in the posttransplant setting: a

distinct type of posttransplant lymphoproliferative disorder? Am J Surg Pathol. 2011;35:807–15.
71. Natkunam Y, Goodlad JR, Chadburn A, de Jong D, Gratzinger D, Chan JK, et al. EBV-positive B-cell proliferations of varied malignant potential: 2015 SH/EAHP workshop report-part 1. Am J Clin Pathol. 2017;147:129–52.
72. O'Neill BP, Vernino S, Dogan A, Giannini C. EBV-associated lymphoproliferative disorder of CNS associated with the use of mycophenolate mofetil. Neuro-Oncology. 2007;9:364–9.
73. Crane GM, Powell H, Kostadinov R, Rocafort PT, Rifkin DE, Burger PC, et al. Primary CNS lymphoproliferative disease, mycophenolate and calcineurin inhibitor usage. Oncotarget. 2015;6:33849–66.
74. Parakkal D, Sifuentes H, Semer R, Ehrenpreis ED. Hepatosplenic T-cell lymphoma in patients receiving TNF-alpha inhibitor therapy: expanding the groups at risk. Eur J Gastroenterol Hepatol. 2011;23:1150–6.

Primary Extranodal Lymphomas of the GI Tract, Lung, CNS, and Skin with Common Mimics

12

Linlin Wang

List of Frequently Asked Questions

1. What are the lymphomas seen in the gastrointestinal (GI) tract?
2. What are the typical morphological findings in the two most common lymphomas of the stomach – MALT lymphoma and DLBCL?
3. What is the workup required for accurate diagnosis of MALT-type extranodal marginal zone lymphoma (i.e., MALT lymphoma)?
4. What are the distinctive features of large cell/aggressive lymphomas (EITL, MEITL, *EBV*+ DLBCL, BL, blastoid MCL) occurring in the intestines?
5. What are the distinctive features of small cell/indolent lymphomas and lymphoproliferative disorders involving the intestines?
6. What are the mimics of common lymphomas in the stomach and intestine?
7. What is primary CNS lymphoma (PCNSL) and which are the common PCNSLs?
8. What are the morphological and immunophenotypic findings in primary DLBCL of the CNS?
9. Which are other aggressive CNS lymphomas with unusual clinicopathological findings?
10. What are the clinicopathological findings in dural and epidural lymphomas?
11. What are the mimics of CNS lymphomas?
12. What is primary pulmonary lymphoma (PPL), and what are the morphological findings in the two most common PPLs – MALT lymphoma and DLBCL?
13. What are the features of lymphomatoid granulomatosis (LYG) in the lung?
14. What types of lymphomas commonly occur in the skin?
15. What are the differences between cutaneous marginal zone lymphoma and extranodal marginal zone lymphoma in other sites?
16. What is the most common type of primary cutaneous B-cell lymphoma?
17. What is the most common cutaneous T-cell lymphoma, and what are its characteristic features?
18. Which disorders are included under primary cutaneous CD30-positive lymphoproliferative disorders, and what are the features of primary cutaneous anaplastic large cell lymphoma?
19. Is lymphomatoid papulosis a lymphoma?
20. What is subcutaneous panniculitis-like T-cell lymphoma (SPTCL) according to WHO (2017) classification, and what are its clinicopathological features?

1. What are the lymphomas seen in the gastrointestinal (GI) tract?

The gastrointestinal tract is the most common site for extranodal lymphomas [1, 2]. Overall, diffuse large B-cell lymphoma is the most common type (50–66%) in the GI tract, followed by extranodal marginal zone lymphoma of mucosa-associated lymphoid tissue (MALT) lymphoma (about 10–25%) [1–5].

- The stomach is the primary site in approximately two thirds of cases of GI lymphoma. MALT lymphoma and DLBCL are the common lymphomas, but other lymphomas listed below can also be seen in the stomach.
- Most of the intestinal lymphoma arises in the small intestine or the ileocecal region [6]. The ileum is more commonly affected than the duodenum and jejunum. The most common type of intestinal lymphoma overall is diffuse large B-cell lymphoma [7]. The other types of lymphomas include B-cell lymphomas such as mantle cell

L. Wang (✉)
Lab Medicine, University of California San Francisco, San Francisco, CA, USA
e-mail: Linlin.Wang@ucsf.edu

E. Wang, A. S. Lagoo (eds.), *Practical Lymph Node and Bone Marrow Pathology*, Practical Anatomic Pathology,
https://doi.org/10.1007/978-3-030-32189-5_12

lymphoma (MCL), MALT lymphoma, Burkitt lymphoma, *EBV*+ large B-cell lymphoma, and intestinal-type follicular lymphoma, as well as T/NK cell processes such as enteropathy-associated T-cell lymphoma, indolent T-cell lymphoproliferative disorder of the GI tract, and NK cell enteropathy.

- It can be challenging to diagnose lymphoma in the GI tract. Most of the specimens are small biopsies with crush artifact and without flow cytometry studies, which limits a complete evaluation. In addition, there are normal/benign lymphocytes and plasma cells in the lamina propria and submucosa throughout the gastrointestinal tract, which may show variable degree of hyperplasia.

2. What are the typical morphological findings in the two most common lymphomas of the stomach – MALT lymphoma and DLBCL?

- MALT lymphoma is a small B-cell lymphoma, composed of lymphoid cells with oval to slightly irregular nuclei, mature chromatin, and inconspicuous nucleoli, often with moderate to abundant clear cytoplasm, with variable number of admixed plasma cells. In some cases, the lymphoid cells have scant cytoplasm. In other cases, the infiltrate is composed predominantly of plasma cells/plasmacytoid cells (Fig. 12.1a, b). In cases with significant coexisting inflammation, the lymphoma cells may

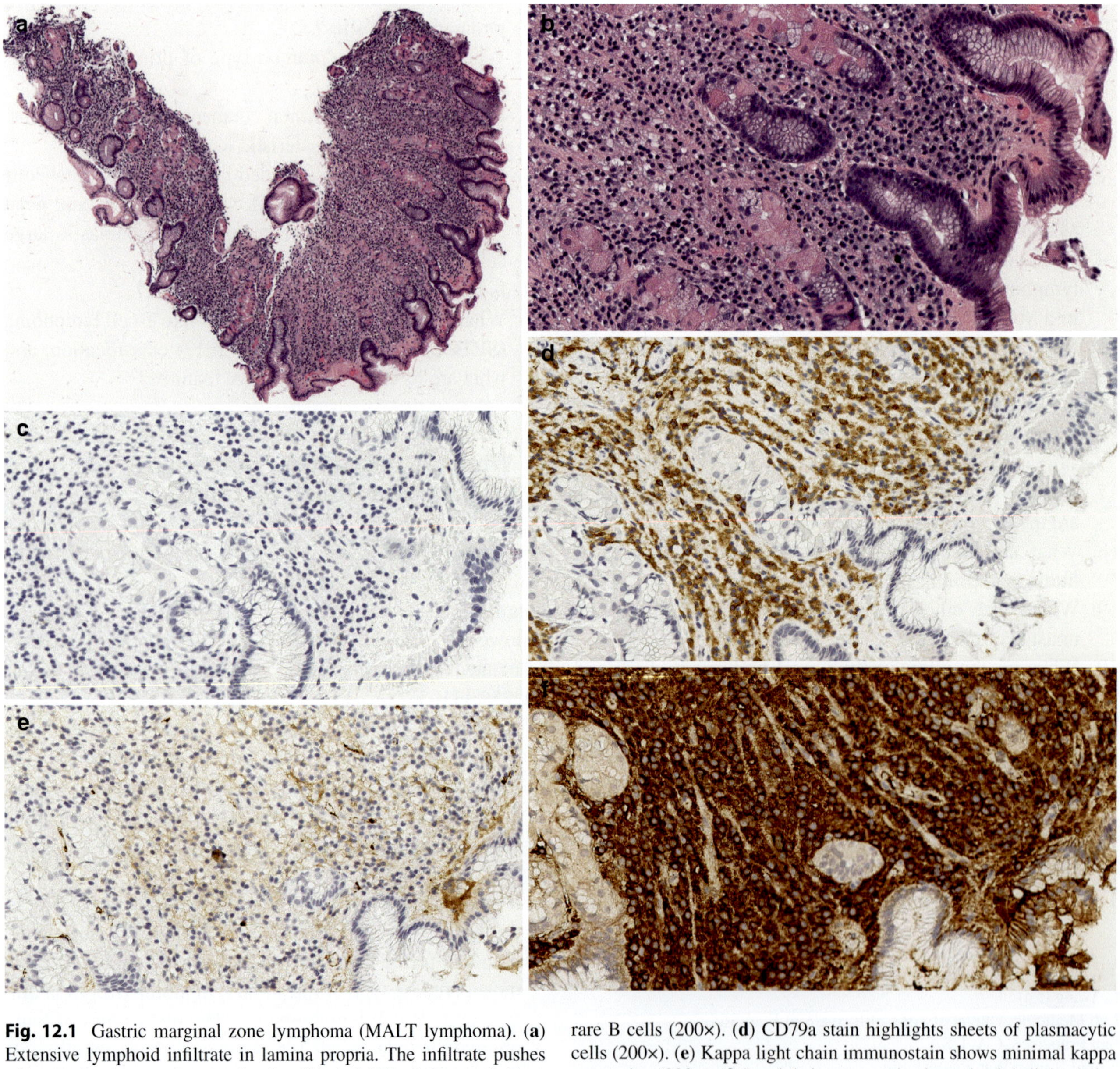

Fig. 12.1 Gastric marginal zone lymphoma (MALT lymphoma). (**a**) Extensive lymphoid infiltrate in lamina propria. The infiltrate pushes adjacent glands apart from each other (40×). (**b**) The infiltrate displays extreme plasmacytic differentiation (200×). (**c**) CD20 stain shows very rare B cells (200×). (**d**) CD79a stain highlights sheets of plasmacytic cells (200×). (**e**) Kappa light chain immunostain shows minimal kappa expression (200×). (**f**) Lambda immunostain shows lambda light chain-restricted plasmacytic cells (200×)

appear larger and/or show degenerative changes, including apparently round or oval nuclei with vesicular chromatin. Variable number of large lymphoma cells may be intermixed in the infiltrate, but a high-grade MALT lymphoma is not recognized in the WHO classification (as opposed to a high-grade follicular lymphoma). Instead, uniform collections of large B cells should be designated as MALT lymphoma with coexisting DLBCL [8].
- The growth pattern is primarily diffuse but may appear nodular due to the presence of reactive follicles. The neoplastic cells surround reactive follicles and often infiltrate into them (follicular colonization).
- Small clusters of neoplastic cells can usually be identified infiltrating and disrupting gastric glands to form lymphoepithelial lesions, a characteristic feature of MALT. The presence of lymphoepithelial lesions is suggestive but not diagnostic of MALT lymphoma, since they could be seen in severe cases of gastritis.
- *Helicobacter pylori* infection is frequently associated with MALT lymphoma in stomach [9].
- DLBCL in the stomach (and elsewhere in the GI tract) usually arises de novo and can extend from the lamina propria to involve the entire thickness of the gastric wall. The diagnosis can be established in most cases based on cytologic atypia, diffuse growth, and expression of pan-B-cell antigens.

3. What is the workup required for accurate diagnosis of MALT- type extranodal marginal zone lymphoma (MALT lymphoma)?

- *Immunophenotyping:* Since flow cytometry is not performed routinely on gastric biopsies, immunohistochemistry (IHC) is essential for the diagnosis of MALT lymphomas in most cases. The majority of cases show an overall increase in B cells expressing CD20 and PAX5. If performed, flow cytometry studies show CD20+, CD5-, CD10-, BCL6-, and light chain-restricted B cells. By IHC, CD20-positive B cells can be in sheet-like collections or at least predominate over reactive T cells.
- BCL2 is commonly positive in the diffuse areas but can be negative in the reactive follicle centers (unless these are colonized by the lymphoma cells). CD10 and CD5 are usually negative. CD21 and CD23 stains highlight follicular dendritic cell meshworks, which may be disrupted or irregular. B cells co-express CD43 in up to 40% of the cases, which is considered as aberrant expression in neoplastic B cells.
- In cases showing marked plasmacytic differentiation, CD20-positive B cells can be few, with the majority of cells being CD138-positive plasmacytic cells (Fig. 12.1c). CD79a can highlight both B cells and plasmacytic cells (Fig. 12.1d). In these cases, the restricted kappa or lambda immunohistochemical staining can demonstrate light chain restriction and thus confirm the neoplastic nature of the infiltrate (Fig. 12.1e, f). However, residual polyclonal plasma cells may be present, and thus polytypic plasma cells in dense B-cell infiltrate do not exclude the diagnosis of MALT lymphoma.
- *Molecular studies:* In difficult cases with more prominent B cells than T cells in the lymphoid infiltrate, but without aberrant CD43 on the B cells or monotypic light chain restriction in plasma cells by immunohistochemical stain, the clonal nature of B cells detected by PCR-based B-cell clonality test is necessary to confirm the diagnosis of MALT lymphoma in those equivocal cases [10].

4. What are the distinctive features of large cell/aggressive lymphomas (EITL, MEITL, *EBV*+ DLBCL, BL, blastoid MCL) occurring in the intestines?

Large cell/aggressive intestinal lymphomas include both T-cell and B-cell lymphomas. The following section primarily deals with those entities which either occur primarily in the GI tract or show certain characteristic findings when they occur in the intestine.

- *EATL and MEITL:* T-cell lymphomas which occur almost exclusively in the intestine and have an aggressive course include two rare but related entities. These are designated enteropathy-associated T-cell lymphoma (EATL) and monomorphic epitheliotropic intestinal T-cell lymphoma (MEITL). Prior to the WHO (2017) classification, these were considered variants of the same lymphoma and were designated as Type I EATL and Type II EATL, respectively, but they have become two separate entities according to the recent WHO classification [11, 12].
  - EATL is a rare T-cell lymphoma that most commonly presents in the small intestine. It has a close association with celiac disease and occurs primarily in patients of North European origin.
  - Monomorphic epitheliotropic intestinal T-cell lymphoma (MEITL) has no association with celiac disease [13], and majority of the cases occurs in Asian and Hispanic population.
  - Both EATL and MEITL occur almost exclusively in adults and are clinically aggressive with poor prognosis.
  - EATL often presents with intestinal perforation or obstruction, and the diagnosis is frequently established on a specimen of intestinal resection rather than an endoscopic biopsy. EATL has broad morphologic spectrum. Most cases of EATL are characterized by a diffuse infiltrate of atypical medium- to large-sized lymphoid cells with moderate nuclear pleomorphism,

round to angulated vesicular nuclei, prominent nucleoli, and moderate amount of pale cytoplasm. The neoplastic cells may display a bizarre anaplastic appearance. The involved intestines are usually associated with ulceration and a variable mixture of inflammatory cells including histiocytes and eosinophils. Changes suggestive of celiac disease, including increased intraepithelial lymphocytes and villous atrophy, are often seen in the mucosa adjacent to the lymphoma (Table 12.1).

Table 12.1 Different features of EATL and MEITL

	EATL	MEITL
Association with celiac disease	Yes	No
Race	Northern Europe	Asian, Hispanic
Morphology	Pleomorphic, with anaplastic morphology	Monomorphic medium-sized cells
Villous morphology	Villous atrophy	Villous expansion
Ulceration and necrosis	Common	Uncommon
Admixed inflammatory cells	Present	Absent
Immunophenotype	CD3+, CD4-, CD8-, CD30+	CD3+, CD4–, CD8+, CD56+
T-cell receptor	Beta	Gamma

– In MEITL, the infiltrate is medium-sized and relatively uniform and have smooth chromatin and clear cytoplasm. The tumor cells extensively infiltrate into the epithelium (epitheliotropism) (Fig. 12.2a, b). The villous architecture is widely expanded (Fig. 12.2c). Areas of necrosis are uncommon, and an inflammatory background is usually absent (Table 12.1).
– EATL and MEITL have distinct immunophenotypic profiles (Table 12.1). In EATL, the neoplastic lymphocytes usually express CD3, CD7, and cytotoxic granule-associated proteins such as TIA1, granzyme B, and perforin. CD5 expression is often lost in neoplastic T cells. In most cases, CD4 and CD8 are both absent (double negative). CD8 may be expressed in 30% cases but CD4 expression is rare. CD30 expres-

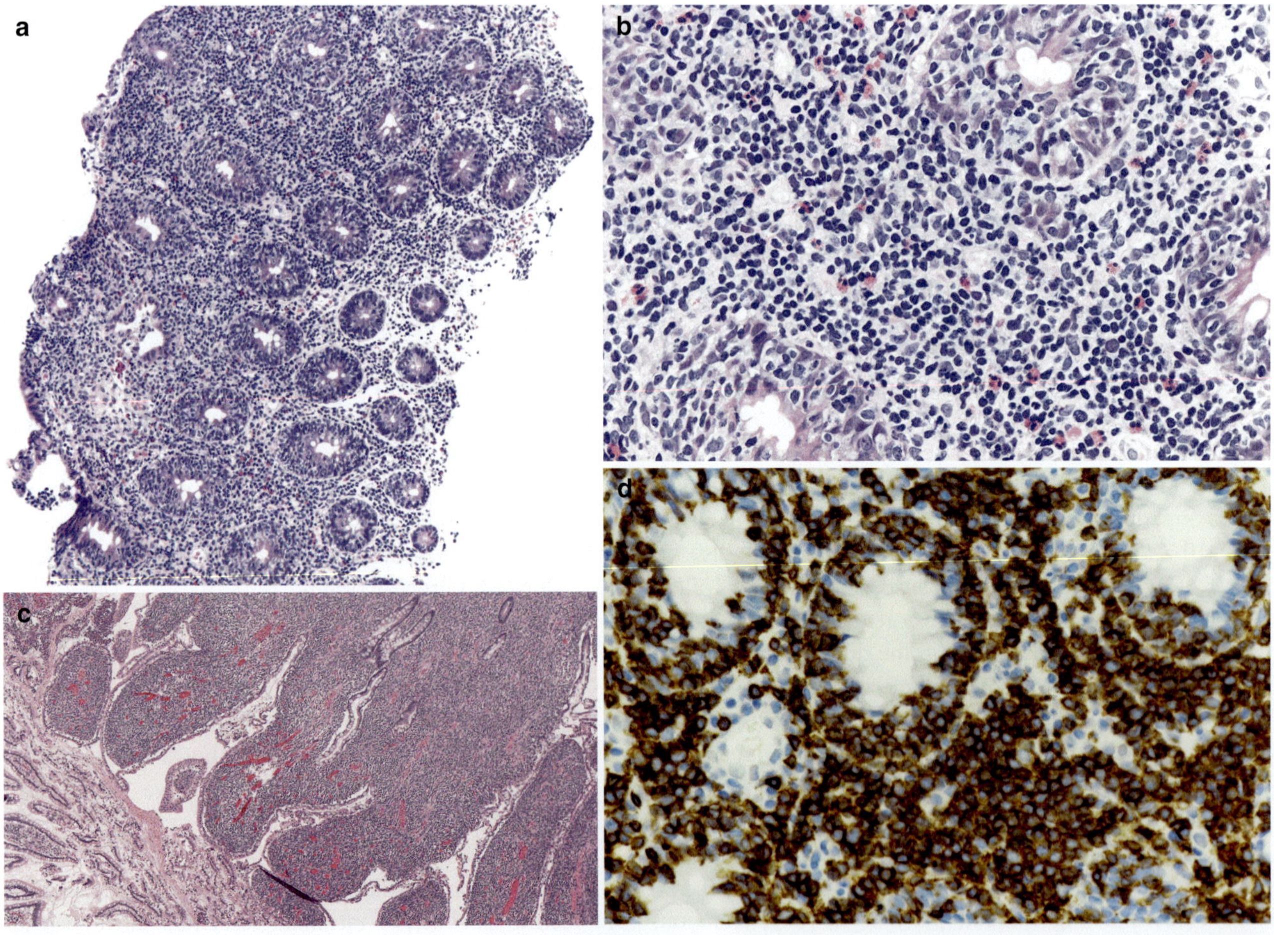

Fig. 12.2 Monomorphic epitheliotropic intestinal T-cell lymphoma (MEITL). (**a**) Mild lymphoid infiltrate in the lamina propria (10×). (**b**) Prominent epitheliotropism and mild lymphoid atypia are present (400×). (**c**) Another case of MEITL shows broadly expanded villous architecture (40×). The lymphoid cells are positive for CD3 (400×) (**d**)

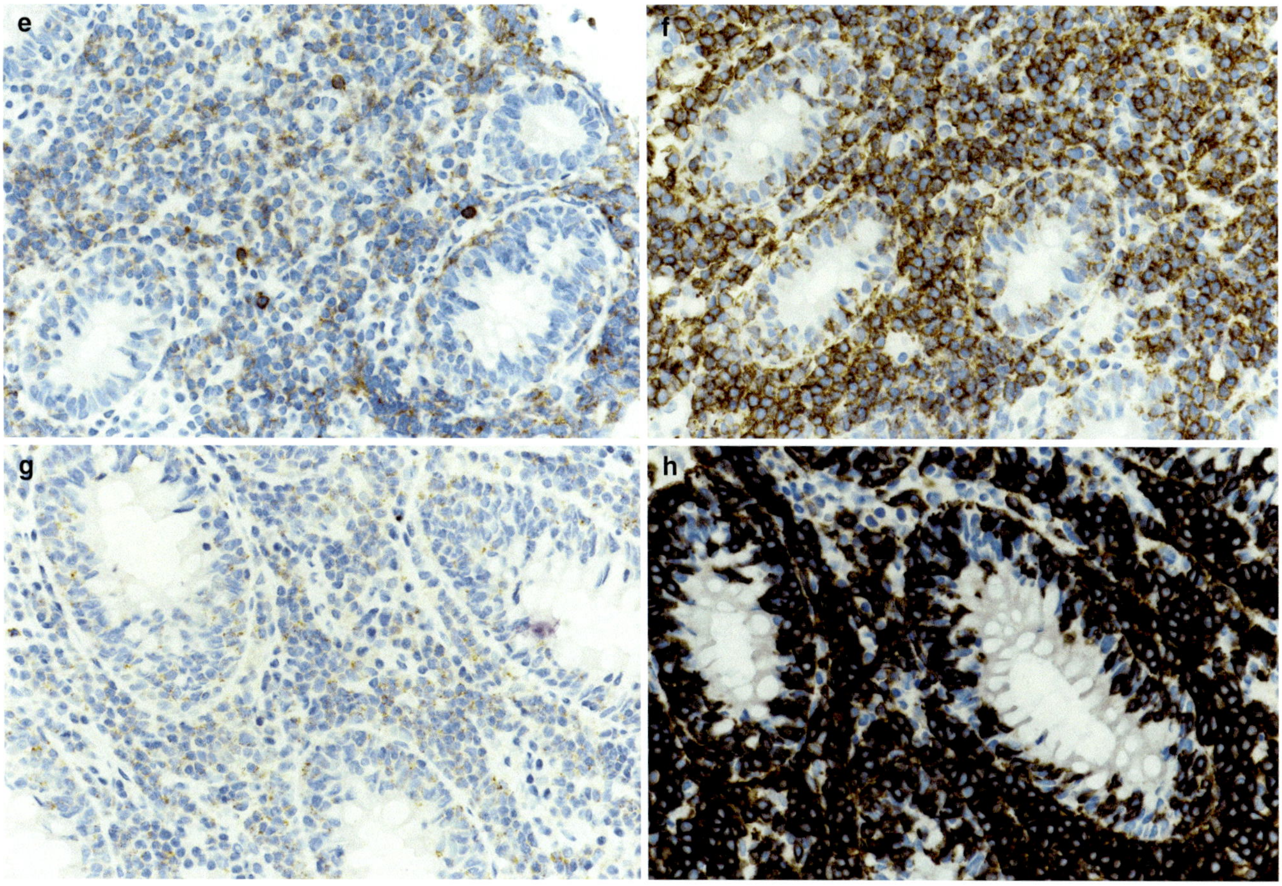

Fig. 12.2 (continued) CD8 (400×) (**e**), CD56 (400×) (**f**), and TIA1 (400×) (**g**). They express T-cell receptor gamma isotype (400×) (**h**)

sion is present in the tumor cells with anaplastic morphology. CD56 is typically not expressed. Most cases are thought to be alpha/beta T cell in origin.

– In MEITL, the tumor cells are usually positive for CD3, CD8, and CD56 (Fig. 12.2d–f). T-cell receptor gamma is often expressed (Fig. 12.2h), and T-cell receptor beta is less frequently expressed. TIA1 is usually positive (Fig. 12.2g). MATK is not commonly used in daily practice but is expressed in more than 80% MEITL, which can be useful to distinguish from EATL.

- *EBV-positive DLBCL:* The gastrointestinal tract is one of the most common extranodal sites of *EBV*-positive DLBCL [14]. This entity was formerly designated as *EBV*-positive DLBCL of the elderly, but it can present over a wide age range. The disease is aggressive in patients older than 45 years; however, in patients younger than 45 years, the disease has an excellent prognosis with complete remission in more than 80% of the patients [15, 16].
  – By morphology, the neoplastic cells may be monomorphous, with a variable number of large atypical lymphoid cells that may have the appearance of immunoblasts or Hodgkin/Reed-Sternberg-like cells (Fig. 12.3a, b). In other cases, the neoplastic cells may be more polymorphic, showing small and larger lymphoid cells, histiocytes, and plasma cells. Geographic necrosis may be present.
  – By immunophenotype, the neoplastic cells are positive for pan-B-cell markers such as CD20 (Fig. 12.3c), PAX5, and CD79a. By definition, *EBV* is present and is positive in large Hodgkin/Reed-Sternberg-like cells as well as smaller B cells (Fig. 12.3d), which is different from Hodgkin lymphoma where the *EBV* is positive only in Hodgkin/Reed-Sternberg-like cells. CD30 is frequently positive but strong expression of CD20 and PAX5, and *EBV* expression pattern can distinguish them from classic Hodgkin lymphoma.
- *Burkitt lymphoma (BL)* is a highly aggressive lymphoma that often presents in extranodal sites. Involvement of the ileocecal region is the most common manifestation of sporadic BL. Sporadic Burkitt lymphoma mainly affects children and young adults, who commonly present with abdominal mass. A typical BL involving the intestine is shown in Fig. 12.4a, b. For a detailed discussion of morphological, immunophenotypic, and molecular features of BL, please see Chap. 6. Here we emphasize the distinctive features seen in BL involving the intestine.

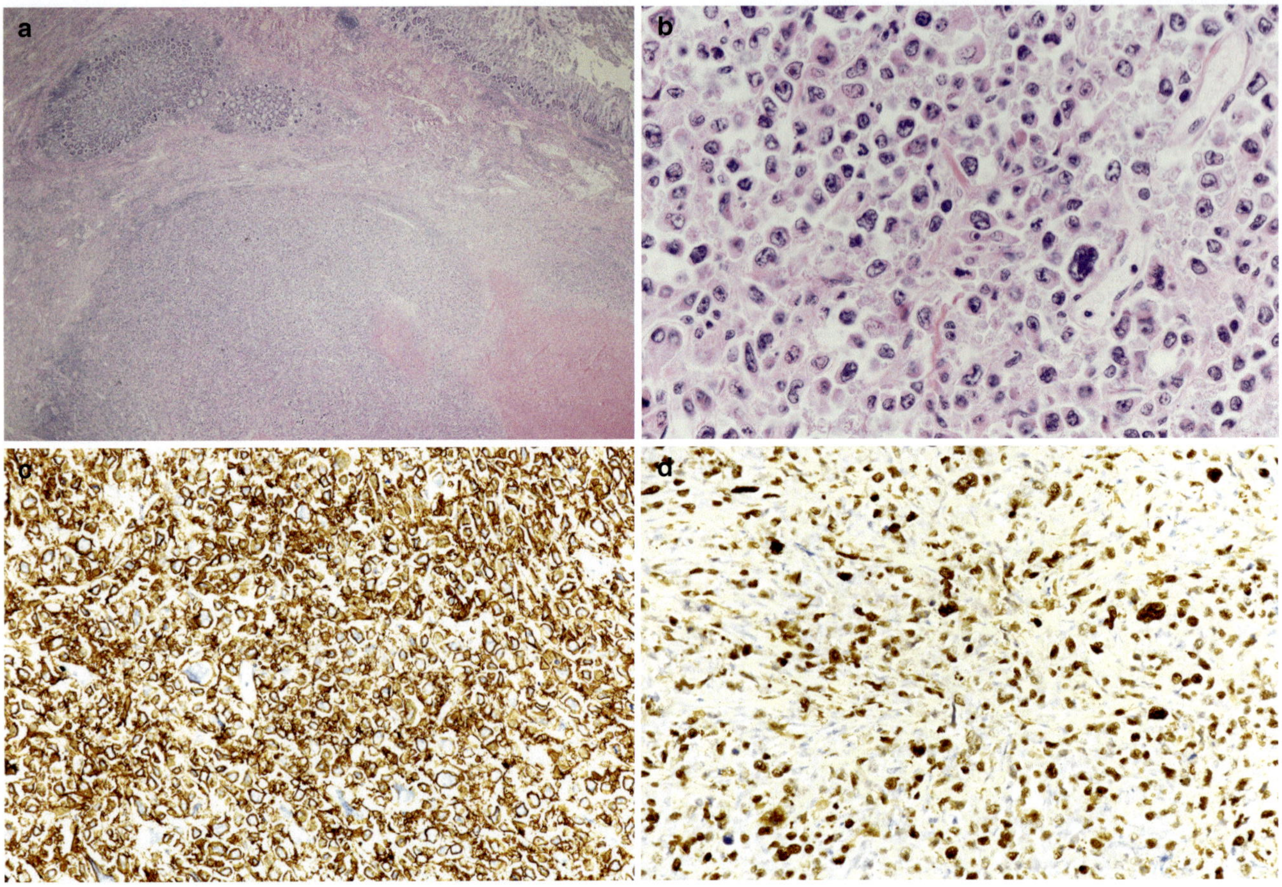

Fig. 12.3 *EBV*-positive large B-cell lymphoma. (**a**) Extensive lymphoid infiltrate in the intestinal wall (20×). (**b**) The lymphoid cells show Hodgkin/Reed-Sternberg-like cell morphology with folded, bilobed, or multilobated nuclei and prominent nucleoli (200×). (**c**) The lymphoid cells are diffusely positive for CD20 (200×). (**d**) EBER in situ hybridization is positive in many lymphoid cells (200×)

- The absence of pleomorphism used to be an important morphologic feature for the diagnosis. However, some cases of BL may show greater nuclear pleomorphism or single prominent nucleoli. The gene expression profile of these cases is similar to BL occurring in other anatomic sites and thus suggests the morphologic spectrum of BL is now broader than previously thought [17].
- Double-hit B-cell lymphoma can have similar morphology, immunophenotype, and translocation as BL. However, additional FISH with *BCL2* or *BCL6* rearrangements can distinguish it from Burkitt lymphoma.
- The GI biopsy specimen is usually small with crush artifact, which can be a challenge to evaluate cell size and pleomorphism. DLBCL can have similar immunophenotype and high proliferation rate and may also show t(8;14) translocation. See Chap. 6 for important distinguishing features between these entities.
- Another scenario is that if the morphologic and immunophenotype is that seen in Burkitt lymphoma but without t(8;14), or less commonly t(8;22), t(2;8) translocation or 11q aberration, it can be classified as a high-grade B-cell lymphoma, NOS.

- *Mantle cell lymphoma (MCL)*, especially the blastoid variant of MCL, involving the intestines has a unique presentation as multiple polyps, referred to as "lymphomatous polyposis." In almost all cases, concurrent involvement of lymph nodes is present, and the morphological and biological properties are the same as nodal MCL (see Chap. 5).

5. What are the distinctive features of small cell/indolent lymphomas and lymphoproliferative disorders involving the intestines?

We will consider the unique features of following indolent B-cell and T/NK-cell entities encountered in the intestines: (1) intestinal MALT lymphoma, (2) follicular lymphoma of GI tract, (3) indolent T-cell lymphoproliferative disorder of the GI tract, and (4) NK-cell enteropathy/lymphomatoid gastropathy.

- *MALT lymphomas in the intestine or immunoproliferative small intestinal disease (IPSID)* or alpha chain dis-

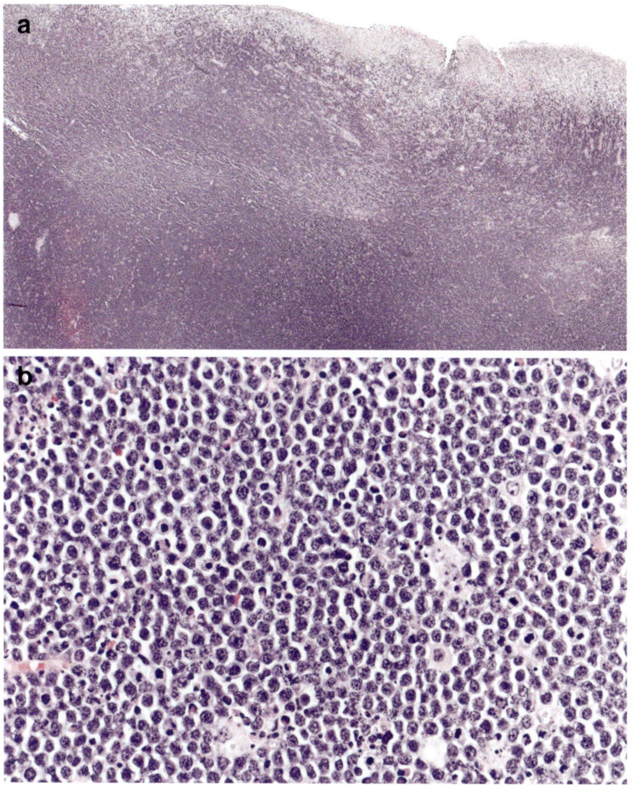

Fig. 12.4 Burkitt lymphoma. (**a**) Diffuse lymphoid infiltrate in the bowel wall showing starry-sky pattern (20×). (**b**) The monotonous lymphoid cells are intermediate in size and show round nuclei, stippled chromatin, and multiple small nucleoli. Frequent apoptotic bodies are seen (400×)

ease has some similarities to *H. pylori*-induced gastric MALT lymphoma. Chronic infection with *Campylobacter jejuni* is suspected to be the cause, but the link is not as clear as in case of *H. pylori* and gastric MALT lymphoma [18].

- The disease is seen most frequently in young males of the Mediterranean region but can also occur elsewhere.
- There are polypoid or flat lesions in the duodenum on upper GI endoscopy and biopsies show blunting or flattening of villi and an infiltrate rich in plasma cells involving the lamina propria. Due to mutations in the area spanning V_{H1} or C_H region of immunoglobulin heavy chain genes, abnormal alpha chains are produced which are incapable of forming the complete immunoglobulin molecule.
- More typical MALT lymphomas most commonly involve the ileocecal area. Of note, the intestinal lamina propria can naturally have sparse to abundant lymphocytes, including focal exuberant lymphoid aggregates, which can mimic MALT lymphoma in a small GI biopsy. Therefore, caution should be exercised to distinguish between intestinal MALT lymphoma and benign lymphoid aggregates. IHC and when necessary molecular studies of B-cell clonality, as described for gastric MALT lymphoma, are necessary for definitive diagnosis.

- *Primary follicular lymphoma (FL) of GI tract:* Most cases occur in the small intestine, usually duodenum [19]. Duodenal-type FL is a specific variant of FL defined by distinct clinical presentations and biological behavior.
  - This disorder is most common in young or middle-aged women and presents as small polyp in the duodenum. Morphologically it shows neoplastic follicles in the mucosa and submucosa. They have typical immunophenotypic features of follicular lymphoma such as CD20+, BCL2+, BCL6+, CD10+, and low proliferation rate by Ki-67 stain.
  - The key features distinguishing these cases from follicular lymphoma arising elsewhere are that they are often localized to the small intestine only, without systemic spread of disease. Survival is excellent even without treatment.
- *Indolent T-cell lymphoproliferative disorder of the GI tract:* This entity is rare and can mimic T-cell lymphomas or inflammatory bowel disease [20–22]. These disorders can involve any site in the GI tract or at multiple sites simultaneously.
  - This T-cell lymphoproliferative disorder typically shows dense infiltrate in the lamina propria displacing but not destroying the mucosal glands (Fig. 12.5a, b). The infiltrate is more often composed of small, mature-appearing CD8+ T cells expressing TIA1, CD3, CD2, CD5, and variable CD7 (Fig. 12.5c, d). The proliferation rate is low (<10%) (Fig. 12.5e). The abnormal T cells usually express alpha/beta T-cell receptor (TCR) and are negative for gamma/delta TCR (Fig. 12.5f). All reported cases have clonal rearrangement of *TCR*.
  - The lesion has indolent clinical course and the patients remain stable without therapy, although they do not respond to chemotherapy.
- *NK-cell enteropathy (lymphomatoid gastropathy):* This is a benign proliferation that has a typical immunophenotype of NK cells (CD56+/TIA-1+/granzyme B+/cCD3+), which displaces but does not invade the glandular epithelium [22, 23].
  - Epstein-Barr virus-encoded RNA in situ hybridization (EBER) is negative, and T-cell receptor gene rearrangement shows no evidence of a clonal process. It has an indolent but sometimes persistent clinical course.
  - This unique entity mimics intestinal and NK−/T-cell lymphomas on endoscopic biopsies and can result in erroneous diagnosis, leading to aggressive chemotherapy. No specific pathogenesis has been described, but cases have been described in association with celiac disease and following chemotherapy for gastric carcinoma.

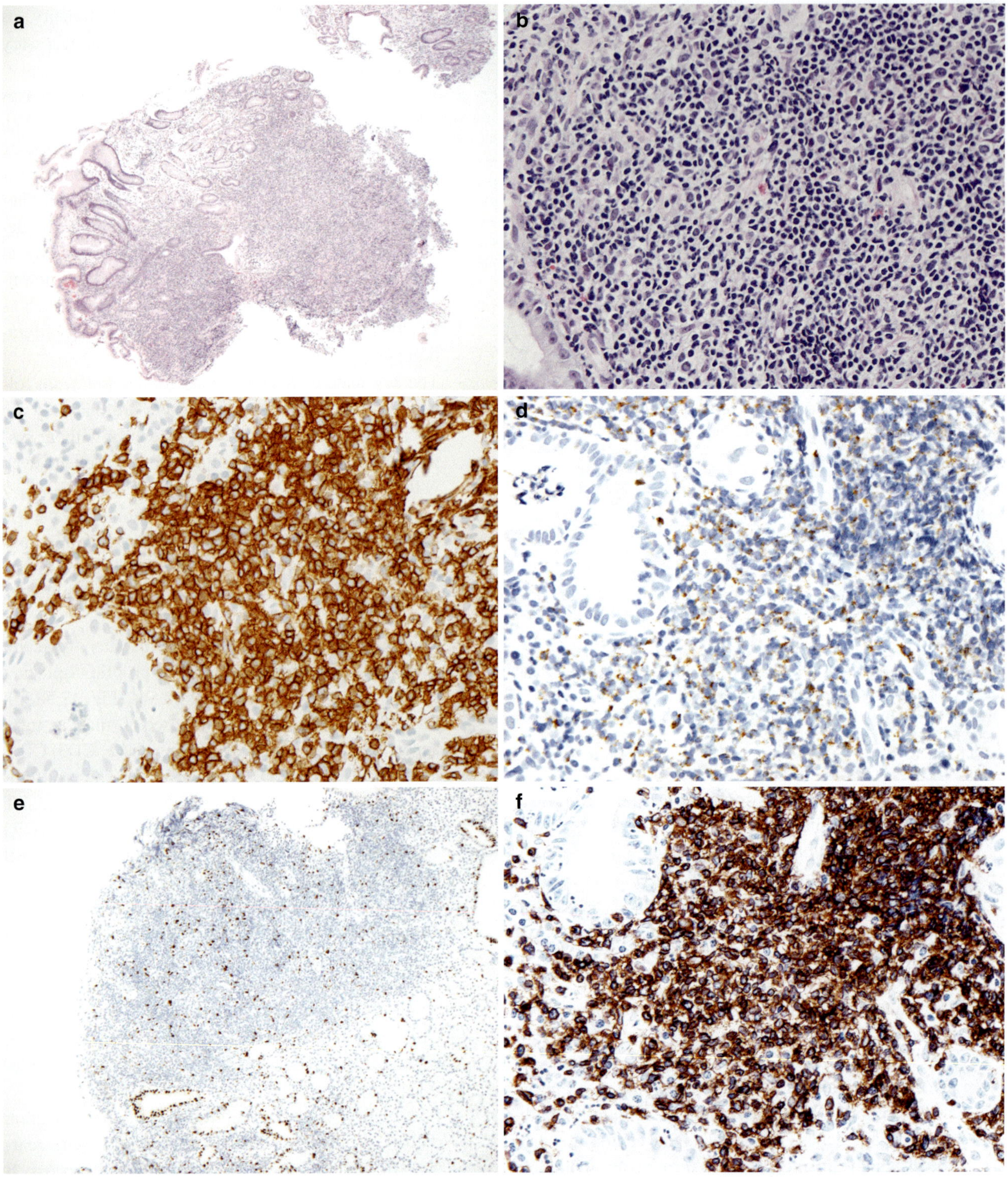

Fig. 12.5 Indolent T-cell lymphoproliferative disorder of the GI tract. (**a**) Dense lymphoid infiltrate in the lamina propria displacing but not destroying the mucosal glands in the stomach (40×). (**b**) The lymphoid cells show mild morphologic atypia (400×). The infiltrate is positive for CD3 (400×) (**c**) and TIA1 (400×) (**d**) with low proliferation rate by Ki-67 staining (400×) (**e**). They express alpha/beta T-cell receptor (400×) (**f**). (The pictures are courtesy of Dr. Yi Xie)

6. What are the mimics of common lymphomas in the stomach and intestine?

Chronic gastritis can mimic MALT lymphoma in the stomach, plasmacytoma may be difficult to differentiate from MALT lymphoma with marked plasmacytic differentiation, and reactive lymphoid hyperplasia may raise suspicion of lymphoma in the intestines. The distinguishing features in these three mimics of GI tract lymphomas are discussed below:

- *Chronic gastritis and gastric MALT lymphoma*: The histological findings in chronic gastritis can mimic and overlap those in gastric MALT lymphoma as both show mixed infiltration of small lymphocytes and plasma cells. When the inflammation is moderate to severe, workup to exclude MALT lymphoma should be considered.
  - Morphologically, MALT lymphomas usually have lymphoepithelial lesions. The infiltrate in MALT lymphoma is usually more extensive, pushing the adjacent glands apart from each other or partially or completely effacing the mucosa architecture. Neutrophils are more commonly seen in gastritis than in MALT lymphoma. The diagnosis is confirmed by ancillary studies as mentioned above (Question 3).
  - Be aware that gastric MALT lymphoma may arise from chronic gastritis, and *H. pylori* infection is associated with both conditions. Therefore, when making a diagnosis of chronic gastritis, particularly one with *H. pylori*, a comment should be included to emphasize the risk of MALT lymphoma in such cases.
- *Plasmacytoma and MALT lymphoma with extensive plasmacytic differentiation:* In either case, the infiltrate can be composed of sheets of plasma cells, and in rare cases, it can be difficult to distinguish MALT lymphoma from plasmacytoma of GI tract [23]. Following points are helpful:
  - MALT lymphoma commonly produces IgM, but it can also be IgG or IgA. On the other hand, plasmacytoma very rarely shows IgM production and should prompt additional workup to rule out MALT lymphoma. While plasmacytoma, but not MALT lymphomas, can be positive for CD56 or cyclin D1, a negative CD56 or cyclin D1 does not favor one diagnosis over the other.
  - Clinical correlation with skeletal survey, serum protein electrophoresis, and bone marrow biopsy can be used to evaluate plasma cell neoplasm. However, an extramedullary solitary plasmacytoma will not show either bone marrow involvement or osteolytic lesions.
- *Benign lymphoid hyperplasia and intestinal lymphoma:* Small intestine has abundant amount of normal lymphoid tissue, such as Peyer's patches. Lymphoid hyperplasia of the GI tract is most often localized to the ileum and occasionally the colon.
  - Young patients have more prominent lymphoid follicles. Diffuse lymphoid hyperplasia can be seen in patients with immunodeficiency [24, 25] or inflammatory bowel disease [26].
  - See Chap. 19 for morphological features which distinguish reactive lymphoid hyperplasia and lymphoma in general.

7. What is primary CNS lymphoma (PCNSL) and which are the common PCNSLs?

- Primary CNS lymphoma is defined as lymphoma that arises in the brain, spinal cord, eyes, or leptomeninges without evidence of previous or concurrent lymphoma outside the CNS system [27]. PCNSL has a worse prognosis than nearly all other primary extranodal lymphomas [28].
- PCNSL develops in two clinical settings: in immunocompetent patients and in immunosuppressed patients. Immunocompetent patients are predominantly older adults with male predominance. Most immunosuppressed patients who develop PCNSL have HIV infection, and they are usually younger.
- Nearly 95% of PCNSLs in western countries are DLBCL. The remaining are rare low-grade B-cell lymphomas, T-cell lymphomas, or Burkitt lymphoma.

8. What are the morphological and immunophenotypic findings in primary DLBCL of the CNS?

- Usually present as single or more, well-circumscribed or ill-defined, infiltrative mass lesions, with displacement of normal structures.
  - In HIV-negative patients, a rare type of PCNSL can have a diffusely infiltrative process without formation of a discrete mass.
  - Radiologically, HIV-associated PCNSLs usually are supratentorial and more often are multiple [29]. The lesions are more often ring enhancing or heterogeneously enhancing. The appearance can mimic that of toxoplasmic encephalitis.
- CNS-DLBCL typically shows patchy, poorly demarcated, angiocentric proliferation that differs from other systemic lymphomas (Fig. 12.6a). They are composed of medium-sized to large pleomorphic cells with oval or irregular

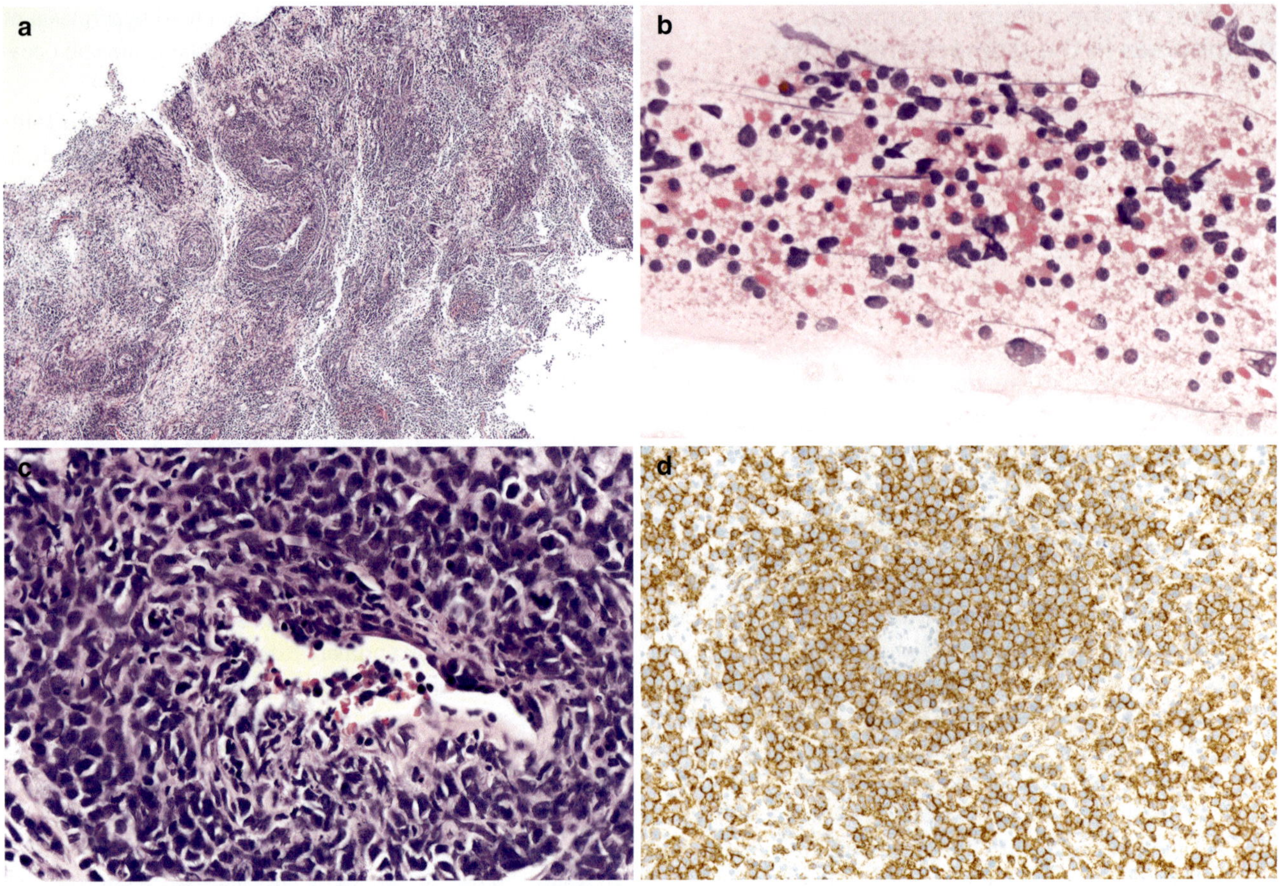

Fig. 12.6 Primary CNS diffuse large B-cell lymphoma. (**a**) Angiocentric lymphoid proliferation (40×). The touch prep (400×) (**b**) and H&E section (400×) (**c**) show large, pleomorphic, and hyperchromatic lymphoid cells with irregular nuclei and prominent nucleoli. They are diffusely positive for CD20 (200×) (**d**)

nuclei, prominent nucleoli, and scant cytoplasm (Fig. 12.6b, c). The morphology may resemble centroblasts. Large area of geographic necrosis is common. Tumor cells can invade parenchyma or subarachnoid spaces from the perivascular cuffs. In some cases, admixed small lymphocytes, macrophages, and reactive glial cells can be prominent and mimic a variety of nonneoplastic inflammatory, infectious, and neurodegenerative disorders. In these cases, the large neoplastic lymphoid cells show an infiltrative pattern.

  - If steroids are administered before biopsy, neoplastic cells may show rapid shrinkage of size or even disappear, resulting in a condition referred to as "vanishing tumor." The areas previously involved by lymphoma may show macrophages and reactive gliosis, which makes the diagnosis challenging. It must be noted that other neoplastic and nonneoplastic disorders can also respond to steroids.

- The neoplastic cells show diffuse positivity for CD20 (Fig. 12.6d) and other B-cell markers such as PAX5, CD19, CD22, and CD79a. They show light chain restriction by flow cytometry. Most cases express BCL6 and MUM1 but are negative for CD138.
  - CD10 is expressed in less than 10% of CNS-DLBCLs, which is a much lower frequency than systemic DLBCL [30]. Therefore, CD10 positivity in CNS-DLBCL should warrant imaging study to exclude systemic lymphoma with secondary involvement of the central nervous system.
- Primary CNS-DLBCL is an aggressive neoplasm. Without therapy, the survival is only a few months, particular in those aged >60, but a long-term survival now has been reported in some cases [31].

9. Which are other aggressive CNS lymphomas with unusual clinicopathological findings?

Two conditions are noteworthy, as they are often difficult to diagnose: lymphomatoid granulomatosis in the brain and intravascular lymphoma with CNS involvement.

- *Lymphomatoid granulomatosis (LYG)* is a systemic, angiocentric, and angiodestructive lymphoproliferative disease involving extranodal sites [32, 33]. It almost

Table 12.2 Histologic grading for LYG

Grade 1	*EBV*-positive B lymphocytes are rare (<5 per HPF) Minimal cellular atypia/large transformed lymphocytes absent Necrosis is absent
Grade II	*EBV*-positive lymphocytes are present (5–20/HPF) Occasional large atypical lymphoid cells present Necrosis is common
Grade III[a]	Many large atypical lymphoid cells and can form large aggregates *EBV*-positive lymphoid cells are numerous (>50/HPF) Extensive necrosis

[a]Differentiating LYG grade 3 from PCNSBL can be difficult as both conditions can have angiocentric growth pattern. However, PCNSBL lacks the angioinvasive/destructive pattern, seen in LYGs, and is usually negative for *EBV*-latency infection

always involves the lungs but also involves the central nervous system in up to 20% of the cases. In addition, rare cases of isolated CNS-LYG have been reported.

- The lesion is composed of *EBV*-positive B -cells admixed with reactive T -cells, with the latter usually predominating [33]. The lesion has a spectrum of histological grade which is related to the proportion of *EBV*- positive B cells relative to reactive lymphocyte in the background, the extent of necrosis (Table 12.2) [34], and the clinical aggressiveness.
- Isolated CNS-LYG seems not to be associated with *EBV* and appears to have a better prognosis than systemic LYG with CNS involvement.
- Brain involvement by LYG manifests as nodular lesions with associated central necrosis. There is an angiocentric and angiodestructive polymorphous lymphoid infiltrate composed of admixed lymphocytes, plasma cells, and histiocytes (Fig. 12.7a–c). Well-formed granulomas are usually not found. *EBV* is usually positive in a variable number of CD20- positive B -cells (Fig. 12.7d, e). The cells show some degree of atypia. They are variably positive for CD30, but negative for CD15. The background lymphocytes are CD3+ T cells.

• *Intravascular lymphoma:* Most intravascular lymphomas are B-lineage and constitute a distinct but rare subtype of extranodal diffuse large B-cell lymphoma characterized by the selective growth of neoplastic cells within the lumens of small blood vessels [35, 36].

- A variety of extranodal sites can be involved and may present in virtually any organ. Commonly involved tissues/organs include the CNS, kidneys, adrenals, lungs, and skin. It has a tendency to spare lymph nodes. The most common clinical presentation is related to CNS involvement including confusion, dementia, and seizure [34, 37].
- On histological sections, small or intermediate blood vessels are filled with and distended by large lymphoid cells with prominent nucleoli, usually with the appearance of centroblasts or immunoblasts (Fig. 12.8a). The involved tissue usually shows intact architecture.
- By immunohistochemistry, these cells express CD45 and CD20 (Fig. 12.8b). CD5 expression is more common than DLBCL.
- Intravascular large B-cell lymphoma is generally aggressive, except for the cases with disease limited to the skin. The poor prognosis is in part due to the delay of timely and accurate diagnosis. Patients promptly diagnosed and treated with chemotherapy have a better prognosis than those who do not receive that therapy.

10. What are the clinicopathological findings in dural and epidural lymphomas?

• *Primary dural lymphomas* are much less common than lymphomas arising in the brain. Dural lymphomas are almost all extranodal marginal zone lymphomas of mucosa-associated lymphoid tissue (MALT lymphomas). Rare cases of DLBCL have been described. Patients are usually middle-aged adults with female preponderance.

- Microscopic examination reveals a perivascular and/or diffuse infiltrate of small lymphoid cells, usually with plasmacytic differentiation. In some cases, remnants of reactive follicles and follicular colonization can be seen. The immunophenotype is similar to that of marginal zone lymphoma in other anatomic sites.

• *Primary spinal epidural lymphoma* is defined as lymphoma occurring in the epidural space in the absence of previously detected lymphoma elsewhere. It is uncommon, accounting for fewer than 10% of all lymphomas in this site. More commonly, the epidural lymphoma involvement occurs in the setting of widespread disease or through direct extension from lymphoma in the vertebral body or the retroperitoneum.

- Patients usually present with symptoms related to extrinsic compression of the spinal cord or cauda equina, depending on the anatomic level of involvement [38].
- Most of these lymphomas are B-cell lymphoma, with DLBCL as the most common type. A few MALT and plasmablastic lymphoma have been described [38].

11. What are the mimics of CNS lymphomas?

Differentiation between primary CNS lymphomas and other brain lesions, including malignant gliomas, infarctions, metastatic brain tumors, demyelinating disease, and inflammatory disease, is often difficult.

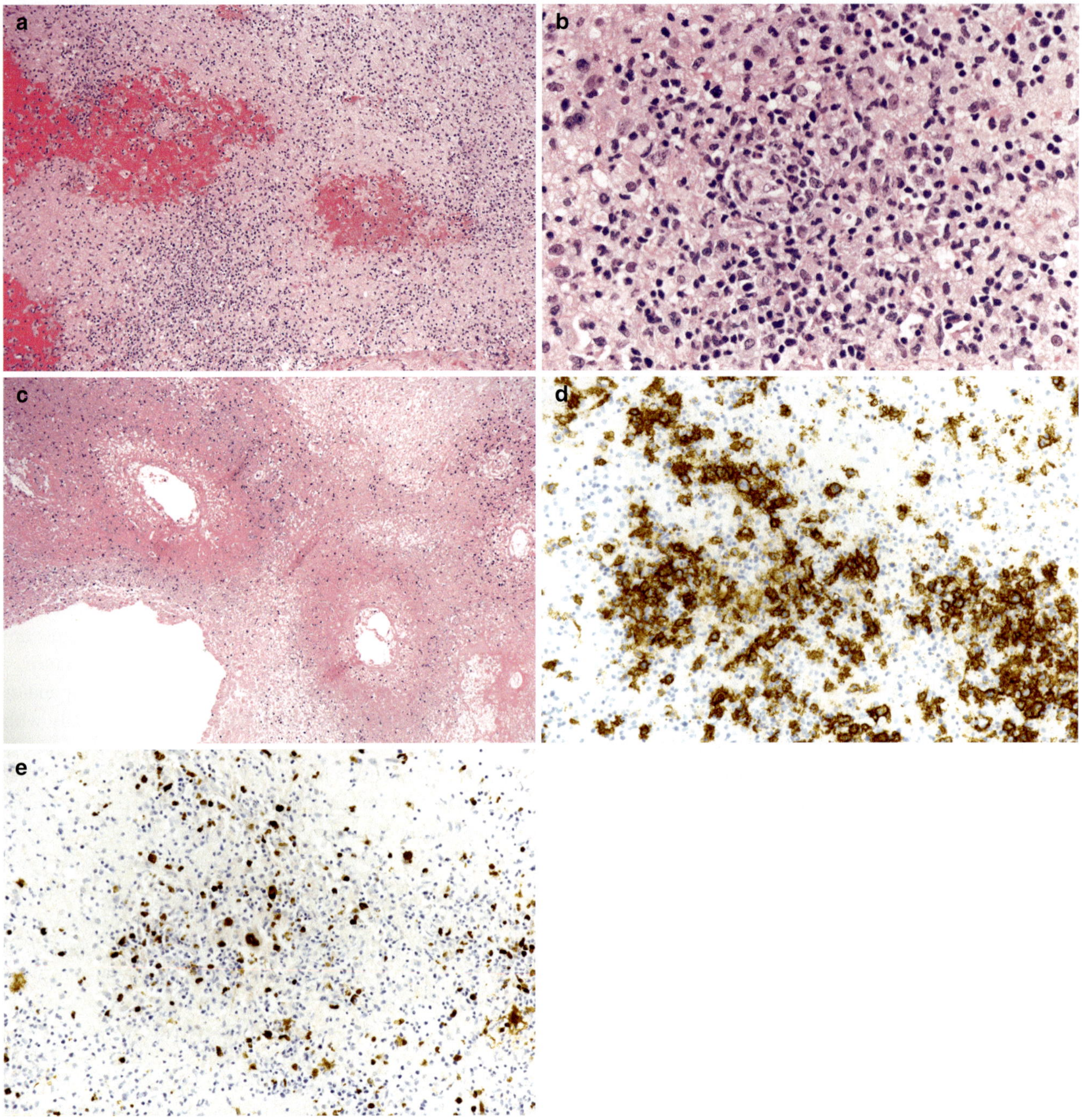

Fig. 12.7 Lymphomatoid granulomatosis (LYG). (**a**) (100×) and (**b**) (400×). Polymorphous lymphoid infiltrate composed of large atypical cells, admixed with lymphocytes and histiocytes. Necrosis is also present. (**c**) The lesion is angiocentric (100×). The large lymphoid cells are highlighted by positive CD20 (200×) (**d**) and positive EBER in situ hybridization (200×) (**e**). This lesion could be graded as grade 2

- Primary CNS lymphomas may be histologically indistinguishable from demyelinating disease because the edge of the lesion often contains demyelination, gliosis, macrophages, and small nonneoplastic perivascular lymphocytes [39]. In cases with corticosteroid administration before the biopsy, the tumor can show rapid shrinkage. In addition, several cases of spontaneous regression of primary CNS lymphomas without steroid administration have been reported [40]. Clinicopathological correlation, especially with history of recent steroid treatment, should be done when the histological findings are equivocal. On the other hand, demyelinating disease and many inflammatory diseases could resemble primary CNS lymphoma clinically and

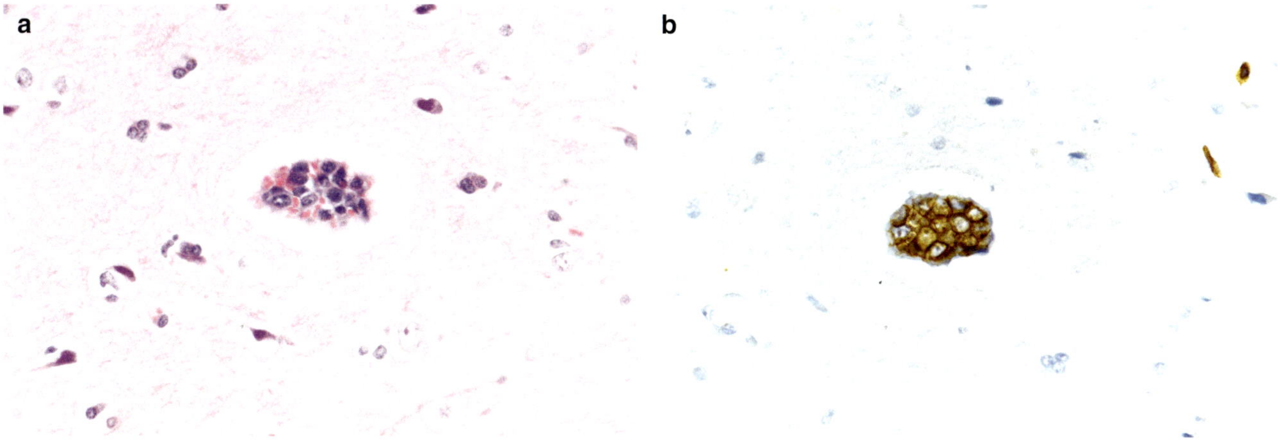

Fig. 12.8 Intravascular lymphoma. (**a**) Small blood vessels in the brain parenchyma are filled with large lymphoid cells with prominent nucleoli (400×). The lymphoid cells are positive for CD20 (400×) (**b**)

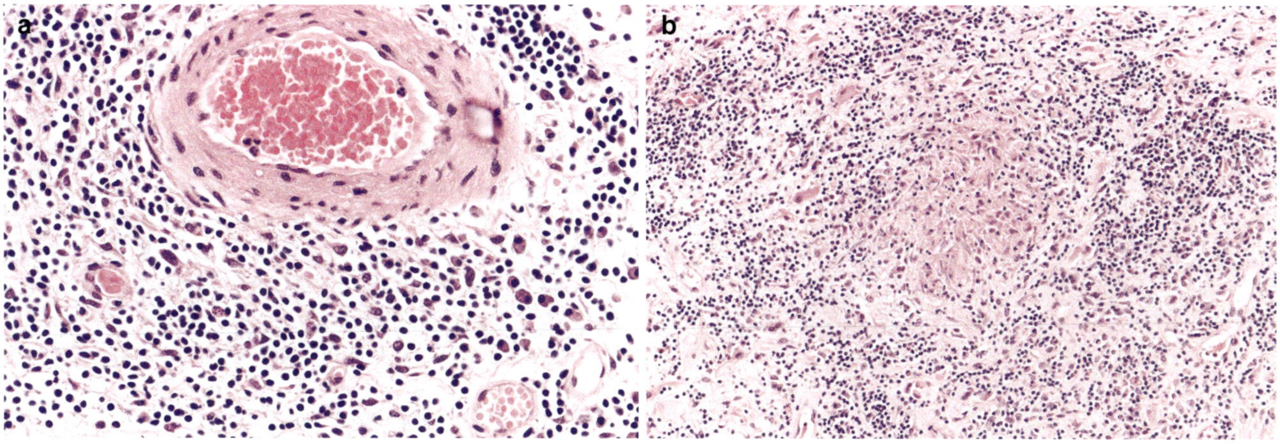

Fig. 12.9 *Brucella* infection in the brain. (**a**) Angiocentric/perivascular lymphoplasmacytic inflammation, mimicking lymphoma. However, morphologic atypia is not present (400×). (**b**) Granulomatous inflammation is present (200×). Microbiology culture suggests *Brucella* infection

histologically because of prominent perivascular lymphocytes and other inflammatory cells (Figs. 12.9, 12.10 and 12.11). However, these lymphocytes do not show significant morphological atypia. Careful morphologic evaluation and special stains for microorganisms are especially important in such cases.

12. What is primary pulmonary lymphoma (PPL) and what are the morphological findings in the two most common PPLs – MALT lymphoma and DLBCL?

- Primary pulmonary lymphoma is traditionally defined as lymphoma that presents as one or more pulmonary lesions with no clinical, pathologic, or radiographic evidence of lymphoma elsewhere at the time of diagnosis or within 3 months following the diagnosis [41].
  - Lymphoma in the lung may be (1) primary pulmonary involvement, (2) hematogenous dissemination of lymphoma, and (3) contiguous spread from hilar or mediastinal nodes. The latter two entities are secondary involvement of lung by lymphoma and are much more common than primary pulmonary involvement.
- Extranodal marginal zone lymphoma is by far the most common type of PPL, accounting for more than 70% of the cases [42, 43], and DLBCL is the second most common type. Other types of lymphoma are rare and include intravascular lymphoma, T- cell lymphomas, and very rarely Hodgkin lymphoma [42, 44]. Video-assisted thoracic surgery (VATS), open wedge biopsy, or lobectomy usually is required for the diagnosis.

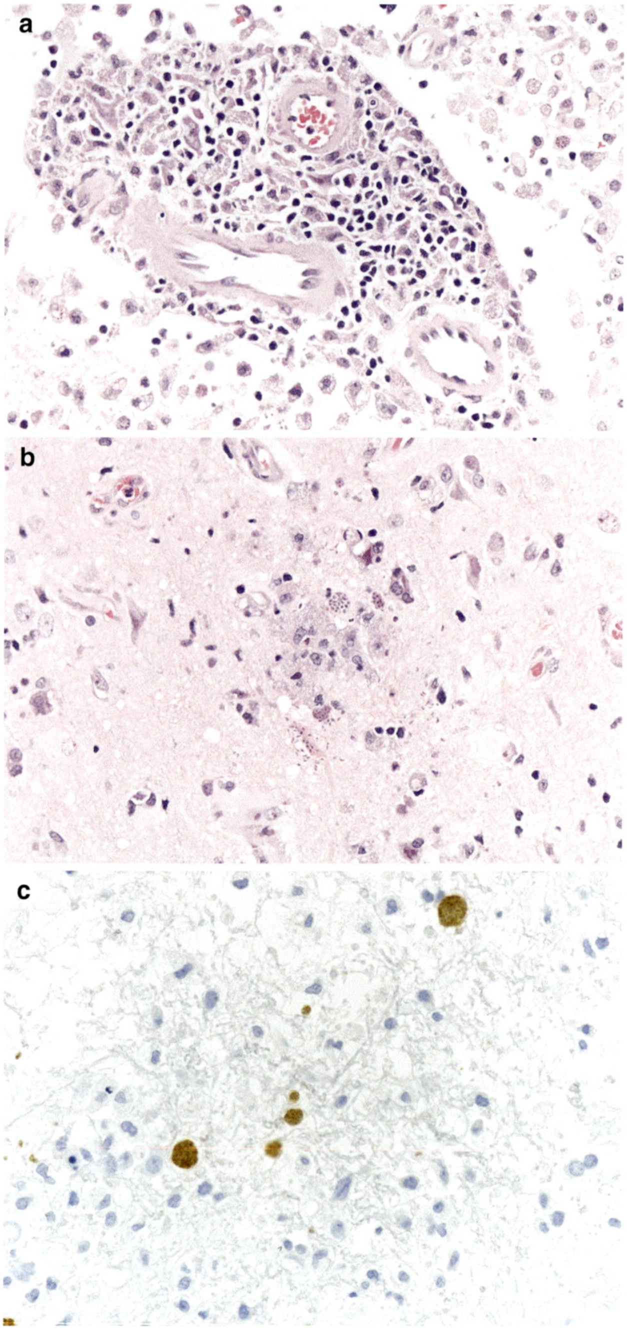

Fig. 12.10 Toxoplasmosis in the brain. (**a**) Angiocentric/perivascular lymphoplasmacytic inflammation, a lymphoma mimic (400×). (**b**) Toxoplasma is identified by morphology and immunostain (400×) (**c**)

- *Extranodal marginal zone lymphoma of MALT type:* This is the most common type of PPL [45, 46]. MALT almost exclusively affects adults of over 30 years old, with a median age of 60 years.
  - Approximately 29% of patients diagnosed with MALT-PPL had a connective tissue disorder, such as Sjögren's syndrome, rheumatoid arthritis, Hashimoto's thyroiditis, and systemic lupus erythematosus, or infections such as hepatitis C and HIV [46, 47]. Patients with Sjögren's syndrome have shown 6.6–44-fold higher risk of developing lymphomas, of which MALT-PPL is the most common type [48].
  - Monoclonal serum paraproteins are relatively common. IgM is the most common type of immunoglobulin. It could also be IgG or IgA. Chest radiographic findings are not specific for MALT-PPL and vary greatly. The most common findings are multiple bilateral lung nodules with air bronchograms or areas of bronchiectasis within larger lesions [49, 50].
  - On gross examination, the lesions are white, white-tan, or gray-pink, unencapsulated, poorly defined mass with a firm, fibrous, or granular cut surface.
  - The histologic and immunophenotypic features are similar to those of marginal zone lymphomas at other anatomic sites. The lymphoma consists of a variable admixture of small lymphocytes, monocytoid cells, plasmacytoid cells, and occasional centrocyte-like cells (Fig. 12.12a, b). Admixed reactive lymphoid follicles are usually present, with at least partially colonized by lymphoma cells. Tumor cells spread in a lymphatic growth pattern along the bronchovascular bundles and interlobular septa. Lymphoepithelial lesions are often present; they may involve bronchial or bronchiolar epithelium and occasional mucous glands. Necrosis is not a feature [51].
  - Amyloid deposition can be seen in 1–6% of the cases, more commonly in older women. The MALT lymphoma with amyloid deposition is more common in the lung [42, 52]. Those lesions usually contain a prominent plasma cell component. The amyloid may be associated with a foreign body giant cell reaction and less often with calcification or even ossification. The amyloid is Congo red positive with apple green birefringence.
  - Immunohistochemical findings are the same as those described earlier for gastric MALT (Question 3). Key IHC findings are shown in Fig. 12.12c, d.
  - *IGH* is clonally rearranged. The t(11;18) (q21;q21) translocation is more commonly found in MALT lymphomas arising in the lung than in all other sites [53–56]. The t(14;18) (q32;q21) (*IGH-MALT1*) and t(1;14) (p22;q32)(*IGH-BCL10*) also have been described in pulmonary MALT lymphoma but are uncommon.
  - Clinical course of MALT-PPL is generally indolent with reported 5-year overall survival rate of greater than 80% [57].

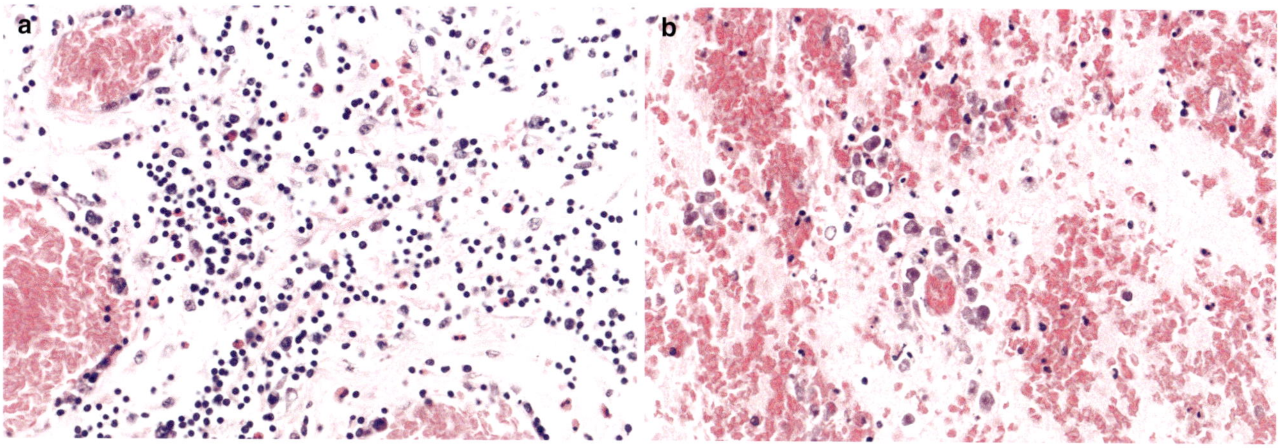

Fig. 12.11 Hemorrhagic amebic organisms. (**a**) Lymphocytic infiltrate in brain parenchyma (400×). (**b**) Other fields show hemorrhagic changes and amebic organisms (400×)

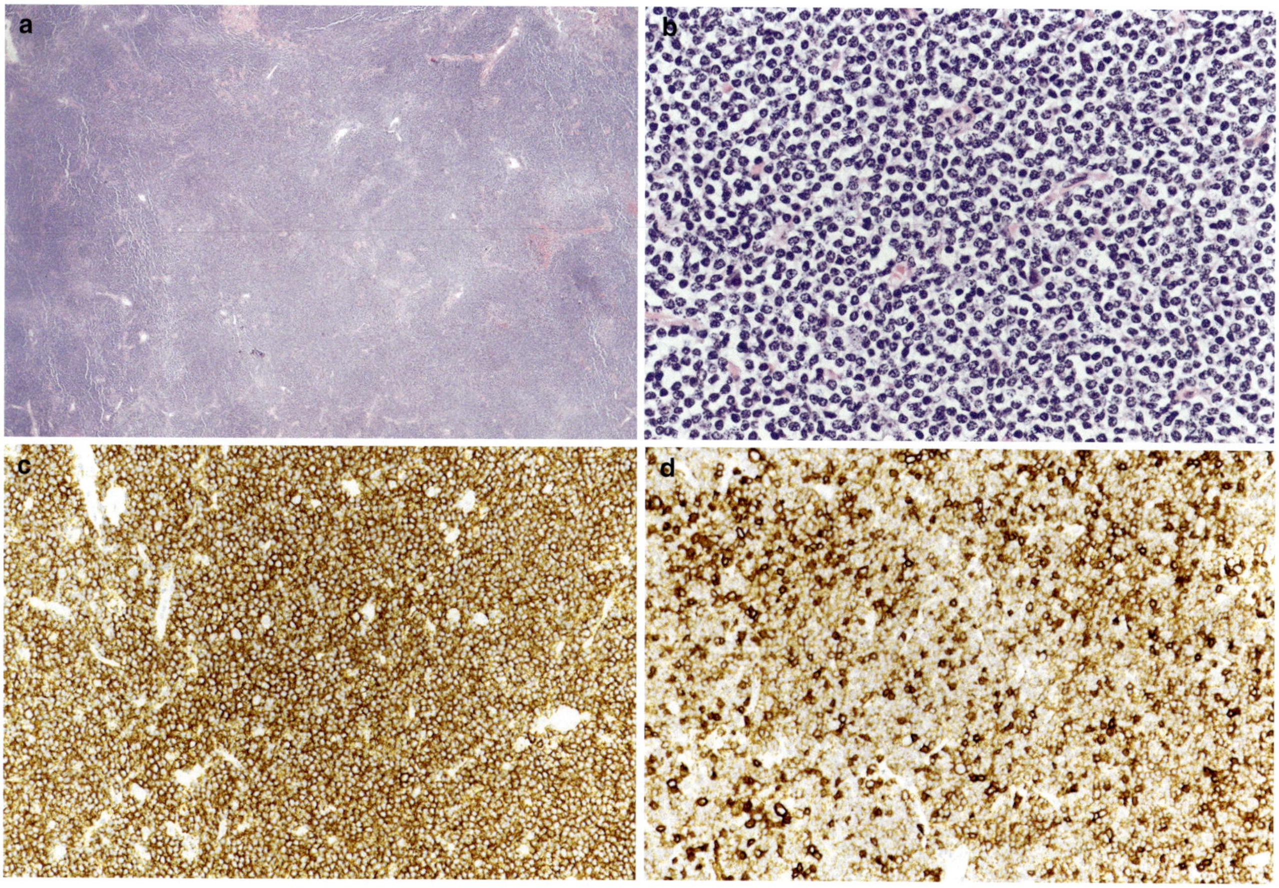

Fig. 12.12 Extranodal marginal zone lymphoma in the lung. (**a**) Diffuse lymphoid infiltrate effaces the lung parenchyma (20×). (**b**) The lymphoid cells are small with mature chromatin and clear cytoplasm (400×). They are positive for CD20 (200×) (**c**). CD43 is weakly positive on the neoplastic B cells and strongly positive on the normal T cells (200×) (**d**)

- *Diffuse large B-cell lymphoma of the lung:* DLBCL is the second most common type of PPL, accounting for 10–20% of PPL [47, 58]. About half of the DLBCL-PPL cases arise de novo and the other half arise from the transformation of the more indolent MALT-PPL. On average, patients with pulmonary DLBCL are slightly younger than those with pulmonary MALT lymphoma.
  - DLBCL-PPL can present as a single or multiple well-defined round solid masses on chest CT. Features of MALT-PPL and DLBCL-PPL can overlap where multiple nodules or areas of consolidation are seen by imaging. Cavitation and/or central necrosis on chest CT is seen in 50% of the cases and is a feature more common and frequent of DLBCL-PPL compared to MALT-PPL [50]. On gross examination, the lymphomas sometimes have areas of necrosis. Biopsy section typically shows sheets of medium-sized to large lymphoid cells with coarse chromatin, distinct nucleoli, and abundant cytoplasm (Fig. 12.13a, b). The immunophenotype (Fig. 12.13c) and molecular findings are similar to nodal DLBCL.

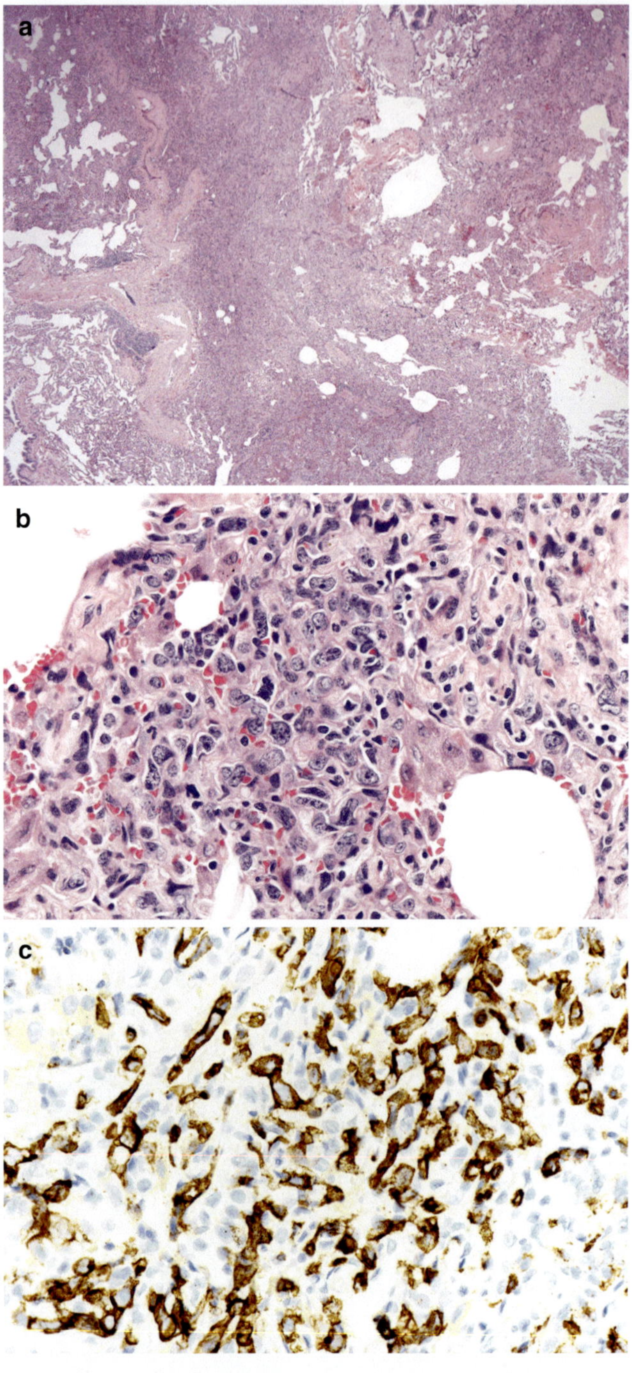

Fig. 12.13 Large B-cell lymphoma in the lung. (**a**) Nodular organizing pneumonia with intra-alveolar fibrin (20×). (**b**) High-power examination shows large atypical lymphoid cells (400×), which are B cells by CD20 stain (400×) (**c**)

13. What are the features of lymphomatoid granulomatosis (LYG) in the lung?

- LYG is a very rare extranodal lymphoproliferative disorder that arises primarily in the lungs [59, 60]. It is an angiocentric and angiodestructive lymphoproliferative disease that is driven by proliferation of *EBV*-positive B cells associated with abundant reactive T cells [58], and pulmonary involvement is by far the most common and most characteristic manifestation [42, 61]. LYG mainly affects adults. Patients often are middle-aged, although older adults and, in rare cases, children are affected as well. LYG characteristically affects immune-compromised patients, such as AIDS, autoimmune disease, post-solid-organ transplantation, and children with certain congenital immunodeficiency syndromes [41, 47]. Rare cases of LYG in immunocompetent patients have also been reported.
- In approximately 80% of the case, the most common radiographic findings on CT are multiple lung nodules ranging from 0.5 to >10 cm [50]. Pulmonary involvement is seen in nearly all cases (more than 90%). Lung lesions are bilateral in nearly 80% of cases.
- On histology, the lesions are composed of a variable admixture of small, intermediate-sized lymphoid cells, histiocytes, plasma cells, and large atypical lymphoid cells (Fig. 12.14a, b). Occasional large bizarre cell reminiscent of Reed-Sternberg cells can be seen. The process is characterized by angiocentric and angiodestructive growth, involving medium-sized to small pulmonary veins and arteries with vasculitis and areas of coagulative necrosis. The surrounding lung parenchyma is usually unremarkable. Despite the name of the disease, well-formed granulomas are not a feature. Eosinophils and neutrophils are inconspicuous.
- Immunophenotyping shows that large atypical cells are B cells with CD20 expression (Fig. 12.14c). They are positive for *EBV*. Large cells may co-express CD30 but they

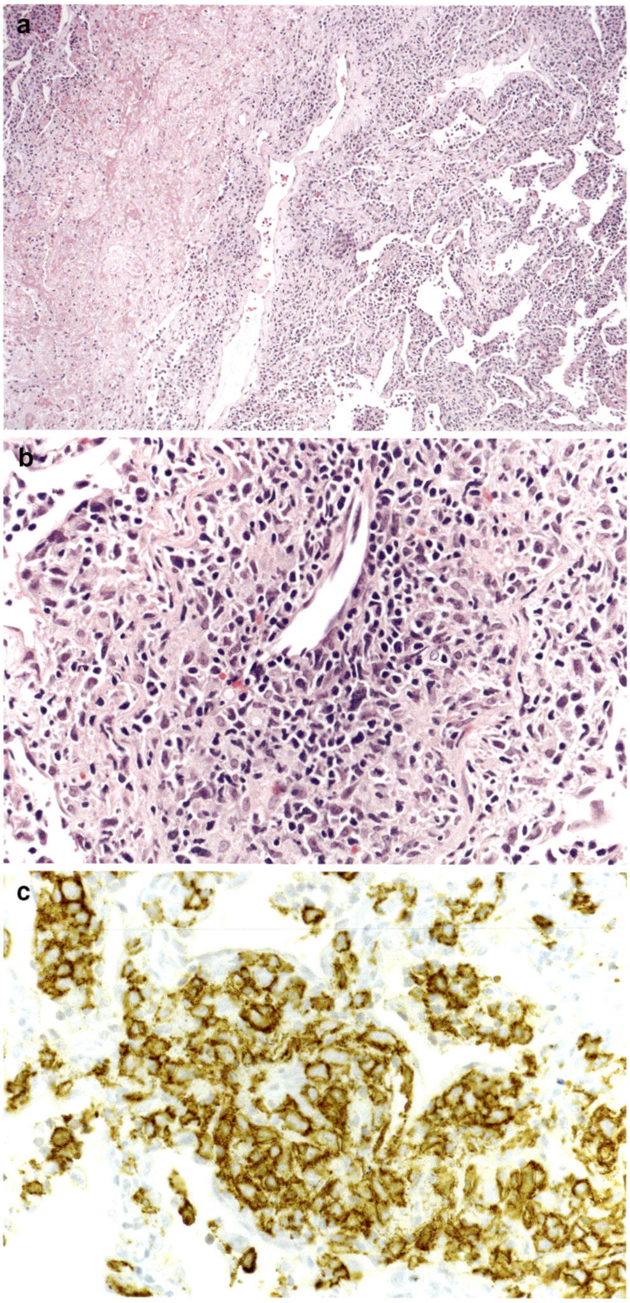

Fig. 12.14 Lymphomatoid granulomatosis in the lung. (**a**) Angiocentric and angioinvasive atypical lymphoid infiltrate (100×). (**b**) The lymphoid infiltrate is composed of admixture of small-, intermediate-sized lymphoid cells, histiocytes, plasma cells, and large atypical lymphoid cells. They show angioinvasive feature (400×). The large cells are highlighted by CD20 stain (400×) (**c**)

are negative for CD15. Small- to medium-sized cells are mainly T cells, most of which are CD4+. The criteria for histologic grading of LYG are shown in Table 12.2.

- Adequate sampling of lung lesion is necessary for the proper diagnosis and histologic grading of LYG. Surgical lung biopsy is the preferred method of tissue sampling if there are not easily accessible sites such as skin involvement. Due to the focal infiltration of *EBV*-positive large cells, biopsy of all accessible sites is recommended [61].
- The disease prognosis of LYG is variable and generally associates with a poor diagnosis with a median survival of approximately 4 years. The clinical course of the disease is related to the proportion of *EBV*-positive large B cells. Grades 2 and 3 have poorer prognosis and higher risk of disseminating to other anatomic sites, such as the lymph nodes, spleen, and BM [61].

14. What types of lymphomas commonly occur in the skin?

In contrast to lymphomas that arise in many other sites, most primary cutaneous lymphomas are T-cell lymphomas, accounting for more than 70% of cases. B-cell lymphomas account for fewer than 30% of cases [62].

- Most cutaneous T-cell lymphomas have distinctive clinical presentations that help differentiate them from histologically similar processes. In contrast, most cutaneous B-cell lymphomas appear clinically similar to one another [63].
- Several types of cutaneous T-cell lymphoma are characterized by epidermotropism, in contrast to cutaneous B-cell lymphomas, in which the tumor cells spare the epidermis and usually are separated from it by the grenz zone of papillary dermis free of the tumor.
- T-cell lymphomas have aberrant T-cell immunophenotype. Loss of pan-T-cell antigens, such as CD2, CD3, or CD5, or loss of both CD4 and CD8 supports a diagnosis of cutaneous T-cell lymphoma. CD7 is expressed on many but not all normal T cells. It might be absent in small portion of CD4+ nonneoplastic T cells. However, a significant loss of CD7 is seen most frequently in cutaneous T-cell lymphoma, particularly mycosis fungoides type.
- Similar to T-cell lymphoma, B-cell lymphoma may have aberrant immunophenotype. The lymphocytes in cutaneous inflammation are mostly T cells; therefore, a diffuse cutaneous infiltrate composed of predominantly B cells is worrisome for B-cell lymphoma. In addition, dense reactive T-cell infiltrates are frequently seen in B-cell lymphoma.

15. What are the differences between cutaneous marginal zone lymphoma and extranodal marginal zone lymphoma in other sites?

- Primary cutaneous marginal zone B-cell lymphoma is an indolent lymphoma composed of small B cells, including lymphocytes, lymphoplasmacytic cells, and plasma cells.

This category includes cases previously designated as primary cutaneous immunocytoma [64] and cases of cutaneous follicular lymphoid hyperplasia with monotypic plasma cells [65]. Primary cutaneous plasmacytoma without underlying multiple myeloma (extramedullary plasmacytoma of the skin) show considerable overlap with PCMZL and are therefore included in this category. It shares many clinical and pathologic features with marginal zone lymphomas arising in other sites but has some distinctive features.

- PCMZLs commonly present as erythematous papules, plaques, or nodules on the trunk or extremities. Occasionally multiple tumors may be seen. PCMZLs have a tendency to recur in the skin, but dissemination to extracutaneous sites is exceedingly rare [64, 66, 67]. In some cases, spontaneous resolution of the skin lesion may be observed. Associated autoimmune diseases are uncommon in PCMZL but rather suggest secondary cutaneous involvement of a systemic lymphoma.
- The lymphoma shows nodular to diffuse infiltrates composed of small lymphocytes with monocytoid or centrocyte-like morphology, lymphoplasmacytoid cells, plasma cells, and admixed reactive T lymphocytes. Reactive germinal centers are frequently observed. Epidermal involvement is rare; the infiltrate usually is separated from the epidermis by a zone of uninvolved papillary dermis. PCMZLs have a spectrum of histologic findings, ranging from most of the neoplastic cells composed of small mature B cells with few plasma cells to sheets of plasma cells without significant mature lymphocytes (Fig. 12.15a, b).
- The marginal zone B cells express CD20, CD79a, and BCL2 but are negative for CD5, CD10, and BCL6, which may be useful in distinction from primary cutaneous follicle center lymphoma. Plasma cells express CD138 and CD79a, but generally not CD20, and monotypic cytoplasmic immunoglobulin light chain expression identified by immunohistochemistry or in situ hybridization (Fig. 12.15c, d).
- Most cutaneous marginal zone lymphomas express class-switched immunoglobulin. IgG is expressed most frequently and IgA, IgE, and IgM less commonly. This is in contrast to marginal zone lymphomas arising in most other sites, in which expression of IgM is the most common.

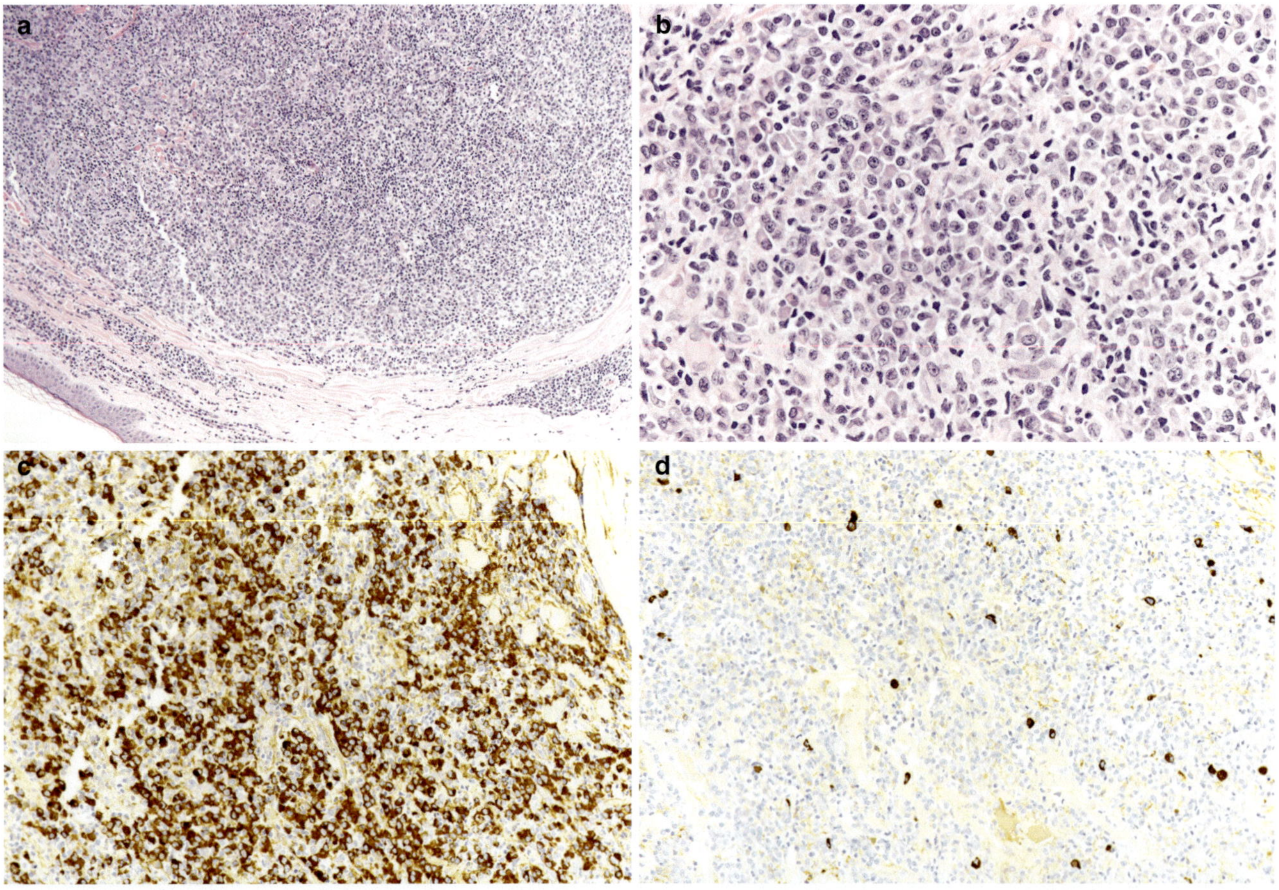

Fig. 12.15 Primary cutaneous marginal zone lymphoma. (**a**) Dermal diffuse lymphoid infiltrate that is separated from the epidermis by a zone of uninvolved papillary dermis (100×). (**b**) The lymphoid cells are composed of small lymphocytes and many admixed plasma cells (40×). The plasma cells are kappa light chain restricted (200×) (**c**) without significant expression of lambda light chain (200×) (**d**)

- Immunoglobulin heavy chain (*IgH*) genes are clonally rearranged. Recent studies suggest the presence of the t(14;18)(q32;q21), involving the *IGH* gene on chromosome 14 and the *MALT* gene on chromosome 18, and t(3;14)(p14.1;q32), involving *IGH* and *FOXP1* genes, in a proportion of PCMZLs [68, 69]. However, other translocations observed in MALT lymphomas at other sites, such as t(11;18)(q21;q21) and t(1;14)(p22;q32), have not been found in PCMZL [70, 71].
- The prognosis of PCMZL is excellent with a 5-year survival close to 100%.

16. What is the most common type of primary cutaneous B-cell lymphoma?

- Primary cutaneous follicle center lymphoma (PCFCL) is the most common type of primary cutaneous B-cell lymphoma; it accounts for about 60% of the cases.
- PCFCLs have a characteristic clinical presentation with solitary or grouped plaques and tumors, preferentially located on the scalp or forehead or on the trunk.
- PCFCLs are characterized by a dermal proliferation of centrocytes and centroblasts in a follicular, follicular and diffuse, or diffuse pattern that often extends into the subcutaneous fat, with almost constant sparing of the epidermis (Fig. 12.16a, b). The neoplastic cells usually assume a growth pattern of expanded, irregularly shaped, lymphoid follicles in the dermis. Numerous admixed small T cells and sclerosis are often present. Histologic grading of primary cutaneous follicle center lymphoma, as done for the nodal counterpart, is not recommended, because it has not been shown to have clinical relevance.
- The neoplastic cells express the B-cell-associated antigens CD20 and CD79a (Fig. 12.16c). PCFCLs consistently express BCL6 (Fig. 12.16d). CD10 expression is particularly observed in cases with follicular growth pattern but is uncommon in PCFCLs with a diffuse growth pattern. The tumor cells do not stain for CD5, CD43, or MUM1/IRF4. Unlike nodal follicular lymphomas, PCFCL does not usually express BCL2 protein, or, if it does, it often shows faint BCL2 staining in a minority of neoplastic B cells (Fig. 12.16e) [72, 73]. Therefore, strong BCL2 staining should prompt a search for a possibility of systemic or nodal follicular lymphoma.
- In most studies, PCFCLs, including cases with a follicular growth pattern, do not show the t(14;18), which is characteristically found in systemic follicular lymphomas [74, 75].
- PCFCLs have an excellent prognosis with a 5-year survival of more than 95% [63, 75].

17. What is the most common cutaneous T-cell lymphoma, and what are its characteristic features?

- Mycosis fungoides (MF) is the most common type of cutaneous T-cell lymphoma (CTCL) and accounts for almost 50% of all primary cutaneous lymphomas. MF typically affects older adults but may occur in children and adolescents [76, 77]. It has indolent clinical course with slow progression over years or sometimes decades. MF primarily involves the skin; however, it may spread to lymph node, blood, and viscera in the later stage of the disease. The skin lesions present as erythematous, round, oval patches, or plaques.
- The characteristic feature of mycosis fungoides is epidermotropism, which is defined as the presence of atypical T cells within the epidermis (Fig. 12.17a) [78]. The neoplastic T cells are small- to medium-sized with mature chromatin and cerebriform nuclear contour (Fig. 12.17b). A clear space or halo around the neoplastic lymphocytes is present. Pautrier microabscess showing intraepidermal aggregates of three or more cytological atypical T cells is a highly characteristic feature. Superficial band-like or lichenoid infiltrates are often present in the early patch lesion (Fig. 12.17c). Rare, large cell transformation of mycosis fungoides to CD30-positive large cell lymphoma may occur, which is associated with a poor prognosis.
- By immunophenotype, the neoplastic T cells are CD4+ and CD8- T cells that also express CD2, CD3, CD5, and alpha-beta T-cell receptor (Fig. 12.17d, e). Rarely, the neoplastic cells can be CD8 positive [79]. Neoplastic T cells often show loss of CD7. Loss of one or more T-cell antigens in addition to loss of CD7 is supportive of a diagnosis of T-cell lymphoma. However, the immunophenotypic features are not specific for mycosis fungoides and may be seen in other T-cell lymphomas. Loss of CD7 only may be seen in some reactive processes with expansion of normal CD4+, CD7− population. Occasional CD30+ large cells can be seen in MF; however, this finding is not specific either, and they can be seen in reactive process or other B- or T-cell lymphoma.
- T-cell receptor gene rearrangement is typically positive in mycosis fungoides, which can be helpful in the diagnosis of T-cell lymphoma without T-cell antigen loss. However, positive TCR results can be seen in some reactive condition; therefore, correlation with not only TCR results but also morphology, immunophenotype, and clinical features is important for the diagnosis of mycosis fungoides.

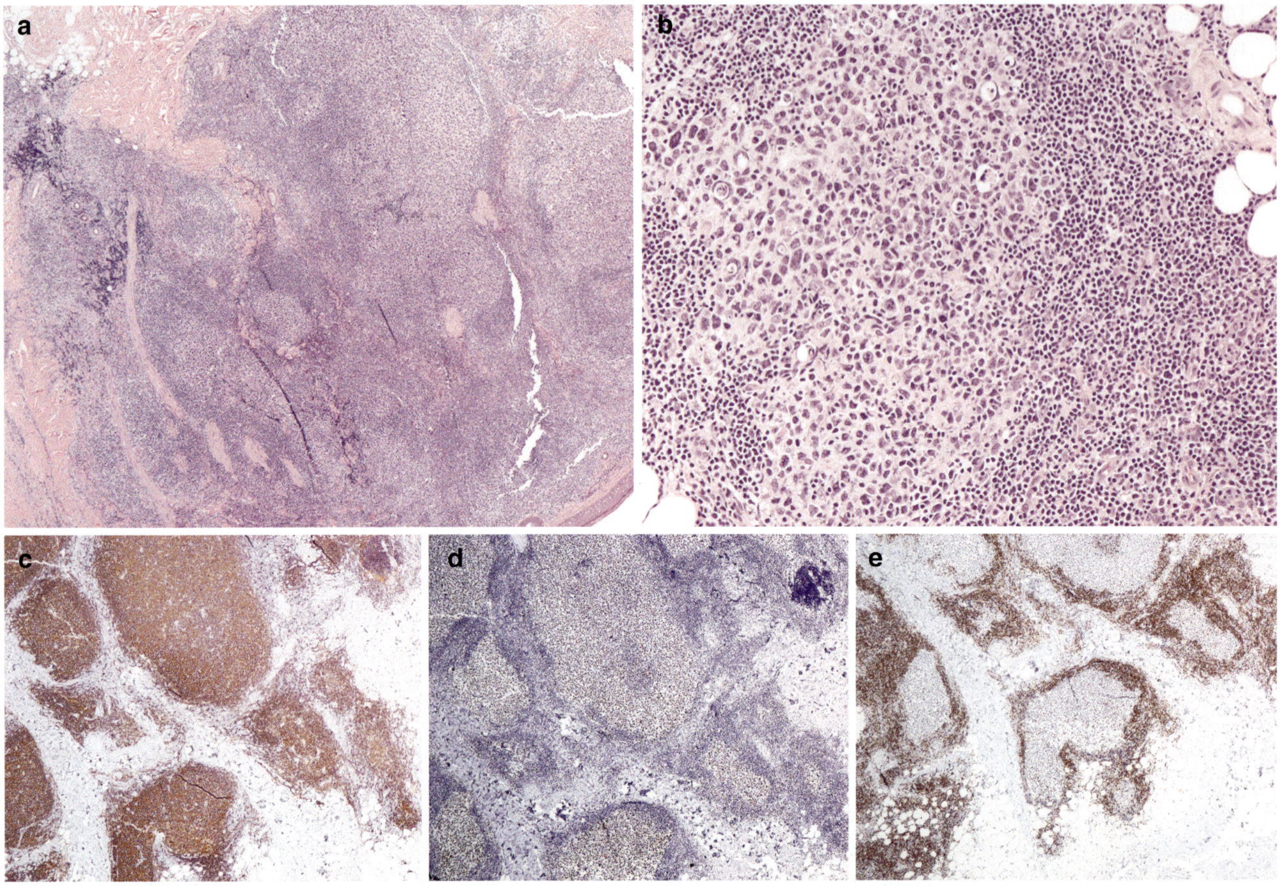

Fig. 12.16 Primary cutaneous follicle center lymphoma. (**a**) Dense dermal lymphoid infiltrate with follicular pattern and sparing of the epidermis (40×). (**b**) The follicle shows proliferation of centrocytes and centroblasts (200×). The lymphoid cells are positive for CD20 (40×) (**c**) and BCL6 (40×) (**d**) and negative for BCL2 (40×) (**e**)

- The cytologic appearance of activated T cells may be similar to the early cerebriform changes of mycosis fungoides. Epidermotropism might be difficult to distinguish from a reactive exocytosis. In early lesion of mycosis fungoides with minimal cytological atypia and the late stage tumors without epidermotropism are the most diagnostically challenging. Mycosis fungoides usually displays a relatively uniform proliferation of CD4+ T cells with rare scattered CD8+ cells. Reactive process usually displays CD8+ cells in the epidermis and CD4+ cells in the dermis. The presence of cytologically atypical CD4+ cells with an aberrant T-cell immunophenotype supports a diagnosis of T-cell lymphoma.
- The prognosis of patients with MF is dependent on stage, in particular the type and extent of skin lesions and the presence of extracutaneous disease [76, 80]. Patients with effaced lymph nodes, visceral involvement, and transformation into a large T-cell lymphoma have an aggressive clinical course.

18. Which disorders are included in primary cutaneous CD30-positive lymphoproliferative disorders, and what are the features of primary cutaneous anaplastic large cell lymphoma?

Primary cutaneous CD30+ lymphoproliferative disorders are the second most common group of CTCLs, accounting for approximately 30% of CTCLs. They are characterized by the presence of CD30+ large cells. This group includes primary cutaneous anaplastic large cell lymphoma (C-ALCL), lymphomatoid papulosis (LyP), and borderline cases. It is now generally accepted that C-ALCL and LyP from a spectrum of

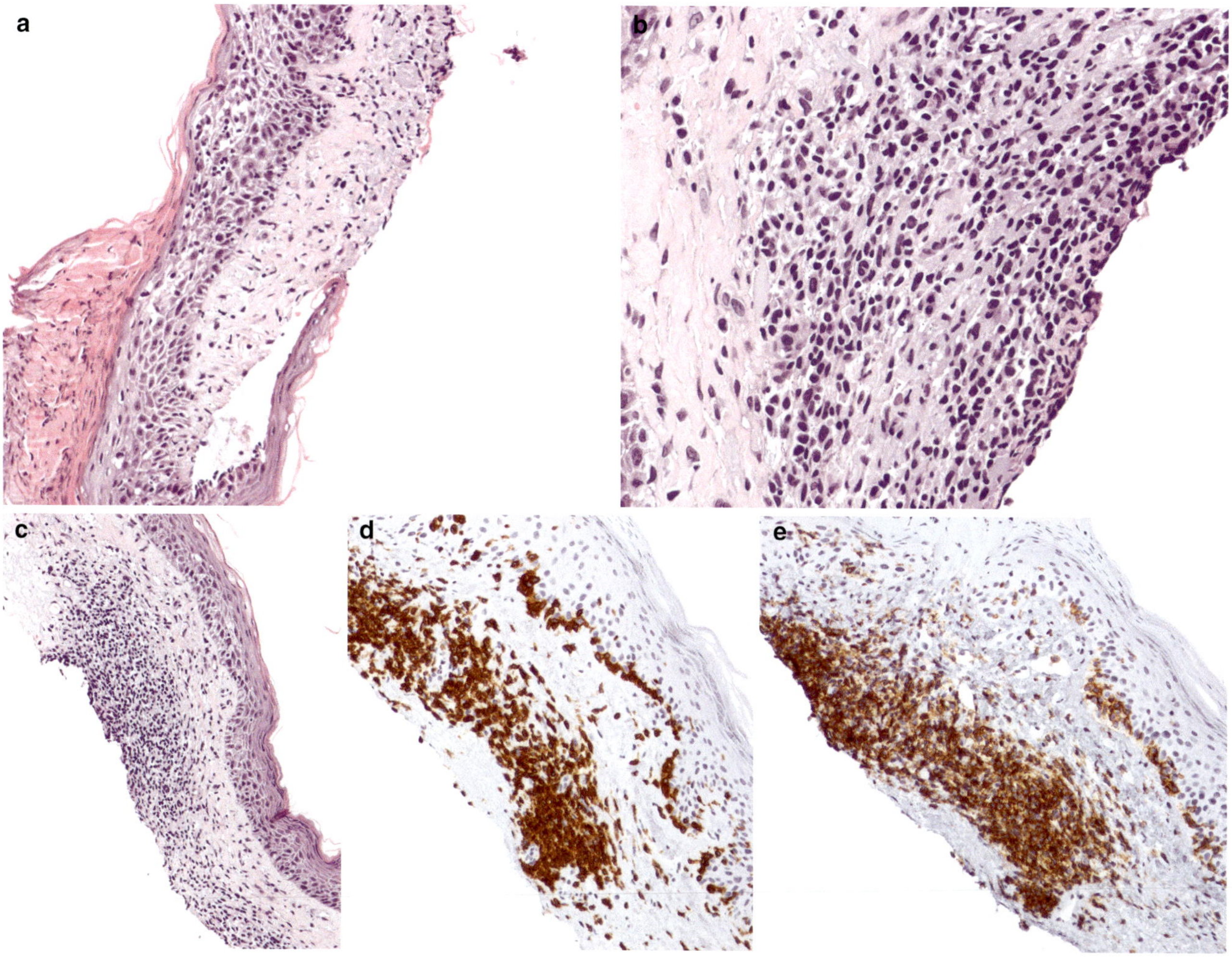

Fig. 12.17 Mycosis fungoides. (**a**) Mild epidermotropism is present (100×). (**b**) The neoplastic T cells are small- to medium-sized with mature chromatin and cerebriform nuclear contour (400×). (**c**) Superficial band-like or lichenoid infiltrates is present, consistent with early patch lesion (200×). The neoplastic cells are positive for CD3 (200×) (**d**) and CD4 (200×) (**e**). Epidermotropism is also highlighted by the stains

disease and that histologic criteria alone are often insufficient to differentiate between these two ends of the spectrum [81, 82].

- Primary cutaneous anaplastic large cell lymphoma (C-ALCL) is composed of large cells with an anaplastic, pleomorphic, or immunoblastic morphology and expression of CD30 antigen by the majority (more than 75%) of the tumor cells. There is no clinical evidence or history of MF.
- Primary cutaneous ALCL usually presents as a solitary cutaneous nodule or localized nodules in patients in the seventh or eighth decade of their lives [83]. The skin lesions may show partial or complete spontaneous regression but undergo frequently relapse in the skin. Extracutaneous dissemination occurs in approximately 10% of the patients and mainly involves the regional lymph nodes.
- This disease must be distinguished from cutaneous involvement by systemic ALCL, which has different clinical and pathologic features. If the patient has a history of MF, a diagnosis of large cell transformation of MF is much more likely than a prognostically favorable primary cutaneous ALCL.
- The histological features of primary cutaneous ALCL include diffuse dermal infiltrate with cohesive sheets of large CD30+ tumor cells (Fig. 12.18a). The tumor cells commonly have anaplastic cell morphology with round, oval, or irregularly shaped nuclei, prominent eosinophilic nucleoli, and abundant cytoplasm (Fig. 12.18b). Binucleated and multinucleated forms are occasionally seen. Reactive lymphocytes are often present at the periphery of the lesions. Epidermotropism is rare.
- The tumor cells of cutaneous ALCL are strongly positive for CD30 (Fig. 12.18c) and show a characteristic

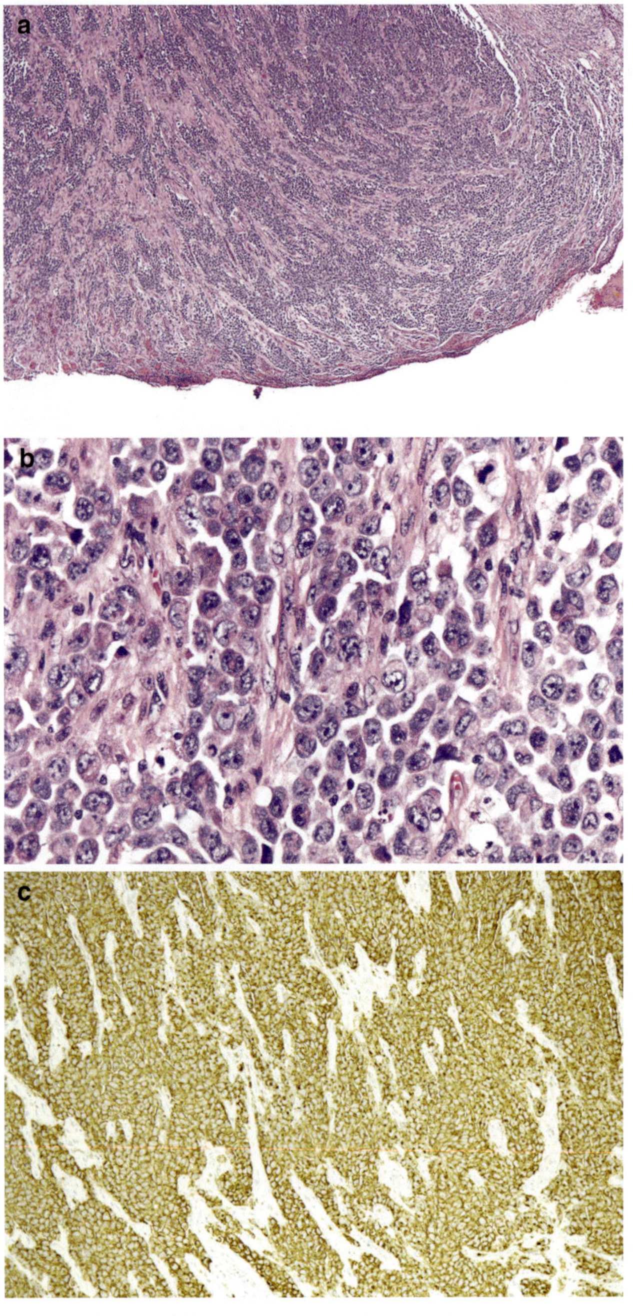

Fig. 12.18 Primary cutaneous anaplastic large cell lymphoma. (**a**) Diffuse dermal infiltrate with cohesive sheets of large lymphoid cells (40×). (**b**) The tumor cells show round, oval, or irregularly shaped nuclei, prominent eosinophilic nucleoli, and abundant cytoplasm (400×). They are strongly positive for CD30 with dot-like Golgi staining pattern (100×) (**c**)

punctate accentuation of staining in the perinuclear Golgi region. The neoplastic cells generally show an activated CD4+ T-cell phenotype with variable loss of CD2, CD5, or CD3 and frequent expression of cytotoxic proteins (granzyme B, TIA-1, perforin). Unlike systemic ALCL, most primary cutaneous ALCLs do not express EMA and ALK. CD56 co-expression is rarely observed.

- Most cases show clonal rearrangement of T-cell receptor genes. The (2;5)(p23;q35) translocation, and its variant, is not present or rarely found in C-ALCL [84].

19. Is lymphomatoid papulosis a lymphoma?

- Lymphomatoid papulosis (LyP) is defined as a chronic, recurrent, self-healing papulonecrotic, or papulonodular skin disease characterized by a dermal lymphoid infiltrate that contains large atypical CD30+ cells scattered in an inflammatory background. LyP is a skin-limited disease that usually occurs in adults but in rare cases may be seen in children. It presents clinically as recurrent erythematous papules and nodules on the proximal extremities and trunk. LyP may be self-limited, lasting only a few months, or may persist for decades [82].
- The histopathologic picture of LyP is extremely variable and in part correlates with the age of biopsied skin lesion. Three major histologic subtypes of LyP (types A, B, and C) have been described, which represent a spectrum with overlapping features [81, 85]. In type A, scattered CD30+ cells, occasionally clustered, are seen in a background of inflammatory cells such as histiocytes, small lymphocytes, neutrophils, and/or eosinophils. Type B is uncommon (less than 10%) and is characterized by an epidermotropic infiltrate of atypical lymphocytes, similar to that seen in MF, but with the clinical features of LyP (Fig. 12.19a). Type C shows a monotonous population of CD30+ cells with few admixed inflammatory cells (Fig. 12.19b). In addition, type D and type E (both CD8+) have also been reported, but those are extremely rare.
- Most of the cells in the infiltrate have a CD4+ phenotype. The large lymphocytes may show loss of some pan-T-cell antigens. The CD30+ large cells in types A and C usually are CD15-. Type B tumor cells have a CD3+, CD4+, CD8- immunophenotype. Clonal rearrangement T-cell receptor genes have been detected in approximately 60–70% of LyP lesions.
- LyP is believed to represent the indolent end of spectrum of cutaneous CD30+ lymphoproliferative disorders and has an excellent prognosis [82]. In up to 20% of patients, LyP may be preceded by, associated with, or followed by another type of malignant cutaneous lymphoma, generally MF, C-ALCL, or Hodgkin lymphoma [82].

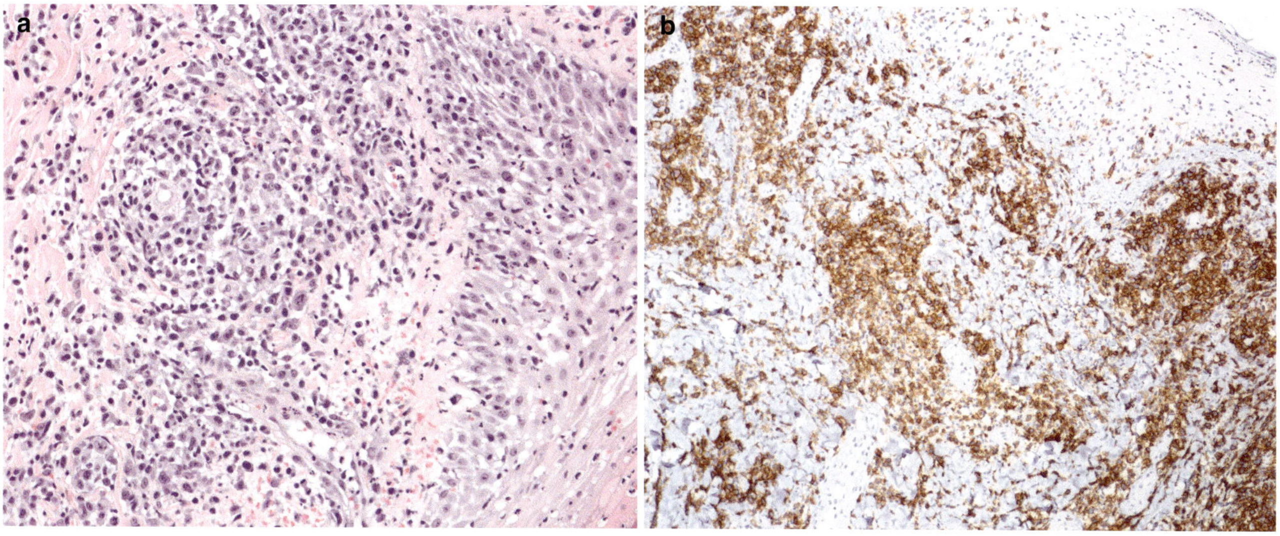

Fig. 12.19 Lymphomatoid papulosis. The patient has multiple papules come and gone. (**a**) The biopsy of the papules shows large lymphoid with few admixed inflammatory cells (200×). The large lymphoid cells are positive for CD30 (100×) (**b**). Based solely on the histopathology, primary cutaneous anaplastic large cell lymphoma would be considered, though clinically more consistent with lymphomatoid papulosis

20. What is subcutaneous panniculitis-like T-cell lymphoma (SPTCL) according to the WHO (2017) classification, and what are its clinicopathological features?

- Subcutaneous panniculitis-like T-cell lymphoma is a cytotoxic T-cell lymphoma of the alpha-beta type that preferentially involves subcutaneous fat.
  - Historically, it included alpha-beta and gamma-delta subtypes. Recent studies suggest that alpha-beta T-cell-type lymphoma differs both morphologically and clinically from those of gamma-delta phenotype [86–88].
  - Cases with an alpha-beta T-cell phenotype are usually CD8+, are restricted to the subcutaneous tissue without dermal or epidermal involvement, and often show an indolent clinical course [86–89].
  - In contrast, cases with a gamma-delta phenotype are typically CD4- and CD8- and often express CD56 and involve the epidermis and/or dermis. They invariably have a very poor prognosis [86–88, 90].
  - As a result, the WHO classification system designate the term "SPTCL" is only applied for the cases with an alpha-beta phenotype, whereas cases with a gamma-delta T-cell phenotype are designated in the category of cutaneous gamma/delta T-cell lymphomas [89].
- SPTCL occurs in adult as well as in young children. Patients generally present with solitary or multiple nodules and plaques, which mainly involve the legs or may be more generalized. The disease may be complicated by a hemophagocytic syndrome, which is generally associated with a rapid progressive course and systemic symptoms [91]; however, hemophagocytic syndrome is more commonly observed in cutaneous gamma-delta T-cell lymphoma. Dissemination to extracutaneous sites is rare.
  - SPTCL is characterized by a subcutaneous infiltrate simulating a panniculitis showing small, medium-sized, or sometimes large pleomorphic T cells with hyperchromatic nuclei and moderate amount of pale cytoplasm. The overlying epidermis and dermis are typically uninvolved. The neoplastic cells form rims around the fat cells, often with associated karyorrhexis and histiocytes filled with karyorrhectic debris and necrosis (Fig. 12.20a).
  - The neoplastic T cells show a TCR of alpha-beta subtype, CD3+, CD4-, or CD8+ T-cell phenotype, with expression of cytotoxic proteins such as TIA1, granzyme B, and/or perforin (Fig. 12.20b–d). CD30 and CD56 are usually negative. *EBV* infection is absent. Clonal rearrangement of T-cell receptor genes can be detected.

Case Presentations

Case 1

Learning Objectives

1. To become familiar with the entity "*EBV*-positive large B-cell lymphoma"
2. To generate differential diagnosis with morphologic Reed-Sternberg-like cells
3. To understand the prognosis

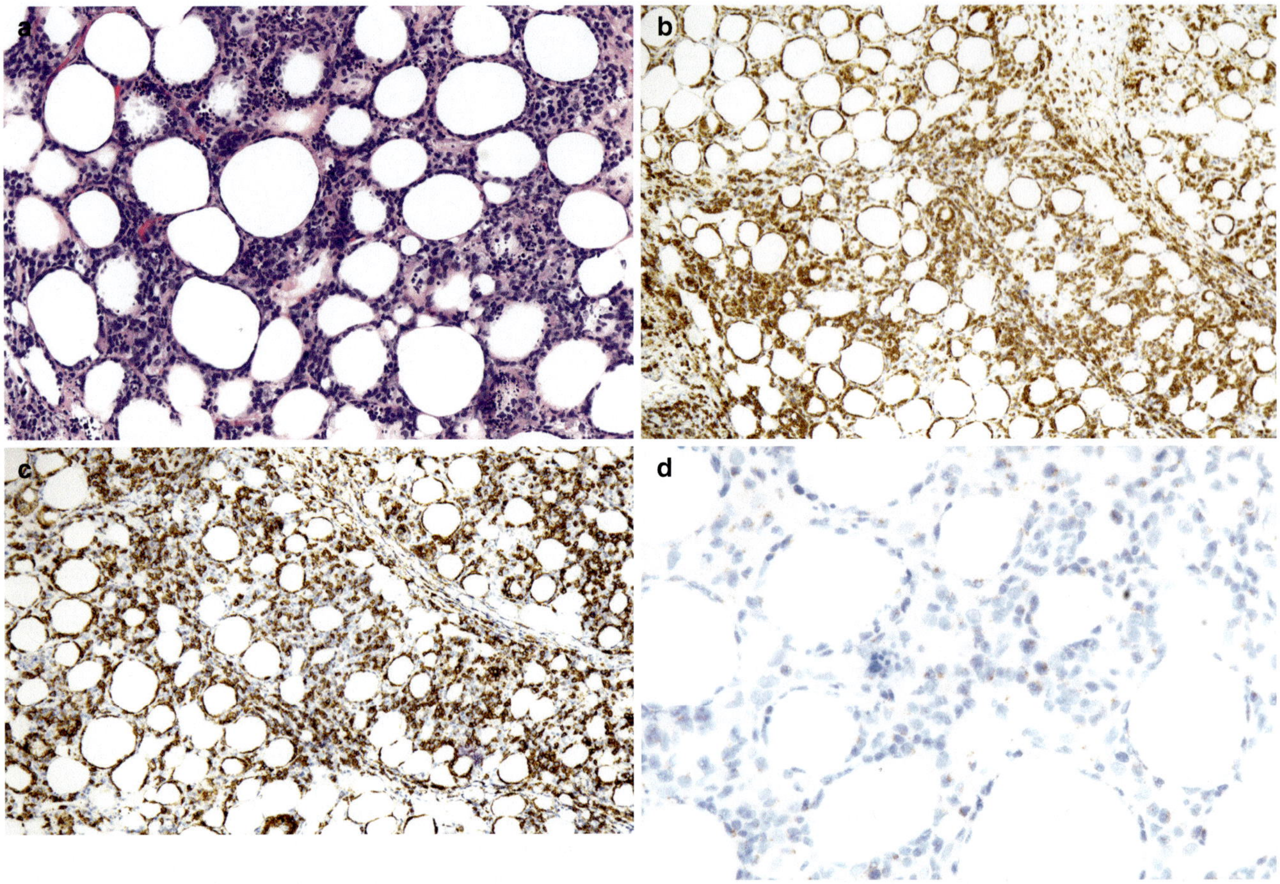

Fig. 12.20 Subcutaneous panniculitis-like T-cell lymphoma. (**a**) Medium-sized pleomorphic neoplastic cells form rims around the fat cells. Associated karyorrhexis and necrosis are present (20×). The neoplastic cells express CD3 (10×) (**b**), CD8 (10×) (**c**), and TIA1 (40×) (**d**)

Case History

A 43-year-old man with a 12 cm jejunal mass

Histologic Findings

- Extensive lymphoid infiltrate in the bowel wall (Fig. 12.3a).
- The lymphoid cells show Hodgkin/Reed-Sternberg-like cell morphology with folded, bilobed, or multilobated nuclei and prominent nucleoli (Fig. 12.3b).

Differential Diagnosis

- Large B-cell lymphoma
- Anaplastic large cell lymphoma
- Classic Hodgkin lymphoma

IHC and Other Ancillary Studies (Fig. 13.3c and d)

- CD20 positive
- *EBV* positive

Final Diagnosis

***EBV*-positive diffuse large B-cell lymphoma (*EBV*-positive DLBCL)**

Take-Home Messages

1. *EBV*-positive DLBCL can present over a wide age range. The disease is aggressive in patients older than 45 years; however, in patients younger than 45 years, the disease has an excellent prognosis with complete remission in more than 80% of the patients.
2. *EBV*-positive large atypical lymphoid cells may have the appearance of Hodgkin/Reed-Sternberg-like cells.
3. *EBV* staining is important in workup for large B-cell lymphoma

References [14–16]

Case 2

Learning Objectives

1. To become familiar close mimics of large cell lymphomas involving the GI tract
2. To become familiar with the IHC feature
3. To generate the differential diagnosis

Case History

A 59-year-old woman presented with 2 weeks of abdominal pain and diarrhea. CT shows 14 cm mass surrounding the ileum and mesentery leading to a partial small bowel obstruction.

Histologic Findings

- Extensive diffuse infiltrate by hematolymphoid cells in the intestinal wall (Fig. 12.21a).
- The neoplastic cells are large in size and show irregular nuclear contour and vesicular chromatin (Fig. 12.21b).

Differential Diagnosis

- DLBCL
- Lymphoblastic leukemia/lymphoma

IHC and Other Ancillary Studies (Fig. 12.21c)

- CD34 is strongly and diffusely positive, in addition to staining for CD33.
- The cells are negative for B-cell and T-cell-specific antigens.

Final Diagnosis

Myeloid sarcoma

Take-Home Messages

1. Leukemia can present as mass lesion or as myeloid sarcoma.
2. In H-E section, the morphology of myeloid sarcoma can mimic aggressive B- or T-cell lymphoma.
3. Precursor hematolymphoid neoplasm is in the differential of aggressive hematolymphoid neoplasm.

References [92–95]

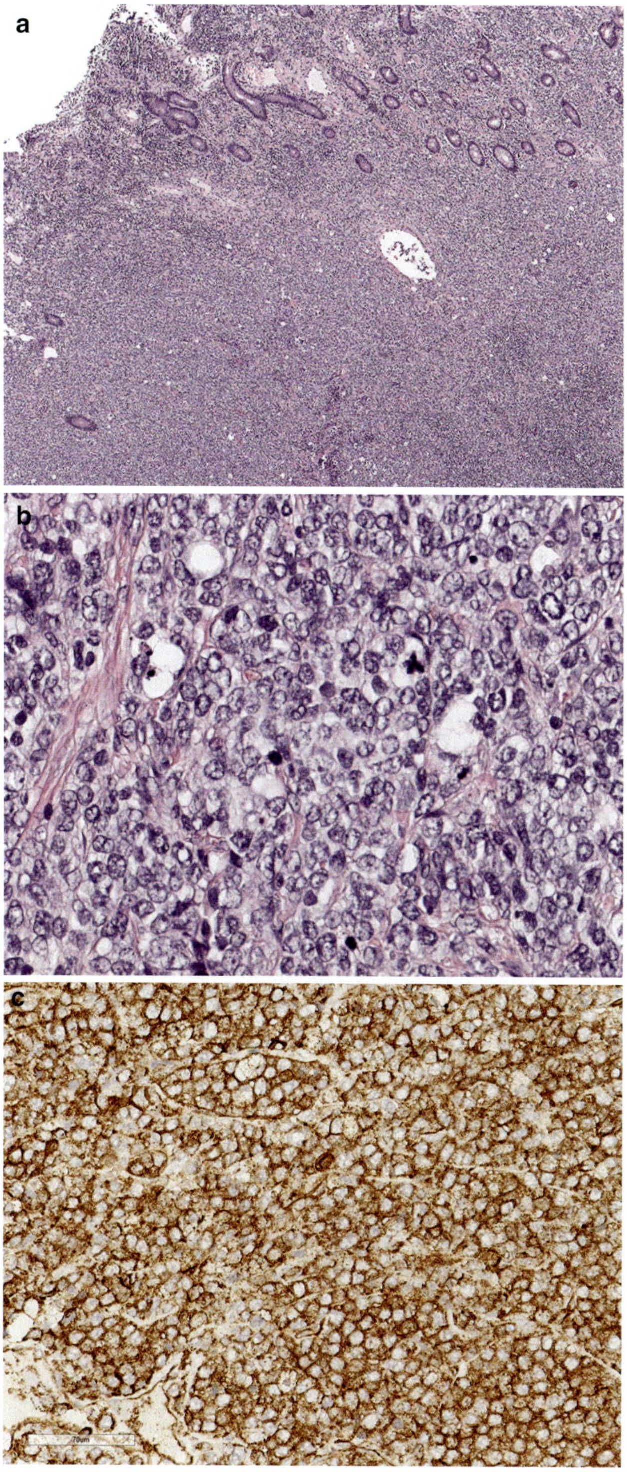

Fig. 12.21 Myeloid sarcoma. (**a**) Extensive diffuse hematolymphoid cells infiltrating the intestinal wall (40×). (**b**) The neoplastic cells are large in size and show irregular nuclear contour and vesicular chromatin (400×). They are diffusely and strongly positive for CD34 (400×) (**c**)

Case 3

Learning Objectives

1. To become familiar with an unusual presentation of DLBCL
2. To become familiar with the IHC features
3. To generate the differential diagnosis

Case History

A 66-year-old man with dementia. Vasculitis needs to be excluded as an underlying cause.

Histologic Findings

- Small blood vessels in the brain parenchyma filled with large lymphoid cells with prominent nucleoli (Fig. 12.8a)

Differential Diagnosis

- Intravascular lymphoma

IHC and Other Ancillary Studies

- CD20 is strongly positive (Fig. 12.8b).
- CD3 is negative.

Final Diagnosis

Intravascular large B-cell lymphoma

Take-Home Messages

1. Intravascular large B-cell lymphoma is now a distinct entity, a rare subtype of extranodal diffuse large B-cell lymphoma characterized by the selective growth of neoplastic cells within the lumens of small blood vessels.
2. A variety of extranodal sites can be involved and may present in virtually any organ, including the CNS, kidneys, adrenals, lungs, and skin but preferentially sparing of lymph nodes.
3. Intravascular large B-cell lymphoma is generally aggressive with a poor prognosis.

References [34–37]

Case 4

Learning Objectives

1. To become familiar with the morphologic features of possible lymphoma in a granulomatous process
2. To become familiar with the IHC features
3. To generate the differential diagnosis

Case History

A 61-year-old man with a cerebellar mass

Histologic Findings

- Polymorphous lymphoid infiltrate composed of large atypical cells, admixed with lymphocytes and histiocytes. Necrosis is also present (Fig. 12.7a, b).
- The lesion is angiocentric (Fig. 12.7c).

Differential Diagnosis

- Large B-cell lymphoma
- NK-T-cell lymphoma

IHC and Other Ancillary Studies (Fig. 12.7d, e)

- CD20 positive in the large cells
- *EBV* positive in the large cells

Final Diagnosis

Lymphomatoid granulomatosis

Take-Home Messages

1. Lymphomatoid granulomatosis (LYG) is an angiocentric and angiodestructive lymphoproliferative disease.
2. The lesion is composed of *EBV*-positive B cells admixed with reactive T cells, which usually predominate over the *EBV*-positive large B cells.
3. The lesion has a spectrum of histological grades and clinical aggressiveness, which is related to the proportion of *EBV*-positive large B cells.

References [32, 33, 60]

Case 5

Learning Objectives

1. To become familiar with the unusual morphologic features of a common lymphoma occurring in the lung
2. To become familiar with the IHC features
3. To generate the differential diagnosis

Case History

A 65-year-old man with reticular and nodular opacities on CT scan who presents with worsening dyspnea and fatigue

Histologic Findings

- Nodular lymphoid proliferation around the bronchovascular bundles and interlobular septa (Fig. 12.22a).
- The lymphoid cells are composed of centrocytes and centroblasts (Fig. 12.22b).

Differential Diagnosis

- Follicular lymphoma
- Chronic lymphocytic leukemia/small lymphocytic lymphoma (CLL/SLL)
- Marginal zone lymphoma
- Mantle cell lymphoma

IHC and Other Ancillary Studies (Fig. 12.22c–e)

- CD20 positive
- BCL6 positive
- BCL2 positive

Final Diagnosis

Follicular lymphoma (FL)

Take-Home Messages

1. Follicular lymphoma in lung can present as nodules around bronchovascular bundles, interlobular septa, and subpleural regions.
2. BCL2 positive in germinal centers is the diagnostic feature of FL.

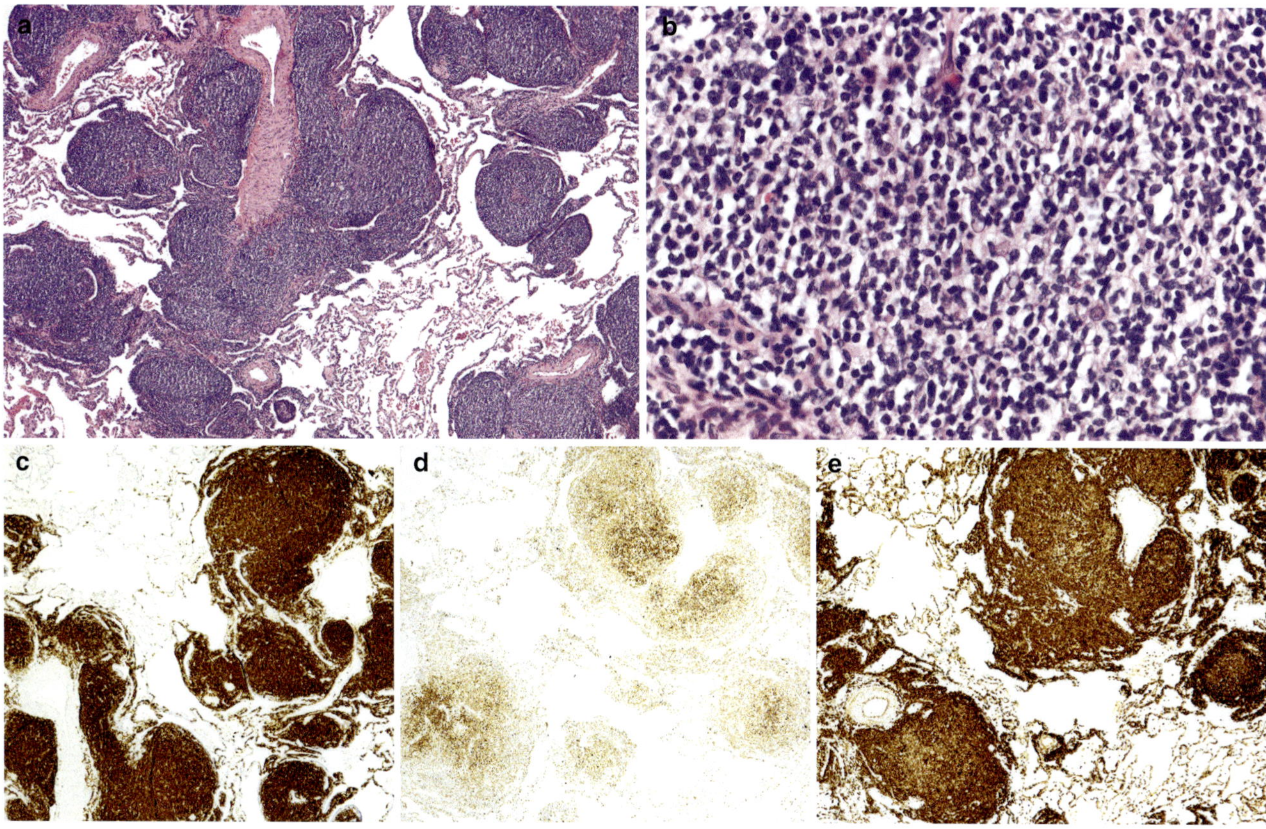

Fig. 12.22 Lung follicular lymphoma. (**a**) Nodular lymphoid proliferation around bronchovascular bundles and interlobular septa (40×). (**b**) The lymphoid cells are composed of centrocytes and centroblasts (400×). They are positive for CD20 (40×) (**c**), BCL6 (40×) (**d**), and BCL2 (40×) (**e**)

3. CD10 can be negative in FL, but other germinal center markers such as BCL6 are positive to demonstrate follicle center origin of the neoplastic cells.

References [96, 97]

Case 6

Learning Objectives

1. To become familiar with the unusual morphologic features of a common lymphoma occurring in the lung
2. To become familiar with the IHC features
3. To generate the differential diagnosis

Case History

A 66-year-old female with a right lung mass and she underwent right middle and upper lobe resection.

Histologic Findings

- Diffuse lymphoid infiltrate along alveolar walls and septa (Fig. 12.23a).
- The lymphoid cells are small with round nuclear and mature chromatin (Fig. 12.23b).

Differential Diagnosis

- Follicular lymphoma
- Chronic lymphocytic leukemia/small lymphocytic lymphoma (CLL/SLL)
- Marginal zone lymphoma
- Mantle cell lymphoma

IHC and Other Ancillary Studies

(Fig. 12.23c–f)

- CD20 positive
- CD5 positive
- CD23 positive
- CD43 positive

Final Diagnosis

Chronic lymphocytic leukemia/small lymphocytic lymphoma (CLL/SLL)

Take-Home Messages

1. CLL/SLL morphology shows small lymphocytes with mature chromatin, round nuclei, and very scant cytoplasm.

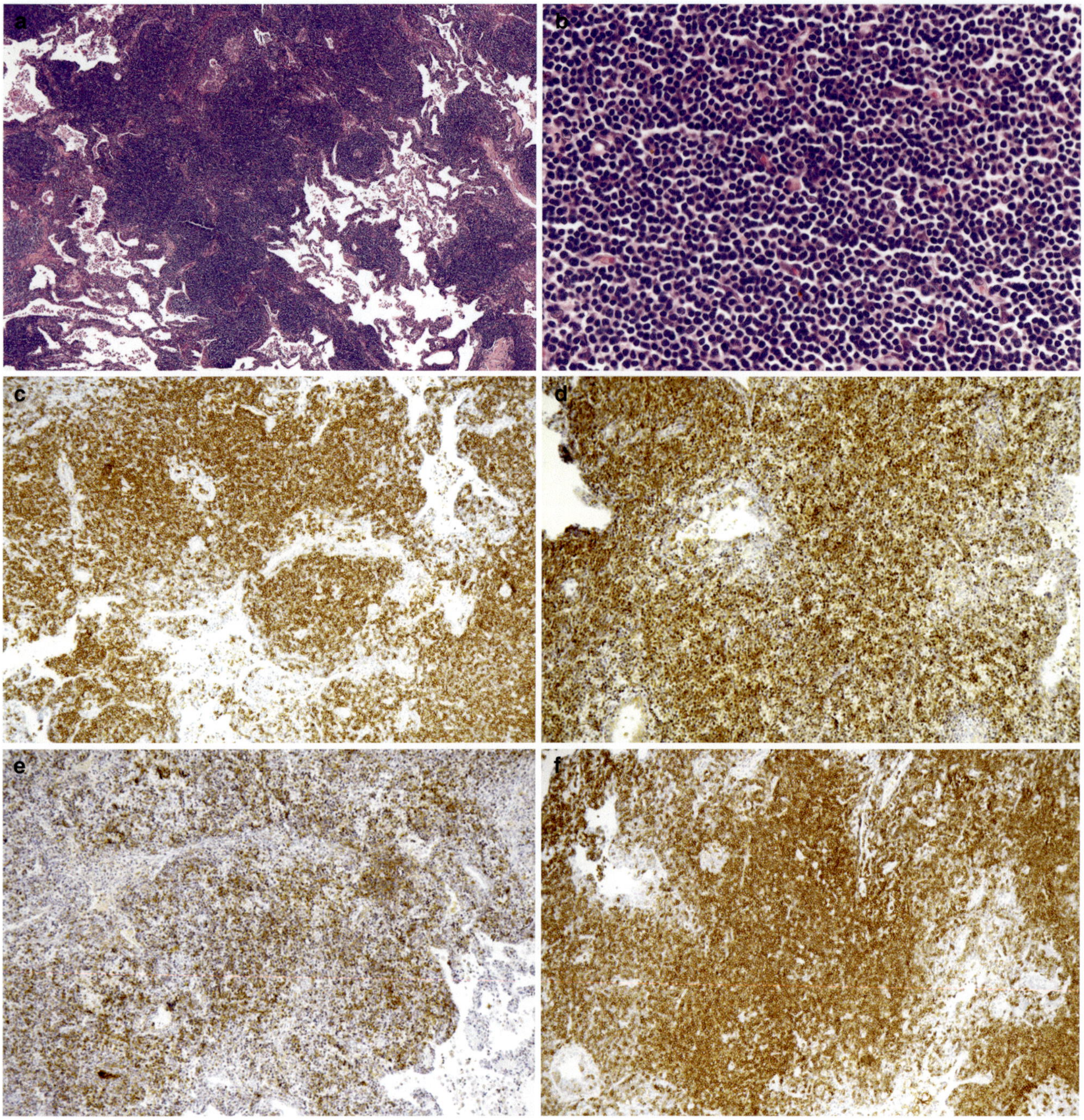

Fig. 12.23 Lung small lymphocytic lymphoma. (**a**) Diffuse lymphoid infiltrate along the alveolar walls and septa (40×). (**b**) The lymphoid cells are small with round nuclear and mature chromatin (400×). The cells are positive for CD20 (100×) (**c**), CD5 (100×) (**d**), CD23 (100×) (**e**), and CD43 (100×) (**f**)

2. CLL/SLL is CD5-positive small B-cell lymphoma with expression of CD23 and negative for BCL1.
3. CD20 usually shows weaker staining, a characteristic feature of CLL/SLL.

References [98–101]

Case 7

Learning Objectives

1. To become familiar with morphologic variation possible in small B-cell lymphomas occurring in the skin
2. To become familiar with the IHC feature
3. To generate the differential diagnosis

Case History

A 63-year-old man with a 5x5mm keloid on the left upper chest with an associated pink papule

Histologic Findings

- Dermal diffuse lymphoid infiltrate that is separated from the epidermis by a zone of uninvolved papillary dermis (Fig. 12.15a).
- The lymphoid cells are composed of small lymphocytes and many admixed plasma cells (Fig. 12.15b).

Differential Diagnosis

- B-cell lymphoma with plasmacytic differentiation
- Plasma cell neoplasm

IHC and Other Ancillary Studies (Fig. 12.15c and d)

- Kappa: positive.
- Lambda: largely negative.
- CD20 is positive.

Final Diagnosis

Primary cutaneous marginal zone B-cell lymphoma

Take-Home Messages

1. MALT lymphoma can have extreme plasmacytic differentiation with majority of the cells are plasma cells.
2. Primary cutaneous marginal zone B-cell lymphoma includes cases previously designated as primary cutaneous immunocytoma.
3. Kappa and lambda immunostains can be used to establish the B-cell clonality in significant proportion of the cases.

References [64–67]

Case 8

Learning Objectives

1. To become familiar with key histologic features of cutaneous T-cell lymphomas required for correct subtyping
2. To become familiar with the IHC feature
3. To generate the differential diagnosis

Case History

A 4-year-old girl presented with firm subcutaneous nodules on the neck, torso, and legs.

Histologic Findings

- Medium-sized pleomorphic neoplastic cells form rims around the fat cells.
- Associated karyorrhexis and necrosis are present (Fig. 12.20a).

Differential Diagnosis

- Subcutaneous panniculitis T-cell lymphoma
- Lupus panniculitis

IHC and Other Ancillary Studies (Fig. 12.20b–d)

- CD3: positive
- CD8: positive
- TIA1: positive
- Beta F1: positive

Final Diagnosis

Subcutaneous panniculitis T-cell lymphoma (SPTCL)

Take-Home Messages

1. SPTCL is characterized by a subcutaneous infiltrate simulating a panniculitis showing small, medium-sized, or sometimes large pleomorphic T cells with hyperchromatic nuclei and moderate amount of pale cytoplasm. The overlying epidermis and dermis are typically uninvolved.
2. The neoplastic cells form rims around the fat cells, often with associated karyorrhexis and histiocytes filled with karyorrhectic debris, and necrosis.
3. The neoplastic T cells show an alpha-beta, CD3+, CD4-, CD8+ T-cell phenotype, with expression of cytotoxic proteins such as TIA1, granzyme B, and/or perforins.

References [86–90]

Acknowledgments I would like to thank Drs. Andrew Bollen, Kirk Jones, Sarah Umetsu, Yi Xie, Melike Pekmezci, Arash Eslami, and Ifeoma Perkins for providing cases.

References

1. Krol AD, le Cessie S, Snijder S, Kluin-Nelemans JC, Kluin PM, Noordijk EM. Primary extranodal non-Hodgkin's lymphoma (NHL): the impact of alternative definitions tested in the Comprehensive Cancer Centre West population-based NHL registry. Ann Oncol. 2003;14(1):131–9.
2. Gou HF, Zang J, Jiang M, Yang Y, Cao D, Chen XC. Clinical prognostic analysis of 116 patients with primary intestinal non-Hodgkin lymphoma. Med Oncol. 2012;29(1):227–34.
3. Carmack SW, Lash RH, Gulizia JM, Genta RM. Lymphocytic disorders of the gastrointestinal tract: a review for the practicing pathologist. Adv Anat Pathol. 2009;16(5):290–306.
4. Howell JM, Auer-Grzesiak I, Zhang J, Andrews CN, Stewart D, Urbanski SJ. Increasing incidence rates, distribution and histological characteristics of primary gastrointestinal non-Hodgkin lymphoma in a North American population. Can J Gastroenterol. 2012;26(7):452–6.
5. Arora N, Manipadam MT, Pulimood A, Ramakrishna BS, Chacko A, Kurian SS, et al. Gastrointestinal lymphomas: pattern of distribution and histological subtypes: 10 years experience in a tertiary centre in South India. Indian J Pathol Microbiol. 2011;54(4):712–9.
6. Koch P, del Valle F, Berdel WE, Willich NA, Reers B, Hiddemann W, et al. Primary gastrointestinal non-Hodgkin's lymphoma: I. anatomic and histologic distribution, clinical features, and survival data of 371 patients registered in the German Multicenter Study GIT NHL 01/92. J Clin Oncol. 2001;19(18):3861–73.
7. O'Malley DP, Goldstein NS, Banks PM. The recognition and classification of lymphoproliferative disorders of the gut. Hum Pathol. 2014;45(5):899–916.
8. Doglioni C, Ponzoni M, Ferreri AJ, Savio A. Gastric lymphoma: the histology report. Dig Liver Dis. 2011;43(Suppl 4):S310–8.
9. Wotherspoon AC, Ortiz-Hidalgo C, Falzon MR, Isaacson PG. Helicobacter pylori-associated gastritis and primary B-cell gastric lymphoma. Lancet. 1991;338(8776):1175–6.
10. Hummel M, Oeschger S, Barth TF, Loddenkemper C, Cogliatti SB, Marx A, et al. Wotherspoon criteria combined with B cell clonality analysis by advanced polymerase chain reaction technology discriminates covert gastric marginal zone lymphoma from chronic gastritis. Gut. 2006;55(6):782–7.
11. Swerdlow SH, Jaffe ES, Brousset P, Chan JK, de Leval L, Gaulard P, et al. Cytotoxic T-cell and NK-cell lymphomas: current questions and controversies. Am J Surg Pathol. 2014;38(10):e60–71.
12. Attygalle AD, Cabecadas J, Gaulard P, Jaffe ES, de Jong D, Ko YH, et al. Peripheral T-cell and NK-cell lymphomas and their mimics; taking a step forward - report on the lymphoma workshop of the XVIth meeting of the European Association for Haematopathology and the Society for Hematopathology. Histopathology. 2014;64(2):171–99.
13. Ensari A. Gluten-sensitive enteropathy (celiac disease): controversies in diagnosis and classification. Arch Pathol Lab Med. 2010;134(6):826–36.
14. Oyama T, Ichimura K, Suzuki R, Suzumiya J, Ohshima K, Yatabe Y, et al. Senile EBV+ B-cell lymphoproliferative disorders: a clinicopathologic study of 22 patients. Am J Surg Pathol. 2003;27(1):16–26.
15. Oyama T, Yamamoto K, Asano N, Oshiro A, Suzuki R, Kagami Y, et al. Age-related EBV-associated B-cell lymphoproliferative disorders constitute a distinct clinicopathologic group: a study of 96 patients. Clin Cancer Res. 2007;13(17):5124–32.
16. Nicolae A, Pittaluga S, Abdullah S, Steinberg SM, Pham TA, Davies-Hill T, et al. EBV-positive large B-cell lymphomas in young patients: a nodal lymphoma with evidence for a tolerogenic immune environment. Blood. 2015;126(7):863–72.
17. Hummel M, Bentink S, Berger H, Klapper W, Wessendorf S, Barth TF, et al. A biologic definition of Burkitt's lymphoma from transcriptional and genomic profiling. N Engl J Med. 2006;354(23):2419–30.
18. Parsonnet J, Isaacson PG. Bacterial infection and MALT lymphoma. N Engl J Med. 2004;350(3):213–5.
19. Misdraji J, Harris NL, Hasserjian RP, Lauwers GY, Ferry JA. Primary follicular lymphoma of the gastrointestinal tract. Am J Surg Pathol. 2011;35(9):1255–63.
20. Egawa N, Fukayama M, Kawaguchi K, Hishima T, Hayashi Y, Funata N, et al. Relapsing oral and colonic ulcers with monoclonal T-cell infiltration. A low grade mucosal T-lymphoproliferative disease of the digestive tract. Cancer. 1995;75(7):1728–33.
21. Ranheim EA, Jones C, Zehnder JL, Warnke R, Yuen A. Spontaneously relapsing clonal, mucosal cytotoxic T-cell lymphoproliferative disorder: case report and review of the literature. Am J Surg Pathol. 2000;24(2):296–301.
22. Perry AM, Warnke RA, Hu Q, Gaulard P, Copie-Bergman C, Alkan S, et al. Indolent T-cell lymphoproliferative disease of the gastrointestinal tract. Blood. 2013;122(22):3599–606.
23. Hussong JW, Perkins SL, Schnitzer B, Hargreaves H, Frizzera G. Extramedullary plasmacytoma. A form of marginal zone cell lymphoma? Am J Clin Pathol. 1999;111(1):111–6.
24. Rubio-Tapia A, Hernandez-Calleros J, Trinidad-Hernandez S, Uscanga L. Clinical characteristics of a group of adults with nodular lymphoid hyperplasia: a single center experience. World J Gastroenterol. 2006;12(12):1945–8.
25. Ardeniz O, Basoglu OK, Gunsar F, Unsel M, Bayraktaroglu S, Mete N, et al. Clinical and immunological analysis of 23 adult patients with common variable immunodeficiency. J Investig Allergol Clin Immunol. 2010;20(3):222–36.
26. Appleman HD. What are the critical histologic features in the diagnosis of ulcerative colitis? Inflamm Bowel Dis. 2008;14(Suppl 2):S164–5.
27. Schlegel U. Primary CNS lymphoma. Ther Adv Neurol Disord. 2009;2(2):93–104.
28. Villano JL, Koshy M, Shaikh H, Dolecek TA, McCarthy BJ. Age, gender, and racial differences in incidence and survival in primary CNS lymphoma. Br J Cancer. 2011;105(9):1414–8.
29. Levy RM, Bredesen DE, Rosenblum ML. Neurological manifestations of the acquired immunodeficiency syndrome (AIDS): experience at UCSF and review of the literature. 1985. J Neurosurg. 2007;107(6):1253–73; discussion 1.
30. Camilleri-Broet S, Criniere E, Broet P, Delwail V, Mokhtari K, Moreau A, et al. A uniform activated B-cell-like immunophenotype might explain the poor prognosis of primary central nervous system lymphomas: analysis of 83 cases. Blood. 2006;107(1):190–6.
31. Pels H, Schmidt-Wolf IG, Glasmacher A, Schulz H, Engert A, Diehl V, et al. Primary central nervous system lymphoma: results of a pilot and phase II study of systemic and intraventricular chemotherapy with deferred radiotherapy. J Clin Oncol. 2003;21(24):4489–95.
32. Takiyama A, Nishihara H, Tateishi U, Kimura T, Wang L, Marukawa K, et al. CNS lymphomatoid granulomatosis with lymph node and bone marrow involvements. Neuropathol. 2008;28(6):640–4.
33. Dunleavy K, Roschewski M, Wilson WH. Lymphomatoid granulomatosis and other Epstein-Barr virus associated lymphoproliferative processes. Curr Hematol Malig Rep. 2012;7(3):208–15.
34. Shimada K, Matsue K, Yamamoto K, Murase T, Ichikawa N, Okamoto M, et al. Retrospective analysis of intravascular large B-cell lymphoma treated with rituximab-containing chemotherapy as reported by the IVL study group in Japan. J Clin Oncol. 2008;26(19):3189–95.
35. Ponzoni M, Ferreri AJ, Campo E, Facchetti F, Mazzucchelli L, Yoshino T, et al. Definition, diagnosis, and management of intravascular large B-cell lymphoma: proposals and perspec-

tives from an international consensus meeting. J Clin Oncol. 2007;25(21):3168–73.
36. Shimada K, Murase T, Matsue K, Okamoto M, Ichikawa N, Tsukamoto N, et al. Central nervous system involvement in intravascular large B-cell lymphoma: a retrospective analysis of 109 patients. Cancer Sci. 2010;101(6):1480–6.
37. Shimada K, Kinoshita T, Naoe T, Nakamura S. Presentation and management of intravascular large B-cell lymphoma. Lancet Oncol. 2009;10(9):895–902.
38. Chahal S, Lagera JE, Ryder J. Kleinschmidt-DeMasters BK. Hematological neoplasms with first presentation as spinal cord compression syndromes: a 10-year retrospective series and review of the literature. Clin Neuropathol. 2003;22(6):282–90.
39. Ohe Y, Hayashi T, Mishima K, Nishikawa R, Sasaki A, Matsuda H, et al. Central nervous system lymphoma initially diagnosed as tumefactive multiple sclerosis after brain biopsy. Intern Med. 2013;52(4):483–8.
40. Okita Y, Narita Y, Miyakita Y, Ohno M, Fukushima S, Maeshima A, et al. Long-term follow-up of vanishing tumors in the brain: how should a lesion mimicking primary CNS lymphoma be managed? Clin Neurol Neurosurg. 2012;114(9):1217–21.
41. Cadranel J, Wislez M, Antoine M. Primary pulmonary lymphoma. Eur Respir J. 2002;20(3):750–62.
42. William J, Variakojis D, Yeldandi A, Raparia K. Lymphoproliferative neoplasms of the lung: a review. Arch Pathol Lab Med. 2013;137(3):382–91.
43. Sirajuddin A, Raparia K, Lewis VA, Franks TJ, Dhand S, Galvin JR, et al. Primary pulmonary lymphoid lesions: radiologic and pathologic findings. Radiographics. 2016;36(1):53–70.
44. Zhang XY, Gu DM, Guo JJ, Su QQ, Chen YB. Primary pulmonary lymphoma: a retrospective analysis of 27 cases in a single tertiary hospital. Am J Med Sci. 2019;357(4):316–22.
45. Nahorecki A, Chabowski M, Straszak E, Teplicki A, Szuba A, Langfort R, et al. Primary pulmonary MALT lymphoma - case report and literature overview. Eur Rev Med Pharmacol Sci. 2016;20(10):2065–9.
46. Borie R, Wislez M, Thabut G, Antoine M, Rabbat A, Couderc LJ, et al. Clinical characteristics and prognostic factors of pulmonary MALT lymphoma. Eur Respir J. 2009;34(6):1408–16.
47. Kligerman SJ, Franks TJ, Galvin JR. Primary extranodal lymphoma of the thorax. Radiol Clin N Am. 2016;54(4):673–87.
48. Borie R, Wislez M, Antoine M, Fleury-Feith J, Thabut G, Crestani B, et al. Clonality and phenotyping analysis of alveolar lymphocytes is suggestive of pulmonary MALT lymphoma. Respir Med. 2011;105(8):1231–7.
49. Cardenas-Garcia J, Talwar A, Shah R, Fein A. Update in primary pulmonary lymphomas. Curr Opin Pulm Med. 2015;21(4):333–7.
50. Hare SS, Souza CA, Bain G, Seely JM, Frcpc, Gomes MM, et al. The radiological spectrum of pulmonary lymphoproliferative disease. Br J Radiol. 2012;85(1015):848–64.
51. Kurtin PJ, Myers JL, Adlakha H, Strickler JG, Lohse C, Pankratz VS, et al. Pathologic and clinical features of primary pulmonary extranodal marginal zone B-cell lymphoma of MALT type. Am J Surg Pathol. 2001;25(8):997–1008.
52. Lim JK, Lacy MQ, Kurtin PJ, Kyle RA, Gertz MA. Pulmonary marginal zone lymphoma of MALT type as a cause of localised pulmonary amyloidosis. J Clin Pathol. 2001;54(8):642–6.
53. Fujii K, Ishibashi KI, Kato J, Kan J, Fujii K, Ito Y, et al. Cellular-level characterization of B cells infiltrating pulmonary MALT lymphoma tissues. Virchows Arch. 2016;469(5):575–80.
54. Remstein ED, Dogan A, Einerson RR, Paternoster SF, Fink SR, Law M, et al. The incidence and anatomic site specificity of chromosomal translocations in primary extranodal marginal zone B-cell lymphoma of mucosa-associated lymphoid tissue (MALT lymphoma) in North America. Am J Surg Pathol. 2006;30(12):1546–53.
55. Okabe M, Inagaki H, Ohshima K, Yoshino T, Li C, Eimoto T, et al. API2-MALT1 fusion defines a distinctive clinicopathologic subtype in pulmonary extranodal marginal zone B-cell lymphoma of mucosa-associated lymphoid tissue. Am J Pathol. 2003;162(4):1113–22.
56. Streubel B, Simonitsch-Klupp I, Mullauer L, Lamprecht A, Huber D, Siebert R, et al. Variable frequencies of MALT lymphoma-associated genetic aberrations in MALT lymphomas of different sites. Leukemia. 2004;18(10):1722–6.
57. Sammassimo S, Pruneri G, Andreola G, Montoro J, Steffanoni S, Nowakowski GS, et al. A retrospective international study on primary extranodal marginal zone lymphoma of the lung (BALT lymphoma) on behalf of International Extranodal Lymphoma Study Group (IELSG). Hematol Oncol. 2016;34(4):177–83.
58. Pina-Oviedo S, Weissferdt A, Kalhor N, Moran CA. Primary pulmonary lymphomas. Adv Anat Pathol. 2015;22(6):355–75.
59. Song JY, Pittaluga S, Dunleavy K, Grant N, White T, Jiang L, et al. Lymphomatoid granulomatosis--a single institute experience: pathologic findings and clinical correlations. Am J Surg Pathol. 2015;39(2):141–56.
60. Katzenstein AL, Doxtader E, Narendra S. Lymphomatoid granulomatosis: insights gained over 4 decades. Am J Surg Pathol. 2010;34(12):e35–48.
61. Borie R, Wislez M, Antoine M, Cadranel J. Lymphoproliferative disorders of the lung. Respiration. 2017;94(2):157–75.
62. Bradford PT, Devesa SS, Anderson WF, Toro JR. Cutaneous lymphoma incidence patterns in the United States: a population-based study of 3884 cases. Blood. 2009;113(21):5064–73.
63. Willemze R, Jaffe ES, Burg G, Cerroni L, Berti E, Swerdlow SH, et al. WHO-EORTC classification for cutaneous lymphomas. Blood. 2005;105(10):3768–85.
64. Rijlaarsdam JU, van der Putte SC, Berti E, Kerl H, Rieger E, Toonstra J, et al. Cutaneous immunocytomas: a clinicopathologic study of 26 cases. Histopathology. 1993;23(2):117–25.
65. Schmid U, Eckert F, Griesser H, Steinke C, Cogliatti SB, Kaudewitz P, et al. Cutaneous follicular lymphoid hyperplasia with monotypic plasma cells. A clinicopathologic study of 18 patients. Am J Surg Pathol. 1995;19(1):12–20.
66. Li C, Inagaki H, Kuo TT, Hu S, Okabe M, Eimoto T. Primary cutaneous marginal zone B-cell lymphoma: a molecular and clinicopathologic study of 24 Asian cases. Am J Surg Pathol. 2003;27(8):1061–9.
67. Bailey EM, Ferry JA, Harris NL, Mihm MC Jr, Jacobson JO, Duncan LM. Marginal zone lymphoma (low-grade B-cell lymphoma of mucosa-associated lymphoid tissue type) of skin and subcutaneous tissue: a study of 15 patients. Am J Surg Pathol. 1996;20(8):1011–23.
68. Streubel B, Vinatzer U, Lamprecht A, Raderer M, Chott A. T(3;14) (p14.1;q32) involving IGH and FOXP1 is a novel recurrent chromosomal aberration in MALT lymphoma. Leukemia. 2005;19(4):652–8.
69. Streubel B, Lamprecht A, Dierlamm J, Cerroni L, Stolte M, Ott G, et al. T(14;18)(q32;q21) involving IGH and MALT1 is a frequent chromosomal aberration in MALT lymphoma. Blood. 2003;101(6):2335–9.
70. Gronbaek K, Ralfkiaer E, Kalla J, Skovgaard GL, Guldberg P. Infrequent somatic Fas mutations but no evidence of Bcl10 mutations or t(11;18) in primary cutaneous MALT-type lymphoma. J Pathol. 2003;201(1):134–40.
71. Hallermann C, Kaune KM, Gesk S, Martin-Subero JI, Gunawan B, Griesinger F, et al. Molecular cytogenetic analysis of chromosomal breakpoints in the IGH, MYC, BCL6, and MALT1 gene loci in primary cutaneous B-cell lymphomas. J Invest Dermatol. 2004;123(1):213–9.
72. Cerroni L, Arzberger E, Putz B, Hofler G, Metze D, Sander CA, et al. Primary cutaneous follicle center cell lymphoma with follicular growth pattern. Blood. 2000;95(12):3922–8.

73. Geelen FA, Vermeer MH, Meijer CJ, Van der Putte SC, Kerkhof E, Kluin PM, et al. bcl-2 protein expression in primary cutaneous large B-cell lymphoma is site-related. J Clin Oncol. 1998;16(6):2080–5.
74. Child FJ, Russell-Jones R, Woolford AJ, Calonje E, Photiou A, Orchard G, et al. Absence of the t(14;18) chromosomal translocation in primary cutaneous B-cell lymphoma. Br J Dermatol. 2001;144(4):735–44.
75. Goodlad JR, Krajewski AS, Batstone PJ, McKay P, White JM, Benton EC, et al. Primary cutaneous follicular lymphoma: a clinicopathologic and molecular study of 16 cases in support of a distinct entity. Am J Surg Pathol. 2002;26(6):733–41.
76. Kim YH, Liu HL, Mraz-Gernhard S, Varghese A, Hoppe RT. Long-term outcome of 525 patients with mycosis fungoides and Sezary syndrome: clinical prognostic factors and risk for disease progression. Arch Dermatol. 2003;139(7):857–66.
77. Wain EM, Orchard GE, Whittaker SJ, Spittle MSMF, Russell-Jones R. Outcome in 34 patients with juvenile-onset mycosis fungoides: a clinical, immunophenotypic, and molecular study. Cancer. 2003;98(10):2282–90.
78. Smoller BR, Santucci M, Wood GS, Whittaker SJ. Histopathology and genetics of cutaneous T-cell lymphoma. Hematol Oncol Clin North Am. 2003;17(6):1277–311.
79. Whittam LR, Calonje E, Orchard G, Fraser-Andrews EA, Woolford A, Russell-Jones R. CD8-positive juvenile onset mycosis fungoides: an immunohistochemical and genotypic analysis of six cases. Br J Dermatol. 2000;143(6):1199–204.
80. van Doorn R, Van Haselen CW, van Voorst Vader PC, Geerts ML, Heule F, de Rie M, et al. Mycosis fungoides: disease evolution and prognosis of 309 Dutch patients. Arch Dermatol. 2000;136(4):504–10.
81. Willemze R, Beljaards RC. Spectrum of primary cutaneous CD30 (Ki-1)-positive lymphoproliferative disorders. A proposal for classification and guidelines for management and treatment. J Am Acad Dermatol. 1993;28(6):973–80.
82. Bekkenk MW, Geelen FA, van Voorst Vader PC, Heule F, Geerts ML, van Vloten WA, et al. Primary and secondary cutaneous CD30(+) lymphoproliferative disorders: a report from the Dutch Cutaneous Lymphoma Group on the long-term follow-up data of 219 patients and guidelines for diagnosis and treatment. Blood. 2000;95(12):3653–61.
83. Liu HL, Hoppe RT, Kohler S, Harvell JD, Reddy S, Kim YH. CD30+ cutaneous lymphoproliferative disorders: the Stanford experience in lymphomatoid papulosis and primary cutaneous anaplastic large cell lymphoma. J Am Acad Dermatol. 2003;49(6):1049–58.
84. DeCoteau JF, Butmarc JR, Kinney MC, Kadin ME. The t(2;5) chromosomal translocation is not a common feature of primary cutaneous CD30+ lymphoproliferative disorders: comparison with anaplastic large-cell lymphoma of nodal origin. Blood. 1996;87(8):3437–41.
85. El Shabrawi-Caelen L, Kerl H, Cerroni L. Lymphomatoid papulosis: reappraisal of clinicopathologic presentation and classification into subtypes A, B, and C. Arch Dermatol. 2004;140(4):441–7.
86. Salhany KE, Macon WR, Choi JK, Elenitsas R, Lessin SR, Felgar RE, et al. Subcutaneous panniculitis-like T-cell lymphoma: clinicopathologic, immunophenotypic, and genotypic analysis of alpha/beta and gamma/delta subtypes. Am J Surg Pathol. 1998;22(7):881–93.
87. Santucci M, Pimpinelli N, Massi D, Kadin ME, Meijer CJ, Muller-Hermelink HK, et al. Cytotoxic/natural killer cell cutaneous lymphomas. Report of EORTC Cutaneous Lymphoma Task Force Workshop. Cancer. 2003;97(3):610–27.
88. Hoque SR, Child FJ, Whittaker SJ, Ferreira S, Orchard G, Jenner K, et al. Subcutaneous panniculitis-like T-cell lymphoma: a clinicopathological, immunophenotypic and molecular analysis of six patients. Br J Dermatol. 2003;148(3):516–25.
89. Massone C, Chott A, Metze D, Kerl K, Citarella L, Vale E, et al. Subcutaneous, blastic natural killer (NK), NK/T-cell, and other cytotoxic lymphomas of the skin: a morphologic, immunophenotypic, and molecular study of 50 patients. Am J Surg Pathol. 2004;28(6):719–35.
90. Takeshita M, Imayama S, Oshiro Y, Kurihara K, Okamoto S, Matsuki Y, et al. Clinicopathologic analysis of 22 cases of subcutaneous panniculitis-like CD56- or CD56+ lymphoma and review of 44 other reported cases. Am J Clin Pathol. 2004;121(3):408–16.
91. Marzano AV, Berti E, Paulli M, Caputo R. Cytophagic histiocytic panniculitis and subcutaneous panniculitis-like T-cell lymphoma: report of 7 cases. Arch Dermatol. 2000;136(7):889–96.
92. Lee JY, Chung H, Cho H, Jang JE, Kim Y, Kim SJ, et al. Clinical characteristics and treatment outcomes of isolated myeloid sarcoma without bone marrow involvement: a single-institution experience. Blood Res. 2017;52(3):184–92.
93. Meireles LC, Lagos AC, Marques I, Serejo F, Velosa J. Myeloid sarcoma of gastrointestinal tract: a rare cause of obstruction. Rev Esp Enferm Dig. 2015;107(5):326–7.
94. Kaygusuz G, Kankaya D, Ekinci C, Topcuoglu P, Kuzu I. Myeloid sarcomas: a clinicopathologic study of 20 cases. Turk J Haematol. 2015;32(1):35–42.
95. Gadage V, Zutshi G, Menon S, Shet T, Gupta S. Gastric myeloid sarcoma--a report of two cases addressing diagnostic issues. Indian J Pathol Microbiol. 2011;54(4):832–5.
96. Graham BB, Mathisen DJ, Mark EJ, Takvorian RW. Primary pulmonary lymphoma. Ann Thorac Surg. 2005;80(4):1248–53.
97. L'Hoste RJ Jr, Filippa DA, Lieberman PH, Bretsky S. Primary pulmonary lymphomas. A clinicopathologic analysis of 36 cases. Cancer. 1984;54(7):1397–406.
98. Hill BT, Weil AC, Kalaycio M, Cook JR. Pulmonary involvement by chronic lymphocytic leukemia/small lymphocytic lymphoma is a specific pathologic finding independent of inflammatory infiltration. Leuk Lymphoma. 2012;53(4):589–95.
99. Berkman N, Polliack A, Breuer R, Okon E, Kramer M. Pulmonary involvement as the major manifestation of chronic lymphocytic leukemia. Leuk Lymphoma. 1992;8(6):495–9.
100. Moore W, Baram D, Hu Y. Pulmonary infiltration from chronic lymphocytic leukemia. J Thorac Imaging. 2006;21(2):172–5.
101. Dear A, Goldstein D, Salem HH. Pulmonary chronic lymphocytic leukemia: difficulty in establishing a tissue diagnosis. Eur J Haematol. 1995;54(2):130–3.

Lymphoid Neoplasms with "Benign" Clinical Course or Unclear Malignant Potential

13

Juehua Gao and Shunyou Gong

List of Frequently Asked Questions

1. What are the diagnostic criteria for monoclonal B-cell lymphocytosis (MBL)?
2. What are the immunophenotypes of MBL?
3. What is a nodal equivalent of MBL?
4. What is in situ follicular neoplasia and how is it diagnosed?
5. What ancillary studies may be considered in ISFN?
6. What are the risks of in situ follicular neoplasia to progress to subsequent follicular lymphoma?
7. What is the difference between in situ follicular neoplasia and partial involvement by follicular lymphoma?
8. What are the types of indolent mantle cell lymphoma?
9. What are the clinical and pathologic features of leukemic non-nodal mantle cell lymphoma?
10. What are the diagnostic pitfalls for leukemic non-nodal mantle cell lymphoma?
11. What is in situ mantle cell neoplasia and how is it diagnosed?
12. What is the differential diagnosis of in situ mantle cell neoplasia?
13. What is the prognosis of in situ mantle cell neoplasia?

J. Gao (✉)
Department of Pathology, Northwestern University Feinberg School of Medicine, Chicago, IL, USA
e-mail: j-gao@northwestern.edu

S. Gong
Hematology and Hematopathology, Department of Pathology, Ann & Robert H. Lurie Children's Hospital, Northwestern University Feinberg School of Medicine, Chicago, IL, USA
e-mail: Shunyou.Gong@Northwestern.edu

1. What are the diagnostic criteria for monoclonal B-cell lymphocytosis (MBL)?

Monoclonal B-cell lymphocytosis is defined by a clonal B-cell proliferation less than 5000/uL in the peripheral blood with no lymphadenopathy, splenomegaly, or other evidence of tissue involvement by a B-cell lymphoproliferative disorder.

- MBL with chronic lymphocytic leukemia (CLL) phenotype can be further separated into low count (less than 500/uL) or high count (>500/uL) based on the absolute number of monotypic B cells in the peripheral blood.
- The low-count MBL has extremely limited, if any, chance of progression and does not require routine follow-up outside of standard medical care.
- The high-count MBL has biologic features similar to low-stage CLL and may progress to overt CLL at an annual rate of 1–2% [1, 2].

2. What are the immunophenotypes of MBL?

- The majority of MBLs have an immunophenotype resembling CLL, characterized by coexpression of CD19, CD5, and CD23, with dim expression of CD20 and surface immunoglobulin light chain.
- Some MBL cases have an atypical CLL phenotype with brighter CD20 or surface immunoglobulin light chain expression.
- Occasional MBL cases with a non-CLL phenotype have also been reported. These cases are characterized by lacking or dim CD5 expression and bright surface immunoglobulin light chain expression.

E. Wang, A. S. Lagoo (eds.), *Practical Lymph Node and Bone Marrow Pathology*, Practical Anatomic Pathology, https://doi.org/10.1007/978-3-030-32189-5_13

3. What is a nodal equivalent of MBL?

While MBL is mostly defined based on the number of circulating monotypic B cells, occasional cases are incidentally identified in lymph node biopsy for other purposes.

- Focal or low level of nodal infiltration by monotypic B cells with CLL phenotype could be considered as a tissue equivalent of MBL rather than overt small lymphocytic lymphoma. However, a precise numeric cutoff between MBL and overt lymphoma involving the lymph node is not defined.
- The B-cell infiltrate does not efface nodal architecture or form significant confluent growth with typical proliferative centers.
- A low level of monoclonal B-cell population is detected often by flow cytometry rather than histologic evaluation.
- The current recommendation is lymphadenopathy less than 1.5 cm on CT [3].

4. What is in situ follicular neoplasia and how is it diagnosed?

In situ follicular neoplasia (ISFN) is defined by monotypic B cells harboring *BCL2* gene rearrangement seen in typical follicular lymphoma with partial or total colonization of the germinal centers without spreading to surrounding structure.

- ISFN is usually an incidental finding and it is not apparent in hematoxylin-eosin-stained tissue sections. The neoplastic follicles have similar size to other reactive follicles and show predominantly centrocyte morphology.
- ISFN is often highlighted by immunohistochemistry for BCL2 which is usually negative in reactive germinal centers but is often strongly positive in the follicle centers affected by ISFN. Caution must be paid to co-distribution of germinal center signature markers, such as CD10 and BCL6, and BCL2 to make sure coexpression of the antigens in the same lymphoid nodules. Primary lymphoid follicles could express BCL2, but they are negative for germinal center signature antigens.
- ISFN may involve reactive lymph node, extranodal site with reactive follicles, or detected in lymphoid tissue with other types of lymphoma [4–6]. Therefore, additional clinical evaluation is needed particularly when the patient has lymphadenopathy.
- Rare cases of coexisting ISFN and in situ mantle cell lymphoma have been reported [7, 8].

5. What ancillary studies may be considered in ISFN?

- The monoclonal B-cell population is often overlooked by routine flow cytometry due to diluting effect of predominant reactive follicles and other polyclonal B-cell population.
- Clonal rearrangement of *IGH/K* gene can be detected by a PCR-based assay on a DNA sample from microdissected BCL2-positive follicle centers. Assays performed on DNA sample from whole tissue extract are often negative for clonal amplicon.
- *IGH/BCL2* fusion can be detected by interphase FISH analysis on a slide with microdissected BCL2-positive follicle centers but may be potentially missed on a whole tissue section.

6. What are the risks of in situ follicular neoplasia to progress to subsequent follicular lymphoma?

- For patients with incidental findings of ISFN with no other evidence of overt follicular lymphoma, the risk of developing subsequent follicular lymphoma is very low [4, 9].

7. What is the difference between in situ follicular neoplasia and partial involvement by follicular lymphoma?

The distinction between ISFN and partial involvement by follicular lymphoma is important as the former has relatively low risks of disease progression. In contrast, partial involvement by follicular lymphoma is considered a form of follicular lymphoma that has clinical significance.

- Partial involvement of follicular lymphoma, although demonstrates similar immunohistochemistry profiles of strong BCL2 and CD10 in the germinal centers, shows partial architecture alteration.
- The affected follicles may appear enlarged or crowded on the hematoxylin-eosin-stained tissue sections.
- Other histologic clues indicating partial follicular lymphoma include attenuated mantle zones surrounding the follicles, variable BCL2 and CD10 staining intensity, CD10 staining outside of the follicles, and a mixture of centrocyte and centroblast morphology in the affected follicles (Table 13.1).

Table 13.1 Diagnostic comparison between in situ follicular neoplasia (ISFN) and partial involvement by follicular lymphoma (FL)

	ISFN	Partial involvement by FL
Clinical presentation	Incidental finding	May have nodal or extranodal enlargement
Lymph node architecture	Preserved nodal architecture with normal-sized follicles	Partial architecture alteration with expanded follicles
Affected follicles	Follicles with monotonous population of centrocytes, in a background of reactive follicles	Follicles with monotonous population of centrocytes and few centroblasts, surrounded by attenuated mantle zones
Immunohistochemistry	Strong coexpression of BCL2 and CD10 confined to the affected follicles	Variable BCL2 and CD10 staining intensity, CD10 staining outside of the follicles
Immunophenotype	Light chain-restricted B cells in a background of more numerous polytypic B cells	Light chain-restricted B cells and variable polytypic B cells
Genetics	t(14;18) translocation with few other genetic alterations	t(14;18) translocation, may have additional genetic alterations
Risks for disease progression	Low risk of progression to overt lymphoma	A form of overt lymphoma, risk of progression according to prognostic scores

- Partial involvement by follicular lymphoma is more often detected by flow cytometry, immunoglobulin gene rearrangement, and interphase FISH analysis for *IGH/BCL2* in preparation from whole tissue sample, while in ISFN the abnormalities are often detected in preparation from micromanipulated specimen.

8. What are the types of indolent mantle cell lymphoma?

Mantle cell lymphoma is generally considered an aggressive lymphoma with a median survival of 3–5 years. However, indolent types of mantle cell lymphoma have been recognized.

- The recently updated WHO Classification of Tumors of Hematopoietic and Lymphoid Tissue included two distinct subtypes of mantle cell lymphoma with indolent clinical behavior.
- Leukemic non-nodal mantle cell lymphoma and in situ mantle cell neoplasia.

9. What are the clinical and pathologic features of leukemic non-nodal mantle cell lymphoma?

Leukemic non-nodal mantle cell lymphoma is characterized by mantle cell lymphoma predominantly involving the peripheral blood, bone marrow, and sometimes spleen without significant lymphadenopathy. This is defined by peripheral lymph nodes less than 2 cm or no lymphadenopathy by CT.

- The lymphocytes may have morphology similar to CLL lymphocytes, and they are more likely to be SOX11-negative and have somatic immunoglobulin hypermutations.
- A small subset of cases may have CD200 expression, another feature overlapping with CLL.
- The CD5 expression may be less common than in typical mantle cell lymphomas.
- The prognosis in this variant is better than nodal mantle cell lymphoma with an overall median survival of 6–7 years.

10. What are the diagnostic pitfalls for leukemic non-nodal mantle cell lymphoma?

The leukemic non-nodal mantle cell lymphoma should be distinguished from leukemic phase of mantle cell lymphoma which is an advanced stage of mantle cell lymphoma with peripheral blood and bone marrow involvement and associated with aggressive clinical course.

- Evaluation for lymphadenopathy and correlation with radiologic findings is helpful to distinguish between the two.
- In some cases of leukemic non-nodal mantle cell lymphoma, the CD5 expression may be negative, and the diagnosis of mantle cell lymphoma may not be considered if a cyclin D1 stain or FISH for t(11;14) *IGH-CCND1* is not included.
- Leukemic non-nodal mantle cell lymphoma may show overlapping clinical, morphologic, or immunophenotypic features with CLL. Cyclin D1 immunostain or FISH for t(11;14) *IGH-CCND1* is recommended for any B-cell lymphoma with peripheral blood and marrow involvement (Table 13.2).

Table 13.2 Diagnostic comparison between leukemic non-nodal mantle cell lymphoma and leukemic phase of typical mantle cell lymphoma

	Leukemic non-nodal mantle cell lymphoma	Leukemic phase of typical mantle cell lymphoma
Clinical presentation	Peripheral blood and bone marrow involvement without significant adenopathy	Nodal or extranodal enlargement; advanced stage may involve peripheral blood and bone marrow
Morphology	More likely to be small, resembling CLL-type lymphocytes	May have greater atypia
Immunophenotype	Less common CD5+, SOX11−, *IGHV* somatic hypermutation	Often CD5+, cyclin D1+, SOX11+
Genetics	Few abnormalities other than t(11;14) translocation	More complex abnormalities in addition to t(11;14) translocation
Clinical course	Indolent	A form of overt lymphoma

Table 13.3 Diagnostic comparison between in situ mantle cell neoplasia and mantle zone pattern of mantle cell lymphoma

	In situ mantle cell neoplasia	Mantle zone pattern of mantle cell lymphoma
Clinical presentation	Incidental finding	May have nodal or extranodal enlargement
Lymph node architecture	Preserved nodal architecture	Partial architecture alteration
Mantle zone of affected follicles	Mantle zone is thin with no or minimal expansion	Mantle zone expansion; nodular or diffuse pattern may be seen in other areas
Immunohistochemistry	Cyclin D1-positive B cells are exclusively restricted to the inner mantle zones	Cyclin D1-positive B cells replace and expand the mantle zones
Immunophenotype	More likely to be CD5-, cyclin D1+, SOX11+/−	Often CD5+, cyclin D1+, SOX11+
Genetics	t(11;14) translocation	t(11;14) translocation
Clinical course	Indolent	A form of overt lymphoma

11. What is in situ mantle cell neoplasia and how is it diagnosed?

In situ mantle cell neoplasia is defined by cyclin D1-positive B cells localized to the mantle zone of reactive lymphoid follicles with otherwise unremarkable histologic features.

- A cyclin D1 stain is helpful to identify in situ mantle cell lymphoma.
- In situ mantle cell neoplasia is often an incidental finding, but in rare cases it may occur with other types of lymphoma [10, 11].
- As in ISFN, in situ mantle cell neoplasia may be missed by flow cytometry and B-cell clonality study of preparation from whole tissue sample.

12. What is the differential diagnosis of in situ mantle cell neoplasia?

In situ mantle cell neoplasia should be differentiated from overt mantle cell lymphoma with a mantle zone growth pattern. The distinction is clinically important as most of the in situ mantle cell lymphoma is considered an indolent lesion which may not require additional treatment.

- Overt mantle cell lymphoma has mantle zone, nodular, or diffuse growth pattern. Careful histologic examination may help identify other histologic pattern and differentiate overt lymphoma from in situ neoplasia.
- In in situ mantle cell neoplasia, the cyclin D1-positive B cells are exclusively restricted to the mantle zone and are typically distributed in the inner mantle zone.
- In mantle cell lymphoma with mantle zone pattern, the cyclin D1-positive B cells often completely replace or expand the mantle zones (Table 13.3).

13. What is the prognosis of in situ mantle cell neoplasia?

In situ mantle cell neoplasia has an indolent clinical course. The patients can achieve long-term survival without treatment. However, rare cases may show disease progression to overt mantle cell lymphoma [10].

Case Presentations

Case 1 (Fig. 13.1)

Learning Objectives

1. To become familiar with the diagnostic criteria for MBL
2. To become familiar with the most common phenotype of MBL

Case History

The patient was an 85-year-old man with a history of persistent lymphocytosis for the past year. CBC reported leukocytosis with an absolute lymphocyte count of 6.2 K/uL. There was

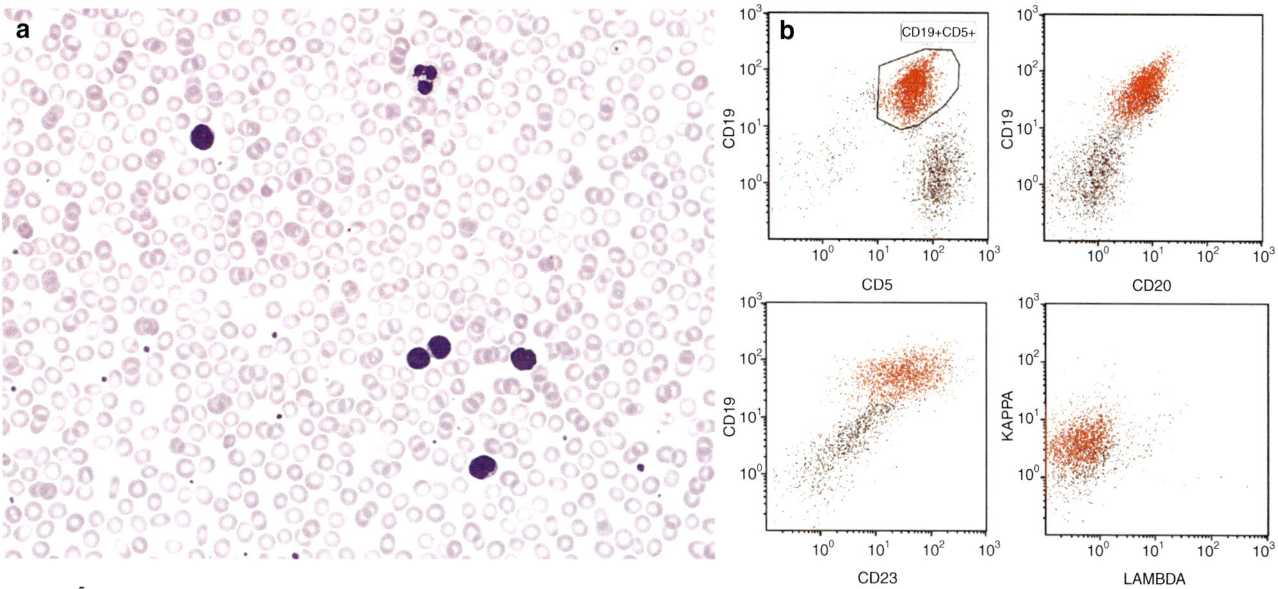

Fig. 13.1 Monoclonal B-cell lymphocytosis. (**a**) The peripheral blood smear reveals increased lymphocytes. The lymphocytes are predominantly small mature appearing with clumped chromatin (Wright-Giemsa, ×600). (**b**) Flow cytometric analysis reports a monotypic B-cell population, that is, CD5+, CD19+, CD20+, CD23+, and CD20 dim+ with dim kappa-restricted surface immunoglobulin light chain expression. These cells are also CD200+, FMC7 dim+, and CD79b dim/negative (not shown)

no anemia or thrombocytopenia. Additional workup revealed no lymphadenopathy, splenomegaly, or other evidence of tissue involvement by a B-cell lymphoproliferative disorder.

Histologic Findings

- The peripheral blood smear revealed increased lymphocytes.
- The lymphocytes consisted of monotonous small- to medium-sized forms with clumped chromatin and scant to moderate cytoplasm.

Differential Diagnosis

- Chronic lymphocytic leukemia
- Monoclonal B-cell lymphocytosis
- Other indolent leukemia/lymphoma

Ancillary Test Results

- Flow cytometric analysis reported 64% of the lymphocytes are B cells.
- There was a monotypic B-cell population, that is, CD5+, CD19+, CD20+, CD23+, and CD20 dim+ with dim surface kappa light chain restriction. These cells were also CD200+, FMC7 dim+, and CD79b dim/negative.
- Based on the absolute lymphocyte count and the fraction of the monotypic B cells (93% of the B-cell population), the absolute monotypic B-cell count was 3.7 K/uL.

Final Diagnosis

Monoclonal B-cell lymphocytosis (MBL) of CLL phenotype

Follow-Up

The patient has been watched and has since showed no disease progression.

Take-Home Messages

1. Flow cytometric analysis is required to make the diagnosis of MBL and to differentiate from overt CLL.
2. The most common type of MBL is CLL-phenotype, but non-CLL phenotype MBL also exists.
3. It is imperative to rule out lymphadenopathy, splenomegaly, or other tissue involvement, as these cases should not be diagnosed as MBL.

Case 2 (Fig. 13.2)

Learning Objective

1. To understand the immunohistochemical staining pattern of in situ follicular neoplasia (ISFN)

Case History

A 53-year-old man underwent colonoscopy for routine colorectal cancer screening. He had no family history of colorectal cancer. There was no past history or current clinical evidence for lymphoma.

Histologic Findings

- The random colon biopsy showed unremarkable colonic mucosa.

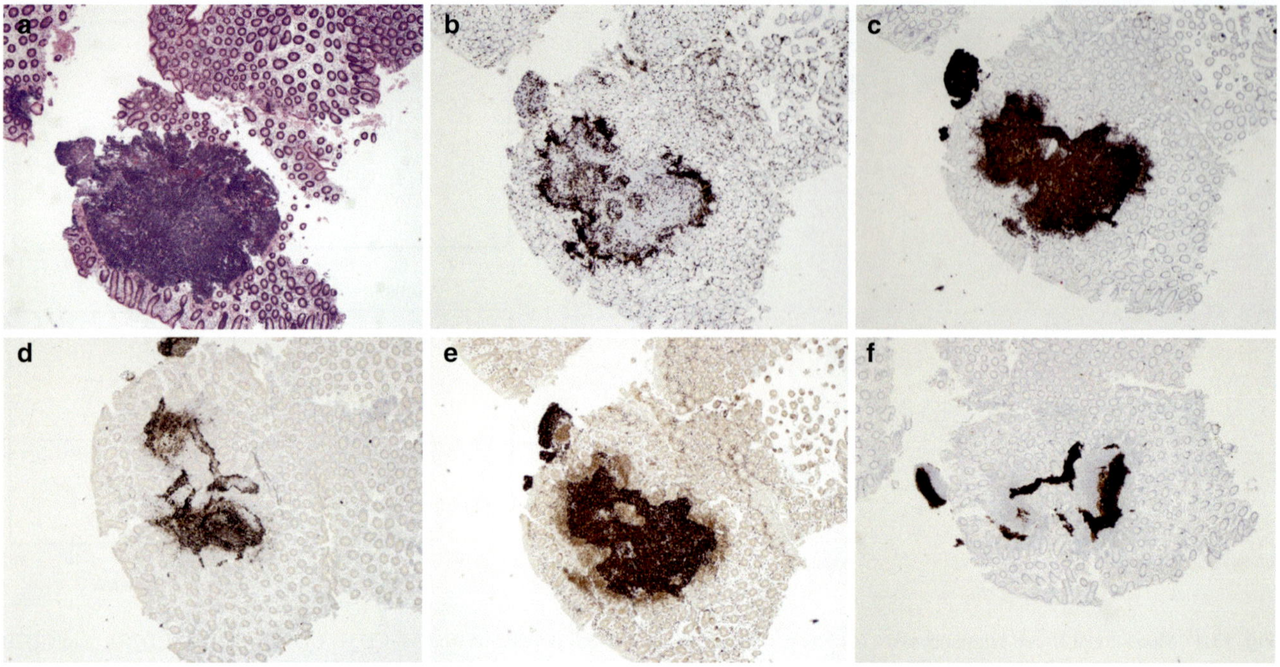

Fig. 13.2 In situ follicular neoplasia. (**a**) Unremarkable colonic mucosa with a well-circumscribed lymphoid aggregate comprising of predominantly small lymphocytes (hematoxylin-eosin, ×200). (**b**) CD3 stains a rim of T cells (peroxidase, ×200). (**c**) CD20 stains a predominance of B cells in the lymphoid aggregates (peroxidase, ×200). (**d**) CD23 highlights dendritic cell meshwork (peroxidase, ×200). (**e**) BCL2 is intensely positive in the B cells, weakly positive in the T cells (peroxidase, ×200). (**f**) CD10 is strongly positive in a subset of B cells (peroxidase, ×200)

- There were scattered lymphoid aggregates noted in the lamina propria; the lymphoid aggregates were well circumscribed without infiltrative borders and comprised of predominantly small lymphocytes admixed with some large cells.

Differential Diagnosis

- Reactive follicular hyperplasia
- Intestinal follicular lymphoma
- In situ follicular neoplasia

Ancillary Test Results

- Immunohistochemical analyses were performed for further characterization of the lymphoid aggregates. Based on the results of immunostains, most of the lymphoid aggregates were reactive follicles.
- One of the lymphoid aggregates demonstrated abnormal immunohistochemical staining pattern with strong BCL2+ and CD10+ B cells within the germinal centers.

Final Diagnosis

In situ follicular neoplasia

Follow-Up

The patient received no additional treatment and has since demonstrated no evidence of lymphoma.

Take-Home Messages

1. In situ follicular neoplasia is often an incidental finding.
2. In situ follicular neoplasia can only be diagnosed with the aid of immunohistochemistry demonstrating strong expression of BCL2 and CD10 within the affected germinal centers.
3. It is crucial to differentiate in situ follicular neoplasia from partial involvement by overt follicular lymphoma.

Case 3 (Fig. 13.3)

Learning Objectives

1. To become familiar with the clinical presentation of leukemia non-nodal mantle cell lymphoma
2. To appreciate the immunophenotypic difference between leukemia non-nodal mantle cell lymphoma and typical mantle cell lymphoma

Case History

The patient was an 82-year-old man who was noted to have lymphocytosis on routine CBC. The absolute lymphocyte count was 5.5 K/uL. There was no evidence of lymphadenopathy or splenomegaly. A bone marrow biopsy was performed for further evaluation.

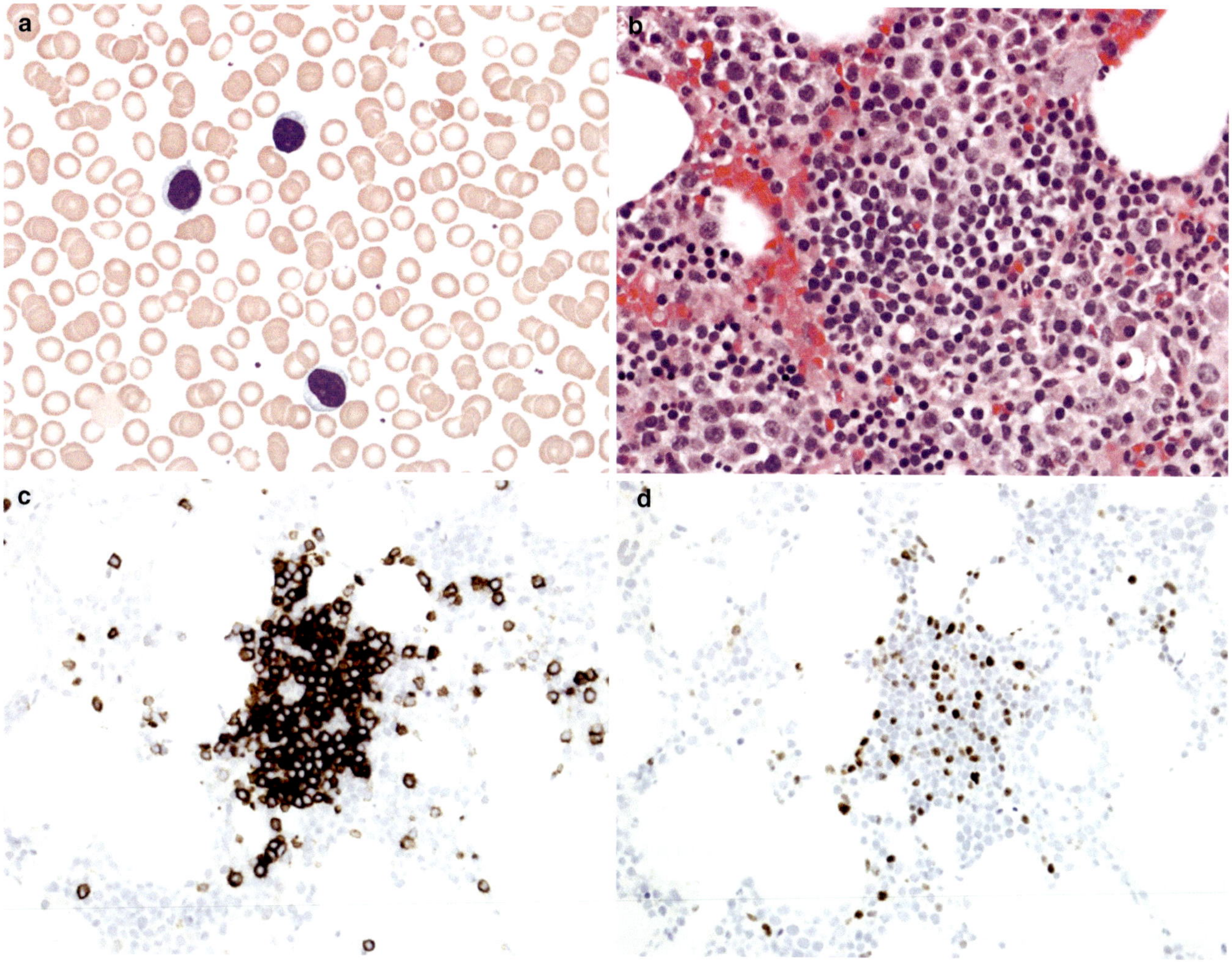

Fig. 13.3 Leukemic non-nodal mantle cell lymphoma. (**a**) Peripheral blood smear shows mildly increased lymphocytes that are small and mature appearing with condensed chromatin (Wright-Giemsa, ×1000). (**b**) Bone marrow core biopsy shows hypercellular marrow with scattered lymphoid aggregates comprising of small mature-appearing lymphocytes (hematoxylin-eosin, ×600). (**c**) CD20 stains a predominance of B cells in the lymphoid aggregates (peroxidase, ×600). (**d**) Some of the lymphocytes are positive for cyclin D1 (peroxidase, ×600), but negative for SOX11 (not shown)

Histologic Findings

- The peripheral blood smear showed mildly increased lymphocytes that were small and mature appearing with condensed chromatin.
- The bone marrow core biopsy showed hypercellular bone marrow with scattered interstitial lymphoid aggregates comprising of small mature-appearing lymphocytes.
- By immunohistochemistry, the lymphoid aggregates were predominantly B cells that were also cyclin D1 positive, but SOX11 negative.

Differential Diagnosis

- Mantle cell lymphoma, usual type
- Leukemic non-nodal mantle cell lymphoma

Ancillary Test Results

- Flow cytometric analysis detected a kappa-restricted monotypic B-cell population that was CD5 partial+, CD19+, CD20+, CD22+, CD23 partial+, CD200 negative, CD79b+, and FMC7 dim.
- FISH analysis of this sample was positive for *IGH/CCND1* fusion.

Final Diagnosis

Peripheral blood and bone marrow involved by leukemic non-nodal mantle cell lymphoma

Follow-Up

The patient was followed clinically, and he died of heart attack 1 year later without overt evidence of the lymphoma progression.

Take-Home Messages

1. Leukemic non-nodal mantle cell lymphoma shows overlapping morphologic and immunophenotypic features with CLL, except for cyclin D1 expression in the former.
2. Cytogenetic and/or FISH studies show the t(11;14), *IGH/CCND1* translocation, the genetic hallmark of mantle cell lymphoma.
3. It is crucial to differentiate leukemic non-nodal mantle cell lymphoma from leukemic phase of mantle cell lymphoma.

Case 4 (Fig. 13.4)

Learning Objectives

1. To become familiar with the immunohistochemical staining pattern of in situ mantle cell lymphoma
2. To appreciate the morphologic features that help differentiate in situ mantle cell lymphoma from mantle zone pattern of mantle cell lymphoma

Case History

A 63-year-old man had chronic cervical lymphadenopathy for the past year. There was no evidence of other lymphadenopathy. CBC was reported within normal limits. He underwent an excisional biopsy of the cervical lymph node to rule out lymphoma.

Histologic Findings

- The excised lymph node showed intact architecture with widely spaced follicles and open sinuses.
- Some of the follicles showed a rim of the mantle zone surrounding reactive-appearing germinal centers.
- A cyclin D1 stain highlighted the inner layer of the mantle zone cells.

Differential Diagnosis

- Reactive follicular hyperplasia
- Mantle cell lymphoma, mantle zone pattern
- In situ mantle cell neoplasia

Final Diagnosis

In situ mantle cell lymphoma

Follow-Up

The patient received no treatment other than excision of lymph node and has been well without clinical and radiologic evidence of lymphoma.

Take-Home Messages

1. In situ mantle cell lymphoma can only be diagnosed with the aid of immunohistochemistry which demonstrates cyclin D1-positive B cells exclusively localized to the mantle zones.
2. It is important to differentiate in situ mantle cell lymphoma from mantle zone pattern of mantle cell lymphoma.

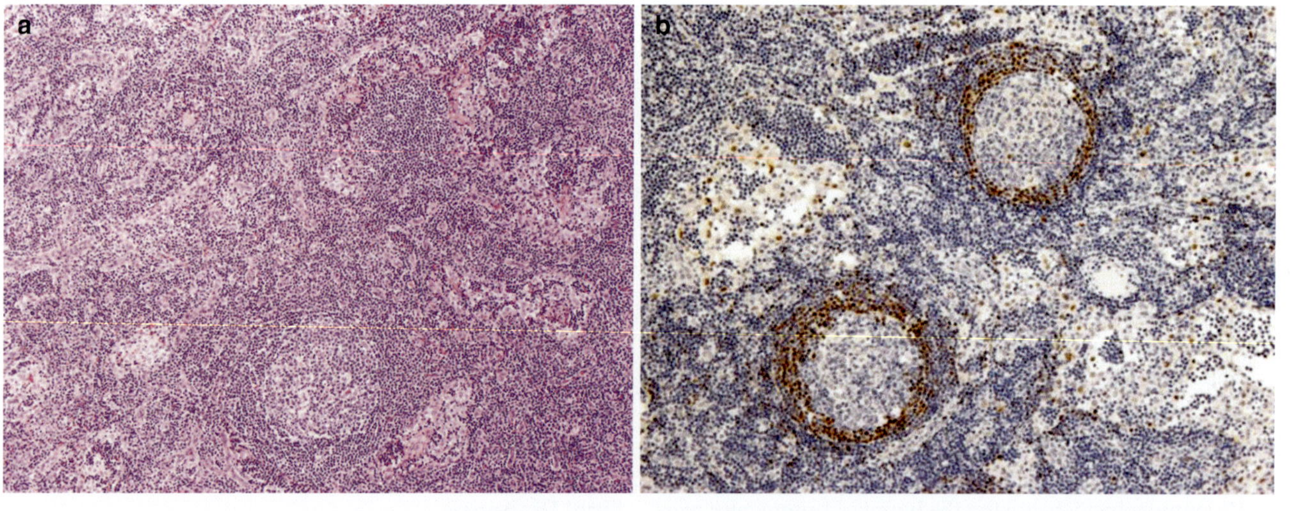

Fig. 13.4 In situ mantle cell lymphoma. (**a**) The lymph node shows intact architecture with widely spaced follicles and open sinuses. Some of the follicles show a rim of the mantle zone surrounding reactive-appearing germinal centers (hematoxylin-eosin, ×200). (**b**) Cyclin D1 stains positive in the mantle zone cells (peroxidase, ×200)

References

1. Fazi C, Scarfo L, Pecciarini L, Cottini F, Dagklis A, Janus A, et al. General population low-count CLL-like MBL persists over time without clinical progression, although carrying the same cytogenetic abnormalities of CLL. Blood. 2011;118(25):6618–25.
2. Rawstron AC, Bennett FL, O'Connor SJ, Kwok M, Fenton JA, Plummer M, et al. Monoclonal B-cell lymphocytosis and chronic lymphocytic leukemia. N Engl J Med. 2008;359(6):575–83.
3. Gibson SE, Swerdlow SH, Ferry JA, Surti U, Dal Cin P, Harris NL, et al. Reassessment of small lymphocytic lymphoma in the era of monoclonal B-cell lymphocytosis. Haematologica. 2011;96(8):1144–52.
4. Jegalian AG, Eberle FC, Pack SD, Mirvis M, Raffeld M, Pittaluga S, et al. Follicular lymphoma in situ: clinical implications and comparisons with partial involvement by follicular lymphoma. Blood. 2011;118(11):2976–84.
5. Montes-Moreno S, Castro Y, Rodriguez-Pinilla SM, Garcia JF, Mollejo M, Castillo ME, et al. Intrafollicular neoplasia/in situ follicular lymphoma: review of a series of 13 cases. Histopathology. 2010;56(5):658–62.
6. Pillai RK, Surti U, Swerdlow SH. Follicular lymphoma-like B cells of uncertain significance (in situ follicular lymphoma) may infrequently progress, but precedes follicular lymphoma, is associated with other overt lymphomas and mimics follicular lymphoma in flow cytometric studies. Haematologica. 2013;98(10):1571–80.
7. Roullet MR, Martinez D, Ma L, Fowler MH, McPhail ED, Judkins A, et al. Coexisting follicular and mantle cell lymphoma with each having an in situ component: a novel, curious, and complex consultation case of coincidental, composite, colonizing lymphoma. Am J Clin Pathol. 2010;133(4):584–91.
8. Carbone A, Gloghini A. Coexisting follicular and mantle cell lymphoma with each having an in situ component. Am J Clin Pathol. 2011;136(3):481–3.
9. Bermudez G, Gonzalez de Villambrosia S, Martinez-Lopez A, Batlle A, Revert-Arce JB, Cereceda Company L, et al. Incidental and isolated follicular lymphoma in situ and mantle cell lymphoma in situ lack clinical significance. Am J Surg Pathol. 2016;40(7):943–9.
10. Carvajal-Cuenca A, Sua LF, Silva NM, Pittaluga S, Royo C, Song JY, et al. In situ mantle cell lymphoma: clinical implications of an incidental finding with indolent clinical behavior. Haematologica. 2012;97(2):270–8.
11. Karube K, Scarfo L, Campo E, Ghia P. Monoclonal B cell lymphocytosis and "in situ" lymphoma. Semin Cancer Biol. 2014;24:3–14.

14 B-Cell Lymphoma in Children or Pediatric Type

Shunyou Gong and Juehua Gao

List of Frequently Asked Questions

1. What is pediatric-type follicular lymphoma (PTFL)?
2. How is PTFL diagnosed?
3. What are the diagnostic criteria for PTFL?
4. What is the differential diagnosis of PTFL?
5. How to distinguish PTFL in adults and usual follicular lymphoma?
6. How to distinguish PTFL and large B-cell lymphoma with *IRF4* rearrangement?
7. What is pediatric nodal marginal zone lymphoma (PNMZL)?
8. How is pediatric nodal marginal zone lymphoma diagnosed?
9. What is the differential diagnosis of pediatric nodal marginal zone lymphoma?
10. What is leukemia variant of Burkitt lymphoma (Burkitt cell leukemia, BCL)?
11. How is Burkitt cell leukemia diagnosed?
12. What is the differential diagnosis of Burkitt cell leukemia?
13. What is Burkitt-like lymphoma with 11q aberration?
14. How is Burkitt-like lymphoma with 11q aberration diagnosed?
15. What is the differential diagnosis of Burkitt-like lymphoma with 11q aberration?

S. Gong (✉)
Hematology and Hematopathology, Department of Pathology, Ann & Robert H. Lurie Children's Hospital, Northwestern University Feinberg School of Medicine, Chicago, IL, USA
e-mail: Shunyou.Gong@Northwestern.edu

J. Gao
Department of Pathology, Northwestern University Feinberg School of Medicine, Chicago, IL, USA

1. What is pediatric-type follicular lymphoma (PTFL)?

- A nodal follicular lymphoma (FL) that occurs primarily in children and young adults, most often involves lymph nodes of the head and neck, less commonly the inguinal and femoral lymph nodes [1–3].
- PTFL almost always presents with localized (stage I–II) disease, and systemic symptoms are usually absent.
- There is a striking male predominance, with male to female ratio approximately 10:1.
- Majority of PTFL cases may be managed by surgical resection alone.

2. How is PTFL diagnosed?

- Excisional biopsy of the involved lymph node is required for diagnosis.
- Histopathologically, the lymph node shows effaced architecture and large expansile follicles with attenuated mantle zones and a serpiginous growth pattern. The follicles are nonpolarized, but a partial starry-sky pattern with tingible-body macrophages may be retained. The lymphoma cells are monotonous, intermediate-sized, and morphologically different from centrocytes or centroblasts seen in adult FL. Instead, they are typically blastic in appearance, with dispersed chromatin and inconspicuous nucleoli.
- Although grading is not required, PTFL usually demonstrates deceivingly high-grade morphology, with frequent mitotic figures and moderate to high proliferation index by Ki-67 staining (30% and above).
- Immunophenotypically, the lymphoma cells express mature B-cell markers (CD20, CD79a, PAX5) and are positive for BCL6 and CD10 (characteristically very strong staining). They are negative or only weakly positive for BCL2, almost always negative for MUM1 and IgD.

E. Wang, A. S. Lagoo (eds.), *Practical Lymph Node and Bone Marrow Pathology*, Practical Anatomic Pathology,
https://doi.org/10.1007/978-3-030-32189-5_14

- By definition, PTFL does not have *BCL2, BCL6*, and *IRF4* gene rearrangements or *BCL2* gene amplification. Immunoglobulin gene is clonally rearranged in almost all cases.

3. What are the diagnostic criteria for PTFL?

To establish a diagnosis of PTFL, the following morphological, immunohistochemical, genetic, and clinical features must be met:

- At least partial effacement of nodal architecture and pure follicular proliferation.
- Lymphoma cells are positive for BCL6 but negative or weakly positive for BCL2, with high proliferation index (≥30%).
- No *BCL2, BCL6, IRF4*, or aberrant immunoglobulin gene rearrangements and no *BCL2* gene amplification.
- Clinically stage I–II nodal disease without extranodal involvement.

4. What is the differential diagnosis of PTFL?

Major differential diagnosis includes:

- Usual follicular lymphoma
- Large B-cell lymphomas with *IRF4* rearrangement
- Reactive follicular hyperplasia, florid variant, if flow cytometry is not performed

A detailed comparison of the clinicopathologic features of the three neoplastic entities is shown in Table 14.1.

5. How to distinguish PTFL in adults and usual follicular lymphoma?

Rare PTFL may occur in adults up to 40 years old, so distinguishing PTFL in adults and usual follicular lymphoma (UFL) is crucial.

- High-grade UFL may be BCL2 weak or negative by immunohistochemistry with the commonly used clone 124 of BCL2 antibody, at least partially due to the mutation of *BCL2* gene [4]. This may resemble PTFL, however:
  - The lymphoma cells in high-grade UFL are centroblastic-looking, not like those in PTFL which are usually round with dispersed chromatin and inconspicuous nucleoli.
  - Expansile/serpiginous follicles are more likely seen in PTFL than UFL.

6. How to distinguish PTFL and large B-cell lymphoma with *IRF4* rearrangement?

- Areas of diffuse large cells are not allowed in PTFL. If present, particularly in this age group, an alternative diagnosis of large B-cell lymphoma (LBCL) with *IRF4* rearrangement should be seriously considered.
- LBCL with *IRF4* rearrangement is also most often seen in children, commonly involving Waldeyer's ring and cervical lymph nodes but unlike PTFL, these patients require chemo-immunotherapy with or without radiation.
- Morphologically it may reveal infiltrate of large cells with follicular, diffuse, or mixed growth patterns, and lymphoma cells are MUM1 positive. *IRF4* rearrangement is always present.

Table 14.1 Clinical, morphologic, immunophenotypic, and genetic features of pediatric-type follicular lymphoma, usual follicular lymphoma, and large B-cell lymphoma with *IRF4* rearrangement

	PTFL [2]	UFL [2]	LBCL with *IRF4* [13]
Median age	14 years (5–21)	24 years (18–28)	12 years (4–79)
M/F	All male	1:2.2	1.2:1
Stage	100% localized	86% localized	84% localized
Head and neck predilection	Yes	No	Yes including Waldeyer's ring
Diffuse areas	Usually absent	Some cases may have	Often
Starry-sky pattern retained	Yes	No	No
CD10 IHC	100% strongly positive	91% variably positive	66% positive
BCL2 IHC	Mostly negative, 18% weakly positive	81% positive	63% positive
MUM1 IHC	Negative	Usually negative	100% positive
FISH for *BCL2* rearrangement	Negative	Positive, usually to IgH locus	Negative
FISH for *IRF4* rearrangement	Negative	Negative	Positive, most commonly translocated to *IGH* locus

7. What is pediatric nodal marginal zone lymphoma (PNMZL)?

- PNMZL has clinical and histologic features distinctive from its adult counterpart.
- Usually presents with localized (stage I in 90% of patients), asymptomatic lymphadenopathy most commonly involving the head and neck areas.
- A marked male predominance was observed (male to female ratio up to 20:1).
- Majority of PNMZL patients were successfully managed by surgical removal and/or local radiation [5].

8. How is pediatric nodal marginal zone lymphoma diagnosed?

- Excisional biopsy is required for diagnosis.
- Morphologic features of PNMZL are similar to adult NMZL, except that the former commonly demonstrates large expanded follicles disrupted by mantle zone cells, resembling progressive transformation of germinal centers (PTGC).
- The atypical B cells in PNMZL are commonly monocytoid, with irregular nuclear contours and pale cytoplasm.
- They often co-express CD43 and may be positive for BCL2, while germinal center B-cell markers (CD10 and BCL6) are usually negative [6]. Light chain restriction is usually demonstrated by flow cytometry and/or immunohistochemistry. The lymphoma cells are negative for IgD, which highlights the expanded mantle zone B cells in PTGC-like follicles.
- Immunoglobulin gene is clonally rearranged.

9. What is the differential diagnosis of pediatric nodal marginal zone lymphoma?

- Nodal atypical marginal zone hyperplasia (AMZH), with frequently skewed light chain expression and association with *Haemophilus influenzae* infection, may morphologically and immunophenotypically resemble PNMZL. However, in contrast to PNMZL, the atypical cells in AMZH are usually IgD positive, and immunoglobulin gene rearrangement reveals polyclonal amplification [7].
- Some PNMZL cases may histologically show prominent nodular appearance due to marked follicular colonization, mimicking pediatric-type follicular lymphoma (PTFL).
- CD279/PD1 may be helpful for the differential diagnosis and reveals many positive cells in the reactive germinal centers of PNMZL but only shows a few positive cells pushed to the periphery of the follicles in PTFL.
- PTGC-like features also favor PNMZL over PTFL [5, 6].

10. What is leukemia variant of Burkitt lymphoma (Burkitt cell leukemia, BCL)?

- Burkitt lymphoma is an aggressive mature B-cell lymphoma with distinctive morphologic, immunophenotypic, and genetic characteristics.
- Microscopically, Burkitt lymphoma cells are medium-sized, with basophilic, often vacuolated cytoplasm, round nuclei, finely clumped chromatin, and multiple small nucleoli. Due to very high growth rate of the tumor, numerous apoptotic bodies and abundant tingible-body macrophages are present, demonstrating a so-called starry-sky pattern.
- The lymphoma cells are germinal center B-cell-derived, positive for pan-B-cell markers and CD10 and BCL6, negative or weakly positive for BCL2, and demonstrating light chain restriction by flow cytometry. Ki-67 reveals nearly 100% proliferation rate.
- Vast majority of Burkitt lymphomas have *C-MYC* gene (chromosome 8) translocated to one of the three immunoglobulin gene loci (heavy chain on chromosome 14, kappa light chain on chromosome 2, and lambda light chain on chromosome 22, respectively).
- While most of Burkitt lymphomas are mass-like lesions of extranodal sites, they occasionally present as purely leukemic phase (Burkitt cell leukemia, BCL), particularly in children. A US study found 14% sporadic BL cases in children presented as Burkitt cell leukemia [8].
- Except for absence of mass lesion, BCL should have similar cytologic, immunophenotypic, and genetic features as its lymphoma counterpart.

11. How is Burkitt cell leukemia diagnosed?

Like Burkitt lymphoma, there is no single morphologic, immunophenotypic, or genetic criteria as a golden standard for diagnosis of BCL. Instead, a multiparametric approach must be used.

- Cytologic features of BL and correct immunophenotype of the tumor cells, as well as clinical presentations, should support such a diagnosis.
- *C-MYC* translocation to one of the immunoglobulin loci is seen in approximately 90% of the cases. The other 10% of the cases may have cryptic *C-MYC* translocation not detectable by regular methods, and/or genetic changes consistent with Burkitt-like lymphoma with 11q aberration, which will be discussed in the next section.
- Cases with otherwise classic morphology and immunophenotype of Burkitt lymphoma but lacking *C-MYC* translocation may need array comparative genomic hybridization (aCGH) for the possibility of Burkitt-like lymphoma with 11q aberration.

12. What is the differential diagnosis of Burkitt cell leukemia?

- The major differential diagnosis is B-lymphoblastic leukemia/lymphoma (B-ALL).
- Rare cases of B-ALL, with otherwise typical immunophenotype of B-lymphoblasts, such as negative CD20, lack of surface immunoglobulin light chain expression, and positive TdT, may carry t(8;14) (q24;q32) with *MYC/IGH* translocation, which may be confused with Burkitt cell leukemia [9, 10].

13. What is Burkitt-like lymphoma with 11q aberration?

- Burkitt-like lymphoma with 11q aberration (BLL11q) is a new provisional entity included in the 2017 WHO classification, with pathologic features closely resembling those of Burkitt lymphoma (BL) but lacking MYC rearrangements. Instead, this entity shows recurrent chromosome 11q alterations, particularly proximal gains and telomeric losses [11].
- Unlike Burkitt lymphoma, this lymphoma more commonly present as nodal disease [12].

14. How is Burkitt-like lymphoma with 11q aberration diagnosed?

To diagnose BLL11q, the lymph node biopsy is subjected to histologic, immunohistochemical, cytogenetic, and molecular studies.

- Histologically, BLL11q shows a diffuse infiltrate of medium- to large-sized lymphoid cells which may resemble Burkitt lymphoma cells but usually demonstrate more cytologic pleomorphism.
- Starry-sky pattern may be prominent and mitotic activity is very high.
- The immunophenotype of the lymphoma cells are similar to Burkitt lymphoma, positive for pan-B-cell markers and germinal center B-cell markers and negative or only weakly positive for BCL2.
- It characteristically lacks *MYC* translocation and demonstrates characteristic chromosome 11q aberration including proximal gain and terminal loss by array CGH.

15. What is the differential diagnosis of Burkitt-like lymphoma with 11q aberration?

- In addition to typical Burkitt lymphoma, other major differential diagnosis includes high-grade B-cell lymphoma, not otherwise specified, and high-grade B-cell lymphoma with *MYC*, *BCL2*, and/or *BCL6* rearrangements (double- or triple-hit lymphoma).
- These two entities may be morphologically and immunophenotypically resembling BLL11q but lack characteristic 11q aberration.
- Notably, double- or triple-hit lymphomas almost never occur in pediatric patients [1].

Case Presentations

Case 1 (Figs. 14.1 and 14.2)

Learning Objectives

1. To be familiar with the pathologic and clinic features of pediatric-type nodal follicular lymphoma
2. To understand how to distinguish PTFL from usual follicular lymphoma, large B-cell lymphoma with *IRF4* rearrangement, and reactive follicular hyperplasia

Case History

The patient was a 13-year-old male with no significant past medical history who presented with an enlarged left cervical lymph node, measuring 3 cm in greatest dimension. He was otherwise asymptomatic.

Histologic Findings

- Sections of the excised lymph node revealed effaced architecture and large expansile nodules with monotonous cellular components.
- The nodules were composed of intermediate-sized, blastoid cells with dispersed chromatin, and inconspicuous nucleoli.
- Mitotic figures were frequent.
- Immunohistochemical stains showed that the lymphoma cells are positive for CD20, BCL6, and CD10 (very strong staining) and negative for BCL2. CD3 highlighted small T cells which nicely delineated the malignant follicles.
- Ki-67 revealed moderate to high proliferative index in the tumor cells.

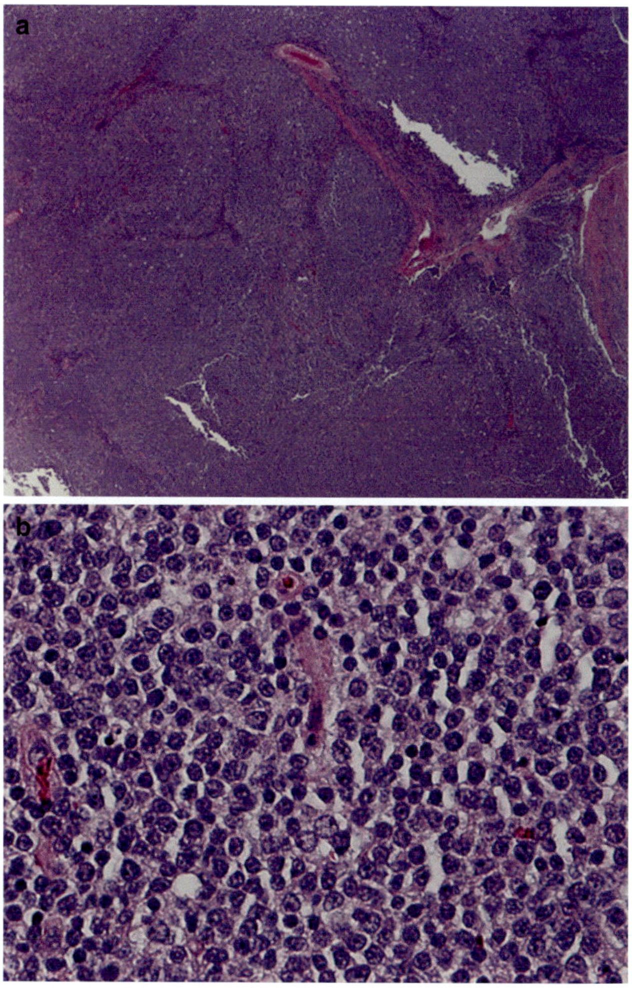

Fig. 14.1 Pediatric-type follicular lymphoma: histopathologic features. (**a**) Sections of the excised lymph node reveal effaced architecture and numerous large expansile nodules with monotonous cellular components (H&E, ×20). (**b**) The nodules are composed of intermediate-sized, blastoid cells with dispersed chromatin and inconspicuous nucleoli. Mitotic figures are frequent (H&E, ×200)

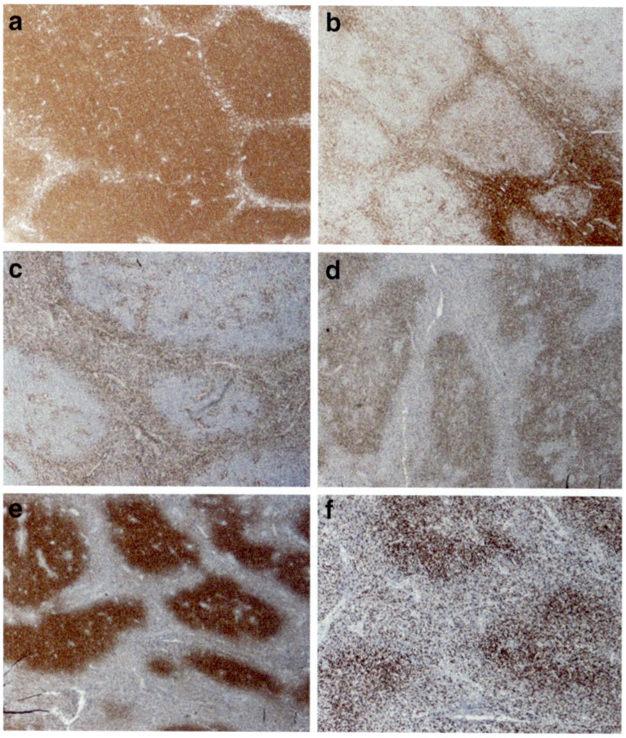

Fig. 14.2 Pediatric-type follicular lymphoma: immunohistochemical findings. Immunohistochemical stains show that the lymphoma cells are positive for CD20 (**a**, ×40), BCL6 (**d**, ×40), and CD10 (**e**, ×40, very strong staining) and negative for BCL2 (**c**, ×40). CD3 (**b**, ×40) highlights small T cells which nicely delineate the malignant follicles. Ki-67 (**f**, ×40) reveals moderate to high proliferative index in the tumor cells. The lymphoma is negative for *BCL2*, *BCL6*, and *IRF4* abnormalities by FISH, and immunoglobulin gene rearrangement by PCR reveals a clonal pattern (not shown)

Differential Diagnosis

- Pediatric-type follicular lymphoma
- Follicular lymphoma, high-grade, usual type
- Reactive follicular hyperplasia
- Large B-cell lymphoma with *IRF4* rearrangement

Ancillary Test Results

- Fluorescence in situ hybridization (FISH) was negative for *BCL2, BCL6*, and *IRF4* gene rearrangements.
- Immunoglobulin gene rearrangement by PCR revealed a clonal pattern.

Final Diagnosis

Pediatric-type follicular lymphoma

Follow-Up

The patient received no additional treatment and has since been doing well without evidence of lymphoma.

Take-Home Messages

1. Pediatric-type follicular lymphoma is a nodal follicular lymphoma primarily in children and young adults, most commonly involving the lymph nodes in the head and neck area, and with a striking male predominance.
2. Correct diagnosis of pediatric-type follicular lymphoma is based on morphologic (large expansile, serpiginous follicles composed of often blastic-appearing cells), immunohistochemical (BCL2 negative or only weakly positive, CD10 strongly positive), and genetic features (clonal immunoglobulin gene rearrangement, no *BCL2, BCL6, and IRF4* gene rearrangements).
3. PTFL has indolent biological behavior.

Case 2 (Figs. 14.3 and 14.4)

Learning Objectives

1. To be familiar with the pathologic and clinic features of pediatric nodal marginal zone lymphoma
2. To be aware of the key features distinguishing pediatric nodal marginal zone lymphoma from pediatric-type follicular lymphoma and atypical marginal zone hyperplasia

Case History

The patient was a 15-year-old male with no significant past medical history who presented with an enlarged right cervical lymph node, measuring 2.5 cm in greatest dimension. He was otherwise asymptomatic.

Histologic Findings

- The lymph node was effaced and contained a few large PTGC-like follicles and atypical infiltrate with a predominantly interfollicular pattern.
- Majority of the atypical cells were small to intermediate, with moderately abundant pale cytoplasm and irregular nuclear contours.
- Occasional large transformed cells were also present.
- By immunohistochemistry, the lymphoma cells were positive for CD20 and BCL2 and negative for CD10.
- CD3 highlighted relatively fewer small T cells in the interfollicular areas, and many of them migrated to the residual follicles, which contained reactive germinal centers outlined by CD10.
- The lymphoma cells were negative for kappa and lambda light chains by immunohistochemical stains.
- No fresh material was available for flow cytometric analysis.

Differential Diagnosis

- Pediatric-type follicular lymphoma
- Pediatric nodal marginal zone lymphoma
- Reactive lymphadenopathy with marginal zone hyperplasia
- Reactive lymphadenopathy with follicular hyperplasia and progressive transformation of germinal centers
- Nodular lymphocyte predominant Hodgkin lymphoma

Ancillary Test Results

- Immunoglobulin gene rearrangement revealed a clonal pattern.

Final Diagnosis

Pediatric nodal marginal zone lymphoma

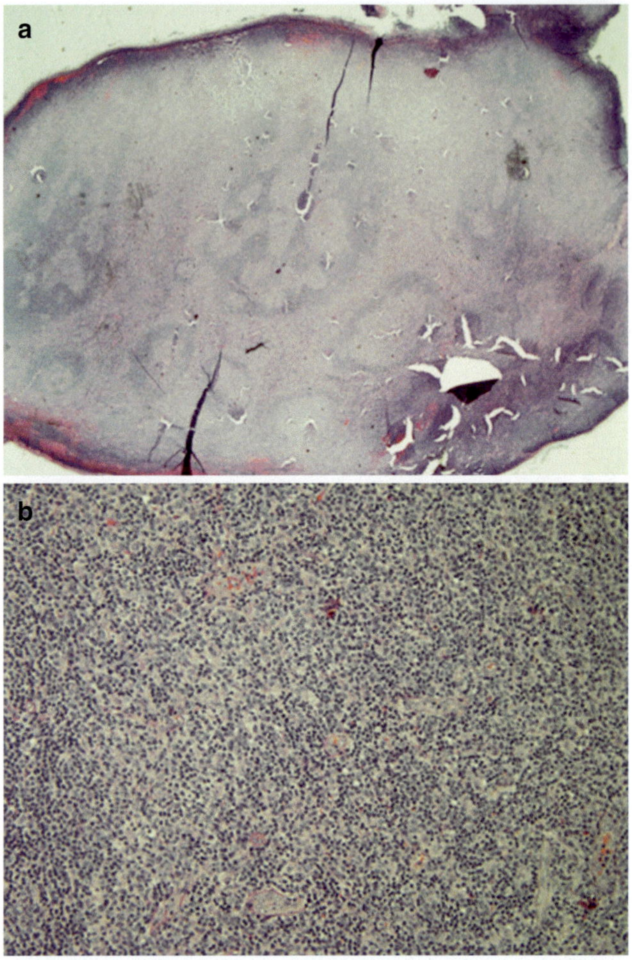

Fig. 14.3 Pediatric nodal marginal zone lymphoma: histopathologic features. (**a**) The lymph node is effaced and contains a few large PTGC-like follicles and atypical infiltrate with a predominantly interfollicular pattern (H&E, ×20). (**b**) Majority of the atypical cells are small to intermediate, with moderately abundant pale cytoplasm and irregular nuclear contours. Occasional large transformed cells are also present (H&E, ×200)

Take-Home Messages

1. Pediatric nodal marginal zone lymphoma is a nodal lymphoma primarily in children and young adults, most commonly involving the lymph nodes in the head and neck area, and with a marked male predominance.
2. Pediatric nodal marginal zone lymphoma commonly has large PTGC-like follicles, a feature not seen in PTFL; it also demonstrates clonal immunoglobulin gene rearrangement, which is generally absent in atypical marginal zone hyperplasia.

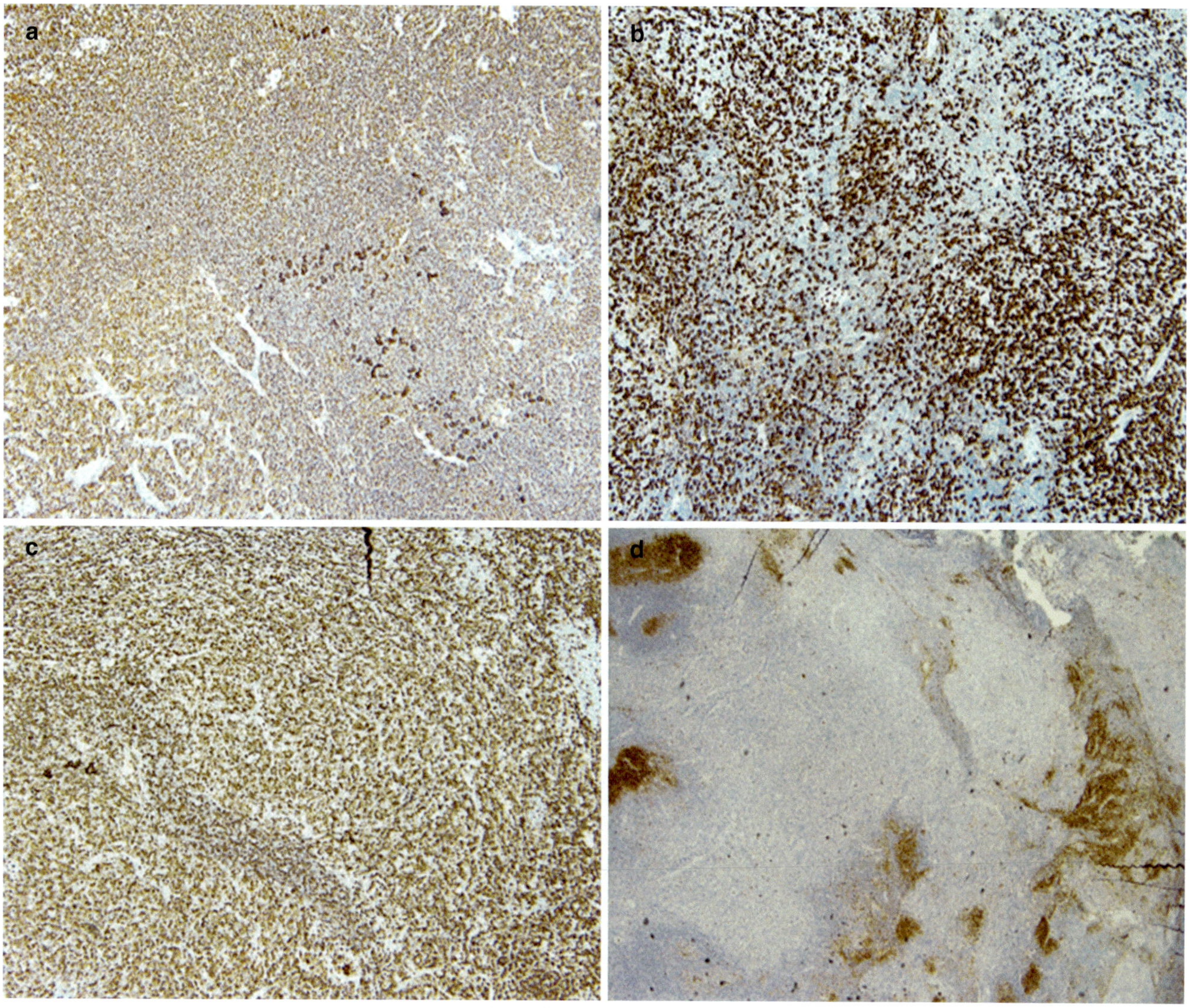

Fig. 14.4 Pediatric nodal marginal zone lymphoma: immunohistochemical findings. Immunohistochemical stains show that the lymphoma cells are positive for CD20 (**a**, ×100) and BCL2 (**c**, ×100) and negative for CD10 (**d**, ×100). CD3 (**b**, ×100) highlights relatively fewer small T cells in the interfollicular areas, and many of them migrate to the residual follicles, which contain reactive germinal centers outlined by CD10 (**d**, ×100). The lymphoma is negative for kappa and lambda light chains by immunohistochemical stains, but immunoglobulin gene rearrangement reveals a clonal pattern (not shown). No fresh material is available for flow cytometric analysis

Case 3 (Figs. 14.5 and 14.6)

Learning Objectives

1. To be aware of the leukemic variant of Burkitt lymphoma (Burkitt cell leukemia)
2. To correctly distinguish Burkitt cell leukemia from B-lymphoblastic leukemia/lymphoma

Case History

The patient was a 5-year-old male with no significant past medical history who presented with diffuse bone pain. CT revealed marrow infiltration process but no localized lesion. Random marrow biopsy was performed.

Histologic Findings

- Marrow aspirate revealed sheets of medium cells with minimal basophilic and vacuolated cytoplasm, round nuclei, dispersed chromatin, and multiple nucleoli.
- The core biopsy revealed largely replaced marrow with monotonous cell infiltrate comprising medium-sized atypical lymphoid cells and frequent tingible-body macrophages forming starry-sky pattern.

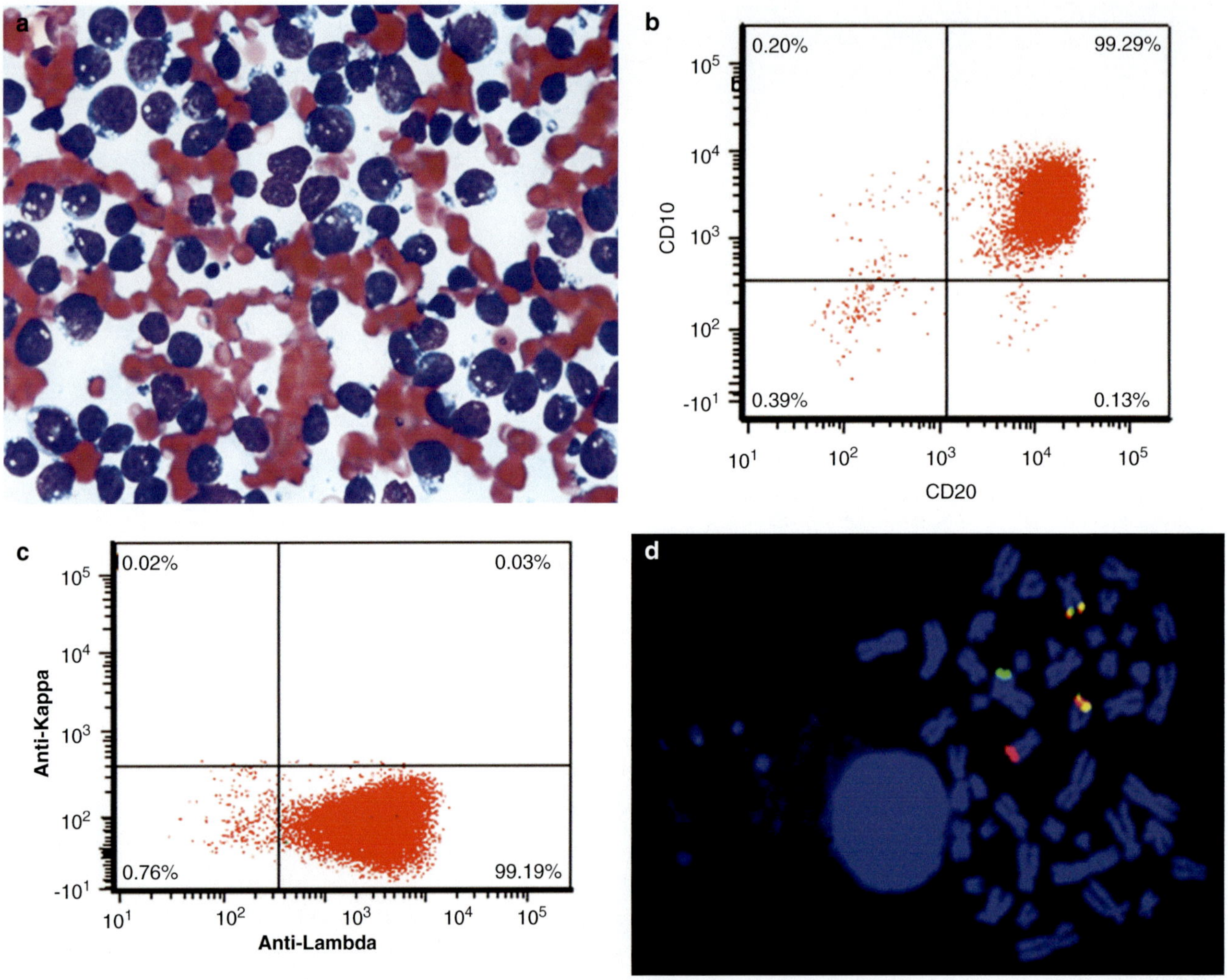

Fig. 14.5 Burkitt cell leukemia: morphology, flow cytometry, and cytogenetics. (**a**) Marrow aspirate reveals sheets of medium cells with minimal basophilic and vacuolated cytoplasm, round nuclei, finely clumped chromatin, and multiple nucleoli (Wright-Giemsa, ×1000). (**b**) Flow cytometry shows that the tumor cells are positive for CD20 and CD10. (**c**) The lymphoma cells express surface light chain and are lambda-restricted. (**d**) Metaphase FISH using *IGH/MYC* dual-color double-fusion probes demonstrates balanced translocation consistent with t(8;14) (q24;q32). (Image courtesy of Katrin Leuer, Ph.D.)

- The lymphoma cells were positive for CD20 and negative for BCL2 and TdT.

Differential Diagnosis

- Leukemic variant of Burkitt lymphoma
- Other high-grade B-cell lymphoma/leukemia
- B-lymphoblastic leukemia

Ancillary Test Results

- Flow cytometry showed that the tumor cells were positive for CD20 and CD10, and the lymphoma cells expressed surface light chain and were lambda-restricted.
- Metaphase FISH using *IGH/MYC* dual-color double-fusion probes demonstrated balanced translocation consistent with t(8;14) (q24;q32).

Final Diagnosis

Leukemic variant of Burkitt lymphoma (Burkitt cell leukemia)

Take-Home Messages

1. Burkitt cell leukemia is a rare variant of Burkitt lymphoma and most commonly seen in children.
2. Except for absence of mass lesion, Burkitt cell leukemia should have similar cytologic, immunophenotypic, and genetic features as its lymphoma counterpart.
3. Burkitt cell leukemia needs to be distinguished from B-lymphoblastic leukemia/lymphoma (B-ALL). Rare cases may carry t(8;14) (q24;q32) with *MYC/IGH* translocation, but otherwise are typical for B-ALL, and should be still diagnosed and treated as B-ALL.

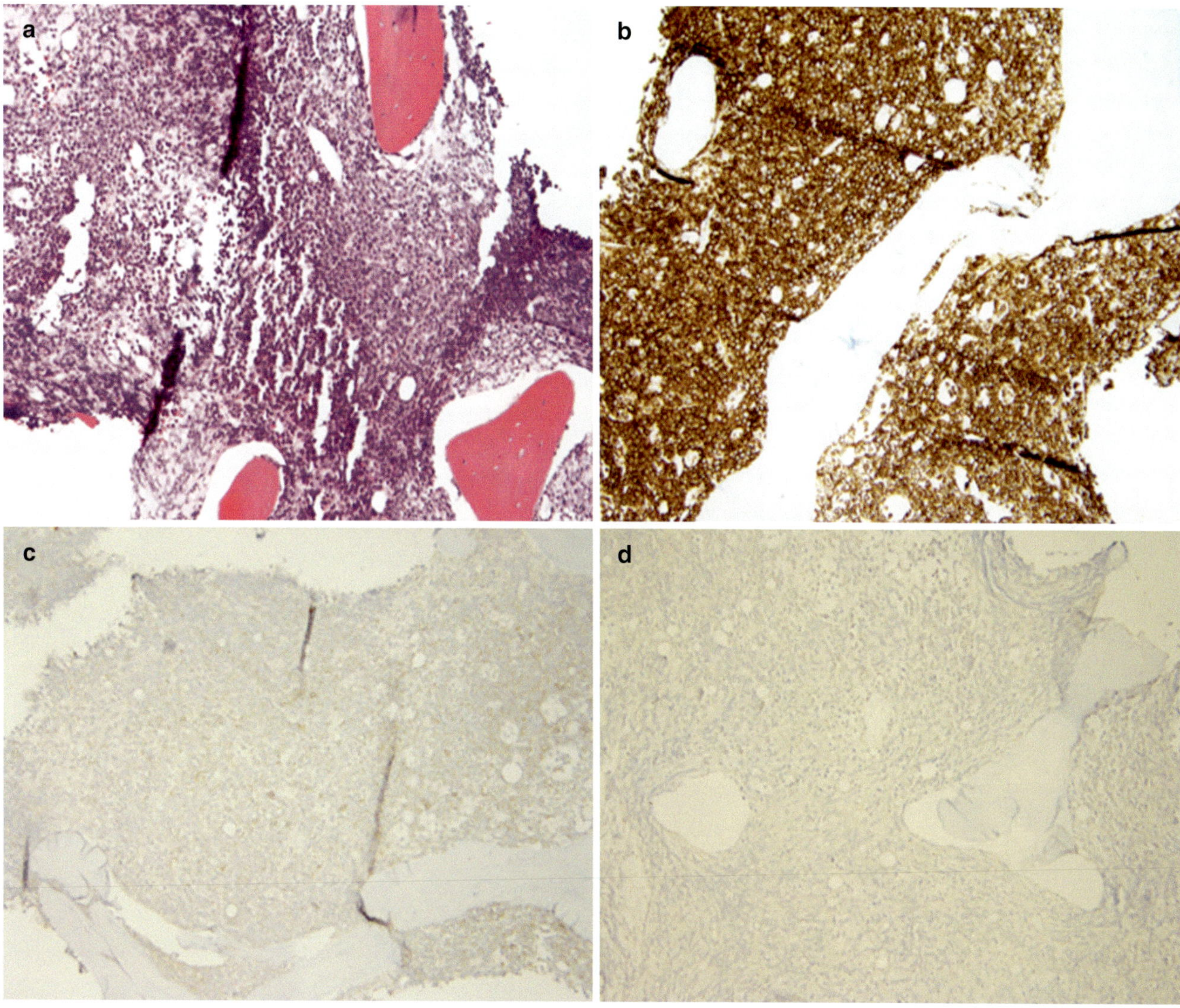

Fig. 14.6 Burkitt cell leukemia: marrow biopsy histology and immunohistochemical findings. (**a**) The core biopsy reveals largely replaced marrow with monotonous cell infiltrate comprising medium-sized atypical lymphoid cells and frequent tingible-body macrophages forming starry-sky pattern. (**b–d**) The lymphoma cells are positive for CD20 (**b**) and negative for BCL2 (**c**) and TdT (**d**)

Case 4 (Figs. 14.7 and 14.8)

Learning Objectives

1. To be familiar with the pathologic and clinic features of Burkitt-like lymphoma with 11q aberration
2. To be aware of the major differential diagnosis of Burkitt-like lymphoma with 11q aberration

Case History

The patient was a 6-year-old female with no significant past medical history who presented with rapidly enlarging left cervical mass. Core biopsy was performed.

Histologic Findings

- Histologic sections showed a diffuse infiltrate of medium to large lymphoid cells with moderate pale cytoplasm, slightly convoluted nuclei, stippled to vesicular chromatin, and inconspicuous to small nucleoli.
- Patchy necrosis, abundant apoptotic bodies, and many mitotic figures were seen in the background.
- The neoplastic cells were positive for CD20 and CD10.
- The cells were negative for BCL2.
- Ki-67 showed a very high proliferative index (>95%).

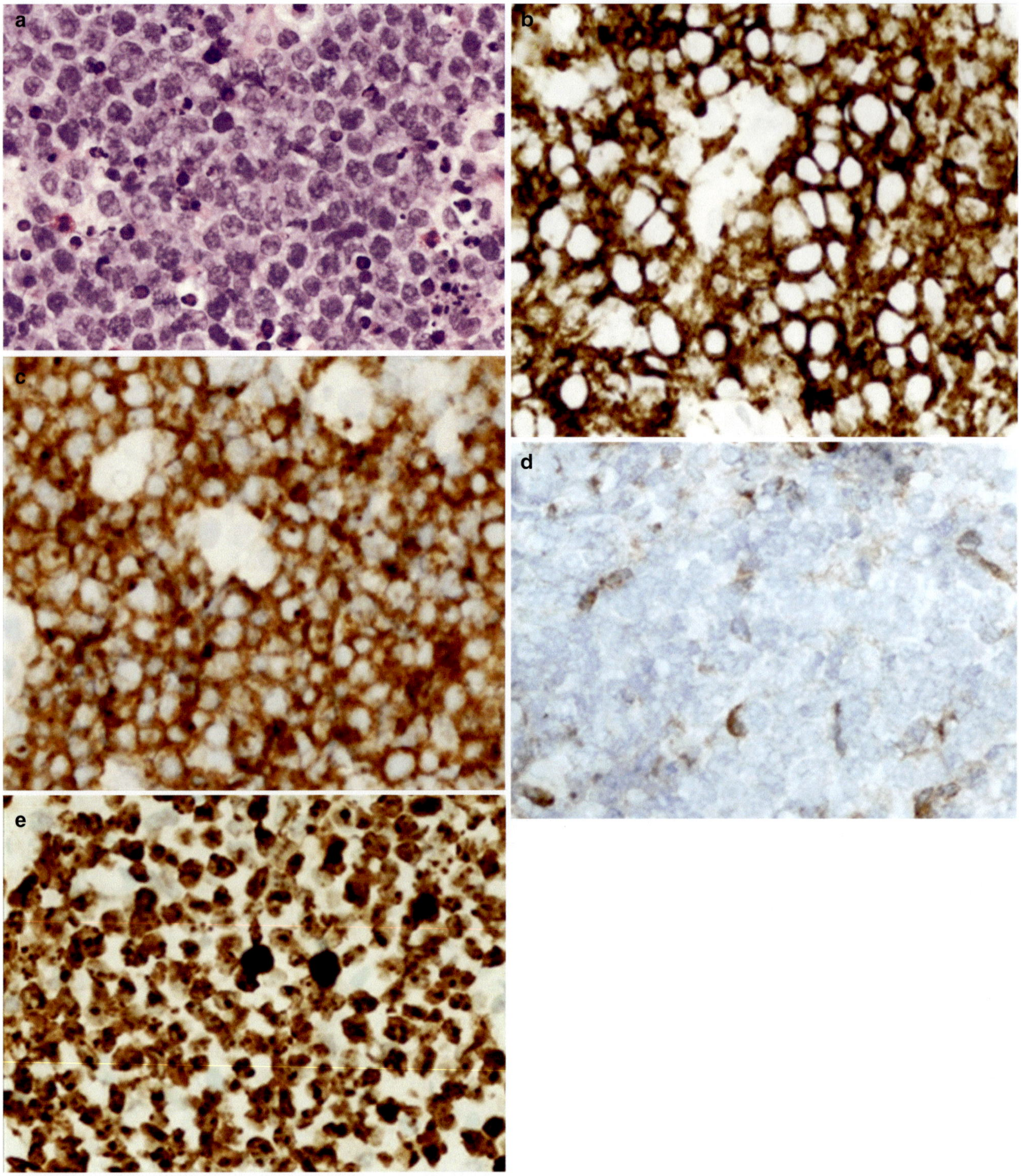

Fig. 14.7 Burkitt lymphoma with 11q aberration: histologic and immunophenotypic features. (**a**) Cervical lymph node, H&E 50X. Histologic sections show a diffuse infiltrate of medium- to large-sized lymphoid cells with moderate pale cytoplasm, slightly convoluted nuclei, stippled to vesicular chromatin, and inconspicuous to small nucleoli. Patchy necrosis, abundant apoptotic bodies, and many mitotic figures are seen in the background. The neoplastic cells are positive for (**b**) CD20 and (**c**) CD10. (**d**) The cells are negative for BCL2. (**e**) Ki-67 shows a very high proliferation index (>95%)

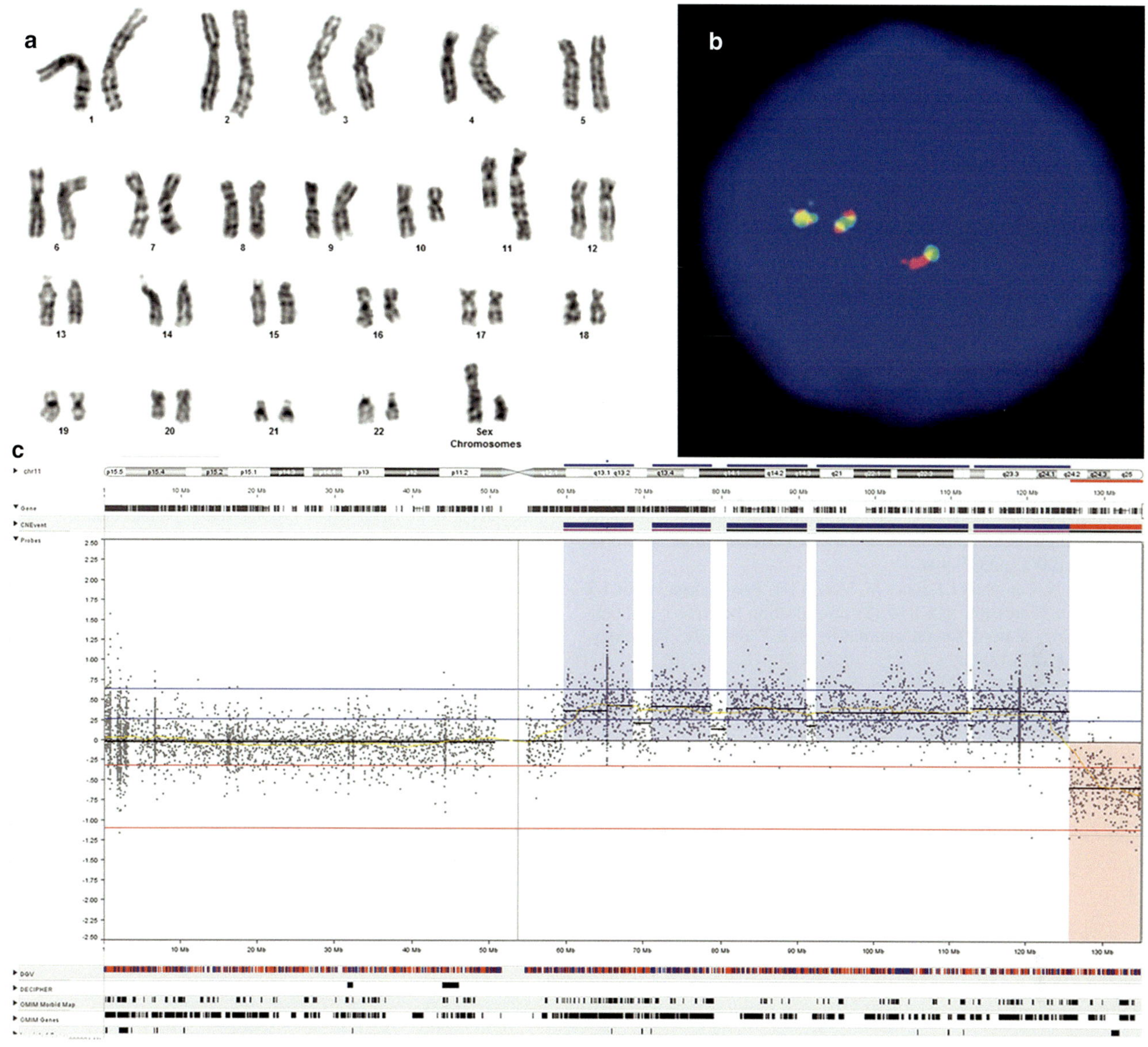

Fig. 14.8 Burkitt lymphoma with 11q aberration: cytogenetic and molecular features. (**a**) Chromosome G-banding analysis reveals 46, der(11)dup(11)(q13q22)dup(11)(q22q23). (**b**) Interphase FISH using dual-color break-apart probe for *MLL* gene rearrangement reveals three MLL copies with no rearrangements (three yellow signals). (**c**) Array CGH shows proximal gains between 11q13-q23 and telomeric losses between 11q24-qter

Differential Diagnosis

- Burkitt lymphoma
- Burkitt-like lymphoma with 11q aberration
- Other high-grade B-cell lymphomas

Ancillary Test Results

- Chromosome G-banding analysis revealed 46, der (11) dup (11) (q13q22) dup (11) (q22q23).
- Interphase FISH using dual-color break-apart probe for *MLL* gene rearrangement revealed three *MLL* copies with no rearrangements (three yellow signals).
- Array CGH showed proximal gains between 11q13-q23 and telomeric losses between 11q24-qter.

Final Diagnosis

Burkitt-like lymphoma with 11q aberration

Take-Home Messages

1. Burkitt-like lymphoma with 11q aberration is a newly described provisional entity in the 2017 WHO and most commonly seen in children, with pathologic features closely resembling those of Burkitt lymphoma (BL) but lacking *MYC* rearrangements. Instead, this entity shows recurrent chromosome 11q alterations, particularly proximal gains and telomeric losses.

2. Major differential diagnosis includes classic Burkitt lymphoma, high-grade B-cell lymphoma, not otherwise specified, and high-grade B-cell lymphoma with *MYC*, *BCL2*, and/or *BCL6* rearrangements (double- or triple-hit lymphoma).

References

1. Swerdlow SH, International Agency for Research on C, World Health O. WHO classification of tumours of haematopoietic and lymphoid tissues. Lyon: International Agency for Research on Cancer; 2017.
2. Liu Q, Salaverria I, Pittaluga S, Jegalian AG, Xi L, Siebert R, et al. Follicular lymphomas in children and young adults: a comparison of the pediatric variant with usual follicular lymphoma. Am J Surg Pathol. 2013;37(3):333–43.
3. Louissaint A Jr, Ackerman AM, Dias-Santagata D, Ferry JA, Hochberg EP, Huang MS, et al. Pediatric-type nodal follicular lymphoma: an indolent clonal proliferation in children and adults with high proliferation index and no BCL2 rearrangement. Blood. 2012;120(12):2395–404.
4. Masir N, Campbell LJ, Jones M, Mason DY. Pseudonegative BCL2 protein expression in a t(14;18) translocation positive lymphoma cell line: a need for an alternative BCL2 antibody. Pathology. 2010;42(3):212–6.
5. Taddesse-Heath L, Pittaluga S, Sorbara L, Bussey M, Raffeld M, Jaffe ES. Marginal zone B-cell lymphoma in children and young adults. Am J Surg Pathol. 2003;27(4):522–31.
6. Quintanilla-Martinez L, Sander B, Chan JK, Xerri L, Ott G, Campo E, et al. Indolent lymphomas in the pediatric population: follicular lymphoma, IRF4/MUM1+ lymphoma, nodal marginal zone lymphoma and chronic lymphocytic leukemia. Virchows Arch. 2016;468(2):141–57.
7. Kluin PM, Langerak AW, Beverdam-Vincent J, Geurts-Giele WR, Visser L, Rutgers B, et al. Paediatric nodal marginal zone B-cell lymphadenopathy of the neck: a Haemophilus influenzae-driven immune disorder? J Pathol. 2015;236(3):302–14.
8. Mbulaiteye SM, Biggar RJ, Bhatia K, Linet MS, Devesa SS. Sporadic childhood Burkitt lymphoma incidence in the United States during 1992–2005. Pediatr Blood Cancer. 2009;53(3):366–70.
9. Li Y, Gupta G, Molofsky A, Xie Y, Shihabi N, McCormick J, et al. B lymphoblastic leukemia/lymphoma with Burkitt-like morphology and IGH/MYC rearrangement: report of 3 cases in adult patients. Am J Surg Pathol. 2018;42(2):269–76.
10. Navid F, Mosijczuk AD, Head DR, Borowitz MJ, Carroll AJ, Brandt JM, et al. Acute lymphoblastic leukemia with the (8;14)(q24;q32) translocation and FAB L3 morphology associated with a B-precursor immunophenotype: the Pediatric Oncology Group experience. Leukemia. 1999;13(1):135–41.
11. Salaverria I, Martin-Guerrero I, Wagener R, Kreuz M, Kohler CW, Richter J, et al. A recurrent 11q aberration pattern characterizes a subset of MYC-negative high-grade B-cell lymphomas resembling Burkitt lymphoma. Blood. 2014;123(8):1187–98.
12. Rimsza L, Pittaluga S, Dirnhofer S, Copie-Bergman C, de Leval L, Facchetti F, et al. The clinicopathologic spectrum of mature aggressive B cell lymphomas. Virchows Arch. 2017;471(4):453–66.
13. Salaverria I, Philipp C, Oschlies I, Kohler CW, Kreuz M, Szczepanowski M, et al. Translocations activating IRF4 identify a subtype of germinal center-derived B-cell lymphoma affecting predominantly children and young adults. Blood. 2011;118(1):139–47.

Indolent T-/NK-Cell Lymphoproliferative Disorders

15

Wenbin Xiao and Huan-You Wang

List of Frequently Asked Questions

1. What is the clinical manifestation of T-cell large granular lymphocytic leukemia (T-LGL leukemia)?
2. What are the key histologic features for T-LGL leukemia?
3. What are the commonly used immunomarkers in T-LGL leukemia?
4. What is the differential diagnosis for T-LGL leukemia?
5. What is the clinical manifestation of chronic lymphoproliferative disorder of NK cells (CLPD-NK)?
6. What are the key histologic features for CLPD-NK?
7. What are the commonly used immunomarkers in CLPD-NK?
8. What is the differential diagnosis for CLPD-NK?
9. What is the clinical manifestation of indolent T-cell lymphoproliferative disorder of the GI tract (iT-LPD of the GI tract)?
10. What are the key histologic features for iT-LPD of the GI tract?
11. What are the commonly used immunomarkers in iT-LPD of the GI tract?
12. What is the differential diagnosis for iT-LPD of the GI tract?
13. What is the clinical manifestation of NK-cell enteropathy?
14. What are the key histologic features of NK-cell enteropathy?
15. What are the commonly used immunomarkers in NK-cell enteropathy?
16. What is the differential diagnosis for NK-cell enteropathy?
17. What is the clinical manifestation of primary cutaneous CD4-positive small/medium T-cell LPD?
18. What are the key histologic features for primary cutaneous CD4-positive small/medium T-cell LPD?
19. What are the commonly used immunomarkers in primary cutaneous CD4-positive small/medium T-cell LPD?
20. What is the differential diagnosis for primary cutaneous CD4-positive small/medium T-cell LPD?
21. What is the clinical manifestation of primary cutaneous acral CD8-positive T-cell lymphoma?
22. What are the key histologic features for primary cutaneous acral CD8-positive T-cell lymphoma?
23. What are the commonly used immunomarkers in primary cutaneous acral CD8-positive T-cell lymphoma?
24. What is the differential diagnosis for primary cutaneous acral CD8-positive T-cell lymphoma?

1. What is the clinical manifestation of T-LGL leukemia?

- T-LGL leukemia is an indolent and rare disease with the incidence of 0.2 cases per 1,000,000 individuals [1], and it accounts for 2–3% of mature small lymphocytic leukemia [2].
- T-LGL leukemia occurs with a median age of 60 years with both male and female roughly equally affected [3].
- Neutropenia and severe anemia are the most common and initial presentations in Western and Asia countries, respectively [3], but thrombocytopenia is not. Approximately 26% and 31% of T-LGL leukemia patients have monoclonal gammopathy of undetermined significance (MGUS) and splenomegaly, respectively [4].

W. Xiao
Department of Pathology, Memorial Sloan Kettering Cancer Center, New York, NY, USA

H.-Y. Wang (✉)
Department of Pathology, University of California San Diego Health System, La Jolla, CA, USA
e-mail: huw003@ucsd.edu

E. Wang, A. S. Lagoo (eds.), *Practical Lymph Node and Bone Marrow Pathology*, Practical Anatomic Pathology,
https://doi.org/10.1007/978-3-030-32189-5_15

- T-LGL leukemia is associated with autoimmune disorders such as rheumatoid arthritis and autoimmune hemolytic anemia in approximately 14% and 6% of patients, respectively [4].
- Certain bone marrow disorders such as myelodysplastic syndrome and pure red cell aplasia are seen in 5.9% and 4.7% of T-LGL, respectively [4]. In a recent multicenter study of 432 cases of T-LGL leukemia patients, 5.1% of T-LGL leukemia patients have an associated B-cell non-Hodgkin lymphoma with T-LGL leukemia occurring either synchronously, preceding, or thereafter [5].
- T-LGL leukemia can rarely occur after solid organ transplant [6].

2. What are the key histologic features for T-LGL leukemia?

- T-LGL leukemia involves the peripheral blood, bone marrow, (Fig. 15.1), spleen, and liver more often than lymph node; thus, peripheral blood smear and bone marrow aspirate smear and/or core biopsy specimens are very important to make the diagnosis of T-LGL leukemia.
- In peripheral blood and bone marrow aspirate smears, T-LGLs are by definition large granular lymphocytes with moderate to abundant cytoplasm containing fine or course azurophilic granules.
- In bone marrow core biopsy, T-LGLs have characteristic infiltration pattern: typically interstitial and/or intrasinusoidal rather than forming aggregates (see Case Presentation).

3. What are the commonly used immunomarkers in T-LGL leukemia?

Flow cytometry and/or immunohistochemistry (IHC) are/is of paramount importance in immunophenotyping T-LGLs in order to distinguish them from the natural killer LGLs (NK-LGLs) and reactive T-cell large granular lymphocytosis.

- For T-cell receptor (TCR) alpha/beta+ T-LGL leukemias, a majority of cases are positive for CD8 with abnormalities of pan-T-cell antigens including CD2, CD3, CD5, and CD7 and with variable expression of CD16, CD56, CD57, and CD94 [7], but negative for CD4. However, CD4+ T-LGL leukemia occurs in rare cases [8].
- TCRgamma/delta+ T-LGL leukemia is extremely rare but does exist: It is typically positive for CD2, CD3, and CD7 but negative for CD4 and CD8, with CD5 being negative to rarely dimly positive [9].
- An important differential diagnosis of TCRgamma/delta+ T-LGL is hepatosplenic T-cell lymphoma [9, 10].

4. What is the differential diagnosis for T-LGL leukemia?

The differential diagnosis for T-LGL leukemia includes reactive T-LGL lymphocytosis, oligo- to clonal T-LGL lymphocytosis/proliferation, and hepatosplenic T-cell lymphoma. To make things even worse, so far there is no agreement with regard to the level of T-LGL needed for an accurate diagnosis of T-LGL leukemia. This is because T-LGL leukemia can be seen in patients with a spectrum of blood T-LGL levels ranging from less than 2×10^9/L to 20×10^9/L (2), which may explain why other terms have been proposed [11].

- *Reactive T-LGL lymphocytosis/proliferation*: This phenomena typically refers to T-LGL less than 0.5×10^9/L, and it can be seen in a variety of clinical settings including but not limited to myelodysplastic syndrome [12], Felty's syndrome [13], inflammatory arthropathy [14], and post allogeneic bone marrow HCT [15, 16]. Please note in some of the situations, *TCR* rearrangement can be monoclonal [12, 14], but there is no *STAT3* mutations in persistent cytotoxic T lymphocyte expansions after allogeneic hematopoietic stem cell transplantation [15].
- *Hepatosplenic T-cell lymphoma:* Since both T-LGL leukemia and hepatosplenic T-cell lymphoma can involve the spleen, liver, and bone marrow, it is critical to distinguish them, especially when T-LGL leukemia manifests γδ-immunophenotype. Table 15.1 summarizes the differences between T-LGL leukemia and hepatosplenic T-cell lymphoma.

Table 15.1 Difference between γδ T-LGL leukemia and hepatosplenic T-cell lymphoma

Features	T-LGL leukemia	Hepatosplenic T-cell lymphoma	References
Clinical behavior	Indolent	Aggressive	[2]
Massive splenomegaly	Absent	Present	[10]
Azurophilic granules	Present	Absent	[10]
Bone marrow infiltrative pattern-sinusoidal	Rare	Often	
T-cell receptor: αβ vs γδ	Majority: αβ Minority: γδ	Majority: γδ Minority: αβ	[2]
Isochromosome 7	Absent	Often	[2]
STAT3 mutations	Often (27–40%)	Rare	[4, 17, 18]
STAT5 mutations	Rare	Often (33–36%)	[4, 17, 18]

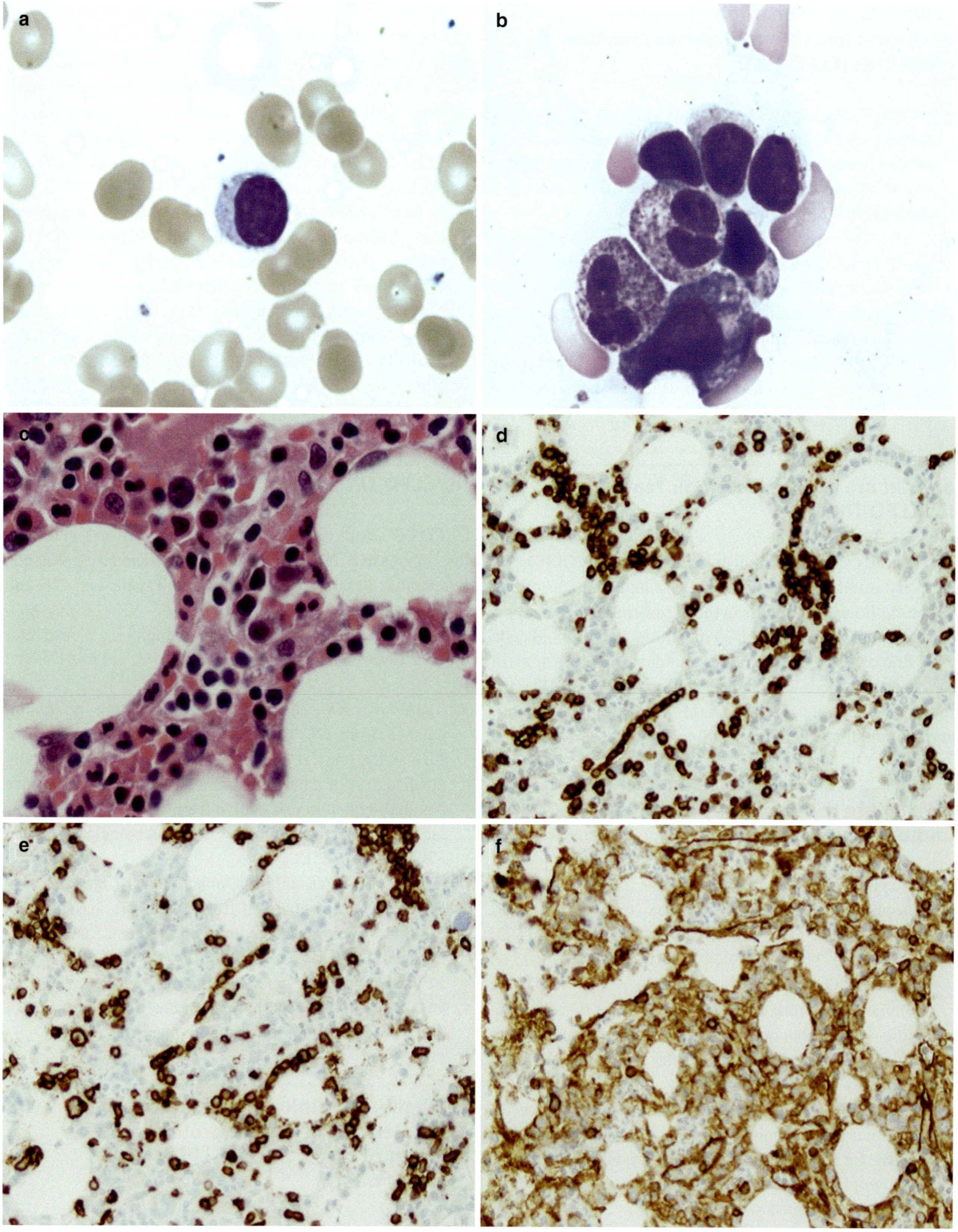

Fig. 15.1 T-cell large granular lymphocytic leukemia. The peripheral blood (**a**) and bone marrow aspirate (**b**) show atypical lymphoid cells with eccentrically located nuclei and few azurophilic granules (**a** & **b**: Wright Giemsa. Original magnifications are 1000× and 1000×, respectively). Bone marrow core biopsy (**c**) shows interstitial lymphoid infiltrate (H&E, 400×). Immunohistochemistry shows interstitial and sinusoidal infiltrate of T-LGL cells by CD3 (**d**), CD8 (**e**), and markedly decreased CD4 (**f**) (original magnifications of **d**, **e**, and **f** are 200×, 200×, and 200×, respectively). Please note CD4 also shows macrophages

5. What is the clinical manifestation of chronic lymphoproliferative disorder of NK cells (CLPD-NK)?

- CLPD-NK is a provisional entity defined by the 2017 revised 4th edition of the WHO [2]. It is defined as a persistent (more than 6 months) increase in the peripheral blood NK cells (usually more than 2×10^9/L) without a clear identified cause [2].
- CLPD-NK is an indolent and very rare disorder, usually asymptomatic, but some patients can present with cytopenias mainly neutropenia and anemia [19] and associated other medical conditions such as vasculitic skin lesions, musculoskeletal symptoms, and peripheral neuropathy [20]. CLPD-NK progression to a massive lymphocytosis with lung infiltration leading to death has been reported from one study [21].

6. What are the key histologic features for CLPD-NK?

The overall cytologic and histologic features of CLPD-NK are very similar to those of T-LGL leukemia described above. Although NK-LGLs in the peripheral blood are typically obvious as medium-sized monotonous lymphoid cells with fine or coarse azurophilic granules, in contrast, as in the cases of T-LGL leukemia, detection of CLPD-NK infiltration in the bone marrow might be subtle and difficult, and immunohistochemistry is often needed (see below).

7. What are the commonly used immunomarkers in CLPD-NK?

- The main NK-cell-associated antigens include CD2, CD3 (cytoplasmic by IHC but not flow cytometry), CD7, CD16, CD56, CD57, CD94, CD161, CD158a, CD158b, and CD158e. The basic NK-cell phenotype is defined as surface CD3−, CD19−, CD56+, and CD45+. Immunophenotyping is absolutely needed in revealing the nature of NK phenotype either by multiparameter flow cytometry or immunohistochemistry or by both. Bearing in mind, by flow cytometry, surface and cytoplasmic CD3 is positive in T-LGL, but negative in NK-LGL; however, by immunohistochemistry, both T-LGL and NK-LGL are positive for CD3 because both T-LGL and NK-LGL possess cytoplasmic CD3-ε chain, which is recognized by immunohistochemistry.
- Comparing to normal NK cells, NK-LGLs from CLPD-NK are positive for CD16 but typically negative or dimly positive for CD56 [21]: in other words, a major reduction in the size of the CD56 (bright) NK-cell subset is a constant feature of CLPD-NK according to one study [22].
- Similarly, CD2, CD7, and CD57 expression in CLPD-NK can be diminished or lost; CD8 expression, on the other hand, can be abnormally expressed uniformly [2]. In addition, altered distribution of CD94+/CD161+/CD162R+ NK-cell subsets is also observed in CLPD-NK [22].
- It was further demonstrated that CLPD-NK patients had increased activating-to-inhibitory killer-cell immunoglobulin-like receptor (KIR) ratio, namely, CD94, and its inhibitory heterodimerization partner NKG2A was homogenously expressed at high levels [23]. With regard to the killing inhibitory KIRs CD158a, CD158B, and CD158e, CLPD-NK cells show either single KIR isoform or lack all tested KIRs [24].

8. What is the differential diagnosis for CLPD-NK?

CLPD-NK needs to be distinguished from NK-cell enteropathy, aggressive NK-cell leukemia, extranodal T-/NK-cell lymphoma, nasal type, *EBV*-positive T cell, and NK-cell lymphoproliferative disease of childhood. *NK-cell enteropathy* will be described in subsequent paragraphs; please refer to those discussions for more details.

- *Aggressive NK-cell leukemia (ANKL)* can be distinguished from CLPD-NK by its frequent positivity for *EBV* and aggressive clinical course [2]. CD56 is typically positive. It is of interest that rare *EBV*-negative aggressive NK-cell leukemia can evolve from CLPD-NK [2] but is indistinguishable clinically and pathologically from *EBV*+ ANKL [25].
- *Extranodal T-/NK-cell lymphoma (ETNKL), nasal type*: ETNKL can be separated from CLPD-NK based on its typical location (nasal cavity), very frequent *EBV* positivity, and CD56 expression [2, 26].
- *EBV-positive T-cell and NK-cell lymphoproliferative disease of childhood.* Again, this is a heterogenous group of diseases with a common feature – positive *EBV*.

9. What is the clinical manifestation of indolent T-cell lymphoproliferative disorder of the GI tract (iT-LPD of the GI tract)?

- Indolent T-LPD of the GI tract is a rare disorder seen in patients ranging in age from 15 years to 77 years. In the study of the largest cohort of 10 patients, the male to female ratio is 6:4. The entire GI tract from the oral cavity to colon can be affected, but the small intestine including the ileum followed by the duodenum is the most commonly affected sites.

- As the name suggests, iT-LPD of the GI tract affects the GI tract; therefore, the associated symptoms are those of the GI tract with no specificities. These symptoms include but are not limited to diarrhea, abdominal pain, rectal bleeding, oropharyngeal ulcers, vomiting, dyspepsia, and food intolerance [27]. Rare patients exhibit chemical imbalance such as hypocalcemia, hypomagnesemia, hypokalemia, and hypozincemia. Among the 10 cases reported, one patient reported to have drenching night sweat [27].
- Endoscopically they present as polyps, erosions, or erythema [27]. iT-LPD of the GI tract has also been reported in patients with Crohn disease [27–29].

10. What are the key histologic features for iT-LPD of the GI Tract?

- The key histologic features of iT-LPD of the GI tract are (1) small mature atypical T cells and (2) involvement of the lamina propria without significant intraepithelial lesion (Fig. 15.2) [27]. In other words, the lymphoid infiltrate mainly resides in the stroma of the lamina propria as opposed to celiac disease (CD) and monomorphic epitheliotropic intestinal T-cell lymphoma (MEITL), both of which show prominent intraepithelial lesion.
- Please note rare cases of iT-LPD of the GI tract can exhibit intraepithelial lesion and villus blunting [27].

11. What are the commonly used immunomarkers in iT-LPD of the GI tract?

- Immunophenotyping in particular IHC plays an important role in the work-ups of this entity. All T-cell-specific (CD3, TCR-BF1) and associated antigens including CD2, CD5, CD7, CD4, CD8, CD56, and CD57 as well as cytotoxic molecules such as TIA-1, granzyme B, and perforin should be employed. In addition, *EBV* by EBER should be included.
- Among the 15 well-documented iT-LPD of the GI tract from English literature [27–30], ~67% (10/15) show CD4−/CD8+, ~27% (4/15) CD4+/CD8−, and only ~6.7% (1/15) CD4−/CD8−. Among the nine cases in which TCR-BF1 was performed [1–3], all were positive. However, among the ten cases and eight cases in which CD56 and *EBV* were tested, respectively [27], none of them was positive for either CD56 or *EBV*.

12. What is the differential diagnosis for iT-LPD of the GI tract?

The differential diagnosis for iT-LPD of the GI tract is wide and includes neoplastic as well as nonneoplastic disorders such as indolent peripheral T-cell lymphoma involving the GI tract [31], NK-cell enteropathy (see below), celiac disease (CD), autoimmune enteritis, tropic sprue, bacterial overgrowth, and food intolerance. The summary of the differential diagnosis is listed in Table 15.2.

13. What is the clinical manifestation of NK-cell enteropathy?

- NK-cell enteropathy affects both male and female with the age ranging from 20s to 70s. In contrast to the patients with aggressive NK- or T-cell lymphoma, these patients are asymptomatic or only present with vague gastrointestinal symptoms including abdominal pain, constipation, diverticulosis, and reflux.
- There is no prior history of celiac disease, inflammatory bowel disease, or malabsorption. There is no clinical evidence of any lymphadenopathy or organomegaly.
- Endoscopic examinations show single or multiple small lesions (mucosal hemorrhages, erosions, or superficial bleeding ulcers approximately 1–2 cm). The lesions can involve single or multiple sites along the gastrointestinal tract. The lesions can be persistent, self-regressed, and/or recurred.

14. What are the key histologic features of NK-cell enteropathy?

- The key histologic features are expansion of the lamina propria by a relatively well-circumscribed but confluent infiltrate of medium-sized cells with irregular nuclei, inconspicuous nucleoli, finely clumped chromatin, and a moderate amount of pale cytoplasm [35, 36]. Eosinophilic granules have been reported in one study [36]. The mucosal glands can be displaced and/or destroyed because of dense atypical cellular infiltrate.
- Epitheliotropism is typically absent. Angiocentricity or angiodestructive pattern of growth is absent. Necrosis can be occasionally seen and if present is usually associated with mucosal ulceration. The muscularis mucosae, if observed, are intact. There is no villous atrophy or crypt hyperplasia. Small reactive lymphoid aggregates and neutrophils may be occasionally found.

- High prevalence of *Helicobacter pylori* infection has been reported by one study [36].

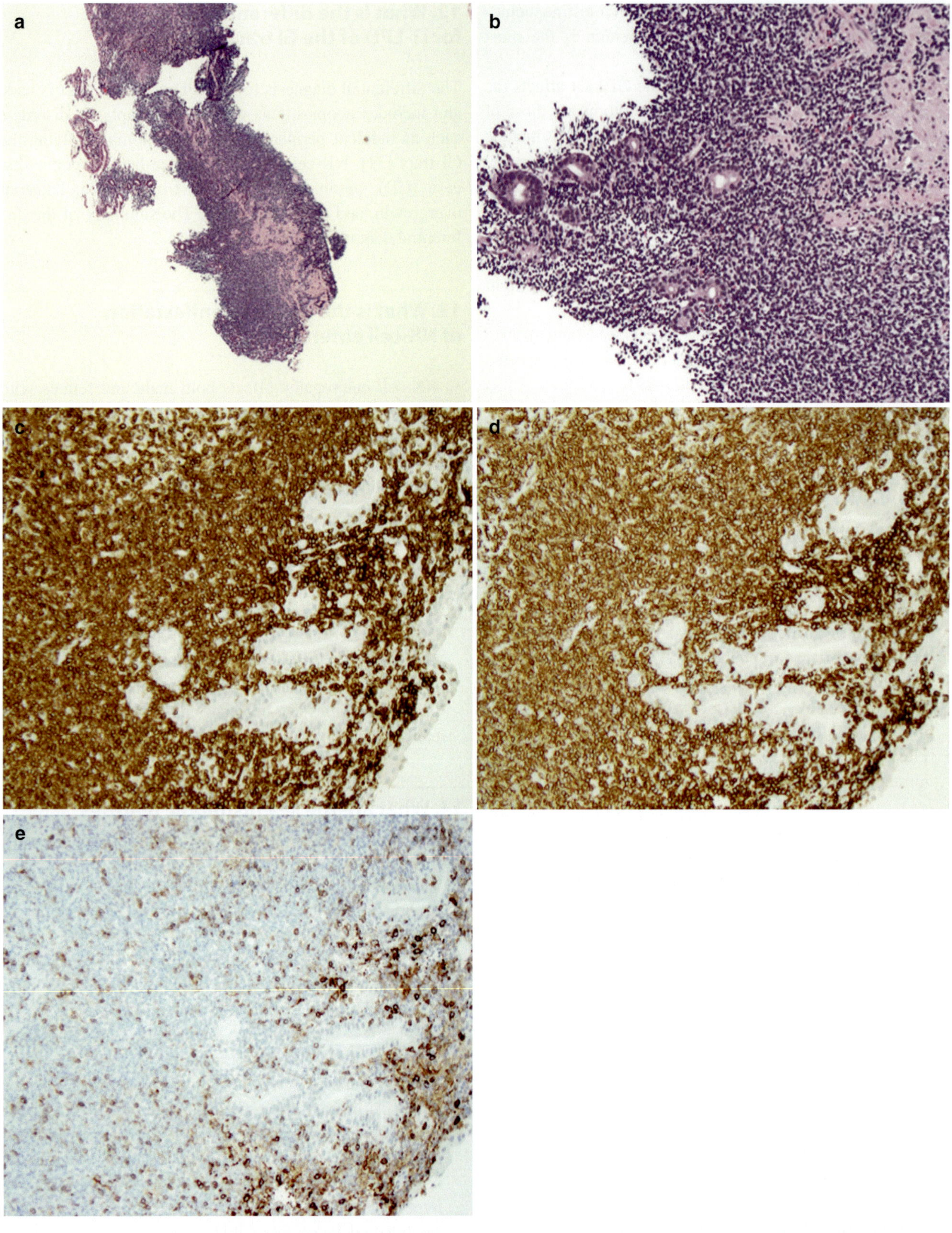

Fig. 15.2 iT-LPD of the GI tract. (**a**) to (**e**) are from a recent stomach biopsy. H&E stained section in **a** and **b** shows dense atypical lymphoid infiltrate expanding the lamina propria with resultant glandular loss but with no increased intraepithelial lymphocytes (the original magnifications of **a** and **b** are 20× and 100×). The atypical cells are cytotoxic T cells as revealed by diffuse and strong positivity by CD3 (**c**) and CD8 (**d**) with no expression of CD4 (**e**) (the original magnification of **c**, **d**, and **e** is 100x)

Table 15.2 Differential diagnosis of iT-LPD of the GI tract

Features	iT-LPD of the GI tract [2]	Celiac disease (CD)	Autoimmune enteropathy [32]	Tropical sprue
Villous blunting/ shortening	Less common	Very common	Can be seen	Mild to moderate villous shortening
Crypt hyperplasia	Rarely	Usually	Rarely	Usually
Increased intraepithelial lymphocytes (IELs)	Typically absent	Present	Can be seen	Can be seen
Expansion of the lamina propria	Usually	Rarely	Can be seen	Can be seen
Monoclonal *TCR* rearrangement	Present	Present in type refractory CD	Absent	Absent
STAT3-JAK2	Present [33]	Absent	Absent	Absent
Serological abnormality	Absent	IgA tissue transglutaminase, IgA endomysial antibodies, and others [34]	Anti-enterocytes or anti-goblet cell antibodies	Absent

15. What are the commonly used immunomarkers in NK-cell enteropathy?

- The atypical cells express CD2, CD56, CD7, cytoplasmic CD3 (positive by IHC, negative by flow cytometry), TIA-1, and granzyme B, but not surface CD3 (by flow cytometry), TCRαβ, TCRγδ, CD5, CD4, CD8, CD10, CD20, CD30, PAX5, CD138, or CD68.
- The proliferative index as determined by MIB-1/Ki-67 is usually low but can be up to 40–50%.
- *EBV* is always negative by *EBV*-LMP immunostain or by in situ hybridization technique using *EBV*-encoded RNA probe.

16. What is the differential diagnosis for NK-cell enteropathy?

The main differential diagnosis includes iT-LPD of the GI tract, extranodal NK/T-cell lymphoma, enteropathy-associated T-cell lymphoma (EATL, type I), monomorphic epitheliotropic intestinal T-cell lymphoma (MEITL, also formerly known as EATL type II), and peripheral T-cell lymphoma, not otherwise specified (PTCL, NOS) (Table 15.3).

17. What is the clinical manifestation of primary cutaneous CD4- positive small/ medium T-cell LPD?

- Primary cutaneous CD4-positive small/medium T-cell LPD involves both male and female with a median age of about 50 years old.
- It usually presents as a solitary slow-growing nodule most commonly located on the head and neck area, followed by the upper trunk [37, 38].
- Patients are asymptomatic and have an indolent clinical course. The cases with widespread and rapid-growing lesions do not belong to this group.

18. What are the key histologic features for primary cutaneous CD4- positive small/ medium T-cell LPD?

- Key histologic features are characterized by non-epidermotropic, diffuse polymorphous infiltrates composed of predominantly small- to medium-sized pleomorphic lymphoid cells involving the entire dermal thickness often with nodular extension into the subcutis [37, 38].
- The atypical cells show mild to moderate atypia and include elongated, hyperchromatic nuclei with indistinct nucleoli. Atypical large cells are less than 30%.
- The pattern of infiltration is mainly perivascular and periadnexal without destruction of these structures. The infiltrate is intermingled with many histiocytes, plasma cells, and some eosinophils.

19. What are the commonly used immunomarkers in primary cutaneous CD4- positive small/medium T-cell LPD?

- The atypical cells are positive for CD3 and CD4 with normal expression of pan-T-cell antigens CD2, CD5, and CD7. They are positive for TCRαβ and do not express CD8, TCRγδ, CD30, CD56, or cytotoxic granules.
- They are also positive for T follicular helper markers such as PD1, CXCL13, BCL6 and less frequently CD10.
- *EBV* is invariably negative. A prominent B-cell component can be demonstrated by CD20. Secondary B-lymphoid follicles are not present. Plasma cells have a polytypic staining pattern by kappa- and lambda-light chain immunohistochemistry but can rarely be light chain restricted.

Table 15.3 Differential diagnosis of NK-cell enteropathy

	NK-cell enteropathy	Indolent T-cell LPD of the GI tract	Extranodal NK/T-cell lymphoma	EATL	PTCL NOS
History of celiac disease	–	–	–	Yes for type I No for type II	–
B symptoms	–	–	+	+	+
Lymphadenopathy	–	–	–	+/–	+
Hepatosplenomegaly	–	–	–	+/–	+
Lesional involvement	Superficial	Superficial	Infiltrative	Infiltrative	Infiltrative
Necrosis	–	–	+	+/–	+/–
Epitheliotropism	–/minimal	–	–	+	–
EBV	–	–	+	–	–
CD56	+	–	+	– in type I + in type II	–
CD3	cyCD3+	sCD3+	cyCD3+	Mostly sCD3+	Mostly sCD3+
CD4	–	+/–	–	+/– in type I – in type II	+/–
CD8	–	+/–	–	+/– in type I + in type II	+/–
TCRαβ	–	+	–	+/–	+/–
TCRγδ	–	–	–	+/–	+/–

Table 15.4 Differential diagnosis of primary cutaneous CD4-positive small/medium T-cell LPD

	Primary cutaneous CD4-positive small/medium T-cell LPD	Mycosis fungoides	Primary cutaneous anaplastic large cell lymphoma	Lymphomatoid papulosis	PTCL NOS
B symptoms	–	–	–	–	+
Skin manifestation	Solitary lesion, head/neck	Patches	Solitary, ulceration	Multiple, waxing, and waning	+
Lymphadenopathy	–	–/+	–/+	–	+
Hepatosplenomegaly	–	–	–	–	+/–
Lesional involvement	Dermis	Epidermis/ dermis	Dermis	Wedge-shaped, dermis	Infiltrative
Necrosis	–	–	–/+	–/+	+/–
Epidermotropism	–	+	–/+	+/–	–
CD30	–	–	+	+	–/scattered
CD3	+	+	+/–	+	+
CD4	+	+/–	+	+/–	+/–
CD8	–	+/–	–	+/–	+/–
TCRαβ	+	+	+	+	+/–
TCRγδ	–	Rarely +	–	–	+/–

20. What is the differential diagnosis for primary cutaneous CD4- positive small/ medium T-cell LPD?

- The main differential diagnosis includes mycosis fungoides, primary cutaneous anaplastic large cell lymphoma, lymphomatoid papulosis (type B), and peripheral T-cell lymphoma, not otherwise specified (PTCL, NOS) (Table 15.4).

21. What is the clinical manifestation of primary cutaneous acral CD8- positive T-cell lymphoma?

- Primary cutaneous acral CD8-positive T-cell lymphoma affects individuals mostly older than 50 years (median age 57 years) with a slight male predominance (M:F 1.7:1).

Table 15.5 Differential diagnosis of primary cutaneous acral CD8-positive T-cell LPD

	Primary acral CD8-positive T-cell lymphoma	Lymphomatoid papulosis	Primary cutaneous CD8-positive aggressive epidermotropic cytotoxic T-cell lymphoma	Primary cutaneous gamma-delta T-cell lymphoma	PTCL NOS
B symptoms	–	–	+	+	+
Skin manifestation	Solitary nodule, ear	Multiple, waxing, and waning	Multiple, necrotic	Multiple, necrotic	+
Lymphadenopathy	–	–	–	–	+
Hepatosplenomegaly	–	–	Uncommon	Uncommon	+/–
Lesional involvement	Superficial	Superficial	Infiltrative	Infiltrative	Infiltrative
Necrosis	–	–	+	+	+/–
Epitheliotropism	–	–	+	+/–	–
CD30	–	+	–	–	–/scattered
CD56	–	–	–	+	–
CD3	+	+	+	+	+
CD4	–	+/–	–	–	+/–
CD8	+	+/–	+	–	+/–
TCRαβ	+	+	+	–	+/–
TCRγδ	–	–	–	+	+/–

- The typical findings are a slow-growing nodule on the ear, but it can involve the nose, the hands, and the feet. Lesions are solitary at presentation; however, bilateral symmetrical disease has been described.
- Patients have no systemic symptoms and show an indolent clinical course with no progression to systemic disease.
- Patients can be managed by topical corticosteroids, radiotherapy, surgical excision, or simple observation, although limited cutaneous relapses may occur.

22. What are the key histologic features for primary cutaneous acral CD8- positive T-cell lymphoma?

- Key histologic features are a dense, diffuse lymphoid infiltration within the dermis without involvement of the epidermis and an uninvolved grenz zone in superficial dermis [39, 40]. Subcutaneous tissues can be occasionally involved, but rimming of adipocytes or nuclear karyorrhexis is not observed.
- The lymphoid infiltration is composed of monomorphous medium-sized cells with an irregular nucleus, small nucleoli, and a small amount of cytoplasm. Large cells are less than 5%. Mitoses were rare. No angiodestruction or necrosis is seen.
- Variably sized collections of small lymphocytes are often present within the neoplastic cell infiltrate with no germinal center or follicular dendritic cell networks. No significant numbers of plasma cells, neutrophils, eosinophils, or histiocytes are seen. Hair follicle and eccrine glands are surrounded and compressed by the lymphoid proliferation but not infiltrated.

23. What are the commonly used immunomarkers in primary cutaneous acral CD8- positive T-cell lymphoma?

- The atypical lymphoid cells are positive for CD3, CD8, CD2, CD5, TIA1, and TCRαβ while negative for CD4, CD30, granzyme B, CD56, CD57, TCRγδ, and TdT. CD7 can be negative. Ki-67 shows a low proliferation index (<10% of cells).
- CD20 and CD79a highlight the small B lymphocytes. *EBV* is negative. One study has reported CD68 expression in these atypical cells but was not able to be confirmed by another study.

24. What is the differential diagnosis for primary cutaneous acral CD8- positive T-cell lymphoma?

- The main differential diagnosis includes lymphomatoid papulosis, primary cutaneous CD8-positive aggressive epidermotropic cytotoxic T-cell lymphoma, primary cutaneous gamma-delta T-cell lymphoma, and peripheral T-cell lymphoma, not otherwise specified (PTCL, NOS) (Table 15.5).

Case Presentations

Case 1 (Fig. 15.1)

Learning Objectives

1. To become familiar with the clinical presentation, histologic features, and immunophenotypic findings of T-cell large granular lymphocytic leukemia
2. To generate the differential diagnosis

Case History

This is a 55-year-old male with absolute neutrophil count of 0.5×10^9/L, hemoglobin of 12 g/dl, and platelet count of 65×10^9/L. The lymphocytes account for 93% of the peripheral blood white blood cells with absolute lymphocytes of $11{,}000 \times 10^9$/L.

Histologic Findings (Fig. 15.1a–c)

- Increased circulating large granular lymphocytes
- Interstitial lymphocytosis in the bone marrow

Differential Diagnosis

- T-LGL leukemia
- Reactive T-cell large granular lymphocytosis
- Chronic lymphoproliferative disorder of NK cells
- Hepatosplenic T-cell lymphoma

IHC and Other Ancillary Studies (Fig. 15.1d–f)

- Positive for CD2, CD3 (D), CD5 (weak), CD7, CD8 (E), TCRαβ, TIA1, and granzyme B
- Negative for CD4 (F), TCRγδ, CD25, CD20, and EBER
- Interstitial T-cell lymphocytosis with sinusoidal infiltrate highlighted by positive stains
- CD8-positive T-cell population with dim CD5 detected by flow cytometry
- Clonal *TCR* gene rearrangements detected

Final Diagnosis

T-LGL leukemia

Take-Home Messages

1. T-LGL leukemia is relatively rare but has recently been diagnosed more frequently than before. It has indolent clinical course and is associated with some autoimmune disorders such as rheumatoid arthritis.
2. Key features are:
   - Patients often present with neutropenia and/or anemia, but thrombocytopenia and lymphadenopathy are usually absent.
   - Peripheral blood smear shows increased large granular lymphocytes.
   - The bone marrow infiltrate is often interstitial with sinusoidal distribution.
   - The cells have CD8+ and TCRα/β T-cell phenotype.
   - Clonal rearrangement of *TCR* gene can be detected.

Case 2 (Fig. 15.2)

Learning Objectives

1. To become familiar with the clinical presentation, histologic features, and immunophenotypic findings of indolent T-cell lymphoproliferative disorder of the GI tract
2. To generate the differential diagnosis

Case History

This is a 44-year-old gentleman who carried a diagnosis of iT-LPD of the GI tract for 7 years since 2011. The disease involves the entire GI tract from the esophagus to the rectum. He has been treated with methotrexate intermittently with no progression of the disease.

Histologic Findings (Fig. 15.2a–c)

- Fragments of the gastric mucosa with a dense lymphoid infiltrate in the lamina propria and submucosa.
- The lymphoid cells are small in size and show no significant morphologic atypia.
- There is minimal epitheliotropism, but necrosis is not identified.

Differential Diagnosis

- Indolent T-LPD of the GI tract
- Celiac disease
- Autoimmune enteropathy
- EATL

IHC and Other Ancillary Studies (Fig. 15.2d, e)

- Positive for CD2, CD3 (D), CD5, CD7, TIA1, and CD8 (E).
- Negative for CD4 (F), CD20, and *EBV* by EBER.
- Ki-67 proliferation index is ~5%.
- *H. pylori* negative.
- Clonal *TCRG* gene rearrangements detected.

Final Diagnosis

Indolent T-cell LPD of the GI tract

Take-Home Messages

1. Indolent T-cell LPD of the GI tract is an extremely rare type of T-cell proliferation occurring in the GI tract, usually presents with chronic GI symptom, and has

indolent clinical course but symptom tends to relapse after treatment.

2. Key features are:
    - Patients have GI symptoms, including abdominal pain, diarrhea, etc., and usually no lymphadenopathy.
    - The infiltrate is often confined to the lamina propria and submucosa, but occasional infiltrate into the muscularis may be focally seen.
    - The cells are monotonous, small with no significant atypia.
    - Epitheliotropism is usually absent but could be focal if present.
    - The cells have T-cell phenotype.

Case 3 (Fig. 15.3)

Learning Objectives

1. To become familiar with the clinical presentation, histologic features, and immunophenotypic findings of NK-cell enteropathy
2. To generate the differential diagnosis

Case History

A 76-year-old female presented with nonspecific dyspepsia for a few years. An upper GI endoscopic examination performed 2 years ago showed multiple superficial ulcers in duodenal and gastric mucosa. A biopsy was performed and

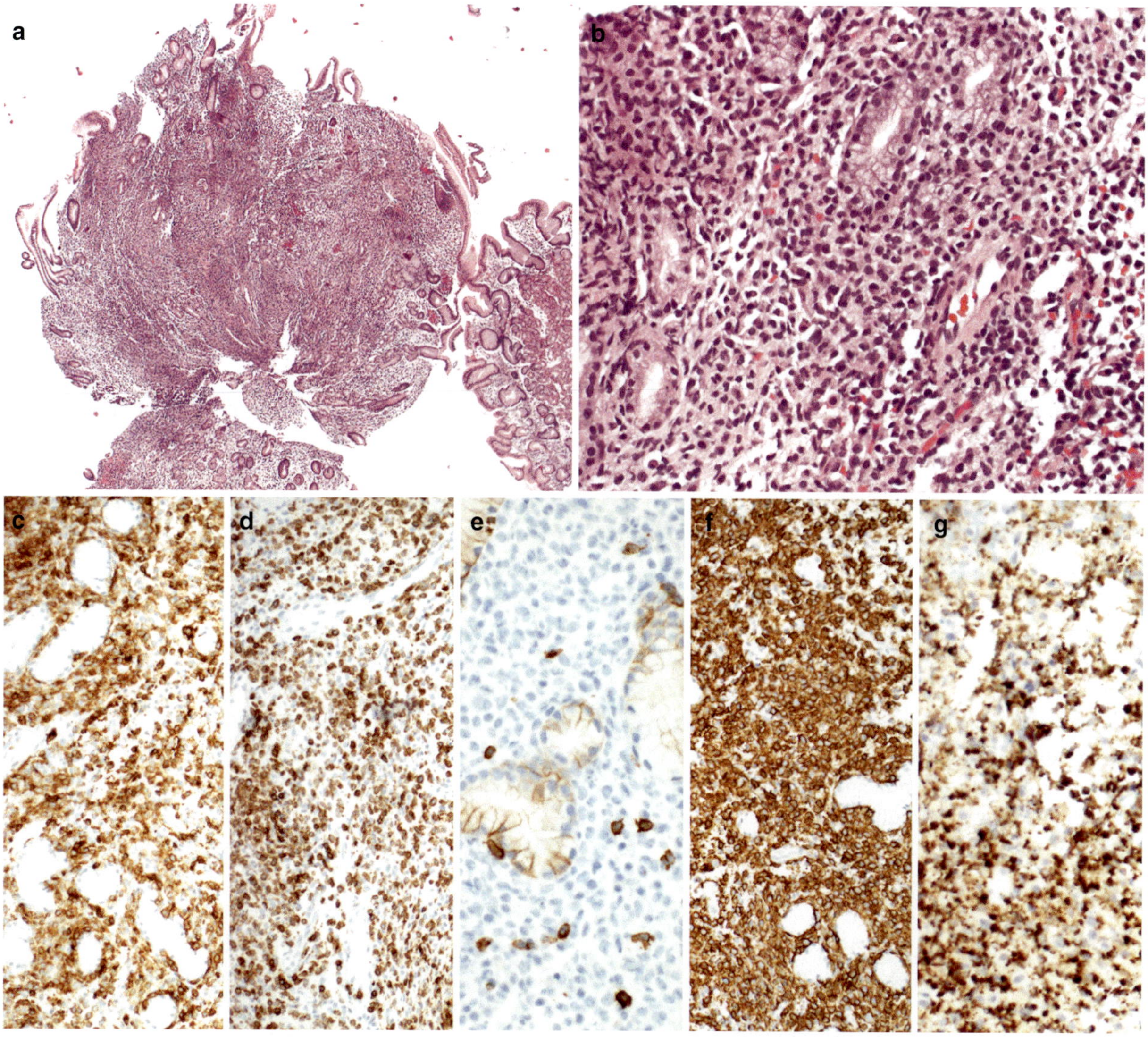

Fig. 15.3 NK-cell enteropathy. (**a**) Low magnification of H&E stain of the gastric biopsy shows a dense lymphoid infiltrate in the lamina propria. (**b**) High magnification of H&E stain shows predominantly small lymphoid cells with minimal atypia and no epitheliotropism. (**c–g**) Immunohistochemical stains show the lymphoid cells are CD2+ (**c**), CD3+ (cytoplasmic pattern, **d**), CD5− (**e**), CD56+ (**f**), and TIA-1+ (**g**)

an NK-cell proliferation was noted. Recently, a repeated upper GI endoscopic examination showed similar findings, and another biopsy was taken. The patient had no lymphadenopathy or B symptoms and PET scan showed no avid uptake.

Histologic Findings (Fig. 15.3a, b)

- Fragments of the gastric mucosa with a dense lymphoid infiltrate in the lamina propria.
- The lymphoid cells are small to medium in size and only show mild atypia.
- There is no necrosis or epitheliotropism.

Differential Diagnosis

- NK-cell enteropathy
- Indolent T-LPD of the GI tract
- Extranodal NK/T-cell lymphoma
- EATL

IHC and Other Ancillary Studies (Fig. 15.3c–g)

- Positive for CD2, CD3 (cytoplasmic), CD56 (strong), TIA1, and granzyme B.
- Negative for CD5, CD4, CD8, TCRαβ, TCRγδ, CD25, CD30, PD1, and EBER.
- Ki-67 proliferation index is 40%.
- *H. pylori* negative.
- No clonal *TCR* gene rearrangements detected.

Final Diagnosis

NK-cell enteropathy

Take-Home Messages

1. NK-cell enteropathy is a rare type of NK-cell proliferation occurring in the GI tract, usually presents with multiple superficial ulcers that can be persistent/recurrent, refractory to treatment and have indolent clinical course.
2. Key features are:
   - Patients have no B symptoms or lymphadenopathy.
   - The infiltrate is superficial.
   - The cells have no significant atypia.
   - The cells have a NK-cell phenotype.
   - *EBV* is negative.

Case 4 (Fig. 15.4)

Learning Objectives

1. To become familiar with the clinical presentation, histologic features, and immunophenotypic findings of primary cutaneous CD4-positive small/medium T-cell LPD
2. To generate the differential diagnosis

Case History

A 55-year-old male presented with a 2-cm slow-growing solitary nodule on the forehead. A biopsy was performed.

Histologic Findings (Fig. 15.4a, b)

- A dense dermal lymphoid infiltrate composed of small- to medium-sized lymphoid cells in a polymorphous background.
- Epidermis is unremarkable.

Differential Diagnosis

- Primary cutaneous CD4-positive small/medium T-cell LPD
- Mycosis fungoides
- Primary cutaneous anaplastic large cell lymphoma
- Lymphomatoid papulosis

IHC and Other Ancillary Studies (Fig. 15.4c–f)

- Positive for CD2, CD3, CD4, CD5, PD1, and BCL6.
- Negative for CD8, CD25, CD30, and *EBV* by EBER.
- Ki-67 proliferation index is 20%.
- Clonal *TCRG* gene rearrangements detected.

Final Diagnosis

Primary cutaneous CD4-positive small/medium T-cell LPD

Take-Home Messages

1. Primary cutaneous CD4-positive small/medium T-cell LPD is a rare type of indolent cutaneous T-cell proliferation.
2. Key features are:
   - Patients are asymptomatic and have no lymphadenopathy.
   - Solitary nodule involving the head/neck or upper trunk.
   - The infiltrate is non-epidermotropic and involves dermis.
   - Large cells are less than 30%.
   - The cells have a TFH phenotype.

Case 5 (Fig. 15.5)

Learning Objectives

1. To become familiar with the clinical presentation, histologic features, and immunophenotypic findings of primary cutaneous acral CD8-positive T-cell lymphoma
2. To generate the differential diagnosis

Case History

A 32-year-old male presented with a 1-cm slowly growing nodule in the left ear.

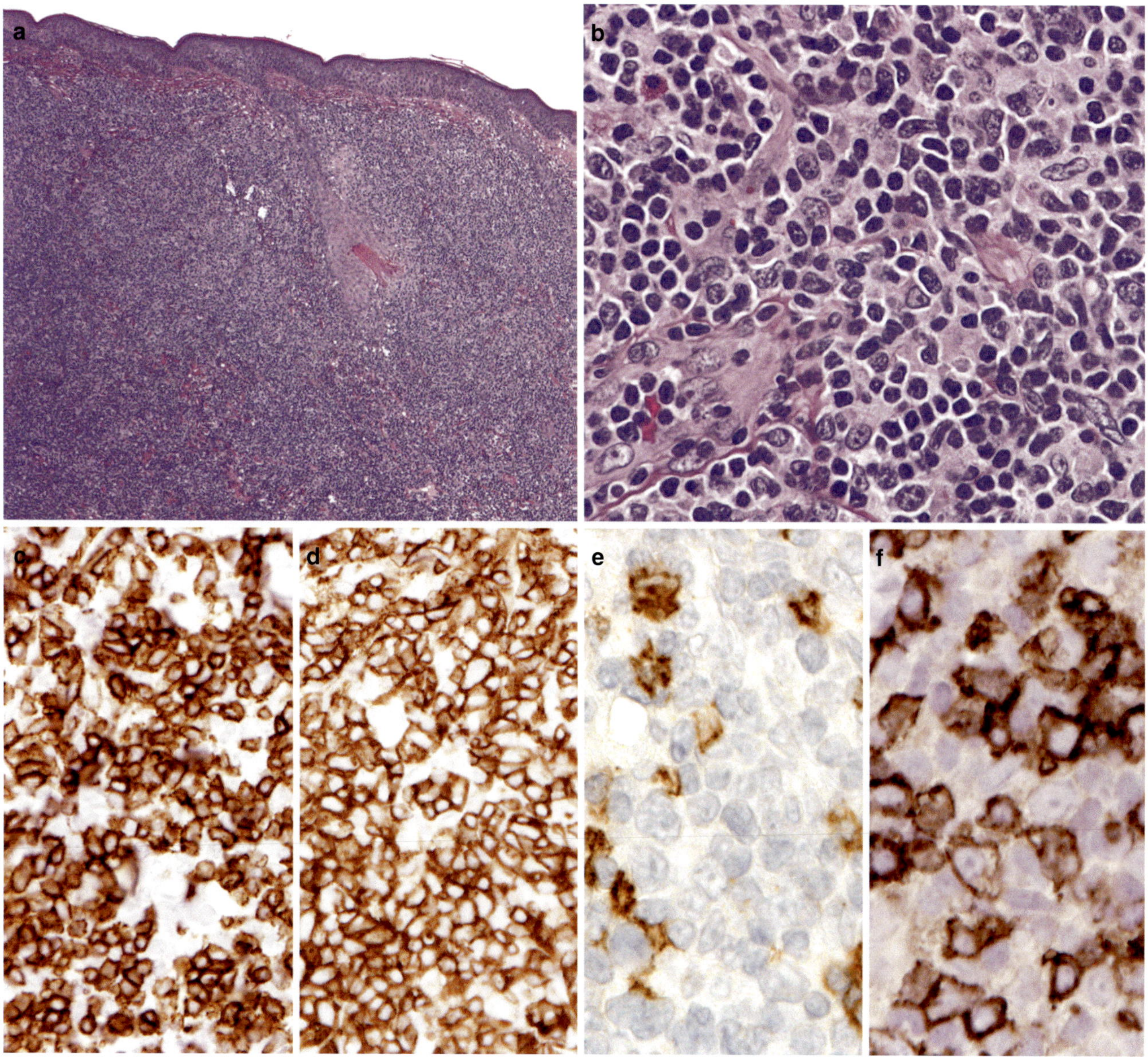

Fig. 15.4 Primary cutaneous CD4-positive small/medium T-cell LPD. (**a**) Low magnification of H&E stain of the skin biopsy shows a dense lymphoid infiltrate in the dermis. (**b**) High magnification of H&E stain shows predominantly small- to medium-sized lymphoid cells with atypia. (**c–f**) Immunohistochemical stains show the lymphoid cells are CD3+ (**c**), CD4+ (**d**), CD8– (**e**), and PD1 (**f**)

Histologic Findings (Fig. 15.5a, b)

- A dense dermal lymphoid infiltrate composed of monomorphic medium- to large-sized atypical lymphoid cells.
- Epidermis is unremarkable.

Differential Diagnosis

- Primary cutaneous acral CD8-positive T-cell lymphoma
- Lymphomatoid papulosis
- Primary cutaneous anaplastic large cell lymphoma
- Primary cutaneous CD8 aggressive epidermotropic cytotoxic T-cell lymphoma

IHC and Other Ancillary Studies (Fig. 15.5c–e)

- Positive for CD3, CD8, CD2, CD5, TIA1, and TCRβ.
- Negative for CD4, granzyme, CD8, CD56, CD7, TCRδ, CD25, CD30, PD1, and EBER.
- Ki-67 proliferation index is 10%.
- Clonal *TCRG* gene rearrangements detected.

Final Diagnosis

Primary cutaneous acral CD8-positive T-cell lymphoma

Take-Home Messages

1. Primary cutaneous acral CD8-positive T-cell lymphoma is a rare type of indolent cutaneous T-cell proliferation.
2. Key features are:
   - Patients are asymptomatic and have no lymphadenopathy.

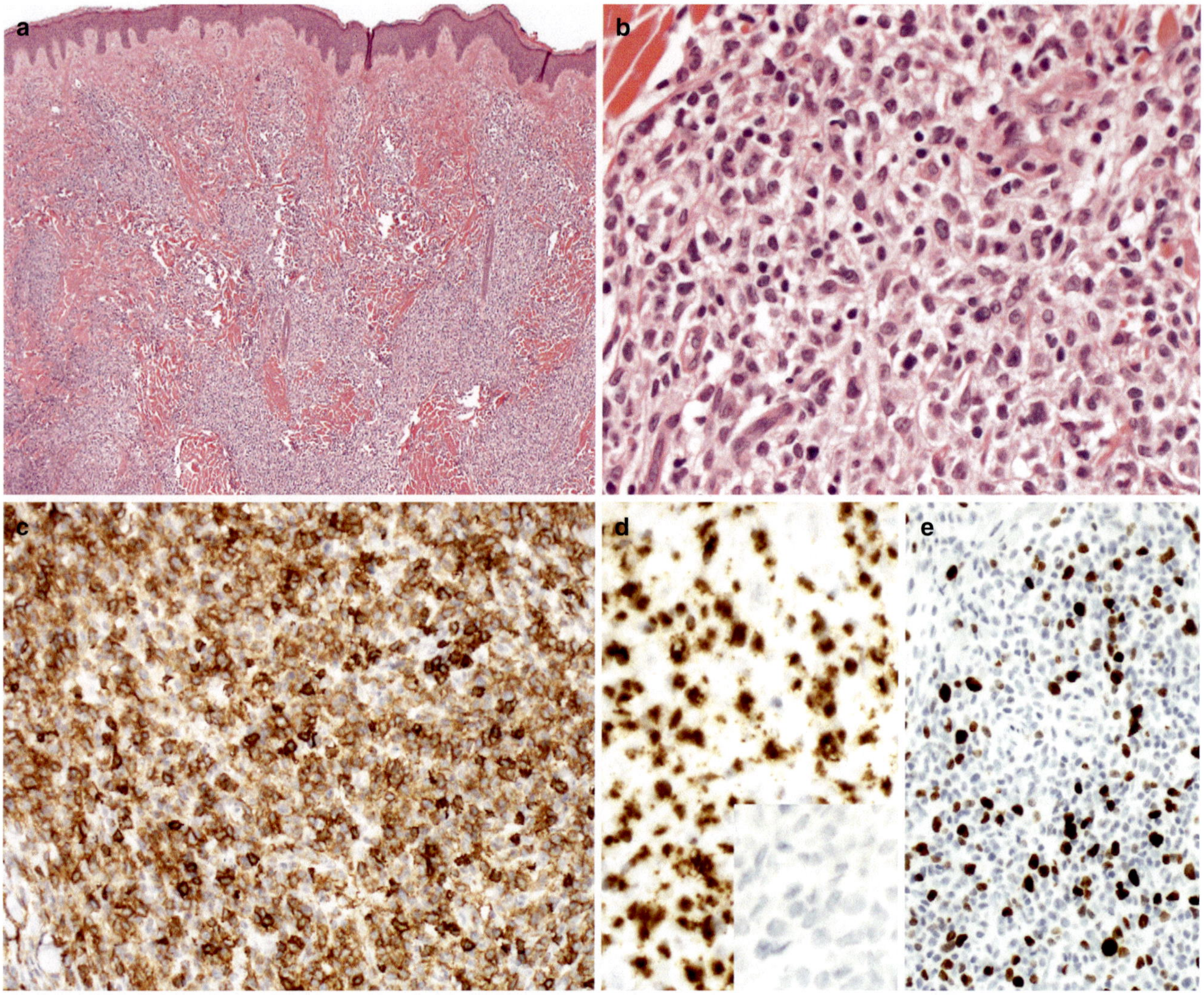

Fig. 15.5 Primary cutaneous acral CD8-positive T-cell lymphoma. (**a**) Low magnification of H&E stain of the skin biopsy shows a dense lymphoid infiltrate in the dermis. (**b**) High magnification of H&E stain shows predominantly small- to medium-sized lymphoid cells with minimal atypia. (**c–e**) Immunohistochemical stains show the lymphoid cells are CD8+ (**c**) and TIA1+ (**d,** inset, granzyme) and have low proliferation index demonstrated by Ki-67 (**e**)

- Solitary nodule involves the ear.
- The infiltrate is non-epidermotropic and involves dermis.
- The cells are CD8 and TIA1 positive but granzyme negative.

References

1. Shah MV, Hook CC, Call TG, Go RS. A population-based study of large granular lymphocyte leukemia. Blood Cancer J. 2016;6:e455.
2. Chan WC, Foucar K, Morice WG, Matutes E. T-cell large granulocytic leukemia. In: Swerdlow SH, Campo E, Harris NL, et al., editors. WHO Classification of tumors of haematopoietic and lymphoid tissue. Revised 4th ed. Lyon: International Agency for Research on Cancer (IARC); 2017.
3. Oshimi K. Clinical features, pathogenesis, and treatment of large granular lymphocyte leukemia. Intern Med. 2017;56:1759–69.
4. Jerez A, Clemente MJ, Makishima H, Koskela H, Leblanc F, Peng Ng K, et al. STAT3 mutations unify the pathogenesis of chronic lymphoproliferative disorders of NK cells and T-cell granular lymphocyte leukemia. Blood. 2012;120:3048–57.
5. Goyal T, Thakral B, Wang SA, Bueso-Ramos CE, Shi M, Jevremovic D, et al. T-cell large granular lymphocytic leukemia and coexisting B-cell lymphomas: A study from the Bone Marrow Pathology Group. Am J Clin Pathol. 2018;149:164–71.
6. Kataria A, Cohen E, Saad E, Atallah E, Bresnahan B. Large granular lymphocytic leukemia presenting later after solid organ transplantation: a case series of four patients and review of the literature. Transplant Proc. 2014;46:3278–81.
7. Lundell R, Hartung L, Hill S, Perkins SL, Bahler DW. T-cell large granular lymphocytes leukemias have multiple phenotypic abnormalities involving pan-T-cell antigens and receptors for MHC molecules. Am J Clin Pathol. 2005;124:937–46.

8. Lima M, Almeida J, Dos Anjos Teixeira M, Alguero Md Mdel C, Santos AH, Balanzategui A, et al. TCRalphabeta(+)/CD4+ large granular lymphocytosis: a new clonal T-cell lymphoproliferative disorder. Am J Pathol. 2003;163:763–71.
9. Chen YH, Chadburn A, Evens AM, Winter JN, Gordon LI, Chenn A, et al. Clinical, morphologic, immunophenotypic, and molecular cytogenetic assessment of CD4-/CD8- γδ T-cell large granular lymphocytic leukemia. Am J Clin Pathol. 2011;136:289–99.
10. Yabe M, Medeiros LJ, Wang SA, Tang G, Bueso-Ramos CE, Jorgensen JL, et al. Distinguishing between hepatosplenic T-cell lymphoma and gd T-cell large granular lymphocytic leukemia: a clinicopathologic, immunophenotypic, and molecular analysis. Am J Surg Pathol. 2017;41:82–93.
11. Singleton TP, Yin B, Teferra A, Mao JZ. Spectrum of clonal large granular lymphocytes (LGLs) of ab T cells: T-cell clones of undetermined significance, T-cell LGL leukemias, and T-cell immunoclones. Am J Clin Pathol. 2015;144:137–44.
12. Zhang X, Sokol L, Bennett JM, Moscinski LC, List A, Zhang L. T-cell large granular lymphocytes proliferation in myelodysplastic syndromes: Clinicopathologic features and prognostic significance. Leuk Res. 2016;43:18–23.
13. Schrenk KG, Krokowski M, Feller AC, Bernhard V, Mügge LO, Oelzner P, et al. Clonal T-LGL population mimicking leukemia in Felty's syndrome-part of a continuous spectrum of T-LGL proliferation? Ann Hematol. 2013;92:985–7.
14. Prochorec-Sobieszek M, Rymkiewicz G, Makuch-Lasica H, Majewski M, Michalak K, Rupiński R, et al. Characteristics of T-cell large granular lymphocytes proliferations associated with neutropenia and inflammatory arthropathy. Arthritis Res Ther. 2008;10:R55.
15. Munoz-Ballester J, Chen-Liang TH, Hurtado AM, Heras I, de Arriba F, García-Malo MD, et al. Persistent cytotoxic T lymphocyte expansion after allogeneic haematopoietic stem cell transplantation: kinetics, clinical impact and absence of STAT3 mutation. Br J Haematol. 2016;172:937–46.
16. Poch Martell M, Hamad N, Shin E, Moon JH, Sohn SK, Uhm J, et al. Distinctive clinical characteristics and favorable outcomes in patients with large granulocytosis after all-HCT: 12-year follow-up data. Eur J Haematol. 2017;99:160–8.
17. Nicolae A, Xi L, Pittaluga S, Abdullaev Z, Pack SD, Chen J, et al. Frequent STAT5 mutations in gd hepatosplenic T-cell lymphomas. Leukemia. 2014;28:2244–8.
18. Koskela HL, Eldfors S, Ellonen P, van Adrichem AJ, Kuusanmäki H, Andersson EI, et al. Somatic STAT3 mutations in large granular lymphocytic leukemia. N Engl J Med. 2012;366:1905–13.
19. Bareau B, Rey J, Hamidou M, Donadieu J, Morcet J, Reman O, et al. Analysis of a French cohort of patients with large granular lymphocyte leukemia: a report on 229 cases. Haematologica. 2010;95:1534–41.
20. Rabbani GR, Phyliky RL, Tefferi A. A long-term study of patients with chronic natural killer cell lymphocytosis. Br J Haematol. 1999;106:96–966.
21. Lima M, Almeida J, Montero AG, Teixeira Mdos A, Queirós ML, Santos AH, et al. Clinicobiological, immunophenotypic, and molecular characteristics of monoclonal CD56−/+dim chronic natural killer cell large granular lymphocytosis. Am J Pathol. 2004;165:1117–27.
22. Pascal V, Schleinitz N, Brunet C, Ravet S, Bonnet E, Lafarge X, et al. Comparative analysis of NK subset distribution in normal and lymphoproliferative disease of granular lymphocytes conditions. Eur J Immunol. 2004;34:2930–40.
23. Epling-Burnetter PK, Painter JS, Chaurasia P, Bai F, Wei S, Djeu JY, et al. Dysregulated Nk receptor expression in patients with lymphoproliferative disease of granular lymphocytes. Blood. 2004;103:3431–9.
24. Morice WG, Kurtin PJ, Leison PJ, Tefferi A, Hanson CA. Demonstration of aberrant T-cell and natural killer-cell antigen expression in all cases of granular lymphocytic leukemia. Br J Haematol. 2003;120:1026–36.
25. Nicolae A, Ganapathi KA, Pham TH, Xi L, Torres-Cabala CA, Nanaji NM, et al. EBV-negative aggressive NK-cell leukemia/lymphoma: clinical, pathologic and genetic features. Am J Surg Pathol. 2017;41:67–74.
26. De Mel S, Li JB, Abid MB, Tang T, Tay HM, Ting WC, et al. The utility of flow cytometry in differentiating NK/T cell lymphoma from indolent and reactive NL cell proliferations. Cytometry B Clin Cytom. 2018;94:159–68.
27. Perry AM, Warnke RA, Hu Q, Gaulard P, Copie-Bergman C, Alkan S, et al. Indolent T-cell lymphoproliferative disease of the gastrointestinal tract. Blood. 2013;122:3599–606.
28. Edison N, BelhancesPeled H, Eitan Y, Guthmann Y, Yeremenko Y, Raffeld M, et al. Indolent T-cell lymphoproliferative disease of the gastrointestinal tract after treatment with adalimumab in resistant Crohn's colitis. Hum Pathol. 2016;57:45–50.
29. Soon G, Wang S. Indolent T-cell lymphoproliferative disease of the gastrointestinal tract in a renal transplant patient: diagnostic pitfalls and clinical challenges. Pathology. 2017;49:547–50.
30. Margolskee E, Jobanputra V, Lewis SK, Alobeid B, Green PH, Bhagat G. Indolent small intestinal CD4+ T-cell lymphoma is a distinct entity with unique biologic and clinical features. PLoS One. 2013;8:e68343.
31. Leventaki V, Manning JT, Luthra R, Mehta P, Oki Y, Romaguera JE, et al. Indolent peripheral T-cell lymphoma involving the gastrointestinal tract. Hum Pathol. 2014;45:421–6.
32. Umetsu SF, Brown I, Langner C, Lauwers GY. Autoimmune enteropathies. Virchows Arch. 2018;472:55–66.
33. Sharma A, Oishi N, Boddicker RL, Hu G, Benson HK, Ketterling RP, et al. Recurrent *STAT3-JAK2* fusions in indolent T-cell lymphoproliferative disorder of the gastrointestinal tract. Blood. 2018;131:2262–6.
34. Chou R, Bougatsos C, Blazina I, Mackey K, Grusing S, Selph S. Screening for celiac disease evidence report and systematic review for the US preventive services task force. JAMA. 2017;317:1258–68.
35. Mansoor A, Pittaluga S, Beck PL, Wilson WH, Ferry JA, Jaffe ES. NK-cell enteropathy: a benign NK-cell lymphoproliferative disease mimicking intestinal lymphoma: clinicopathologic features and follow-up in a unique case series. Blood. 2011;117:1447–52.
36. Takeuchi K, Yokoyama M, Ishizawa S, Terui Y, Nomura K, Marutsuka K, et al. Lymphomatoid gastropathy: a distinct clinicopathologic entity of self-limited pseudomalignant NK-cell proliferation. Blood. 2010;116:5631–7.
37. Garcia-Herrera A, Colomo L, Camós M, Carreras J, Balague O, Martinez A, et al. Primary cutaneous small/medium CD4+ T-cell lymphomas: a heterogeneous group of tumors with different clinicopathologic features and outcome. J Clin Oncol. 2008;26:3364–71.
38. Grogg KL, Jung S, Erickson LA, McClure RF, Dogan A. Primary cutaneous CD4-positive small/medium-sized pleomorphic T-cell lymphoma: a clonal T-cell lymphoproliferative disorder with indolent behavior. Mod Pathol. 2008;21:708–15.
39. Petrella T, Maubec E, Cornillet-Lefebvre P, Willemze R, Pluot M, Durlach A, et al. Indolent CD8-positive lymphoid proliferation of the ear: a distinct primary cutaneous T-cell lymphoma? Am J Surg Pathol. 2007;31:1887–92.
40. Kluk J, Kai A, Koch D, Taibjee SM, O'Connor S, Persic M, et al. Indolent CD8-positive lymphoid proliferation of acral sites: three further cases of a rare entity and an update on a unique patient. J Cutan Pathol. 2016;43:125–36.

16 Composite Lymphoma

Rohit Gulati and Jiehao Zhou

List of Frequently Asked Questions

1. What is composite lymphoma and what is the incidence of composite lymphoma?
2. Are the components of composite lymphoma clonally related?
3. What is the utility of assessment of clonality in composite lymphoma?
4. What are the hypotheses explaining the pathogenesis of composite lymphoma?
5. What are the major subtypes of composite lymphoma?
6. What are the typical morphological findings in composite lymphoma?
7. What are the main ancillary studies and their role in diagnosis of composite lymphoma?
8. What findings are suggestive for composite lymphoma diagnosis?
9. What are the main mimics of composite lymphoma?
10. What is an appropriate sample to diagnose composite lymphoma?
11. What is an appropriate reporting format of composite lymphoma?
12. What are the treatment considerations for composite lymphoma?

R. Gulati · J. Zhou (✉)
Department of Pathology and Laboratory Medicine, Indiana University School of Medicine, Indianapolis, IN, USA
e-mail: zhouji@iupui.edu

1. What is composite lymphoma and what is the incidence of composite lymphoma?

- *Definition:* Composite lymphoma (CL) is simultaneous presence of multiple distinct lymphoma types at the same anatomic site.
- The term "composite lymphoma" (CL) was coined by Custer in 1954 to describe "the occurrence of more than one histological pattern of lymphoma in a single patient" [1]. This entity was further defined by Kim and colleagues to only include cases with two or more distinct types of lymphoma involving the same organ or tissue in 1977 [2]. The latter definition was eventually adopted by the Working Formulation of NHL in 1982 [3].
- CL is currently not an entity defined in the WHO classification of hematopoietic neoplasia (2017) [4]. The inclusion criteria for CL remain a matter of debate.
  - It should be noted that some clinicians use the term "CL" in a less specific manner to include all cases of multiple lymphomas in a patient, even though occurring at different anatomical locations or at different times. However, most pathologists believe that the former should be called as simultaneous lymphoma and the latter as sequential lymphoma, respectively [5].
- In this chapter, for practical purpose, we adopt the definition used by many pathologists to define CL as simultaneous presence of multiple distinct lymphoma types at the same anatomic site.
- It is well documented that low-grade lymphomas can transform to a higher-grade process as part of the natural course of disease. For example, chronic lymphocytic leukemia/small lymphocytic lymphoma (CLL/SLL) can transform into diffuse large B-cell lymphoma (DLBCL) [4] or classic Hodgkin lymphoma (CHL) [6]; follicular lymphoma (FL) and other low-grade B-cell lymphoma can transform into DLBCL [4]; indolent mycosis fungoides (MF) can have histological large cell transformation, defined by the presence of >25% large lymphoid cells in the dermal infiltrates [7].

E. Wang, A. S. Lagoo (eds.), *Practical Lymph Node and Bone Marrow Pathology*, Practical Anatomic Pathology,
https://doi.org/10.1007/978-3-030-32189-5_16

  - Occasionally, the lower-grade lymphoma co-exists with its transformed higher-grade counterpart in the same tissue biopsy. By strict definition, it is arguable that this represents a form of composite lymphoma. However, details of lymphoma transformation/progression will not be discussed in this chapter but are considered in other chapters of this book. The current chapter will focus on CL other than lymphoma with transformation.
- *Incidence:* CL represents 1–4.7% of all lymphomas based on published data. Though initially thought to be a rare entity, the six decades following the first report have witnessed a steady rise in number of CL. This progressive increase in incidence may be attributed to the widespread utilization of ancillary diagnostic modalities including immunohistochemistry, flow cytometry, cytogenetics, and molecular studies.
- Lymph node is the most common organ involved by CL. Spleen, gastrointestinal tract, lung, salivary glands, skin, bone, liver, and bone marrow are common extranodal sites which have been affected by CL [8, 9].

2. Are the components of composite lymphoma clonally related?

- CL components can be either clonally related or independent. Initially it was thought that the components of a CL would be clonally independent, given the different morphology and immunophenotype. However, recent investigations using molecular methods have confirmed that a significant proportion of these distinct lymphomas within CL are clonally related [10–14], although there are more cases of CL containing clonally independent components [15, 16].
- The clonal relationship of CL components varies significantly among different CL subtypes and will be discussed further in this chapter. The take-home message by the currently acceptable definition is that CL should be used as a descriptive term and includes both clonally related and unrelated lymphomas.

3. What is the utility of assessment of clonality in composite lymphoma?

- Diagnostic role: proof of clonality of each lymphoma component may act as supportive evidence for diagnosis of each component and thus establish the diagnosis of CL.
- Understanding the biology behind the development of CL.
- Evaluation of clonality of each component helps to investigate clonal relationship of CL components.

4. What are the hypotheses explaining the pathogenesis of composite lymphoma?

A number of hypotheses have been suggested to explain the existence of composite lymphomas [17–20].

- Simple coincidence
- Malignant transformation of a common stem cell with the capacity to differentiate into different lymphomas
- Genetic predisposition leading to simultaneous but independent development of two lymphomas
- Immune dysregulation and immunodeficiency associated with propensity to develop mixed neoplastic clones
- Exposure to chemotherapy for one tumor inducing secondary neoplasms
- The presence of one lymphoma causing reduced capacity to overcome the lymphomagenic effect of pre-established viral infection such as *EBV*, or enhanced carcinogenic effects of new viral infection or other carcinogens

5. What are the major subtypes of composite lymphoma?

The morphology of CL can be very diverse depending on the two (or more) lymphomas comprising the CL. Many different combinations of lymphomas have been described in CL. The most commonly reported cases comprise two or more B-cell non-Hodgkin lymphoma (NHL) or a B-cell NHL with a Hodgkin lymphoma (HL) [21]. There are five major subtypes of CL based on the lymphoma composition.

- *Two or more B-cell NHL:* This is a common subtype of CL and in theory can encompass all possible combinations of B-cell NHL defined in WHO classification.
  - The most common form is a combination of low-grade B-cell lymphoma with a higher-grade B-cell lymphoma, often DLBCL. This subtype of CL usually represents a B-cell lymphoma with transformation [22] which will be discussed in other chapters.
  - Other forms of CL within this subtype include different combinations of low-grade B-cell lymphomas including but not restricted to mantle cell lymphoma (MCL), CLL/SLL, FL, and marginal zone lymphoma (MZL) [10, 23, 24].
  - Cases of co-existence of two or more high-grade B-cell lymphoma are rare but have been reported [25].
  - The lymphoma components in CL comprising a low-grade and high-grade B-cell lymphoma are often clonally related, although clonally unrelated cases have been reported [26]. CL composed of two low-grade B-cell lymphomas or two high-grade B-cell lymphomas are less likely to be clonally related. More combinations of CL in this subtype are listed in Table 16.1.

Table 16.1 Summary of composite lymphomas reported in literature

		B-NHL
B-NHL	DLBCL	CLL/SLL FL LPL[17,36] SMZL MALT NMZL MCL[37] BL
	FL	DLBCL MCL[38] CLL[39] BL NMZL
	CLL/SLL	DLBCL MCL FL[39] BL PCN[40]
	MCL	FL CLL BL PBL SMZL NMZL[41] PCN[42] DLBCL[37]
	PCN	LPL NMZL[43] CLL[12] MCL

		B-NHL
HL	CHL	CLL/SLL LPL[44,45] SMZL NMZL[46] MALT[46] FL[11,44] MCL[12] DLBCL[13,44] TCRBCL BL PMBL
	NLPHL	FL[47] DLBCL BL Heavy Chain Disease-gamma

		B-NHL
T-NHL	AITL	DLBCL[49,50] PCN
	MF	MALT[51] CLL[51,52] DLBCL
	PTCL	CLL[17] MALT NMZL Small B cell lymphoma[17] DLBCL[53,54]
	Sezary syndrome	Small B-cell Lymphoma
	ATLL	DLBCL[55]

		T-NHL
HL	CHL	PTCL ATLL T-PLL CTCL MF
	NLPHL	PTCL[48]

		T-NHL
T-NHL	MF	PTCL ALCL, ALK-

		HL
HL	CHL	NLPHL

AITL **angioimmunoblastic T-cell lymphoma,** *ALCL* **anaplastic large cell lymphoma,** *ATLL* **adult T-cell leukemia/lymphoma,** *BL* **Burkitt lymphoma,** *CHL* **classic Hodgkin lymphoma,** *CLL/SLL* **chronic lymphocytic leukemia/small lymphocytic lymphoma,** *CTCL* **cutaneous T-cell lymphoma,** *DLBCL* **diffuse large B-cell lymphoma,** *FL* **follicular lymphoma,** *LPL* **lymphoplasmacytic lymphoma,** *MALT* **extranodal marginal zone B-cell lymphoma of MALT,** *NHL* **non-Hodgkin lymphoma,** *MCL* **mantle cell lymphoma,** *MF* **mycosis fungoides,** *NLPHL* **nodular lymphocyte-predominant Hodgkin lymphoma,** *NMZL* **nodal marginal zone lymphoma,** *PBL* **plasmablastic lymphoma,** *PCN* **plasma cell neoplasm,** *PTCL* **peripheral T-cell lymphoma,** *SMZL* **splenic marginal zone lymphoma,** *TCRBCL* **T-cell/histiocyte-rich large B-cell lymphoma,** *T-PLL* **T-cell prolymphocytic leukemia**

- *HL with NHL:* This subtype of CL is well published, and the most common combination is CHL with a NHL of B-cell lineage, either indolent or aggressive.
  - B-cell lymphoma components include CLL/SLL, FCL, MZL, MCL, DLBCL, NOS, T-cell-rich large B-cell lymphoma (TCRBCL), and primary mediastinal large B-cell lymphoma (PMBL) [11, 12, 14, 27–29]. Despite a distinct morphology and immunophenotypic difference between HL and NHL, the HL and NHL in CL are frequently clonally related.

It should be noted that when a CHL co-exists with a CLL, it usually represents transformation of CLL [18, 30]. Similarly, nodular lymphocyte-predominant Hodgkin lymphoma (NLPHL) co-presenting with DLBCL represents a high-grade transformation of the NLPHL [31].

  - A few cases of CHL with a T-cell NHL have been also reported, and the T-cell lymphoma components in CL include peripheral T-cell lymphoma (PTCL) NOS, T-cell prolymphocytic leukemia (T-PLL), and cutaneous T-cell lymphoma (CTCL) [32].
  - Please refer to Table 16.1 for more combinations of CL within this subtype.
- *B-cell NHL with T-cell NHL:* The incidence of this CL subtype is very low with fewer than 100 reported cases [21, 33].
  - The most common B-cell NHL identified in this subtype is DLBCL. Other types of B-cell NHL in this type of CL include FL, MCL, lymphoplasmacytic lymphoma (LPL), hairy cell leukemia (HCL), MALT lymphoma, and CLL/SLL.
  - PTCL, NOS and angioimmunoblastic T-cell lymphoma (AITL) are the most frequently identified T-cell NHL component. Other types of T-cell lymphoma include hepatosplenic T-cell lymphoma, T-cell large granular cell leukemia, anaplastic large cell lymphoma (ALCL), and CTCL.
  - Components in this subtype of CL are usually clonally unrelated.
- *Two T-cell NHLs:* This subtype is rare. The reported combinations of two T-cell NHLs include MF with PTCL, NOS and MF with ALK-ALCL [34]. Due to extremely low incidence of this CL subtype, the clonal relationship of CL components remains to be determined although some cases appear to be clonally related.
- *CHL with NLPHL:* This combination is extremely rare. Molecular analyses on isolated tumor cells have proved that the NLPHL and CHL in CL are clonally related [35]. In addition, often only the CHL component but not the NLPHL harbored *EBV* if EBER in situ hybridization is positive in CL.

6. What are the typical morphological findings in composite lymphoma?

- Effacement of the underlying nodal and extranodal architecture.
- Morphology of CL varies significantly due to different combinations of lymphoma components.
- Each component of CL may individually present the morphologic features as described in WHO classification:
  - Cytomorphologic features of neoplastic lymphoid cells such as irregular nucleus, abnormal chromatic texture, and aberrant nuclear/cytoplasmic ratio can be identified.
  - Morphologic features of each individual lymphoma component are present. For example, CLL commonly presents as diffuse infiltrates of monotonous small round lymphocytes with mature chromatin; FL shows nodular proliferation of small centrocytes with cleaved nucleus admixed with few scattered large centroblasts; DLBCL demonstrates diffuse proliferation of large atypical lymphoid cells with either centroblastic or immunoblastic morphology; CHL manifests as scattered Reed–Sternberg (RS) cells and variant Hodgkin cells in a background of mixed infiltrates.
  - The topographic distribution of each neoplastic component is variable, from indisputably evident to highly subtle. Some cases may show clear-cut demarcation between different lymphoma components, whereas others show uneven distribution with one component overshadowing the other one. Occasionally, one lymphoma component may intermingle within the other component. Therefore, the diagnosis of CL based solely on histomorphologic findings is very challenging. Thus, application of ancillary studies is indispensable in essentially all CL diagnosis.

7. What are the main ancillary studies and their role in diagnosis of composite lymphoma?

According to the current World Health Organization classification, lymphomas are defined by their morphology, immunophenotype, cytogenetics, and clinical features [4]. Thus, ancillary tests are critically important tools in diagnosing CL.

- The ancillary studies used in diagnosis of CL are the same as those used in diagnosis of single lymphoma and include flow cytometry analysis, immunohistochemistry, cytogenetics/FISH, and *IGH/TCR* gene rearrangement study. The decision on which of the ancillary tests are to be used depends on the clinical and morphologic features of the individual cases. The following ancillary work-ups are of great importance in diagnosing CL.
  - Flow cytometry analysis and immunohistochemistry: Immunophenotyping by flow cytometry analysis and/or immunohistochemistry is essential in CL diagnosis. The diagnosis of CL can be achieved based on morphology evaluation and flow cytometric immunophenotyping when the lymphoma components in CL show evidently diverse morphology and two phenotypically different, monotypic B-cell populations are detected.

- T-cell clonality is more difficult to determine by flow cytometry. The demonstration of an abnormal phenotype on a large percentage of T-cells is a useful, albeit indirect indicator of T-cell clonality. Despite its infrequent application, some labs use restricted TCR repertoire (V-beta analysis) to establish T-lymphocyte clonality [56].
- In addition to confirming lymphocyte clonality, flow cytometry analysis can determine detailed immunophenotype in cells of interest to further categorize the lymphoma types, particularly B-cell lymphomas, as described in earlier chapters. The possibility of an atypical antigen expression pattern, such as CD10-negative FL, CD5-negative MCL, CD5-positive LPL, etc., can add another level of complexity in diagnosing CL cases.
- There is potential pitfall of flow cytometry analysis for immunophenotyping. In about 15–25% of DLBCL flow cytometry analysis results may be nondiagnostic due to the abundance of nonviable cells or fragile cells that are lost during the processing.
- Some lymphomas such as Hodgkin lymphoma and T-cell-rich B-cell lymphoma frequently show nondiagnostic flow cytometry result due to low number of neoplastic cells. In the absence of a positive flow cytometry result, if morphology supports, immunohistochemistry should be employed to characterize the cells of interest. Immunohistochemistry study can provide the spatial and distribution information of individual components of CL.

- Cytogenetics and FISH studies: Both conventional cytogenetics by karyotyping and FISH study are used to demonstrate the characteristic recurrent cytogenetic abnormalities found in certain lymphomas. FISH performed on FFPE sections can be particularly valuable if the divergent results correlate with morphologically distinct areas.
  - It should be noted that the identification of certain abnormal cytogenetics is not sufficient by itself to diagnose a specific lymphoma. Instead, it is suggestive of a particular diagnosis. For example, t(14;18)(*IGH/BCL2*) is commonly seen in FL. However, a subset of DLBCL can also harbor the same cytogenetics abnormality. Therefore, cytogenetics/FISH study result should be interpreted under an appropriate clinical and morphologic setting.
- Immunoglobulin and *TCR* gene rearrangement: Gene rearrangement of immunoglobulin and *TCR* by PCR, and more recently by next generation sequencing technology, which provides increased sensitivity and specificity compared to PCR [57], have replaced older methods of Southern blot analysis to determining clonality of B cells and T cells, respectively (see Chap. 2).
  - In practice, these ancillary studies are frequently used in CL diagnosis when morphology and immunophenotypic work-up fail to establish a convincing evidence of lymphocyte clonality. Sometimes, tissue microdissection is required to prevent contamination in diagnostic work-up for CL.
  - These DNA-based tests, in particular the NGS method, are also used to establish clonal relationship between different components in CL.
- Gene mutational study by sequencing: Of the many genes analyzed by next generation sequencing (NGS) (Table 16.2), two genes particularly stand out in strong association with specific lymphomas and are useful when analyzing the components of CL.
  - *BRAF* V600E mutation has proved to be very sensitive and specific for hairy cell leukemia (HCL) diagnosis within mature B-cell lymphoproliferative disorders [58, 59]. The positive and negative predictive value is estimated at ~97%, respectively. Only rare unclassifiable splenic B-cell lymphoma and rare CLL showed *BRAF* V600E mutation. On the other hand, only small subset of hairy cell leukemia lacks *BRAF* V600E mutation, particularly those HCLs expressing *IGHV4-34*. Therefore, V600E mutation study is a very useful diagnostic tool for HCL, particularly for those HCLs with atypical morphology and immunophenotypical features.
  - *MYD88* L265P is present in approximately 91% of patients with LPL and absent in multiple myeloma and rarely present in other low-grade B-cell lymphomas including splenic MZL, CLL, and HCL [60]. Although not entirely specific, the presence of *MYD88* L265P is a very helpful tool to differentiate LPL from other lymphoproliferative disorders, particularly plasma cell neoplasm, the most important differential diagnosis of LPL.

    Of note, *MYD88* L265P is relatively common in a subset of DLBCL with an activated B-cell-like immunophenotype, primary DLBCL of the central nervous system and primary cutaneous DLBCL, leg type. These large B-cell lymphomas can be easily separated from low-grade B-cell lymphoma based on morphology features.

8. What findings are suggestive for composite lymphoma diagnosis?

Any finding which cannot be readily explained by one single lymphoma entity should raise a differential for CL. These findings can be clinical presentation, laboratory parameters, morphology, immunophenotypes, cytogenetics, and molecular abnormalities. Here are some examples:

Table 16.2 Common genetic abnormalities in lymphomas [61–63]

Lymphoid neoplasia	Genetic alteration	Mechanism/significance
Diffuse large B-cell lymphoma	*EZH2* mutation	Almost exclusive in GC-type DLBCL Histone methyltransferase activity
	GNA13 mutation *MYD88* mutation	Almost exclusive in GC-type DLBCL Associated with activated B-cell type NF-kB pathway
	CARD11 mutation	Associated with activated B-cell type NF-kB pathway
	CD79B mutation	Associated with activated B-cell type BCR-subunit
	CREBBP mutation *E300* mutation *KMT2D* mutation	Histone acetylation Histone acetylation Histone methyltransferase activity
	MEFB2 mutation *TBL1XR1-TP63* fusion	Histone acetylation activity Disruption of p53 tumor suppressor pathway
Follicular lymphoma	*EZH2* mutation *CREBBP* mutation *E300* mutation *KMT2D* mutation *MEFB2* mutation *TBL1XR1-TP63* fusion	Histone methyltransferase activity Histone acetylation activity Histone acetylation activity Histone methyltransferase activity Histone acetylation activity Disruption of p53 tumor suppressor pathway
Classic Hodgkin lymphoma	*CIITA* fusions	MHC class II transactivator Promiscuous fusion partners
	STAT6 mutation *TP53* mutation	JAK–STAT signal transduction pathway Disruption of p53 tumor suppressor pathway
Primary mediastinal large B-cell lymphoma	*CIITA* fusions	MHC class II transactivator Fuses with PD1 ligand genes in 50% of cases
	STAT6 mutation	JAK–STAT signal transduction pathway
Chronic lymphocytic leukemia	*NOTCH1* mutation *MYD88* mutation *XPO1* mutation *KLHL6* mutation *SF3B1* mutation	Associated with unmutated IGH Associated with mutated IGH Associated with unmutated IGH Associated with mutated IGH Member of RNA splicing machinery Associated with disease progression
Splenic B-cell marginal zone lymphoma	*NOTCH2* mutation	Gain of function mutation targeting the PEST domain
Hairy cell leukemia	*BRAF* V600E mutation *CDKN1B* mutation	MAPK pathway Highly sensitive and specific Disruption of tumor suppressor pathway
Lymphoplasmacytic lymphoma	*MYD88* mutation *ARID1A* mutation	NF-kB pathway activation Loss of function mutations
Mantle cell lymphoma	*NOTCH1* mutation	Associated with poor clinical outcome
Peripheral T-cell lymphoma	*DUSP22-FRA7H* fusion *TP63* fusions	Identified in ALCL, ALK-negative Identified in PTCL, NOS and ALCL, ALK-negative; disruption of p53 tumor suppressor pathway

- Clinically, a patient with chronic stable lymphadenopathy who presented with sudden enlargement of lymph node may suggest a high-grade transformation or coexistence of a high-grade lymphoma.
- The presence of two monoclonal proteins with different heavy chain or different light chain expression by serum protein electrophoresis and/or immunofixation electrophoresis may suggest more than one B-cell lymphoproliferative disorders.
- Divergent morphology/immunophenotypic features suggestive of more than one lymphoma component such as low-grade component co-existing with a high-grade component or NHL co-existing with an HL.
- Coexistence of multiple distinct cytogenetics abnormalities which are a hallmark of different lymphomas. For example, detection of both t(11;14) of *CCND1* translocation and t(14:18) of *BCL2* translocation in the same biopsy suggests a composite mantle cell lymphoma and follicular lymphoma.
- Coexistence of both clonal *IGH* and *TCR* rearrangement in the same tissue biopsy should raise a concern for composite B- and T-cell lymphoma. See also Chap. 2 for caveats when using presence clonal rearrangements of Ig or TCR genes as evidence of cell lineage.

It should be emphasized that the diagnosis of CL requires a high degree of suspicion based on prior experience followed by a comprehensive approach to prove or rule out the suspected "second" lymphoma. Any one of aforementioned findings alone is not sufficient for CL diagnosis.

9. What are the main mimics of composite lymphoma?

CL exhibits a diverse morphological spectrum based on its components. Hence, the diagnostic mimics are also different for each subtype.

- Mimics for the composite lymphoma with two B-NHL:
  - Low-grade B-cell lymphoma with areas of atypical architecture or cytomorphology may mimic composite lymphoma of two B-NHLs. For example, it was estimated that follicular colonization can be present in 14–44% of MZL, whereas a prominent monocytoid lymphocyte proliferation can be observed in ~9% of follicular lymphoma [64, 65]. Thus, both FL with marginal zone differentiation and MZL with follicular colonization are not uncommon. These morphologic variants are morphologic mimics of composite follicular lymphoma and marginal zone lymphoma.

    Ancillary studies including flow cytometry analysis, immunohistochemistry, and sometimes FISH may help make this distinction. Compared to true composite follicular and marginal zone lymphoma, these mimics usually demonstrate one monoclonal B-cell population by flow cytometry analysis. FL with marginal differentiation usually still retains germinal center B-cell immunophenotype such as positivity for CD10, BCL6, HGAL, and LMO2, whereas marginal zone lymphoma is negative for these markers. *IGH/BCL2* translocation is identified in majority of follicular lymphoma even it shows extensive marginal zone differentiation.
- Mimics for composite lymphoma with HL and B-NHL:
  - Low-grade B-cell lymphoma with RS-like cells: Not infrequently, CLL, MZL, and FL may contain large atypical cells, morphologically compatible with RS cells, interspersed within the neoplastic population [66, 67].

    In CLL, these RS-like cells may display an activated B-cell immunophenotype with expression of CD20 and CD30, and commonly *EBV+*.

    In the setting of follicular lymphomas, RS-like cells may be few or numerous and can be seen between or within the neoplastic follicles and are usually *EBV−*. In fact, in some cases, these RS-like cells may be immunophenotypically identical to RS cells in CHL. In the absence of an appropriate background/microenvironment, a diagnosis of CHL should not be rendered. The current data indicates that presence of RS-like cells alone does not change the diagnosis or confer a more aggressive clinical course.
  - Large B-cell lymphoma with RS-like cells: Scattered and sometimes clusters of pleomorphic cells resembling RS cells can be identified in large B-cell lymphoma, especially in *EBV*-positive DLBCL, NOS. These cells are usually positive for CD30 and occasionally co-express CD15. However, compared to CHL, these lymphoma cells are positive for CD20, CD79a, and PAX5 (strong). The expression of EBER is more uniform than CHL, highlighting both RS-like cells and smaller cells.
  - B-cell lymphoma, unclassifiable, with features intermediate between DLBCL and CHL: This large B-cell lymphoma shows morphologic and immunophenotypic features of both diffuse large B-cell lymphoma and classic Hodgkin lymphoma; the immunophenotype of both entities is characteristically expressed by same neoplastic cells (one abnormal population) [4]. In contrast, a composite lymphoma contains separate cell populations, where one population meets the morphologic and immunophenotypic criteria for DLBCL and the other population meets diagnostic criteria for CHL.
- Mimics for composite lymphoma with HL and T-NHL:
  - T-cell lymphomas such as PTCL, NOS, and AITL can also contain RS-like cells which can morphologically mimic CL [68, 69].
  - Rare cases of RS-like cells with T-cell lineage were reported in the literature. However, as previously described, the lack of the correct immunophenotype and/or the appropriate background essentially excludes classic Hodgkin lymphoma.

10. What is an appropriate sample to diagnose composite lymphoma?

- Excisional biopsy is the preferred sample. Because morphology and distribution pattern of CL varies significantly from case to case, it is conceivable that a minor component in CL may not be well represented if the submitted sample is limited. Therefore, the tissue must be adequately sampled.
- Neither fine needle aspiration nor small core biopsy is the suitable methodology to provide adequate sample for CL diagnosis. However, both FNA and core biopsy may provide the first diagnostic clue which may raise a suspicion for CL, particularly when the morphologic evaluation is coupled with immunophenotypic ancillary studies.
- Evaluation of excisional biopsy with at least flow cytometric analysis or immunohistochemical work-up is almost invariably required for establishing the diagnosis of CL beyond reasonable doubt.

11. What is an appropriate reporting format of composite lymphoma?

- Each individual component of CL should be listed in the diagnosis line.
- The term "composite lymphoma" is not required in the diagnosis line, but for the purpose of clarity and conveying the clinical significance of diagnosis, the relative percentage of each component should be reported as it may influence the treatment plan.

12. What are the treatment considerations for composite lymphoma?

- There is no consensus treatment guideline for CL although treatment is commonly aimed at the more aggressive component.
  - The general treatment strategy is to consider each component. The published data suggest that each component of a composite lymphoma behaves similarly to the respective entity alone.
  - Most clinicians opt to treat the patient against the more aggressive component of CL with the consideration of the other component in CL. Therefore, accurate diagnosis of CL will help the patient receive the most appropriate treatment.

Case Presentations

Case 1

Learning Objectives

1. To be familiar with the composite lymphoma subtype composed of two distinct B-cell lymphomas
2. To understand the divergent immunophenotypic finding as a clue for composite lymphoma diagnosis
3. To confirm diagnosis by immunohistochemical study and more definitively by FISH study when applicable

Case History

A 66-year-old female with extensive retroperitoneal and mesenteric adenopathy. Core biopsy of periaortic lymph node with flow cytometry analysis was performed.

Histologic Findings (Fig. 16.1)

- Effacement of normal lymphoid tissue architecture by nodular proliferation composed of predominantly small atypical lymphoid cells with irregular nuclei.
- The mitosis and apoptosis rate was not high.
- The lymphoid nodules lacked normal polarization and tingible body macrophages.

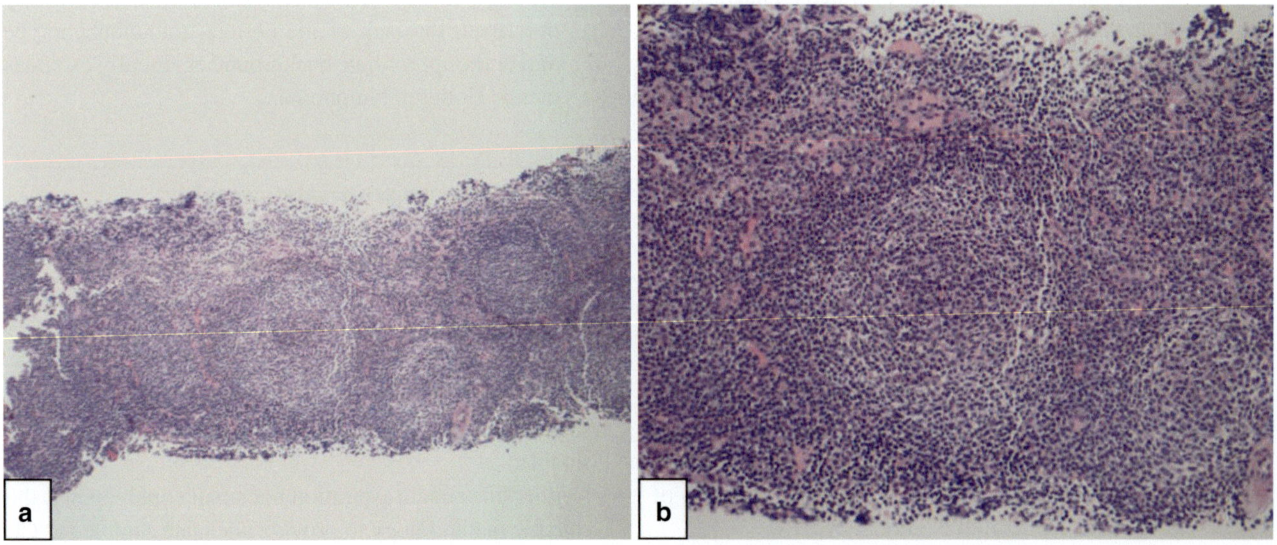

Fig. 16.1 Histology of lymph node core biopsy. (**a**) 40×; (**b**) 200×

Morphologic Diagnosis

- Lymphoma with small mature lymphoid cells and nodular pattern with follicular lymphoma as top differential diagnosis

Flow Cytometry Analysis (Fig. 16.2)

- Two monoclonal B-cell populations were identified by flow cytometry analysis. One was CD10+ monoclonal B-cell population with lambda light chain expression. The other one was CD5+ monoclonal B-cell population with kappa light chain expression. This finding raised a possibility of composite lymphoma of two monoclonal B-cell populations.

Immunohistochemical Stains (Fig. 16.3)

- Immunohistochemical stains show majority of atypical lymphoid cells were positive for PAX5, BCL6, and BCL2. In combination of nodular proliferation and CD10+ positivity by flow cytometry analysis, the finding was consistent with follicular lymphoma. Due to small size of core biopsy, a grade could not be adequately assessed.
- Subset of lymphocytes was also positive for cyclin D1, predominantly in the mantle zone and interfollicular region, which raised a possibility of mantle cell lymphoma.

FISH Study (Fig. 16.4)

- FISH study was positive for t(11;14), *CCND1/IGH* translocation, confirming the diagnosis of mantle cell lymphoma.

Final Diagnosis

Mantle cell lymphoma and follicular lymphoma

Take-Home Messages

1. The presence of two distinct monoclonal B-cell populations detected by flow cytometry analysis should raise a possibility of composite lymphoma composed of two B-cell NHLs.
2. Further work-up including immunohistochemistry and targeted FISH is employed to confirm the diagnosis.

Case 2

Learning Objectives

1. To learn that rarely a lymphoplasmacytic lymphoma coexists with plasma cell neoplasm

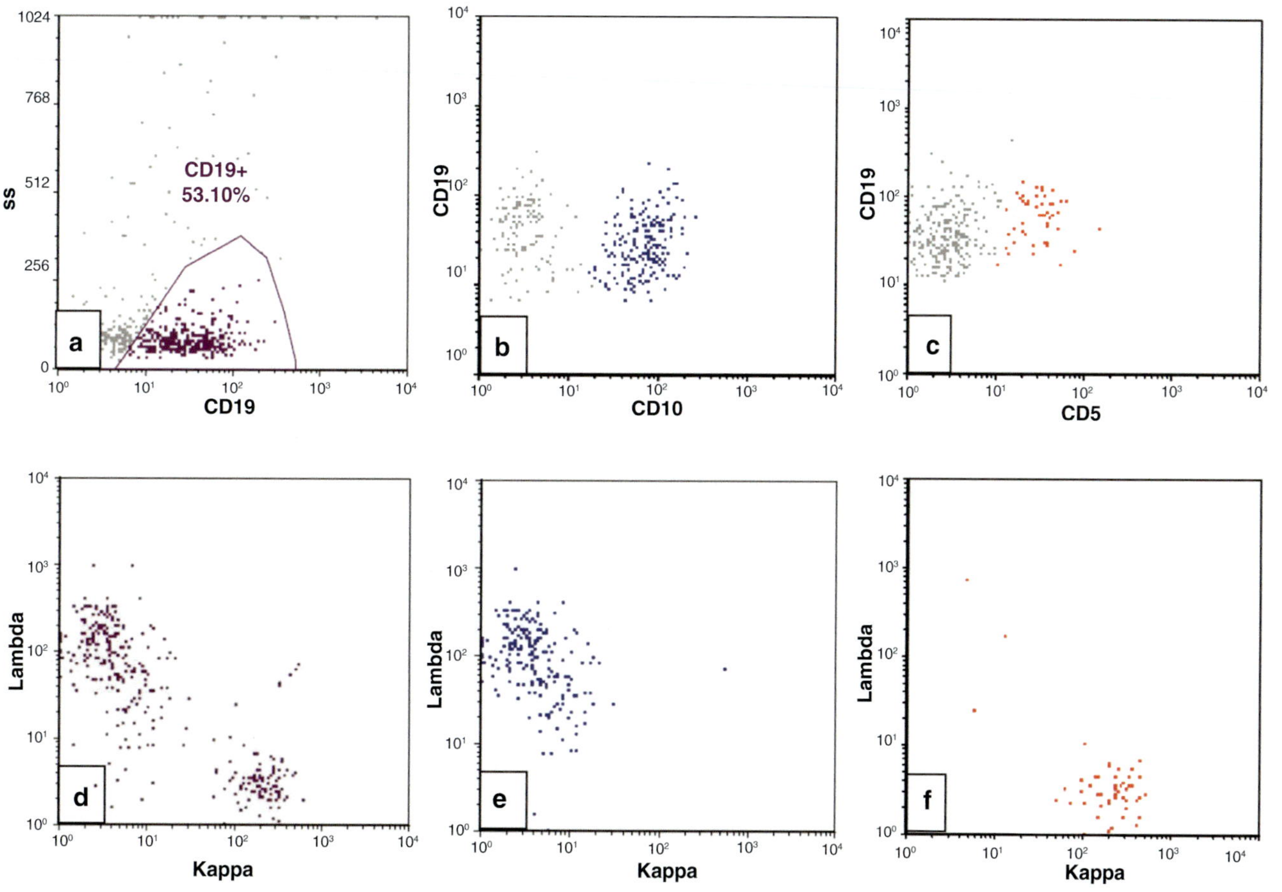

Fig. 16.2 Flow cytometry analysis of lymph node core biopsy

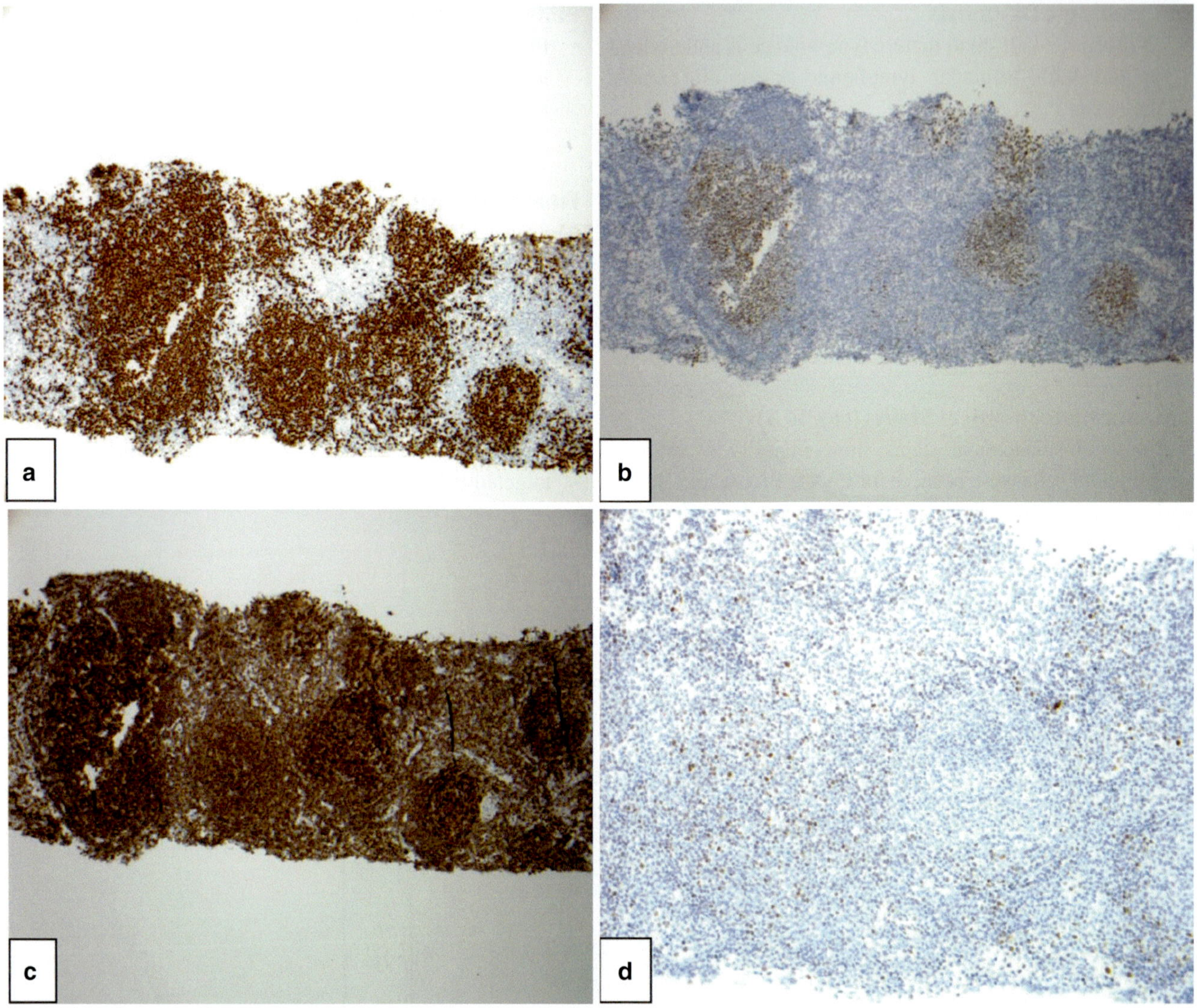

Fig. 16.3 Immunohistochemical work-up of lymph node core biopsy. (**a**) PAX5; (**b**) BCL6; (**c**) BCL2; (**d**) cyclin D1

2. To learn that the presence of multiple distinct monoclonal protein is a clue of composite lymphoid malignancy with immunoglobulin production
3. To learn that appropriate ancillary studies are required to confirm the diagnosis

Case History

A 76-year-old male presented with acetabular fracture. X-ray showed lytic lesion in the right pelvis. There was no lymphadenopathy and splenomegaly. Bone marrow biopsy is performed.

Laboratory Finding (Fig. 16.5)

- Serum protein electrophoresis and immunofixation electrophoresis showed one IgM kappa band and two IgA kappa bands. The presence of multiple monoclonal proteins with two different types of heavy chain suggested more than one clonal process.

Histologic Findings

- There were dense lymphoplasmacytic infiltrates in the bone marrow biopsy. Foci of plasma cell enrichment were present.

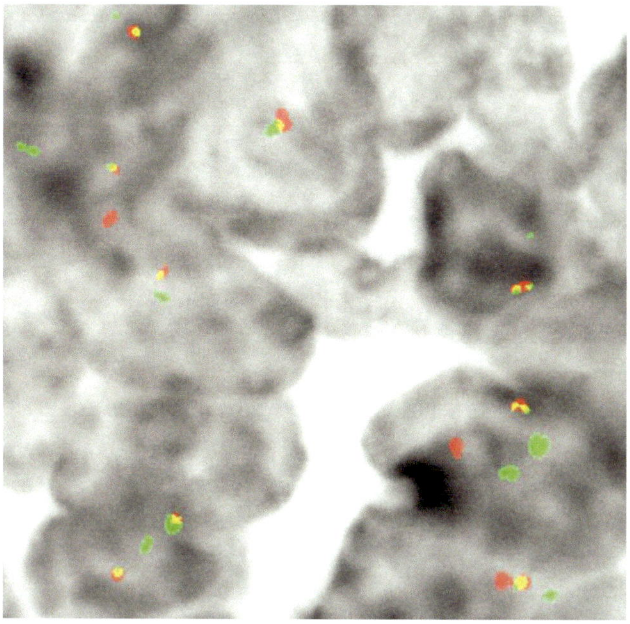

Fig. 16.4 FISH of core biopsy with *CCND1/IGH* translocation using *CCND1/IGH* dual color dual fusion translocation probe. The *IGH* probe is green and the *CCND1* probe is red. The abnormal cells show fused yellow signal

Morphologic Diagnosis

- B-cell lymphoma with plasmacytic differentiation or B-cell lymphoma co-existing with a plasma cell neoplasm

Flow Cytometry Analysis (Fig. 16.6)

- A kappa light chain restricted CD5-/CD10- monoclonal B-cell population and a kappa light chain restricted plasma cell population were identified by flow cytometry analysis.

Immunohistochemical Stains (Fig. 16.7)

- Immunohistochemical stains showed that majority of atypical lymphoid cells were B lymphocytes with positive CD20. The plasma cells were positive for CD138 and exclusively expressed kappa light chain. These plasma cells were also positive for cyclin D1 (nuclear staining brown) and IgA (cytoplasmic and red).

FISH Study

- FISH study was positive for t(11;14), *CCND1/IGH* translocation in plasma cell enriched smear, confirming the diagnosis of plasma cell neoplasm.

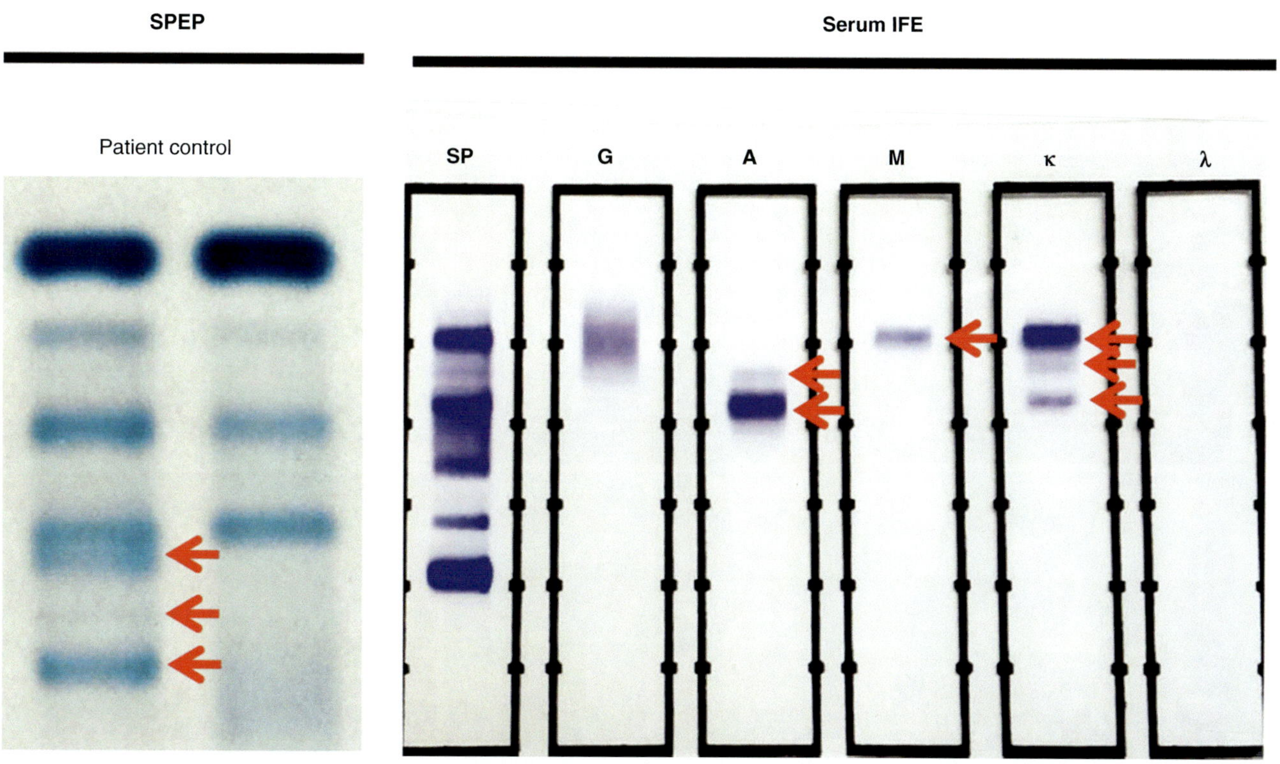

Fig. 16.5 Serum protein electrophoresis and immunofixation electrophoresis

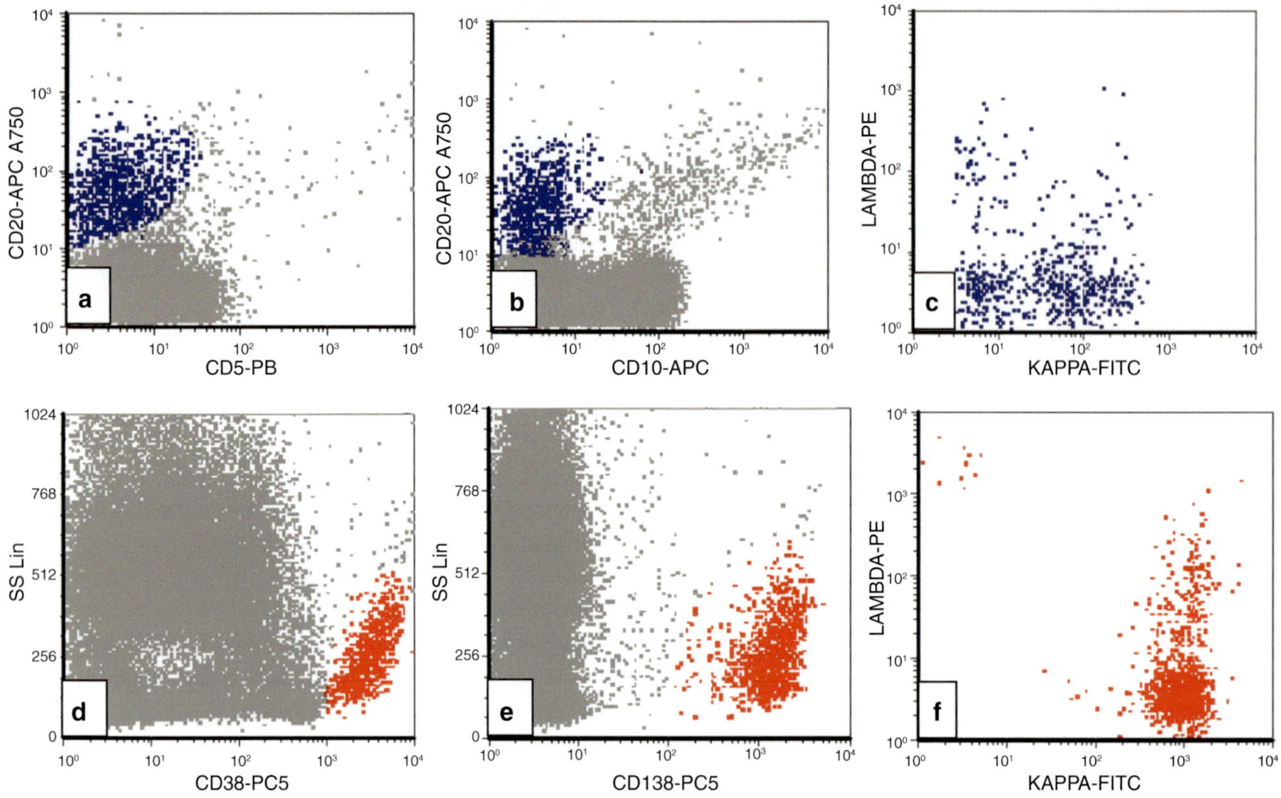

Fig. 16.6 Flow cytometry analysis of bone marrow aspirate

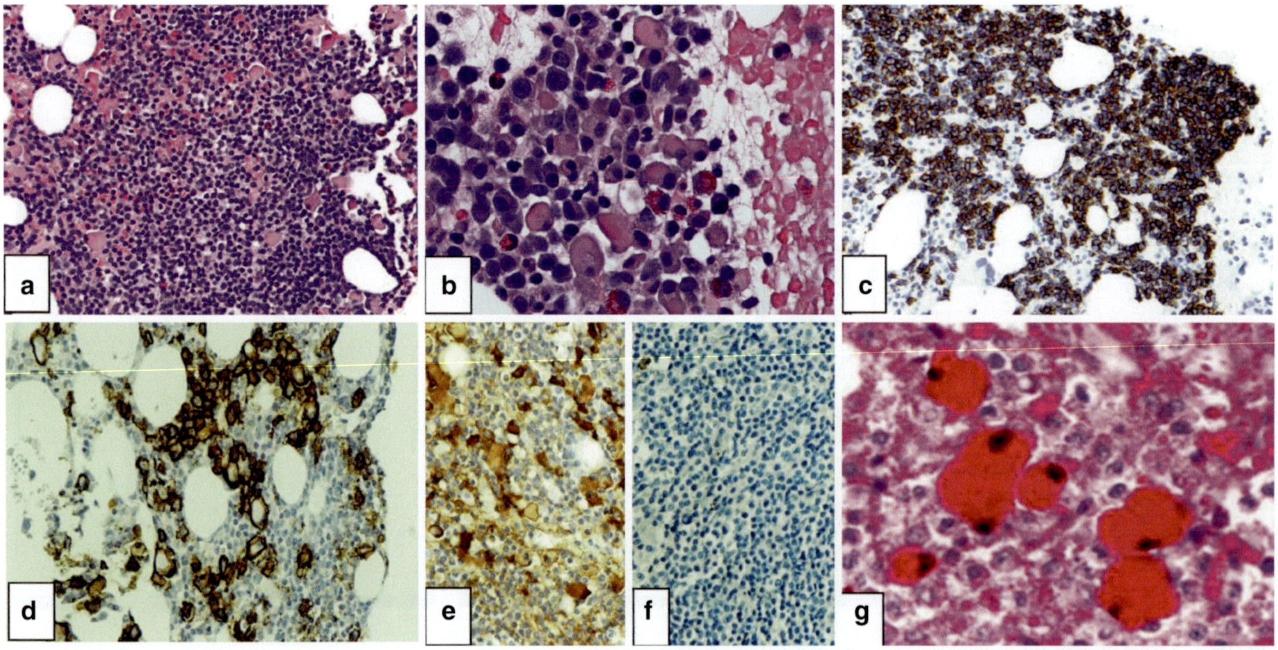

Fig. 16.7 Histology and immunohistochemical work-up of bone marrow aspirate clot section. (**a**) H&E 100×; (**b**) H&E 400×; (**c**) CD20; (**d**) CD138; (**e**) Kappa; (**f**) lambda; (**g**) cyclin D1(brown)/IgA (red)

Mutational Study

- *MYD88* L265P mutation is detected, consistent with lymphoplasmacytic lymphoma.

Final Diagnosis

Plasma cell myeloma and lymphoplasmacytic lymphoma

Take-Home Messages

1. The presence of multiple distinct monoclonal proteins with different light chain restriction or heavy chain isotypes should raise a possibility of composite lymphoma comprising two distinct neoplastic B-cell components.
2. Co-existing lymphoplasmacytic lymphoma and plasma cell neoplasm are rarely reported in the presence of double M proteins detected by SPEP/IFE. Both *MYD88* mutational assay and myeloma associated cytogenetics/FISH abnormality are useful for accurate diagnosis.

Case 3

Learning Objectives

1. To learn that diffuse large B-cell lymphoma can co-exist with classic Hodgkin lymphoma
2. To learn that the presence of multiple morphologies is a diagnostic clue of composite lymphoma
3. To learn to confirm diagnosis by immunohistochemical work-up

Case History

A 29-year-old female presented with 2 months of enlarged left neck lymph node and unintentional weight loss. CT scan showed left neck, mediastinal, and hilar adenopathy measuring up to 8 cm in conglomerate. Left neck lymph node excisional biopsy was performed.

Histologic Findings (Fig. 16.8)

- There were two demarcated areas in the biopsy.
- One showed diffuse proliferation of large neoplastic lymphoid cells with irregular nucleus and distinct nucleolus. Increased mitosis and apoptosis were present.
- The other one showed mixed inflammatory infiltrates admixed with few large mononuclear or binuclear cells with vesicular nucleus and prominent nucleoli, morphologically compatible with Reed–Sternberg cells or Hodgkin cells. The background mixed inflammatory cells included small lymphocytes, plasma cells, histiocytes, and a few eosinophils.

Morphologic Diagnosis (Figs. 16.9 and 16.10)

- Diffuse large B-cell lymphoma with RS-like cells versus composite diffuse large B-cell lymphoma and classic Hodgkin lymphoma

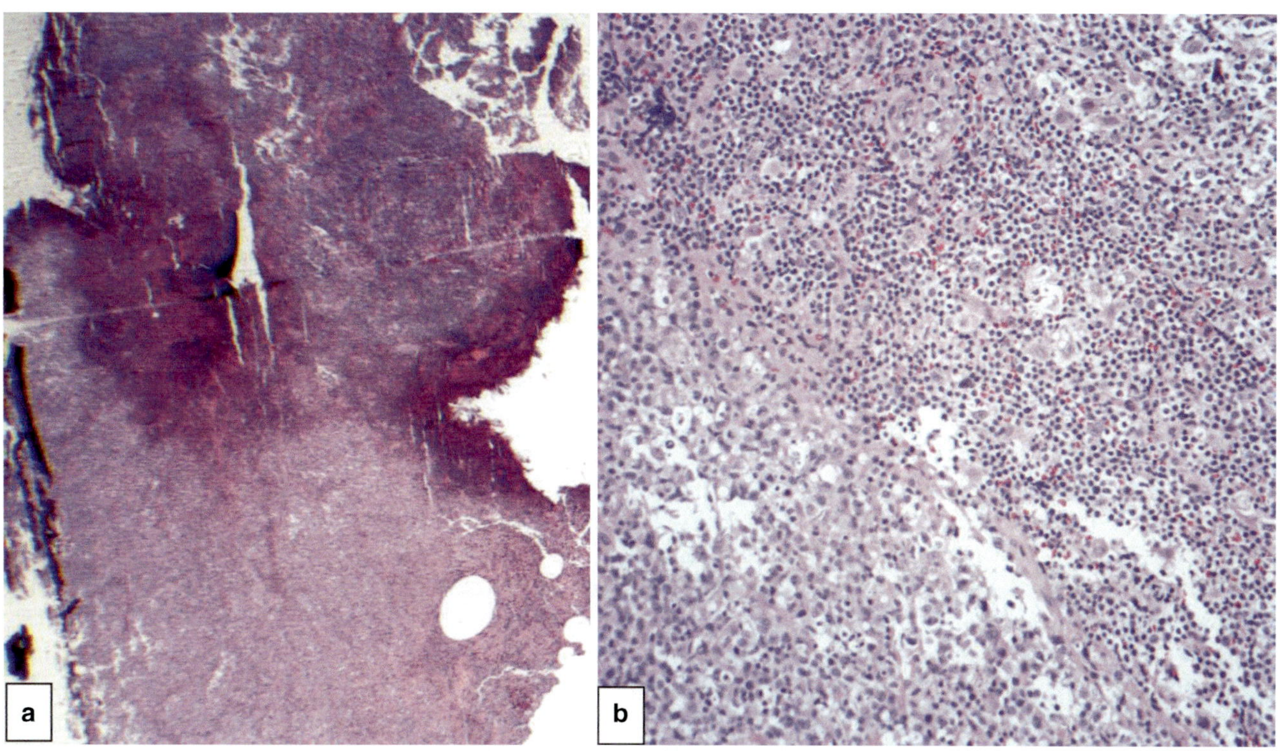

Fig. 16.8 Histology of lymph node excisional biopsy. (**a**) H&E, 40×; (**b**) H&E, 200×

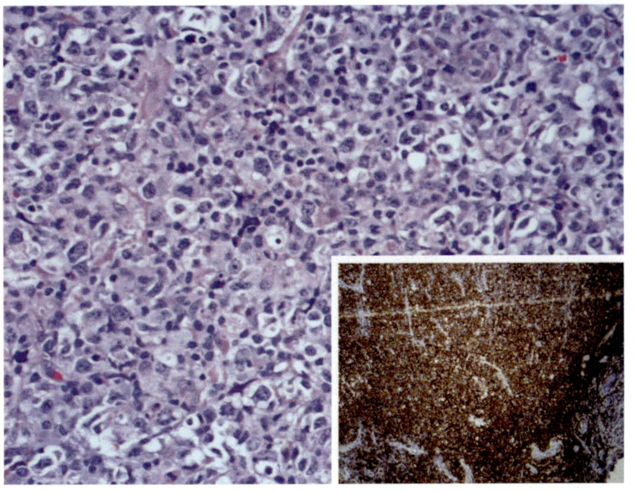

Fig. 16.9 High power morphology (H&E, 400×) of diffuse area and immunohistochemical study of CD20 (*inset*)

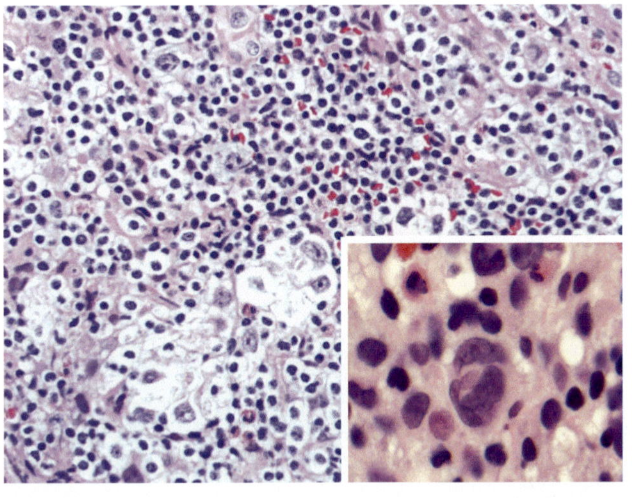

Fig. 16.10 High power morphology (H&E, 400×) of area with mixed inflammatory infiltrates. *Inset* (H&E, 1000×) shows an atypical binucleated cell

Flow Cytometry Analysis

- Not contributory

Immunohistochemical Stains (Fig. 16.11)

- Immunohistochemical stains show large cells in diffuse area were positive for CD20. Additional immunohistochemical stains (not shown) demonstrate these cells were positive for BCL6 and MUM1, but negative for CD10. This finding was compatible with DLBCL.
- On the other hand, the scattered atypical cells within the mixed inflammatory background were positive for CD30, CD15, and PAX5 (weak) and negative for CD20, CD3, and CD45. This portion of tissue was consistent with diagnosis of classic Hodgkin lymphoma.

Final Diagnosis

Diffuse large B-cell lymphoma, NOS, ABC-type and classic Hodgkin lymphoma

Take-Home Messages

1. The presence of two well-demarcated distinct morphologies within same tissue biopsy is a diagnostic clue for composite lymphoma.
2. Additional ancillary studies such as immunohistochemistry are indispensable in confirmation of diagnosis.

Case 4

Learning Objectives

1. To learn that it is not uncommon that cells morphologically resembling Reed–Sternberg cells (RS-like cells) can be identified in an otherwise typical non-Hodgkin lymphoma
2. To learn how to differentiate RS-like cells from RS cells in the classic Hodgkin lymphoma

Case History

A 75-year-old male presented with mesenteric lymphadenopathy. Abdominal excisional biopsy was performed.

Histologic Findings (Fig. 16.12)

- Effacement of normal lymphoid tissue architecture by nodular proliferation composed of predominantly small atypical lymphoid cells with irregular nucleus. Other inflammatory infiltrates including eosinophils, plasma cells, and histiocytes were essentially absent.
- There were scattered large atypical lymphoid cells with occasional double nucleus; vesicular chromatin, prominent nucleus, and ample cytoplasm are identified. These cells were located predominantly within the lymphoid nodules with a small subset showing internodular localization.

Flow Cytometry Analysis (Fig. 16.13)

- A CD10+ monoclonal B-cell population with kappa light chain restriction was identified.

Morphologic Diagnosis

- Low-grade lymphoma with RS-like cells vs composite lymphoma with CHL as one component

Immunohistochemical Stains (Figs. 16.14 and 16.15)

- Immunohistochemical stains show majority of atypical lymphoid cells were positive for PAX5, BCL6 (not shown), and BCL2. In combination of nodular proliferation and CD10+ positivity by flow cytometry analysis, the finding was consistent with follicular lymphoma. The

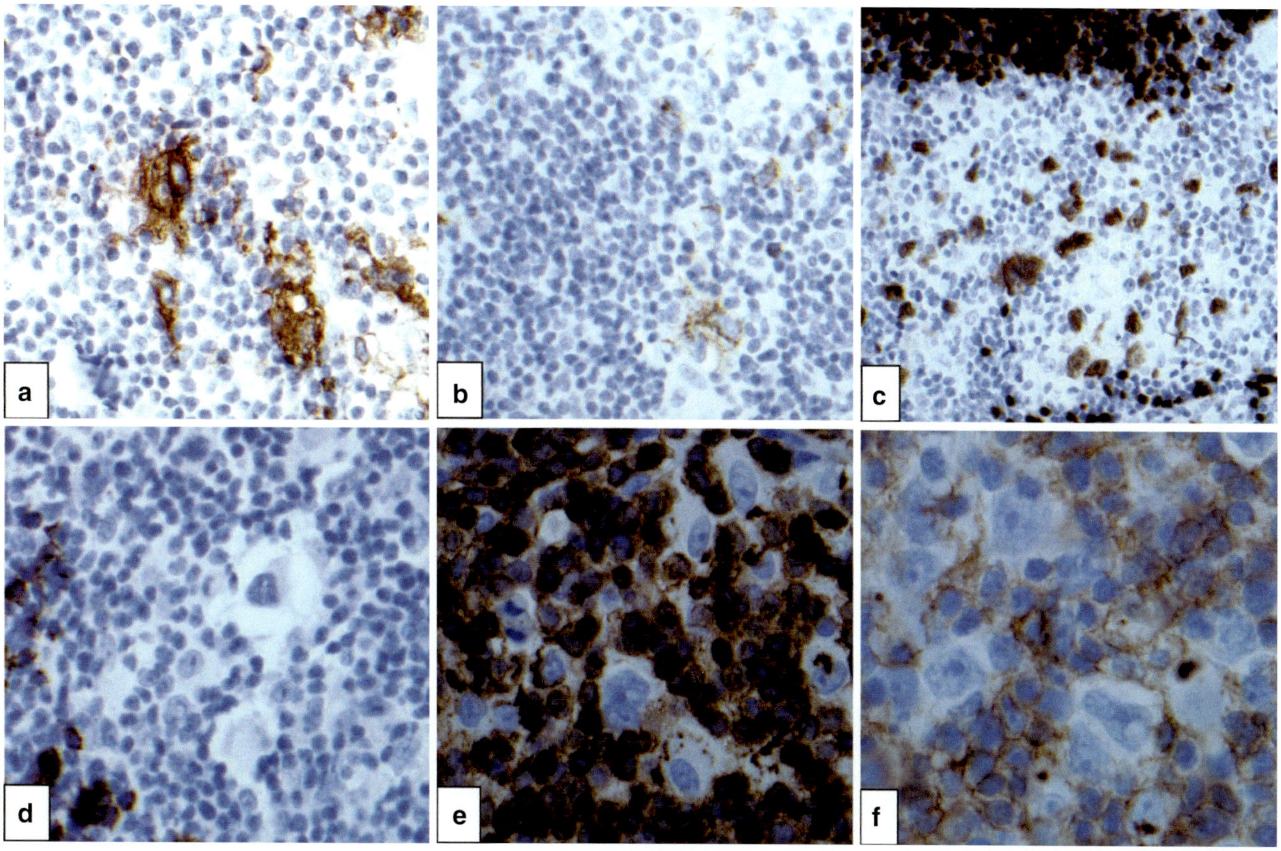

Fig. 16.11 Immunohistochemical work-up of area with mixed inflammatory infiltrates. (**a**) CD30; (**b**) CD15; (**c**) PAX5; (**d**) CD20; (**e**) CD3; (**f**) CD45

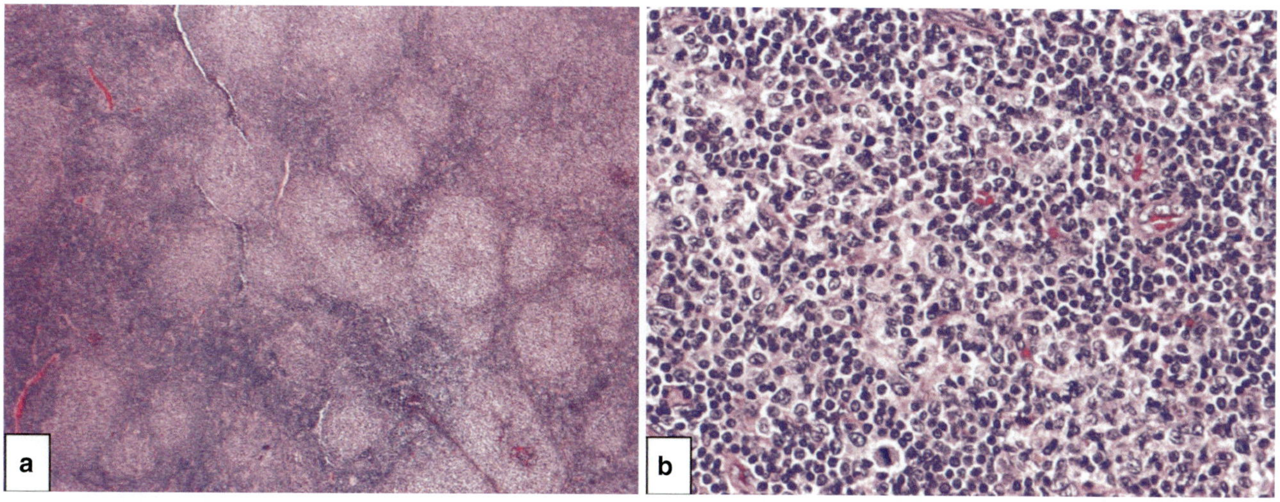

Fig. 16.12 Histologic findings of lymph node biopsy. (**a**) H&E, 40×, (**b**) H&E, 200×

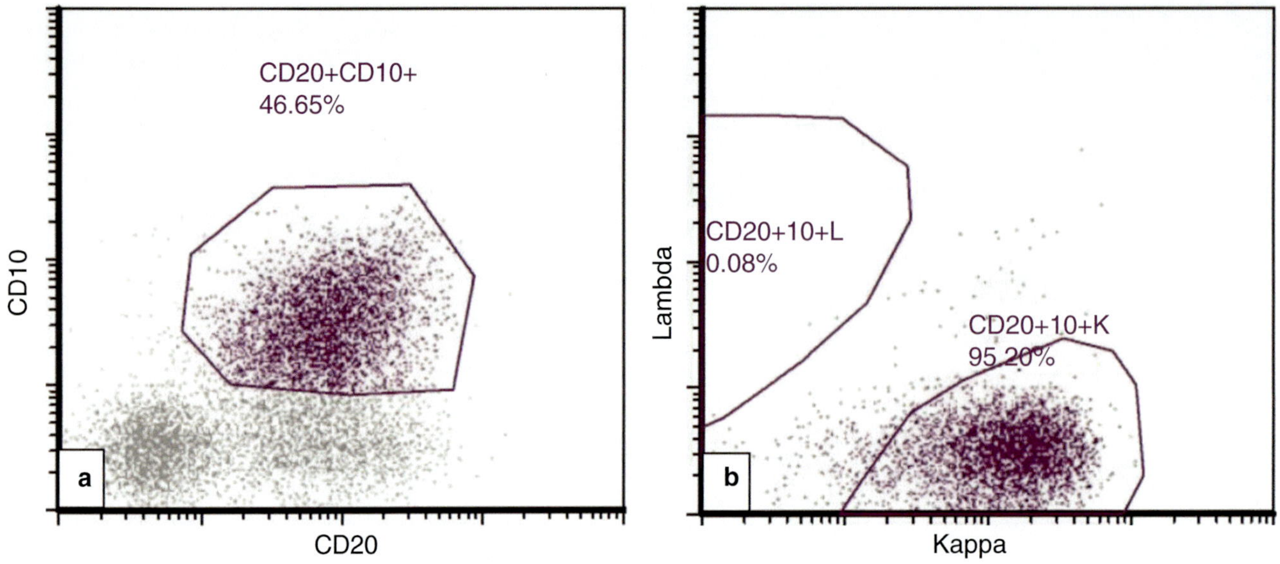

Fig. 16.13 Flow cytometry analysis of lymph node biopsy

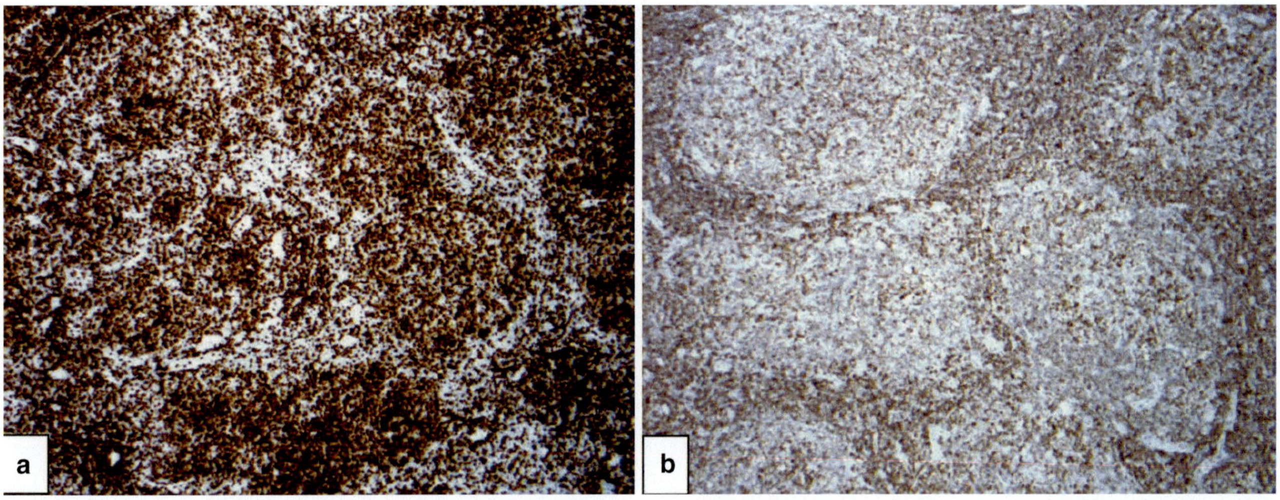

Fig. 16.14 Immunohistochemical work-up of lymph node biopsy. (**a**) PAX5; (**b**) BCL2

large atypical cells were positive for CD30, PAX5 (strong), BCL6 (not shown), and CD45 (not shown), but negative for CD15.

Final Diagnosis

Follicular lymphoma, grades 1–2, follicular pattern with RS-like cells

Take-Home Messages

1. The low-grade B-cell lymphomas such as FL can uncommonly contain cells morphologically compatible with RS cells which introduce the differential diagnosis of composite lymphoma.
2. The main findings that can differentiate RS-like cells from RS cells in CHL include:

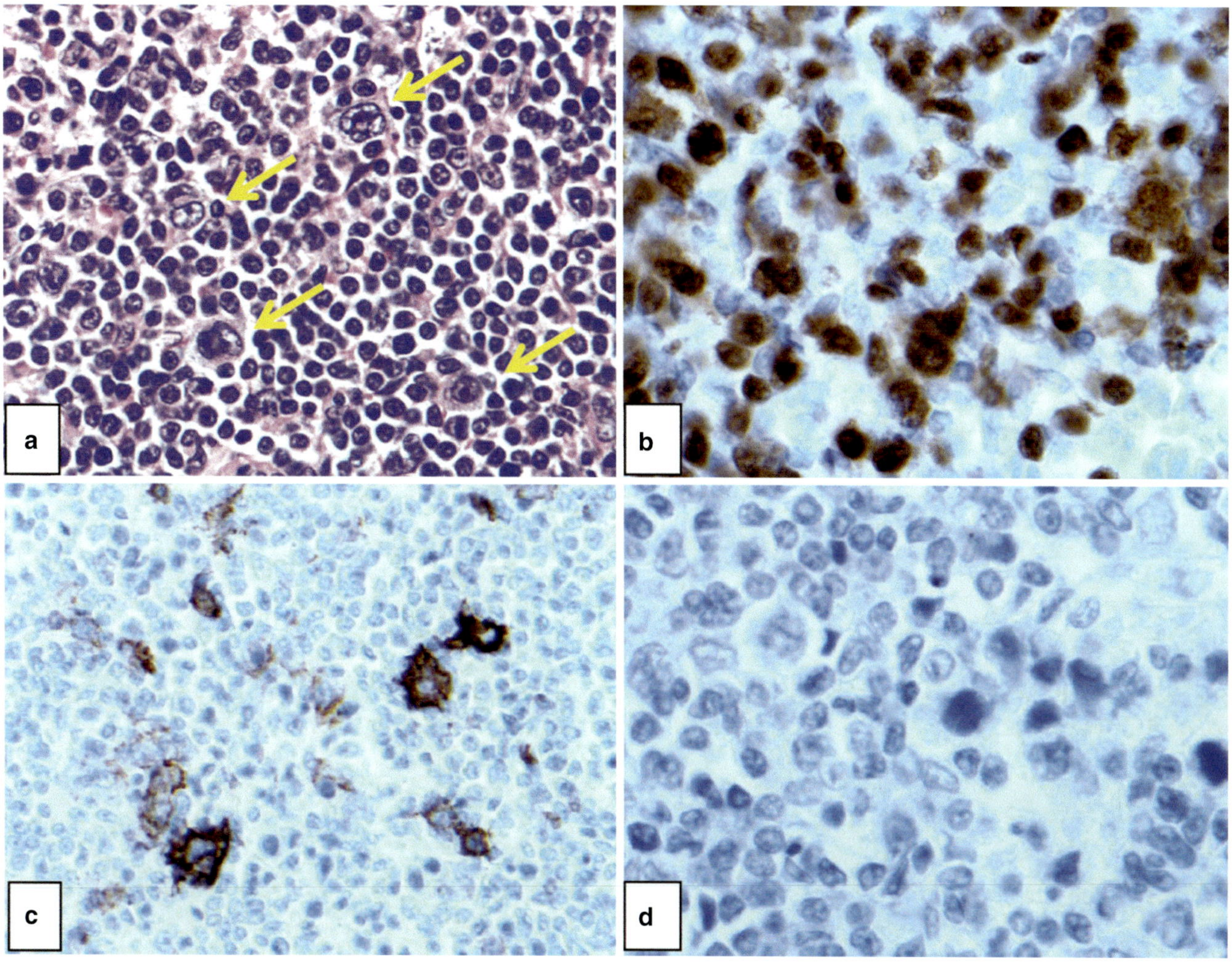

Fig. 16.15 Morphology and immunohistochemical work-up of occasional scattered large cells (*yellow arrows*) identified in the biopsy. (**a**) H&E, 400×; (**b**) PAX5; (**c**) CD30; (**d**) CD15

- RS-like cells lack appropriate background infiltrates commonly seen in CHL.
- The immunophenotype of these RS-like cells can be different from although sometimes identical to RS cells in the CHL.

Case 5

Learning Objectives

1. To learn that a T-cell NHL can co-exist with a B-cell NHL
2. To learn that the diagnosis requires comprehensive evaluations including morphology, immunophenotyping by flow cytometry/immunohistochemistry, and clonal analysis by *IGH/TCR*

Case History

A 57-year-old female presented with bilateral cervical lymphadenopathy. PET scan revealed increased uptake in the neck, pelvis, and retroperitoneal lymph nodes. Left neck core biopsy was taken for evaluation.

Histologic Findings

- Core biopsy showed effacement of normal lymphoid tissue architecture.
- There were two distinct morphologies of atypical lymphoid proliferation. One showed diffuse large lymphocytic proliferation. The other one showed mixed small lymphocytes and few large lymphocytes. Prominent vasculature was identified in this area.

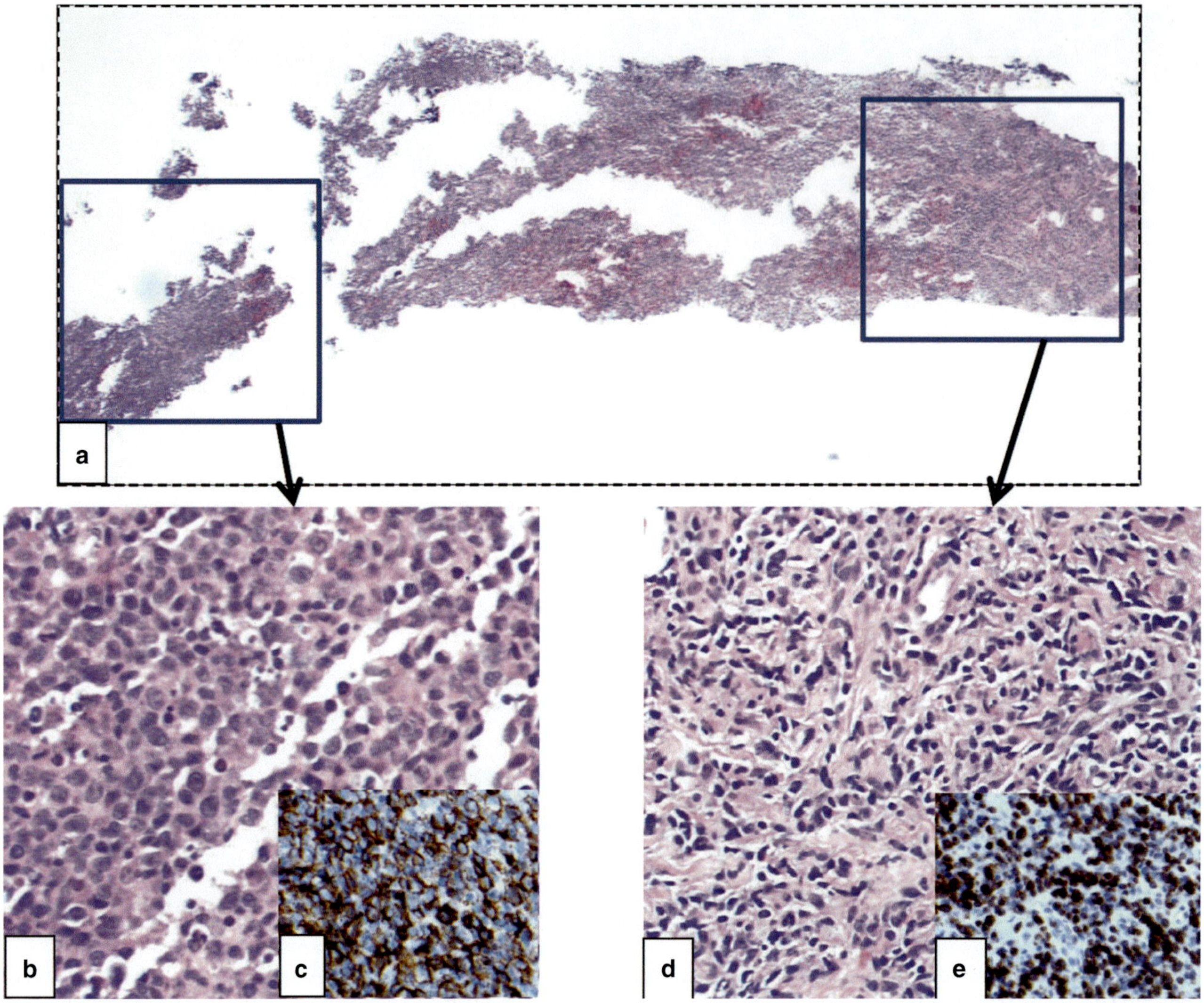

Fig. 16.16 Morphology evaluation and immunohistochemical work-up of the core biopsy. (**a**) H&E, 20×; (**b**) H&E, 400×; (**c**) CD20; (**d**) H&E, 400×; (**e**) CD3

Morphologic Diagnosis (Fig. 16.16)

- Large cell lymphoma and foci suggestive of second neoplastic lymphoid proliferation.
- Alternatively, the second area could be a reactive background.

Flow Cytometry Analysis (Fig. 16.17)

- Atypical CD19+/CD20+ B cells without definitive surface light chain expression compatible with a monoclonal B-cell population.
- A predominant CD8+/CD3+ T-cell population showed aberrant loss of CD5 expression.
- These findings suggested a composite B-cell and T-cell process.

Immunohistochemical Stains

- Immunohistochemical stains show the large cells in diffuse area were positive for CD20 and BCL6 (not shown) and negative for CD10 (not shown) and MUM1 (not shown).
- The cells in the area composed of mixed infiltrates were predominantly positive for CD3. Additional stains (not shown) demonstrated these cells are positive for CD2 and BCL6 and negative for CD10, PD1, and CXCL13.
- EBER in situ hybridization was negative.

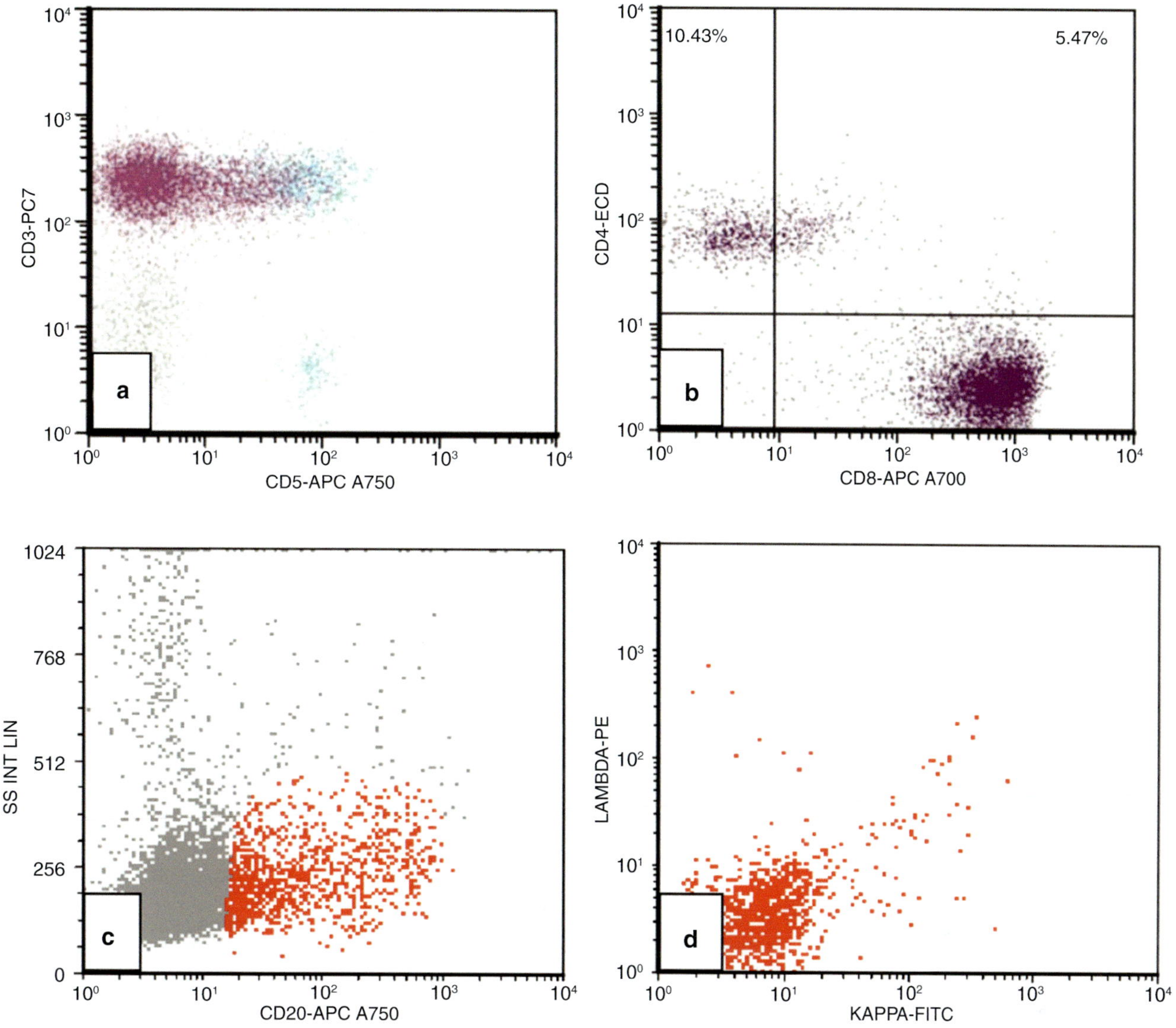

Fig. 16.17 Flow cytometry analysis

IgH and TCR Gene Rearrangement (Fig. 16.18)

- Clonal *IGH* and clonal *TCR* rearrangements were identified by PCR.

Final Diagnosis

Peripheral T-cell lymphoma, NOS and DLBCL, NOS, GCB type

Take-Home Messages

1. Composite lymphomas consisting of concurrent B-cell and T-cell lymphomas are rare, and the diagnosis can be very challenging.
2. In addition to morphology, multiple ancillary studies are critical for establishing a definitive diagnosis. These ancillary studies include flow cytometry analysis, immunohistochemistry, and clonal analysis of IgH and TCR genes.

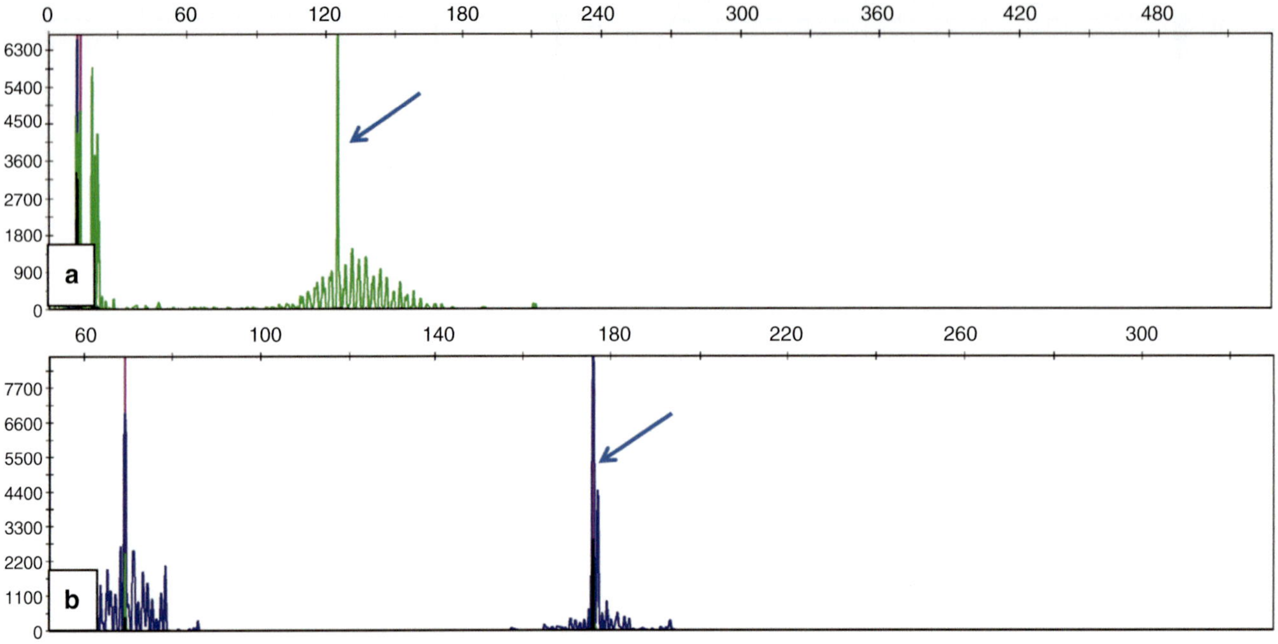

Fig. 16.18 *IGH* and *TCRG* clonal analysis by PCR. (**a**) *IGH*; (**b**) *TCRG*

References

1. Custer R. Pitfalls in the diagnosis of lymphoma and leukemia from the pathologist's point of view. In: Proceedings from the 2nd national cancer conference: American Cancer Society; 1954. 1: p. 554–7.
2. Kim H, Hendrickson R, Dorfman RF. Composite lymphoma. Cancer. 1977;40(3):959–76.
3. National Cancer Institute sponsored study of classifications of non-Hodgkin's lymphomas: summary and description of a working formulation for clinical usage. The Non-Hodgkin's lymphoma pathologic classification project. Cancer. 1982;49(10):2112–35.
4. Swerdlow SH, Campo E, Harris NL, Jaffe ES, Pileri SA, Stein H, Theile J, editors. WHO Classification of Tumours of Haematopoietic and Lymphoid Tissues. Revised 4th ed. Lyon: IARC Press; 2017.
5. Jaffe ES, Zarate-Osorno A, Medeiros LJ. The interrelationship of Hodgkin's disease and non-Hodgkin's lymphomas--lessons learned from composite and sequential malignancies. Semin Diagn Pathol. 1992;9(4):297–303.
6. Brecher M, Banks PM. Hodgkin's disease variant of Richter's syndrome. Report of eight cases. Am J Clin Pathol. 1990;93(3):333–9.
7. Kadin ME, Hughey LC, Wood GS. Large-cell transformation of mycosis fungoides-differential diagnosis with implications for clinical management: a consensus statement of the US Cutaneous Lymphoma Consortium. J Am Acad Dermatol. 2014;70(2):374–6.
8. Hoppe RT. Histologic variation in non-Hodgkin's lymphomas: commentary. Cancer Treat Rep. 1981;65(11–12):935–9.
9. Mokhtar NM. Review article composite lymphoma. J Egypt Natl Canc Inst. 2007;19(3):171–5.
10. Wang S, Tzankov A, Xu-Monette ZY, Hoeller S, Wang SA, Richards KL, et al. Clonally related composite follicular lymphoma and mantle cell lymphoma with clinicopathologic features and biological implications. Hum Pathol. 2013;44(12):2658–67.
11. Brauninger A, Hansmann ML, Strickler JG, Dummer R, Burg G, Rajewsky K, et al. Identification of common germinal-center B-cell precursors in two patients with both Hodgkin's disease and non-Hodgkin's lymphoma. N Engl J Med. 1999;340(16):1239–47.
12. Tinguely M, Rosenquist R, Sundström C, Amini RM, Küppers R, Hansmann ML, et al. Analysis of a clonally related mantle cell and Hodgkin lymphoma indicates Epstein-Barr virus infection of a Hodgkin/Reed-Sternberg cell precursor in a germinal center. Am J Surg Pathol. 2003;27(11):1483–8.
13. Huang Q, Wilczynski SP, Chang KL, Weiss LM. Composite recurrent Hodgkin lymphoma and diffuse large B-cell lymphoma: one clone, two faces. Am J Clin Pathol. 2006;126(2):222–9.
14. Kerl K, Girardet C, Borisch B. A common B-cell precursor in composite lymphomas. N Engl J Med. 1999;341(10):764–5.
15. Thomas RK, Wickenhauser C, Kube D, Tesch H, Diehl V, Wolf J, et al. Repeated clonal relapses in classical Hodgkin's lymphoma and the occurrence of a clonally unrelated diffuse large B cell non-Hodgkin lymphoma in the same patient. Leuk Lymphoma. 2004;45(5):1065–9.
16. Caleo A, Sánchez-Aguilera A, Rodríguez S, Dotor AM, Beltrán L, de Larrinoa AF, et al. Composite Hodgkin lymphoma and mantle cell lymphoma: two clonally unrelated tumors. Am J Surg Pathol. 2003;27(12):1577–80.
17. Campidelli C, Sabattini E, Piccioli M, Rossi M, De Blasi D, Miraglia E, et al. Simultaneous occurrence of peripheral T-cell lymphoma unspecified and B-cell small lymphocytic lymphoma. Report of 2 cases. Hum Pathol. 2007;38(5):787–92.
18. Muller-Hermelink HK, Zettl A, Pfeifer W, Ott G. Pathology of lymphoma progression. Histopathology. 2001;38(4):285–306.
19. Kuppers R, Duhrsen U, Hansmann ML. Pathogenesis, diagnosis, and treatment of composite lymphomas. Lancet Oncol. 2014;15(10):e435–46.
20. Schmitz R, Renné C, Rosenquist R, Tinguely M, Distler V, Menestrina F, et al. Insights into the multistep transformation process of lymphomas: IgH-associated translocations and tumor suppressor gene mutations in clonally related composite Hodgkin's and non-Hodgkin's lymphomas. Leukemia. 2005;19(8):1452–8.
21. Wang E, Papavassiliou P, Wang AR, Louissaint A Jr, Wang J, Hutchinson C. et al. Composite lymphoid neoplasm of B-cell

and T-cell origins: a pathologic study of 14 cases. Hum Pathol. 2014;45(4):768–84.
22. Matolcsy A, Schattner EJ, Knowles DM, Casali P. Clonal evolution of B cells in transformation from low- to high-grade lymphoma. Eur J Immunol. 1999;29(4):1253–64.
23. Fend F, Quintanilla-Martinez L, Raffeld M. Composite lymphoma. Hum Pathol. 2000;31(5):626–7.
24. Sun Y, Wang SA, Sun T. Composite mantle cell lymphoma and chronic lymphocytic leukemia/small lymphocytic lymphoma. Cytometry B Clin Cytom. 2018;94(1):148–50.
25. Horing E, Staiger AM2,3, Lenze D4, Horn H2, Vöhringer M1, Steurer W, et al. Burkitt lymphoma and diffuse large B-cell lymphoma: a unique case of a composite lymphoma of different clonal origin. Leuk Lymphoma. 2018;59(1):249–52.
26. Mansour AT, Shandiz AE, Zimmerman MK, Roth TD, Zhou J. Concomitant lymphoplasmacytic lymphoma and plasma cell myeloma, a diagnostic challenge. Am J Blood Res. 2017;7(2):10–7.
27. de Leval L, Vivario M, De Prijck B, Zhou Y, Boniver J, Harris NL, et al. Distinct clonal origin in two cases of Hodgkin's lymphoma variant of Richter's syndrome associated With EBV infection. Am J Surg Pathol. 2004;28(5):679–86.
28. Traverse-Glehen A, Pittaluga S, Gaulard P, Sorbara L, Alonso MA, Raffeld M, et al. Mediastinal gray zone lymphoma: the missing link between classic Hodgkin's lymphoma and mediastinal large B-cell lymphoma. Am J Surg Pathol. 2005;29(11):1411–21.
29. Khan U, Hadid T, Ibrar W, Sano D1, Al-Katib A. Composite lymphoma: opposite ends of spectrum meet. J Clin Med Res. 2017;9(3):213–5.
30. Venkatraman L, Catherwood M, Benson G, Drake M. Hodgkin transformation of small lymphocytic lymphoma: gene usage, mutational status and clonal relationship. Histopathology. 2007;51(6):866–8.
31. Miettinen M, Franssila KO, Saxen E. Hodgkin's disease, lymphocytic predominance nodular. Increased risk for subsequent non-Hodgkin's lymphomas. Cancer. 1983;51(12):2293–300.
32. Brown JR, Weng AP, Freedman AS. Hodgkin disease associated with T-cell non-Hodgkin lymphomas: case reports and review of the literature. Am J Clin Pathol. 2004;121(5):701–8.
33. Suefuji N, Niino D, Arakawa F, Karube K, Kimura Y, Kiyasu J, et al. Clinicopathological analysis of a composite lymphoma containing both T- and B-cell lymphomas. Pathol Int. 2012;62(10):690–8.
34. Kang SK, Chang SE, Choi JH, Sung KJ, Moon KC, Koh JK. Coexistence of CD30-positive anaplastic large cell lymphoma and mycosis fungoides. Clin Exp Dermatol. 2002;27(3):212–5.
35. Jaffe ES, Zarate-Osorno A, Kingma DW, Raffeld M, Medeiros LJ. The interrelationship between Hodgkin's disease and non-Hodgkin's lymphomas. Ann Oncol. 1994;5(Suppl 1):7–11.
36. Sekikawa T, Takahara S, Suzuki H, Takeda N, Yamada H, Horiguchi-Yamada J. Diffuse large B-cell lymphoma arising independently to lymphoplasmacytic lymphoma: a case of two lymphomas. Eur J Haematol. 2007;78(3):264–9.
37. Mohammad F, Garcia G, Kedia S, Ding J, Hurford M, Bershadskiy A. Composite diffuse large B-cell and mantle cell lymphoma: a case report. Cureus. 2017;9(1):e963.
38. Wang HW, Yang W, Wang L, Lu YL, Lu JY. Composite diffuse large B-cell lymphoma and classical Hodgkin's lymphoma of the stomach: case report and literature review. World J Gastroenterol. 2013;19(37):6304–9.
39. Copur MS, Ledakis P, Novinski D, Fu K, Hutchins M, Frankforter S, et al. An unusual case of composite lymphoma involving chronic lymphocytic leukemia follicular lymphoma and Hodgkin disease. Leuk Lymphoma. 2004;45(5):1071–6.
40. Aktan M, Akkaya A, Doğan O, Dincol G. Chronic lymphocytic leukemia and multiple myeloma in the same patient: case report. Leuk Lymphoma. 2003;44(8):1421–4.
41. Rodig SJ, Healey BM, Pinkus GS, Kuo FC, Dal Cin P, Kutok JL. Mantle cell lymphoma arising within primary nodal marginal zone lymphoma: a unique presentation of two uncommon B-cell lymphoproliferative disorders. Cancer Genet Cytogenet. 2006;171(1):44–51.
42. Cachia AR, Diss TC, Isaacson PG. Composite mantle-cell lymphoma and plasmacytoma. Hum Pathol. 1997;28(11):1291–5.
43. Saito H, Oka K, Nakamura N, Nagayama R, Hakozaki H, Mori N. A common clonal origin of nodal marginal zone B-cell lymphoma and plasma cell myeloma demonstrating different immunophenotypes: a case report of composite lymphoma. Diagn Mol Pathol. 2004;13(2):75–80.
44. Gonzalez CL, Medeiros LJ, Jaffe ES. Composite lymphoma. A clinicopathologic analysis of nine patients with Hodgkin's disease and B-cell non-Hodgkin's lymphoma. Am J Clin Pathol. 1991;96(1):81–9.
45. Rosales CM, Lin P, Mansoor A, Bueso-Ramos C, Medeiros LJ. Lymphoplasmacytic lymphoma/Waldenstrom macroglobulinemia associated with Hodgkin disease. A report of two cases. Am J Clin Pathol. 2001;116(1):34–40.
46. Zettl A, Rüdiger T, Marx A, Müller-Hermelink HK, Ott G. Composite marginal zone B-cell lymphoma and classical Hodgkin's lymphoma: a clinicopathological study of 12 cases. Histopathology. 2005;46(2):217–28.
47. Dargent JL, Lespagnard L, Meiers I, Bradstreet C, Heimann P, De Wolf-Peeters C. Composite follicular lymphoma and nodular lymphocyte predominance Hodgkin's disease. Virchows Arch. 2005;447(4):778–80.
48. Delabie J, Greiner TC, Chan WC, Weisenburger DD. Concurrent lymphocyte predominance Hodgkin's disease and T-cell lymphoma. A report of three cases. Am J Surg Pathol. 1996;20(3):355–62.
49. Xu Y, McKenna RW, Hoang MP, Collins RH, Kroft SH. Composite angioimmunoblastic T-cell lymphoma and diffuse large B-cell lymphoma: a case report and review of the literature. Am J Clin Pathol. 2002;118(6):848–54.
50. Alperovich A, Vlachostergios PJ2, Binder A3, Oliff AH4, Balmiki RL5, Dufresne F1. Composite angioimmunoblastic T-cell and diffuse large B-cell lymphoma. Hematol Oncol Stem Cell Ther. 2015;8(3):136–7.
51. Barzilai A, Trau H, David M, Feinmesser M, Bergman R, Shpiro D, et al. Mycosis fungoides associated with B-cell malignancies. Br J Dermatol. 2006;155(2):379–86.
52. Volk AL, Vannucci SA, Cook W, Thompson KA, Listinsky CM. Composite mycosis fungoides and B-cell chronic lymphocytic leukemia. Ann Diagn Pathol. 2002;6(3):172–82.
53. Hirose Y, Fukushima T, Masaki Y, Shimoyama K, Karasawa H, Ogawa N, et al. Epstein-Barr virus-associated composite lymphoma composed of peripheral T-cell lymphoma and an anaplastic variant of a diffuse large B-cell type of non-Hodgkin's lymphoma and strongly expressing p53 protein. Int J Hematol. 2004;79(3):260–5.
54. Abou-Elella AA, Nifong TP. Composite EBV negative peripheral T-cell lymphoma and diffuse large B-cell lymphoma involving the ileum: a case report and a systematic review of the literature. Leuk Lymphoma. 2006;47(10):2208–17.
55. Tobinai K, Ohtsu T, Hayashi M, Kinoshita T, Matsuno Y, Mukai K, et al. Epstein-Barr virus (EBV) genome carrying monoclonal B-cell lymphoma in a patient with adult T-cell leukemia-lymphoma. Leuk Res. 1991;15(9):837–46.
56. Tembhare P, Yuan CM, Xi L, Morris JC, Liewehr D, Venzon D, Janik JE, et al. Flow cytometric immunophenotypic assessment of T-cell clonality by Vbeta repertoire analysis: detection of T-cell clonality at diagnosis and monitoring of minimal residual disease following therapy. Am J Clin Pathol. 2011;135(6):890–900.
57. Ladetto M, Brüggemann M, Monitillo L, Ferrero S, Pepin F, Drandi D, et al. Next-generation sequencing and real-time quantita-

tive PCR for minimal residual disease detection in B-cell disorders. Leukemia. 2014;28(6):1299–307.
58. Falini B, Martelli MP, Tiacci E. BRAF V600E mutation in hairy cell leukemia: from bench to bedside. Blood. 2016;128(15):1918–27.
59. Tiacci E, Trifonov V, Schiavoni G, Holmes A, Kern W, Martelli MP, et al. BRAF mutations in hairy-cell leukemia. N Engl J Med. 2011;364(24):2305–15.
60. Treon SP, Xu L, Yang G, Zhou Y, Liu X, Cao Y, et al. MYD88 L265P somatic mutation in Waldenstrom's macroglobulinemia. N Engl J Med. 2012;367(9):826–33.
61. Slack GW, Gascoyne RD. Next-generation sequencing discoveries in lymphoma. Adv Anat Pathol. 2013;20(2):110–6.
62. Zhang J, Grubor V, Love CL, Banerjee A, Richards KL, Mieczkowski PA, et al. Genetic heterogeneity of diffuse large B-cell lymphoma. Proc Natl Acad Sci. 2013;110(4):1398–403.
63. Davis RE, Ngo VN, Lenz G, Tolar P, Young RM, Romesser PB, et al. Chronic active B-cell-receptor signalling in diffuse large B-cell lymphoma. Nature. 2010;463(7277):88–92.
64. Naresh KN. Nodal marginal zone B-cell lymphoma with prominent follicular colonization - difficulties in diagnosis: a study of 15 cases. Histopathology. 2008;52(3):331–9.
65. Isaacson PG, Wotherspoon AC, Diss T, Pan LX. Follicular colonization in B-cell lymphoma of mucosa-associated lymphoid tissue. Am J Surg Pathol. 1991;15(9):819–28.
66. Gomez-Gelvez JC, Smith LB. Reed-Sternberg-Like Cells in Non-Hodgkin Lymphomas. Arch Pathol Lab Med. 2015;139(10):1205–10.
67. Shin SS, Ben-Ezra J, Burke JS, Sheibani K, Rappaport H. Reed-Sternberg-like cells in low-grade lymphomas are transformed neoplastic cells of B-cell lineage. Am J Clin Pathol. 1993;99(6):658–62.
68. Quintanilla-Martinez L, Fend F, Moguel LR, Spilove L, Beaty MW, Kingma DW, et al. Peripheral T-cell lymphoma with Reed-Sternberg-like cells of B-cell phenotype and genotype associated with Epstein-Barr virus infection. Am J Surg Pathol. 1999;23(10):1233–40.
69. Nicolae A, Pittaluga S, Venkataraman G, Vijnovich-Baron A, Xi L, Raffeld M, et al. Peripheral T-cell lymphomas of follicular T-helper cell derivation with Hodgkin/Reed-Sternberg cells of B-cell lineage: both EBV-positive and EBV-negative variants exist. Am J Surg Pathol. 2013;37(6):816–26.

Histiocytic/Dendritic Cell Neoplasms: Primary and Transdifferentiated

17

Chen Zhao and Zenggang Pan

List of Frequently Asked Questions

1. What are the major subtypes of histiocytic/dendritic cell neoplasms?
2. What are the typical morphological findings in histiocytic/dendritic cell neoplasms
3. What are the mimics and what is the clinical relevance of misinterpretation between the true diagnosis and mimics with reference to mistreatment and/or wrong prognosis?
4. What is the minimal and optimal ancillary work-up for diagnosis and subclassification of histiocytic/dendritic cell neoplasms?
5. Which ancillary test results are diagnostic, are suggestive of diagnosis, are unreliable for diagnosis, or rule out the diagnosis?
6. What is the work-up to provide prognostic and therapeutic target information?
7. What should be the approach to provide maximum, but defensible information, from limited specimen or work-up? What is a descriptive diagnosis appropriate in such situations?
8. When is a diagnostic comment necessary and what should be discussed in the diagnostic comment for this entity?
9. Transdifferentiation or dedifferentiation?
10. When it is appropriate to seek external consultation for this entity?

C. Zhao (✉)
Department of Pathology, Carver College of Medicine, University of Iowa, Iowa City, IA, USA
e-mail: chen-zhao@uiowa.edu

Z. Pan
Department of Pathology, Yale University School of Medicine, New Haven, CT, USA

1. What are the major subtypes of histiocytic/dendritic cell neoplasms?

According to the updated 2017 *WHO Classification of Tumours of Haematopoietic and Lymphoid Tissues*, the following entities are included in this category:

1. Histiocytic sarcoma
2. Langerhans cell histiocytosis/sarcoma
3. Indeterminate dendritic cell tumor
4. Interdigitating dendritic cell sarcoma
5. Follicular dendritic cell sarcoma (and its variant inflammatory pseudotumor-like follicular/fibroblastic dendritic cell sarcoma)
6. Fibroblastic reticular cell tumor
7. Disseminated juvenile xanthogranuloma
8. Erdheim-Chester disease

2. What are the typical morphological findings in histiocytic/dendritic cell neoplasms?

In this chapter, we will focus on several relatively frequently encountered entities, including histiocytic sarcoma, Langerhans cell histiocytosis/sarcoma, follicular dendritic cell sarcoma, and interdigitating dendritic cell sarcoma.

A. *Histiocytic sarcoma*
   - Based on pathogenesis, histiocytic sarcoma can be separated into three groups:
     - De novo histiocytic sarcoma
     - Histiocytic sarcoma associated with mediastinal non-seminomatous germ cell tumors with shared isochromosome 12p
     - Histiocytic sarcoma clonally related to a B-cell lymphoma that either concurs or preexists
   - Histiocytic sarcoma most often affects adults with a wide age range. Patients present with either nodal

E. Wang, A. S. Lagoo (eds.), *Practical Lymph Node and Bone Marrow Pathology*, Practical Anatomic Pathology,
https://doi.org/10.1007/978-3-030-32189-5_17

(e.g., cervical and axillary lymph nodes) or extranodal (e.g., gastrointestinal tract, skin, and soft tissue) mass.
- Microscopically, the tumor cells are usually large (>20 μm) with round or elongated folded nuclei, vesicular chromatin, and abundant eosinophilic cytoplasm, diffusely infiltrating nodal or extranodal architecture.
- Occasionally, sarcomatoid changes, multinucleated tumor cells, and hemophagocytosis can be observed.
- A variable number of reactive cells including small lymphocytes, neutrophils, plasma cells, benign histiocytes, and eosinophils are present in the background.

B. *Langerhans cell histiocytosis (LCH)*
- A clonal proliferation of Langerhans-type cells in bone or, less frequently, other organs/tissues.
- In early stage of LCH, lymph nodes are usually focally involved, and the tumor cells tend to be located in the sinuses.
- More extensive involvement is seen in the later stage of LCH, which expands most of the sinuses and spreads into the paracortex and effaces normal nodal architecture.
- Langerhans cells are oval to spindled shaped, about 10–15 μm in diameter, with characteristic coffee bean-like grooved, folded, indented nuclei, dispersed chromatin, inconspicuous nucleoli, thin nuclear membranes, and ample pinkish cytoplasm.
- The diagnostic and characteristic Birbeck granules can be demonstrated in Langerhans cells by electromicroscopic examination.
- Langerhans cell proliferation is also associated with other neoplasms (e.g., classic Hodgkin lymphoma), which has been named as "tumor-associated LCH." It should be noted that the Langerhans cells in tumor-associated LCH are non-clonal, in contrast with LCH associated with AML, in which LCH is clonally related to AML.
- Marked pleomorphism, overt nuclear atypia, necrosis, and increased mitotic activity (more than 50 per 10 high-power fields) are features of a Langerhans cell sarcoma.

C. *Follicular dendritic cell (FDC) sarcoma*
- FDC sarcoma derives from mesenchymal FDCs, exhibiting fascicular or storiform growth pattern.
- The neoplastic cells are usually spindle, with oval nuclei, small nucleoli, moderate to abundant eosinophilic cytoplasm, and indistinct cell borders.
- Occasionally, tumor cells are highly atypical, binucleated, or multinucleated resembling Warthin-Finkeldey giant cells.
- Foci of coagulative necrosis, fluid-filled cystic spaces (reminiscent of thymoma), epithelioid morphology, clear cells, oncocytic cells, myxoid stroma, prominent fibrovascular septa, and osteoclast-looking giant cells can be observed.
- FDC sarcoma usually has an inflammatory background. The prominent plasmacytic reaction has been found to be positive for IgG4 [1].
- In cases of mediastinal FDC sarcoma, TdT+ immature T lymphocytes may present [2].
- A portion of FDC sarcoma arises within the context of preexisting hyaline vascular or plasmacytic variant of Castleman disease.
- FDC sarcoma may metastasize to lymph nodes, lungs, liver, etc.
- Inflammatory pseudotumor-like variant FDC sarcoma almost exclusively occurs in the spleen or liver, is positive for Epstein-Barr virus (*EBV*), and may or may not express FDC markers.
- Large tumor size (>6 cm), intra-abdominal location, coagulative necrosis, substantial cytologic atypia, and a high proliferation index herald a poorer prognosis.

D. *Interdigitating dendritic cell sarcoma*
- Mainly occurs in cervical and axillary lymph nodes. Other lymph nodes and extranodal sites (skin, soft tissue, gastrointestinal tract, liver, and spleen) can also be involved.
- Paracortical expansion of spindle or epithelioid cells with vesicular or hyperchromatic chromatin, small nucleoli, abundant eosinophilic cytoplasm, and indistinct cell borders arranged in a whorled or storiform pattern is characteristic.

3. What are the mimics and what is the clinical relevance of misinterpretation between the true diagnosis and mimics with reference to mistreatment and/or wrong prognosis?

- It is important to differentiate the entities under histiocytic/dendritic cell neoplasm category. As these tumors originate from common monocytic progenitors (excluding mesenchymal derived tumors, e.g., FDC sarcoma), they share some morphological features, which make the differentiation between them heavily reliant on immunohistochemical staining.
- The key point here is to distinguish benign lesions from sarcoma as the therapeutic regimens are different. For example, differentiate LCH from dermatopathic lymphadenopathy, tumor-associated LCH, and Langerhans cell sarcoma.
- Differentiation of histiocytic/dendritic cell tumor from other lineage tumors. For example, histiocytic sarcoma should be differentiated from AML with monocytic differentiation involving an extramedullary site (myeloid

sarcoma). Peripheral blood and bone marrow examination may resolve this issue.

- Other non-histiocytic mimickers are diffuse large B-cell lymphoma, ALK+/– anaplastic large cell lymphoma, spindle cell carcinoma, undifferentiated tumor, melanoma, and thymoma.
- Another pitfall is due to the inadequate specimen. For example, in a small needle biopsy specimen, FDC sarcoma cells can be outnumbered by background reactive cell infiltrate. Detailed clinical information, cytologic atypia, mitosis, and immunohistochemical staining will differentiate these lesions.

4. What is the minimal and optimal ancillary work-up for diagnosis and subclassification of histiocytic/dendritic cell neoplasms?

Immunohistochemistry is the mainstay for diagnosis and differentiation of these histiocytic/dendritic cell neoplasms from other non-histiocytic tumors, e.g., large cell lymphoma, melanoma, and carcinoma. In a case of neoplastic proliferation with histiocytoid morphology, a minimal immunohistochemical work-up should include the following stains: CD163, CD68, lysozyme, CD1a, S100, CD4, CD21, CD23, MPO, CD3, CD20, CD45, and pancytokeratin.

A. *Immunophenotype of histiocytic sarcoma:*
  - Most histiocytic sarcoma cells are positive for one or more histiocytic markers: CD163 (membranous and cytoplasmic), CD68 (cytoplasmic granular), PU.1 (nuclear), lysozyme (cytoplasmic granular, accentuated in the Golgi region), and CD4.
  - Some histiocytic sarcoma is positive for CD31, CD56 (rare), S100 (usually variable), CD15 (weak), B-cell transcription factor OCT2 (in cases of histiocytic sarcoma that arises from previously diagnosed B-cell lymphoma), but not PAX5 [3].
  - CD45, CD45RO, and HLA-DR are usually positive.
  - The proliferation index (Ki-67+) varies from 10% to 90%.
  - By definition, histiocytic sarcoma cells are negative for pan-B-cell (CD19, CD20, CD79a), pan-T-cell (CD3), Langerhans cell (CD1a, langerin), follicular dendritic cell (CD21, CD23, CD35), melanoma (HMB45), and epithelial (EMA and keratin) and myeloid cell (MPO) markers.
  - There is no evidence of *EBV* infection.

B. *Immunophenotype of Langerhans cell histiocytosis/sarcoma:*
  - LCH cells express S100, CD1a, langerin (CD207), CD68, and vimentin.
  - Some cases express lysozyme (weakly), CD4, and CD14.
  - Unlike normal or hyperplastic Langerhans cells, LCH cells are commonly positive for cyclin D1 [4].
  - Langerhans cell sarcomas are also variably positive for langerin (at least focally), S-100, CD1a, CD68, lysozyme, and PD-L1 [5].
  - B-cell and T-cell lineage markers (except for CD4), CD30, and follicular dendritic cell markers are absent.

C. *Immunophenotype of follicular dendritic cell (FDC) sarcoma:*
  - FDC sarcoma cells are positive for CD21, CD23, CD35, clusterin, D2-40/podoplanin, CXCL13, CD4 (weak), S-100 (focal), CD68 (weak), and PD-L1 (~50%).
  - EMA is variably positive in FDC sarcoma but not in normal FDC cells.
  - FDC sarcoma cells are negative for CD1a, CD207/langerin, CD10, CD19, CD79a, CD30, CD31, CD34, CD163, lysozyme, BCL6, cyclin D1, MPO, pan-T-cell antigens, HMB45, and keratins.
  - It should be noted that FDC markers CD21 and CD23 are not specific and may be expressed by Reed-Sternberg and Hodgkin cells.
  - Ki-67 labeling ranges from 1% to 25%.

D. *Immunophenotype of interdigitating dendritic cell sarcoma:*
  - These sarcoma cells are consistently positive for S-100 (moderate to strong), vimentin, and fascin and are variably positive for CD45 and CD68.
  - They are usually negative for CD4, CD14, CD163, and lysozyme with rare exceptions.
  - They are negative for CD1a, CD207, follicular dendritic cell markers (CD21, CD23, and CD35), pan-B- and T-cell antigens, CD30, CD34, MPO, clusterin, D2-40/podoplanin, EMA, and cytokeratins.
  - The proliferation index (Ki-67+) is low (10–20%).

5. Which ancillary test results are diagnostic, suggestive of diagnosis, unreliable for diagnosis, or rule out the diagnosis?

In practice, if the histiocytic/dendritic cell neoplasm is in the differential diagnosis, S100, CD1a, CD207/langerin, CD163, CD21, CD35, and keratin can be ordered initially to differentiate the most common type of histiocytic/dendritic cell tumors (Table 17.1):

- Histiocytic sarcoma (CD163+)
- Follicular dendritic cell sarcoma (CD21+, CD35+)

Table 17.1 Basic markers required for differentiation of histiocytic/dendritic cell neoplasms

Marker / Tumor	CD163	S100	CD1a	CD207/langerin	CD21	CD35	Keratin
Histiocytic sarcoma	+	–/+	–	–	–	–	–
Langerhans cell histiocytosis/sarcoma	–	+	+	+	–	–	–
Follicular dendritic cell sarcoma	–	–	–	–	+	+	–
Interdigitating dendritic cell sarcoma	–	+	–	–	–	–	–
Indeterminate dendritic cell tumor	–	+	+	–	–	–	–
Fibroblastic reticular cell tumor	–	–	–	–	–	–	+

- Langerhans cell histiocytosis/sarcoma (S100+, CD1a+, langerin+)
- Interdigitating dendritic cell sarcoma (S100+)
- Fibroblastic reticular cell tumor (keratin+)
- Indeterminate dendritic cell tumor (S100+, CD1a+, CD207−)
- Immunostaining results in combination with B-cell, T-cell, and melanoma markers, PU.1, lysozyme, CD68, EMA, vimentin, and smooth muscle actin will reach a definitive diagnosis.

6. What is the work-up to provide prognostic and therapeutic target information?

- In general, the tumor size, cytologic atypia, proliferation index, and the organ involved (localized vs systemic) are relevant to prognosis.
- Activating *BRAF* mutation or activation of *MEK*, *ERK*, and *MAP2K1* has been variably detected in Langerhans cell histiocytosis/sarcoma, histiocytic sarcoma, follicular dendritic cell sarcoma, and interdigitating dendritic cell sarcoma along with benign histiocytic lesion (e.g., Erdheim-Chester disease).
- Targeting BRAF therapy is under clinical investigation.

7. What should be the approach to provide maximum, but defensible information, from limited specimen or work-up? What is a descriptive diagnosis appropriate in such situations?

- If the specimen is limited, distinguishing benign reactive hyperplasia with sarcoma is the first goal.
- If tissue biopsy is small with processing artifact, it would cause a limitation of immunohistochemical work-up. In this situation, providing the differential diagnoses with recommendation for a re-biopsy would be appropriate.
- The key point is "do not over-diagnose."

8. When is a diagnostic comment necessary and what should be discussed in the diagnostic comment for this entity?

- When a definitive diagnosis cannot be reached, either due to limited specimen or equivocal ancillary work-up, a diagnostic comment with important differential diagnosis and proper recommendation should be provided.
- For example, before diagnosis of histiocytic sarcoma, a bone marrow study to rule out an extramedullary proliferation of acute monoblastic leukemia (myeloid sarcoma) should be recommended.

9. Transdifferentiation or dedifferentiation?

- Some patients with B-cell lymphoma/leukemia subsequently or simultaneously develop clonally related myeloid tumors, including histiocytic sarcoma (most common), interdigitating dendritic cell sarcoma, Langerhans cell histiocytosis/sarcoma, and acute myeloid leukemia [6–8].
- These converted myeloid tumors contain identical clonal immunoglobulin gene rearrangement or the hallmark of follicular lymphoma, t(14;18) [3, 9, 10].
- Rarely, LCH cells with the leukemia-associated T-cell receptor gene rearrangement in patient with T-lymphoblastic leukemia have also been identified [11].
- As B-myeloid conversion is observed across different types of lymphomas, including follicular lymphoma, chronic lymphocytic leukemia/small lymphocytic lymphoma, diffuse large B-cell lymphoma, marginal zone lymphoma, and acute lymphoblastic leukemia, and not limited to a specific subtype of lymphoma, some common underlying mechanisms must be shared.
- The lymphoid to myeloid conversion has been considered through transdifferentiation in the literature, which implies that a mature neoplastic lymphocyte can become a neoplastic myeloid cell as a result of genetic or epigenetic changes, which differ from dedifferentiation or origin from a shared progenitor cell.

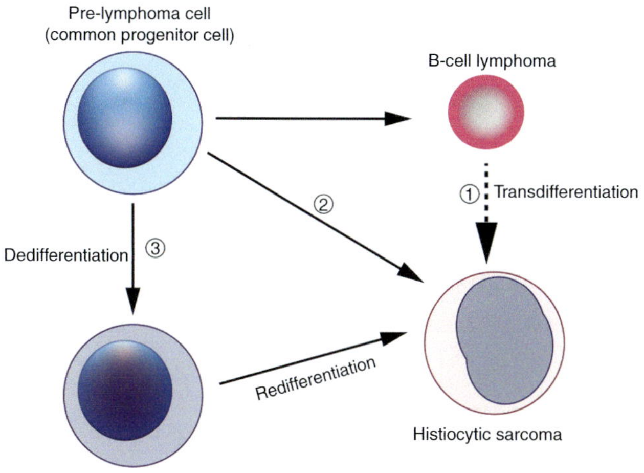

Fig. 17.1 Routes of B-myeloid conversion. Currently, the underlying mechanisms of B-cell lymphoma transformation into histiocytic sarcoma are still unclear. Transdifferentiation (route 1) has been used frequently in the literature. However, recent clonal tracing indicates the evolution from a common progenitor cell/pro-lymphoma cell (route 2). Our unpublished genetic data strongly suggest that B-myeloid conversion is through dedifferentiation from a pro-lymphoma cell/common progenitor cell, followed by redifferentiation (route 3)

- Recent clonal tracing analysis demonstrated that histiocytic sarcoma derives from the common progenitor cells identified in the follicular lymphoma (Fig. 17.1) [12, 13].
- Our unpublished data (manuscript in preparation) suggest that the lymphoma-initiating cells (or pro-lymphoma cells, which function as common progenitor cells), but not overt transformed lymphoma cells, have the potential to convert to myeloid tumor through dedifferentiation but not transdifferentiation (Fig. 17.1).
- As the process of dedifferentiation is transient, it is impossible for pathologists to capture this process.
- In addition to phenotyping the two neoplasms, proof of clonal relationship between the primary B-cell neoplasm and converted secondary tumors would be the key to make the diagnosis. Because the secondary tumor often inherits the clonally rearranged immunoglobulin gene from the primary B-cell neoplasm, detecting identical amplicons with the same break points would provide evidence of clonal relationship between the two neoplasms. Since introduction of NGS analysis for B-cell clonality in many molecular diagnostic laboratories, this goal will be achieved spontaneously, without undergoing multiple steps to sequence the PCR products as was done previously. For some B-cell lymphomas with specific cytogenetic changes, such as *IGH/BCL2* fusion in follicular lymphoma, interphase FISH analysis could be performed on section with converted secondary tumor. If the change is identified, the clonal relationship would be established.
- These patients typically present with advanced disease and poor prognosis. Due to diagnostic difficulties and lack of standard therapeutic regimens, understanding the underlying mechanisms will have significant clinical relevance for treating these uncommon, but fatal diseases.

10. When it is appropriate to seek external consultation for this entity?

- When the specimen is adequate but the immunohistochemical results are equivocal, consultation with hematopathology colleagues and/or pathologists with expertise in soft tissue pathology is necessary to establish the final diagnosis.
- Particularly challenging are those lesions that have overlapped morphologic and immunohistochemical features. For example, electron microscopy is the only way to differentiate spindle cell melanoma with interdigitating dendritic cell sarcoma [14]. Therefore, detailed clinical information and expert's opinion are required.
- Histiocytic/dendritic neoplasms are rare tumors, and many medical institutes often have only few each year. For those who do not have sufficient experience with the diagnosis, it may be prudent to lower the threshold to send for external expertise consult.

Case Presentations

Case 1

Learning Objectives

1. To become familiar with the histologic features of histiocytic sarcoma
2. To become familiar with the immunohistochemical features of histiocytic sarcoma
3. To generate the differential diagnosis

Case History

A 53-year-old male presented with fever, weight loss, and a solitary mass (5.0 cm in diameter) on the trunk.

Histologic Findings

- Large atypical cells with round or elongated folded nuclei, vesicular chromatin, and abundant eosinophilic cytoplasm (Fig. 17.2a) diffusely infiltrate the soft tissue.
- The neoplastic cells are obscured by an extensive inflammatory cell infiltrate including many neutrophils. These features make it mimic an inflammatory lesion (Fig. 17.2b).
- Tumor cell necrosis (Fig. 17.2c) is present in focal areas.

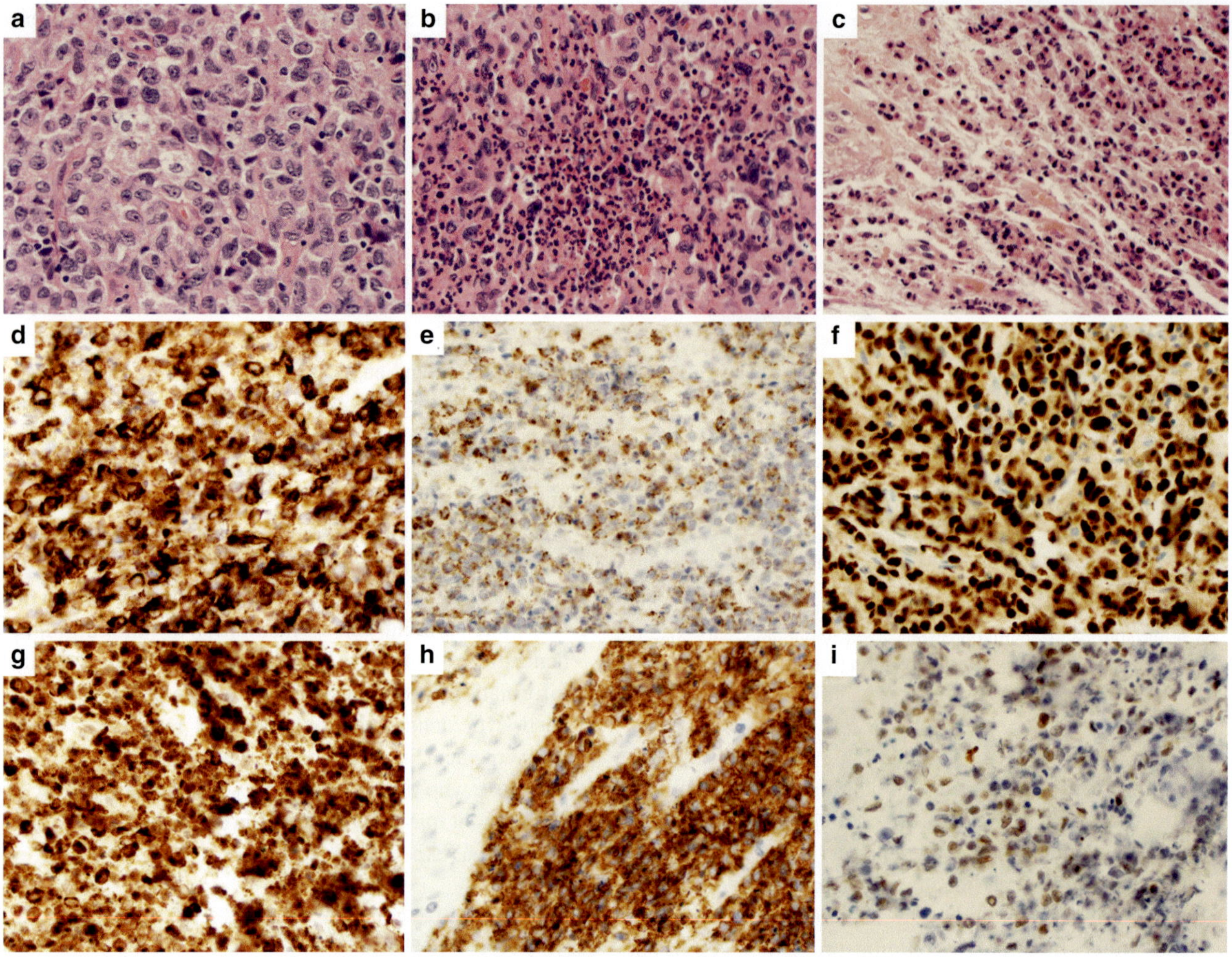

Fig. 17.2 Histiocytic sarcoma. The section of biopsy shows proliferation of histiocytoid cells that are large and atypical with round or elongated folded nuclei, vesicular chromatin, and abundant eosinophilic cytoplasm (**a**). Neutrophil infiltration (**b**) and tumor cell necrosis (**c**) present in focal area. The neoplastic cells are strongly positive for histiocytic markers CD163 (**d**), CD68 (**e**), PU.1 (**f**), and lysozyme (**g**). Tumor cells are positive for CD56 (**h**) and B-cell transcription factor OCT2 (subset) (**i**). **a–i**, 500×

Differential Diagnosis

- Inflammatory lesion
- Langerhans cell histiocytosis/sarcoma
- Anaplastic large cell lymphoma
- Large B-cell lymphoma
- Myeloid sarcoma
- Malignant melanoma

IHC and Other Ancillary Studies

- Tumor cells are strongly positive for histiocytic markers CD163 (Fig. 17.2d), CD68 (Fig. 17.2e), PU.1 (Fig. 17.2f), and lysozyme (Fig. 17.2g).
- Rare tumor cells are positive for CD56 (Fig. 17.2h) and B-cell transcription factor OCT2 (subset) (Fig. 17.2i).
- CD20, CD3, MPO, S100, CD1a, CD21, HMB45, and cytokeratin stains are essentially negative in tumor cells.

Final Diagnosis

Histiocytic sarcoma

Take-Home Messages

1. Histiocytic sarcoma can mimic inflammatory lesion.
2. Diagnosis of histiocytic sarcoma relies on the morphologic examination and immunohistochemical analysis to rule out other neoplastic entities.
3. Histiocytic sarcoma is an aggressive neoplasm.

Case 2

Learning Objectives

1. To become familiar with the histologic features of Langerhans cell histiocytosis

2. To become familiar with the immunohistochemical features of Langerhans cell histiocytosis
3. To generate the differential diagnosis

Case History

A 14-year-old boy presented with a solitary pelvic bone lesion (8.2 cm in diameter) with inguinal lymphadenopathy, but without systemic syndrome.

Histologic Findings

- Biopsy of an enlarged regional lymph node shows nodal architecture effaced by proliferation of histiocytoid cells.
- Tumor cells have folded and grooved nuclei.
- Many multinucleated giant histiocytes are identified in this case.
- Numerous small lymphocytes, plasma cells, and eosinophils are present in the background (Fig. 17.3a, 100×; Fig. 17.3b, 400×).

Differential Diagnosis

- Dermal dendritic cell hyperplasia
- Giant cell tumor of tendon sheath and related entities.
- Histiocyte-rich lymphomas and leukemias
- Rosai-Dorfman disease

IHC and Other Ancillary Studies

- Tumor cells are strongly positive for S100 (Fig. 17.3c, 400×) and CD1a (Fig. 17.3d, 400×) and CD207/langerin (not shown).
- Tumor cells are negative for CD163, lysozyme, MPO, CD21, CD20, CD3, and CD30.

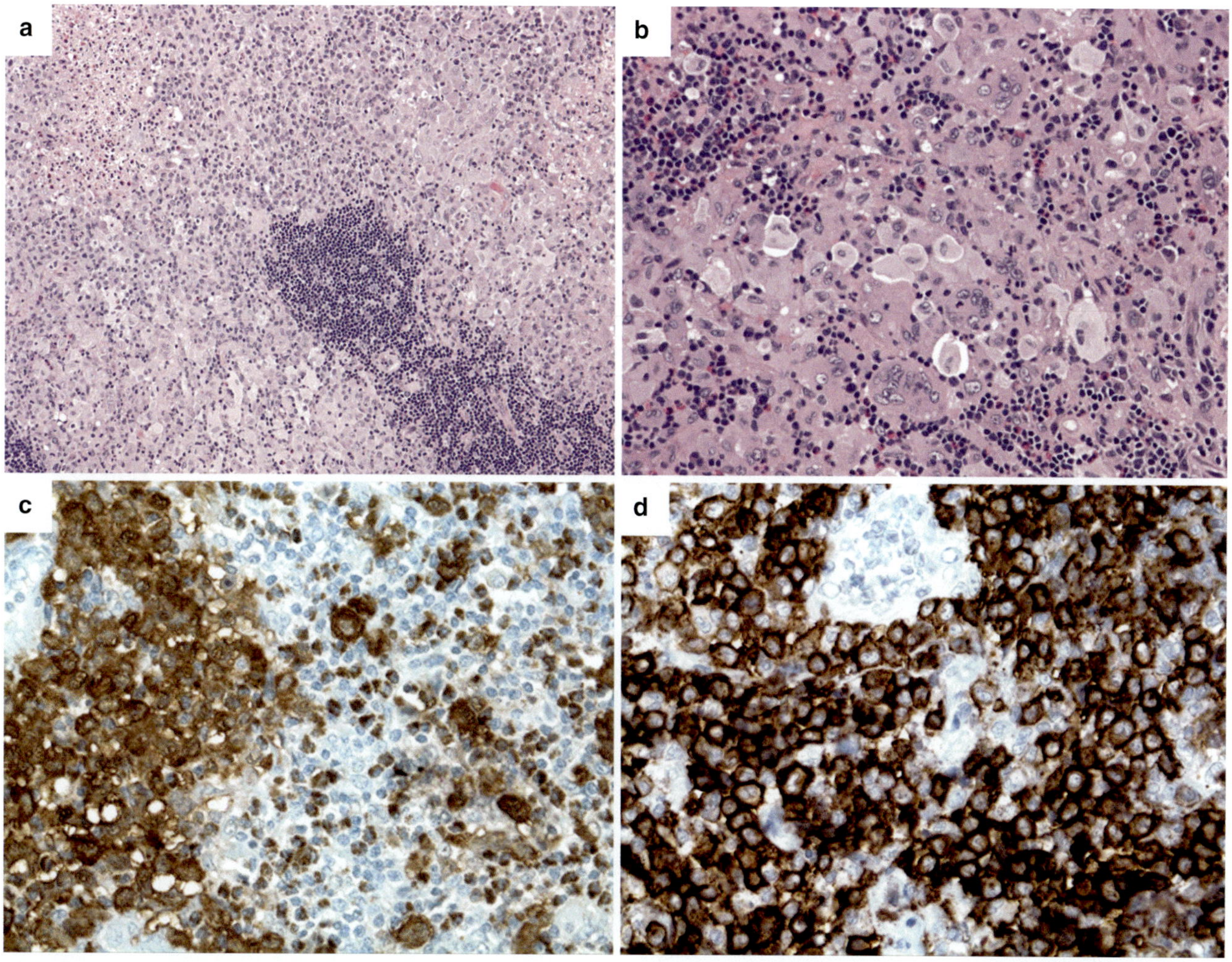

Fig. 17.3 Langerhans cell histiocytosis. The biopsy of inguinal lymph node shows effaced nodal architecture by histiocytoid cells that have folded and grooved nuclei. Many multinucleated giant histiocytes are identified in this case. Numerous small lymphocytes, plasma cells, and eosinophils are present in the background (**a**, 100×; **b**, 400×). Immunohistochemical staining shows that neoplastic cells are strongly positive for S100 (**c**, 400×) and CD1a (**d**, 400×) and CD207/langerin (not shown)

- Ultrastructure study demonstrates typical Birbeck granules in tumor cells.

Final Diagnosis

Langerhans cell histiocytosis

Take-Home Messages

1. Langerhans cell histiocytosis should be distinguished from other histiocytic/dendritic cell neoplasm.
2. Langerhans cell histiocytosis often occurs in pediatric patients and presents with bone lesion.
3. EM study can identify Birbeck granules in Langerhans cell histiocytosis.

Case 3

Learning Objectives

1. To become familiar with the histologic features of follicular dendritic cell sarcoma
2. To become familiar with the immunohistochemical features of follicular dendritic cell sarcoma
3. To generate the differential diagnosis

Case History

A 47-year-old female presented with enlarged cervical lymph node (3.5 cm in diameter).

Histologic Findings

- H&E sections of lymph node biopsy (Fig. 17.4a, 100×; Fig. 17.4b, 400×) show the nodal architecture effaced by proliferation of whorling bundles and fascicles of spindle-shaped tumor cells with bland nuclei and indistinct cytoplasmic borders.
- Admixed are many small lymphocytes throughout.

Differential Diagnosis

- Thymoma
- Interdigitating dendritic cell sarcoma
- Spindle cell carcinoma
- Melanoma

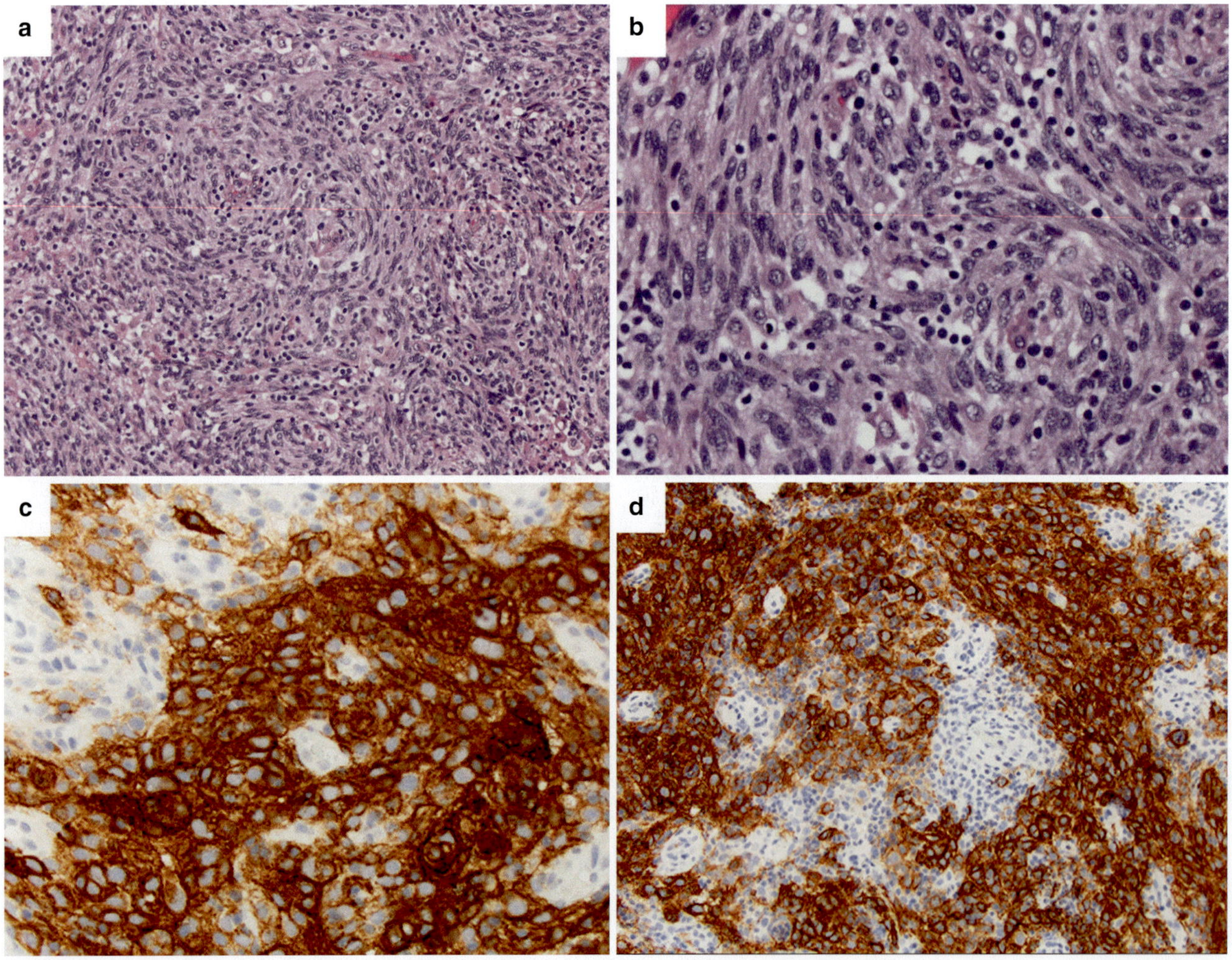

Fig. 17.4 Follicular dendritic cell sarcoma. H&E sections of excised cervical lymph node (**a**, 100×; **b**, 400×) show whorling bundles and fascicles of spindle-shaped tumor cells with bland nuclei and indistinct cytoplasmic borders admixed with numerous small lymphocytes. Tumor cells are strongly positive for CD21 (**c**, 400×) and CD23 (**d**, 400×)

IHC and Other Ancillary Studies

- Tumor cells are strongly positive for CD21 (Fig. 17.4c, 400×) and CD23 (Fig. 17.4d, 400×).
- Tumor cells are negative for CD163, lysozyme, MPO, S100, CD1a, HMB45, CD20, CD3, and pancytokeratin.

Final Diagnosis

Follicular dendritic cell sarcoma

Take-Home Messages

1. Follicular dendritic cell sarcoma should be distinguished from other histiocytic/dendritic cell neoplasm and other tumors with spindled morphology.
2. Follicular dendritic cell sarcoma often presents in lymph node, though extranodal lesions are also seen. Occasionally it is seen in lymph nodes involved by hyaline vascular type Castleman disease.
3. The diagnosis relies on morphologic examination and immunohistochemical analysis.

Case 4

Learning Objectives

1. To become familiar with the clinical presentation and pathologic diagnosis of histiocytic sarcoma arising from follicular lymphoma
2. To become familiar with the application of genetic or molecular diagnostic tests to determine the clonal relationship between primary follicular lymphoma and subsequent histiocytic sarcoma
3. To be familiar with the pathogenesis and clinical significance of transdifferentiation in follicular lymphoma or other B-cell neoplasms

Case History

A 67-year-old female with remote history of follicular lymphoma presented with bilateral enlarged cervical lymph node and lytic bone lesions in cervical vertebra. Cervical lymph node biopsy was performed to rule out large B-cell lymphoma transformed from the preexisting follicular lymphoma.

Histologic Findings

- H&E sections of lymph node biopsy excised many years ago showing typical low-grade follicular lymphoma within one neoplastic follicle (Fig. 17.5a).
- Section of the recent biopsy of cervical lymph node demonstrated the nodal architecture effaced by proliferation of large cells with abundant cytoplasm that are reminiscent of histiocytoid or dendritic cells.
- Admixed are scattered neutrophils and small lymphocytes throughout (Fig. 17.5b).

Differential Diagnosis

- Recurrent follicular lymphoma
- Diffuse large B-cell lymphoma transformed from follicular lymphoma
- De novo diffuse large B-cell lymphoma
- De novo histiocytic/dendritic cell sarcoma
- Other hematolymphoid neoplasm
- Metastatic tumors

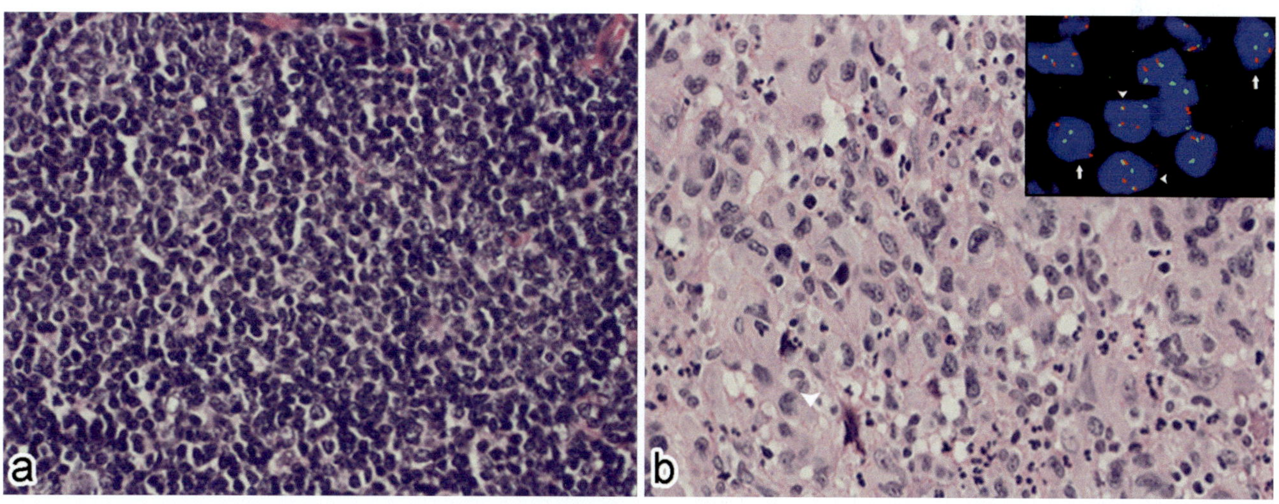

Fig. 17.5 Histiocytic sarcoma arising from preexisting follicular lymphoma. (**a**) H&E section of remote lymph node biopsy showing the low-grade follicular lymphoma at high magnification. 500×. Note the centrocyte morphology without significant number of centroblasts. (**b**) H&E section of cervical lymph node biopsy demonstrating histiocytic sarcoma. 500×. *Inset:* interphase FISH analysis shows evidence of *IGH/BCL2* fusion on section with histiocytic sarcoma in this particular patient with two metachronous neoplasms. Arrowheads indicate the nuclei with typical dual fusions, *IGH/BCL2* and reciprocal fusion genes, respectively; isolated red signal represents intact allele of *BCL2* gene, and isolated green signal represents intact *IGH* gene. *Arrows* indicated the nuclei without the fusion gene (all the probes are separated; two intact *IGH* and two intact *BCL2* genes)

IHC and Other Ancillary Studies

- Tumor cells are strongly positive for CD163, lysozyme, CD4, and CD68.
- Tumor cells are negative for MPO, S100, CD1a, CD21, CD23, HMB45, CD20, CD79a, CD3, and pancytokeratin.
- *IGH* gene rearrangement analysis was positive for clonal rearrangement of the gene, which is identical in amplicon size and breakpoint sequences to that detected in the patient's prior follicular lymphoma.
- Interphase FISH analysis demonstrates *IGH/BCL2* fusion in 61% of the total nuclei on the section of histiocytic sarcoma (Fig. 17.5b, inset).

Final Diagnosis

Histiocytic sarcoma transdifferentiated from preexisting follicular lymphoma

Take-Home Messages

1. Follicular lymphoma or other B-cell neoplasms could transform to histiocytic/dendritic cell neoplasm in rare occasions.
2. The conversion is named as "transdifferentiation," given the event that does not follow the conventional route of lineage differentiation.
3. The diagnosis relies on morphologic examination and immunohistochemical analysis as well as determination of clonal relationship between the morphologically and phenotypically distinct neoplasms.

References

1. Choe JY, Go H, Jeon YK, Yun JY, Kim YA, Kim HJ, et al. Inflammatory pseudotumor-like follicular dendritic cell sarcoma of the spleen: a report of six cases with increased IgG4-positive plasma cells. Pathol Int. 2013;63(5):245–51.
2. Hartert M, Ströbel P, Dahm M, Nix W, Marx A, Vahl CF. A follicular dendritic cell sarcoma of the mediastinum with immature T cells and association with myasthenia gravis. Am J Surg Pathol. 2010;34(5):742–5.
3. Chen W, Lau SK, Fong D, Wang J, Wang E, Arber DA, et al. High frequency of clonal immunoglobulin receptor gene rearrangements in sporadic histiocytic/dendritic cell sarcomas. Am J Surg Pathol. 2009;33(6):863–73.
4. Shanmugam V, Craig JW, Hornick JL, Morgan EA, Pinkus GS, Pozdnyakova O. Cyclin D1 is expressed in neoplastic cells of Langerhans cell histiocytosis but not reactive Langerhans cell proliferations. Am J Surg Pathol. 2017;41(10):1390–6.
5. Gatalica Z, Bilalovic N, Palazzo JP, Bender RP, Swensen J, Millis SZ, et al. Disseminated histiocytoses biomarkers beyond BRAFV600E: frequent expression of PD-L1. Oncotarget. 2015;6(23):19819–25.
6. Takahashi E, Nakamura S. Histiocytic sarcoma: an updated literature review based on the 2008 WHO classification. J Clin Exp Hematop. 2013;53(1):1–8.
7. Stoecker MM, Wang E. Histiocytic/dendritic cell transformation of B-cell neoplasms: pathologic evidence of lineage conversion in differentiated hematolymphoid malignancies. Arch Pathol Lab Med. 2013;137(6):865–70.
8. Steussy B, Lekostaj J, Qian Q, Rosenthal N, Holman CJ, Syrbu S, et al. Leukemic transdifferentiation of follicular lymphoma into an acute histiocytic leukemia in a 52-year-old caucasian woman. Lab Med. 2016;47(2):155–7.
9. Feldman AL, Arber DA, Pittaluga S, Martinez A, Burke JS, Raffeld M, et al. Clonally related follicular lymphomas and histiocytic/dendritic cell sarcomas: evidence for transdifferentiation of the follicular lymphoma clone. Blood. 2008;111(12):5433–9.
10. Wang E, Papalas J, Hutchinson CB, Kulbacki E, Huang Q, Sebastian S, et al. Sequential development of histiocytic sarcoma and diffuse large b-cell lymphoma in a patient with a remote history of follicular lymphoma with genotypic evidence of a clonal relationship: a divergent (bilineal) neoplastic transformation of an indolent B-cell lymphoma in a single individual. Am J Surg Pathol. 2011;35(3):457–63.
11. Feldman AL, Berthold F, Arceci RJ, Abramowsky C, Shehata BM, Mann KP, et al. Clonal relationship between precursor T-lymphoblastic leukaemia/lymphoma and Langerhans-cell histiocytosis. Lancet Oncol. 2005;6(6):435–7.
12. Brunner P, Rufle A, Dirnhofer S, Lohri A, Willi N, Cathomas G, et al. Follicular lymphoma transformation into histiocytic sarcoma: indications for a common neoplastic progenitor. Leukemia. 2014;28(9):1937–40.
13. Green MR, Alizadeh AA. Common progenitor cells in mature B-cell malignancies: implications for therapy. Curr Opin Hematol. 2014;21(4):333–40.
14. Stowman AM, Mills SE, Wick MR. Spindle cell melanoma and interdigitating dendritic cell sarcoma: do they represent the same process? Am J Surg Pathol. 2016;40(9):1270–9.

Typical Morphologic Patterns of Infectious and Other Reactive Lymphadenopathies

18

Maria (Ria) Vergara-Lluri and Rosemary She

Abbreviation

AITL	Angioimmunoblastic T-cell lymphoma
ALCL	Anaplastic large cell lymphoma
ANA	Antineutrophil antibody
anti-CCP	Anti-citrullinated peptide/protein antibody
anti-dsDNA	Anti-double-stranded deoxyribonucleic acid
anti-Sm	Anti-Smith antibody
AOSD	Adult-onset Still's disease
cHL	Classic Hodgkin lymphoma
CF	Complement fixation
CLL/SLL	Chronic lymphocytic leukemia/small lymphocytic lymphoma
CMV	Cytomegalovirus
CRP	C-reactive protein
DAT	Direct antiglobulin test/direct Coombs test
DLBCL	Diffuse large B-cell lymphoma
EBER ISH	*EBV*-encoded RNA in situ hybridization
EBV	Epstein Barr virus
EBV-IM	*EBV*-related infectious mononucleosis
EIA	Enzyme immunoassay
ESR	Erythrocyte sedimentation rate
FDC	Follicular dendritic cell
FRFH	Florid reactive follicular hyperplasia
GC	Germinal center
HIV/AIDS	Human immunodeficiency virus/acquired immunodeficiency syndrome
HHV8	Human herpesvirus 8
HLH	Hemophagocytic lymphohistiocytosis/hemophagocytic syndrome
HRS	Hodgkin/Reed-Sternberg
HSV	Herpes simplex virus
HTN	Hypertension
HV	Hyaline vascular
IBD	Inflammatory bowel disease
IFH	Interfollicular hyperplasia
IFH/DFH	Interfollicular hyperplasia/diffuse hyperplasia
IgG4-RD	IgG4-related disease
IgG4-R-LAD	IgG4-related lymphadenopathy
IHC	Immunohistochemistry
IPT	Inflammatory pseudotumor
KFD	Kikuchi-Fujimoto disease
LA	Latex agglutination
LAD	Lymphadenopathy/lymphadenitis
LCH	Langerhans cell histiocytosis
LDH	Lactate dehydrogenase
LFA	Lateral flow assay
LN	Lymph node
LPL	Lymphoplasmacytic lymphoma
MAI	Mycobacterium avium intracellulare
MCD	Multicentric Castleman disease
MCL	Mantle cell lymphoma
MF	Mycosis fungoides
MTB	Mycobacterium tuberculosis
MZL	Marginal zone lymphoma
NAAT	Nucleic acid amplification test
NHL	Non-Hodgkin lymphoma
NLPHL	Nodular lymphocyte predominant Hodgkin lymphoma
NOS	Not otherwise specified
NTM	Non-tuberculous/atypical mycobacteria
PB	Peripheral blood
PC	Plasma cell
POEMS	Polyneuropathy, organomegaly, endocrinopathy, monoclonal gammopathy, and skin changes
PTCL	Peripheral T-cell lymphoma
PTGC	Progressive transformation of germinal centers
PTLD	Post-transplant lymphoproliferative disorder
RA	Rheumatoid arthritis
RDD/SHML	Rosai-Dorfman-Destombes/sinus histiocytosis with massive lymphadenopathy
RF	Rheumatoid factor
RFH	Reactive follicular hyperplasia
SLE	Systemic lupus erythematosus
TCHRLBL	T-cell histiocyte-rich large B-cell lymphoma
TTP	Thrombotic thrombocytopenic purpura
UCD	Unicentric Castleman disease
VCA	Viral capsid antigen

M. (Ria) Vergara-Lluri (✉)
Clinical Pathology, Hematopathology Service, Department of Pathology, LAC+USC Medical Center, Keck School of Medicine of USC (University of Southern California), Los Angeles, CA, USA
e-mail: Maria.Vergara-Lluri@med.usc.edu

R. She
Clinical Pathology, Department of Pathology, Keck School of Medicine of USC (University of Southern California), Los Angeles, CA, USA

E. Wang, A. S. Lagoo (eds.), *Practical Lymph Node and Bone Marrow Pathology*, Practical Anatomic Pathology,
https://doi.org/10.1007/978-3-030-32189-5_18

List of Frequently Asked Questions

1. What are the major histologic patterns of infectious and other reactive lymphadenopathies?
2. What are typical findings in reactive follicular hyperplasia (RFH)?
3. What is the differential diagnosis (DDx) for RFH?
4. As a very typical entity that can display RFH, what other morphologic features can HIV/AIDS-related LAD exhibit?
5. Are histologic features alone sufficiently diagnostic for HIV/AIDS-related LAD?
6. What ancillary testing can help establish the diagnosis of HIV/AIDS-related LAD?
7. If RFH is not due to HIV/AIDS-related LAD, then what other histologic features could suggest another reactive entity (i.e., what else is in the DDx)?
8. What is the minimal histopathologic work-up in RFH?
9. What clinical and epidemiologic features are present in *Toxoplasma* LAD?
10. What are typical histologic and immunophenotypic findings for *Toxoplasma* LAD?
11. What ancillary testing can help establish the diagnosis of *Toxoplasma* LAD?
12. What clinical and epidemiologic features are present in lymphadenopathy associated with rheumatoid arthritis (RA-related LAD) and other autoimmune disorders?
13. What are typical histologic and immunophenotypic findings in RA-LAD and other autoimmune disorders?
14. What ancillary testing can help establish the diagnosis for RA-LAD?
15. What are clinical and epidemiologic features of unicentric Castleman disease (UCD)?
16. What are typical histologic findings in UCD?
17. What minimal histopathologic work-up and relevant clinical information can I use to avoid diagnostic pitfalls in UCD (like misdiagnosing HHV8-related multicentric Castleman disease [HHV8+ MCD] and early stage AITL)?
18. What clinical and epidemiologic features are present in progressive transformation of germinal centers (PTGC), another example of RFH?
19. What typical histologic findings are seen in PTGC?
20. What is the major DDx to consider and the minimal histopathologic work-up when PTGC is observed?
21. Considering all the entities in the DDx, what is the clinical relevance of misinterpretation in RFH?
22. In RFH, what information can be conveyed to the clinician? When is a diagnostic comment necessary? What is an adequate specimen?
23. When is consultation necessary in RFH?
24. What are typical findings in paracortical/interfollicular hyperplasia and diffuse hyperplasia (IFH/DH)?
25. What is the DDx in IFH/DH?
26. As a very typical entity that can display IFH/DH, what additional morphologic features does *EBV*-IM LAD exhibit?
27. Are immunohistologic features alone sufficiently diagnostic for *EBV*-IM-LAD?
28. What ancillary testing can help establish the diagnosis of *EBV*-IM-LAD?
29. If IFH/DH is not due to *EBV*-IM LAD, then what other histologic features could suggest another reactive entity (i.e., what else is in the DDx)?
30. What is the minimal histopathologic work-up in IFH/DH?
31. What clinical and epidemiologic features are present in adult-onset Still's disease (AOSD), another entity which can present with IFH/DH?
32. As a very typical entity that can display IFH/DH, what other morphologic features does AOSD exhibit?
33. What ancillary testing can help establish diagnosis of AOSD?
34. Considering entities in the DDx, what is the clinical relevance of misinterpretation in IFH/DH?
35. In IFH/DH, what information can be conveyed to the clinician? When is a diagnostic comment necessary? What is an adequate specimen?
36. When is consultation necessary in IFH/DH?
37. What are the typical morphologic findings in the major subtype of granulomatous and/or histiocyte-rich lymphadenopathy (G/H-LAD)?
38. What is the differential diagnosis for G/H-LAD patterns?
39. What is the minimal histopathologic and ancillary work-up for G/H-LAD?
40. As a very typical entity that displays necrotizing and/or non-necrotizing granulomatous LAD, what are salient clinical features in *Mycobacterium tuberculosis* complex lymphadenitis (MTBC LAD) and atypical mycobacterial/non-tuberculous mycobacterial lymphadenitis (NTM LAD)?
41. What histologic and special stain features suggest that a necrotizing and/or non-necrotizing granulomatous LAD is due to MTBC or NTM?
42. Are histologic and special stain findings alone sufficiently diagnostic for MTBC and NTM LAD?
43. What ancillary testing can help establish the diagnosis for MTBC and NTM LAD?

44. If necrotizing and/or non-necrotizing granulomas are not secondary to MTB or NTM, then what other histologic and special stain features could suggest another infectious entity (i.e., what else is in the DDx of infectious etiologies)?
45. What ancillary testing can help establish the specific infectious organism in fungal LAD?
46. What infectious organisms induce suppurative LAD?
47. What are typical histologic and immunophenotypic findings in suppurative LAD?
48. What ancillary testing can help establish the specific infectious organisms that induce suppurative LAD (includes *Bartonella* spp., *Staphylococcus*, *Streptococcus*, *Lymphogranuloma venereum*, *Francisella*, *Brucella*, *Yersinia*)?
49. After an exhaustive infectious disease work-up for etiologies of non-necrotizing (and even necrotizing and suppurative) granulomatous LAD, what else is in the DDx?
50. What clinical and epidemiologic features are present in sarcoid LAD?
51. What are typical histologic and special stain findings in sarcoid LAD?
52. What ancillary testing can help establish the diagnosis of sarcoid LAD?
53. Aside from sarcoidosis, what other non-infectious reactive agents can lead to non-necrotizing granulomatous LAD? What clinical and morphologic features allow their recognition?
54. As a very typical entity that can display prominent foamy macrophage and/or epithelioid histiocyte-rich inflammatory LAD, what are the salient clinical and morphologic features in *Mycobacterium avium-intracellulare* complex (MAC) vs. *M. leprae* (Hansen's disease)?
55. What ancillary testing can help establish the diagnosis for MAC, NTM, or Hansen's disease?
56. If prominent foamy macrophages and/or histiocyte-rich lymphadenitis is not due to mycobacterial infections (like MAC/NTM or leprosy), then what other etiologies should be considered (i.e., what else is in the DDx)? Are there clues to distinguishing one from another?
57. What morphologic features, immunohistochemical findings, and genetic/molecular studies would allow distinction of sinus histiocytosis from Rosai-Dorfman-Destombes disease and other neoplastic entities?
58. As an entity that can display massive necrosis and numerous histiocytes, what is Kikuchi-Fujimoto disease (KFD)? How does it typically present clinically?
59. What are typical histologic and immunophenotypic findings in KFD?
60. What is the minimal histopathologic work-up for KFD?
61. What ancillary testing can help establish the diagnosis of KFD?
62. KFD and SLE (one of its histologic patterns) have nearly identical histologic and immunophenotypic findings. What features will allow distinction between KFD and SLE?
63. To summarize G/H-LAD: what would be the clinical relevance of misinterpretation?
64. What information can be conveyed to the clinician? When is a diagnostic comment necessary? What is an adequate specimen?
65. When is external consultation in G/H-LAD necessary?
66. What are the typical morphologic findings in the major subtype of plasma cell-rich lymphadenopathy (PC-rich LAD)?
67. As a very typical entity that can display PC-rich LAD, what clinical and epidemiologic features does syphilitic (luetic) lymphadenitis exhibit?
68. What are typical histologic and immunophenotypic findings for syphilitic LAD?
69. What ancillary testing can support the diagnosis of syphilitic LAD?
70. What is the clinical relevance of not recognizing syphilitic LAD?
71. As a typical entity demonstrating PC-rich LAD, how does IgG4-related LAD (IgG4-R-LAD) present clinically?
72. What are typical histologic and immunophenotypic findings in IgG4-R-LAD and the minimal histopathologic work-up when suspected?
73. What clinical information and ancillary testing are highly suggestive of IgG4-RD and would support IgG4-R-LAD?
74. In LAD cases with increased IgG4+ plasma cells, what information can be conveyed to the clinician? When is a diagnostic comment necessary? What are the clinical implications of the diagnosis?
75. What is an adequate specimen in reactive LAD with increased IgG4+ plasma cells?
76. As another typical entity that displays PC-rich LAD, what salient clinical and epidemiologic features do multicentric Castleman Disease (MCD) exhibit?
77. What are typical histologic and immunophenotypic findings in MCD?
78. What is the clinical relevance of misinterpretation of PC-rich LAD?

79. What information can be conveyed to the clinician in LAD with features of plasma cell-rich Castleman disease? When is a diagnostic comment necessary?
80. What is an adequate specimen in LAD with MCD-like histopathology?
81. When is external consultation necessary in LAD with MCD-like histopathology?
82. What are the typical entities in the major subtype of LAD with prominent spindled cell proliferations?
83. What are some selected entities displaying spindled morphology and how does one establish their diagnoses?
84. What is the clinical relevance of misinterpretation in this group of intranodal vascular/spindle cell proliferations?
85. When is consultation necessary in LAD with prominent spindled proliferation?

Introduction

In this chapter, we describe the key histopathologic features in needle core, incisional, and/or (optimally) excisional biopsies, to be able to distinguish benign from malignant lymphadenopathy (LAD). Multiple schemata have been proposed by several authors to follow a pattern-based approach to the diagnosis of lymph node (LN) pathology [1, 2]. We adapt similar principles here. It is important to recognize that histologic features in any given diagnostic entity will vary based on whether LN was biopsied early or late into the time course of disease. Thus, patterns may overlap, or one pattern may predominate over another depending on the timing for any given disease.

The following are general histologic and immunohistochemical features that can be used to favor benign/reactive etiologies over malignant processes in LNs (Fig. 18.1):

- Nodal architectural preservation with generally well-spaced lymphoid follicles throughout
- Germinal centers exhibiting polarization
- Patent sinuses which may contain cytologically bland histiocytes
- Absence of overt cytologic atypia
- Admixture of B-lymphoid follicles and interfollicular T-cells
- Admixture of B- and T-immunoblasts in an immunoblastic proliferation
- Sinus and perisinusoidal expansion by many monocytoid B cells (medium-sized cells with oval to slightly irregular nuclear contours, moderately clumped chromatin, and abundant clear cytoplasm), at times admixed with neutrophils
- Lack of capsular fibrosis
- Sparse to absent extranodal lymphoid extension

Some of these features may also be seen in neoplastic conditions (e.g., patent sinuses can be seen in angioimmunoblastic T-cell lymphoma and lymphoplasmacytic lymphoma) or are directly contradicted by reactive conditions (e.g., one of the hallmark features in syphilitic lymphadenitis is capsular fibrosis). Thus, thoughtful review and consideration of neoplastic mimics is of utmost importance.

If ancillary studies are pursued, flow cytometric analysis will confirm absence of clonality in B- and T-cells; polyclonal peaks on B-cell and T-cell receptor gene rearrangement studies can support benignity. However, it is also well-documented that clonal (and pseudoclonal) B- and T-cell populations can be demonstrated by flow cytometry, FISH, and/or by molecular studies even in histologically reactive lymphoid proliferations. Thus, interpretation of ancillary data must be made with careful consideration of the histology [3–5].

It is possible to recognize reactive hyperplasia by assessment of histopathology alone. However, the pathologist adds value by proposing a focused differential diagnostic list (based on morphologic features) that clinicians can assess in their subsequent evaluation. Furthermore, knowledge of the patient's clinical presentation, pertinent laboratory studies, and imaging data all prove invaluable in rendering a specific diagnosis, or at least in suggesting a differential diagnosis and work-up that the treating physician can pursue.

Special Notes on Specimen Adequacy

In the case of reactive lymphadenopathy/lymphadenitis (LAD), an excisional biopsy is optimal for evaluation. However, less and less tissue is being procured using ever smaller caliber core needle biopsies (CNBx). Even fine needle aspiration (FNA) biopsy material can be received from a wide range of clinical providers including (but not limited to) surgeons, radiologists, general practitioners, and our cytopathology colleagues. Proponents of FNA sampling for LAD point to a body of literature advocating its utility as a first-line diagnostic technique, particularly in immunocompromised hosts and in regions with high prevalence of infec-

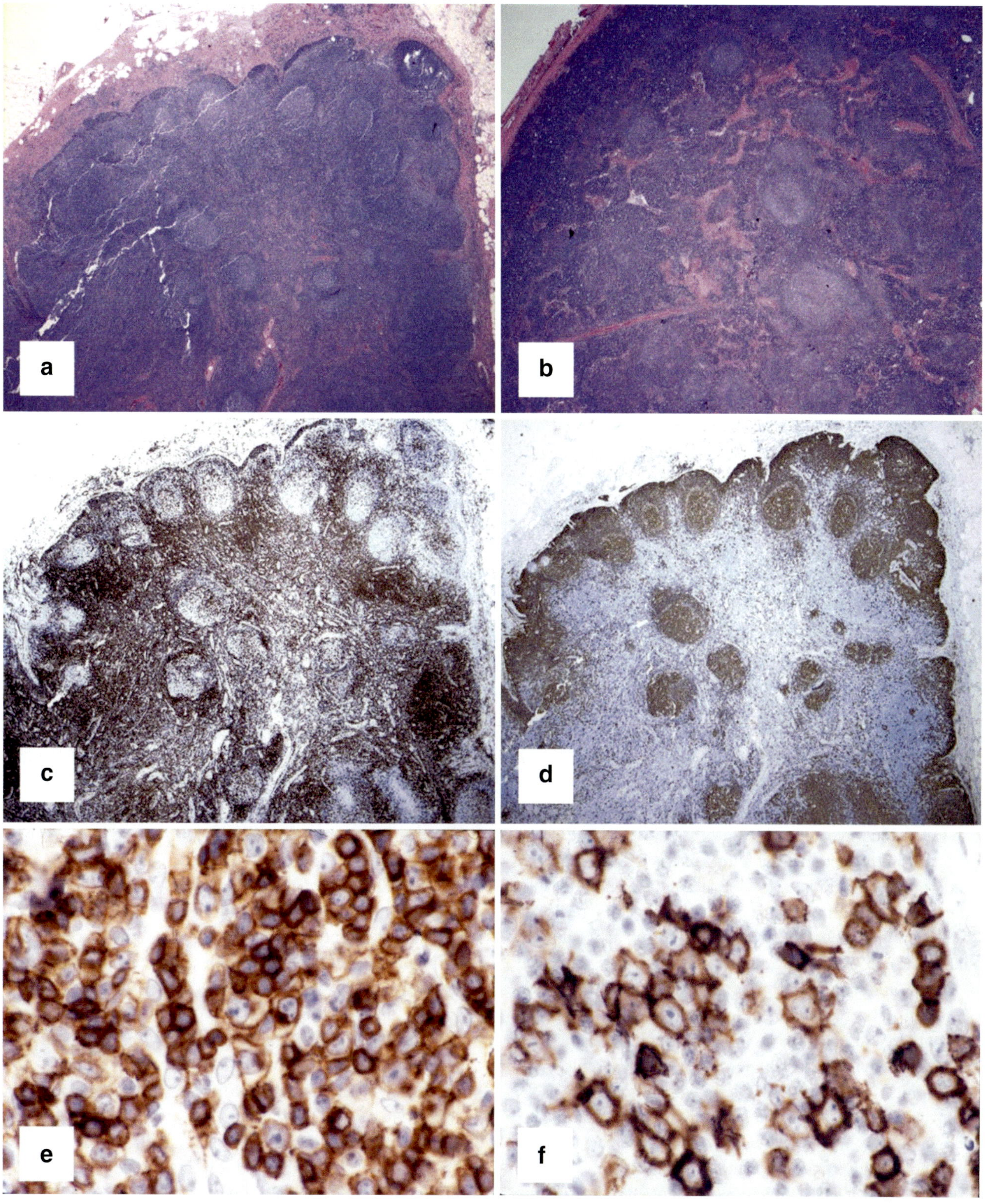

Fig. 18.1 Histologic and immunohistochemical features favoring benign/reactive etiology for lymphadenopathy. (**a**) Nodal architectural preservation is observed on low power, with generally well-spaced primary and secondary follicles throughout. Lymphocytes are largely confined within the nodal capsule. (**b**) Patent sinuses are apparent in this section. Cytologically bland histiocytes typically fill patent sinuses. Immunohistochemical stains serve to highlight nodal architectural preservation, showing numerous interfollicular T-cells by CD3 IHC (**c**) in between well-spaced B-lymphoid follicles by CD20 IHC (**d**). In immunoblastic proliferations, the admixture of CD3+ T-cell (**e**) and CD20+ B-cell (**f**) immunoblasts (i.e., large reactive transformed lymphocytes; apparent here by large size and nucleoli) favors a reactive process

tious disease. As compared to excisional biopsies, FNAs and CNBx have been reported to be safer and much less invasive procedures, simple to perform, less costly, easier to access in resource-limited settings, valuable in lymph nodes containing malignancy, useful in monitoring and staging patients with known malignancies, and a necessary alternative in surgically inaccessible sites and in patients unable to tolerate a surgical procedure.

Having said this, some investigators acknowledge that uncovering the etiology of reactive LAD in FNA/CNBx may prove more difficult in immunocompetent/HIV-negative patients and could ultimately require an excisional biopsy for definitive diagnosis.

Thus, if the etiology of an infectious LAD can be appropriately diagnosed by FNA (such as tuberculous LAD or coccidioidomycosis) because of the presence of characteristic infectious morphologic features (e.g., neutrophil-rich infiltrate, necrotizing granulomas, etc.) *and* ample sampling for confirmatory microbiologic studies, then FNA could be considered adequate and would not require further biopsy. Barring such diagnostic conditions in FNA, however, it is our practice to say "lymphoid tissue present" rather than "reactive lymphadenitis" in FNA biopsies even when no overt cytologic atypia nor flow cytometric abnormalities are detected. The rationale is that nodal architectural preservation (an essential measure for evaluation and arguably one of the topmost criteria for determining benignity) cannot be appropriately assessed on FNA sampling alone.

Our practice is to carefully review all clinical, laboratory, and radiologic studies whenever available to appreciate the degree of suspicion for malignancy. In the diagnostic comment, we indicate that limited FNA sampling in isolation precludes unequivocal exclusion of malignancy and/or prevents definitive characterization of a reactive process. Therefore, if clinical concern persists and the lesion of interest grows and/or fails to regress, we recommend a more generous sampling such as excisional biopsy, particularly in superficial and surgically accessible LNs.

Nodal architectural preservation can be observed on CNBx. In some cases, the etiology of a reactive process can be even uncovered on CNBx when diagnostic features are present (like paracortical hyperplasia, necrosis, and typical CMV-infected cells in CMV lymphadenitis). If the LN is well-sampled and CNBx appears to demonstrate reactive changes, it may well be considered adequate, particularly if a "reactive" interpretation fits the clinical picture.

On the other hand, if any atypical histopathologic features are worrisome for (yet not diagnostic of) a lymphoproliferative disorder, we append a diagnostic comment (similar to FNA) that an excisional biopsy is strongly advised [6–9].

1. What are the major histologic patterns of infectious and other reactive lymphadenopathies?

Table 18.1 gives a broad overview of the topics that will be discussed in this chapter. The major subtypes are divided into pattern-based constructs, with predominant reactive morphologic features separated in columns exhibiting:

- Reactive follicular hyperplasia (RFH)
- Paracortical/interfollicular hyperplasia to sometimes diffuse hyperplasia (IFH/DH)
- Granulomatous (non-necrotizing, necrotizing, and suppurative) and histiocyte-rich inflammatory infiltrates (G/H-LAD)
- Plasma cell-rich infiltrates (PC-rich LAD)
- Prominent spindled cell proliferations

The differential diagnosis is then further subclassified into infectious versus non-infectious etiologies, with a final row showing neoplastic mimics for these morphologic patterns. Many cases will display a mixture of patterns, so this classification is not inviolate, but can serve as a guide (Table 18.1) [2, 10, 11].

Reactive Follicular Hyperplasia (RFH), DDx Including LAD Secondary to HIV/AIDS, Toxoplasma, Rheumatoid Arthritis, HV-CD, PTGC

2. What are typical findings in reactive follicular hyperplasia (RFH)?

- RFH is characterized by an increase in number and/or size of lymphoid follicles leading to enlargement of LN, without architectural effacement.
- Typically, follicles are widely spaced (rather than back-to-back), contain intact surrounding mantle zones, and display polarized germinal centers (i.e., with light zone of centrocyte-rich cells toward the capsule and dark zone of centroblasts toward the medulla) with scattered tingible body macrophages and brisk mitotic activity.
- In contrast to neoplastic follicles in follicular lymphoma (FL), reactive follicles exhibit histologic polarization, absence of BCL2 expression, and gradation of proliferative activity on Ki-67 immunostaining (Fig. 18.2).
- RFH is the most common reactive morphologic finding encountered in clinical practice. It is thought to occur

Table 18.1 Predominant morphologic patterns and diagnostic entities/etiologies classified by infectious and non-infectious causes and neoplastic mimics

	Reactive follicular hyperplasia (RFH)	Reactive interfollicular to diffuse (immunoblastic) hyperplasia (IFH/DH)	Granulomatous and/or histiocyte-rich lymphadenopathy (G/H-LAD)		Plasma cell rich (PC-rich LAD)	Prominent spindled cell proliferations
			Well-formed granulomas [Non-necrotizing#, necrotizing*, suppurative^]	Foamy or epithelioid histiocyte-rich or foreign body granuloma		
Infectious	Bacterial LAD with RFH, NOS HIV/AIDS (acute/early stage) Toxoplasmosis Primary or secondary syphilis CMV HSV	*EBV*/infectious mononucleosis CMV HSV HHV6 Parasitic (*Wuchereria bancrofti*, *Onchocerca volvulus*, *Brugia malayi*, *Strongyloides*)	BACTERIA/MYCOBACTERIA *M. tuberculosis** NTM including *M. leprae**,# *Mycobacteria avium-intracellulare* (MAI) *Chlamydia*/LGV#,^ *Bartonella henselae*^ (Cat-scratch disease) *Yersinia* spp.^ *Brucella* spp.*,# *Francisella* spp.*,# *Treponema pallidum* (syphilis) FUNGAL *Histoplasma capsulatum**,# *Cryptococcus neoformans/C. gattii** *Blastomyces dermatitidis** *Coccidioides immitis*, *C. posadasii**,# *Aspergillus* spp.* PARASITIC *Leishmania* spp.	Whipple disease (*Tropheryma whipplei*) NTM including *M. leprae**,#, *Mycobacteria avium-intracellulare* (MAI) *Toxoplasma gondii* (toxoplasmosis) *Histoplasma capsulatum*	Syphilis MCD, HHV8+ HIV/AIDS (intermediate/ chronic stage) HHV8+ germinotropic lymphoproliferative disorder	Mycobacterial spindle cell pseudotumor Bacillary angiomatosis (*Bartonella* spp.) MCD, HHV8+
Non-infectious	FRFH, NOS (idiopathic) PTGC IgG4-RD (follicular hyperplasia- and PTGC-like patterns) SLE RA AOSD UCD, HV variant MCD, PC variant Kimura disease Drugs, chemicals, environmental exposure	IFH, NOS Dermatopathic Kimura disease SLE AOSD Exposure to environmental pollutants, chemicals Drug-related (Dilantin) Postvaccinial administration Churg-Strauss disease (allergic granulomatous angiitis) IgG4-R-LAD (interfollicular hyperplasia pattern) Mucocutaneous LN syndrome (Kawasaki disease)	Sarcoidosis# Crohn disease# Granulomatosis with polyangiitis SLE*,# KFD Kimura disease Drug-related immune reaction	RDD/SHML HLH SLE AOSD KFD Joint prosthesis associated Foreign body granulomas (e.g., talc, suture, lipid) Lipogranulomas from lymphangiogram	RDD/SHML iMCD = MCD, PC variant RA AOSD IgG4-R-LAD PC CD-like pattern SLE	Vascular transformation of LN sinuses Angiomyomatous hamartoma Palisaded myofibroblastoma Inflammatory pseudotumor IgG4-RD (inflammatory-pseudotumor-like pattern)

	Reactive follicular hyperplasia (RFH)	Reactive interfollicular to diffuse (immunoblastic) hyperplasia (IFH/DH)	Granulomatous and/or histiocyte-rich lymphadenopathy (G/H-LAD)		Plasma cell rich (PC-rich LAD)	
			Well-formed granulomas [Non-necrotizing#, necrotizing*, suppurative^]	Foamy or epithelioid histiocyte-rich or foreign body granuloma		Prominent spindled cell proliferations
Neoplastic mimics	Follicular lymphoma (typical and floral variant) NLPHL MZL with follicular colonization Mantle cell lymphoma with mantle zone pattern AITL cHL with interfollicular involvement	TCHRLBL DLBCL cHL ALCL MF involvement of LN AITL Myeloid/lymphoid neoplasms associated with eosinophilia	cHL with necrosis*,^ Infarcted malignant neoplasms (carcinomas, lymphomas, etc.)* ALCL, neutrophil rich*,^ Follicular dendritic cell sarcoma and indeterminate cell sarcoma Lymphoepithelioid variant of PTCL (Lennert lymphoma) Indolent B-cell lymphomas secreting abnormal proteins that incite granulomatous reaction	LCH/Langerhans cell sarcoma Erdheim-Chester disease ALCL Lymphoepithelioid variant of PTCL (Lennert lymphoma) Metastatic carcinoma Indolent B-cell lymphomas secreting abnormal proteins that incite granulomatous reaction	cHL AITL *EBV*+ polymorphic PTLD B-cell lymphoma with plasmacytic differentiation (e.g., nodal MZL, LPL) Nodal involvement of plasma cell neoplasm	Kaposi sarcoma Angiosarcoma Metastatic sarcomatoid carcinoma Metastatic sarcoma

ALCL anaplastic large cell lymphoma, *AOSD* adult onset Still's disease, *AITL* angioimmunoblastic T-cell lymphoma, *cHL* classic Hodgkin lymphoma, *CMV* cytomegalovirus, *DLBCL* diffuse large B-cell lymphoma, *EBV* Epstein Barr virus, *FRFH* florid reactive follicular hyperplasia, *HIV/AIDS* human immunodeficiency virus/acquired immunodeficiency syndrome, *HLH* hemophagocytic lymphohistiocytosis/hemophagocytic syndrome, *HSV* herpes simplex virus, *HV* hyaline vascular, *IgG4-R-LAD* IgG4-related lymphadenopathy, *KFD* Kikuchi-Fujimoto disease, *LAD* lymphadenopathy, *LCH* Langerhans cell histiocytosis, *LN* lymph node, *LPL* lymphoplasmacytic lymphoma, *NTM* non-tuberculous/atypical mycobacteria, *MCD* multicentric Castleman disease, *MF* mycosis fungoides, *MTB* Mycobacterium tuberculosis, *MZL* marginal zone lymphoma, *NOS* not otherwise specified, *NLPHL* nodular lymphocyte predominant Hodgkin lymphoma, *PC* plasma cell, *PTCL* peripheral T-cell lymphoma, *PTGC* progressive transformation of germinal centers, *PTLD* post-transplant lymphoproliferative disorder, *RA* rheumatoid arthritis, *RDD/SHML* Rosai-Dorfman-Destombes/sinus histiocytosis with massive lymphadenopathy, *SLE* systemic lupus erythematosus, *TCHRLBL* T-cell histiocyte-rich large B-cell lymphoma, *UCD* unicentric Castleman disease

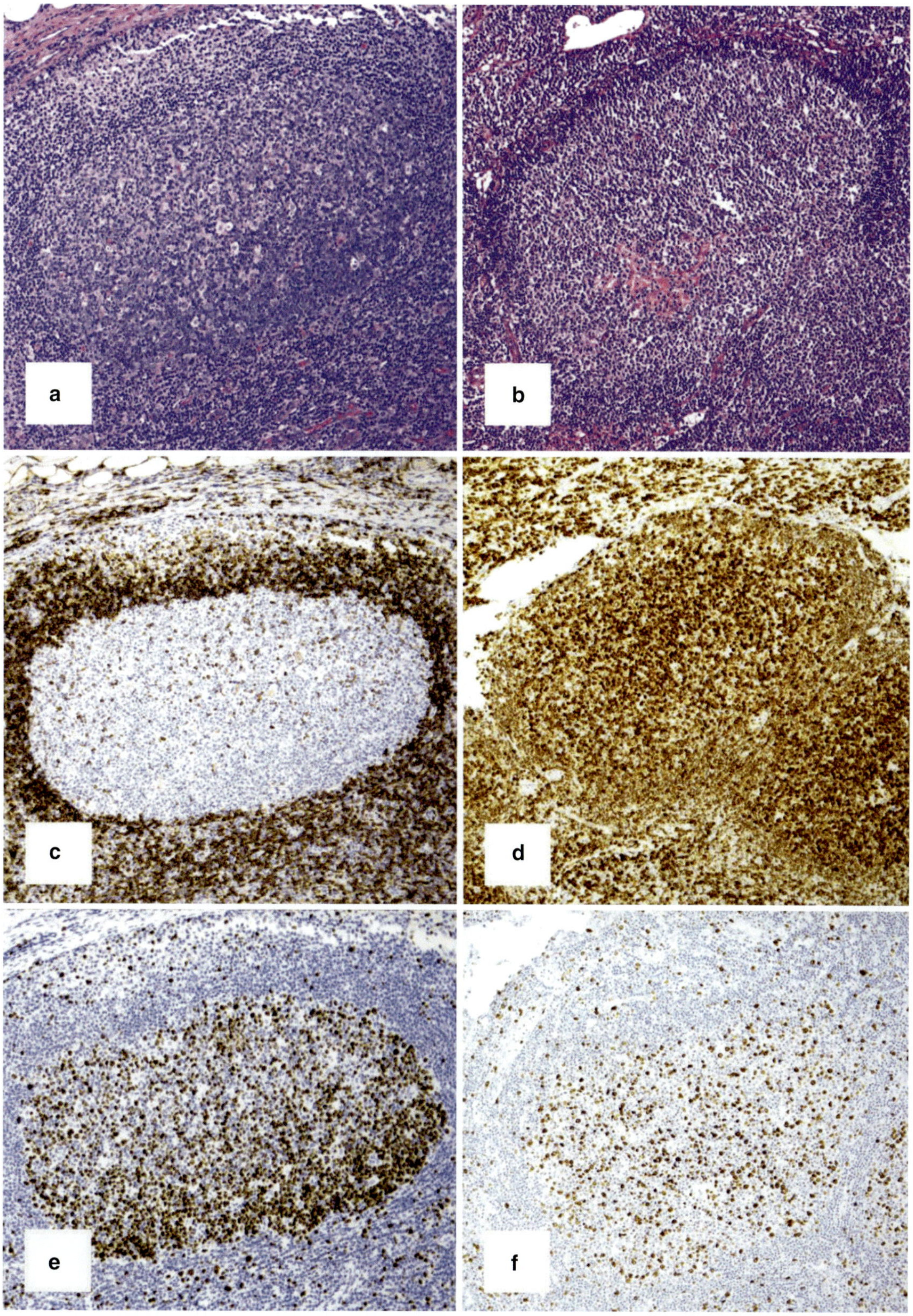

Fig. 18.2 Comparison between reactive follicular hyperplasia (RFH – **a**, **c**, **e**) and follicular lymphoma (FL – **b**, **d**, **f**). (**a**) Germinal center demonstrating polarization, with centroblasts in the dark zone (bottom of follicle, toward medulla) and centrocytes (top of follicle, toward capsule). (**b**) FL: despite having an intact (albeit attenuated) mantle zone overlying follicle, polarization is not easily observed. Cells appear randomly distributed throughout. (**c**) RFH: BCL2 is absent in reactive germinal center, yet present in all the other surrounding lymphocytes. (**d**) FL: BCL2 is aberrantly upregulated in neoplastic follicle. (**e**) RFH: Ki-67 demonstrates polarization, with gradation of proliferative activity, from most centroblasts positive in the dark zone (bottom of follicle) to fewer centrocytes positive in the light zone (top of follicle). (**f**) FL: Ki-67 pattern in the follicle of this FL is positive throughout, without polarization

most commonly with bacterial infections. Viral infections, autoimmune disorders, and exposure to drugs, chemicals, and environmental pollutants can also lead to RFH. More often than not, however, a specific etiology cannot be uncovered.

3. What is the differential diagnosis (DDx) for RFH?

- Table 18.2 summarizes infectious and non-infectious etiologies of RFH and neoplastic mimics.
- Select entities in the DDx of RFH will be discussed further.

4. As a very typical entity that can display RFH, what other morphologic features can HIV/AIDS-related LAD exhibit?

- There are three phases of HIV/AIDS-related lymphadenopathy, which has also been called persistent generalized lymphadenopathy (PGL) [12–15]. Described below are typical histologic findings in each phase of disease.
- Early or acute stage (pattern type A or grade 1) (Fig. 18.3)
  - Florid reactive follicular hyperplasia (FRFH) with geographic enlargement of highly proliferative germinal centers, creating large, irregular to serpiginous shapes.
  - Follicular lysis (i.e., fragmentation of follicles, intrafollicular hemorrhage, and infiltration of small lymphocytes).
  - Attenuation or loss of mantle zones, interfollicular polytypic plasmacytosis, multinucleated giant cells (a.k.a. Warthin-Finkeldey-like cells), and monocytoid B-cell clusters.
- Intermediate or chronic stage (pattern type B or grade 2)
  - Mixed pattern of follicular hyperplasia and involution.
  - Combination of hyperplastic and regressed follicles, interfollicular plasmacytosis, and vascular proliferation with sometimes hyalinized vessels.
  - Can mimic plasma cell variant and/or mixed pattern multicentric Castleman disease.
- Burnt out or advanced stage (pattern type C or grade 3)
  - Striking lymphocyte depletion.
  - Regressed follicles observed frequently.

Table 18.2 Differential diagnosis of reactive follicular hyperplasia and its neoplastic mimics

Infectious	Non-infectious	Neoplastic mimics
Bacterial infections HIV/AIDS Toxoplasmosis CMV[a] HSV[a] Primary or secondary syphilis[b] HHV8+ multicentric Castleman disease, PC variant[b]	PTGC UCD, HV variant HHV8-negative, multicentric Castleman disease, PC variant[b] IgG4-R-LAD[b] SLE[b] RA AOSD[a] Kimura disease[a] Drugs, chemicals, environmental exposure	Follicular lymphoma (typical and floral variant) NLPHL Marginal zone lymphoma with follicular colonization Mantle cell lymphoma with mantle zone pattern AITL cHL with interfollicular involvement

[a]Discussed further in IFH/DH section
[b]Discussed further in plasma cell-rich section

5. Are histologic features alone sufficiently diagnostic for HIV/AIDS-related LAD?

- To be brief, no. As with many reactive entities, only careful integration of all data leads to definitive diagnosis.
- Table 18.3 compares the morphologic, immunophenotypic, and ancillary study results that are reliably diagnostic, suggestive of the diagnosis, unreliable for the diagnosis, and can rule out the diagnosis. DDx is also included for each stage.
- One of HIV retrovirus' main actions is to infect and debilitate CD4+ T-cells, monocytes, and dendritic cells.
  - Leads to progressive weakening of the immune system, resulting in opportunistic infections and uncontrolled neoplasms

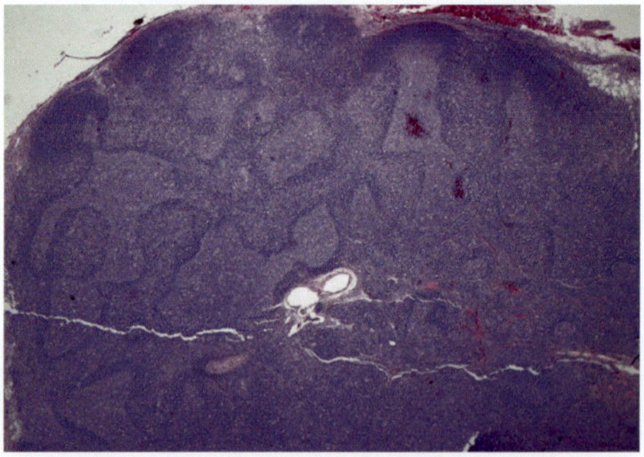

Fig. 18.3 Early phase of HIV-related lymphadenopathy. This acute/early phase of HIV-related LAD is characterized by florid reactive follicular hyperplasia, with large geographic and serpentine expansions of germinal centers. Surrounding mantle zones are attenuated, but still present

Table 18.3 Histomorphologic, immunophenotypic, and ancillary work-up of reactive persistent generalized lymphadenopathy in HIV/AIDS

	Reliably diagnostic	Suggestive of diagnosis	Unreliable for diagnosis	Rule out diagnosis	Differential diagnosis (DDx)
Early/acute stage					
Morphologic	None	Florid reactive follicular hyperplasia Follicular lysis and hemorrhage	H&E features alone, as it can mimic other entities in DDx	n/a	Lymphadenitis due to: *EBV*/infectious mononucleosis CMV HSV *Toxoplasma* Rheumatoid arthritis/adult-onset Still's disease
Immunophenotypic	None	Decreased numbers of CD4+ T-cells	n/a	Clonal B-cell or plasma cell population	
Ancillary work-up	HIV serology (+) HIV viral load (+)	Low CD4+ counts	HIV serology (−), especially in the first 2–3 weeks of acute HIV infection	Absence of HIV viral load	
Intermediate/chronic stage					
Morphologic	None	Co-existence of opportunistic infections	H&E features alone, as it can mimic other entities in DDx	n/a	Multicentric Castleman disease, HHV8-related or idiopathic
Immunophenotypic	None	None	n/a	n/a	
Ancillary work-up	HIV serology (+) HIV viral load (+)	Low CD4 counts	n/a	HIV serology (−) HIV viral load (−)	
Burnt out/advanced stage					
Morphologic	None	Co-existence of opportunistic infections and Kaposi sarcoma	H&E features alone, as it can mimic other entities in DDx	n/a	Multicentric Castleman disease, HHV8-related or idiopathic
Immunophenotypic	None	None	n/a		
Ancillary work-up	HIV serology (+) HIV viral load (+)	Low CD4+ counts	n/a	HIV serology (−) HIV viral load (−)	

- Not uncommon for other pathologic findings to co-exist (some of which are AIDS-defining), like lymphomas, Kaposi sarcoma, and opportunistic infections (e.g., cryptococcosis, mycobacterial infection, Herpes zoster, etc.)

6. What ancillary testing can help establish the diagnosis of HIV/AIDS-related LAD?

- Histopathologic findings in isolation in a patient without an established diagnosis of HIV are insufficient for diagnosis. Serologic testing must be performed to establish HIV infection [12, 53].
  - In acute HIV infection, there is a window period in which a serologic response is not yet detectable. Tests relying solely on antibody detection are frequently negative in the first 2–3 weeks after infection.
  - Addition of HIV p24 antigen detection to fourth- and fifth-generation assays narrows this window period to <2 weeks. HIV viral loads are usually very high during early infection and are recommended to be performed when serologic tests are non-reactive in suspected acute infection.

7. If RFH is not due to HIV/AIDS-related LAD, then what other histologic features could suggest another reactive entity (i.e., what else is in the DDx)?

- (i) RFH with (ii) monocytoid B-cell nodules and (iii) epithelioid granulomas encroaching upon and/or involving germinal centers = classic triad is thought to be highly predictive of acute *Toxoplasma* LAD.
  - Monocytoid B-cell hyperplasia is a special type of marginal zone hyperplasia, wherein clusters/aggregates of bland monocytoid cells are found just adjacent to follicles and/or perisinusoidal regions. The abundance of their clear cytoplasm and reniform nuclei lead to their resemblance to peripheral blood monocytes (Fig. 18.4).
  - It is not infrequent to see neutrophils admixed in monocytoid cell clusters, and when found, further suggest a reactive process.
  - Monocytoid B-cell hyperplasia can be seen in entities other than acute toxoplasmosis (Table 18.4). A specific etiology is usually elusive, however.
- RFH with increased plasma cells: consider (i) autoimmune disease like rheumatoid arthritis (RA) [14, 16, 17],

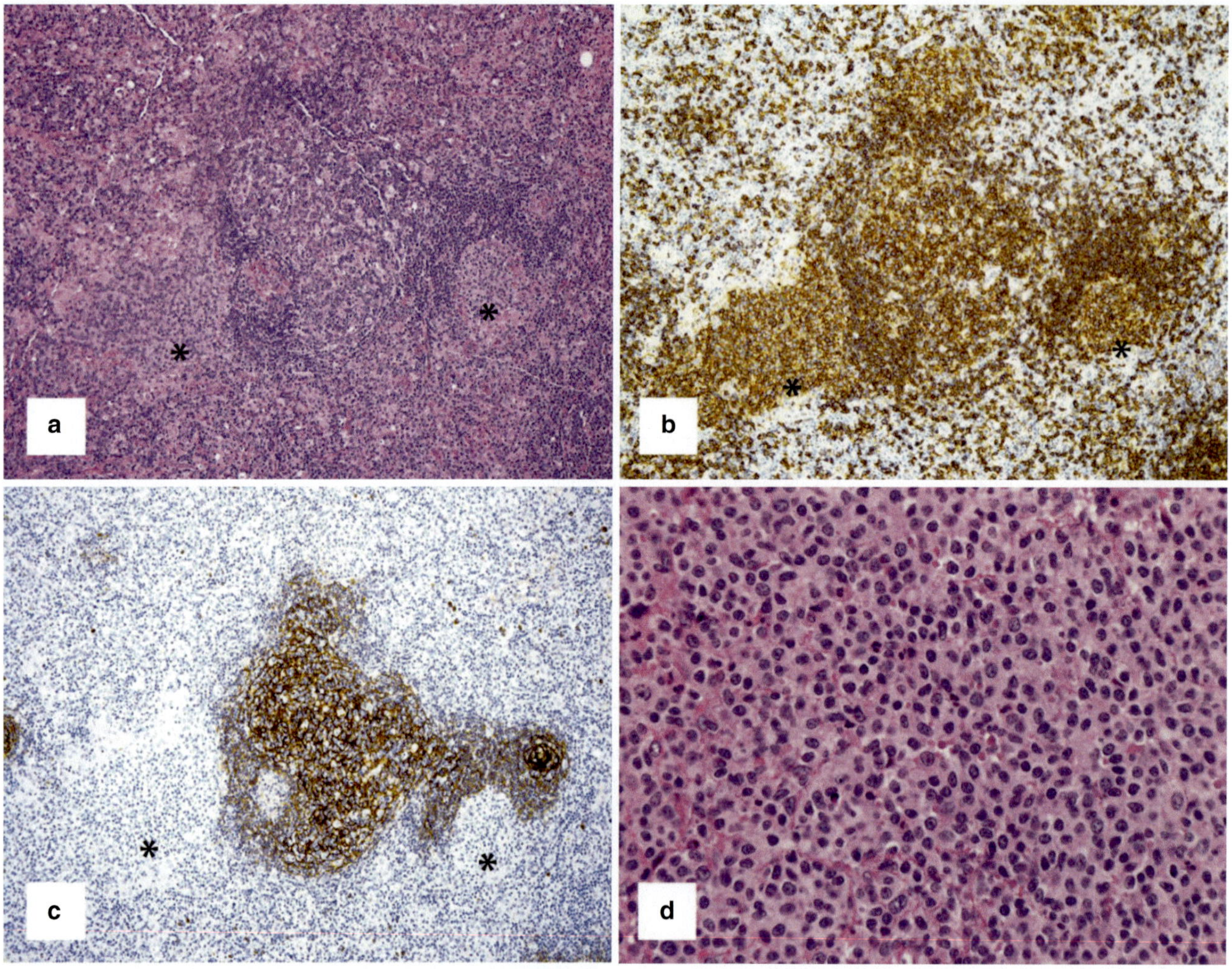

Fig. 18.4 Monocytoid B-cell hyperplasia. A special type of marginal zone hyperplasia – monocytoid B-cell hyperplasia – can manifest as numerous cells distending sinuses or as nodules/aggregates located near sinusoids or, at times, adjacent to germinal centers (GCs). Two monocytoid B-cell nodules (asterisks [*] denote their presence in (**a**)) flank a germinal center. The B-cell lineage of the monocytoid B-cell clusters is highlighted by CD20 (**b**). CD21 staining is confined to the follicular dendritic cell network of the GC (**c**) and spares the monocytoid B-cell clusters (asterisks [*] denote their presence). High magnification of the nodules displays monomorphic cells with abundant pale eosinophilic cytoplasm and reniform nuclear contours (**d**). See text for significance and differential diagnosis

Table 18.4 Entities that can show marginal zone/monocytoid B-cell hyperplasia

Bacterial
Cat-scratch disease (*Bartonella henselae*, *B. quintana)*
Lymphogranuloma venereum (*Chlamydia trachomatis*)
Parasitic
Toxoplasmosis (*Toxoplasma gondii*)
Filaria (including *Wuchereria bancrofti*, *Onchocerca volvulus*, *Brugia malayi*)
Viral
CMV-related lymphadenopathy
EBV-related infectious mononucleosis
HIV-related lymphadenopathy
HSV-related lymphadenopathy

systemic lupus erythematosus (SLE)), (ii) syphilitic LAD, and (iii) IgG4-related LAD → discussed further in Questions 12, 62, 67, and 73, respectively.

- RFH with interfollicular hyperplasia: viral LAD, such as *EBV*-related infectious mononucleosis, CMV LAD, and HSV LAD → discussed further in Question 26 and Table 18.10.
- RFH with "lollipop" vessels and "onion-skinning" mantle zones: think unicentric Castleman disease and exclude angioimmunoblastic T-cell lymphoma (AITL) → see Question 16.
- RFH with progressive transformation of germinal centers (PTGC): main consideration is excluding the possibility of nodular lymphocyte predominant Hodgkin

lymphoma (NLPHL) → for further discussion, see Questions 19 and 20.

- Table 18.5 provides a summary of select entities with RFH.
- Even with all these features, the etiology for RFH may not be uncovered.

8. What is the minimal histopathologic work-up in RFH?

- Depends on what findings are prominent and what one entertains in DDx
- CD3 and CD20: Confirms histologic impression of nodal architectural preservation
- If interfollicular hyperplasia is also prominent:
  - CMV and HSV IHC, and/or EBER ISH: Assesses for viral inclusions
- If plasma cells are increased:
  - CD138, kappa, lambda: Determines degree of plasmacytosis; establishes polytypic staining pattern
  - IgG4, IgG: Conveys whether IgG4-positive plasma cells are significantly increased
  - *Treponema* IHC: Establishes syphilitic LAD
  - HHV8: Assesses for HHV8-related multicentric Castleman disease
- If the classic triad suggestive of *Toxoplasma* LAD is considered:
  - *Toxoplasma* IHC commercially available and could be performed
- If follicular lymphoma is of concern (see Fig. 18.2):

Table 18.5 Clinical, histomorphologic, immunophenotypic, and ancillary work-up in select entities with reactive follicular hyperplasia

	HIV/AIDS-related LAD and other viral LAD	*Toxoplasma* LAD	Bacterial LAD, NOS	Unicentric Castleman disease	Rheumatoid arthritis (and other autoimmune disorders)
Etiology	Different viruses, including (but not limited to) *EBV*, CMV, HSV	Protozoan *Toxoplasma gondii*	Many bacterial agents, including, but not limited to, *Staphylococcus*, *Streptococcus*, *Bartonella* spp.	Unknown	Autoimmune disorder
Clinical setting	Immunocompromised pt	Immunocompetent pt.: localized LAD, no other symptoms Immunocompromised pt.: can be disseminated, involving multiple organs (toxoplasmosis)	Depends on organism	Typically localized/regional LAD Can be asymptomatic Manifests if affected LNs compress nearby structures causing symptoms	Polyarthritis of ≥3 joints Disease duration >6 weeks
Epidemiology	Depends on specific infectious agent (see Table 18.10)	Exposure to cats (parasitic host)	Depends on organism	Variable	F > M affected
Typical morphology	3 stages with florid RFH in acute stage (see Table 18.3)	Triad: RFH Monocytoid B-cell hyperplasia Epithelioid granulomas	RFH; nonspecific findings	Regressed germinal centers Interfollicular vascular proliferation "Lollipop sign" "Onion-skinning"	RFH Interfollicular polytypic plasmacytosis
Most useful histopathologic work-up to establish Dx	Depends on specific infectious agent (see Table 18.10)	*Toxoplasma* IHC (commercially available)	Can attempt bacterial gram stains if suppurative LAD present; however, low yield	Characteristic morphology combined with radiologic findings Carefully exclude early AITL	None
Most useful ancillary testing to establish Dx	HIV serology (+) HIV viral load (+)	Acute and convalescent serologic testing with IgG and IgM antibodies to toxoplasma by IFA or EIA	Microbiologic bacterial cultures Supportive clinical history	Supportive histopathology with appropriate clinical history and isolated/regional LAD	Clinical history and supportive labs: (+) RF, anti-CCP, and elevated CRP or ESR
Appropriate therapy	Treat with appropriate HIV/AIDS drugs	Self-limited, if immunocompetent Antibiotics, if necessary	Usually self-limited Antibiotics, if necessary	Complete excision curative	Disease-modifying anti-rheumatic drug therapy

  - Obtain CD10, BCL6, BCL2: To reveal CD10+/BCL2-/BCL6+ germinal centers

    Note: BCL2 expression may sometimes be lost in high-grade (i.e., grade 3) FL; therefore, absence of BCL2 in an expanded follicle does not completely exclude FL and should be interpreted in the context of the other findings.
  - Ki-67: To demonstrate polarization and high proliferation rate of reactive germinal centers
- If PTGC is prominent:
  - Obtain CD3, CD20, PD1, CD21, CD23, IgD: Evaluates possibility of NLPHL
  - IgG4, IgG: Conveys whether IgG4-positive plasma cells are significantly increased

9. What clinical and epidemiologic features are present in *Toxoplasma* LAD?

- Caused by protozoan *Toxoplasma gondii* [21].
- History of exposure to cat (parasitic host).
- In immunocompetent children and young adults: asymptomatic localized LAD (most common manifestation)
- In immunocompromised patients: disseminated, multi-organ infection (toxoplasmosis)
- Self-limited infection in immunocompetent patients

10. What are typical histologic and immunophenotypic findings for *Toxoplasma* LAD?

- The classic histologic triad for toxoplasmosis (so-called Piringer-Kuchinka LAD) is:
  1. Follicular hyperplasia
  2. Monocytoid B-cell hyperplasia [and/or marginal zone hyperplasia]
  3. Epithelioid histiocytes encroaching upon a reactive germinal center (Fig. 18.5)
- Absence of necrosis.
- No multinucleated giant cells seen (unlike sarcoidosis, e.g.).
- *Toxoplasma* pseudocyst containing bradyzoites is a very rare finding in LAD.
- *Toxoplasma* IHC stain is commercially available.

11. What ancillary testing can help establish the diagnosis of *Toxoplasma* LAD?

Minimal Ancillary Work-Up:

- Serology confirms suspicion of *Toxoplasma* as cause of LAD [23].
  - IgG and IgM antibodies to toxoplasma by IFA or EIA should be tested.
  - Negative IgM helps exclude recent infection but may be falsely negative in immunocompromised patients.
  - Positive IgM has low specificity.
- Both acute and convalescent serologic testing are often necessary to provide sufficient data for interpretation.
- Interpretive information available from CDC website: https://www.cdc.gov/dpdx/toxoplasmosis/dx.html.
- Unlike with toxoplasmal infections at other sites, organism DNA is not reliably detected by PCR of affected lymph nodes [22, 23].

12. What clinical and epidemiologic features are present in lymphadenopathy associated with rheumatoid arthritis (RA-related LAD) and other autoimmune disorders?

- Manifests as a polyarticular inflammatory arthritis of >6 weeks' duration.
- Painless LAD (typically axillary, cervical, supraclavicular).
- Felty syndrome: a severe form of RA with splenomegaly and neutropenia.
- A rheumatologist should be involved in the care of patients with autoimmune disorders. Early intervention with disease-modifying anti-rheumatic drug therapy (DMARD) is strongly recommended by experts for better outcomes.

13. What are typical histologic and immunophenotypic findings in RA-LAD and other autoimmune disorders?

- Untreated RA: RFH and interfollicular polytypic plasmacytosis are characteristic (Fig. 18.6a, b).
- PAS+, Congo red-negative eosinophilic hyaline material may be present and may contain dystrophic calcification.
- Plasma cells can be quite abundant and may contain large, intracytoplasmic immunoglobulin inclusions (so-called Russell bodies).

14. What ancillary testing can help establish the diagnosis for RA-LAD?

- About 60% of patients demonstrate elevated serum rheumatoid factor (RF).
- RF elevation is also seen in other autoimmune disorders → not a sole reliable diagnostic marker.
- Other supportive laboratory tests include positive titers for anti-citrullinated peptide/protein antibody (anti-CCP)

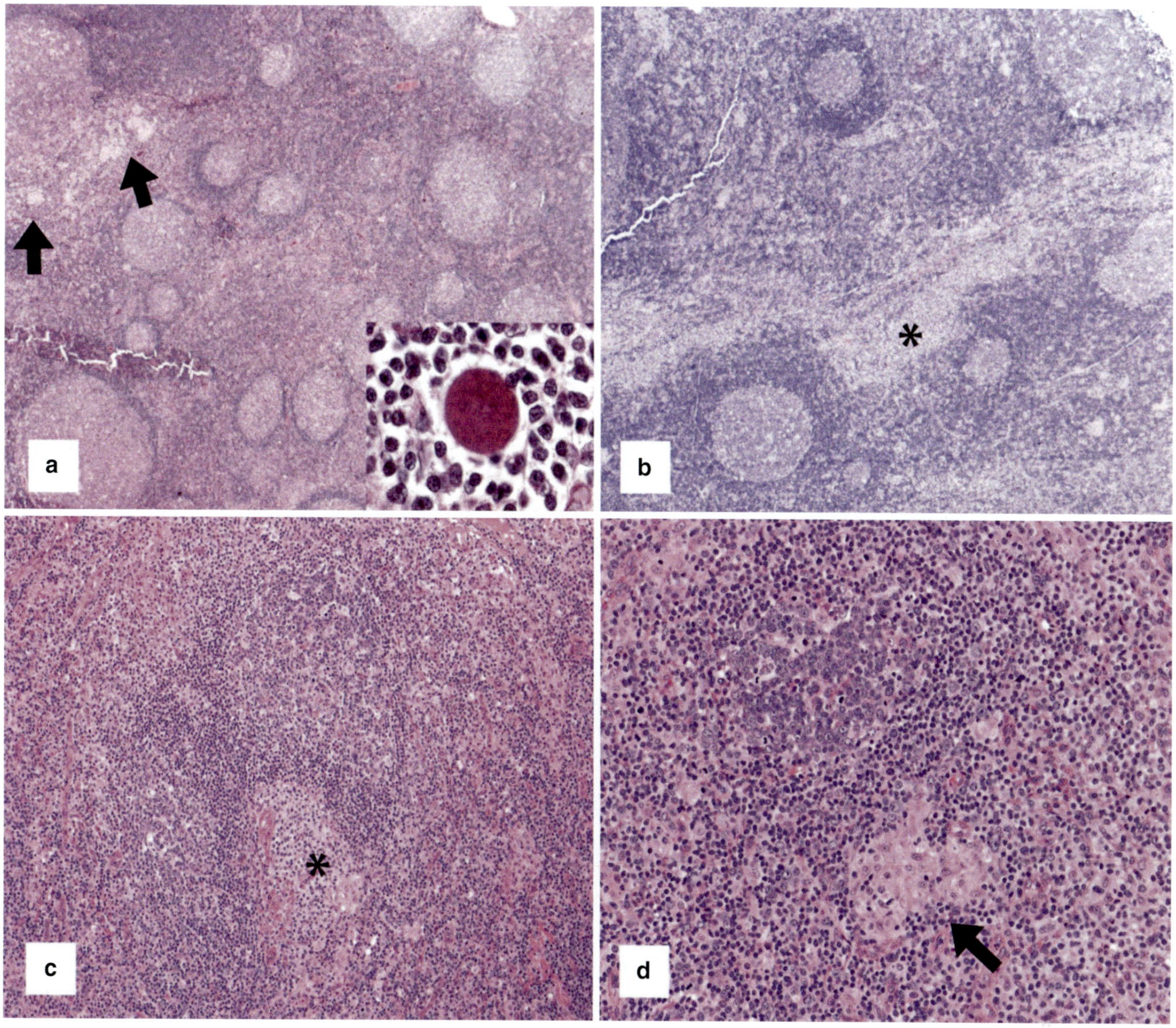

Fig. 18.5 *Toxoplasma* lymphadenitis. This is another example of LAD with prominent RFH. In addition to an increase in the number of variably sized lymphoid follicles, epithelioid macrophages (underscored by arrows) are seen encroaching upon germinal centers [low magnification in (**a**); high magnification in (**d**)]. Monocytoid B-cell hyperplasia (denoted by asterisks, ∗) is also evident: on intermediate power distending sinuses (**b**) and on high power (**c**). The findings of RFH, epithelioid granulomas invading GCs, and monocytoid B-cell hyperplasia constitute the classic triad of toxoplasma LAD. The toxoplasma pseudocyst containing numerous bradyzoites is a very rare finding [shown on H&E, inset for (**a**)], but IHC for *Toxoplasma gondii* can be utilized to decorate rare pseudocysts

and elevated C-reactive protein (CRP) or erythrocyte sedimentation rate (ESR).

Comparison of RA with adult-onset Still's disease and systemic lupus erythematosus is found in Table 18.6.

15. What are clinical and epidemiologic features of unicentric Castleman disease (UCD)?

- Tumefactive lesions resulting in localized/regional LAD.
- Usually incidental and asymptomatic.
- Occasional enlarged LNs lead to compression of nearby structures and associated symptoms.
- Typically involves young adults.
- Complete excision curative.

16. What are typical histologic findings in UCD?

- Three histologic types of UCD: a) hyaline vascular variant (UCD-HV), b) plasma cell variant (UCD-PC), and c) mixed HV and PC variant (UCD-mixed HV/PC) [2, 10].
- UCD-HV:

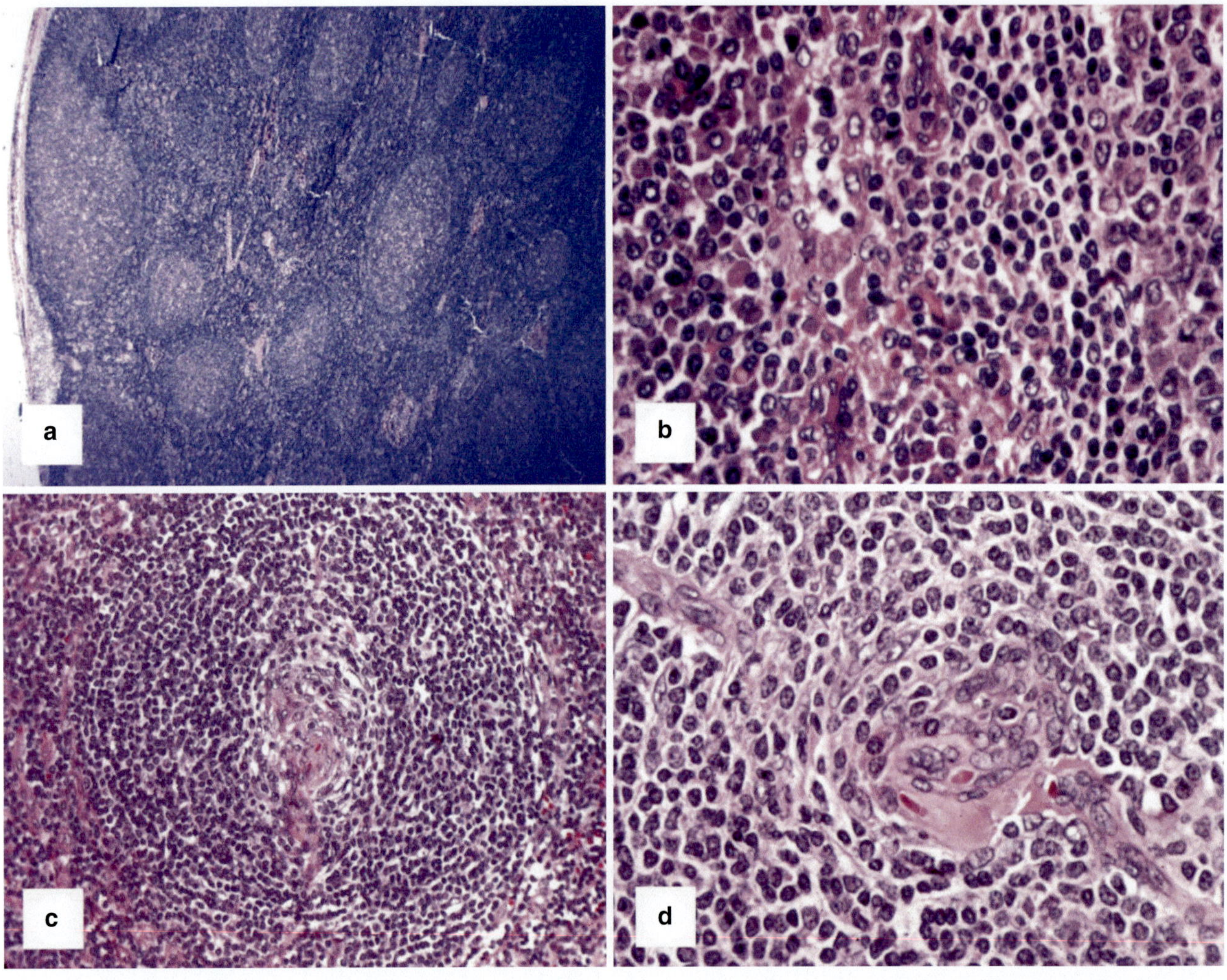

Fig. 18.6 Other causes of RFH: rheumatoid arthritis (**a** and **b**) and unicentric Castleman disease (**c** and **d**). RFH is seen, with many, well-spaced, and variably sized lymphoid follicles, as well as patent sinuses in this example of untreated rheumatoid arthritis-related LAD (**a**). High magnification reveals numerous plasma cells within interfollicular regions (**b**). Characteristic findings in the hyaline vascular variant of unicentric Castleman disease are shown. The "onion skinning" in (**c**) pertains to concentric layers of mantle zone lymphocytes surrounding atretic GCs, resembling many layers of an onion when viewed on its bisected cut surface. The "lollipop sign" (**d**) refers to GCs that are radially penetrated by hyalinized blood vessels, with the blood vessel representing the stick to the GC "lollipop"

  - Numerous variably sized follicles, some hyperplastic (as in RFH).
  - Prominent regressed (atretic/atrophic) germinal centers (GCs).
  - GCs penetrated by hyalinized blood vessels ("lollipop" sign).
  - GC surrounded by concentric layers of mantle zone lymphocytes ("onion skinning") (Fig. 18.6c, d).
- UCD-PC:
  - Vascular proliferation between follicles may be increased.
  - Plasma cells and immunoblasts are typically not abundant in UCD; however, there are some cases of UCD which are plasma cell-rich and HHV8-negative (around 10% of localized/unicentric CD).
- UCD-mixed HV/PC: combination of features
  - "Twinning": Two germinal centers surrounded by same group of mantle zone lymphocytes (useful feature in CD).
  - No "water clear" lymphoma cells (as seen in angioimmunoblastic T-cell lymphoma (AITL)) or cytologically abnormal lymphocytes.
  - Some investigators have described follicular dendritic cells in CD as "dysplastic" → suggests a precursor lesion for follicular dendritic cell neoplasms.

Table 18.6 Useful histopathologic findings, clinical features, and laboratory clues to diagnosis of LAD associated with select autoimmune rheumatologic conditions

Autoimmune/rheumatologic disease	Typical histologic features	Most useful histologic features suggestive of diagnosis	Useful IHC stains	Typical clinical signs/ symptoms	Useful laboratory work-up supportive of diagnosis	Most reliable diagnostic feature
Rheumatoid arthritis (RA)	Florid follicular hyperplasia Interfollicular polytypic plasmacytosis	RFH + plasmacytosis	None	Inflammatory arthritis of ≥3 joints Disease duration >6 weeks	(+) RF (+) anti-CCP Elevated CRP or ESR	Clinical presentation and supportive lab results
Adult onset still's disease (adult-onset systemic juvenile idiopathic arthritis)	One of the following four patterns: a) Atypical paracortical hyperplasia b) Massive sinus histiocytosis c) Exuberant immunoblastic proliferation d) Follicular hyperplasia	Retention of follicular architecture (to prevent misdiagnosis of lymphoma)	None	Fever Arthralgias/arthritis Characteristic rash [see Table 18.12] Sore throat LAD Organomegaly	ANC ≥ 8 K/μL (−) ANA (+) RF Abnormal AST, ALT Elevated LDH	Clinical presentation and supportive lab results
Systemic lupus erythematosus	IFH/DH Necrosis	Hematoxylin bodies Azzopardi phenomenon Plasma cells Neutrophils	None	[See Table 18.20 for details] Acute or chronic cutaneous lupus Nonscarring alopecia Oral or nasal ulcers Joint disease Serositis Renal abnormalities Neurologic abnormalities Hemolytic anemia Leukopenia or lymphopenia Thrombocytopenia	(+) ANA (+) anti-dsDNA (+) anti-Sm (+) antiphospholipid work-up Low complement (+) DAT	Hematoxylin bodies Azzopardi phenomenon Clinical presentation and supportive lab results

ANA antineutrophil antibody, *anti-CCP* anti-citrullinated peptide/protein antibody, *anti-dsDNA* anti-double stranded deoxyribonucleic acid, *CRP* C-reactive protein, *DAT* direct antiglobulin test/direct Coombs test, *ESR* erythrocyte sedimentation rate, *IFH/DFH* interfollicular hyperplasia/diffuse hyperplasia, *LDH* lactate dehydrogenase, *RF* rheumatoid factor, *anti-Sm* anti-Smith antibody

17. What minimal histopathologic work-up and relevant clinical information can be used to avoid diagnostic pitfalls in UCD (like misdiagnosing HHV8-related multicentric Castleman disease [HHV8+ MCD] and early stage AITL)?

- H&E findings can be so characteristic for UCD-HV type that IHC may seem extraneous.
- If desired: CD3, CD10, CD20, CD21, CD23, BCL2, and Ki-67 should demonstrate normal immunoarchitecture and cellular composition in UCD.
  - In contrast to UCD, AITL (early involvement/pattern 1) would show:
    - "Water clear" lymphoma cells = follicular helper T-cells with co-expression of CD10, BCL6, PD1, and/or CD4 in neoplastic T-cells
    - FDC network expansion beyond B-lymphoid follicles → highlight with CD21, CD23
    - *EBV*+ B-immunoblasts by EBER ISH
- If plasma cells prominent: CD138, kappa, lambda, and HHV8 will highlight numerous interfollicular polytypic plasma cells and *absence* of HHV8 in UCD-PC.
  - In contrast to UCD-PC, HHV8+ MCD would show:
    - HHV8+ plasmablasts scattered around mantle zone layers
    - Lambda light chain restricted plasmablasts
- Notably, UCD clinically presents as asymptomatic, localized/regional LAD. In contrast, AITL and MCD have a constellation of significant clinical and laboratory findings, including:
  - Multi-organ/systemic involvement, generalized LAD, and/or hepatosplenomegaly
  - Constitutional symptoms (including fevers, night sweats)
  - Diffuse skin rash
  - Polyclonal hypergammaglobulinemia

18. What clinical and epidemiologic features are present in progressive transformation of germinal centers (PTGC), another example of RFH?

- Usually presents as a localized LAD.
- Young males more commonly affected than females.
- PTGC can occur in isolation but can also appear at the time of patient's diagnosis of lymphoma (in the same node as lymphoma or separate node unaffected by lymphoma).
- PTGC also can be seen *before* lymphoma diagnosis or emerge even *after* lymphoma diagnosis (most commonly, nodular lymphocyte predominant Hodgkin lymphoma (NLPHL) [2, 10, 24–27].
- Etiology unknown.
- Self-limited disease.

19. What typical histologic findings are seen in PTGC?

- PTGC are markedly enlarged lymphoid nodules compared to admixed GCs (>2x the size of hyperplastic follicles) [26, 27].
- Enlarged GCs infiltrated by numerous small, mantle zone-type B-cells.
- Absence of cytologically abnormal "LP" cells (also called "L&H" or "popcorn" cells of NLPHL).
- Can sometimes exhibit hyaline vascular Castleman disease-like morphology.

20. What is the major DDx to consider and the minimal histopathologic work-up when PTGC is observed?

- Because of the association of PTGC with NLPHL, an adequate specimen for excluding lymphoma would be an excisional biopsy.
  - If only a needle core biopsy is obtained, the clinician should be advised to pursue excisional biopsy.
  - At a minimum, perform immunostains for CD3, CD10, CD20, PAX5, CD21, CD23, BCL2, and BCL6. The addition of IgD and PD1 can prove particularly useful.

Table 18.7 presents useful immunoarchitectural features to help distinguish PTGC from NLPHL [26], while Figs. 18.7 and 18.8 illustrate these features.

- If cHL and FL are strongly considered:

Table 18.7 Distinguishing features between PTGC and NLPHL

Parameter	PTGC	NLPHL
Morphologic features	No atypical "LP" cells	Presence of *atypical "LP" cells* (i.e., popcorn cells), uniformly CD20+
CD21	CD21 staining shows intact, *dense* FDC meshwork with *sharp borders*	CD21 staining shows FDC with *irregular borders* and abundant "*holes*" where LP cells are located
PD1	PD1+ T-cells *scattered singly* throughout germinal center	PD1+ T-cells present as *rosettes, rimming "LP" cells*
IgD	IgD highlights *smooth, round borders* of FDC meshwork	IgD highlights FDC meshwork has *moth-eaten and irregular* borders

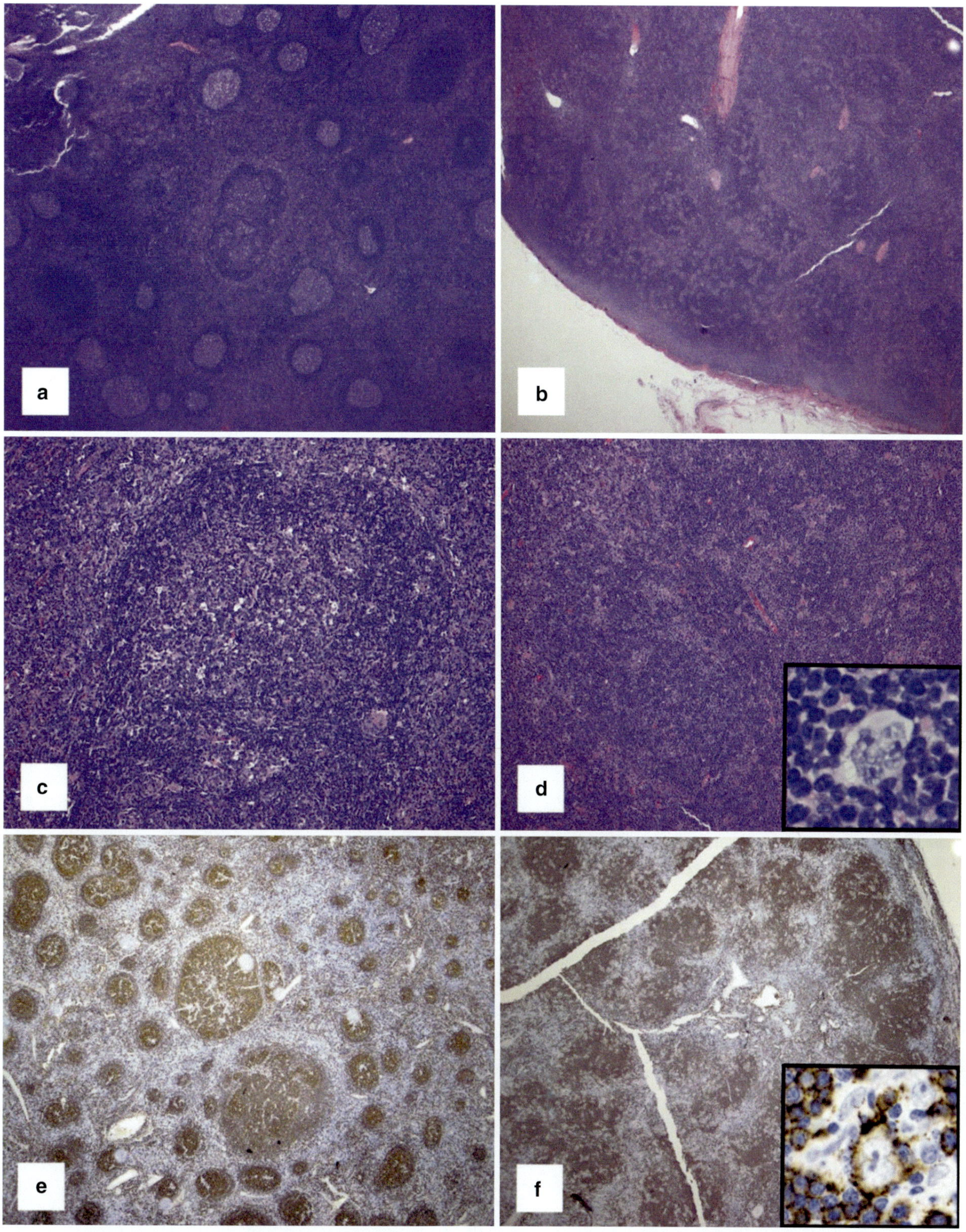

Fig. 18.7 Immunomorphologic comparison between progressive transformation of germinal centers (PTGC) (left-hand side of the panel: **a**, **c**, **e**) and nodular lymphocyte predominant Hodgkin lymphoma (NLPHL) (right-hand side: **b**, **d**, **f**), part 1. Nodal architecture is retained in PTGC. The hyperplastic follicle in the center is much larger than 2x the size of surrounding GCs (**a**). In contrast, neoplastic nodules in NLPHL efface nodal architecture (**b**). Intermediate magnification view in (**c**) displays PTGC with numerous small lymphocytes infiltrating into a reactive GC. By comparison, a similar intermediate-power magnification view of NLPHL (**d**) exhibits a moth-eaten appearance due to histiocytes and/or large neoplastic B-cells. Normal reactive follicles are not seen. The characteristic "LP" (for lymphocyte predominant) cell is very large, with lobulated nuclear contours, vesicular chromatin, and multiple nucleoli, resembling a popped kernel of corn (hence the alternate name "popcorn cell") [inset for (**d**)]. CD20 IHC highlights the reactive lymphoid follicles in PTGC (**e**) and the irregular neoplastic nodules in NLPHL (**f**). The neoplastic "LP" cell is uniformly CD20 positive and surrounded by many small B-cells [inset for (**f**)]

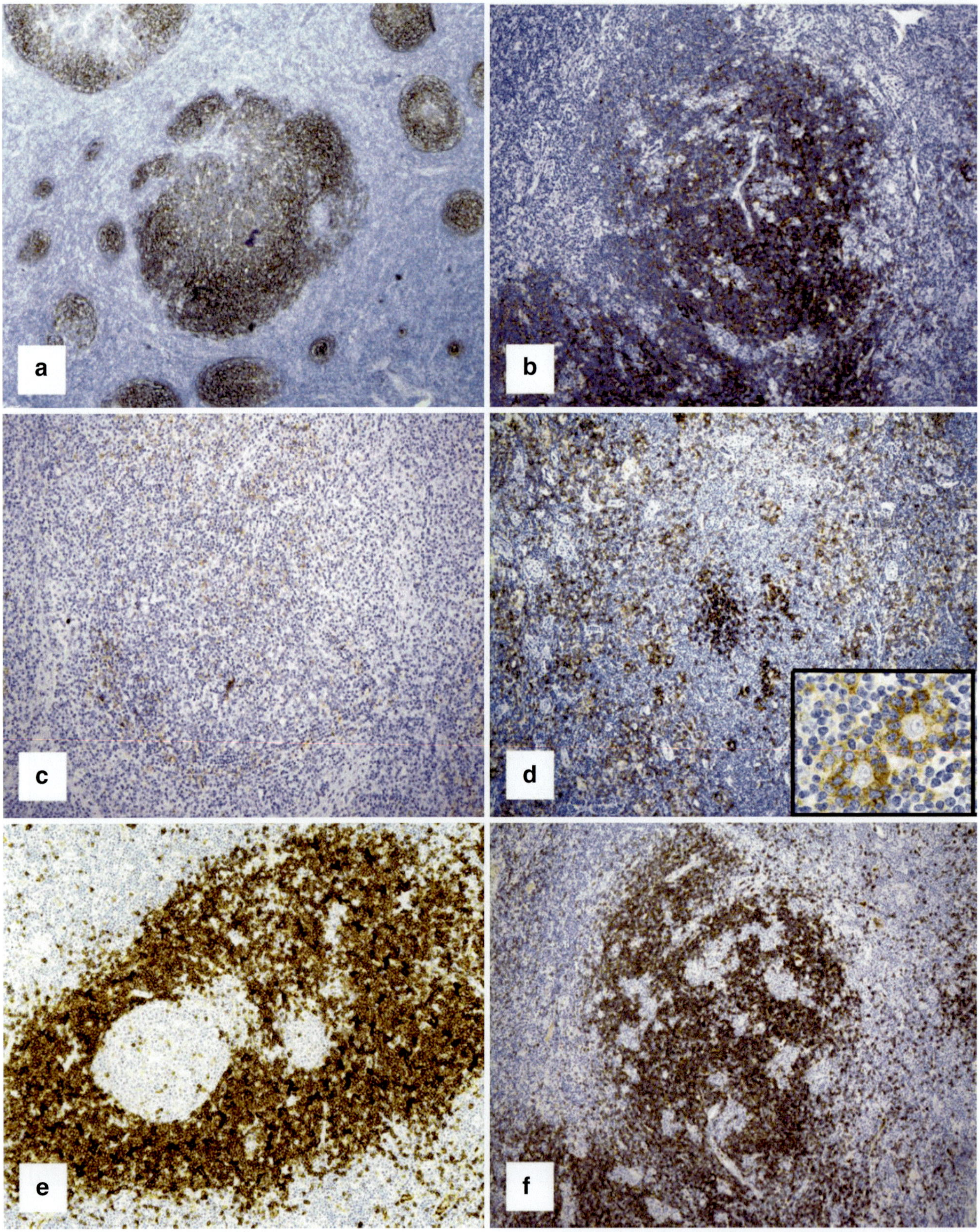

Fig. 18.8 Comparison between PTGC (left-hand side of the panel: **a**, **c**, **e**) and NLPHL (right-hand side: **b**, **d**, **f**), part 2. CD21 IHC highlights intact, dense follicular dendritic cell (FDC) meshwork with sharp borders in PTGC (**a**). In contrast, CD21 stain in NLPHL displays "holes" created by neoplastic LP cells in the FDC meshwork (**b**). PD1 IHC in PTGC shows scattered, relatively uniform dispersal of T-follicular helper cells in reactive follicles (**c**). In sharp contrast, PD1 stain in NLPHL shows clusters visible on intermediate power (**d**), which are PD1+ T-follicular helper cells rosetting neoplastic cells [inset for (**d**)]. IgD IHC reveals smooth and round FDC meshwork borders with IgD+ mantle zone lymphocytes infiltrating a reactive GC in PTGC (**e**), whereas IgD stain in NLPHL displays a "moth-eaten" appearance and irregular FDC meshwork borders, created by the neoplastic LP cells (**f**)

   - Additional stains (like CD15, CD30, CD45, and PAX5 for cHL and CD20, CD10, BCL2, BCL6, and Ki-67 for FL) may be pursued.
- IgG4-related LAD:
   - PTGC is one of the five recognized LN patterns for this entity.
   - Perform IgG and IgG4 stains to evaluate for increase in IgG4+ plasma cells (discussed later in Question 73).

21. Considering all the entities in the DDx, what is the clinical relevance of misinterpretation in RFH?

- Misinterpreting RFH as lymphoma (see neoplastic DDx in Table 18.2):
   - Majority of cases of NLPHL and even some FL cases are indolent → some managing physicians choose a "watch and wait" approach.
   - If it is an aggressive case of NLPHL or FL, however, misclassification as RFH deprives patient of appropriate treatment for lymphoma.
   - Failure to diagnose cHL or AITL denies patient of appropriate treatment and can prove fatal.
- Not suggesting the correct reactive etiology for RFH:
   - May not be as clinically devastating as misdiagnosis of lymphoma.
   - However, can result in diagnostic and treatment delays (e.g., not treating early acute HIV or previously undiagnosed RA) and lead to additional unnecessary biopsies (e.g., in IgG4-related LAD).

22. In RFH, what information can be conveyed to the clinician? When is a diagnostic comment necessary? What is an adequate specimen?

- Depends on the most likely diagnostic possibilities.
- If RFH is florid, alerting clinician to the prime possibility of infection, whether bacterial or viral (like HIV), may prove vital, particularly in patients who do not disclose a history of high-risk exposures [53].
- Suggesting an autoimmune disorder may also prompt a more thorough rheumatologic work-up.
- Example of diagnostic comment:
   - "The findings are non-specific for etiology. These are commonly seen in bacterial infections and other viral infections [e.g., HIV, *EBV*/infectious mononucleosis, HSV, CMV], toxoplasmosis, and autoimmune diseases [e.g., rheumatoid arthritis]. Correlation with pertinent clinical history with integration of additional laboratory studies (including serologic and other microbiologic studies) is required."
- If PTGC findings predominate and/or cytologic atypia exists, example diagnostic comments:
   - Only CNBx obtained: "If clinical concern persists, excisional biopsy is recommended for complete and definitive assessment for malignancy."
   - Excisional biopsy obtained: "Reactive changes (particularly PTGC) are observed. There is no evidence of malignancy on this LN sampling. Close clinical follow-up is advised. If lymphadenopathy and/or clinical concern persist, we recommend additional excisional biopsies of affected LNs to further characterize the condition."

23. When is consultation necessary in RFH?

- Prudent to show cases to colleagues and/or expert consultants whenever histologic findings are discordant with particularly worrisome clinical findings and/or when morphologic atypia is seen.

Interfollicular to Diffuse Hyperplasia (IFH/DH), DDx Including LAD Secondary to *EBV*-Infectious Mononucleosis, Adult Onset Still's Disease

24. What are typical findings in paracortical/interfollicular hyperplasia and diffuse hyperplasia (IFH/DH)?

- Paracortical/interfollicular hyperplasia (IFH) = expansion of paracortical/interfollicular zones by a variety of cellular elements.
- Expansion can be exuberant and create architectural distortion; however, lymphoid follicles persist.
- Diffuse hyperplasia (DH) = much more extensive proliferation than IFH with seemingly subtotal nodal effacement; retention of lymphoid follicles is evidence of architectural preservation.
- Cellular composition of IFH/DH depends on etiology. Can contain variable numbers of:
   - Small- to medium-sized lymphocytes
   - Immunoblasts (i.e., larger, transformed reactive lymphocytes)
   - Plasma cells
   - Eosinophils
   - Histiocytes (sometimes pigment-laden)
   - Langerhans cells
   - Interdigitating dendritic cells
- Morphologic features are shown in Fig. 18.9.
- IFH/DH often co-exists with RFH ("mixed hyperplasia").
- Occasionally, nodules of T-cells are the culprits of the interfollicular expansion ("nodular paracortical T-cell hyperplasia").
- Histiocyte-rich and plasma cell-rich expansions will be discussed in later sections (see Questions 37 and 67, respectively).

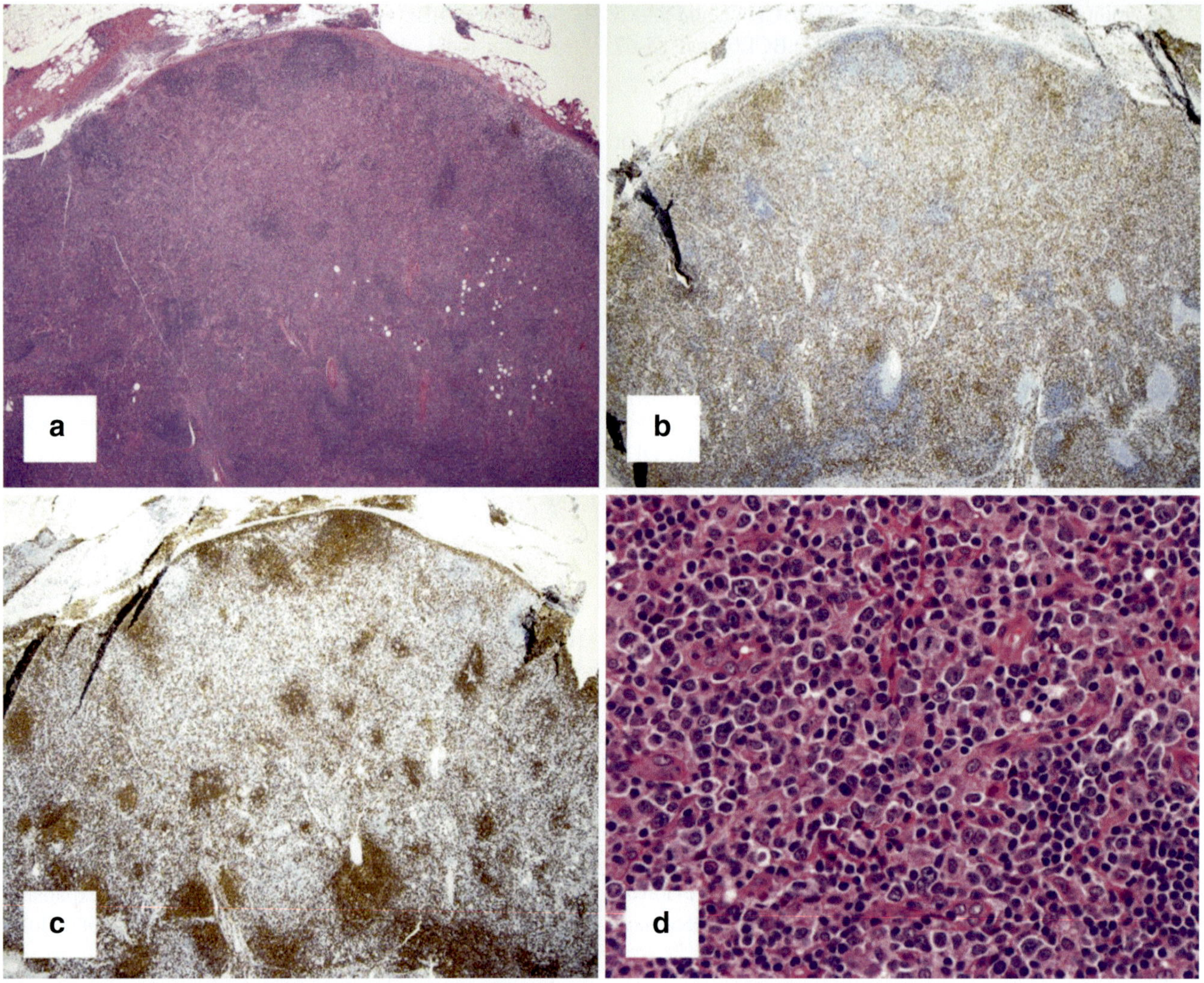

Fig. 18.9 Interfollicular/paracortical to diffuse hyperplasia, not otherwise specified. Low magnification of this enlarged lymph node shows a striking expansion of the interfollicular/paracortical zones, seen as pale sheets (**a**). Immunostains for CD3 and CD20, however, demonstrate retention of nodal architecture by the presence of numerous CD3+ T-cells in interfollicular zones (**b**) and variably sized B-cell follicles (**c**). High magnification (**d**) reveals a polymorphous cellular composition of the interfollicular expansion, with an admixture of small lymphocytes, histiocytes, plasma cells, and larger transformed lymphocytes (i.e., immunoblasts). The morphologic features favor benignity over malignancy

25. What is the DDx in IFH/DH?

- Table 18.8 summarizes infectious and non-infectious etiologies of IFH/DH and its neoplastic mimics [2, 10].
- Select entities in the DDx of IFH/DH will be discussed further.

26. As a very typical entity that can display IFH/DH, what additional morphologic features does *EBV*-IM LAD exhibit?

- Paracortical to diffuse expansion with prominent vascularity and "mottling" (due to presence of scattered immunoblasts).
- May be "mixed pattern" hyperplasia (RFH + IFH/DH).
- Polymorphous lymphoid cells in paracortical expansion with full spectrum of maturation:
  - From small- to medium-sized, reactive-appearing lymphocytes, to
  - Plasmacytoid cells, to
  - Plasma cells, to
  - Immunoblasts (larger transformed cells), to
  - Cells resembling Hodgkin/Reed-Sternberg cells, so-called HRS-like cells
- High endothelial venules proliferate.
- Immunoblastic component can predominate → can be a challenging DDx with large cell lymphoma.
- Monocytoid B-cell hyperplasia can be seen (see Table 18.4 for DDx).
- Sinuses patent; may contain immunoblasts.
- Characteristic IHC:

Table 18.8 Differential diagnosis of paracortical/interfollicular and diffuse hyperplasia and its neoplastic mimics

Infectious	Non-infectious	Neoplastic mimics
EBV/infectious mononucleosis CMV HSV HHV6 Parasitic LAD (*Wuchereria bancrofti*, *Onchocerca volvulus*, *Brugia malayi*, *Strongyloides*)	Reactive interfollicular hyperplasia, NOS Dermatopathic LAD Kikuchi-Fujimoto disease[a] SLE[a] Kimura disease Postvaccinial administration Drug-related (e.g., Dilantin) Environmental pollutants, chemicals Churg-Strauss vasculitis (also known as allergic granulomatous angiitis) IgG4-related LAD (interfollicular pattern) Mucocutaneous LN syndrome (Kawasaki disease)	Polymorphic B-lymphoproliferative disorder, *EBV*+, occurring in setting of immunodeficiency (like PTLD) T-cell/histiocyte-rich large B-cell lymphoma MF involvement of LN DLBCL cHL ALCL AITL PTCL

AITL angioimmunoblastic T-cell lymphoma, *ALCL* anaplastic large cell lymphoma, *cHL* classic Hodgkin lymphoma, *DLBCL* diffuse large B-cell lymphoma, *LAD* lymphadenopathy, *LN* lymph node, *MF* mycosis fungoides, *PTCL* peripheral T-cell lymphoma, *SLE* systemic lupus erythematosus

[a]Discussed further in histiocyte-rich section of granulomatous/histiocytic lymphadenitides

  - Nodal architectural preservation with CD3+ T-cell-rich interfollicular regions and CD20+ B-cell-rich lymphoid follicles.
  - Persistence of follicular dendritic cell (FDC) networks by CD21 and/or CD23.
  - Immunoblasts:
    - Admixture of B- and T-cells.
    - Polytypic kappa and lambda light chain expression.
    - CD30+/CD15-/CD45+ (unlike HRS cells which are CD30+/CD15+/CD45-).
  - Background lymphocytes predominantly CD8+ cytotoxic T-cells.
  - EBER ISH decorates not only immunoblasts and HRS-like cells but also small lymphocytes (in cHL/NHL: EBER ISH expression *only* in large neoplastic cells).
- Histomorphologic findings are illustrated in Fig. 18.10.
- Because of the difficulty in the DDx of *EBV* IM LAD with classic Hodgkin lymphoma, non-Hodgkin lymphoma, and IM-like PTLD (post-transplant lymphoproliferative disorder)/PTLD-like, see Table 18.9 for the clues to correct diagnosis [2, 25, 28–32].

27. Are immunohistologic features alone sufficiently diagnostic for *EBV*/IM-LAD?

- In brief, no. As with many reactive lymphadenitides, the histology must be correlated with clinical context. Characteristic presentation for acute infection includes:
  - Adolescents and young adults typical.
  - Fever.
  - Pharyngitis.
  - Fatigue.
  - Cervical lymphadenopathy (usually of posterior LN chain).
  - Splenomegaly may also be observed.
- Histopathologic features coupled with the appropriate sign-symptom complex (ancillary tests below) will lead to the correct diagnosis.
- Some cases may be quite challenging and require further investigation.

28. What ancillary testing can help establish the diagnosis of *EBV*/IM-LAD?

- Peripheral blood (PB) CBC, smears, and/or serology
  - Leukocytosis with >10% atypical lymphocytes (so-called Downey type II cells).
  - Positive heterophile antibody test (e.g., Monospot)
    - Note: heterophile antibody testing less reliable in children; not recommended for those <4 years old due to excessive false negativity.
- PB flow cytometry
  - Expansion of CD8+ T-cells (average CD4:CD8 ratio = 1:4)
    - CD8+ T-cells will display activation markers, HLA-DR and CD38.
    - Downregulation of CD7 (common) and CD5 (uncommon) [31]
    - Note: Careful clinical and morphologic correlation required to avoid pitfall of diagnosing T-cell lymphoma in PB.
  - CD4+ T-cells and polytypic CD19+ B-cells within normal ranges.
- LN/tissue ancillary studies

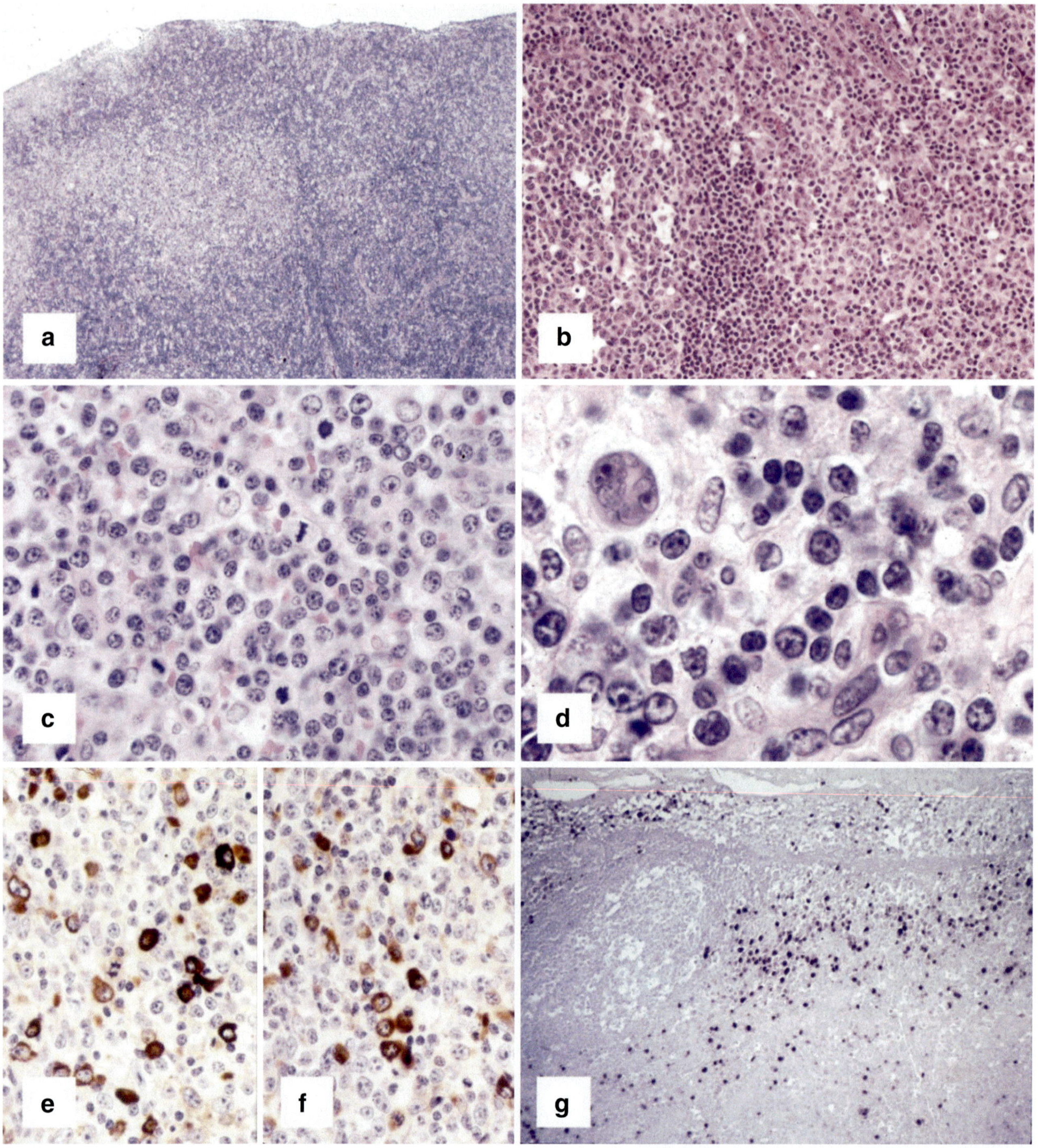

Fig. 18.10 Lymphadenopathy secondary to *EBV* infectious mononucleosis: an entity displaying interfollicular/paracortical hyperplasia. This low-power magnification of an enlarged lymph node demonstrates an ill-defined, pale, paracortical expansion (**a**). IHC stains for CD3 and CD20 demonstrate nodal architectural preservation (not illustrated here). (**b**) Polymorphous paracortical hyperplasia and prominent vasculature (seen on the right-hand side of the photomicrograph) are noted adjacent to the reactive germinal center and mantle zone (seen on the left-hand side). The cellular composition is an admixture of small lymphocytes, histiocytes, plasma cells, and immunoblasts. (**c**) A focus of interfollicular expansion with striking increase in mitotic activity and many immunoblasts can raise concern for lymphoma. (**d**) Hodgkin/Reed-Sternberg (HRS)-like cell (left upper corner of photomicrograph) admixed with lymphocytes showing a spectrum of morphology, from small lymphocytes to plasma cells to immunoblasts. Immunoblast-rich region with IHC stains for CD3 (**e**) and CD20 (**f**) revealing an admixture of T- and B-cell immunoblasts, respectively. (**g**) EBER ISH stain decorates many variably sized *EBV*-infected cells (small lymphocytes to large immunoblasts) in the paracortex; this contrasts with EBER positivity confined to neoplastic cells only in lymphomas

Table 18.9 Morphologic, immunophenotypic, and clinical features which can aid in distinction of *EBV* infectious mononucleosis from large cell non-Hodgkin lymphoma and classic Hodgkin lymphoma and PTLD/PTLD-like lesions

Feature	*EBV* infectious mononucleosis	Large cell non-Hodgkin lymphoma	Classic Hodgkin lymphoma	Infectious mononucleosis-like PTLD/PTLD-like lesions	Additional notes
Clinical setting	Typically adolescent, young adult	Typically older individuals	Bimodal age distribution (affects adolescents/young adults and older adults)	Immunocompromised patient (i.e., post-transplant, iatrogenic immunosuppression, etc.)	Occurrence of IM in older and/or immunocompromised pt. can be challenging
Monospot test	Positive	Negative	Negative	Negative	Around 18–28% of *EBV*-related IM cases can be negative
Lymph node architecture	Partial involvement, with some preservation of architecture	Diffuse effacement by an abnormal large cell proliferation	Occasionally can be partial effacement or subtle interfollicular involvement	Preserved in IM-like PTLD Effaced in polymorphic B-LPD	*One of most important distinguishing features of reactive vs neoplastic*
Sinuses	Patent, sometimes filled with reactive immunoblasts	Typically obliterated	Typically obliterated	Can be patent or obliterated	
Monocytoid B-cell proliferation	Can be present	Absent	Absent	Can be present	
Cellular composition	Polymorphous lymphoid infiltrate with spectrum of maturation (from small lymphocytes to plasmacytoid lymphocytes to plasma cells to immunoblasts), histiocytes, and occasionally HRS-like cells	Typically monomorphic neoplastic infiltrate or cytologic atypia in small and large lymphoid cells	HRS cells admixed with reactive inflammatory infiltrate (including small lymphocytes, neutrophils, eosinophils, plasma cells, and/or histiocytes)	Polymorphous lymphoid infiltrate with spectrum of maturation (from small lymphocytes to plasmacytoid lymphocytes to plasma cells to immunoblasts), histiocytes, and occasionally HRS-like cells	Polymorphous composition very helpful feature against NHL and cHL → caveat is *EBV*+ DLBCL and PTLD/PTLD-like lesions can be polymorphic and/or closely mimic *EBV*-IM histologically
Immunoblastic proliferation interface	Merging of immunoblastic proliferation with reactive follicles and paracortex	Diffuse immunoblastic proliferation with complete effacement of architecture	Uncommon to have a prominent immunoblastic component	Merging of immunoblastic proliferation with reactive follicles and paracortex	
IHC staining					
CD3 and CD20	Mixture of T- and B-immunoblasts	Large cells uniformly strongly express CD3 or CD20	Variable expression and intensity of CD20 in HRS cells	Mixture of T- and B-immunoblasts	Admixture strongly suggestive of reactive etiology
CD4/CD8 in T-cells	Predominance of CD8+ cytotoxic T-cells	Depends on T-cell lymphoma type	Predominance of CD4+ T-helper cells		
CD15	RS-like cells (−)	RS-like cells (−)	HRS cells (+)	RS-like cells (−)	Note that significant subset of cHL can be CD15 negative
CD30	Immunoblasts and RS-like cells (variably +)	Immunoblasts (variably +)	HRS cells (uniformly +)	Immunoblasts, RS-like cells (variably +)	Intensity and distribution of staining can be a helpful feature
CD45	RS-like cells (+)	Positive	HRS cells (−)	RS-like cells (+)	Useful feature
Kappa and lambda	Immunoblasts polytypic	May show light chain restriction in B-cell NHL	Plasma cells polytypic	Immunoblasts polytypic	Polytypic expression supports reactive dx
OCT-2/BOB.1	+/+	+/+ in B-cell NHL	+/− or −/−	+/+	Retained B-cell program expression speaks against cHL
EBER ISH	RS-like cells and small lymphocytes (+)	Large neoplastic cells only (+)	Only neoplastic HRS cells (+)	RS-like cells and small lymphocytes (+)	Expression in variably sized cells strongly favors *EBV*-IM and/or PTLD/PTLD-like over NHL/cHL

– Flow cytometry: Polytypic surface immunoglobulin light chain expression in B-cells.
– Clonality studies for T- and B-cell receptor gene rearrangement can be additionally pursued in problematic cases. The absence of clonal peaks can help reassure and/or confirm one's suspicion of a reactive IM.
- In immunocompromised patients or when first-line testing is negative, serologic test panels may be diagnostically useful [30].
  – Anti-*EBV* viral capsid antigen (VCA) IgG and IgM typically elevated in acute infection.
  – IgG against *EBV* nuclear antigen (EBNA) is not detectable until weeks after primary acute infection period.
  – Note: *EBV* PCR is not established as a method to diagnose IM.
  – If *EBV* laboratory tests are negative, consider ruling out causes of IM-like syndrome, which include HIV, CMV, HHV-6, and toxoplasmosis.
- Table 18.10 summarizes immunohistologic clues and characteristic clinical settings in the most commonly encountered viral lymphadenitides.

Table 18.10 Immunohistologic, clinical, and laboratory findings to the more commonly seen viral lymphadenitides

Virus	Morphology of viral inclusions on H&E stain	IHC/ISH available?	Additional helpful histologic features	Ancillary studies	Typical clinical setting
EBV	None seen	*EBV* LMP IHC; EBER ISH	Exuberant immunoblastic paracortical hyperplasia, can mimic large cell lymphoma +/– Monocytoid B-cell hyperplasia	Acute primary infection: Positive monospot test PB lymphocytosis with "atypical lymphocytes" Immunocompromised patient (or when first-line test negative): Anti-*EBV* VCA IgG, IgM elevated (see text for further details)	Primary infection: Immunocompetent young adult with flu-like symptoms, LAD, and splenomegaly. Immunosuppressed patients: Have undergone BM or solid organ transplantation can have PTLD
CMV	Single large intranuclear eosinophilic inclusion and multiple basophilic cytoplasmic inclusions	CMV IHC	+/– Monocytoid B-cell hyperplasia	PB lymphocytosis with "atypical lymphocytes" Immunocompetent individual: Paired CMV IgG and IgM serology → collect 10–14 days apart to observed seroconversion in primary acute infection Immunocompromised individual: CMV viral load	Rare, typically affects immunocompromised patient Several presentations, but most common mimics *EBV* infectious mononucleosis (i.e., CMV mononucleosis = IM-like syndrome)
HSV	+ Large eosinophilic inclusion leading to margination of chromatin to nuclear membrane margins ["ground glass" or smudgy chromatin] +/– Nuclear molding +/– Multinucleation	HSV IHC	Necrosis +/– Monocytoid B-cell hyperplasia	Pursue HSV NAAT (nucleic acid amplification testing) from mucocutaneous lesion Culture or DFA (direct fluorescence antigen) are options, albeit less sensitive If case is atypical, above testing negative, or mucocutaneous lesion not apparent: Try type-specific HSV IgG serology	Immunocompromised patient Can be primary infection or reactivation LAD associated with mucocutaneous lesions, e.g., genital ulcers (usually HSV type 2), cold sores (usually HSV type 1) Sometimes seen in patients with CLL/SLL and MCL
HHV8	None seen	HHV8 IHC	+ Interfollicular polytypic plasmacytosis + Vascular proliferation +/– "lollipop" sign in follicles and/or "onion-skinning" of mantle zones (if mixed hyaline vascular and plasma cell morphology of MCD)		HIV+ patient HHV8+ MCD patients can be significantly ill: + constitutional symptoms + polyclonal hypergammaglobulinemia + LAD +/– splenomegaly

CLL/SLL chronic lymphocytic leukemia/small lymphocytic lymphoma; *CMV* cytometgalovirus; *EBER ISH EBV* encoded RNA in-situ hybridization; *EBV* Epstein Barr virus; *HHV8* human herpesvirus 8; *HSV* herpes simplex virus; *IHC* immunohistochemistry; *LAD* lymphadenopathy; *MCD* multicentric Castleman disease; *MCL* mantle cell lymphoma; *NAAT* nucleic acid amplification test; *PB* peripheral blood; *VCA* viral capsid antigen

29. If IFH/DH is not due to *EBV*-IM LAD, then what other histologic features could suggest another reactive entity (i.e., what else is in the DDx)?

- See Table 18.8 for the DDx.
  - If IFH/DH + RFH + monocytoid B-cell clusters:
    Recall DDx of monocytoid B-cell clusters (see Table 18.4), which includes LAD due to viral infections (HIV, *EBV*, CMV, HSV), toxoplasmosis, bacterial infections (cat scratch, LGV, etc.)
- Viropathic change in CMV LAD = CMV-infected cell has a single huge acidophilic intranuclear inclusion + multiple small, granular cytoplasmic inclusions (Fig. 18.11a, b) [2, 33, 36].
- Viropathic change in HHV6 LAD = prominent eosinophilic intranuclear inclusion contained within large atypical lymphoid cells, with marked paracortical hyperplasia, necrosis, vascular proliferation [76].
- HSV LAD [20, 30, 34–36]
  - Necrosis (whether focal or extensive) very commonly seen.
  - Viropathic change in HSV LAD = Large acidophilic inclusion → margination of chromatin to the nuclear

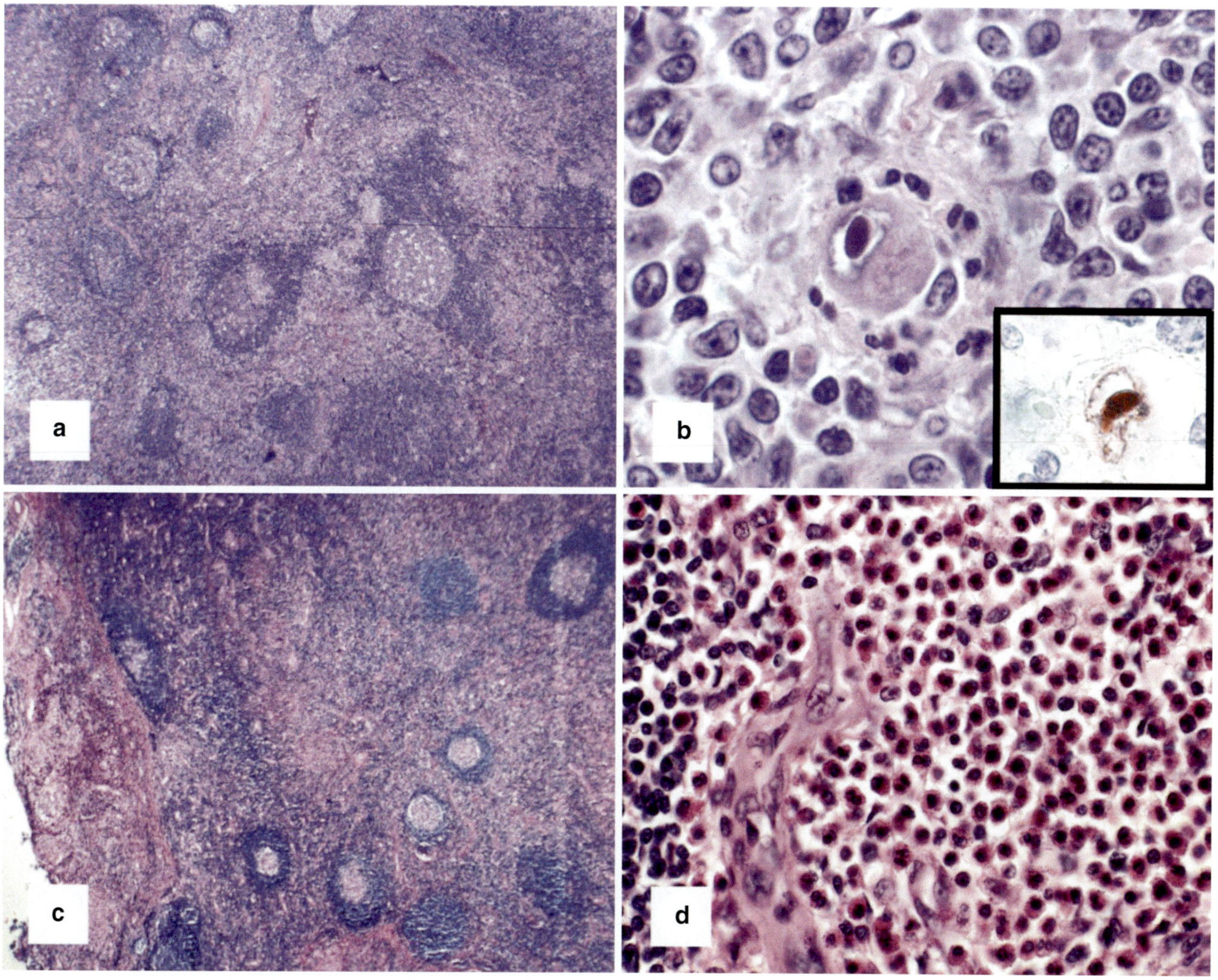

Fig. 18.11 Other entities displaying interfollicular/paracortical hyperplasia: CMV lymphadenitis (**a** and **b**) and eosinophil-rich lymphadenitis due to Kimura disease (**c** and **d**). Cases of IFH/DH can have marked interfollicular expansion, but will invariably show retention of reactive lymphoid follicles, as seen in both (**a**) and (**c**). In this case of CMV lymphadenitis, RFH and IFH are evident on low magnification (**a**). Monocytoid B-cell hyperplasia can also be seen in this entity. The characteristic viropathic changes in a CMV-infected cell are seen in (**b**), with a single huge acidophilic intranuclear viral inclusion as well as multiple small, granular cytoplasmic basophilic inclusions. CMV IHC stain [inset for (**b**)] highlights this mononuclear Hodgkin-like cell, whereas true HRS cells would be negative. In this lymph node of an adolescent Asian male with Kimura disease, fibrosis is present and nodal architecture preserved (**c**). Though vascular proliferation is present, no cuboidal or hypertrophic endothelial cells are seen (vs. cuboidal endothelial cells of angiolymphoid hyperplasia with eosinophilia, also known as epithelioid hemangioma). Eosinophilic microabscesses can be readily identified (**d**). LAD in eosinophil-rich lymphadenitis is heavily dependent on clinical history and laboratory data

membrane, resulting in "ground glass" or smudgy chromatin; multinucleation; nuclear molding.
  - If epithelioid granulomas encroaching on germinal centers seen with IFH/DH + RFH + monocytoid B-cell clusters: think toxoplasmosis (see Question 10).
  - If interfollicular infiltrate is plasma cell-rich, consider:
    - IgG4-related LAD (see further discussion in Question 72): can also have RFH, PTGC, Castleman-like features, and increased interfollicular eosinophils.
    - Castleman disease, plasma cell variant (see Question 77).
    - Autoimmune disorders: RA (Question 13), AOSD (Question 32), SLE (Question 62).
  - If interfollicular infiltrate is eosinophil-rich, consider:
    - Kimura disease (Fig. 18.11c, d).
    - Parasitic infections.
    - Post-vaccinial administration.
    - Environmental/drug/chemical exposure.
    - Allergic granulomatous vasculitis (Churg-Strauss vasculitis).
    - IgG4-related LAD.

    For summary on DDx and distinguishing features of eosinophil-rich LAD, see Table 18.11 [37–39].
  - If massive necrosis and numerous macrophages present, consider:
    - Kikuchi-Fujimoto disease vs SLE (see further discussion, Question 62)
  - If pigmented macrophages present with nodular paracortical T-cell hyperplasia, consider:
    - Dermatopathic LAD – morphologic findings in Fig. 18.12.

30. What is the minimal histopathologic work-up in IFH/DH?

- Depends on what findings are prominent.
- CD3 and CD20: Confirms histologic impression of nodal architectural preservation.
- If lymphoma is of concern, whether because of architectural or cytologic atypia:
  - CD21, CD23: Confirms preserved FDC networks confined to lymphoid follicles.
  - BCL2, BCL6: Underscores absence of BCL2 staining in reactive germinal centers.
  - EBER ISH: Highlights quantity and sparse staining of variably sized *EBV*+ cells (in contrast to frequent positivity in neoplastic cells only).
  - CD30, CD15, CD45, PAX5:
    - Emphasizes the typical CD30+/CD45+ and CD15-negative reactive immunoblast phenotype (in contrast to HRS cell phenotype in cHL).
    - Weak and variable CD30 expression in reactive immunoblasts distinguishes uniform intense staining in cHL and ALCL.
  - T-cell markers (e.g., CD2, CD4, CD5, CD8, CD10): Lack of overt aberrancies in CD8+ cytotoxic T-cell predominant infiltrate favors reactive IFH/DH (in contrast to follicular CD4+ T-helper phenotype of lymphoma cells in AITL).
- If IFH/DH + RFH + monocytoid B-cell clusters:
  - CMV and HSV IHC and/or EBER ISH: Assesses for viral inclusions.
  - *Bartonella* IHC commercially available and could be performed for cat-scratch disease.
- If IFH/DH + RFH + monocytoid B-cell clusters + epithelioid granulomas (classic triad):
  - *Toxoplasma* IHC commercially available and could be performed.
- If plasma cells are increased:
  - CD138, kappa, lambda: Determines degree of plasmacytosis; establishes polytypic staining pattern.
  - IgG4, IgG: Conveys whether IgG4-positive plasma cells are significantly increased.
  - HHV8: Assesses for HHV8-related MCD.
- If eosinophil-rich:
  - S100, CD1a, langerin: Absence of staining excludes LCH (Langerhans cell histiocytosis).
  - T-cell markers and others: Examines possibility of AITL.
  - Reactive entities are largely dependent on clinical history and laboratory data for specific diagnosis (Table 18.11).
- If no infectious etiology, additionally consider autoimmune disorders (see Table 18.6)
  - No additional IHC to suggest.
- Work-up depends on clinical setting for dermatopathic changes:
  - No history of malignancy, no further work-up required.
  - History of mycosis fungoides (MF) or cutaneous T-cell lymphoma (CTCL):
    - Pursue extensive work-up with IHC (T-cell markers, including CD2, CD3, CD4, CD5, CD7, CD8, CD30, TIA1, PD1), flow cytometry, and molecular studies (i.e., clonality studies for T-cell gene receptor rearrangements) to determine nodal involvement of MF/CTCL (also see Fig. 18.12)
  - If histiocytes with nuclear grooves and eosinophils seen: Evaluate for possibility of LCH with S100, CD1a, langerin (all positive in LCH).

Table 18.11 Summary table of differential diagnosis for lymphadenopathy with prominent eosinophilic infiltrates and useful diagnostic features (bolded text indicates most useful features)

	Proliferation	Typical clinical/radiologic/laboratory features	Morphologic features	IHC/special stain
Infectious	Filarial LAD (due to parasitic worms), like *Wuchereria bancrofti*, *Brugia malayi*, *Onchocerca volvulus* *Strongyloides* and other parasitic worms (*Ascaris*, *Trichuris*, *Enterobius*, etc.)	Depends on endemic region, infection duration, etc. Some present with LAD and elephantiasis from parasitic infestation of lymphatics (due to *W. bancrofti* or *B. malayi*) *O. volvulus* causes river blindness *Strongyloides* infection asymptomatic in immunocompetent individuals; but severe and systemic in immunocompromised pts	RFH, monocytoid B-cell hyperplasia (early stage) Granulomas, fibrosis/sclerosis, calcification (mid to late stages) Eosinophil- and neutrophil-rich microabscesses with **degenerated worms** **Infectious disease pathology expert can be sought for classification of microfilaria**	None
Non-infectious	Kimura disease (AHLE/epithelioid hemangioma, below, was formerly thought to be the same entity as Kimura disease)	Chronic inflammatory condition in young males of Asian ancestry Deep head and neck LAD **Serum IgE and blood eosinophilia common**	Florid RFH with IFH, c/o lymphocytes, eosinophils, plasma cells, mast cells Significant fibrosis, +/− polykaryocytes **No cuboidal endothelium or vascular proliferation**	**IgE IHC stains deposits in germinal centers**
	Postvaccinial LAD	**History of vaccine administration critical to diagnosis** Involved LN drains site of vaccine	Diffuse IFH with mottled ("moth-eaten") appearance, composed of variable admixture of lymphocytes, eosinophils, histiocytes, immunoblasts	None
	LAD due to allergic/drug-induced hypersensitivity syndrome	**History of exposure to drug (like diphenylhydantoin), chemicals** **Blood eosinophilia,** atypical **lymphocytosis** Cessation of exposure results in LAD resolution within weeks	Like most IFH, admixture of lymphocytes, eosinophils, histiocytes, immunoblasts plus HRS-like cells	None
	IgG4-related LAD	Older male (>50 years old) Elevation in serum IgG4 and IgE levels IgG4-RD manifestations in other organs, like pancreas	RFH, PTGC, IFH, MCD-like, IPT-like lesions and intragerminal center plasmacytosis Interfollicular eosinophilia is a useful finding favoring plasma cell-rich LAD over other entities (like iMCD)	**IgG4, IgG**
	Churg-Strauss vasculitis (also known as allergic granulomatous angiitis)	**Systemic vasculitis** affecting small to medium-sized vessels Asthma and skin involvement common Less frequent manifestations: cardiovascular, renal, GI, and nervous systems	Leukocytoclastic vasculitis in addition to eosinophilic abscesses	None
Neoplastic	Angiolymphoid hyperplasia with eosinophilia (AHLE, also known as epithelioid hemangioma)	**Benign vascular neoplasm** in Caucasian females Erythematous overlying skin with superficial LAD No IgE elevations or blood eosinophilia	Prominent, thick-walled vascular proliferation with sparse eosinophils **Cuboidal/hypertrophic endothelial cells**	Vascular IHC highlights vessels
	AITL	**Constitutional symptoms**, skin rash Systemic manifestations, hepatosplenomegaly Polyclonal hypergammaglobulinemia	**Lymphoma cells with "water-clear" morphology** **Exuberant vascular proliferation** **FDC meshwork expansion/"bridging"** +/− *EBV*+ B-cell immunoblasts	**Neoplastic cells with follicular T-helper phenotype**
	LCH	Bony lesions and LAD Infants have severe systemic manifestations (fever, cytopenias)	**Neoplastic Langerhans cells** admixed with many eosinophils	**S100+, CD1a+, Langerin+**
	PTCL	Constitutional symptoms, regional to systemic LAD	**Nodal architectural effacement by lymphoma cells**; eosinophils admixed **Cytologically and immunophenotypically abnormal T-cells**	**Neoplastic T-cell phenotype**
	cHL	Constitutional symptoms Confluent supraclavicular/mediastinal LAD	Nodal architectural effacement Scattered **HRS cells admixed with polymorphous reactive inflammatory cells**	**HRS cells with characteristic phenotype**

AITL angioimmunoblastic T-cell lymphoma, *cHL* classic Hodgkin lymphoma, *HRS* Hodgkin/Reed-Sternberg, *IFH* interfollicular hyperplasia, *IgG4-RD* IgG4-related disease; *IPT* inflammatory pseudotumor, *LAD* lymphadenopathy/lymphadenitis, *LCH* Langerhans cell histiocytosis, *MCD* multicentric Castleman disease, *PTCL* peripheral T-cell lymphoma, *PTGC* progressive transformation of germinal centers, *RFH* reactive follicular hyperplasia

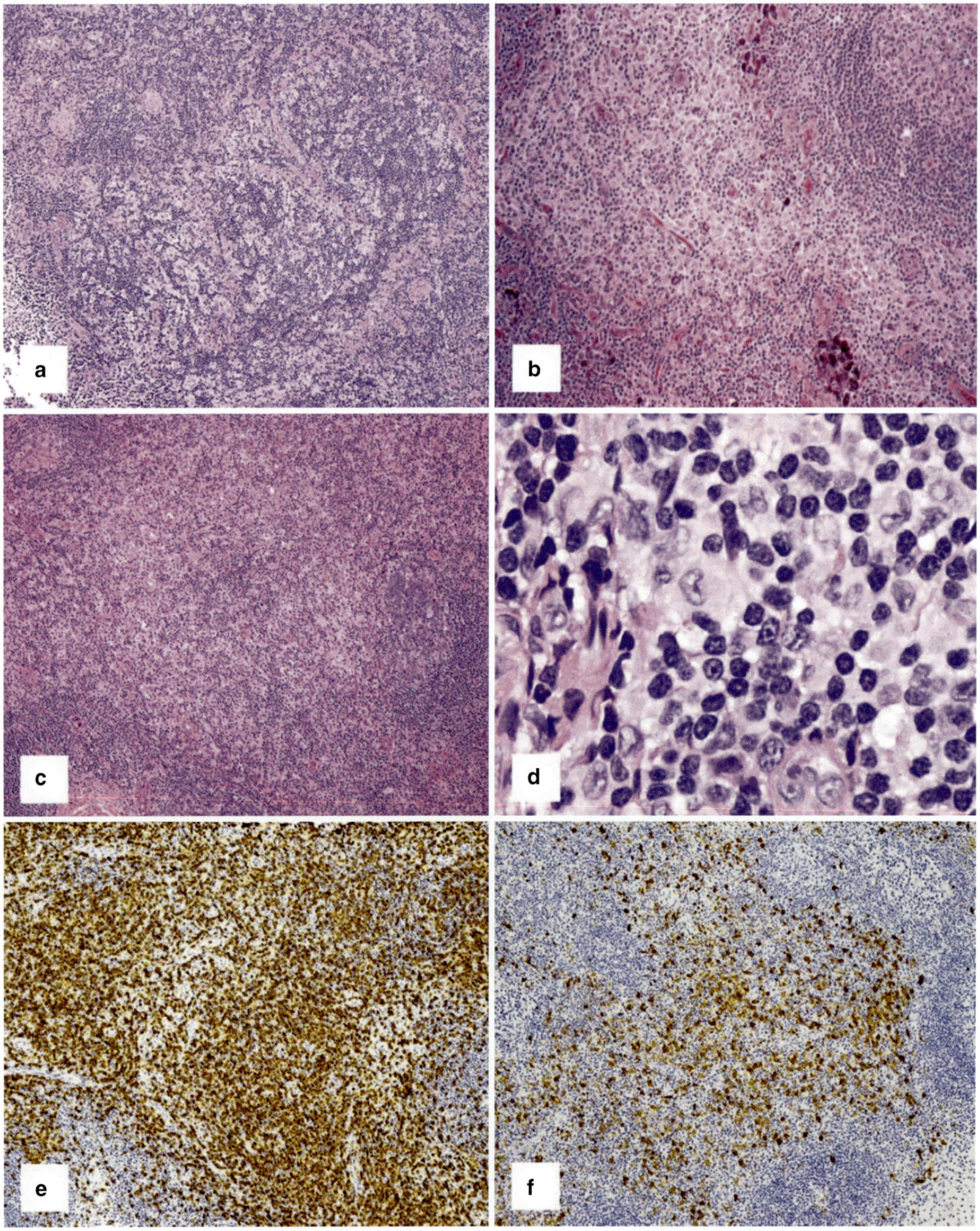

Fig. 18.12 Dermatopathic lymphadenopathy (DLA): another entity in the IFH/DH DDx. Dermatopathic changes leading to DLA are commonly seen in reactive LNs of patients with chronic inflammatory skin disorders (like eczematous dermatitides), as well as patients with cutaneous T-cell lymphomas (CTCL, like mycosis fungoides, MF). (**a**) Nodularity and mottling in the paracortex can be easily appreciated in this LN from a patient with psoriasis; in the absence of pigmented macrophages, this can be characterized as a nodular paracortical T-cell hyperplasia (NPTCH). (**b**) The presence of pigmented macrophages (in lower and upper right of photomicrograph) – as well as many pale histiocytes, Langerhans cells (LCs), and interdigitating dendritic cells (IDCs) adjacent to this germinal center – meet criteria for dermatopathic changes/DLA. This set of photomicrographs (**c-f**) is from a patient with a history of MF. Note the remarkable similarity of (**c**) with (**a**). It is notoriously difficult to distinguish DLA from nodal involvement by CTCL, even on careful H&E and IHC examination. High magnification of DLA displays scattered IDCs and LCs with twisted to elongated nuclei with vesicular chromatin and abundant pale cytoplasm (**d**). CD3 stain shows the predominance of T-cells (**e**), while S100 stain highlights many IDCs and LCs (**f**) in this NPTCH, in the same region as shown in (**c**). PCR clonality studies of T-cell gene rearrangements uncovered identical clonal peaks between the skin biopsy with biopsy-proven MF and this LN sample. Only then could a diagnosis of LN involvement by MF and dermatopathic lymphadenopathy be confidently rendered

31. What clinical and epidemiologic features are present in adult-onset Still's disease (AOSD), another entity which can present with IFH/DH?

- "Still's disease" first described in children → became associated with systemic juvenile idiopathic arthritis (JIA).
- "Adult-onset Still's disease" was later recognized in adults → clinical findings resembled those of pediatric systemic JIA, but *did not* fulfill diagnostic criteria for classic rheumatoid arthritis.
- AOSD is a diagnosis of exclusion: requires careful integration of clinical and laboratory features; no single gold standard laboratory test for diagnosis.
- Several diagnostic classification schema are available for the diagnosis of AOSD.
  - Yamaguchi criteria most widely used classification scheme (has highest sensitivity) → requires five positive features, with at least two major diagnostic criteria (Table 18.12) [41].
  - Presence of infectious, malignant, and other rheumatologic disease mimics of AOSD precludes diagnosis.

32. As a very typical entity that can display IFH/DH, what other morphologic features does AOSD exhibit?

- Jeon and colleagues described the following four histologic patterns of LAD in AOSD [40]:
  - Atypical paracortical hyperplasia with prominent vascular proliferation (most common), with scattered B- and T-immunoblasts, small- to medium-sized lymphocytes, and other inflammatory cells.
  - Paracortical hyperplasia with massive sinus histiocytosis.
  - Exuberant immunoblastic reaction with patchy or diffuse infiltration of highly proliferative large T-immunoblasts.
  - Follicular hyperplasia.
- Table 18.13 shows DDx to consider in AOSD based on histologic patterns.

Table 18.12 Yamaguchi criteria for the diagnosis of adult-onset Still's disease

Major criteria	Minor criteria
Fever ≥39 °C (102.2 °F) lasting ≥1 week	Sore throat
Arthralgias/arthritis ≥2 weeks	Lymphadenopathy
Non-pruritic macular or maculopapular skin rash Salmon colored Usually in the trunk or extremities Usually appears during febrile episodes	Hepatomegaly or splenomegaly
Neutrophilic leukocytosis (ANC ≥ 8 K/microliter)	Abnormal liver function studies, particularly AST, ALT, and LDH elevations
	Negative tests for ANA (anti-nuclear antibody) and RF (rheumatoid factor)

Note: Diagnosis requires 5 positive features, with at least 2 major criteria fulfilled [41]

Table 18.13 Differential diagnosis (DDx) and work-up for adult-onset Still's disease (AOSD) based on histologic pattern

Histologic pattern	Reactive/indeterminate DDx	Neoplastic DDx	IHC work-up	Useful ancillary data
Atypical paracortical hyperplasia	*EBV*-IM Post-vaccinial LAD Kikuchi necrotizing lymphadenitis (proliferative phase) SLE LAD Drug-related LAD (e.g., Dilantin) HHV6 LAD	PTCL AITL TCHRLBL	CD3, CD4, CD8, CD10, CD20, CD21, CD23, BCL6, PD1, TIA1, Ki-67, PAX5, EBER ISH	Clinical information ID work-up negative in AOSD B-cell and T-cell receptor gene rearrangement studies negative for clonality in AOSD
Paracortical hyperplasia with massive sinus histiocytosis	RDD/SHML	Langerhans cell histiocytosis ALCL Metastatic malignancy (like carcinoma, melanoma, etc.)	CD3, CD20, S100, CD1a, Pancytokeratin	Clinical information Subset of RDD/SHML have *BRAF* mutations
Exuberant immunoblastic reaction	*EBV*-IM	Peripheral T-cell lymphoma	CD3, CD4, CD8, CD20, CD21, CD23, PD1, TIA1, Ki-67, EBER ISH	Clinical information T-cell receptor gene rearrangement studies negative for clonality in AOSD
Follicular hyperplasia	Rheumatoid arthritis	Follicular lymphoma	CD3, CD20, BCL2, BCL6, Ki-67	Clinical information

ALCL anaplastic large cell lymphoma, *AITL* angioimmunoblastic T-cell lymphoma, *EBV-IM EBV*-related infectious mononucleosis, *ID* infectious disease, *LAD* lymphadenopathy, *PTCL* peripheral T-cell lymphoma, *RDD/SHML* Rosai-Dorfman-Destombes disease (sinus histiocytosis with massive lymphadenopathy), *SLE* systemic lupus erythematosus, *TCHRLBL* T-cell histiocyte-rich large B-cell lymphoma

33. What ancillary testing can help establish diagnosis of AOSD?

- In a patient presenting with fever, arthritis, and rash, supportive laboratory data include:
  - Neutrophilia (ANC >8 K/microliter).
  - Absence of antineutrophil antibody (ANA).
  - Positive rheumatoid factor (RF).
  - Elevations in the liver enzymes AST and ALT and increased LDH (see Table 18.12).

34. Considering entities in the DDx, what is the clinical relevance of misinterpretation in IFH/DH?

- Misinterpreting IFH/DH as lymphoma (see neoplastic DDx in Table 18.8):
  - Misdiagnosing IFH/DH as cHL, AITL, DLBCL, or other lymphoma leads to unwarranted chemotherapy and/or radiation treatment and additional morbidity/mortality.
- Not suggesting the correct reactive etiology for RFH:
  - May not be as clinically devastating as misdiagnosis of lymphoma.
  - Confusion with other viral lymphadenitides should not present as a large problem, taking clinical and laboratory features into account.
  - However, significant morbidity may result in diagnostic and treatment delays (e.g., not recognizing and treating AOSD or SLE) [40–42] and/or lead to additional unnecessary biopsies (e.g., in IgG4-related LAD).

35. In IFH/DH, what information can be conveyed to the clinician? When is a diagnostic comment necessary? What is an adequate specimen?

- Limited sampling with CNBx can be diagnostic pitfall and lead to misdiagnosis.
- If possible, insist on excisional biopsy for complete and adequate evaluation of nodal architecture to adequately exclude malignancy (unless CNBx findings are concordant with clinical/laboratory/radiologic features).

36. When is consultation necessary in IFH/DH?

- Consultation is prudent in atypical cases, as misdiagnosis of large cell lymphoma in IFH/DH (particularly *EBV*-related IM) is a well-documented occurrence. Consider consultation in the following settings:
  - Clinical presentations and/or nodal sites unusual for IM.
  - Histomorphologic features mimicking lymphoma, including:
    - Necrosis
    - Sheets of large mononuclear lymphoma-like cells
    - HRS-like cells
    - Immunoblasts within sinuses mimicking ALCL
  - Ancillary studies (e.g., flow cytometry, molecular, genetics) with results discordant with histopathology.
  - In NCBx and/or poorly sampled incisional biopsy cases where excisional biopsy cannot/will not be obtained.

Granulomatous, Suppurative, and Histiocyte-rich LAD (G/H-LAD), DDx Including LAD Secondary to Mycobacterial, Bacteria, and Fungal Infections; Sarcoidosis; Rosai-Dorfman-Destombes Disease, Kikuchi-Fujimoto Disease; Systemic Lupus Erythematosus

37. What are the typical morphologic findings in the major subtype of granulomatous and/or histiocyte-rich lymphadenopathy (G/H-LAD)?

- Histiocytes/macrophages can have variable morphology [43, 44]. Definitions of granulomatous and/or histiocyte-rich LAD:
  - Histiocytes = non-activated macrophages with well-defined cell borders, reniform nuclei, clear to pale eosinophilic cytoplasm.
  - Epithelioid histiocytes = macrophages with ill-defined borders, oval/elongated "epithelioid" nuclei, abundant granular eosinophilic cytoplasm.
  - "Foreign body"-type giant cells = multinucleated giant cells (MNGCs) with nuclei dispersed evenly throughout the entire giant cell.
  - Langhans-type MNGCs = MNGCs with peripherally located nuclei. They can be elicited as a reaction to foreign material, such as talc, suture, joint prosthesis material, etc. Both types of MNGCs can occur in any granulomatous reaction, whether foreign body, immune, or infectious (Fig. 18.13a, b).
  - Granulomatous inflammation with well-formed granulomas = can be "foreign body" giant cell granulomas or immune granulomas, within which falls:
    1. Necrotizing granulomas
       - Sometimes called "caseating" because of gross pathologic appearance of cheese-like consistency of a cavitary lesion.
       - Have central necrotic core encompassed by a peripheral rim of epithelioid histiocytes, MNGCs, sometimes with an outer perimeter of lymphohistiocytic infiltrate.
       - Neutrophils not prominent, apoptosis and karyorrhexis seen.
    2. Non-necrotizing granulomas

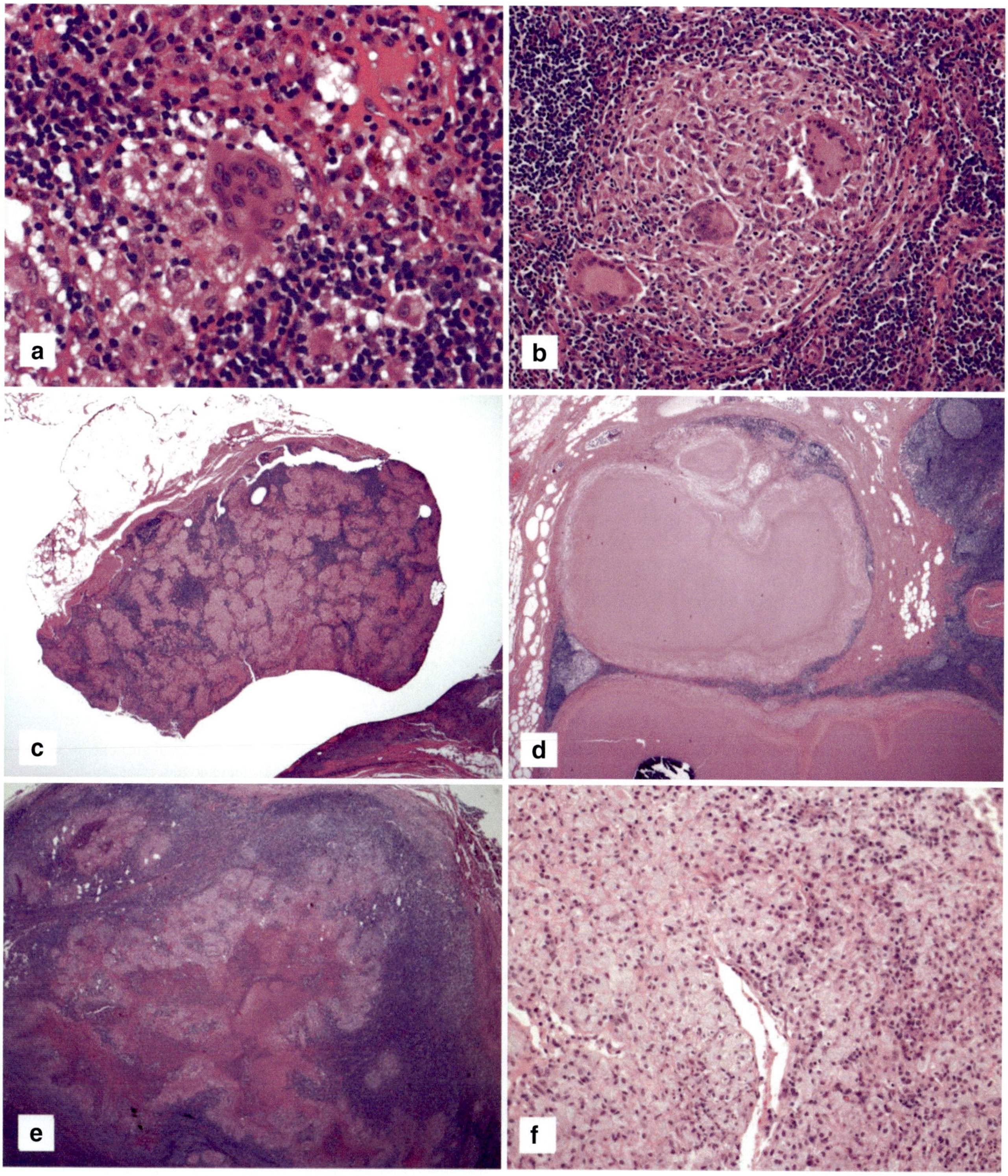

Fig. 18.13 Morphologic spectrum of granulomatous and histiocyte-rich lymphadenitides. "Foreign body"-type giant cells (**a**) are multinucleated giant cells (MNGCs) with evenly dispersed nuclei throughout the entire giant cell, whereas Langhans MNGCs (**b**) have peripherally located nuclei. Both types can occur in any granulomatous reaction, whether immune, infectious, or due to foreign body. Non-necrotizing granulomas can, as in this case of sarcoidosis (**c**), efface nodal architecture. Necrotizing granulomas (**d**) have a central necrotic core, encompassed by a peripheral rim of epithelioid histiocytes, MNGCs, and lymphocytes. Neutrophils are not prominent. In comparison, suppurative granulomas (**e**) are extensively necrotic, neutrophil-, and neutrophilic debris-rich. The low-power view demonstrates finger-like projections, giving it the name stellate microabscess/granuloma; this is a case of cat-scratch disease due to *Bartonella henselae* infection. Foamy macrophages and/or epithelioid histiocytic infiltrates (**f**) are typical of *Mycobacterium avium-intracellulare* complex (MAC) lymphadenitis, depicted here

  - "Naked" non-necrotizing granulomas = devoid of necrosis; have a diminished or absent lymphohistiocytic border.
3. Suppurative granulomas = necrotizing granulomas with exuberant neutrophilic (microabscess) core
   - Low-power morphology of granuloma can sometimes have stellate projections (thus, "stellate microabscess" or "stellate granuloma").
   - Centrally neutrophil-rich and necrotic.
   - Peripheral palisading of histiocytes.
- Figure 18.13 provides a panel of histologic pictures of the G/H-LAD granulomatous/histiocyte-rich patterns.

38. What is the differential diagnosis for G/H-LAD patterns?

- Table 18.14 summarizes infectious and non-infectious etiologies of LAD with prominent granulomatous and/or histiocyte-rich patterns and its neoplastic mimics.
- As with most reactive conditions, the morphologic findings are a spectrum and will depend on disease phase/stage. For example, though suppurative granulomas can be characteristically seen in cat-scratch LAD (i.e., *Bartonella* spp.), granulomas diminish and disappear in later stages of disease as infection resolves.

Table 18.14 Differential diagnosis of granulomatous and/or histiocyte-rich lymphadenopathy and its neoplastic mimics

Morphologic patterns	Infectious		Non-infectious	Neoplastic mimics
Well-formed granulomas (necrotizing and non-necrotizing)	BACTERIA/ MYCOBACTERIA *M. tuberculosis* NTM, including *M. leprae*, MAI *Chlamydia*/LGV *Bartonella henselae* (Cat-scratch disease) *Yersinia* spp. *Brucella* spp. *Francisella* spp.	Syphilis (*Treponema pallidum*) FUNGAL *Histoplasma capsulatum* *Cryptococcus neoformans/C. gattii* *Blastomyces dermatitidis* *Coccidioides immitis, C. posadasii* *Aspergillus* spp. PARASITIC *Leishmania* spp.	Sarcoidosis Crohn disease Granulomatosis with polyangiitis SLE KFD Kimura disease Drug-related immune reaction Foreign body granulomas (e.g., talc, suture, lipid) Lipogranulomatous from lymphangiogram	TCHRLBL DLBCL cHL ALCL MF involvement of LN AITL Lymphoepithelioid variant of PTCL (Lennert lymphoma) Indolent B-cell lymphomas secreting abnormal proteins that incite granulomatous reaction
Neutrophil-rich/ suppurative granulomas	Gram-positive bacteria (*Strep, Staph*) Gram-negative bacteria *Bartonella henselae*/ cat-scratch	NTM Fungal organisms *Yersinia* spp. *Brucella* spp. *Francisella* spp.	SLE KFD	cHL and NHL Infarcted malignant neoplasms (carcinomas, lymphomas, etc.)
Histiocyte-rich (foamy or epithelioid histiocytes)	NTM/MAI Toxoplasmosis	Whipple disease (*Tropheryma whipplei*) Leprosy	RDD/SHML HLH Dermatopathic LAD SLE KFD Joint prosthesis associated Foreign body granulomas (e.g., talc, suture, lipid) Lipogranulomatous from lymphangiogram	LCH/Langerhans cell sarcoma Erdheim-Chester disease ALCL Lymphoepithelioid variant of PTCL (Lennert lymphoma) Metastatic carcinoma Indolent B-cell lymphomas secreting abnormal proteins that incite granulomatous reaction

ALCL anaplastic large cell lymphoma, *AITL* angioimmunoblastic T-cell lymphoma, *cHL* classic Hodgkin lymphoma, *DLBCL* diffuse large B-cell lymphoma, *HLH* hemophagocytic lymphohistiocytosis/hemophagocytic syndrome, *KFD* Kikuchi Fujimoto disease, *LCH* Langerhans cell histiocytosis, *LN* lymph node, *MAI* Mycobacterium avium intracellulare, *MF* mycosis fungoides, *NHL* non-Hodgkin lymphoma, *NTM* non-tuberculous/atypical mycobacteria, *PTCL* peripheral T-cell lymphoma, *RDD/SHML* Rosai-Dorfman-Destombes disease/sinus histiocytosis with massive lymphadenopathy, *SLE* systemic lupus erythematosus, *TCHRLBL* T-cell/histiocyte rich large B-cell lymphoma

- Suppurative, necrotizing, and non-necrotizing granulomatous LAD will be described together, as these findings can be seen in any single entity (at the same time or at different stages of infection) – some are more commonly associated with suppurative (like lymphogranuloma venereum) or necrotizing (like MTB LAD) inflammation, while others are more commonly non-necrotizing (like sarcoidosis).
- Select entities in the DDx of G/H LAD will be discussed further.

39. What is the minimal histopathologic and ancillary work-up for G/H-LAD?

- Work-up is remarkably similar in granulomatous and histiocyte-rich LAD, despite myriad infectious and non-infectious etiologies:
  - Do AFB and GMS special stains, recognizing that these may not reveal organisms.
  - If leprosy is a possibility, add modified AFB Fite-Faraco stain.
  - One could consider more special stains, as needed, including PAS, mucicarmine, Fontana-Masson, Giemsa, Congo red, Warthin-Starry silver stain, Brown-Brenn gram stain, etc. Special stains will be mentioned in subsequent sections, as they pertain to certain entities.
- Microbiologic cultures are a must!

40. As a very typical entity that displays necrotizing and/or non-necrotizing granulomatous LAD, what are salient clinical features in *Mycobacterium tuberculosis* complex lymphadenitis (MTBC LAD) and atypical mycobacterial/non-tuberculous mycobacterial lymphadenitis (NTM LAD)?

- MTBC and NTM organisms may produce a granulomatous reaction, both necrotizing and non-necrotizing [1, 44–47].
- *Mycobacterium tuberculosis* complex (MTBC)
  - Substantial global health-care burden and communicable infectious disease
  - Most commonly presents as pulmonary disease
  - Extrapulmonary presentation (including TB lymphadenitis) more frequent in HIV-infected patients, particularly those with CD4+ cell count <200/μL
  - In developed countries, immigrants from regions where tuberculosis is endemic also more commonly affected
- Non-tuberculous mycobacterial infections (NTM)
  - Infections from so-called atypical mycobacteria.
  - Arise from opportunistic organisms, listed in Table 18.15.
  - These infect primarily immunocompromised individuals (such as HIV/AIDS patients and those with solid organ transplants).

41. What histologic and special stain features suggest that a necrotizing and/or non-necrotizing granulomatous LAD is due to MTBC or NTM?

- MTBC LAD presents most commonly with necrotizing granulomas but can also have non-necrotizing granulomas.
  - Acid-fast bacillus (AFB) stains, like Fite and Kinyoun, will typically contain only rare to few positive organisms in MTBC LAD.
  - Bacilli with "beaded" morphology (Fig. 18.14a, b)
- Presence of beaded AFB+ organisms is not specific for MTB complex organisms, as it can be seen in NTM, albeit with typically greater numbers of organisms in NTM (Fig. 18.14c, d).
- Reportedly, a hallmark of NTM LAD is simultaneous appearance of suppurative and non-necrotizing granulomatous inflammation. Regardless, definitive speciation must be deferred to further ancillary studies (below).

42. Are histologic and special stain findings alone sufficiently diagnostic for MTBC and NTM LAD?

- Finding of AFB+ organisms in a LN with necrotizing and/or non-necrotizing granulomas indicates mycobacterial LAD.
- However, *exact* speciation of mycobacterium (whether MTBC or NTM) must be established by further ancillary microbiologic/molecular testing.

43. What ancillary testing can help establish the diagnosis for MTBC and NTM LAD?

Minimal Work-Up:

- As previously mentioned, "beaded" acid-fast bacilli can be seen in both MTBC and NTM LAD; therefore, AFB culture is essential.
- AFB culture remains the gold standard for definitive diagnosis and should, in all suspect cases, be taken via sterile conditions on the LN tissue specimen at the time of initial grossing and/or frozen section, core needle biopsy procedure, and/or FNA.

Table 18.15 Summary table of mycobacteria [14]

	Organisms	Typical clinical setting	Histologic features							Special stain performance*			
			Well-formed granulomas (necrotizing; suppurative, etc.)	Epithelioid macrophages and giant cells	Foamy macrophages	Capsular thickening	Follicular changes	Fibrosis	Lepra cells	Ziehl-Neelsen or Kinyoun stain (AFB)	Fite-Faraco stain (Modified AFB)	PAS stain	Auramine-rhodamine (fluorescent stain)
Tuberculous LAD	*M. tuberculosis*	Pt in endemic region	+++	+++	–	++	+/–	+	–	+	+	–	+
Lepromatous leprosy	*M. leprae*	Hansen's disease (multibacillary)	–	–	+++	+++	++	+	++/+++	–	+	–	+
Tuberculoid leprosy	*M. leprae*	Hansen's disease (paucibacillary)	+++	+++	–	++	+/–	+	–	–	+	–	+
MAI LAD	*M. avium-intracellulare*	HIV/immunocompromised	–	–	+++	–	–	–	–	+	+	+	+
NTM	*M. abscessus* *M. bohemicum* *M. celatum* *M. chelonae* *M. fortuitum* *M. genavense* *M. gordonae* *M. kansasii* *M. interjectum* *M. malmoense* *M. scrofulaceum* *M. tusciae*	Depends on specific NTM *Usually opportunistic in immunocompromised pt. *Pulmonary involvement common	+/–	+/–	+/–	+/–	+/–	+/–	–	+/–	+	–/+	+/–

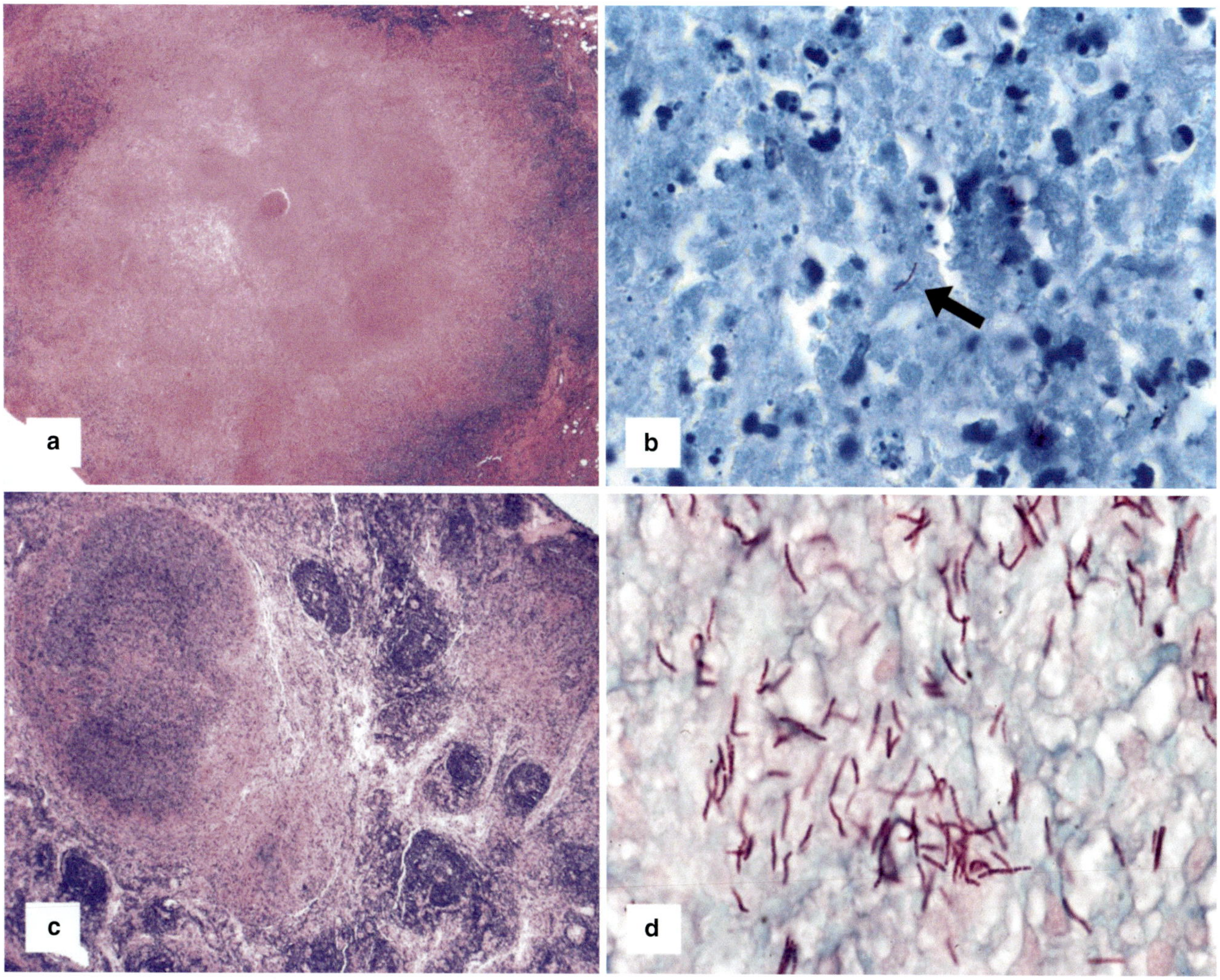

Fig. 18.14 MTB (*Mycobacterium tuberculosis*) and NTM (non-tuberculous mycobacteria, also known as atypical mycobacteria). Typical necrotizing granulomatous inflammation extensively involving LN (**a**) with only very rare acid-fast "beaded" bacillus (highlighted by arrow) on a careful review of the AFB stain (**b**). Necrotizing granulomatous lymphadenitis, this time due to an opportunistic infection of *Mycobacterium kansasii* (**c**), an NTM. In contrast to MTB, this NTM shows frequent AFB+ organisms upon AFB staining (**d**)

- Cultures allow for antimicrobial susceptibility testing to identify resistant strains and guide therapy.
- PCR amplification for MTBC in LN aspirate, fresh tissue, or even FFPE tissue is available and can be informative, even in paucibacillary cases [48, 49].
- Similarly, for NTM, broad-range mycobacterial PCR and sequence analysis are available in some reference laboratories.

Ancillary Work-Up:

- It is helpful to see if there has been an evaluation for active pulmonary tuberculosis, which is performed on 3 sputum specimens by AFB smear and culture and MTB PCR on the first 1–2 specimens; positive results of these additional tests may well correlate with the histologic suspicion of MTB LAD.
- A special note on PPD placement or interferon-gamma release assays:
  - Tests are intended to provide evidence for *latent*, not active, TB.
  - Despite this fact, these are frequently ordered to obtain additional clinical context especially when DDx is broad or when extrapulmonary TB is a possibility.

44. If necrotizing and/or non-necrotizing granulomas are not secondary to MTB or NTM, then what other histologic and special stain features could suggest another *infectious* entity (i.e., what else is in the DDx of *infectious* etiologies)?

- Fungal organisms can induce these granulomas (select examples below).
- Fungal agents discussed here typically affect immunocompromised individuals [53].

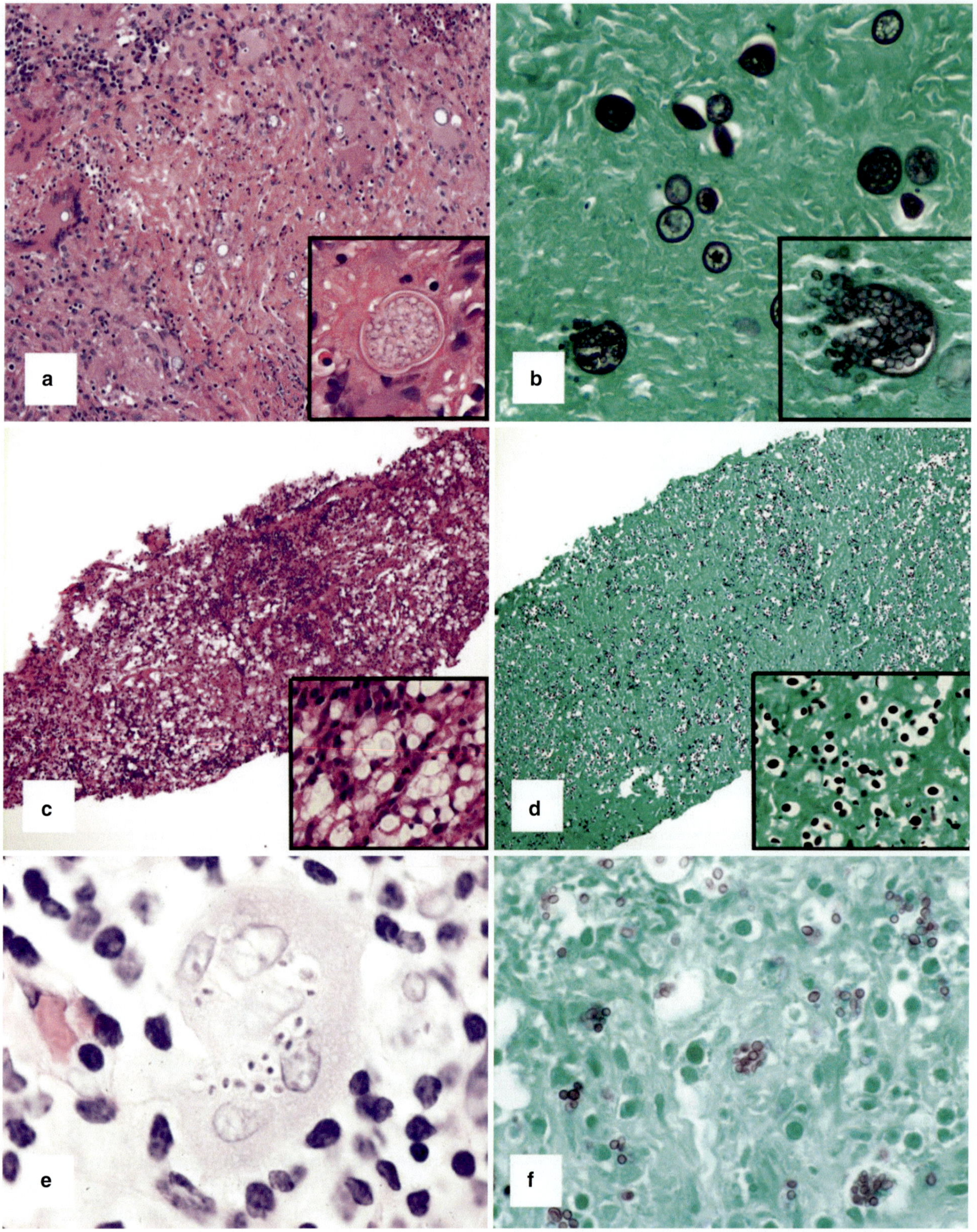

Fig. 18.15 Fungal infections inducing non-necrotizing and/or necrotizing granulomatous LAD. Coccidioides LAD provokes a necrotizing and non-necrotizing granulomatous inflammation with dense fibrosis and sclerosis with numerous characteristic coccidioidal organisms easily recognized on H&E stains (**a**), which are large spherules jam-packed with abundant endospores [inset for (**a**)]. The organisms stain with GMS (**b**) and inset for (**b**). *Cryptococcus* LAD (**c**) incites extensive involvement of the LN with extracellular and intracellular organisms seen as clear spaces on low power; organisms are small and round with refractile capsules [inset for (**c**)]. GMS highlights organisms (**d**) underscoring the characteristic narrow-based budding in cryptococcosis [inset for (**d**)]. Histoplasma infection stimulates epithelioid histiocyte-rich, non-necrotizing granulomatous inflammation, which may become necrotic. On H&E sections, small, intracytoplasmic, round to oval organisms are seen (**e**), whose narrow-based budding are further decorated by GMS stains (**f**)

Table 18.16 Ancillary serologic tests to aid in diagnosis of fungal lymphadenitis

Fungal organism	Ancillary test	Specimen	Test utility	Limitations
Aspergillus species	*Aspergillus* Galactomannan EIA	Serum	Aids in diagnosis of invasive aspergillosis; sensitivity ~70%	Cross-reactivity issues with other molds, various antibiotics, and other substances
Blastomyces dermatitidis	*Blastomyces* antigen EIA	Urine	76–93% sensitive in active disease	Cross-reactivity with blastomycosis, paracoccidioidomycosis, and penicilliosis
	Serology (EIA, CF, or ID)	Serum	Not recommended	Not recommended
Coccidioides immitis/posadasii	Serology (EIA, CF, or ID)	Serum	Aids in diagnosis of active disease and in following response to therapy	May be negative in early infection, limited pulmonary disease, and immunocompromised patients
Cryptococcus neoformans/gattii	Cryptococcal antigen (LA, LFA, EIA)	Serum CSF	Sensitive and rapid test for active disease	Low titer positives by LFA are of uncertain clinical significance
Histoplasma capsulatum/ duboisii	*Histoplasma* antigen EIA	Urine	~80–90% sensitive in acute pulmonary and progressive disseminated infection Not sensitive in chronic pulmonary infection	Cross-reactivity with blastomycosis, paracoccidioidomycosis, and penicilliosis
	Serology (EIA, CF, or ID)	Serum	Sensitive for or chronic and subacute infections, including mediastinal lymphadenitis	Serologic response requires 4–6 weeks

Abbreviations: *CF* complement fixation, *EIA* enzyme immunoassay, *ID* immunodiffusion, *LA* latex agglutination, *LFA* lateral flow assay

- Coccidioides (Fig. 18.15a, b)
  - H&E:
    - Characteristic large spherules (10–100 μm size) teeming with numerous endospores (2–5 μm size).
    - Organisms variably embedded in dense fibrosis or within MNGCs.
    - Capsule is thin, in contrast to thicker capsules of *Blastomyces*.
  - GMS and PAS stains further emphasize organisms.
- *Cryptococcus* (Fig. 18.15c–e)
  - H&E:
    - Nodal infiltration by numerous intra- and extracellular organisms.
    - Non-necrotizing granulomas may also be evident.
    - Round 2–5 μm organisms with refractile capsules.
  - Mucicarmine and PAS stains: organismal capsules stain pink/red.
  - GMS and Fontana-Masson stains: narrow-based budding organisms stain black.
  - India ink stain (performed on CSF): highlight organismal spheres.
- Histoplasma (Fig. 18.15f, g)
  - H&E:
    - Inflammation can be epithelioid histiocyte-rich, non-necrotizing granulomatous, necrotizing granulomatous, or a combination of the above.
    - Round to oval, small, 2–4 μm, organisms.
  - GMS and PAS stains: narrow-based budding organisms

45. What ancillary testing can help establish the specific infectious organism in fungal LAD?

Minimal Ancillary Work-Up:

- While *Cryptococcus* and dimorphic fungal organisms may demonstrate their classic features on histopathologic examination, fungal culture is critical for definitive identification of most fungi.
- Routine bacterial cultures may still isolate fungi, but by themselves they are inappropriate for ruling out fungal disease.

Additional Ancillary Work-Up:

- If cultures were not performed or are uninformative, directed PCR is most commonly available for *Aspergillus* spp. and the *Zygomycetes* from fresh or FFPE tissue.
- Broad-range fungal PCR and sequencing of the ribosomal RNA gene loci (i.e., D1/D2 or ITS regions) could also be requested to determine identification of fungal hyphae visualized in tissue.
- Special note on PCR-based testing: From FFPE, yield of PCR-based tests varies according to the fungal burden present and quality of fungal DNA in the tissue block. It is generally not recommended to perform such testing on FFPE if fungal elements are not visualized by microscopy due to lowered yield, inability to correlate results with morphology, and potential for contamination during the non-sterile processing involved in FFPE tissues.

- Serologic testing can also provide much needed diagnostic evidence for a fungal etiology (Table 18.16).

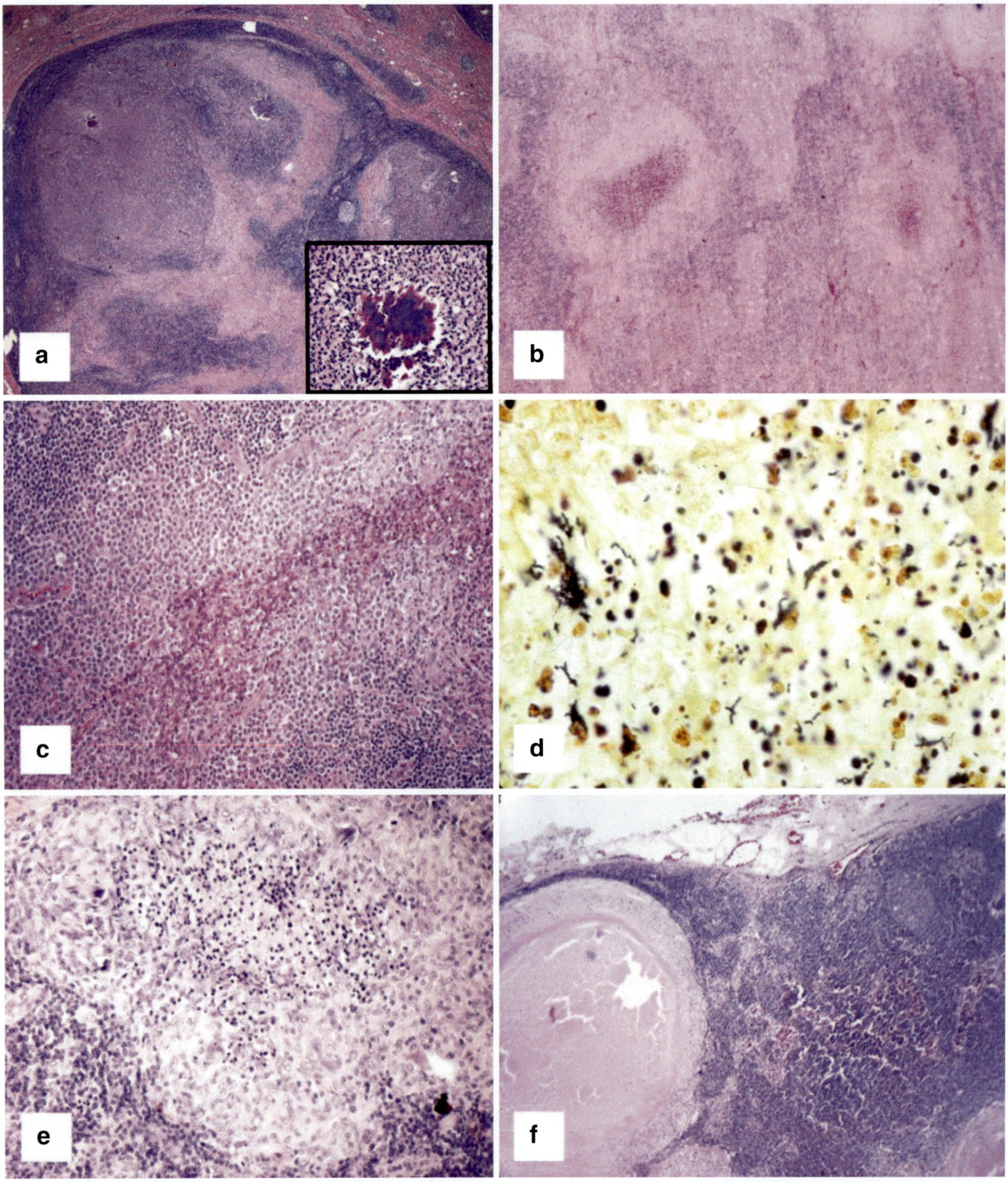

Fig. 18.16 Suppurative LAD due to infection by *Actinomyces* (**a**), *Bartonella henselae* (**b–d**), *Chlamydia trachomatis* (**e**), and *Brucella* (**f**). Exuberant neutrophil-rich abscesses and suppurative granulomas are seen in this actinomycotic infection (**a**); the dense fibrous bands indicate long-standing infection. The distinctive organisms are bacterial colonies with radiating filaments surrounded by numerous neutrophils [inset for (**a**)], corresponding to so-called sulfur granules (yellow to yellow-brown nodules with a foul odor on gross examination). Cat-scratch disease secondary to *Bartonella henselae* infection activates a suppurative granulomatous reaction, with neutrophil- and neutrophil debris-rich pink central core, surrounded by pale palisading epithelioid histiocytes (**b**) and (**c**). Stellate microabscesses and monocytoid B-cell hyperplasia could also be observed (not shown here). Warthin-Starry stain could highlight pleomorphic organisms (**d**), though these are challenging to interpret given the high background/nonspecific staining with this method. IHC, PCR, and/or serologies for *Bartonella* can be pursued instead. (**e**) Another example of granulomatous inflammation and central necrosis is lymphogranuloma venereum due to *Chlamydia trachomatis*. (**f**) Brucellosis manifests as necrotizing granulomatous LAD partially effacing nodal architecture, which is morphologically indistinguishable from MTB LAD

46. What infectious organisms induce suppurative LAD?

- Suppurative lymphadenitides are caused by many different microorganisms, mainly bacteria.
- Clinical presentation varies depending on organism.
  - LGV (lymphogranuloma venereum) caused by *C. trachomatis* (serovars L1, L2, L3) classically presents with a concomitant genital ulcer or papule.
  - Cat-scratch disease (CSD; *Bartonella* spp.).
  - Bacteria, *Staph* and *Strep*.
  - *Yersinia*, *Brucella*, *Francisella*.
  - Selected bacterial organisms that cause lymphadenopathy are illustrated in Fig. 18.16.
  - Summary table of clinical, histologic, stain characteristics, and diagnostic properties is presented in Table 18.17.

47. What are typical histologic and immunophenotypic findings in suppurative LAD?

- Neutrophilic microabscesses dominate in active disease.
- Necrosis may be extensive.
- Later phase of infection: "stellate microabscesses" = necrotic and neutrophil-rich central core surrounded by palisading epithelioid macrophages.
- Preceding overt suppurative reaction (particularly in CSD and LGV), follicular hyperplasia, prominence of tingible body macrophages, and monocytoid B-cell hyperplasia seen.

48. What ancillary testing can help establish the specific infectious organisms that induce suppurative LAD (includes *Bartonella* spp., *Staphylococcus, Streptococcus, Lymphogranuloma venereum, Francisella, Brucella, Yersinia*)?

- Cat-scratch disease (also for bacillary angiomatosis) – *Bartonella* spp [51, 52].
- *Minimal Ancillary Work-Up:*
  - Culture for *Bartonella* spp. = not widely available and insensitive.
  - Diagnosis rests on serology and PCR. Laboratory evaluation should include serologic testing or PCR amplification from fresh (preferred) or FFPE tissue.
  - Serologic testing commonly used to confirm diagnosis when clinical impression is strong.
    - Single high titers typically associated with acute infection.
    - Most (~90%) cases of cat-scratch disease will have detectable antibodies.
  - Reference serologic method is indirect immunofluorescence (IFA). One study demonstrated that IgG titers >1:50 corresponded to *Bartonella* infection, whereas titers >1:800 indicated endocarditis.
  - Important Notes:
    - Serologic response is not reliably detected in immunocompromised patients.
    - Cross-reactivity is reported between *Bartonella* species (*B. henselae* and *B. quintana*).
- *Additional Ancillary Work-Up*:
  - PCR amplification of affected tissues (fresh or FFPE) is commercially available and is particularly useful when serologic testing is negative.
- Suppurative bacterial infection from *Staphylococcus*, *Streptococcus*
- *Minimal Ancillary Work-Up*:
  - Routine bacterial cultures for isolation of staphylocci, streptococci, and less common causes of bacterial LAD.
  - Allows for *both* identification of pathogen and performance of antimicrobial susceptibility testing for guiding therapy.
- *Additional Ancillary Work-Up*:
  - Only if cultures are not performed or show no growth in the face of typical histopathology should molecular testing be considered.
  - *16 s rRNA* gene PCR and sequence analysis can be performed on fresh or FFPE tissue to identify bacteria present in tissue.
  - Results in these cases should be carefully correlated with histopathology and Gram stain findings.
- Lymphogranuloma venereum (LGV) caused by Chlamydia trachomatis [20]
- *Minimal Ancillary Work-Up:*
  - Testing genital ulcer/lesion, tissue, or aspirate from involved LN for *C. trachomatis* by culture, nucleic acid amplification, or direct immunofluorescence → offers strongest direct evidence.
  - For general diagnosis of chlamydial genitourinary infection, nucleic acid amplification testing of female urine, vaginal swab, or endocervical swab, or male urine or urethral swab is recommended.
  - Rectal swabs should also be submitted in appropriate high-risk populations such as men who have sex with men.
- *Additional Ancillary Work-Up*:
  - Serologic testing for L1, L2, or L3 serovars is available at reference laboratories, however:
    - Assays are not standardized.
    - Cross-reactivity between serotypes and chlamydial species complicates interpretation.
  - PCR specifically for LGV serotypes is also available for testing of genitourinary sources, but not necessarily required for clinical management.
- *Brucella*, *Francisella*, *Yersinia* spp [50].
- *Minimal Ancillary Work-Up*:

Table 18.17 Important clinical, histologic, special stain, ancillary study, and diagnostic properties to aid in definitive diagnosis of selected microorganisms

Bacterial, fungal, and mycobacterial organisms (alphabetical order)	Classic clinical presentation and nodal involvement	Predominant morphologic pattern on H&E	Organism morphology on positive stains	Organism size	Gram stain (Brown-Hopps)	GMS	Warthin-Starry	PAS	AFB (Fite, Kinyoun, or Ziehl-Neelsen	IHC and/or ISH stain available?	Useful ancillary study and/or laboratory data	Diagnostic ancillary study	Additional/cautionary notes
Aspergillus	Lung infection (most common) Can be disseminated in immunosuppressed patients	Frequent angioinvasion Exuberant suppurative granulomas	Septated hyphae with dichotomous 45° branching	3–6-μm-wide hyphae	–	+	–	+	–	Yes, but not widely available	*Aspergillus* serum Galactomannan EIA (some cross-reactivity issues)	*Aspergillus* serum Galactomannan EIA	Septation may allow differentiation from *Zygomycetes*
Bartonella henselae	Cat exposure Skin lesions Affected LNs: axillary, cervical, epitrochlear	Necrotizing granulomas Suppurative granulomas with central stellate microabscess	Small, pleomorphic, curved bacilli Clumps or single "L-shaped" forms In vessel walls or necrotic foci	0.3–1.7 μm	+/– [gram-negative]	–	+/–	–	–	Yes, but not widely available	*Bartonella henselae* PCR of affected tissues (fresh or FFPE) High titers serology associated with acute infection	B. henselae **PCR of affected tissues (fresh or FFPE)** **High titers serology associated with acute infection**	Serologic testing may have cross-reactivity between *Bartonella* species
Blastomyces – yeast	Endemic in the US Great Lakes region Lung and skin infections (most common) LAD in systemic dz	Necrotizing granulomas Suppurative granulomas with central stellate microabscess	"Broad-based" budding yeast form	8–20 μm	–	+	–	+	+/–	Yes, but not widely available	Urine *Blastomyces* antigen EIA (76–93% sensitive in active disease) Congo red+	Urine *Blastomyces* antigen EIA (76–93% sensitive in active disease)	Cross-reactivity issues with paracoccidioides, penicilliosis Serum serologic testing is NOT recommended
Brucella ***SELECT*** agent – inform lab if clinically suspected	Acute febrile systemic illness Workers exposed to contaminated milk or animals	Necrotizing granulomas Can be non-necrotizing	Infamously difficult to ID on routine preparations	0.6–1.5 μm	+ (difficult to visualize)	–	–	–	–	Yes, but not widely available	Paired serology for IgG and IgM shows four-fold rise in titers from acute to convalescent stage	**Blood cultures from febrile patients informative**	Direct specimen PCR available at some public health labs and CDC (second line diagnostic test)
Chlamydia/LGV	Sexually transmitted disease	Necrotizing granulomas Suppurative granulomas with central stellate microabscess	Organisms form a clump or a peripheral rim in intrahistiocytic vacuoles	<2 μm	+/– Gram-negative	–	+/–	–	–	Yes, but not widely available	Serology Nucleic acid detection	Intracytoplasmic inclusion bodies best seen on **Giemsa+**	
Coccidioides (*C. immitis*, *C. posadasii*) – dimorphic fungus	Endemic in Western USA, California, Mexico Lung infection (most common) LAD when disseminated	Necrotizing and non-necrotizing granulomas	Mature thin-walled spherules containing numerous endospores	Spherules 10–100 μm Endospores 2–4 μm	–	+	–	–	–	No	Serology (EIA, CF, ID)		May be negative in early infection, limited pulmonary disease, and immunocompromised patients

Cryptococcus (*C. neoformans*, *C. gattii*) – yeast	HIV/AIDS/ immune-compromised patient Pulmonary involvement May involve CNS May be disseminated LNs: cervical, axillary, hilar, inguinal, others	Necrotizing and non-necrotizing granulomas	Prominently encapsulated yeast, within clear spaces in granulomas and macrophages Round yeast forms If budding, narrow-based	4–10 μm	–	+	–	+	–	Yes, but not widely available	Mucicarmine + Fontana-Masson + India Ink + Cryptococcal antigen (LA, LFA, EIA) in serum or CSF Culture Serology	**Cryptococcal antigen (LA, LFA, EIA) in serum or CSF – sensitive and rapid**	
Francisella and *Yersinia* ***SELECT*** agents	Tularemia caused by *Francisella tularensis* Plague from *Yersinia pestis*	Necrotizing and non-necrotizing granulomas Suppurative granulomas	coccobacillus positive on **methylene blue stain** **Yersinia: "bipolar safety pin"**	*Francisella*: 0.2–0.7 μm *Yersinia*: 0.5–2.0 μm	+ gram [Gram-negative]	–	–	–	–	Yes, but not widely available	Paired serology for IgG and IgM shows four-fold rise in titers from acute to convalescent stage		PCR not widely available Inform lab if clinically suspected
Histoplasma capsulatum – dimorphic fungus (both yeast and mold forms)	Immunocompetent: asymptomatic Immunocompromised: pulmonary infection or disseminated LNs: hilar; other nodes involved in disseminated	Necrotizing and non-necrotizing granulomas AND/OR Histiocyte-rich (without well-formed granuloma) response	Intracellular yeast form Narrow based budding Thin cell wall	2–5 μm	–	+	–	+	–/+	No	**Giemsa +**	**Urine Histoplasma antigen EIA** Serologic testing – read details in Table 14	Differentiate from *Leishmania* spp. by: slightly larger size, absence of kinetoplast, ability to stain with GMS
Leishmania spp.	Typically disseminated; fever, hepatosplenomegaly, pancytopenia, LAD	Suppurative granulomas OR Necrotizing and non-necrotizing granulomas (can be stellate)	Numerous intrahistiocytic amastigotes. Organism has 2 basophilic dots (1 kinetoplast; 1 nucleus)	Amastigotes are 2–4 μm	–	–	–	–	–	Yes, but not widely available	**Giemsa +**		Differentiate from *Histoplasma* spp. by: slightly smaller size, kinetoplast+, GMS-
Mycobacterium avium complex	HIV or immunocompromised patient	Foamy histiocytes packed with numerous bacilli	Numerous AFB+ bacilli	<2 μm	+	+	–	+	+	Yes, but not widely available	Microbiologic cultures	NTM PCR of FFPE	
Mycobacterium tuberculosis	Exposure to TB LNs: cervical, axillary, mediastinal	Necrotizing granulomas	Beaded (?) acid-fast bacilli	2–4 μm	–	–	–	–	+	Yes, but not widely available	Microbiologic cultures (long TAT) IFN-gamma release assay serum test Tuberculin skin test	MTB complex PCR of FFPE	

(continued)

Table 18.17 (continued)

Bacterial, fungal, and mycobacterial organisms (alphabetical order)	Classic clinical presentation and nodal involvement	Predominant morphologic pattern on H&E	Organism morphology on positive stains	Organism size	Gram stain (Brown-Hopps)	GMS	Warthin-Starry	PAS	AFB (Fite, Kinyoun, or Ziehl-Neelsen	IHC and/or ISH stain available?	Useful ancillary study and/or laboratory data	Diagnostic ancillary study	Additional/cautionary notes
Non-tuberculous mycobacteria	Opportunistic infections	Variable from necrotizing, non-necrotizing granulomas to foamy histiocytes	Acid-fast bacilli	Varies	–	–	–	–	+	Yes, but not widely available			
Paracoccidioides brasiliensis – dimorphic fungus	Endemic in South and Central America Lung infection (most common) LN/spleen in disseminated dz	Necrotizing and non-necrotizing granulomas	"Mariner's wheel"	Yeast form (10–30 μm) with daughter yeasts budding around larger form	–	+	–	+	–	Yes, but not widely available			Prognosis poor in patients with disseminated dz
Pneumocystis jirovecii (formerly *P. carinii*)	Immunosuppressed individuals (esp. HIV/AIDS) Lung infection (most common) LN/spleen in disseminated dz	Necrotizing granulomas and macrophage aggregates	Nodules of foamy/frothy material Trophozoites and cysts ("crushed ping-pong balls" or "helmets" or "ball in cup"	Trophozoites 2–4 μm Cysts 5–8 μm	–	+	–	–	–	Yes, but not widely available	Giemsa + Papanicolaou +		

- Perform bacterial cultures on affected tissues/body fluids during acute disease.
- Blood cultures may be informative in febrile patients, particularly in brucellosis and plague.
- *Brucella*, *Francisella*, and *Yersinia* spp. are "select agents," so it is important to inform the microbiology laboratory when clinically suspected, to prevent laboratory-acquired infections.

- *Additional Ancillary Work-Up*:
  - Direct specimen PCR for *Brucella* is available at some public health laboratories and the CDC as a second-line diagnostic test.
  - PCR for *Francisella* and *Yersinia* spp. is not widely available.
  - IgG and IgM antibodies to all three agents could be considered to aid in diagnosis.
    - Diagnosis based on a thorough serologic evaluation would be largely retrospective.
    - Ideally, paired sera drawn to analyze for a fourfold rise in titer from the acute to convalescent stage:
      - 2–4 weeks apart for brucellosis (*Brucella*)
      - At least 4 weeks apart for tularemia (*Francisella*)
      - 4–6 weeks apart for plague (*Yersinia*)
    - A single-point serologic titer that is highly elevated is suggestive of a diagnosis in the appropriate clinical setting.
    - Serologic testing is limited by the known cross-reactivity between *Brucella*, *Francisella*, and *Yersinia* spp. antibodies.

49. After an exhaustive infectious disease work-up for etiologies of non-necrotizing (and even necrotizing and suppurative) granulomatous LAD, what else is in the DDx?

- Note: Despite failure to demonstrate organisms by special stains, an infectious organism continues to be the most likely culprit of granulomatous LAD; microbiologic culture and serologies would be necessary to complete exclude this. After an exhaustive work-up, the cause may be idiopathic.
- Entities in the differential diagnosis:
  - Sarcoidosis (further discussion, Question 50 below).
  - Granulomatosis with polyangiitis.
  - Crohn disease.
  - Joint prosthesis associated.
  - Foreign body granulomas (e.g., talc, suture).
  - Lipogranulomas from lymphangiograms.
  - Note of caution:
  - Non-necrotizing granulomas can appear in the setting of malignancies, even though LN may or may not show neoplastic involvement!
  - Non-necrotizing granulomas in the setting of metastatic carcinoma or other non-hematolymphoid malignancies.
  - Indolent B-cell lymphomas (e.g., lymphoplasmacytic lymphoma, marginal zone lymphoma, follicular lymphoma, etc.)
    - Could induce a giant cell reaction against abnormal proteins secreted by neoplastic B-cells.
    - If morphology suggestive, confirm amyloid-induced granulomatous reaction with Congo red stain.
  - T-cell lymphoma, such as lymphoepithelioid variant of peripheral T-cell lymphoma (Lennert lymphoma).

50. What clinical and epidemiologic features are present in sarcoid LAD?

- Sarcoidosis leads to systemic granulomatous inflammation and frequently involves LNs and multiple organ systems.
- Etiology remains unknown and is thought to arise from immune dysregulation or autoimmunity.
- Presentation depends on organ systems involved:
  - Most common: Pulmonary involvement, ocular, cutaneous
  - Hilar LNs most frequently affected
- Diagnosis rests on constellation of histopathologic examination, radiographic findings, clinical presentation, and laboratory evaluation.
- Treatment involves steroids or supportive care.

51. What are typical histologic and special stain findings in sarcoid LAD?

- Partial to complete effacement of nodal architecture by non-necrotizing granulomas that are often coalescent.
- Lymphoid follicles, when present, are usually compressed to periphery of LN.
- Langhans-type multinucleated giant cells frequent.
- Schaumann bodies and/or asteroid bodies present.
- Necrosis typically absent.
- Fibrosis may be present.
- Lymphocytes are mainly T-cells with increased CD4-to-CD8 ratio; B-cells and plasma cells are polytypic.
- Reed-Sternberg cells or other atypical cells absent.
- AFB, GMS, and any other special stains negative for microorganisms (Fig. 18.17).

52. What ancillary testing can help establish the diagnosis of sarcoid LAD?

- Serum polyclonal hypergammaglobulinemia.
- Urine hypercalciuria.
- Elevated ACE (angiotensin-converting enzyme) levels.
- Staining or cultures negative for mycobacteria or fungi.

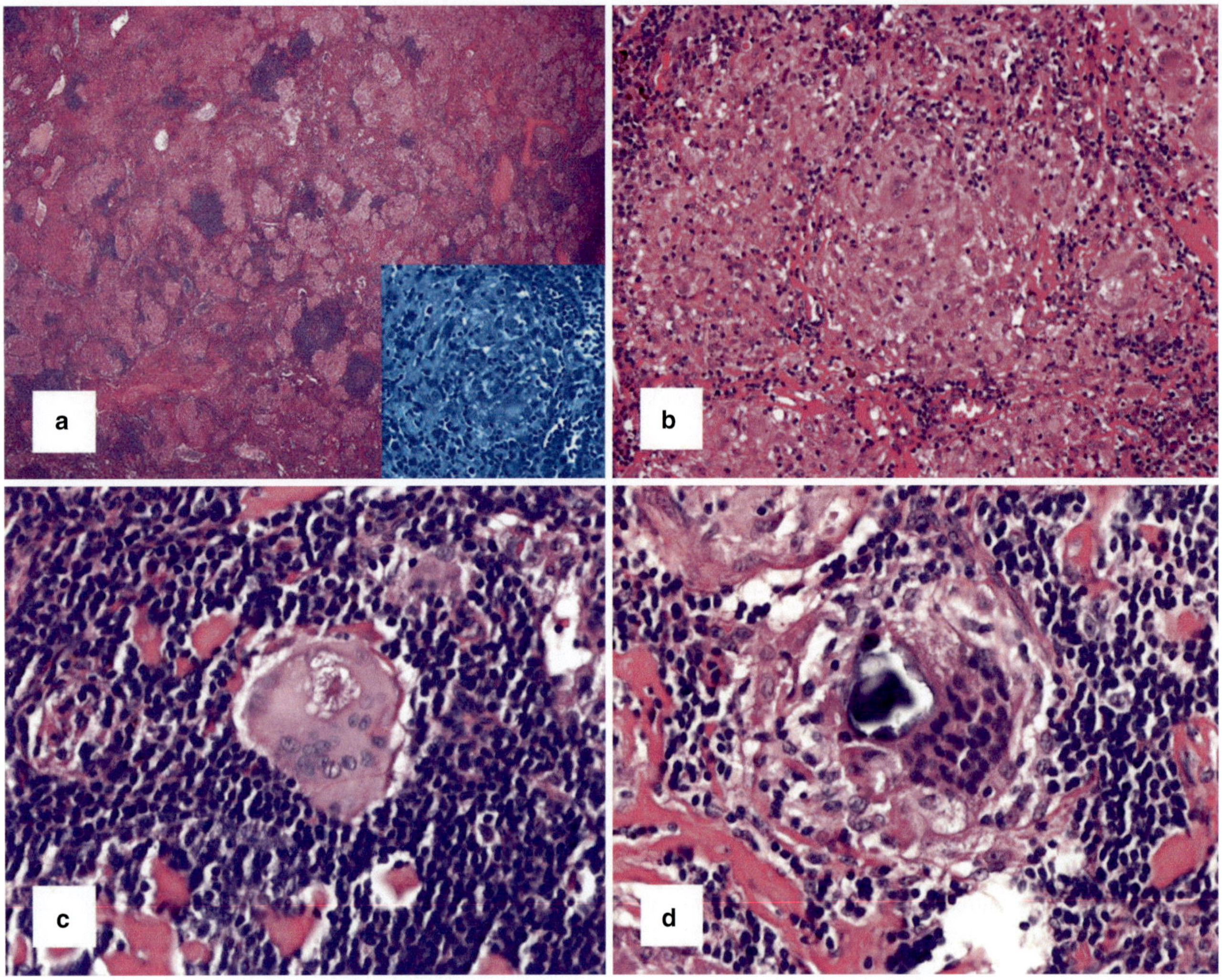

Fig. 18.17 Sarcoidosis. (**a**) Low magnification of near complete nodal effacement by non-necrotizing granulomas. AFB stain (inset for (**a**)] and GMS (not shown) stains are characteristically negative for microorganisms. (**b**) Non-necrotizing granulomas on high magnification display epithelioid macrophages and scattered multinucleated giant cells (combination of "foreign body-type" and "Langhans-type" giant cells). (**c**) Asteroid body. This MNGC contains a delicate, eosinophilic, stellate body = an asteroid body. (**d**) Schaumann body. This MNGC contains a calcific concretion and at times can show concentric lamellations = a Schaumann body. Asteroid and Schaumann bodies are not entirely specific, but are typically reported in the literature in cases of sarcoidosis

53. Aside from sarcoidosis, what other non-infectious reactive agents can lead to non-necrotizing granulomatous LAD? What clinical and morphologic features allow for their recognition?

- Etiology: foreign body-type agents from joint prosthesis, lymphangiogram, and exposure to other foreign materials (talc, sutures, etc.).
- Useful clinical history:
  - Orthopedic prosthesis, cosmetic implantation, contrast medium injection, tattoos, etc.
  - Presents with regional lymphadenopathy.
- Histologic findings (Fig. 18.18):
  - Sinuses and/or paracortex expanded by macrophages with abundant eosinophilic cytoplasm.
  - Aggregates of xanthomatous macrophages and multinucleated giant cells often present.
  - Foreign materials sometimes identified within macrophages or giant cells:
    - Debris and cementing material (e.g., polyethylene, metal) that may have sloughed off a joint prosthesis may appear under polarizing light as birefringent matter.
  - Reed-Sternberg cells or diffuse large cell proliferation is absent.

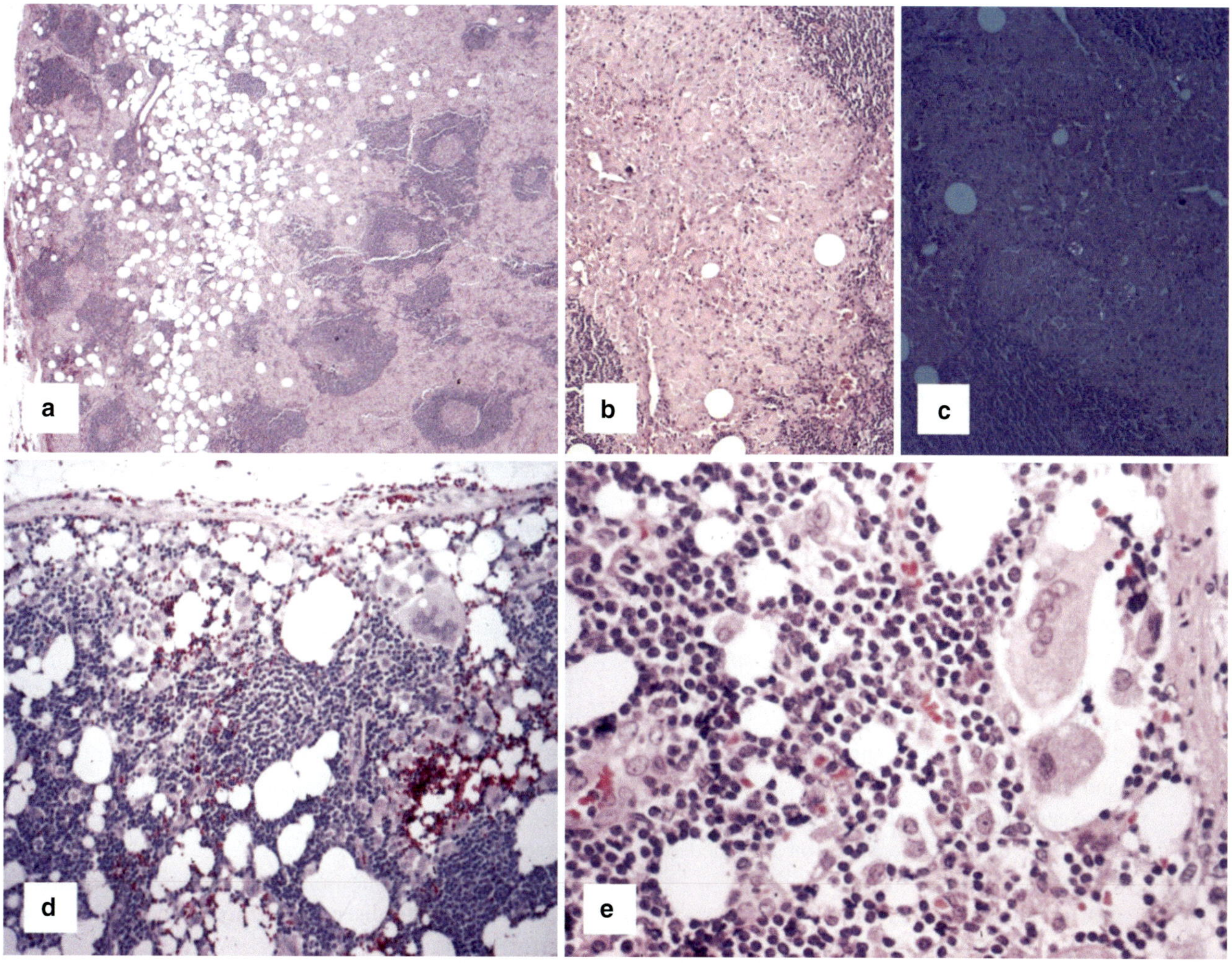

Fig. 18.18 Granulomatous and/or histiocyte-rich LAD due to joint prosthesis (**a**–**c**) and lymphangiogram (**d**, **e**). The nodal paracortex is extensively replaced by a florid histiocytic proliferation (**a**) in this enlarged pelvic LN from a patient who had undergone total hip arthroplasty. The histiocytes display bland nuclei and abundant eosinophilic cytoplasm (**b**), some of which may contain ill-defined, translucent to dark granular material. Examination under polarizing light can uncover scattered shards of birefringent material (**c**). Lymphangiogram effect noted in (**d**) and (**e**) exemplifies lipid-associated LAD, wherein nodal sinuses are distended by lipid, from endogenous (e.g., hyperlipidemia) or exogenous sources (e.g., oil-based radiopaque material used in lymphangiograms, total parenteral nutrition). Numerous fat droplets are seen, as are scattered Langhans-type multinucleated giant cells (**e**)

54. As a very typical entity that can display prominent foamy macrophage and/or epithelioid histiocyte-rich inflammatory LAD, what are the salient clinical and morphologic features in *Mycobacterium avium-intracellulare* complex (MAC) and *M. leprae* (Hansen's disease)?

- MAC infection [14]
  - Disseminated infection affects immunocompromised individuals (e.g., HIV/AIDS).
  - Histology:
    - Histiocyte-rich proliferation effacing LN architecture.
    - Foamy histiocytes with well-defined cellular borders.
    - Small, oval, bland nuclei with abundant cytoplasm.
    - AFB stain uncovers numerous acid-fast bacilli in virtually all macrophages.
    - **PAS stain positive with numerous bacilli (in contrast to PAS negativity in MTB and *M. leprae*).**
- Hansen's disease (leprosy) [54]
  - Due to *Mycobacterium leprae* infection.
  - Mode of transmission unclear; individuals in endemic areas at risk.
  - Chronic infection affects nerves, skin, eyes, and nasal mucosa.
  - Affected skin may have color changes (e.g., lighter, darker, red).
  - Left untreated, nerve damage and paralysis result.
    - Advanced cases can include lymphadenopathy; "saddle nose" deformity; non-healing ulcers; apparent loss of eyebrows, fingers, and toes; and blindness.

- Histology
  - Lepromatous leprosy is multibacillary = contains loads of mycobacteria.
    - Histiocyte-rich proliferation effacing LN architecture.
    - Depleted to replaced follicles.
    - Capsular thickening.
    - Nearly identical cytomorphology to MAC infection (above).
    - Foamy histiocytes termed "lepra" cells.
    - AFB stain must be modified Fite-Faraco rather than Ziehl-Neelsen.
      - Numerous acid-fast bacilli seen in modified Fite-Faraco.
      - Possibly bacilli are not well-highlighted in Ziehl-Neelsen because of more aggressive decolorization during processing.
    - **PAS stain negative.**
  - Tuberculoid leprosy is paucibacillary = only sparse numbers of mycobacteria.
    - As the name suggests, it bears greater resemblance to MTB granulomatous disease (or silicone-related LAD) than MAC infection.
    - Discrete to confluent epithelioid macrophages and giant cells.
    - Also can result in non-necrotizing granulomatous.
    - Only rare organisms positive on modified AFB Fite-Faraco stain.
    - See morphology in Fig. 18.19 and summary table of mycobacteria in Table 18.15.

55. What ancillary testing can help establish the diagnosis for MAC/NTM, or Hansen's disease?

- MAC/NTM
- *Minimal Ancillary Work-Up*:
  - AFB culture remains the gold standard to provide definitive pathogen identification and antimicrobial susceptibility profiling.
  - A portion of fresh LN tissue or aspirate should be reserved for AFB smear and culture if mycobacterial lymphadenitis is suspected.
- *Additional Ancillary Work-Up*:
  - If cultures were not performed, or while results are pending, PCR-based testing of LN aspirate or biopsy material can provide relatively rapid information.
  - PCR for *M. avium* complex and broad-range mycobacterial PCR and sequence analysis are available in some reference laboratories.
- Hansen's disease (leprosy) due to *M. leprae* [54]
- *Minimal Ancillary Work-Up*:
  - Diagnosis depends upon clinical findings and histopathologic evaluation of affected skin or nerve biopsies.
- *Additional Ancillary Work-Up*:
  - In difficult cases, specialized testing, such as PCR, can be sought from the National Hansen's Disease Program.
  - **AFB culture is not useful as the organism cannot be cultivated by routinely used methods**. Serologic testing is not recommended.

56. If prominent foamy macrophages and/or histiocyte-rich lymphadenitis is not due to mycobacterial infections (like MAC, NTM, or leprosy), then what else is in the DDx? Are there clues to distinguishing one from another?

- Sinus histiocytosis: Relatively common reactive finding in enlarged lymph nodes, sometimes found in lymph node sites draining non-hematopoietic malignancies.
- Exposure to foreign body-type agents from joint prosthesis, lymphangiogram, and other foreign materials (talc, sutures, etc.) (see Question 53 above for further discussion)
- *Tropheryma whipplei* (Whipple disease) (Fig. 18.20a–c)
- *Histoplasma capsulatum*
- Toxoplasmosis
- RDD/SHML (see Question 57 for further discussion)
- Kikuchi-Fujimoto disease (KFD) (see Questions 58–62 for further discussion)
- Systemic lupus erythematosus (SLE) (see Question 62 for further discussion)

57. What morphologic features and immunohistochemical findings would allow distinction of sinus histiocytosis from Rosai-Dorfman-Destombes disease and other neoplastic entities?

- Sinus histiocytes distend sinuses and are cytologically bland with oval to reniform nuclei, absent nucleoli, and abundant pale to clear cytoplasm.
- Phagocytosis of intracytoplasmic nuclear debris can be seen in these histiocytes.
- In sharp contrast, histiocytes in RDD/SHML are "atypical":
  - Larger cells with round nuclei with prominent single nucleoli.
  - Well-defined cytoplasmic borders.
  - Frequently contain intact intracytoplasmic lymphocytes (so-called emperipolesis) (Fig. 18.20d–f).
  - The above findings are never seen in the more common sinus histiocytosis.

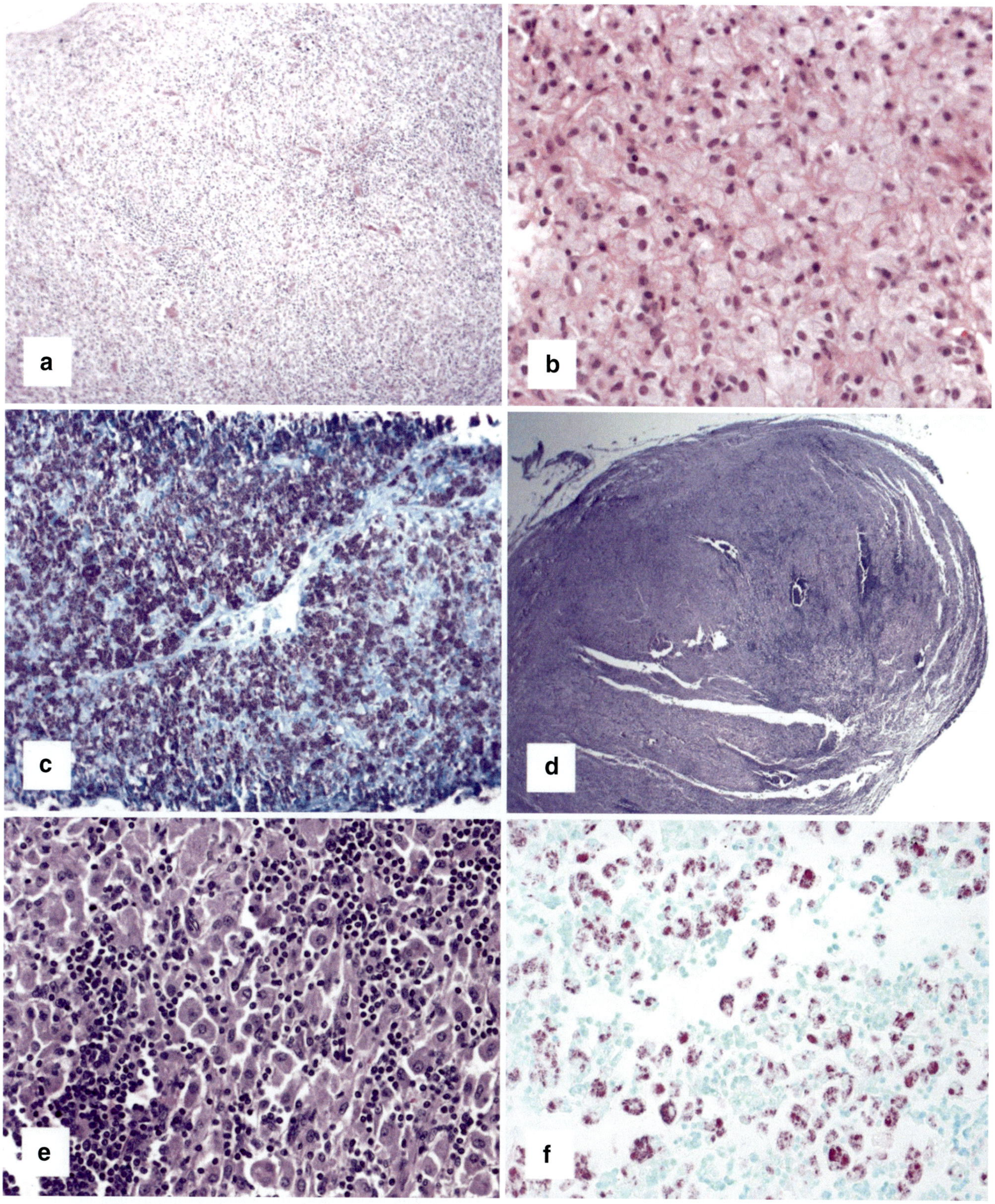

Fig. 18.19 LAD due to *Mycobacterium avium-intracellulare* (MAI – **a–c**) and *M. leprae* (**d–f** – courtesy of Dr. Dennis O'Malley). The extensive nodal involvement and histiocyte-rich cytomorphology for both disseminated MAI infection (**a** and **b**) and lepromatous leprosy from *M. leprae* (**d** and **e**) on H&E and on positive AFB Ziehl-Neelsen (**c**) and AFB Fite-Faraco modified (**f**) stains, respectively, are remarkably similar. Note that the modified Fite-Faraco must be used in uncovering AFB+ lepra cells (foamy macrophages packed with mycobacteria) in leprosy as the Ziehl-Neelsen may be negative. Clinical history would far better distinguish the two entities (with lepromatous skin and nerve involvement being distinct for *M. leprae* infection). AFB culture is the gold standard for definitive pathogen identification for MTB, MAI, and other NTMs; however, *M. leprae* cannot be cultivated by routine methods

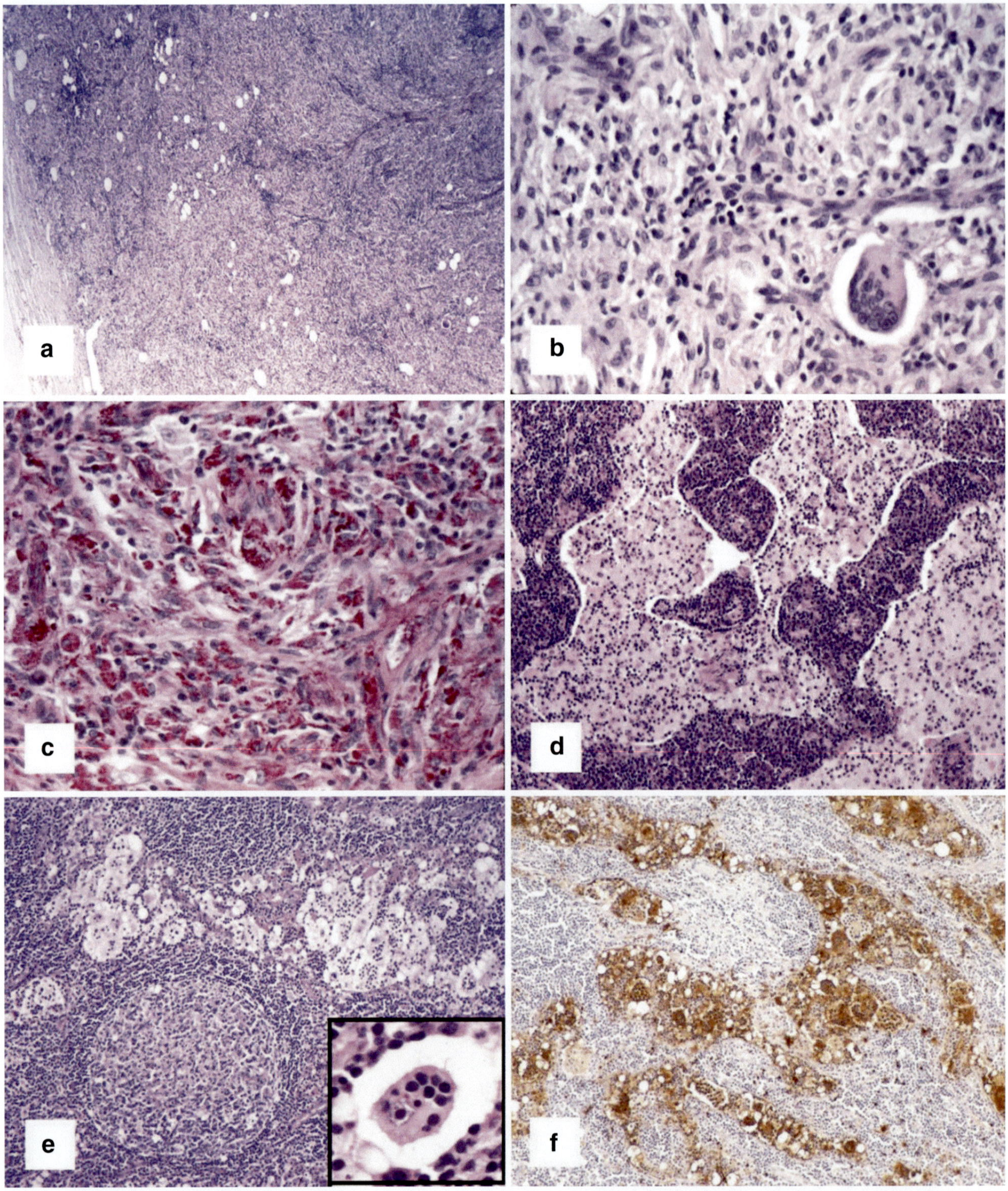

Fig. 18.20 Histiocyte-rich proliferations – Whipple disease (**a–c**) and Rosai-Dorfman-Destombes disease/sinus histiocytosis with massive lymphadenopathy [RDD/SHML] (**d–f**). LAD due to *Tropheryma whipplei* – are extremely rare. Typical clinical presentation is that of a farmer with severe abdominal pain, diarrhea, steatorrhea, and marked abdominal LAD. The histiocyte-rich proliferation subtotally replaces the LN (**a**). The histiocytes are round to elongated with clear to foamy eosinophilic cytoplasm; occasional MNGCs are seen (**b**). In contrast to mycobacterial infections, Whipple disease is AFB-negative, but shows numerous diastase-resistant PAS+ bacilli (**c**). Sinusoidal involvement of "atypical" RDD/SHML histiocytes is observed in (**d**) and (**e**); at times, distention is striking, as seen in (**d**). The infiltrate in RDD/SHML includes not only intrasinusoidal histiocytes, but also lymphocytes, plasma cells, and occasional eosinophils. The RDD/SHML histiocytes are larger than typical sinus histiocytes, with nuclei having prominent macronucleoli and abundant eosinophilic cytoplasm containing several small lymphocytes ("emperipolesis") [inset for (**e**)]. Positive staining by S100 accentuates the presence of intrasinusoidal RDD/SHML histiocytes (**f**)

- If the typical morphologic features of sinus histiocytosis are observed on H&E, no further work-up is necessary.
- If RDD/SHML is suspected on H&E sections, a limited panel of IHC stains for the RDD/SHML histiocytes will have the following profile: S100+/CD1a-/CD68+/CD163+ (as opposed to typical histiocytes, which are S100-/CD1a-/CD68+/CD163+).
- If there is any other concern for cytologic atypia and/or the patient has a history of malignancy, it would be worthwhile to follow-up with IHC:
  - Epithelial (e.g., AE1/AE3) and melanoma (e.g., S100, HMB-45, etc.) markers, because cytologically bland metastatic carcinoma or melanoma cells may have subtle sinusoidal nodal involvement.
  - If cohesive-appearing, cytologically abnormal cells with sinusoidal involvement lack cytokeratin and melanocytic expression:
    - A prime consideration should be anaplastic large cell lymphoma (ALCL).
    - ALCL tumor cells uniformly and strongly express CD30.
    - If CD30-positive, then further IHC work-up should be pursued.

58. As an entity that can display massive necrosis and numerous histiocytes, what is Kikuchi-Fujimoto Disease disease (KFD)? How does it typically present clinically?

- Also called histiocytic necrotizing lymphadenitis. [55, 56]
- Most commonly seen in individuals of Asian ancestry.
- Typical patient:
  - Young Asian.
  - Unilateral, tender/painful lymphadenopathy within the posterior triangle of the neck.
  - Reports 2–3 weeks of upper respiratory symptoms.
  - Low-grade fever and/or night sweats.
- Trigger for KFD not entirely established.
- Has been speculated to be of viral, infectious, and/or autoimmune etiology, although extensive infectious disease work-ups have not consistently nor definitively identified a culprit.

59. What are typical histologic and immunophenotypic findings in KFD?

- Preserved (or at least partially) nodal architecture with reactive lymphoid follicles.
- Irregular patchy zones of coagulative necrosis, particularly in early and mid-stages, result in partial architectural effacement.
- In regions of extensive necrosis: variable numbers of karyorrhectic debris and "crescentic" phagocytic histiocytes (phagocytic histiocytes with C-shaped nuclei).
- Neutrophils and plasma cells scarce to absent (contrast with SLE).
- At the interface of necrotic and viable areas: numerous immunoblasts, moderate numbers of mitoses → findings can be so worrisome as to raise DDx of non-Hodgkin lymphoma.
- Thrombosed vessels near areas of necrosis.
- Predominant features will depend on the stage of disease:
  - Proliferative (early)/lymphohistiocytic stage (Fig. 18.21b)
    - Lymphocytes, immunoblasts, and crescentic (C-shaped) histiocytes dominate.
    - Plasmacytoid dendritic cells (PDCs) increased.
    - Fewer foci of necrosis and apoptosis (compared to other stages).
    - Easily mistaken for lymphoma.
  - Necrotic (mid) stage (Fig. 18.21a)
    - Most commonly seen.
    - Large patchy areas of coagulative necrosis evident.
  - Xanthomatous (late) stage

    Foamy histiocytes predominate as necrotic foci regress.
- Immunophenotypic features:
  - General nodal preservation demonstrated by CD3 and CD20.
  - In necrotic foci: CD8+/TIA-1+ cytotoxic T-cells and T-immunoblasts predominate; B-cells are relatively rare.
  - Histiocytes have unusual staining profile: CD68+, MPO+, lysozyme+.
  - Clusters of PDCs best highlighted by CD123.

60. What is the minimal histopathologic work-up for KFD?

- To establish nodal architectural preservation: CD3 and CD20 should be performed at a minimum.
- Given extensive (albeit, non-neutrophilic) necrosis: AFB and GMS stains.
- If immunostains are desired to further support diagnosis, the following panel can be performed (for reasons discussed above): CD4, CD8, TIA-1, CD68/CD163, CD123, MPO, lysozyme, and Ki-67.
- Note that immunoarchitectural profile is essentially identical to that of SLE and will not distinguish between KFD and SLE.

61. What ancillary testing can help establish the diagnosis of KFD?

Minimal Ancillary Studies

- If there is concern for T- and/or B-cell non-Hodgkin lymphoma, but necrosis is extensive:
  - Cannot reliably interpret most IHC markers, so IHC work-up is likely to be low yield.

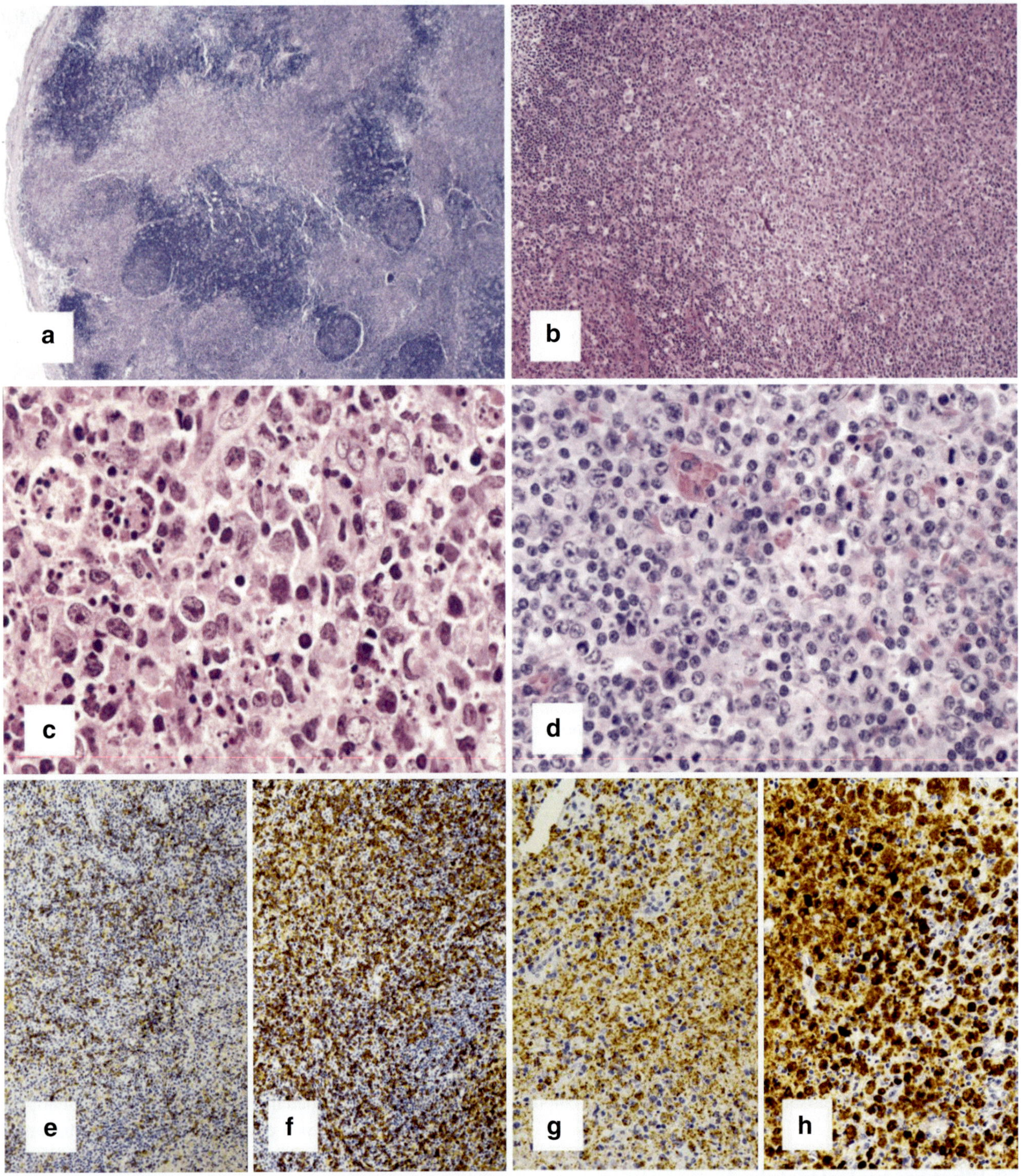

Fig. 18.21 Kikuchi-Fujimoto disease. Large paracortical regions are pale-staining at low magnification, corresponding to irregular patchy zones of coagulative necrosis (**a**). The stage of KFD in (**b**) represents the early proliferative/lymphohistiocytic stage, with relatively sparse foci of necrosis. The mottling is due to increased numbers of tingible body macrophages, reminiscent of the "starry sky" frequently associated with Burkitt lymphoma. Crescentic/C-shaped histiocytes, many of which contain nuclear debris, are readily appreciated in this necrotic focus (**c**). This high magnification view (**d**) displays increased numbers of immunoblasts and mitotic figures, raising concern for a large cell lymphoma. Nodal architectural preservation is present, underscored by CD3 and CD20 stains, with relative paucity of B-cells (not shown). (**e**) and (**f**) demonstrate the T-cell-rich composition of the lymphocytes, with scattered small CD4+ T-cells and weakly positive histiocytes (**e**) and predominance of CD8+ T-cells (**f**). Numerous histiocytes are weakly myeloperoxidase (**g**) and lysozyme (**h**) positive

- CD20 is a fairly robust marker and shows expression even in "ghost" necrotic cells of large B-cell lymphoma → if negative, can be more confident that necrosis does not represent a necrotic B-cell lymphoma (though caution is still advised).
- Consider pursuing T- and B-cell receptor gene rearrangements → though caution advised in interpretation.
- Though not necessary for establishing diagnosis, typical laboratory studies for a patient with KFD include:
  - Slightly increased ESR.
  - Mild neutropenia with reactive lymphocytosis.
  - Increased LDH AST, ALT.
  - Polyclonal gammopathy.
  - Negative infectious disease work-up.

62. KFD and SLE (one of its histologic patterns) have nearly identical histologic and immunophenotypic findings. What features will allow distinction between KFD and SLE?

- Some consider KFD a "forme fruste" of SLE (systemic lupus erythematosus), meaning that it is believed by some authors to be a manifestation of SLE, showing *some but not all* of the diagnostic SLE features.
- Literature suggests that co-occurrence of KFD and SLE appears too frequent to be considered to occur by chance alone and that the two entities must be linked [55, 58].
- 2012 SLICC (Systemic Lupus International Collaborating Clinics) Criteria is one of the most widely used schema to diagnose individuals with SLE (Table 18.18) [57].
- Enlarged LNs affect about 50% of SLE patients.
- Typically involve cervical, axillary, and inguinal nodes.
- SLE LAD can show a variety of histologic patterns:
  - One pattern is a combination of nonspecific RFH (reactive follicular hyperplasia), vascular proliferation, and polytypic plasmacytosis with intragerminal and/or interfollicular plasma cells.
  - Interfollicular immunoblastic hyperplasia may also be seen.
  - Another pattern is strikingly similar to Kikuchi-Fujimoto disease (KFD) [see Question 61 above].
    - Coagulative necrosis extensive.
    - Numerous karyorrhectic bodies, crescentic histiocytes, small lymphocytes, immunoblasts, and clusters of plasmacytoid dendritic cells.
    - Viable immunoblasts may predominate, displaying lymphoma-like foci.
    - Immunoprofile of cellular component is identical to KFD.
- KFD displays non-neutrophilic necrosis; in contrast, SLE LAD can contain neutrophils and neutrophilic debris. The histologic findings thought to distinguish SLE from KFD are:
  - Presence of plasma cells, which can be abundant in SLE.
  - Azzopardi phenomenon = encrustation of degenerated DNA material onto vessels with fibrinoid necrosis.
  - Hematoxylin bodies = acellular and deeply hematoxyphilic globular material, believed to be degenerated nuclear material that has reacted with antinuclear antibodies; most commonly seen in subcapsular sinuses and paracortex.
  - While diagnostic and specific for SLE, unfortunately, these findings are rare (Fig. 18.22).
- Clinical history and serologic studies will also aid in distinction of SLE from KFD:
  - SLE patients experience more indicators of systemic disease (e.g., lupus-related lesions in the skin, mucosal sites, joints, kidney, CNS; cytopenias).
  - Serologic studies favoring SLE over KFD:
    - (+) ANA
    - (+) anti-dsDNA
    - (+) anti-Sm
    - (+) antiphospholipid work-up
    - Low complement
    - (+) DAT
  - See Table 18.18 for details of SLE clinical and laboratory diagnostic criteria.

63. To summarize G/H-LAD: what would be the clinical relevance of misinterpretation?

- Misinterpreting G/H-LAD as lymphoma or other malignancy (see neoplastic DDx in Table 18.14):
  - Misdiagnosing G/H-LAD entities (like KFD) as cHL, AITL, DLBCL, or other lymphoma leads to unwarranted chemotherapy and/or radiation treatment and increases risk of morbidity/mortality.
- Conversely, failure to recognize lymphomatous involvement in G/H-LAD (like lymphoepithelioid variant of PTCL or granulomatous inflammation secondary to B-cell lymphoma) deprives patient of appropriate oncologic treatment and follow-up.
- Not suggesting the correct reactive etiology for G/H-LAD:
  - May not be as clinically devastating as misdiagnosis of lymphoma.
  - Majority of entities are likely due to infections – it may not be possible on histopathologic evaluation alone to isolate exact etiology and will need to rely on other clinical and other ancillary study results.

Table 18.18 Diagnostic criteria for systemic lupus erythematosus based on 2012 Systemic Lupus International Collaborating Clinics (SLICC) Criteria [diagnosis requires 4 of 17 criteria met, including at least 1 clinical criterion PLUS 1 immunologic criterion *or* biopsy-proven lupus nephritis] [57]

Clinical criteria		Immunologic criteria	
Criterion	Definition	Criterion	Definition
1. Acute cutaneous lupus	Lupus malar rash; bullous lupus; toxic epidermal necrolysis variant of SLE; maculopapular lupus rash; photosensitive lupus rash [*w/o^* dermatomyositis] Subacute cutaneous lupus (nonindurated psoriasiform and/or annular polycyclic lesions that resolve without scarring, although occasionally with post-inflammatory dyspigmentation or telangiectasias)	1. ANA	ANA level above laboratory reference range
2. Chronic cutaneous lupus	Classic discoid rash; localized (above the neck); generalized (above and below the neck); hypertrophic (verrucous) lupus; lupus panniculitis (profundus); mucosal lupus; lupus erythematosus tumidus; chilblains lupus Discoid lupus/lichen planus overlap	2. Anti-dsDNA	Anti-dsDNA antibody level above laboratory reference range (or > two-fold the reference range if tested by ELISA)
3. Non-scarring alopecia	Diffuse thinning or hair fragility with visible broken hairs (*w/o^* alopecia areata, drugs, iron deficiency, and androgenic alopecia)	3. Anti-Sm	Presence of antibody to Sm nuclear antigen
4. Oral or nasal ulcers	Palate, buccal, tongue ulcers Nasal ulcers (*w/o^* vasculitis, Behcet disease, infection (herpesvirus), IBD, reactive arthritis, and acidic foods)	4. Antiphospholipid	Antiphospholipid positivity as determined by any of the following: (+) result for lupus anticoagulant (+) results for RPR Medium or high titer anticardiolipin antibody level (IgA, IgG, or IgM) (+) result for anti-beta 2-glycoprotein I (IgA, IgG, or IgM)
5. Joint disease	Synovitis involving 2 or more joints, characterized by swelling or effusion Tenderness in 2 or more joints and at least 30 minutes of morning stiffness		
6. Serositis	Typical pleurisy for more than 1 day, pleural effusions, or pleural rub Typical pericardial pain for more than 1 days, pericardial effusion, rub, or pericarditis by EKG (*w/o^* infection, uremia, and Dressler syndrome)		
7. Renal	Urine protein-to-creatinine ratio (or 24-hour urine protein) representing 500 mg protein/24 hours Red blood cell casts	5. Low complement	Low C3; Low C4 *OR* Low CH50
8. Neurologic	Seizures, psychosis, mononeuritis complex (*w/o^* primary vasculitis); myelitis; peripheral or cranial neuropathy (*w/o^* diabetes) Acute confusional state (in absence of other causes including toxic/metabolic, uremia, drugs)	6. Direct antiglobulin test (direct Coombs test)	Direct antiglobulin test in absence of hemolytic anemia
9. Hemolytic anemia	Hemolytic anemia		
10. Leukopenia or lymphopenia	Leukopenia (<4 K/μL at least once) [in absence of other known causes, such as Felty syndrome, drugs, portal HTN] Lymphopenia (<1 K/μL at least once) [*w/o^* glucocorticoids, drugs, and infection]		
11. Thrombocytopenia	Thrombocytopenia (<100 K/μL at least once) [*w/o^* drugs, portal HTN, TTP]		

HTN hypertension, *IBD* inflammatory bowel disease), *TTP* thrombotic thrombocytopenic purpura, *w/o^* without = "in the absence of other known causes, such as…"

– Failing to suggest that a more extensive work-up for autoimmune disease (as in SLE) can result in delays in appropriate patient management and treatment.
– Not identifying the exact non-infectious etiology for granulomatous/histiocytic reaction (e.g., granulomas induced by talc vs TPN vs gold) may not be clinically relevant.

64. What information can be conveyed to the clinician? When is a diagnostic comment necessary? What is an adequate specimen?

- The vast majority of entities with granulomatous disease (whether necrotizing, non-necrotizing, or suppurative) and many cases of foamy histiocyte-rich infiltrates are associated with infection.

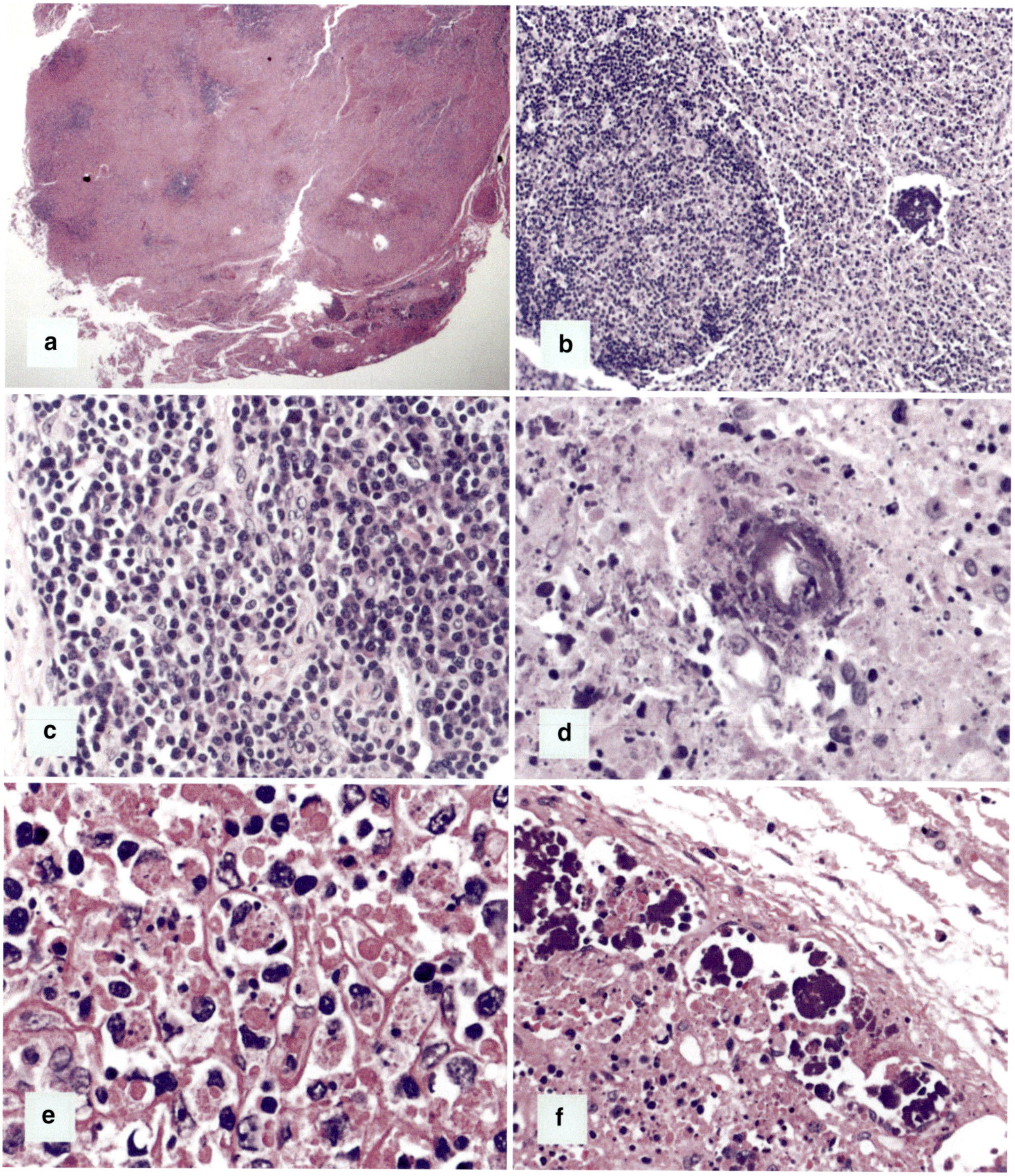

Fig. 18.22 Systemic lupus erythematosus. Very similar to the necrotic stage of KFD illustrated in Fig. 18.21, large paracortical regions are pale-staining at low magnification, corresponding to irregular patchy zones of coagulative necrosis (**a**) in this case of SLE. The immunoprofile is identical to KFD with nodal architectural preservation, only rare B-cells, predominance of cytotoxic CD8+ T-cells, and histiocytes with unusual phenotype (not shown). Deeply basophilic material is present in the necrotic paracortex to the right of the germinal center (**b**) on intermediate magnification. Interfollicular plasmacytosis can be observed in SLE (**c**), in sharp contrast to absence of plasma cells in KFD. On high-power view of (**b**), the deeply basophilic material represents the Azzopardi phenomenon: nuclear remnant encrustation onto a necrotic vessel wall (**d**). Crescentic histiocytes (**e**) are observed in both KFD and SLE. Hematoxylin bodies are deeply hematoxyphilic, globular, acellular material in sinuses (**f**); their presence is said to distinguish SLE from KFD. However, both Azzopardi effect and hematoxylin bodies are very rare findings

- Thus, diagnosis can be descriptive, particularly when no organisms are uncovered by routine histopathologic and special stain evaluation.
- Comments should note that failure to identify organisms on routine evaluation should not preclude diagnosis of infectious lymphadenitis; close correlation with infectious disease work-up is required.
- Even when organisms seen on H&E and special stains, still appropriate to defer final organism speciation to pending microbiologic cultures, serologic, and appropriate ancillary studies (i.e., molecular testing), and correlation with clinical history.

- G/H-LAD reactive pattern is the most likely (of all the histologic patterns) to be deemed "adequate" with limited biopsy sampling, given:
  - Ample cytomorphologic representation (+/– successful discovery of organisms).
  - Appropriate material sent for further microbiologic studies.
  - No clinical, radiologic, or cytomorphologic concern for malignancy.
    - Perfect example of an adequate biopsy: FNA showing numerous spherules containing endospores as well as granulomas (histopathologic features highly suggestive of coccidioidomycosis) PLUS appropriately collected material for fungal culture/sensitivity testing sent to microbiology laboratory.
- In contrast, if only CNBx received and there are clinical or histologic features worrisome for lymphoma (i.e., due to necrosis, exuberant immunoblastic proliferation) → an excisional biopsy is mandatory for complete evaluation.

65. When is external consultation in G/H-LAD necessary?

- Consultation not usually medically necessary given fairly benign disease.
- Consultation can be pursued for medical interest to uncover the cause of the foreign body-type granulomatous LAD.

Plasma Cell Rich Lymphadenopathy (PC-rich LAD), DDx Including LAD Secondary to Syphilis, IgG4-related Disease, Multicentric Castleman Disease

66. What are the typical morphologic findings in the major subtype of plasma cell-rich lymphadenopathy (PC-rich LAD)?

- Differential diagnosis (DDx) for PC-rich LAD
  - Table 18.19 summarizes infectious and non-infectious etiologies of PC-rich LAD and its neoplastic mimics.
  - Select entities in the DDx of PC-rich LAD will be discussed further.
- Minimal histopathologic work-up in cases with PC-rich LAD, depends on DDx based on aggregate histologic (and clinical/radiologic/laboratory) findings:
  - CD3, CD20: Confirms nodal preservation.
  - CD138, kappa, lambda: Highlights plasma cell distribution and polytypic light chain expression.
  - IgG, IgG4: Assesses number of IgG4+ plasma cells.
  - *Treponema* IHC: Evaluates for possibility of syphilitic LAD.
  - HHV8: Verifies HHV8 immunoreactivity in cases with MCD-like histopathology.

67. As a very typical entity that can display PC-rich LAD, what clinical and epidemiologic features do syphilitic (luetic) lymphadenitides exhibit?

- Caused by infection by gram negative spirochete, *Treponema pallidum*.
- LAD manifests in the first and second of three stages of syphilis [59, 60].
  - Primary syphilis (1st stage):
    - Occurs with direct contact of infected sites, as transpires with sexual contact.
    - Once skin is infected, it develops into a painless ulcer called chancre.
    - Spirochetes enter LNs draining primary site → results in LAD.

Table 18.19 Differential diagnosis of plasma cell-rich LAD and its neoplastic mimics

Infectious	Non-infectious	Neoplastic mimics
Syphilitic MCD, HHV8+ HIV/AIDS[b] (intermediate/chronic stage) HHV8+ germinotropic lymphoproliferative disorder	RDD/SHML[a] iMCD = MCD, PC variant Rheumatoid arthritis (RA)[b]/Adult-onset Still's disease[c]/Sjogren syndrome IgG4-RD (Castleman disease-like pattern) SLE[a]	cHL AITL *EBV*+ polymorphic post-transplant lymphoproliferative disorder (PTLD) B-cell lymphoma with plasmacytic differentiation (e.g., nodal marginal zone lymphoma, lymphoplasmacytic lymphoma) Nodal involvement of plasma cell neoplasm

[a]Discussed more extensively in the granulomatous/histiocyte-rich proliferation section
[b]Discussed more extensively in the reactive follicular hyperplasia section
[c]Discussed more extensively in the interfollicular hyperplasia section

- Secondary syphilis (2nd stage):
  - Proceeds within weeks to months after presentation of untreated primary syphilis.
  - Chancre heals.
  - Generalized LAD in vast majority of patients.
  - Fever, malaise, and maculopapular rash can be observed in many patients.
- Tertiary syphilis (3rd stage):
  - Characterized by severe neurologic deficits, cardiovascular disease, and/or gummatous (tumor-like lesion) formation.
  - Striking paucity of organisms.

68. What are typical histologic and immunophenotypic findings for syphilitic LAD?

- Characteristic findings found in both 1st and 2nd stages (Fig. 18.23):
  - Reactive follicular hyperplasia (RFH).
  - Interfollicular polytypic plasmacytosis.
  - Capsular fibrosis.
  - Vasculitis, venulitis, phlebitis (with variable numbers of neutrophils, plasma cells, and lymphocytes infiltrating damaged blood vessels), particularly within paracortex and medulla.
- Though histologic findings are nonspecific in isolation, the combination should put syphilitic LAD at the top of DDx.
- A rare, nodal inflammatory pseudotumor-like (IPT-like) variant in syphilitic LAD has also been described.
- In the appropriate histologic context, demonstration of *Treponema* spirochetes by commercially available IHC stain is diagnostic of syphilitic LAD.
  - Numerous spirochetes concentrated around inflamed and/or obliterated vessels.
  - Warthin-Starry stain can show treponemal organisms, but can be challenging to interpret with high nonspecific background staining.

69. What ancillary testing can support the diagnosis of syphilitic LAD?

Minimal Ancillary Work-Up:

- Serologic testing – the conventional test algorithm starts with a non-treponemal test which, when positive, is confirmed by a treponemal test. The alternative reverse sequence algorithm (treponemal followed by non-treponemal test for positives) is also acceptable and has recently been applied in many laboratories for workflow considerations. Sensitivity of various serologic assays is near 100% in secondary syphilis. During primary syphilis, their sensitivity is cited to be in the range of 70–100% [18–20].
  - Non-treponemal tests: Most commonly used is rapid plasma reagin (RPR), but others include toluidine red unheated serum test (TRUST) and unheated serum (USR). For CSF, Venereal Disease Research Laboratory (VDRL) test is recommended.
  - Treponemal tests: fluorescent treponemal antibody absorbed (FTA-ABS) test, *T. pallidum* passive particle agglutination (TP-PA) assay, enzyme immunoassay, chemiluminescence immunoassays, or microhemagglutination (MHA-TPA).

Additional Ancillary Tests:

- Dark field microscopy of lymph node aspirate can provide rapid and direct etiologic evidence, especially in early syphilis when serologic tests may be falsely negative. Drawbacks are that the procedure is not widely available, slides must be examined immediately for valid results, and sensitivity is ~75%. PCR of lymph node tissue for *T. pallidum* is not widely available.

70. What is the clinical relevance of not recognizing syphilitic LAD?

- If not considered in DDx, one may fail to perform the *T. pallidum* IHC and/or Warthin-Starry stains, which would have flagged an unsuspecting clinician to confirm the histologic findings.
- Deprives patient of relatively benign antimicrobial therapy (e.g., penicillin) → can lead to devastating progression into tertiary syphilis.

71. As a typical entity demonstrating PC-rich LAD, how does IgG4-related LAD (IgG4-R-LAD) present clinically?

- IgG4-related disease (IgG4-RD) is a multisystemic immune-mediated disorder whose unifying pathophysiology was recognized in the early to mid-2000s [61–67]. Prior to that, a wide range of seemingly unrelated disorders in various organs existed in the literature, for example: autoimmune pancreatitis, sclerosing cholangitis, idiopathic retroperitoneal fibrosis, etc.

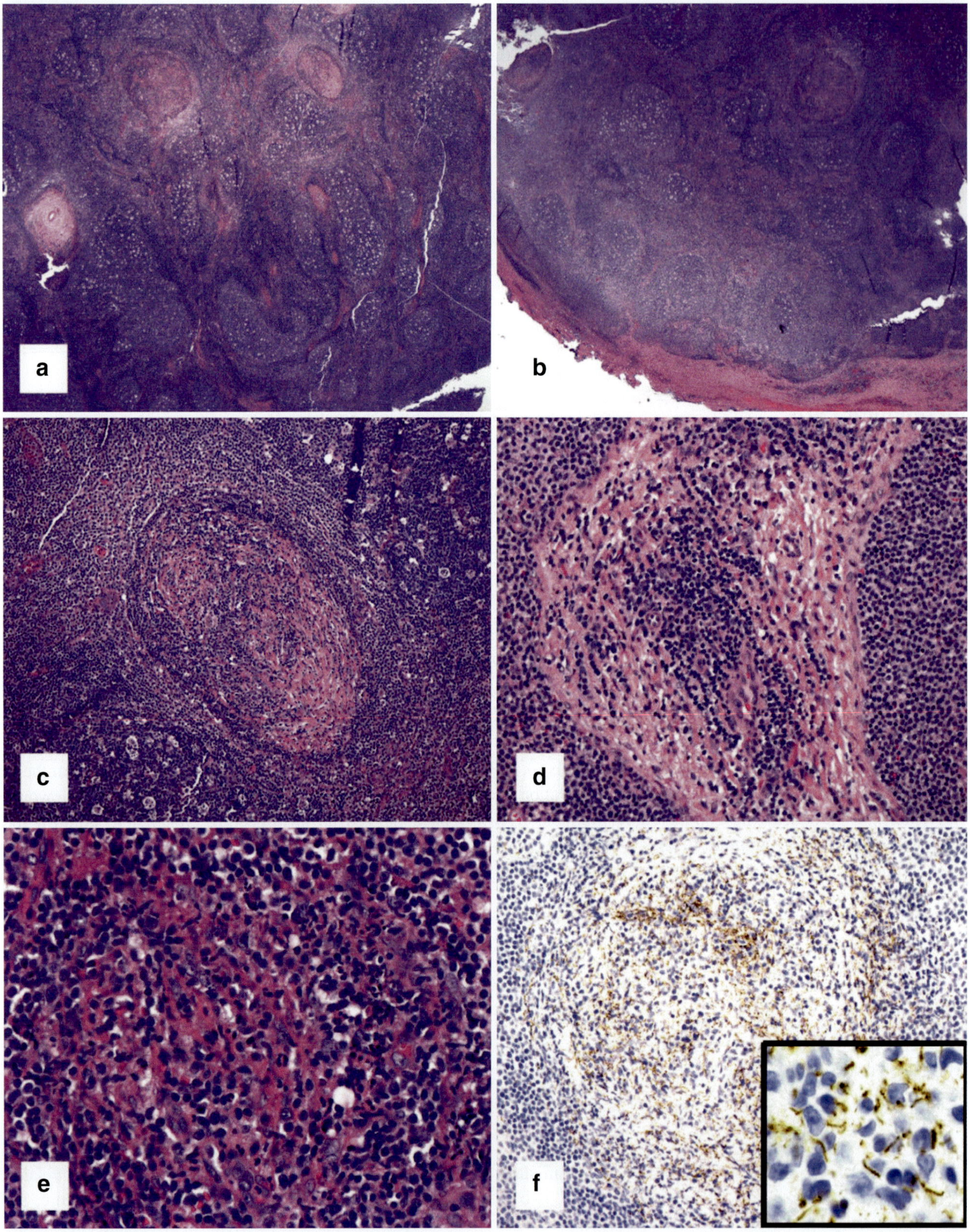

Fig. 18.23 Syphilitic (luetic) LAD due to *Treponema pallidum.* Low magnification views of this enlarged LN display florid reactive follicular hyperplasia; even on low power, obliterative and sclerotic changes are observed in the medullary vessels (**a**), as is a thickened, fibrotic capsule (**b**). Obliterative vasculitis is seen (**c**). Interfollicular regions typically have numerous plasma cells. Many plasma cells are embedded in this fibrous trabeculum (**d**). Vasculitis is evident, with luminal obliteration, dense lymphoplasmacytic infiltration, and frequent neutrophils (**e**). It is at these vasculitic foci that spirochete organisms with corkscrew morphology abound (**f** *and inset*)

- Kamisawa and colleagues posited that these seemingly unrelated disorders in extranodal sites had in common the following histopathologic findings, unifying them into a single pathologic entity of IgG4-RD:
  - Tumefactive (mass-forming) lesions composed variably of lymphoplasmacytic infiltrates with an excess of IgG4-positive plasma cells (PCs).
  - Ability to incite a fibrosing/sclerosing process, resulting in a whorling/storiform fibrosis.
  - Presence of obliterative phlebitis.

72. What are typical histologic and immunophenotypic findings in IgG4-R-LAD and the minimal histopathologic work-up when suspected?

- The diagnostic triad of IgG4-RD [(a) lymphoplasmacytic infiltrate with significant increase in IgG4+ plasma cells; (b) storiform fibrosis; and (c) obliterative phlebitis] is seen in *extranodal* sites, while LN involvement may not display all features (except for pattern 5, inflammatory pseudotumor-like histology).
- Consensus statement on the pathology of IgG4-RD proposed different cut-off values of numbers that would be considered significant for IgG4+ PCs, based on organ, sampling, and other histologic features. For example:
- Pancreas or bile duct with ≥2 pathology features:
  - Biopsy: >10 IgG4+ PCs/high power field (hpf) → considered "histologically highly suggestive of IgG4-RD."
  - Surgical specimen: >50 IgG4+ PCs/hpf → considered "probable histologic features of IgG4-RD."
- Salivary gland
  - With >2 pathology features: >100 IgG4+ PCs/hpf → considered "histologically highly suggestive of IgG4-RD. "
  - With 1 pathology feature: >100 IgG4+ PCs/hpf → considered "probable histologic features of IgG4-RD. See [67] for more examples of proposed diagnostic schema.
- In any site, IgG4-to-IgG ratio > 40% is mandatory for diagnosis.
- Regarding LNs, proposal by consensus group: either >50 or > 100 IgG4+ PCs/hpf would be cutoff for "probable histologic features of IgG4-RD."
- Understanding clinical and laboratory context is key to diagnosis
- There are 5 widely recognized histologic patterns of IgG4-R-LAD:
  - Castleman disease (MCD)-like (pattern 1)
  - Florid follicular hyperplasia (pattern 2; most common) (Fig. 18.24)
  - Interfollicular hyperplasia (pattern 3) (Fig. 18.25)
  - PTGC (pattern 4) (Fig. 18.26)
  - Inflammatory pseudotumor-like (pattern 5) (Fig. 18.27)

Table 18.20 summarizes the patterns, differential diagnostic categories, and reliable discriminators for diagnosis in IgG4-R-LAD.

73. What clinical information and ancillary testing are highly suggestive of IgG4-RD and would support IgG4-R-LAD?

- Clinical history:
  - Older male (>50 years) with any of the 5 histologic patterns.
  - Symptoms are not severe and/or systemic (unlike in MCD) [74, 75].
- Lab results:
  - Elevated serum IgG4 levels
    - Often, but not always elevated.
    - Sensitivity or specificity depends on cutoff level.
    - Can be normal, even in patients with biopsy-proven, active IgG4-RD.
  - Elevated serum IgE level
- Other testing:
  - Possibly peripheral blood flow cytometry to evaluate for markedly increased numbers of plasmablasts ($CD19^{dim}$/CD38+/CD20-/CD27+ [63] → needs further clinical vetting in the literature)

74. In LAD cases with increased IgG4+ plasma cells, what information can be conveyed to the clinician? When is a diagnostic comment necessary? What are the clinical implications of the diagnosis?

- A few comments to consider before examining clinician communication:
  - There are known LAD cases with significantly increased IgG4+ PCs that do *not* represent IgG4-related disease.

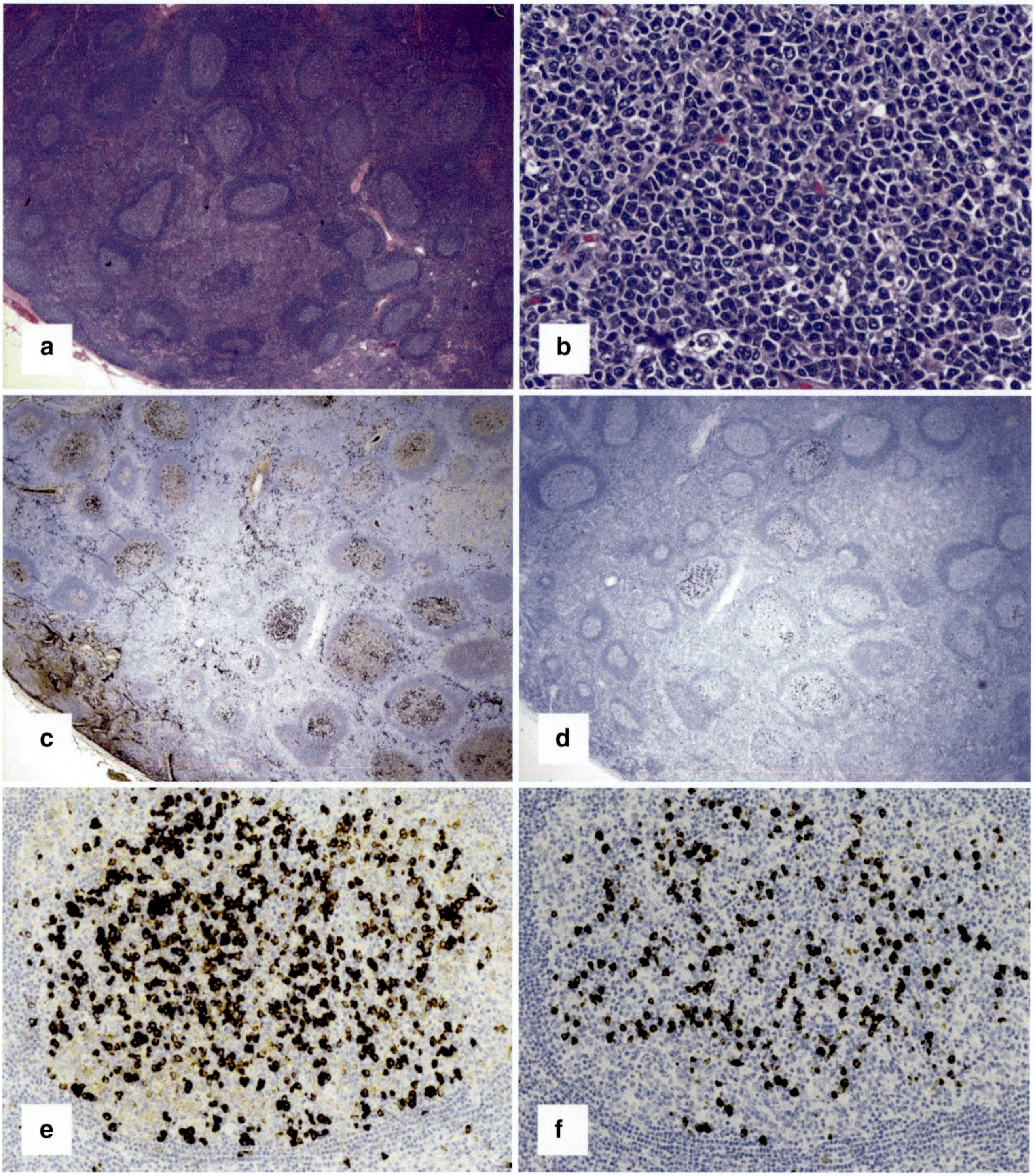

Fig. 18.24 IgG4-related lymphadenopathy (IgG4-R-LAD) pattern: Reactive follicular hyperplasia pattern (pattern 2). The most common of the five histologic patterns of IgG4-R-LAD is reactive follicular hyperplasia with plasmacytosis (**a**). On high magnification, the presence of intrafollicular plasma cells (PCs) (**b**) is a clue to further investigate for an increase in IgG4+ PCs, as well as interfollicular plasmacytosis and eosinophilia. Low-power view of IgG (**c**) and IgG4 staining (**d**) reveals patchy distribution of increased IgG4+ PCs; in this example (**d**) only three reactive follicles have increased IgG4+ PCs, underscoring that IgG4-R-LAD may be missed by limited core needle biopsies. Evaluation for the number of IgG4+ PCs and IgG4:IgG ratio must be performed in "hot spots," with >50 IgG4+ PCs per hpf and > 40% ratio, respectively, qualifying as increased IgG4+ PCs in LN. IgG staining highlights numerous PCs within the germinal center (**e**), while IgG4 is positive in a significant percentage of intrafollicular PCs (**f**)

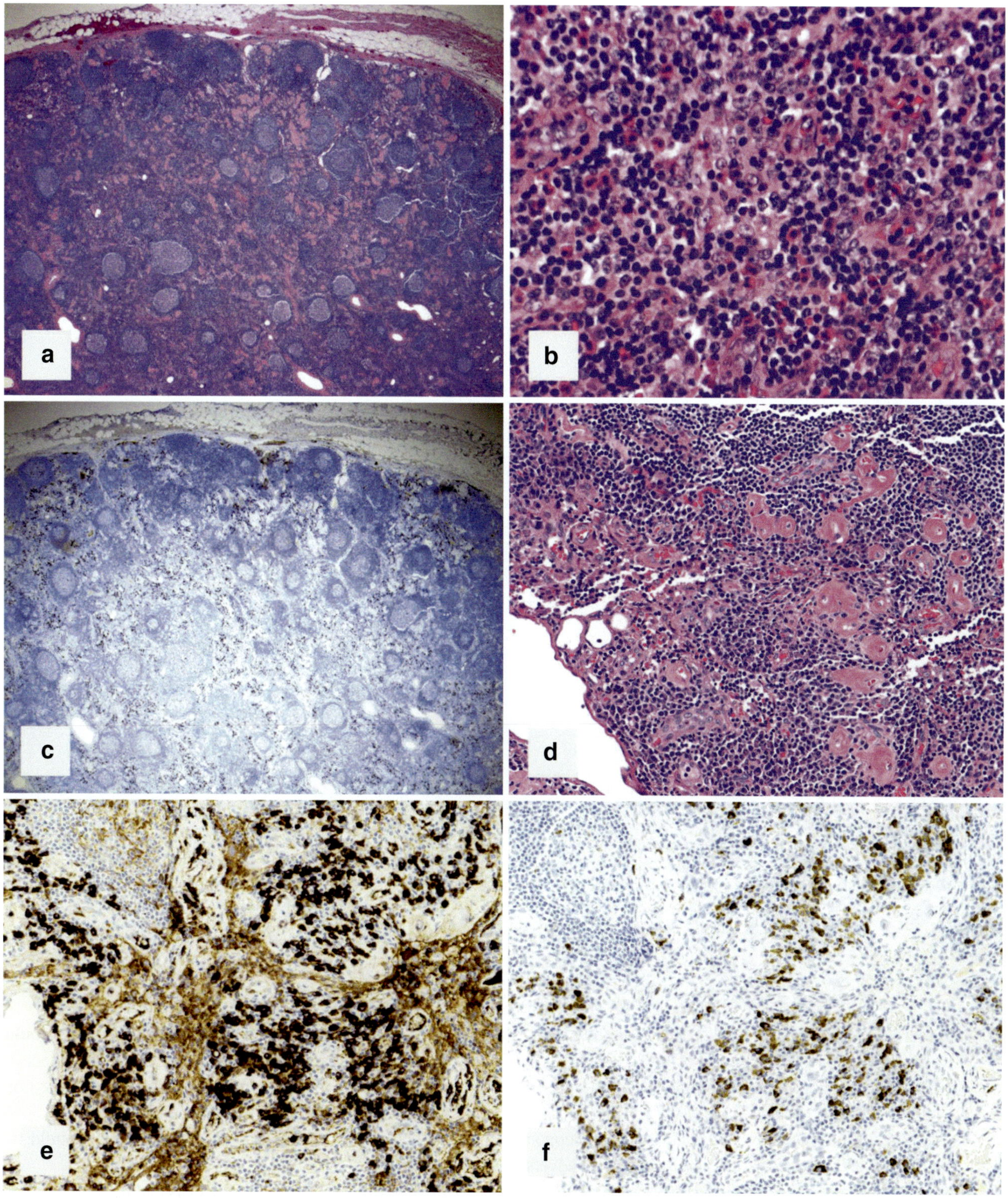

Fig. 18.25 IgG4-R-LAD pattern: Interfollicular plasmacytosis (pattern 3). This pattern also displays reactive follicular hyperplasia (**a**) and increased numbers of eosinophils (**b**). However, the plasmacytosis and IgG4+ PCs are concentrated within interfollicular zones, with sparing of lymphoid follicles, as demonstrated by this low magnification view of IgG4 staining (**c**). Along with hyalinized blood vessels, numerous interfollicular PCs are seen in this region (**d**), also reminiscent of the plasma cell variant of multicentric Castleman disease; many of these PCs are positive for IgG (**e**) with a significant proportion also staining with IgG4 (**f**) (>50 IgG4+ PCs per hpf and > 40% IgG4-to-IgG ratio)

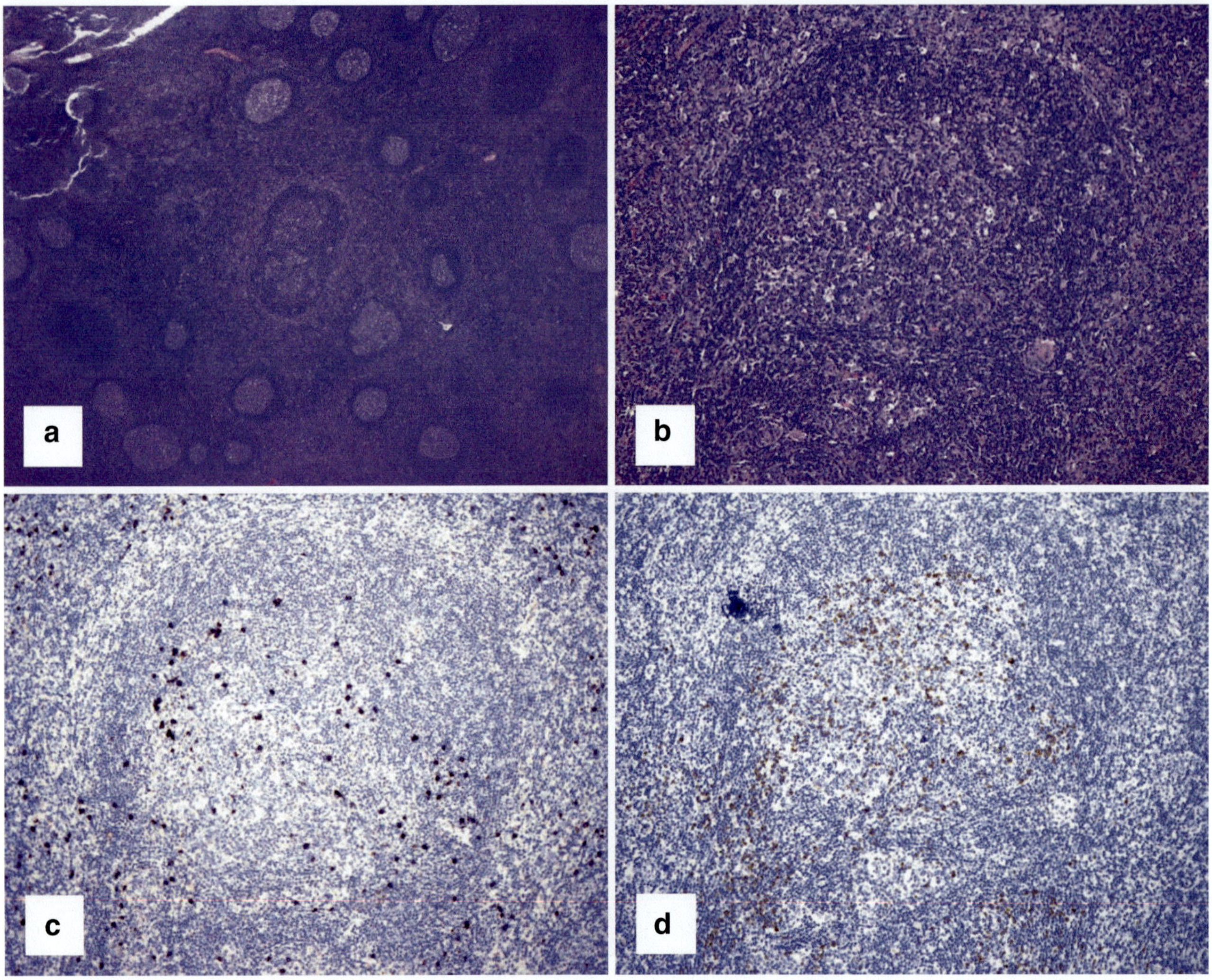

Fig. 18.26 IgG4-R-LAD pattern: Progressive transformation of germinal centers (PTGC) pattern (pattern 4). This low magnification view of a reactive lymph node demonstrates follicular hyperplasia, as well as an enlarged follicle with PTGC (**a**). High magnification view of the affected PTGC lymphoid follicle illustrates small mantle zone-type lymphocytes "transforming"/infiltrating the germinal center and breaking up the sheets of centroblasts and centrocytes into several pale foci (**b**). PCs are increased in germinal centers and interfollicular zones. A subset of PCs is positive for IgG (**c**) and an even greater number stain for IgG4 (**d**) (>50 IgG4+ PCs per hpf and > 40% IgG4-to-IgG ratio)

  - Increased IgG4+ plasma cells, as an isolated finding, is insufficient for a diagnosis of IgG4-R-LAD.
  - Dx is a sign-symptom complex and should be approached as such.
- Overdiagnosis of "IgG4-related LAD" without supportive clinical and laboratory data can have several adverse implications (as detailed by Cheuk and Chan [64]):
  - Incorrectly labels patient with a definitive diagnosis of systemic disease.
  - May lead to inappropriate investigations that could result in increased risk of morbidity (e.g., unnecessary tissue biopsies in extranodal sites that are not radiologically concerning).
  - Thus, definitive diagnosis in this context should be avoided.
- Any of the five histologic patterns can be seen in other disorders → exclusion of these entities is essential (see Table 18.20).

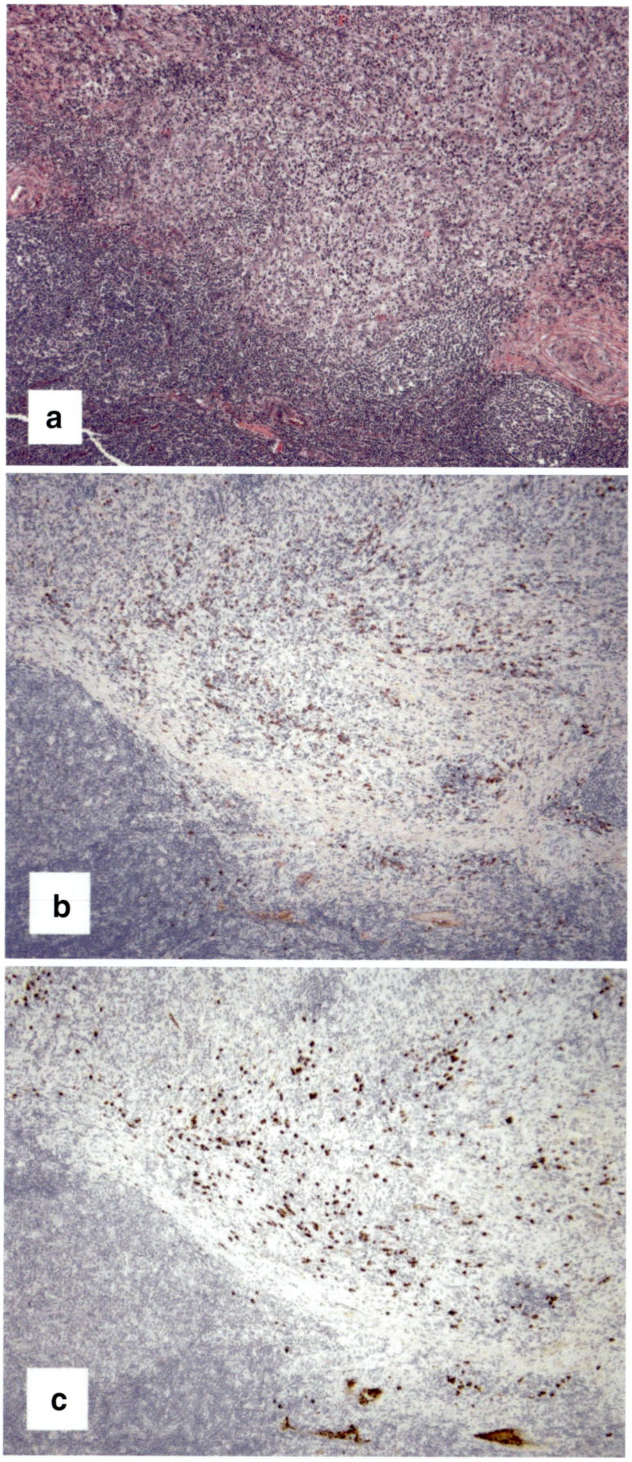

Fig. 18.27 IgG4-R-LAD pattern: Inflammatory pseudotumor-like (IPT-like) pattern (pattern 5) [courtesy of Dr. D. O'Malley]. This rare pattern of IgG4-LAD is similar morphologically to nodal inflammatory pseudotumors, exhibiting at least partial effacement of architecture by a dense fibrotic lesion (**a**) with variable numbers of plasma cells (PCs), eosinophils, lymphocytes, and histiocytes. PCs are positive for IgG (**b**) with nearly all of them showing strong reactivity to IgG4 (**c**) (>50 IgG4+ PCs per hpf and > 40% IgG4-to-IgG ratio)

- Several recommended approaches when a reactive lymph node is found to have increased IgG4+ plasma cells with an IgG4/IgG ratio of >40%:
  - In the setting of documented IgG4-related disease in extranodal sites:

    Diagnostic comment: "The histopathologic findings are consistent with IgG4-related lymphadenopathy."
  - In the setting of systemic lymphadenopathy without previous history of IgG4-RD:

    Diagnostic comment: "In an older patient with systemic lymphadenopathy, these histologic findings are highly worrisome for, though not diagnostic of, IgG4-related LAD. Other autoimmune disorders presenting with systemic adenopathy should also be considered. Close correlation with the serologic IgG4 and IgE levels as well as clinical follow-up by Rheumatology service is warranted. Some patients with these findings may develop subsequent extranodal involvement by IgG4-RD."
  - In the setting of localized lymphadenopathy without previous history of IgG4-RD:
    - Likely the most common setting.
    - Final diagnosis: "Reactive lymphoid hyperplasia with increased IgG4+ plasma cells; See Comment."
    - Diagnostic comment: "The histopathologic findings are not entirely specific, and their significance is unclear in localized lymphadenopathy. Thus, careful correlation with corroborating clinical information (e.g., known IgG4-related disease in another site, history of rheumatoid arthritis?), laboratory data (e.g., serum immunoglobulin levels, including IgE, IgG4, etc.), and imaging studies (localized versus systemic lymphadenopathy?) is required. More detailed history and specific questions directed toward manifestations of IgG4-related disease are recommended to guide management."
- When correctly diagnosed, appropriate therapy for IgG4-RD (like corticosteroids and/or immunosuppressants) should be instituted, with management of patients designated to physicians with expertise/specialized training in treating this entity (e.g., rheumatologists).

75. What is an adequate specimen in reactive LAD with increased IgG4+ plasma cells?

- Needle core biopsy could be sufficient if well-developed findings supporting significant IgG4+ plasmacytosis are present.
- Recommend excisional biopsy if clinical concern for malignancy persists.

Table 18.20 Patterns of IgG4-related lymphadenopathy, morphologic mimics (sometimes with increased numbers of IgG4 plasma cells), and suggestive/reliable discriminators to aid in diagnosis

Variant/ subtype	Histologic pattern of IgG4	Differential diagnostic considerations	Discriminator
I/1	Multicentric Castleman disease (MCD)-like pattern of IgG4-R-LAD	MCD, HHV8-related	HHV8 IHC+ diagnostic of HHV8+ MCD Severe systemic disease with elevated IL-6, CRP supports HHV8+ MCD Lambda monotypic plasma cells sometimes seen in HHV8+ MCD Increased eosinophils in LN favor MCD-like IgG4-LAD Unusual sites of involvement, like orbital, salivary gland, pancreas favor MCD-like IgG4-LAD
		MCD, HHV8-negative (idiopathic MCD)	Severe systemic disease with elevated IL-6, CRP
II/2	Florid follicular hyperplasia (most common) pattern of IgG4-R-LAD	Syphilitic (luetic) LAD	*Treponema pallidum* IHC + in syphilis
		Autoimmune disease (i.e., SLE, RA, Still's disease)	Supportive clinical and laboratory results (e.g., ANA/RF+ or arthralgias/splenomegaly) for autoimmune disease
III/3	Interfollicular hyperplasia pattern of IgG4-R-LAD	AITL	"Water clear" lymphoma cells with T-follicular helper phenotype, *EBV*+ B-immunoblasts, and FDC meshwork bridging in AITL
IV/4	PTGC pattern of IgG4-R-LAD	NLPHL	Perifollicular granulomas surrounding PTGC are rare, but supposedly highly specific manifestation for IgG4-R-LAD
V/5	Inflammatory pseudotumor-like pattern of IgG4-R-LAD	Rosai-Dorfman-Destombes disease (RDD)	S100+/CD1a-negative histiocytes in RDD
		Inflammatory myofibroblastic tumor (IMT) and idiopathic intranodal pseudotumors	ALK IHC+ in IMT

76. As another typical entity that displays PC-rich LAD, what salient clinical and epidemiologic features does multicentric Castleman Disease disease (MCD) exhibit?

- Unicentric CD has been previously discussed (see Question 15).
- MCD is a heterogeneous, multisystemic disease [25, 68].
- Typically severe clinical manifestations due to excessive cytokine production, with serum IL-6 elevations, making MCD amenable to anti-IL-6 drug therapy (e.g., siltuximab, tocilizumab).
- Simplistic distinction in MCD is that of HHV8 status in histologically suggestive LN biopsies: HHV8-related (HHV8+ MCD) vs HHV8-negative (idiopathic MCD = iMCD).
- Clinical presentation similar for both HHV8+ MCD and iMCD:
  - Constitutional symptoms, severely ill.
  - Diffuse skin rash.
  - Polyclonal hypergammaglobulinemia.
  - Body cavity effusions.
  - Widespread lymphadenopathy.
  - Hepatosplenomegaly.
  - Cytopenias.
- HIV+ patients more commonly have HHV8+ MCD rather than iMCD.
- Conversely, iMCD patients are more commonly HIV-negative.

Table 18.21 presents international, evidence-based, consensus diagnostic criteria for HHV8-negative/idiopathic MCD [68].

- As seen in Table 18.21, MCD (whether HHV8-related or iMCD):
  - Is a sign-symptom complex.
  - Requires careful clinicopathologic and laboratory correlation.
  - Is a diagnosis of exclusion: other entities (infectious, autoimmune, neoplastic, etc.) that could simulate MCD must be systemically excluded before diagnosis can be made.
- Recently described paraneoplastic phenomena in patients with MCD include:
  - TAFRO syndrome
    - Acronym stands for **T**hrombocytopenia, **A**nasarca, bone marrow **F**ibrosis, **R**enal dysfunction, and **O**rganomegaly.
  - POEMS syndrome
    - Acronym for **P**olyneuropathy, **O**rganomegaly, **E**ndocrinopathy, **M**onoclonal gammopathy, **S**kin changes.
    - Paraneoplastic syndrome associated with plasma cell neoplasm, osteosclerosis, and frequent LAD with histologic features of plasma cell variant of Castleman disease

Table 18.21 Consensus diagnostic criteria for idiopathic multicentric Castleman disease (iMCD), HHV8-negative (Adapted from Fajgenbaum et al. *Blood* 2017 [68])

Major criteria (NEED BOTH)	Minor criteria (need at least 2 of 11 criteria with at least 1 laboratory criterion)	Exclusion criteria (must rule out each of these iMCD disease mimics)
Histopathologic LN features consistent with iMCD spectrum. Regressed/atrophic/atretic GCs with "onion skinning" mantle zones FDC prominence Vascularity often with prominent endothelium in interfollicular space and vessels penetrating GCs ("lollipop" sign) Sheetlike, polytypic interfollicular plasmacytosis Hyperplastic GCs	*Laboratory* 1. Elevated CRP 2. Anemia 3. Thrombocytopenia 4. Hypoalbuminemia 5. Renal dysfunction or proteinuria 6. Polyclonal hypergammaglobulinemia	*Malignant lymphoproliferative disorders* 1. Lymphoma 2. Multiple myeloma 3. Primary LN plasmacytoma 4. FDC sarcoma 5. POEMS syndrome
Enlarged LNs (≥1 cm in short axis diameter) in ≥2 LN stations	*Clinical* 1. Constitutional symptoms (night sweats, fever, weight loss, fatigue) 2. Large spleen and/or liver 3. Fluid accumulation: edema, anasarca, ascites, pleural effusion 4. Eruptive cherry hemangiomatosis or violaceous papules 5. Lymphocytic interstitial pneumonitis	*Autoimmune/autoinflammatory disorders* 1. SLE 2. RA 3. Adult-onset Still's disease 4. Juvenile idiopathic arthritis 5. Autoimmune lymphoproliferative syndrome *Infection Related Disorders* HHV8 *EBV*-lymphoproliferative disorders Inflammation and adenopathy caused by other uncontrolled infections

CRP = C-reactive protein, FDC = follicular dendritic cell; GC = germinal center; LN = lymph node; POEMS = polyneuropathy, organomegaly, endocrinopathy, monoclonal gammopathy, and skin changes; RA = rheumatoid arthritis; SLE = systemic lupus erythematosus

77. What are typical histologic and immunophenotypic findings in MCD?

- Most cases of iMCD closely parallel findings in HHV8+ MCD, with the obvious difference being lack of HHV8 positivity in iMCD.
- Characteristic histology is a morphologic spectrum of the following (Fig. 18.28):
  - Regressed/atrophic/atretic germinal centers with "onion skinning" mantle zones.
  - Vascularity often with prominent endothelium in interfollicular space and vessels penetrating germinal centers ("lollipop" sign).
  - Sheet-like, polytypic interfollicular plasmacytosis.
  - Follicular dendritic cell prominence.
  - Hyperplastic germinal centers.
  - Plasmablasts variably present along outer rim of lymphoid follicle (within mantle zone layers) → some cases show aggregates of plasmablasts, previously designated "microlymphomas."
- IHC:
  - Both iMCD and HHV8-related MCD share the following phenotype:
    - Sheets of plasma cells (PCs) with positivity for CD138, MUM1, cIgA, and polytypic light chain expression; PCs negative for cIgM and HHV8.
    - IgG4+ plasma cells can be increased (thus integration of all available data is necessary).
    - EBER ISH negative (in contrast: HHV8+ germinotrophic lymphoproliferative disorder, in which plasmablasts – partially or completely – efface germinal centers and are positive for both HHV8 and EBER ISH).
  - Staining is identical between HHV8+ MCD and iMCD except:
    - HHV8+MCD 'plasmablasts' can have the following phenotype:
      - HHV8 LANA1 positivity – stippled nuclear staining pattern
      - Lambda monotypic light chain expression
      - Strong cIgM
      - CD20+/−, CD138-, PAX5-, CD27-

78. What is the clinical relevance of misinterpretation of PC-rich LAD?

- Misinterpreting PC-rich LAD as lymphoma (see neoplastic DDx in Table 18.21):
  - Misdiagnosing PC-rich LAD entities like MCD, syphilitic LAD, and IgG4-R-LAD as cHL, AITL, B-cell lymphoma with plasmacytic differentiation, and

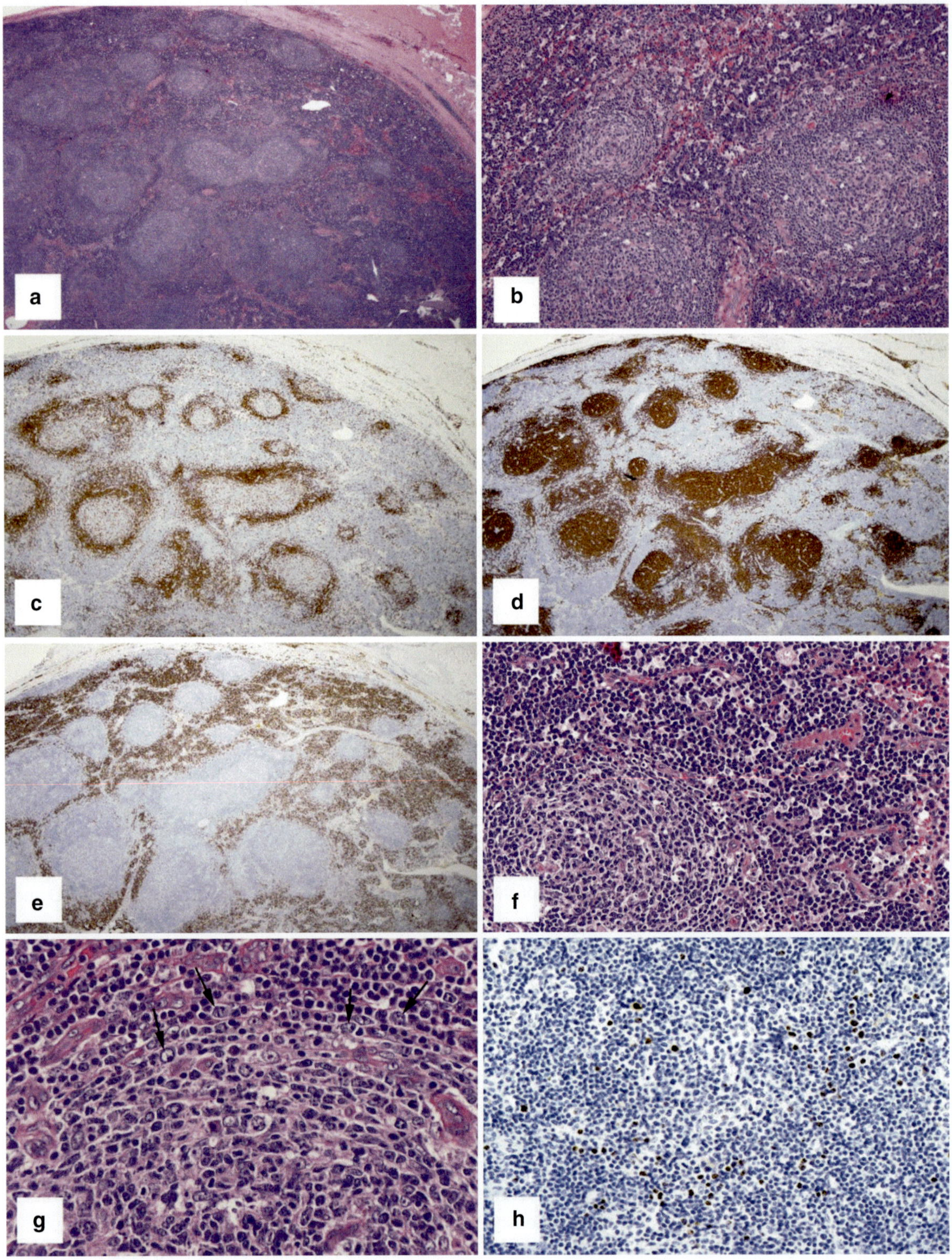

Fig. 18.28 HHV8-related multicentric Castleman disease. In this remarkable example of a PC-rich LAD, general preservation of nodal architecture is observed, with well-spaced lymphoid follicles (**a**). Two germinal centers appear to be encompassed by a single layer of mantle zone lymphocytes (so-called twinning). Intermediate magnification view shows three germinal centers, one of which is atretic/atrophic and displays "onion-skinning" (**b**), as well as a robust interfollicular plasmacytosis and vascular proliferation. CD3 (**c**) and CD20 (**d**) stains highlight the relative retention of normal nodal architecture, while CD138 staining underlines the exuberant plasmacytosis (**e**). Intermediate magnification once again highlights sheets of plasma cells in the interfollicular region (**f**); a "mottled" appearance is observed, due to scattered, yet frequent tingible body macrophages. Large transformed lymphocytes (plasmablasts/immunoblasts – arrows) are seen along the peripheral rim/mantle zone layers of the lymphoid follicle on this high magnification view (**g**). HHV8 immunostain highlights these plasmablasts (**h**), which also display lambda light chain restriction (not shown), in contrast to the polytypic expression of interfollicular plasma cells

nodal involvement of plasma cell neoplasm can lead to unwarranted chemotherapy and/or radiation treatment and additional morbidity/mortality.

- Not suggesting IgG4-RD as the correct reactive etiology for PC-rich LAD:
  - Results in diagnostic and treatment delays (e.g., not treating with corticosteroids/immunosuppressants) and/or leads to additional unnecessary biopsies:
    - Simulated patient example: Older male with multiple tumor-like lesions in nodal and extranodal sites, which have been diagnosed as polytypic plasma cell-rich infiltrates on excisional biopsies of salivary gland, meninges, and lymph nodes attributed to "chronic inflammation" → once again undergoing a repeat (4th) biopsy of lymph node to "rule out lymphoma"
- Not suggesting MCD as the correct reactive etiology for PC-rich LAD:
  - Unlikely scenario to miss MCD when there is close communication with treating physicians → because of the typically severe disease manifestations, clinicians usually eagerly inquire about these critically ill patients before H&E stains available to view.
  - Nevertheless, if histology is seen by the pathologist in isolation (with no provided clinical history), many other reactive conditions with MCD-like morphology could be entertained.

79. What information can be conveyed to the clinician in LAD with features of plasma cell-rich Castleman disease? When is a diagnostic comment necessary?

- If no clinical history is provided and HHV8 stain is negative:
  - Best to render a descriptive, rather than definitive, diagnosis, such as "Features of Castleman disease, plasma cell variant" with diagnostic comment.
  - Comment can raise the possibility of iMCD if multiple LNs are enlarged, but also explain that a broad range of other conditions can display and/or give rise to MCD-like morphology, including, but not limited to, SLE, IgG4-R-LAD, acute HIV and *EBV* infections, lymphomas, hemophagocytic lymphohistiocytosis, adult-onset Still's disease, autoimmune lymphoproliferative syndrome, etc [68]. Clinical correlation is mandatory.
- If clinical and histologic features of MCD are present, alongside HHV8 immunoreactivity:
  - Definitive diagnosis can be rendered: "Multicentric Castleman disease, HHV8-related"
  - Because of the potential severity of disease, it is prudent to have a discussion of implications of diagnosis with treating physician.

80. What is an adequate specimen in LAD with MCD-like histopathology?

- NCBx sampling is adequate if it contains sufficiently diagnostic material (like in the case of HHV8-related MCD).
- As with all reactive LAD, if clinical concern for malignancy persists and enlarged LN continues to grow and/or fails to regress, excisional biopsy should be recommended.

81. When is external consultation necessary in LAD with MCD-like histopathology?

- If correctly recognized, consultation is generally superfluous in this histologically distinctive reactive entity.
- However, consultation may be warranted if there is clinical and/or histologic concern for malignancy.

LAD with Prominent Spindle Cell Proliferation

82. What are the typical entities in the major subtype of LAD with prominent spindled cell proliferations?

- Distinct from the other reactive histologic patterns, this is a heterogeneous group of intranodal proliferations with spindled morphology yet varied (often non-hematopoietic) differentiation.
- Owing to their relative rarity, only a few are discussed briefly below.
- Table 18.22 lists infectious, non-infectious, and neoplastic DDx in this group [60, 69–73].
- Table 18.23 summarizes selected entities with spindled morphology and helpful diagnostic features to consider.

Table 18.22 Differential diagnosis of reactive nodal vascular/spindled proliferations and their neoplastic mimics

Infectious	Non-infectious	Neoplastic mimics
Mycobacterial spindle cell pseudotumor Bacillary angiomatosis (*Bartonella* spp.) MCD, HHV8+	Vascular transformation of sinuses Angiomyomatous hamartoma Palisaded myofibroblastoma Inflammatory pseudotumor IgG4-R-LAD (inflammatory-pseudotumor-like pattern)	Kaposi sarcoma Angiosarcoma Metastatic sarcomatoid carcinoma Metastatic sarcoma Follicular dendritic cell and interdigitating cell sarcoma

Table 18.23 Summary table of select nodal spindle cell/vascular proliferations and useful diagnostic features

	Proliferation	Clinical/radiologic	Differentiation	Histology: Architecture and localization within LN	Histology: Cellular Composition	Special stains and/or IHC (*italicized* stain = unique to entity)	Most useful diagnostic features (*italicized* = unique to entity)
Infectious	Bacillary angiomatosis	Exposure to cats: *Bartonella* infection	Vascular proliferation secondary to infection	Multinodular growth Vascular proliferation	Bland appearing, epithelioid endothelium Neutrophils +	*Bartonella* +	*Warthin-Starry + Serologic titers and PCR for Bartonella +*
	Mycobacterial spindle cell pseudotumor	HIV and Immunocompromised individuals; MAC infections	Histiocytic proliferation with spindled appearance due to MAC	Multinodular growth Storiform pattern	Spindled histiocytes	AFB+, PAS +	*AFB, PAS; AFB microbiologic cultures*
Non-infectious proliferation	Vascular transformation of sinuses	Concurrent malignancy (LN draining malignancy) or thrombotic region	Lymphatic and vascular	Subcapsular and medullary LN sinuses with prominent anastomosing vessels	Bland-appearing endothelial cells	ERG+, WT-1+, Factor VIII+, CD31+, CD34+, HHV8-	*Morphology*
	Idiopathic inflammatory pseudotumor	Unknown etiology; infectious etiology in small subset	Reactive inflammatory process with fibroblastic reticulum cells or histiocytes	Storiform pattern	Mixed inflammatory infiltrate Neutrophils +/−	Vimentin+, SMA+/−, CD68+/−	*Small vessel proliferation with luminal obliteration*
	Angiomyomatous hamartoma	Painful inguinal LAD	Benign smooth muscle and vascular proliferation	Intraparenchymal, haphazard smooth muscle fibers a/w vessels	Bland appearing cytology in vessels and smooth muscle	SMA+, Desmin +/−, D2–40+, HMB-45−	*Smooth muscle stains+* *Ruling out PEComa*
Neoplastic	Kaposi sarcoma, node based	HIV/AIDS patient	Malignant HHV8-related neoplasm	Multinodular growth Capsular-based lesion	Cytologic atypia, intracytoplasmic hyaline globules	*HHV8+*	*HHV8+, atypia, capsular involvement*
	Lymphangioleiomyoma	Females Some have tuberous sclerosis complex and other PEComa-type lesions	Belongs to Perivascular epithelioid cell tumor (PEComa) family	Extranodal extension, subcapsular localization, intralymphatic growth, branching lymphatic channels,	Plump cell shape, foamy cytoplasm	*SMA*+, Desmin +/−, D2–40+, *HMB-45*+, S100+, Cathepsin *K*+, *MiTF*	*Immunoreactivity with both smooth muscle and melanocytic markers*
	Metastatic sarcomatoid carcinoma	H/O known primary carcinoma	Epithelial malignancy	Variable focal to diffuse LN involvement	Cytologic atypia, increased mitotic activity	*Pancytokeratin*+, *EMA*+	*IHC, cytologic atypia, mitotic figures*
	Metastatic melanoma with spindled morphology	H/O known primary melanoma	Melanocytic malignancy	Variable focal to diffuse LN involvement	Cytologic atypia, increased mitotic activity	*S100+, HMB45+, Melan-A+, Mart-1+*	*IHC, cytologic atypia*
	Follicular dendritic cell sarcoma		FDC malignancy	Storiform pattern	Slight atypia	*CD21+, CD23+, CD35+*	*IHC, admixed small lymphocytes*
	Palisaded myofibroblastoma	Rare Localized, painful LAD Typically inguinal LN	Benign smooth muscle and vascular proliferation	Diffuse effacement with hemorrhagic foci	Spindled cells palisading around an eosinophilic collagenous center (so called amianthoid fibers)	*Beta-catenin*+, cyclin D1, SMA+, Vimentin +, FXIII+ Desmin−, S100−, FVIII−	*Amianthoid fibers, smooth muscle stains+*

83. What are some selected entities displaying spindled morphology and how does one establish their diagnosis?

- Mycobacterial spindle cell pseudotumor (Fig. 18.29a, b)
  - Mycobacterial infection, usually of *Mycobacterium avium-intracellulare* complex.
  - Histiocyte-rich proliferation exhibiting uncommon pseudosarcomatous morphology, with spindled, elongated macrophages with bland oval nuclei and abundant clear cytoplasm.
  - As with other MAI infections, the patients affected are typically immunocompromised (most commonly with HIV/AIDS).
  - Diagnostic work-up identical to mycobacterial infections with histiocytic-rich morphology, discussed previously (see Question 54).
  - Treatment with antimycobacterial and/or antimicrobial drugs (like clarithromycin, ethambutol, streptomycin, etc.) effective.
- Vascular transformation of sinuses (Fig. 18.29c, d)
  - Benign vasoproliferation whereby LN sinuses are "transformed" from simple vascular channels into complex, anastomosing lymphovascular, endothelial-lined channels.
  - Typically incidental finding in staging lymph nodes for malignancy, most often in abdomen.
  - Histology:
    - Four architectural patterns described: cleft-like spaces (most common), rounded vascular channels, solid foci of spindled cells interspersed with collagen, and plexiform patterns.
    - Cytologically bland spindled vessels distending sinuses.
    - No capsular involvement nor cytologic atypia (compared to Kaposi sarcoma).
  - IHC
    - Positive for SMA, vimentin, ERG, WT1, CD31 (most cases +), CD34 (subset of cases +)
    - Negative for HHV8 (unlike Kaposi sarcoma)
  - Excision curative.
- Palisaded myofibroblastoma (Fig. 18.29e, f)
  - Benign smooth muscle and vascular neoplasm.
  - Very rare tumor with male predominance.
  - Localized, painful inguinal LN.
  - Also referred to as "intranodal hemorrhagic spindled proliferation with amianthoid fibers."
  - Histology:
    - Cytologically bland spindled cells with fascicular, storiform growth.
    - Hemorrhagic foci common, with extravasated RBCs between spindled cells.
    - Amianthoid fibers = morphologically distinct nodules with centrally acellular core of fine, eosinophilic, radially projecting collagen fibers palisaded by cytologically bland spindled nuclei.
    - Bears histologic resemblance to schwannoma.
  - IHC:
    - Positive for beta catenin, cyclin D1, and smooth muscle markers (SMA, desmin, caldesmon).
    - Negative for S100 (unlike schwannoma).
  - Excision curative.
- Angiomyomatous hamartoma (AMH) (Fig. 18.30a–e)
  - Benign smooth muscle and vascular proliferation.
  - Extensive intraparenchymal localization, with involvement of medulla and cortex.
  - No subcapsular nor extracapsular extension.
  - Long-standing inguinal LAD, typically in males.
  - Histology:
    - Variably sized thick-walled blood vessels embedded in collagenous stroma.
    - Haphazard arrangement of smooth muscle cells intimately associated with vessels.
    - Bland, elongated spindled cells without atypia.
  - IHC:
    - Muscular component positive for smooth muscle markers (SMA, desmin, etc.).
    - Vascular component positive for CD31, CD34.
    - Negative for melanocytic markers (HMB-45, MiTF, cathepsin K), unlike lymphangioleiomyomatosis (a PEComa).
  - Treatment with surgical excision, though some cases of recurrence reported.
- Inflammatory pseudotumor (IPT) (Fig. 18.30f)
  - Benign inflammatory reaction to different postulated infectious antigens, though most commonly idiopathic.
  - Histology:
    - Pale-staining stromal proliferation localized to capsule, trabecula, and hilum.
    - Can have storiform growth pattern.
    - Mixed inflammatory infiltrate includes plasma cells (variable in number and can be quite numerous), eosinophils, histiocytes, and small lymphocytes.
    - Vascular proliferation presents with occasional obliteration of lumina.
    - Vasculitis common.
    - When lymphoid architecture still present, reactive follicular hyperplasia can be prominent.
    - No cytologic atypia, increased mitotic activity, or necrosis.
  - IHC/ancillary studies:
    Positive for myoid markers (desmin, SMA)
    Negative for S100, CD31, CD34, ALK (unlike ALK immunoreactivity in 50% of inflammatory myofibroblastic tumors)
    No evidence of clonality
  - IPT morphology should also raise the possibilities of IPT-like variants/patterns in syphilitic lymphadenitis,

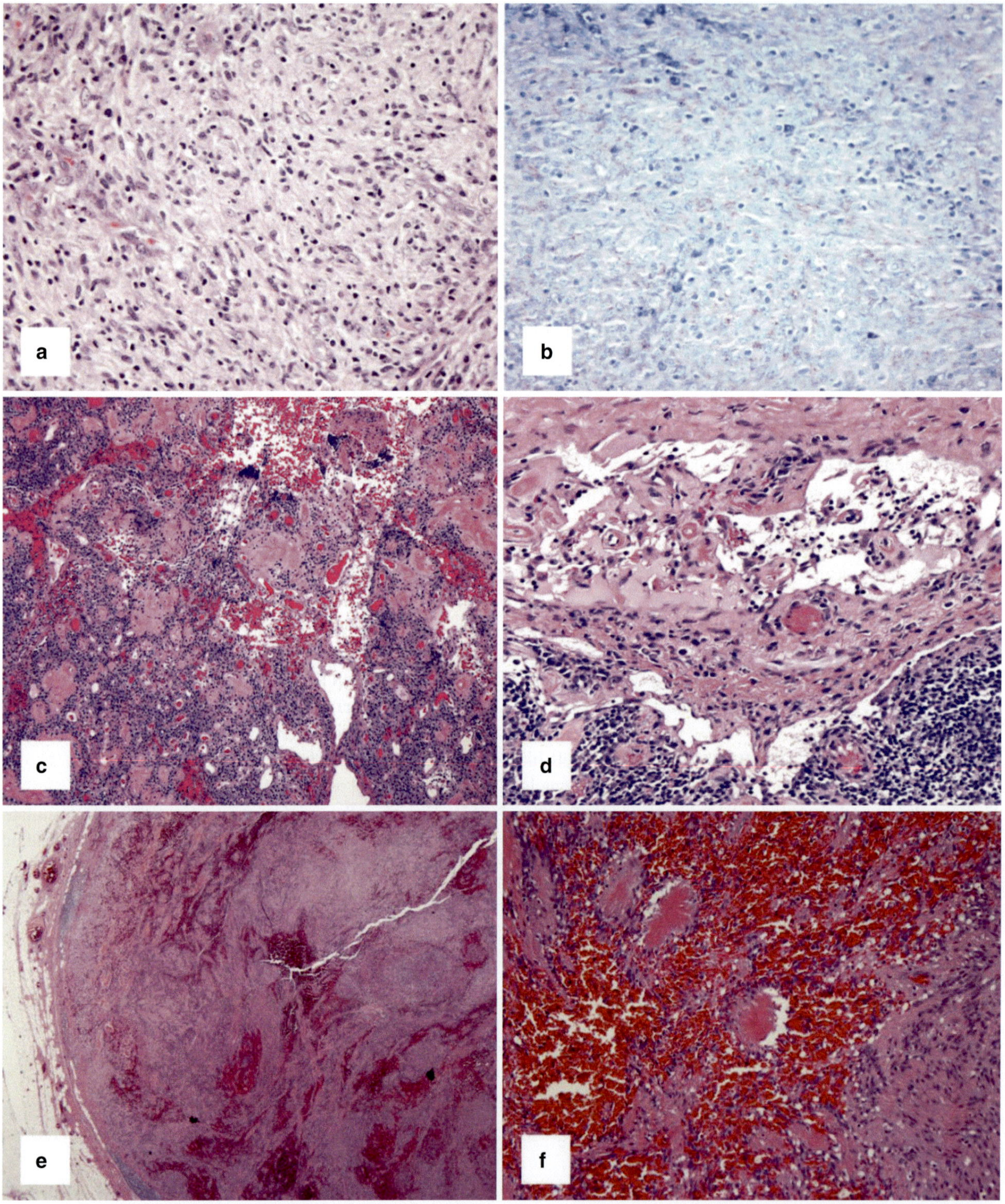

Fig. 18.29 Vascular/stromal nodal proliferations, part 1: Mycobacterial spindle cell pseudotumor (**a**, **b**; courtesy of Dr. D. O'Malley), vascular transformation of sinuses (**c**, **d**), and palisaded myofibroblastoma (**e**, **f**; courtesy of Dr. D. O'Malley). A fibroblastic-appearing pseudosarcomatous proliferation, mycobacterial spindle cell pseudotumor can efface nodal architecture (**a**); it is composed of CD163+ histiocytes (not shown) with elongated nuclei and copious pale eosinophilic cytoplasm. AFB stain (**b**) reveals the abundance of acid-fast bacilli diagnostic for this entity. Photomicrographs for (**c**) and (**d**) show an example of vascular transformation of sinuses, wherein nodal sinuses are "transformed" into complex, anastomosing, endothelial-lined lymphovascular channels. The cells are cytologically bland and frequently involve subcapsular and medullary sinuses, but without capsular extension. Palisaded myofibroblastoma is occasionally referred to as intranodal benign hemorrhagic spindle cell tumor with amianthoid fibers, and these photomicrographs (**e**, **f**) display all elements of this name to spectacular fashion. Note the characteristic amianthoid fibers (striking eosinophilic nodules with acellular cores with radially projecting filaments and palisading bland spindled nuclei) as well as the hemorrhagic nature of this proliferation (**f**). It is reminiscent of schwannoma; however, it lacks S-100 staining and instead exhibits positivity for beta-catenin and cyclin D1 (not shown)

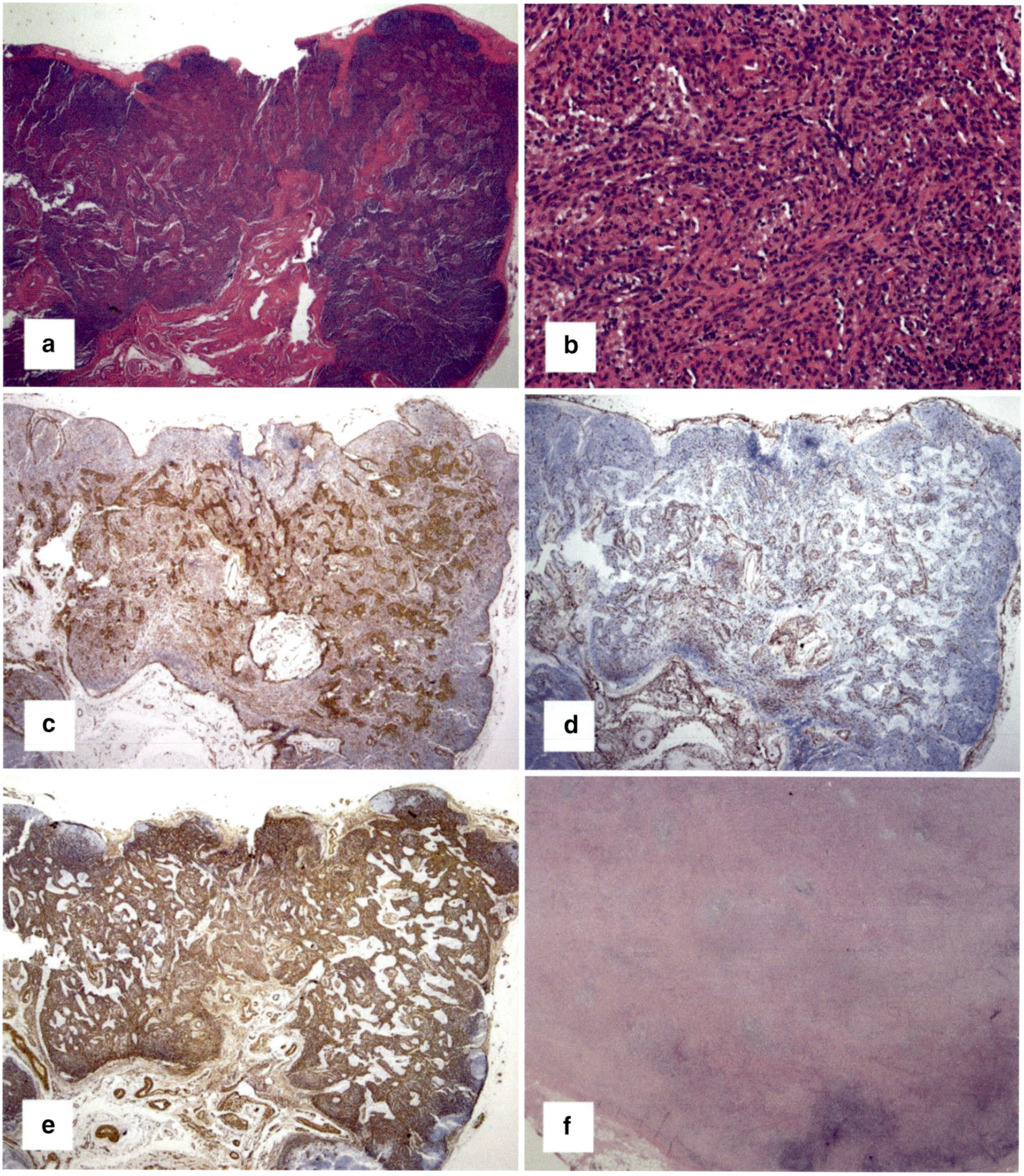

Fig. 18.30 Vascular/stromal nodal proliferations, part 2: Angiomyomatous hamartoma (**a–e**) and nodal inflammatory pseudotumor (**f**; courtesy of Dr. D. O'Malley). An extensive stromal/vascular proliferation occupying >80% of the nodal parenchyma (**a**), this angiomyomatous hamartoma (AMH) exhibits numerous variably sized, thickened blood vessels in collagenous stroma, with closely associated smooth muscle cells (**b**), as confirmed immunohistochemically by uniform SMA positivity (**e**). Though widespread, AMH does not display extracapsular invasion, subcapsular involvement, nor cytologic atypia. The lymphovascular elements are highlighted by CD31 (**c**) and CD34 (**d**) expression. Another example of stromal/vascular proliferation is an intranodal inflammatory pseudotumor (**f**) which is composed of pale eosinophilic spindled stromal cells with an admixture of variable numbers of plasma cells, lymphocytes, and eosinophils. This benign proliferation would exhibit positivity for vimentin, SMA, and/or CD68, but would lack ALK staining (not shown)

IgG4-related lymphadenopathy, and rheumatoid arthritis

Diagnostic work-up should address these possibilities.

- Complete excision curative

84. What is the clinical relevance of misinterpretation in this group of intranodal vascular/spindled cell proliferations?

- Misinterpreting benign entities for malignancy (see neoplastic DDx in Tables 18.22 and 18.23):
  - Misdiagnosing benign spindled proliferations as sarcomas and other malignancies (e.g., sarcomatoid carcinoma) can lead to unwarranted chemotherapy and/or radiation treatment and additional morbidity/mortality.
- Not suggesting the correct reactive etiology for vascular/spindled cell proliferation:
  - May not be as clinically devastating as misdiagnosis of lymphoma.
  - However, significant morbidity may result in diagnostic and treatment delays and/or lead to additional unnecessary biopsies (e.g., in IgG4-related LAD).
    - As an example, if other entities that show IPT-like morphology have not been considered (like IPT-like variant of syphilitic LAD or undiagnosed rheumatoid arthritis), potential for missed opportunity for appropriate patient management.

85. When is consultation necessary in LAD with prominent spindled proliferation?

- Owing to their relative rarity, consultation with colleagues and/or expert consultants would be prudent to ensure accurate diagnosis, particularly in difficult-to-classify proliferations (i.e., whether proliferation has malignant potential).

Case Presentations

Case 1

Learning Objectives

1. To recognize the presence of multiple pathologic findings in an individual sample.
2. To increase awareness of co-existing disorders in patients with HIV/AIDS.
3. To initiate the appropriate work-up for a nodal spindled/vascular proliferation based on histologic features.

Case History

A 25-year-old man with HIV presents with multiple enlarged non-tender cervical LNs. He complains of fevers, night sweats, fatigue, and unintentional 20 lb. weight loss, within the past 3–4 months. FNA and NCBx performed 2 months prior to current presentation were insufficient. He now undergoes excisional LN biopsy.

Histologic Findings (Fig. 18.31a–e)

- Cellular region with several widely spaced, enlarged, and highly proliferative lymphoid follicles with attenuated mantle zones (florid follicular hyperplasia).
- Another region shows marked lymphoid depletion, with only scattered lymphoid follicles.
- Follicles separated by broad dense, collagenous bands.
- Widespread stromal/vascular proliferation with extension from capsule to trabecular and medullary regions.
- On high power, stromal/vascular proliferation shows numerous vascular channels with mild nuclear atypia. Channels contain many red blood cells. Occasional complex vessels demonstrate intracytoplasmic hyaline globules.

Differential Diagnosis

- Mixed stages of HIV-related LAD, with areas of florid RFH and lymphoid depletion
- HHV8-related multicentric Castleman disease
- Burkitt lymphoma, focal
- Classic Hodgkin lymphoma (because of broad dense collagenous bands)
- Vascular transformation of sinuses
- Kaposi sarcoma
- Inflammatory pseudotumor
- Luetic lymphadenitis

IHC and Other Ancillary Studies

- No HRS cells highlighted by CD30, CD15, and PAX5
- HHV8 positivity confined to abnormal spindled/vascular proliferation, negative in lymphoid component (Fig. 18.31f)
- *Treponema* stain negative for spirochetes

Final Histopathologic Diagnosis

- **Kaposi sarcoma**
- **Areas of florid reactive follicular hyperplasia and lymphoid depletion**

Diagnostic Comment

"The combined findings are diagnostic of HIV/AIDS-associated lymphadenopathy."

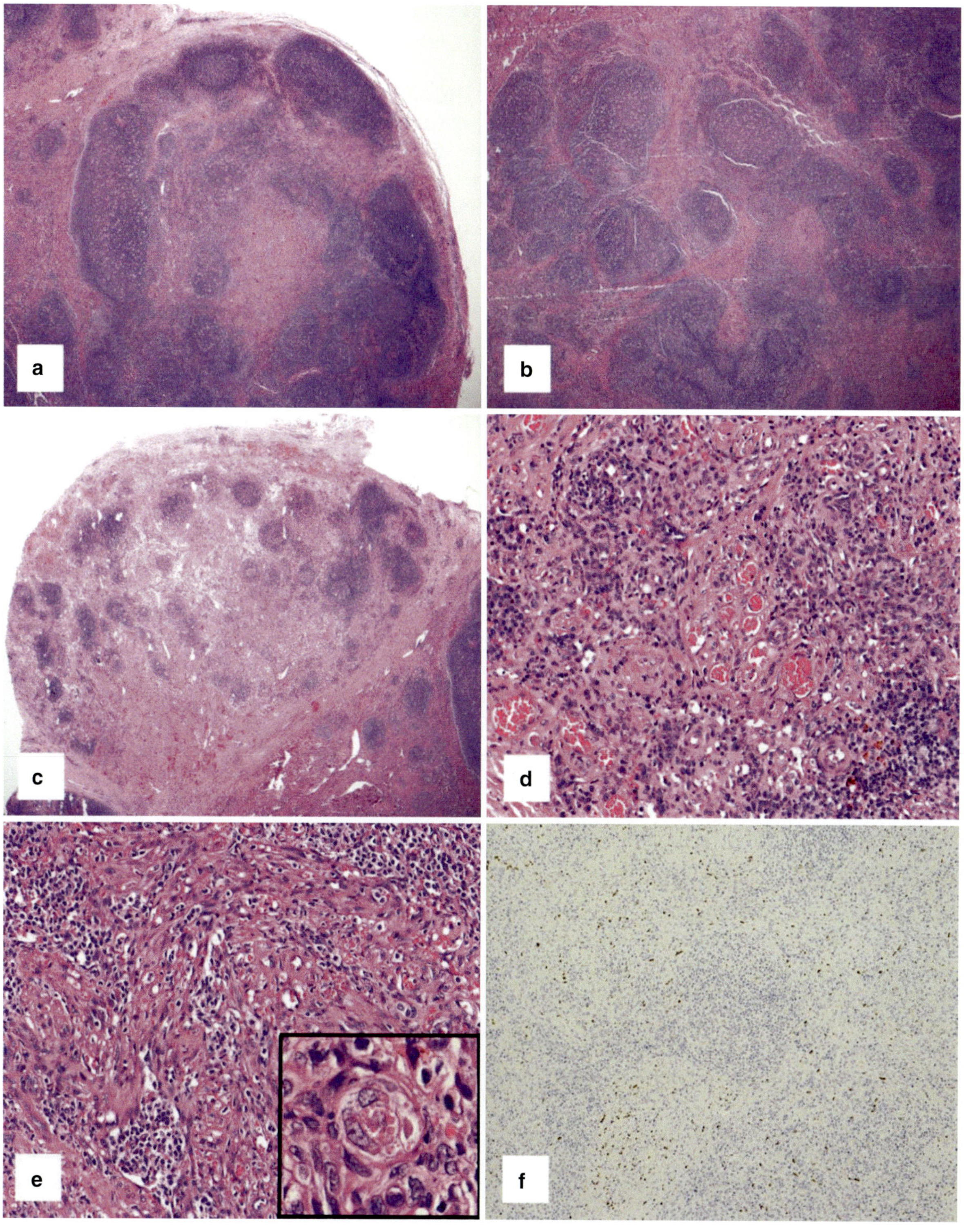

Fig. 18.31 Case 1. This markedly enlarged LN displays several areas of interest. Both (**a**) and (**b**) exhibit florid reactive follicular hyperplasia (FRFH), with variably sized hyperplastic follicles, some that are fairly enlarged. Despite FRFH, however, the interfollicular zones contain dense fibrosis. An ill-defined central vascular proliferation is also notable in (**a**). This photomicrograph view is interesting (**c**) because of striking interfollicular lymphoid depletion, representing markedly diminished T-cells, yet retention of nodal architecture with small, well-spaced B-lymphoid follicles. Multiple foci of ill-defined vascularity are noted (visible on low magnification by dilated vessels containing numerous red blood cells), particularly around the medulla with extension into the nodal capsule. Many plasma cells can be seen (**d**). The vascular proliferation is characterized by numerous back-to-back, slit-like vessels with cytologic atypia, extravasated red blood cells (**d**, **e**), and eosinophilic hyaline globules [inset for (**e**)]. HHV8 staining is positive solely in the vascular proliferation, confirming the morphologic impression of Kaposi sarcoma (**f**). No additional HHV8 staining was seen in the lymphoid component. Thus, this case illustrates HIV/AIDS-related LAD with concurrent nodal Kaposi sarcoma

Take-Home Messages

1. Be vigilant about other pathologic findings, such as malignancy and/or opportunistic infections, particularly in HIV/AIDS patients.
2. LN pathology may exhibit different stages of disease evolution.

Case 2

Learning Objectives

1. To recognize the presence of mixed features in a reactive lymphoid hyperplasia.
2. To be familiar with histopathologic characteristics of IgG4-related LAD.
3. To initiate appropriate work-up for a nodal follicular hyperplasia with PTGC and plasmacytosis based on histologic features.

Case History

A 60-year-old man presents with an 8-year history of persistent/recurrent inguinal lymphadenopathy, and recent demonstration of multistation adenopathy (including cervical, axillary, retroperitoneal, and inguinal lymph nodes). Although he discloses swelling in his inguinal region, he does not report severe constitutional symptoms (i.e. he does not complain of fevers, night sweats, fatigue, etc). Prior needle core biopsies of lymph node reported from another institution showed reactive follicular hyperplasia, focal PTGC, and no immunophenotypic evidence of lymphoma. The patient undergoes an excisional biopsy of inguinal LN.

Excisional Biopsy Histologic Findings (Figs. 18.32 and 18.33a)

- Widely spaced lymphoid follicles, indicating nodal architectural preservation.
- Secondary lymphoid follicles display polarization and preserved mantle zones.
- Progressive transformation of germinal centers.
- Marked plasmacytosis, within germinal centers and interfollicular regions.
- Perifollicular granulomas.
- Tissue eosinophilia.
- Capsular fibrosis with frequent plasma cells.
- Obliterative vasculitis.

Differential Diagnosis

- IgG4-related lymphadenopathy
- Syphilitic lymphadenitis
- *Toxoplasma* LAD and other infection inciting granulomas
- Autoimmune lymphadenopathy, including SLE, RA, adult-onset Still's disease
- Multicentric Castleman disease, HHV8-related or HHV8-negative (iMCD)
- RFH due to bacterial or viral infections, drug/chemical exposures, vs unknown etiology

IHC and Other Ancillary Studies (Fig. 18.33b–f)

- CD3 and CD20 highlight nodal architectural preservation. CD138, kappa, lambda demonstrate exuberant polytypic plasmacytosis (not shown)
- IgD underscores PTGC.
- IgG and IgG4 show significantly increased IgG4+ plasma cells in many "hot spots," including within germinal centers, PTGC, and perifollicular granulomas.
- Treponema IHC negative (not shown).
- AFB, GMS, Warthin-Starry stains negative (not shown).

Final Clinicopathologic Integrated Diagnosis

Reactive lymphoid hyperplasia with significantly increased IgG4+ plasma cells

Diagnostic Comment

"In the setting of systemic lymphadenopathy, the histopathologic findings are more likely to represent IgG4-R-LAD. Correlation with serologic IgG4 and IgE levels is advised. Consultation with Rheumatology and clinical follow-up are strongly recommended, as some patients may develop subsequent extranodal involvement by IgG4-RD."

Take-Home Messages

1. Histologic pattern/variants in IgG4-related lymphadenopathy (IgG4-RL): interfollicular eosinophilia admixed with polytypic plasmacytosis, PTGC, RFH with intragerminal plasma cells, multicentric Castleman disease-like foci, IPT-like morphology.
2. Features that should prompt more thorough investigation for IgG4-RL: adult male >50 years of age and elevated serum IgG4 and IgE levels.
3. Because of focality of disease, IgG4-R-LAD may be missed on NCBx; if clinical suspicion is high, advocate for excisional biopsy of LN and/or other affected tumefactive extranodal site (like salivary gland, etc.) to provide histologic support for diagnosis.
4. Promote clinical follow-up with physician specialist who has training/expertise in treating patients IgG4-RD (like rheumatologists) to ensure appropriate management.

Case 3

Learning Objectives

1. To generate DDx for LAD with prominent IFH/DH histology.
2. To use pertinent clinical information and laboratory data to arrive at the best possible integrated diagnosis.

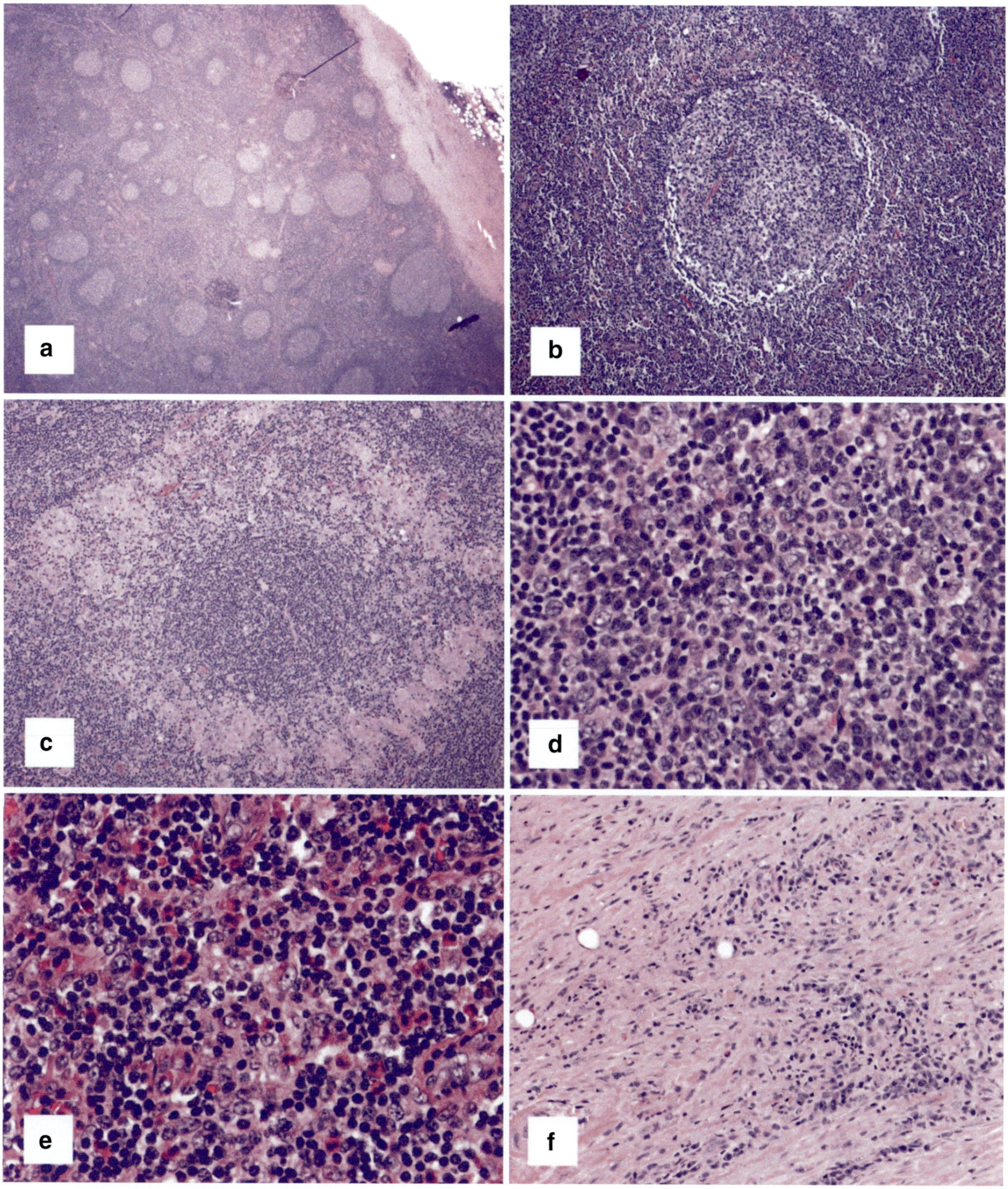

Fig. 18.32 Case 2, part 1 – H&E photomicrographs. Nodal enlargement in this case is characterized by reactive follicular hyperplasia and interfollicular expansion; capsular fibrosis is also evident (**a**). A focus of PTGC is noted (**b**). Unusual perifollicular granulomas (i.e., epithelioid histiocytes rimming germinal center) are apparent in (**c**). This germinal center contains numerous plasma cells (**d**). Tissue eosinophilia is present in this photomicrograph (**e**); note that eosinophils are also increased in (**c**), particularly around the perifollicular granulomas. High magnification view of the capsule reveals significant plasma cell infiltration (**f**). These aggregate should trigger work-up for a plasma cell and histiocyte-rich LAD

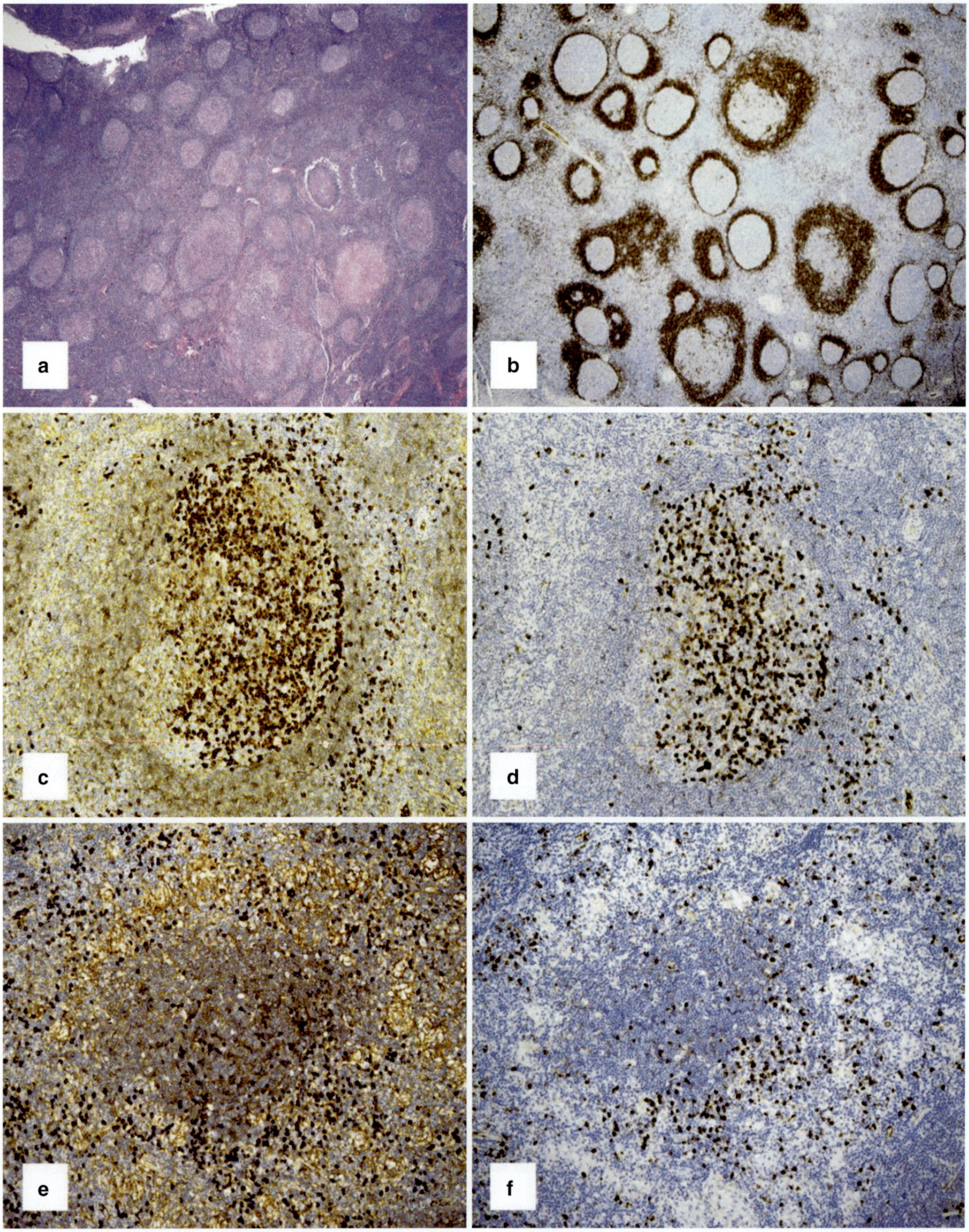

Fig. 18.33 Case 2, part 2 – select slides of IHC work-up. H&E photomicrograph displays follicular hyperplasia, PTGC, as well as obliterative vasculitis, with a deeply sclerotic pale pink nodule along the lower right-hand side (**a**). The histologic findings (RFH, obliterative vasculitis, plasmacytosis, capsular fibrosis), thus far, should prompt performance of *Treponema* IHC stain; this was negative (not shown). Low magnification view of IgD stain (**b**), highlighting several follicles with PTGC, whereby IgD+ mantle zone lymphocytes invade into the germinal centers. Paired IgG and IgG4 stains on a lymphoid follicle with intragerminal plasma cells (**c** and **d**, respectively) and follicle with perifollicular granulomas (**e** and **f**, respectively). Note that the numbers of IgG4+ plasma cells are nearly as high as IgG+ plasma cells. The overall findings are immunomorphologically compatible with IgG4-R-LAD, given supportive clinical and laboratory data

Case History

- HPI: A 40-year-old woman presents with a 2-month history of fevers, chills, skin rash, joint pains, and 10 lb. unintentional weight loss. Physical examination revealed palpable lymphadenopathy and splenomegaly.
- Pertinent laboratory data: WBC 20 × 10^3/mm^3 with neutrophilia (90% neutrophils; ANC 18 × 10^3/mm^3) and abnormally elevated AST and ALT values.
- She undergoes excision of an enlarged (3 × 2 × 1 cm) supraclavicular lymph node.

Histologic Findings (Fig. 18.34a–d)

- Extensive paracortical to diffuse hyperplasia with focal preservation of nodal architecture.
- "Mottling" secondary to scattered tingible body macrophages (resembling "starry sky" in Burkitt lymphoma).
- High magnification views in many areas show polymorphous admixture of small lymphocytes, histiocytes, plasma cells, and scattered immunoblasts.
- Focal high-power view with more prominent immunoblastic proliferation, high mitotic activity.

Differential Diagnosis Based on H&E Findings

- Viral lymphadenitides (like *EBV*-infectious mononucleosis, HIV/AIDS-related LAD, etc)
- Autoimmune disorder
- Non-Hodgkin lymphoma

IHC and Other Ancillary Studies (Figs. 18.34e, f and 18.35)

- Nodal architectural preservation by CD3, CD20, CD21
- Scattered CD30+ immunoblasts with an admixture of CD3+ T- and CD20+ B-immunoblasts
- Intermediate to high proliferation rate by Ki-67
  - Clonality studies for B-cell and T-cell receptor rearrangements negative for clonality

Final Histopathologic Diagnosis

Reactive paracortical/interfollicular hyperplasia
No evidence of malignancy

Diagnostic Comment

"Histologic findings are relatively nonspecific for etiology. However, given the significant clinical history and laboratory data, the features raise concern for lymphadenopathy secondary to an autoimmune disorder, such as adult-onset Still's disease. Consultation with Rheumatology service is strongly recommended."

Take-Home Messages

1. Although initially worrisome on H&E sections, demonstration of nodal architectural preservation by FDC markers and admixture of B- and T-immunoblasts favors reactive etiology.
2. Often, a specific diagnosis for reactive LAD cannot be rendered on histologic examination alone. However, indicating the absence of malignancy can be quite helpful to the managing/treating physician.
3. Additional value can be added by the pathologist if pathologic findings are integrated with clinical and laboratory data to narrow down a rather broad differential diagnostic list.

Case 4

Learning Objectives

1. To generate DDx and appropriate work-up for LAD with suppurative granulomas.
2. To aid treating physicians in pursuing pertinent clinical information, laboratory data, and ancillary testing to arrive at the best possible integrated diagnosis.

Case History

A 15-year-old immigrant boy from El Salvador presents with a 3-week history of fever, fatigue, and multiple enlarged and tender cervical lymph nodes. He undergoes a needle core biopsy of one of the affected LNs.

Histologic Findings (Fig. 18.36a–c)

- Geographic necrosis with neutrophil-rich infiltrate, necrobiosis, surrounded by epithelioid macrophages (stellate granuloma).
- Histiocytic/epithelioid macrophage border is surrounded by many plasma cells.

Differential Diagnosis

- Bacterial infections such as cat-scratch disease, LGV, etc.
- Classic Hodgkin lymphoma with extensive necrosis.
- *Toxoplasma* lymphadenitis.

IHC and Other Ancillary Studies (Fig. 18.36d, e)

- CD3 and CD20 show nodal architectural preservation.
- GMS and AFB stains negative for organisms (not shown).
- Warthin-Starry and Gram stains negative for bacteria, despite careful search (not shown).

Histologic Diagnosis and Comment on Needle Core Biopsy

Necrotizing/suppurative lymphadenitis

Diagnostic Comment

"Special stains for AFB, GMS, Warthin-Starry, and Gram did not uncover organisms in histologic sections. However, inability to highlight organisms by special stains does not imply absence of infection. In this case, suppurative granulo-

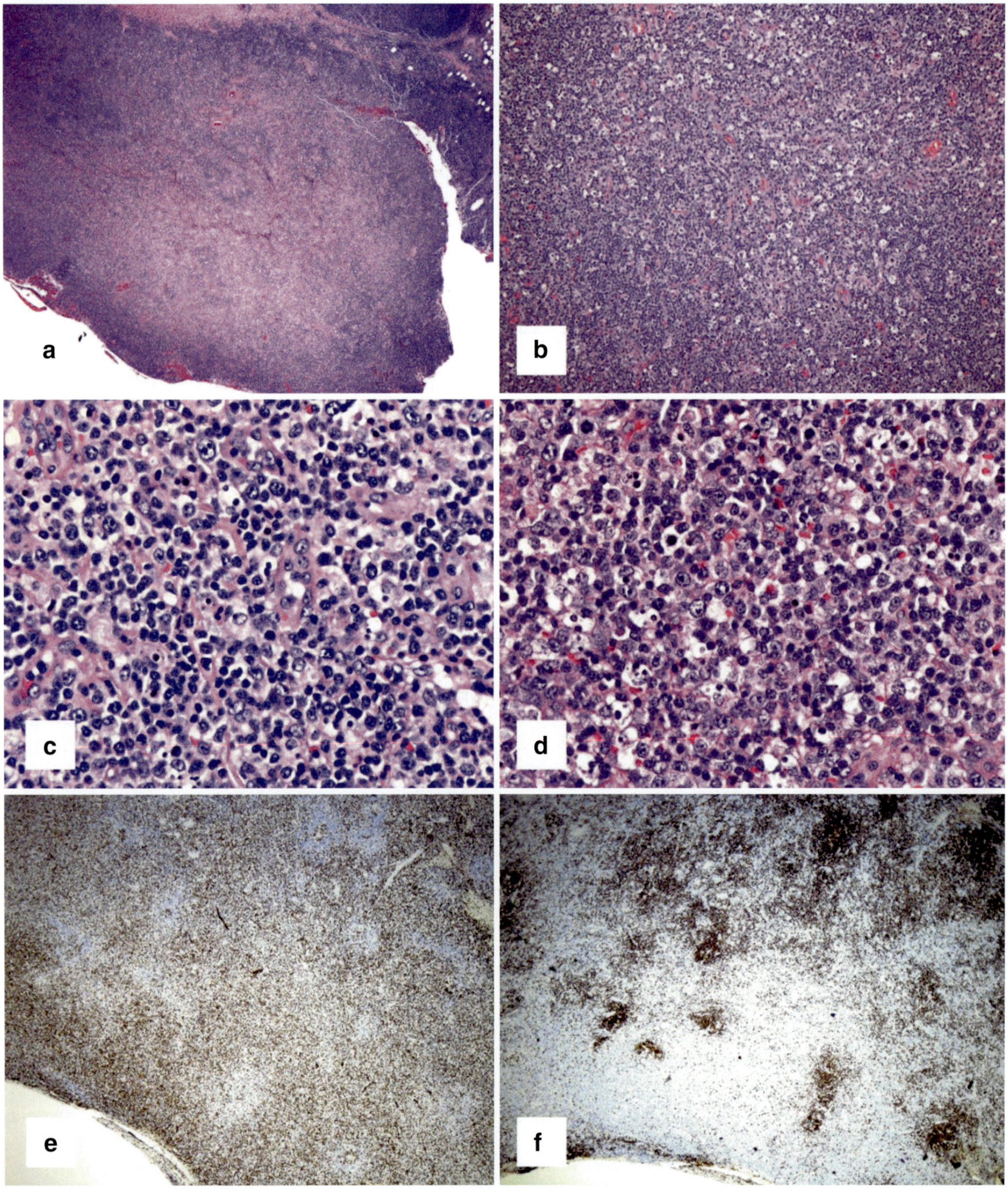

Fig. 18.34 Case 3, part 1 [courtesy of Dr. R. K. Brynes]. A striking interfollicular to diffuse proliferation is observed; rare scattered lymphoid follicles are detected, though subtle (**a**). This intermediate-power view (**b**) features a "mottled" appearance due to increased numbers of tingible body macrophages, reminiscent of the oft-mentioned "starry sky" pattern associated with Burkitt lymphoma. This region (**c**) displays a polymorphous mixture of small lymphocytes, histiocytes, plasma cells, and scattered immunoblasts (large transformed lymphocytes), a finding that is reassuring and would favor a reactive process. Rare foci with more prominent increase in immunoblasts are seen and would likely raise concern for lymphoma (**d**). Fortunately, subsequent IHC staining is helpful in suggesting a reactive etiology, as demonstrated by nodal architectural preservation by CD3 (**e**) and CD20 (**f**)

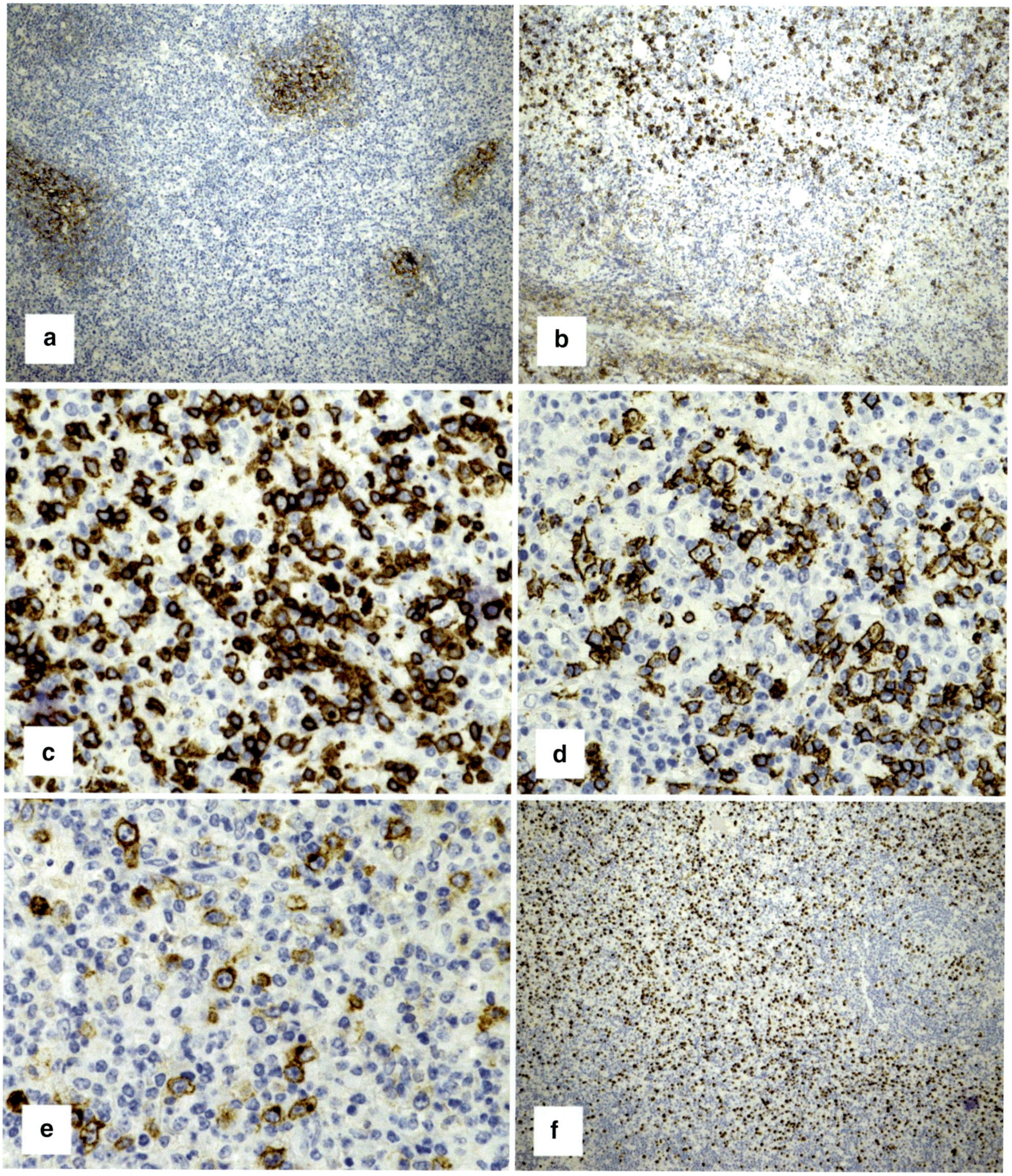

Fig. 18.35 Case 3 [courtesy of Dr. R. K. Brynes]. CD21 stain shows intact follicular dendritic cell networks that are largely confined to lymphoid follicles (**a**), making a diagnosis of angioimmunoblastic T-cell lymphoma (AITL) unlikely. Scattered CD138+ plasma cells are highlighted (**b**). The composition of lymphocytes are revealed to be more T- than B-cells, with an admixture of T- and B-immunoblasts on CD3 (**c**) and CD20 (**d**) stains, respectively. CD30 also serves to highlight predominantly mononuclear immunoblasts, and show variable weak to intense positivity (**e**), unlike the intense and uniform staining expected from binucleated Hodgkin/Reed-Sternberg cells. Despite the non-neoplastic nature of this LAD, Ki-67 reveals a high proliferation rate (**f**): a reminder that not a single finding (such as high Ki-67 staining) should determine a diagnosis of malignancy. PCR studies for B-cell and T-cell receptor gene rearrangements proved to be negative for clonality. Appropriate clinical history and laboratory work-up revealed this case to represent the atypical paracortical hyperplasia pattern of adult-onset Still's disease

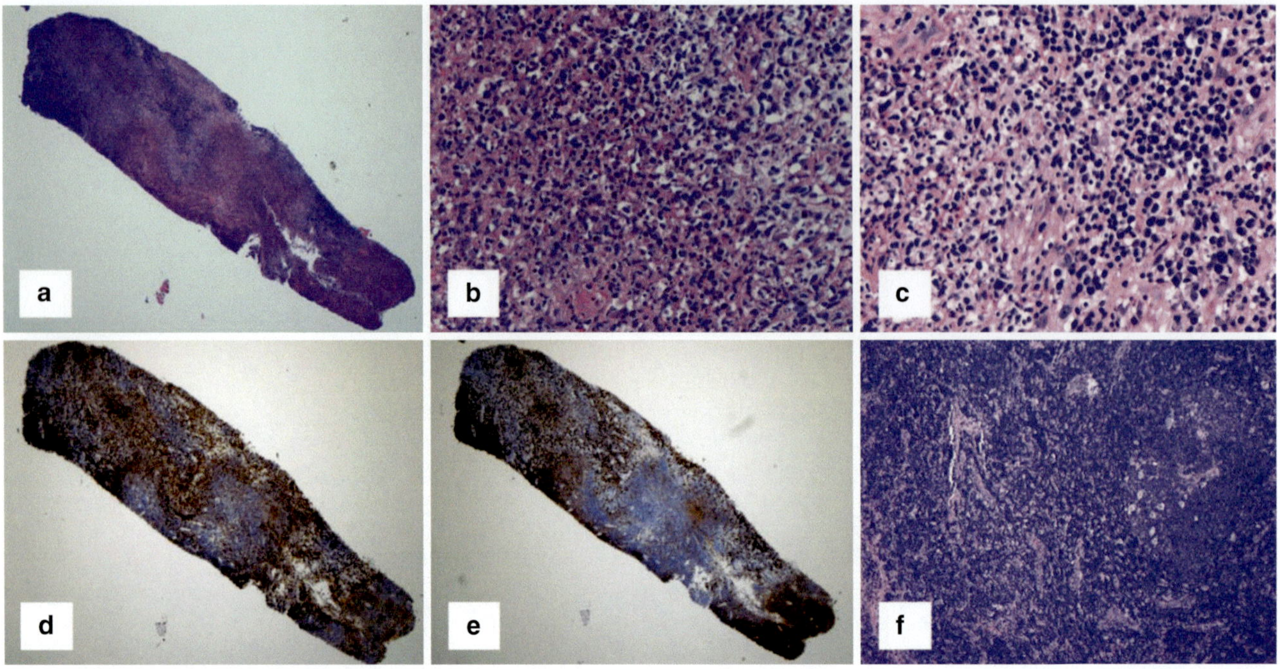

Fig. 18.36 Case 4. Needle core biopsy of a tender cervical lymph node reveals a partial view of an irregularly shaped, deeply eosinophilic lesion surrounded by an outer pale pink peripheral rim (**a**). This corresponds to a so-called stellate microabscess/granuloma. High magnification view of the deep eosinophilic center shows an exuberant neutrophil- and neutrophilic debris-rich necrotic infiltrate (**b**) with the pale outer rim of histiocytes with abundant clear cytoplasm (evident on the upper right-hand corner of the photomicrograph). At the interface of the outer rim of this suppurative granuloma, histiocytes and plasma cells are also numerous (**c**). Architectural preservation is evident from the CD3 (**d**) and CD20 (**e**) immunostained slides. GMS, AFB, and Brown-Brenn (gram) stains were negative (not shown). Warthin-Starry stain was inconclusive, with nonspecific staining (not shown). An excisional biopsy performed 1 month after the needle core biopsy displayed only reactive follicular hyperplasia (**f**), underscoring the fact that histologic findings vary depending on timing/duration/stage of disease. This suppurative lymphadenitis was ultimately attributed to cat-scratch disease (*Bartonella* infection) – see text for further details

mas are highly suggestive of an infectious process, including (but not limited to) *Bartonella* spp. (cat-scratch disease), *Chlamydia trachomatis* (LGV), *Francisella tularensis* (tularemia), *Listeria monocytogenes* (listeriosis), etc. Please correlate with pending microbiologic and serologic studies."

Post-biopsy Clinical Follow-Up

- *Bartonella* IHC not available and was not performed at referring and consulting institutions.
- Microbiologic cultures (i.e., bacterial, fungal, AFB) showed no growth at 6 weeks.
- Based on histopathologic DDx, pediatric housestaff was able to elicit history of the patient caring for several stray cats.
- Repeat excisional biopsy 1 month after the initial core biopsy showed only a reactive follicular hyperplasia (Fig. 18.36f).
- Serologic titers were remarkable for markedly elevated titers for *Bartonella henselae*.
- Based on additional clinical history of cat exposure and histopathologic findings, serum PCR studies for *Bartonella henselae* infection were sent and confirmed positivity.
- Patient was prescribed azithromycin, although parents admit not giving antibiotics since symptoms resolved within 2 weeks of biopsy (5 weeks from start of symptoms).

Final Clinicopathologic Integrated Diagnosis

Suppurative lymphadenitis, due to cat-scratch disease (*Bartonella henselae*)

Take-Home Messages

1. Special stains for microorganisms are not as sensitive for detection as microbiologic/serologic studies.
2. Although a definitive diagnosis of cat-scratch disease cannot be reached by histology alone, offering a differential diagnostic list can help managing physicians to focus their work-up on the most likely etiology.
3. A better history of high-risk exposures (such as close contact with cats, as in this case) might be elicited after histopathology suggests certain diagnostic entities.
4. Histologic findings depend on several factors, including (but not limited to) stage/phase and duration of the reactive process. In this case, exuberant suppurative granulomas were appreciated during the active phase of disease, while RFH observed at excisional biopsy is concordant with the clinical resolution phase of LAD.
5. Cat-scratch disease is typically self-limited.

Case 5

Learning Objectives

1. To generate DDx and initiate the appropriate diagnostic work-up for LAD with plasma cell-rich infiltrates.
2. To exemplify utility of incorporating essential clinical information to arrive at the best possible diagnosis.

Case History

A 43-year-old HIV-negative man presents with fevers, skin rash, and a 5-month history of multistation lymphadenopathy. CT imaging shows multiple enhancing lymph nodes in chest wall, axilla, supraclavicular and mediastinal regions, and pelvis (measuring up to 4 cm in greatest dimension). He undergoes excisional biopsy of a 4-cm ovoid LN with tan, fleshy, homogenous cut surface.

Histologic Findings (Fig. 18.37a–c)

- Nodal architectural preservation with widely spaced follicles, some atretic.
- Follicles display "lollipop sign" with penetrating hyalinized vessels and "onion skinning" mantle zone.
- Exuberant vascular proliferation and interfollicular plasmacytosis.
- Some atretic follicles display prominent follicular dendritic cells.

Differential Diagnosis

- IgG4-related lymphadenopathy
- Nodal involvement by plasma cell neoplasm
- Angioimmunoblastic T-cell lymphoma (AITL)
- Multicentric Castleman disease (HHV8-positive vs HHV8-negative)

IHC and Other Ancillary Studies (Fig. 18.37d–i)

- Absence of FDC expansion and abnormal T-follicular helper cells (excludes AITL)
- Polytypic plasmacytosis (not shown)
- No significant increase in IgG4-positive plasma cells (excludes IgG4-related LAD)
- Not HHV8-related, based on IHC stains

Final Histologic Diagnosis

Castleman disease, plasma cell variant, HHV8-negative

Additional Diagnostic Comments

"Pursue further work-up to better characterize disease, including thorough investigation for plasma cell myeloma (with SPEP/UPEP/IFE and bone marrow biopsy) and evidence of POEMS syndrome (i.e., a paraneoplastic syndrome associated with a plasma cell neoplasm, fibrosis and osteosclerosis in bone trabeculae, LN changes resembling plasma cell variant of Castleman disease, characterized by polyneuropathy, organomegaly, endocrinopathy, monoclonal gammopathy, and skin changes)."

Post-biopsy Clinical Hematology Work-Up

- Additional clinical history elicited:
  - No polyneuropathy endorsed
  - No cutaneous abnormalities on physical exam
- BMBx:
  - Normocellular bone marrow with 6% polyclonal HHV8 negative plasma cells.
  - No significant fibrosis or osteosclerotic bone changes.
- Pertinent Labs:
  - SPEP/UPEP/IFE: faint homogeneous band in the gamma protein region (unquantifiable) as IgA/lambda
  - Serum free light chain ratio within normal range: 1.65 (reference range: 0.26–1.65)
  - IgA and IgG elevated, IgM normal
  - β2-Microglobulin: 2.94 mg/L (reference range: 0.8–2.2 mg/L)
  - ESR and CRP elevated
  - LDH within reference range
  - No other significantly positive rheumatologic markers
- Imaging:
  - Persistent widespread lymphadenopathy
  - Bilateral pleural effusion
  - No osteosclerotic lesions
  - No organomegaly

Clinician Integration of Post-biopsy Data

- No evidence of plasma cell myeloma, POEMS syndrome, infections, autoimmune/inflammatory disorders, and malignant/lymphoproliferative diseases.
- LN histopathology, multiple enlarged LNs, polyclonal hypergammaglobulinemia, thrombocytopenia, and pleural effusion (with exclusion criteria evaluated) qualify for iMCD

Final Integrated Diagnosis

Idiopathic multicentric Castleman disease, HHV8-negative

Take-Home Messages

1. Given the characteristic histologic features, discussion with the treating physician on the most likely diagnostic possibilities can be quite useful especially in the setting of a patient with moderate to severe systemic clinical manifestations.
2. When appropriate, providing suggestions on possible further work-up (like additional bone marrow biopsies, if warranted) can be quite useful for clinical colleagues and in arriving at the best possible integrated diagnosis.

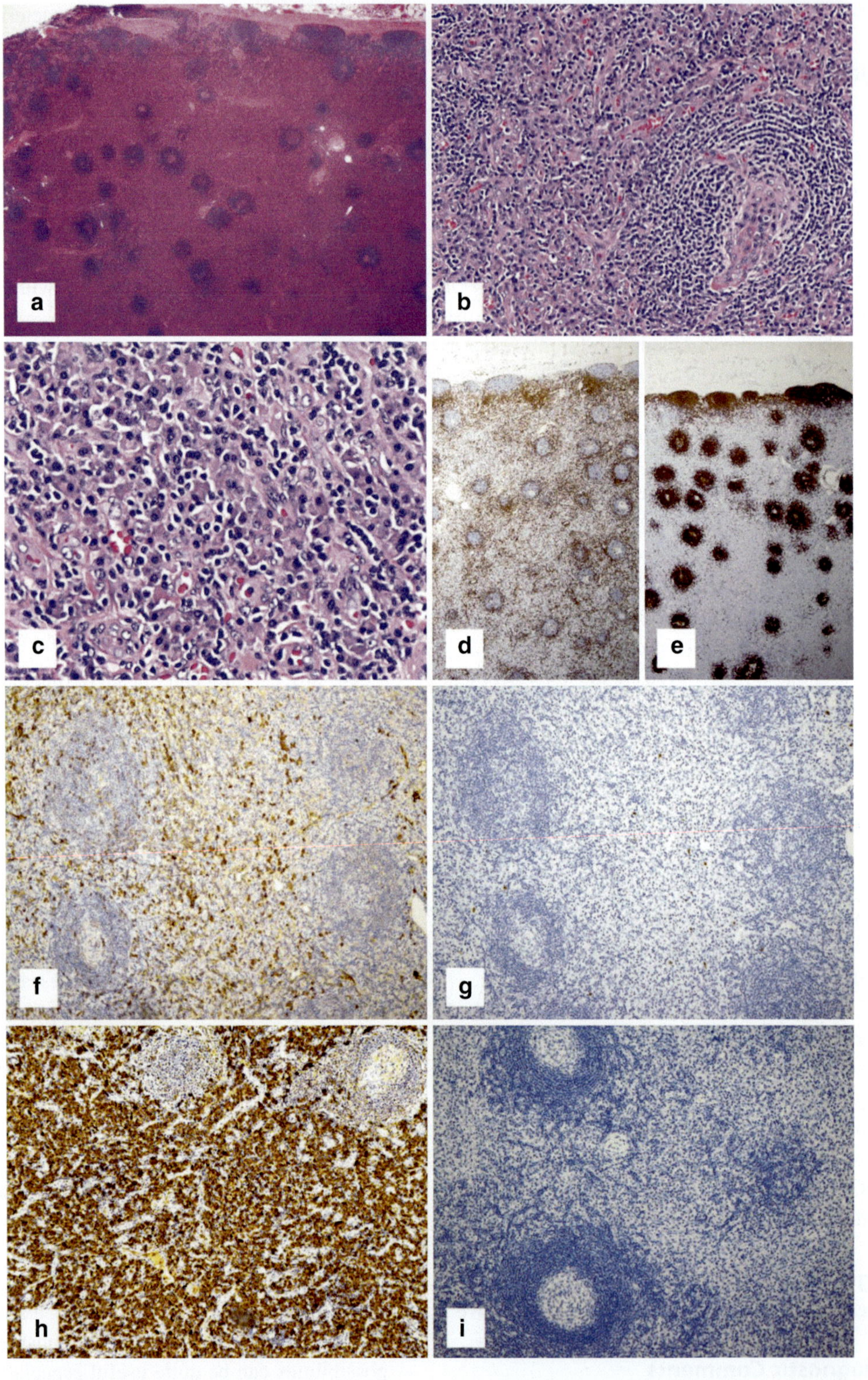

Fig. 18.37 Case 5. This striking case of lymphadenopathy features an exuberant interfollicular expansion with retention of nodal architecture (**a**), as evidenced by multiple, well-spaced lymphoid follicles. Some appear quite small/atrophic. High magnification (**b**) reveals the characteristic "lollipop sign" (hyalinized vessel piercing germinal center), atretic/regressed germinal center with follicular dendritic cell prominence, "onion skinning" of mantle zone-type lymphocytes around the germinal center, and exuberant vascular proliferation in the interfollicular zone. Numerous plasma cells and scattered small lymphocytes are present, embedded in the hypervascular stroma of the interfollicular region (**c**). CD3 (**d**) and CD20 (**e**) confirm architectural preservation and reveal fairly sparse interfollicular T-cells and B-cells largely confined to follicles, respectively. IgG (**f**) and IgG4 (**g**) stains show no prominent IgG4+ plasma cell population. The extensive plasmacytosis is highlighted by this CD138 stain (**h**). Kappa and lambda immunostaining shows polytypic light chain expression (not shown). Given the combined morphologic findings, an HHV8 stain was performed, which is devoid of any HHV8 expression (**i**). Thus, this case appears to represent HHV8-negative, multicentric Castleman disease (idiopathic MCD), particularly in light of the history of disseminated LAD and supportive clinical and laboratory data

Acknowledgments We would like to thank Dr. Russell Brynes for generously sharing his extensive photomicroscopy slide collection, which supplied several of the figures in this chapter. We are also very grateful to Dr. Dennis O'Malley for kindly sharing photomicrographs from his collection of relatively rare entities.

References

1. Tzankov A, Dirnhofer S. A pattern-based approach to reactive lymphadenopathies. Semin Diagn Pathol. 2018;35(1):4–19.
2. Hsi E, Schnitzer B. Reactive lymphadenopathies. In: Jaffe E, Arber D, Campo E, Harris N, Quintanilla-Martinez L, editors. Hematopathology. 2nd ed. Philadelphia: Elsevier; 2017. p. 153–77.
3. Kussick SJ, Kalnoski M, Braziel RM, Wood BL. Prominent clonal B-cell populations identified by flow cytometry in histologically reactive lymphoid proliferations. Am J Clin Pathol. 2004;121(4):464–72.
4. Hoeve MA, Krol AD, Philippo K, Derksen PW, Veenendaal RA, Schuuring E, et al. Limitations of clonality analysis of B cell proliferations using CDR3 polymerase chain reaction. Mol Pathol. 2000;53(4):194–200.
5. Langerak AW, Molina TJ, Lavender FL, Pearson D, Flohr T, Sambade C, et al. Polymerase chain reaction-based clonality testing in tissue samples with reactive lymphoproliferations: usefulness and pitfalls. A report of the BIOMED-2 concerted action BMH4-CT98-3936. Leukemia. 2007;21(2):222–9.
6. Fontanilla JM, Barnes A, von Reyn CF. Current diagnosis and management of peripheral tuberculous lymphadenitis. Clin Infect Dis. 2011;53(6):555–62.
7. Reddy DL, Venter WD, Pather S. Patterns of lymph node pathology; fine needle aspiration biopsy as an evaluation tool for lymphadenopathy: a retrospective descriptive study conducted at the largest hospital in Africa. PLoS One. 2015;10(6):e0130148.
8. Oh KH, Woo JS, Cho JG, Baek SK, Jung KY, Kwon SY. Efficacy of ultrasound-guided core needle gun biopsy in diagnosing cervical lymphadenopathy. Eur Ann Otorhinolaryngol Head Neck Dis. 2016;133(6):401–4.
9. Allin D, David S, Jacob A, Mir N, Giles A, Gibbins N. Use of core biopsy in diagnosing cervical lymphadenopathy: a viable alternative to surgical excisional biopsy of lymph nodes? Ann R Coll Surg England. 2017;99(3):242–4.
10. Reactive lymphadenopathies. In: Medeiros L, editor. Diagnostic pathology: lymph nodes and spleen with extranodal lymphomas. Canada: Amirsys; 2011. p. 3-2 to 3-117.
11. Ohgami RS, Zhao S, Ohgami JK, Leavitt MO, Zehnder JL, West RB, et al. TdT+ T-lymphoblastic populations are increased in Castleman disease, in Castleman disease in association with follicular dendritic cell tumors, and in angioimmunoblastic T-cell lymphoma. Am J Surg Pathol. 2012;36(11):1619–28.
12. Alexander TS. Human immunodeficiency virus diagnostic testing: 30 years of evolution. Clin Vaccine Immunol. 2016;23(4):249–53.
13. Barrionuevo-Cornejo C, Duenas-Hancco D. Lymphadenopathies in human immunodeficiency virus infection. Semin Diagn Pathol. 2018;35(1):84–91.
14. O'Malley D, George T, Orazi A, Abbondanzo S. Benign and reactive conditions of lymph node and spleen. Washington, D.C.: ARP Press; 2009.
15. Infectious causes of lymphadenitis. In: Medeiros L, editor. Diagnostic pathology: lymph nodes and spleen with extranodal lymphomas. Canada: Amirsys; 2011. p. 2–103.
16. Gru AA, O'Malley DP. Autoimmune and medication-induced lymphadenopathies. Semin Diagn Pathol. 2018;35(1):34–43.
17. Moreland L, Cannella A. General principles of management of rheumatoid arthritis in adults. In: JR OD, editor. Waltham: UpToDate, Inc.; 2019.
18. Cantor AG, Pappas M, Daeges M, Nelson HD. Screening for syphilis: updated evidence report and systematic review for the US Preventive Services Task Force. JAMA. 2016;315(21):2328–37.
19. Romanowski B, Forsey E, Prasad E, Lukehart S, Tam M, Hook EW. Detection of Treponema pallidum by a fluorescent monoclonal antibody test. Sex Transm Dis. 1987;14(3):156–9.
20. Workowski KA, Bolan GA, CfDCa P. Sexually transmitted diseases treatment guidelines, 2015. MMWR Recomm Rep. 2015;64(RR-03):1–137.
21. Montoya JG, Liesenfeld O. Toxoplasmosis. Lancet. 2004;363(9425):1965–76.
22. Weiss LM, Chen YY, Berr Warnke RA. Infrequent detection of Toxoplasma gondii genome in toxoplasmic lymphadenitis: a polymerase chain reaction study. Hum Pathol. 1992;23(2):154–8.
23. DPDx – laboratory identiof public health concern: toxoplasmosis. Atlanta [updated August 2015; cited July 2018]. Available from: https://www.cdc.gov/dpdx/toxoplasmosis/index.html.
24. Jegalian AG, Eberle FC, Pack SD, Mirvis M, Raffeld M, Pittaluga S, et al. Follicular lymphoma in situ: clinical implications and comparisons with partial involvement by follicular lymphoma. Blood. 2011;118(11):2976–84.
25. Swerdlow S, Campo E, Harris N, Jaffe E, Pileri S, Stein H, et al., editors. WHO classification of tumours of haematopoietic and lymphoid tissues. Revised 4th ed. Lyon: IARC; 2017.
26. Hartmann S, Winkelmann R, Metcalf RA, Treetipsatit J, Warnke RA, Natkunam Y, et al. Immunoarchitectural patterns of progressive transformation of germinal centers with and without nodular lymphocyte-predominant Hodgkin lymphoma. Hum Pathol. 2015;46(11):1655–61.
27. Chang CC, Osipov V, ns SL. Follicular hyperplasia, follicular lysis, and progressive transformation of germinal centers. A sequential spectrum of morphologic evolution in lymphoid hyperplasia. Am J Clin Pathol. 2003;120(3):322–6.
28. Childs CC, Parham DM, Berard CW. Infectious mononucleosis. The spectrum of morphologic changes simulating lymphoma in lymph nodes and tonsils. Am J Surg Pathol. 1987;11(2):122–32.
29. Louissaint A Jr, Ferry JA, Soupir CP, Hasserjian RP, Harris NL, Zukerberg LR. Infectious mononucleosis mimicking lymphoma: distinguishing morphological and immunophenotypic features. Modern Pathol. 2012;25(8):1149–59.
30. Luzuriaga K, Sullivan JL. Infectious md. 2010;362(21):1993–2000.
31. Weisberger J, Cornfield Dgulation of pan-T-cell antigens, particularly CD7, in acute infectious mononucleosis. Am J Clin Pathol. 2003;120(1):49–55.
32. Aguilera N, Auerbach A. Epstein-Barr virus (EBV) associated reactive and indeterminate lymphoid proliferations in the lymph node. Semin Diagn Pathol. 2018;35(1):54–60.
33. Rushin JM, Riordan GP, Heaton RB, Sharpe RW, Cotelingam JD, Jaffe ES. Cytomegalovirus-infected cells express Leu-M1 antigen. A potential source of diagnostic error. Am J Pathol. 1990;136(5):989–95.
34. Goodell SE, Quinn TC, Mkrtichian E, Schuffler MD, Holmes KK, Corey L. Herpes simplex virus proctitis in homosexual men. Clinical, sigmoidoscopic, and histopathological features. N Engl J Med. 1983;308(15):868–71.
35. Miliauskas JR, Leong AS. Localized herpes simplex lymphadenitis: report of three cases and review of the literature. Histopathology. 1991;19(4):355–60.
36. Horwitz CA, Henle W, Henle G, Snover D, Rudnick H, Balfour HH, et al. Clinical and laboratory evaluation of cytomegalovirus-

induced mononucleosis in previously healthy individuals. Report of 82 cases. Medicine (Baltimore). 1986;65(2):124–34.
37. Taylor MJ, Hoerauf A, Bockarie M. Lymphatic filariasis and onchocerciasis. Lancet. 2010;376(9747):1175–85.
38. Echols RM, Palmer DL, Long GW. Tissue eosinophilia in human coccidioidomycosis. Rev Infect Dis. 1982;4(3):656–64.
39. DPDx – laboratory identification of parasitic diseases of public health concern: lymphatic filariasis. Atlanta. Available from: https://www.cdc.gov/dpdx/lymphaticfilariasis/index.html.
40. Jeon YK, Paik JH, Park SS, Park SO, Kim YA, Kim JE, et al. Spectrum of lymph node pathology in adult onset Still's disease; analysis of 12 patients with one follow up biopsy. J Clin Pathol. 2004;57(10):1052–6.
41. Yamaguchi M, Ohta A, Tsunematsu T, Kasukawa R, Mizushima Y, Kashiwagi H, et al. Preliminary criteria for classification of adult Still's disease. J Rheumatol. 1992;19(3):424–30.
42. Mandl LA. Treatment of adult Still's disease. In: O'Dell JR, editor. . Waltham: UpToDate, Inc.; 2019.
43. Shah KKPB, Alexander MP. Histopathologic review of granulomatous inflammation. J Clin Tubercul Other Mycobact Dis. 2017;7:1–12.
44. Egan C, Jaffe ES. Non-neoplastic histiocytic and dendritic cell disorders in lymph nodes. Semin Diagn Pathol. 2018;35(1):20–33.
45. Houben RM, Dodd PJ. The global burden of latent tuberculosis infection: a re-estimation using mathematical modelling. PLoS Med. 2016;13(10):e1002152.
46. Nahid P, Dorman SE, Alipanah N, Barry PM, Brozek JL, Cattamanchi A, et al., Official American Thoracic Society/Centers for Disease Control and Prevention/Infectious Diseases Society of America. Clinical practice guidelines: treatment of drug-susceptible tuberculosis. Clin Infect Dis. 2016;63(7)e147–95.
47. Miranda RN, Khoury JD, Medeiros LJ. Atlas of lymph node pathology. xix, 530 p.
48. Baek CH, Kim SI, Ko YH, Chu KC. Polymerase chain reaction detection of Mycobacterium tuberculosis from fine-needle aspirate for the diagnosis of cervical tuberculous lymphadenitis. Laryngoscope. 2000;110(1):30–4.
49. Hillemann D, Galle J, Vollmer E, Richter E. Real-time PCR assay for improved detection of Mycobacterium tuberculosis complex in paraffin-embedded tissues. Int J Tuberc Lung Dis. 2006;10(3):340–2.
50. Centers for Disease Control and Prevention. Brucellosis reference guide: exposures, testing, and prevention. In: Centers for Disease Control and Prevention, editor. 2017. p. 1–34.
51. Regnery RL, Olson JG, Perkins BA, Bibb W. Serological response to "Rochalimaea henselae" antigen in suspected cat-scratch disease. Lancet. 1992;339(8807):1443–5.
52. Yanagihara M, Tsuneoka H, Tanimoto A, Otsuyama KI, Nishikawa J, Matsui T, et al. Bartonella henselae DNA in seronegative patients with cat-scratch disease. Emerg Infect Dis. 2018;24(5):924–5.
53. Kaplan JE, Benson C, Holmes KK, Brooks JT, Pau A, Masur H, et al. Guidelines for prevention and treatment of opportunistic infections in HIV-infected adults and adolescents: recommendations from CDC, the National Institutes of Health, and the HIV Medicine Association of the Infectious Diseases Society of America. MMWR Recomm Rep. 2009;58(RR-4):1–207; quiz CE1-4.
54. Hansen's disease (leprosy). Atlanta [updated Feb 2017; cited July 2018]. Available from: https://www.cdc.gov/leprosy/index.html.
55. Cramer J, Schmiedel S, Alegre NG, Schafer H, Burchard GD, Merz H. Necrotizing lymphadenitis: Kikuchi-Fujimoto disease alias lupus lymphadenitis? Lupus. 2010;19(1):89–92.
56. Guilabert A, Miquel R, Campo E. Enigmatic Kikuchi-Fujimoto disease: a comprehensive review. Am J Clin Pathol. 2004;122(1):141–52.
57. Petri M, Orbai AM, Merrill JT, Fortin PR, et al. Derivation and validation of the systemic lupus international collaborating clinics classification criteria for systemic lupus erythematosus. Arthritis Rheum. 2012;64(8):2677–86.
58. Kojima M, Motoori T, Asano S, Nakamura S. Histological diversity of reactive and atypical proliferative lymph node lesions in systemic lupus erythematosus patients. Pathol Res Pract. 2007;203(6):423–31.
59. Nyatsanza F, Tipple C. Syphilis: presentations in general medicine. Clin Med. 2016;16(2):184–8.
60. Facchetti F, Incardona P, Lonardi S, Fisogni S, Legrenzi L, Chioda C, et al. Nodal inflammatory pseudotumor caused by luetic infection. Am J Surg Pathol. 2009;33(3):447–53.
61. Kamisawa T, Egawa N, Nakajima H. Autoimmune pancreatitis is a systemic autoimmune disease. Am J Gastroenterol. 2003;98(12):2811–2.
62. Kamisawa T, Nakajimuruta K, Okamoto A. IgG4-related sclerosing disease incorporating sclerosing pancreatitis, cholangitis, sialadenitis and retroperitoneal fibrosis with lymphadenopathy. Pancreatology. 2006;6(1–2):132–7.
63. Stone JH, Brito-Zeron P, Bosch X, Ramos-Casals M. Diagnostic approach to the complexity of IgG4-related disease. Mayo Clin Proc. 2015;90(7):927–39.
64. Cheuk W, Chan JK. Lymated disease: an underdiagnosed and overdiagnosed entity. Semin Diagn Pathol. 2012;29(4):226–34.
65. Bookhout CE, Rolllobulin G4-related lymphadenopathy. Surg Pathol Clin. 2016;9(1):117–29.
66. Wick MR, O'Malley DP. Lymphadenopathy associated with IgG4-related disease: diagnosis & differential diagnosis. Semin Diagn Pathol. 2018;35(1):61–6.
67. Deshpande V, Zen Y, Chan JK, Yi EE, Sato Y, Yoshino T, et al. Consensus statement on the pathology of IgG4-related disease. Modern Pathol. 2012;25(9):1181–92.
68. Fajgenbaum DC, Uldrick TS, Bagg A, Frank D, Wu D, Srkalovic G, et al. International, evidence-based consensus diagnostic criteria for HHV-8-negative/idiopathic multicentric Castleman disease. Blood. 2017;129(12):1646–57.
69. Moh M, Sangoi AR, Rabban JT. Angiomyomatous hamartoma of lymph nodes, revisited: clinicopathologic study of 21 cases, emphasizing its distinction from lymphangioleiomyomatosis of lymph nodes. Hum Pathol. 2017;68:175–83.
70. Xu ML, O'Malley D. Lymph node stromal and vascular proliferations. Semin Diagn Pathol. 2018;35(1):67–75.
71. Basha BM, Hsi ED. Immunohistochemical analysis of endothelial cells in vascular transformation of lymph node sinuses: vascular or lymphatic differentiation? Appl Immunohistochem Mole Morphol. 2019;27(6):482–9.
72. Chan JK, Warnke RA, Dorfman R. Vascular transformation of sinuses in lymph nodes. A study of its morphological spectrum and distinction from Kaposi's sarcoma. Am J Surg Pathol. 1991;15(8):732–43.
73. Chen KT. Mycobacterial spindle cell pseudotumor of lymph nodes. Am J Surg Pathol. 1992;16(3):276–81.
74. Sato Y, Kojima M, Takata K, Morito T, Mizobuchi K, Tanaka T, Inoue D, Shiomi H, Iwao H, Yoshino T. Multicentric Castleman's disease with abundant IgG4-positive cells: a clinical and pathological analysis of six cases. J Clin Pathol. 2010;63(12):1084–9.
75. Sato Y, Kojima M, Takata K, Morito T, Asaoku H, Takeuchi T, Mizobuchi K, Fujihara M, Kuraoka K, Nakai T, Ichimura K, Tanaka T, Tamura M, Nishikawa Y, Yoshino T. Systemic IgG4-related lymphadenopathy: a clinical and pathologic comparison to multicentric Castleman's disease. Mod Pathol. 2009;22(4):589–99.
76. Balakrishna JP, Bhavsar T, Nicolae A, Raffeld M, Jaffe ES, Pittaluga S. Human Herpes Virus 6 (HHV-6)–associated Lymphadenitis. Am J Surg Pathol. 42(10):1402–8.

HHV8-Associated Lymphoproliferative Disorders

19

Wei Wang and L. Jeffrey Medeiros

List of Frequently Asked Questions

1. What is HHV8?
2. What are the major types of HHV8-positive lymphoproliferative disorders (LPDs)?
3. What are other HHV8-positive LPDs besides these major types?
4. What are the typical morphological findings in this category?
5. What are the typical immunophenotypic findings in this category?
6. How does one distinguish between the major subtypes of HHV8-associated LPD?
7. How do we distinguish HHV8-LPDs from other lymphomas with a similar morphology?
8. When to perform a HHV8 immunostain?
9. What are the treatment options for patients with HHV8-associated LPDs?

1. What is HHV8?

Human herpesvirus 8 (HHV8), also known as Kaposi sarcoma herpesvirus (KSHV), belongs to herpes virus family. In addition to causing Kaposi sarcoma, HHV8 is associated with a spectrum of lymphoproliferative disorders.

2. What are the major types of HHV8-positive lymphoproliferative disorders (LPDs)?

There are four major subtypes including:

- HHV8-positive germinotropic lymphoproliferative disorder (GLPD).
- HHV8-positive multicentric Castleman disease (MCD).
- HHV8-positive diffuse large B-cell lymphoma (DLBCL), NOS.
- Primary effusion lymphoma (PEL). Although PEL most often presents as an effusion, it also can present as an extranodal mass [1].

3. What are other HHV8-positive LPDs besides these major types?

- HHV8-positive LPDs are a spectrum, and there are cases that show features intermediate between those major subtypes described above, which makes them difficult to subclassify.
- HHV8-positive MCD and its associated DLBCL are usually negative for *EBV*-encoded small RNA (EBER), but cases positive for both HHV8 and EBER have been reported [2–5].
- Similarly, there have been cases of HHV8-positive, EBER-positive LPD that showed some morphological features of MCD, but these patients had no immunosuppression history and no IgM lambda expression, and the disease was localized; these features are rather commonly seen in GLPD [6].
- There are also some cases that have distinct pathological features that are not seen in the major subtypes. Examples include HHV8-positive, *EBV*-positive Hodgkin lymphoma-like large B-cell lymphoma and HHV8-positive intravascular large B-cell lymphoma [7, 8].

W. Wang (✉) · L. J. Medeiros
Department of Hematopathology, The MD Anderson Cancer Center, Houston, TX, USA
e-mail: WWang13@mdanderson.org; ljmedeiros@mdanderson.org

E. Wang, A. S. Lagoo (eds.), *Practical Lymph Node and Bone Marrow Pathology*, Practical Anatomic Pathology,
https://doi.org/10.1007/978-3-030-32189-5_19

- HHV8-related reactive lymphoid hyperplasia has also been described in about 1/3 of HIV-associated reactive lymphadenitis, and in these cases, the HHV8-positive cells are often scattered [9].

4. What are the typical morphological findings in this category?

Although the neoplastic cells show a different distribution pattern in different subtypes of HHV8-positive LPD, the cells commonly share a similar cytomorphology with plasmablasts/immunoblasts as a major component. These cells are large, with moderate to large amounts of cytoplasm, round to slightly irregular nuclei, and central prominent nucleoli (Fig. 19.1). Representative cases and pathological features of HHV8-positive GLPD and MCD are shown in Figs. 19.2 and 19.3.

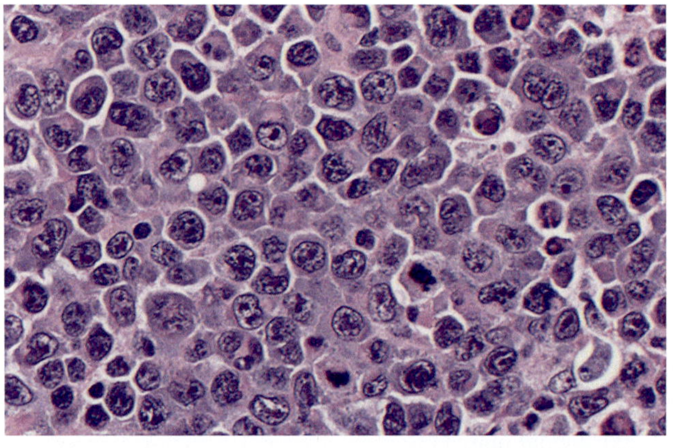

Fig. 19.1 Cytomorphology of HHV8-positive LPDs. Most cells show plasmablastic/immunoblastic morphology manifested as large cells with prominent central nucleoli. Occasional cells show anaplastic morphology. Mitotic figures and apoptosis are abundant. H&E stain, 400×

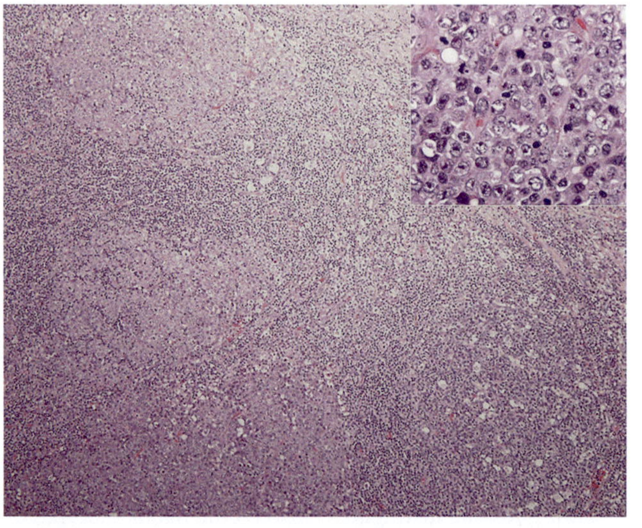

Fig. 19.2 A case of GLPD. The section shows the nodal architecture altered by a vague nodular proliferation. Germinal centers (left) are replaced by sheets of plasmablasts/immunoblasts. A reactive germinal center is present in the right lower corner. H&E stain, 40×. *Inset*: high-power view of germinal centers occupied by immunoblasts/plasmablasts. H&E stain, 400×

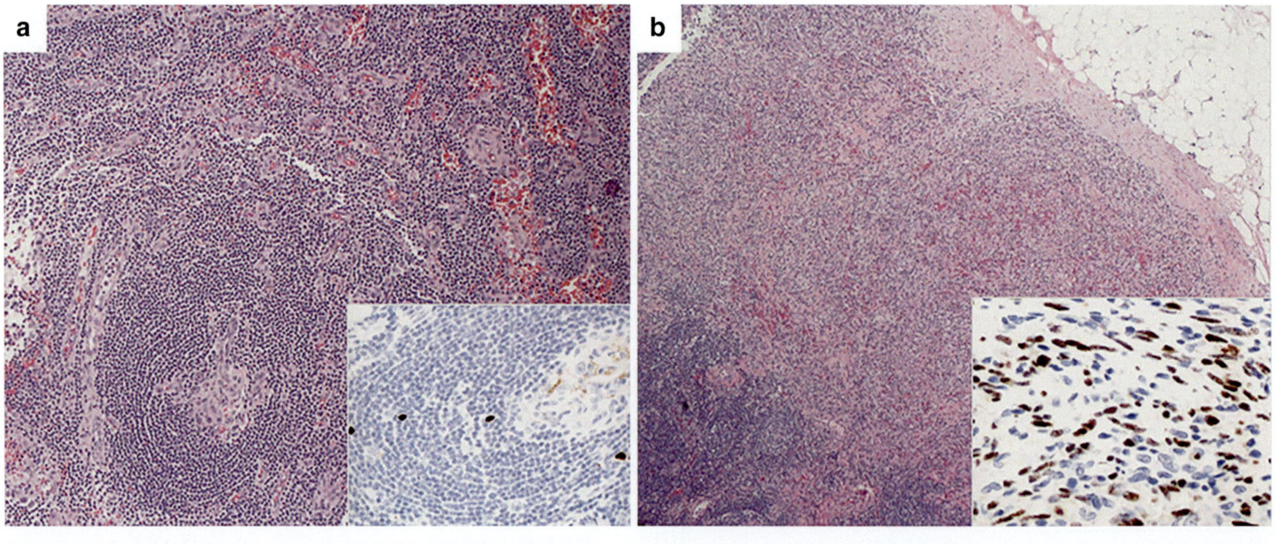

Fig. 19.3 A case of HHV8-positive MCD with concurrent Kaposi sarcoma. (**a**) Low-power view shows a regressed germinal center surrounded by onion skin-like mantle zone cells. The interfollicular areas show prominent vascular proliferation. H&E stain, 40×. *Inset:* HHV8 immunostain highlights scattered large cells in mantle zones.100×. (**b**) An area with Kaposi sarcoma composed of spindle cell proliferation (H&E stain, 40×) with positive HHV8 staining (*inset,* 100×)

5. What are the typical immunophenotypic findings in this category?

- By definition, the cells are positive for HHV8.
- The cells often demonstrate absence of pan-B-cell markers such as CD19, CD20, and CD79a; The majority of the reported cases are positive for MUM1. CD38 and CD138 are variably expressed.
- Aberrant expression of T-cell markers can be seen in some cases.
- EBER is characteristically positive in GLPD and PEL, but is usually negative in HHV8-positive MCD and DLBCL.

6. How does one distinguish between these major subtypes of HHV8-associated LPDs?

- The major clinicopathological features for each subtype and their differential points are listed in Table 19.1. We should be aware that HHV8-positive LPDs represent a spectrum and can have overlapping features.
- For GLPD, although considered to be localized with no tendency to progress, one case was shown to transform into HHV8-positive, *EBV*-positive DLBCL [10]. Although often occurring in immunocompetent patients with the concurrent expression of both HHV8 and *EBV*, cases of GLPD with negative *EBV* and cases of GLPD in HIV-positive patients have been described [9].
- In addition, HHV8-positive DLBCL and extracavitary variant PEL can be challenging to distinguish in some cases (Fig. 19.4). Although *EBV* is often positive in PEL and is usually negative in HHV8-positive DLBCL, both PEL cases that are negative for *EBV* and HHV8-positive DLBCL cases that are positive *EBV* have been described. Of note, due to their poor prognosis and lack of effective therapy, distinguishing between these two entities in this rare scenario may be less critical.

7. How do we distinguish HHV8-LPDs from other lymphomas with a similar morphology?

- In addition to the four HHV8-positive entities described above, there are other neoplasms sharing similar plasmablastic/immunoblastic morphology. These neoplasms include:
  - Diffuse large B-cell lymphoma, immunoblastic variant
  - Plasmablastic lymphoma
  - Plasmablastic myeloma
  - ALK-positive large B-cell lymphoma
- Immunophenotypic analysis is valuable in discriminating between these entities (Fig. 19.5). Positive pan-B-cell markers, such as CD19, CD20, and PAX5, will justify the diagnosis of DLBCL, immunoblastic variant. If pan-B-cell markers are negative, the next step would be to evaluate plasma cell-related markers and other non-lineage associated hematopoietic markers. The absence of these antigens will raise the possibility of T-cell lymphoma especially anaplastic large cell lymphoma (ALCL) or non-hematopoietic disease such as melanoma. The positive (even partial) expression will trigger the workup for ALK1, HHV8, and *EBV*, and based on their positivity, cases can be further subclassified into different entities as shown in Fig. 19.5.
- In addition to their immunophenotypic differences, the clinical and laboratory features can also offer clues in differential diagnosis. ALK-positive large B-cell lymphoma occurs more often in younger patients without a history of immunosuppression and tends to involve lymph nodes, especially in the cervical areas.

Table 19.1 The differential diagnosis of HHV8-positive lymphoproliferative disorders

	MCD	DLBCL	GLPD	PEL
Immunosuppression	+	+	–	+
Presentation	Generalized	Generalized	Localized	Generalized
Prognosis	Poor	Poor	Good	Poor
Microscopy	PB/IB in mantle zones	PB/IB, diffuse	PB/IB within germinal centers	PB/IB in fluid or extracavitary sites
Castleman features	+	+ or –	–	–
HIV status	+/–	+/–	–	+/–
HHV8	+	+	+	+
EBV	–	–	+	+
CD138	–/+	–/+	–/+	+
CD20	–/+	–	–	–
Ig	IgM, λ	Monotypic	Monotypic	–
Molecular (*IGH*)	Polyclonal	Clonal	Polyclonal	Clonal

Note: *MCD* multicentric Castleman disease, *DLBCL* diffuse large B-cell lymphoma, *GLPD* germinotropic lymphoproliferative disorder, *PEL* primary effusion lymphoma, *PB/IB* plasmablastic/immunoblastic

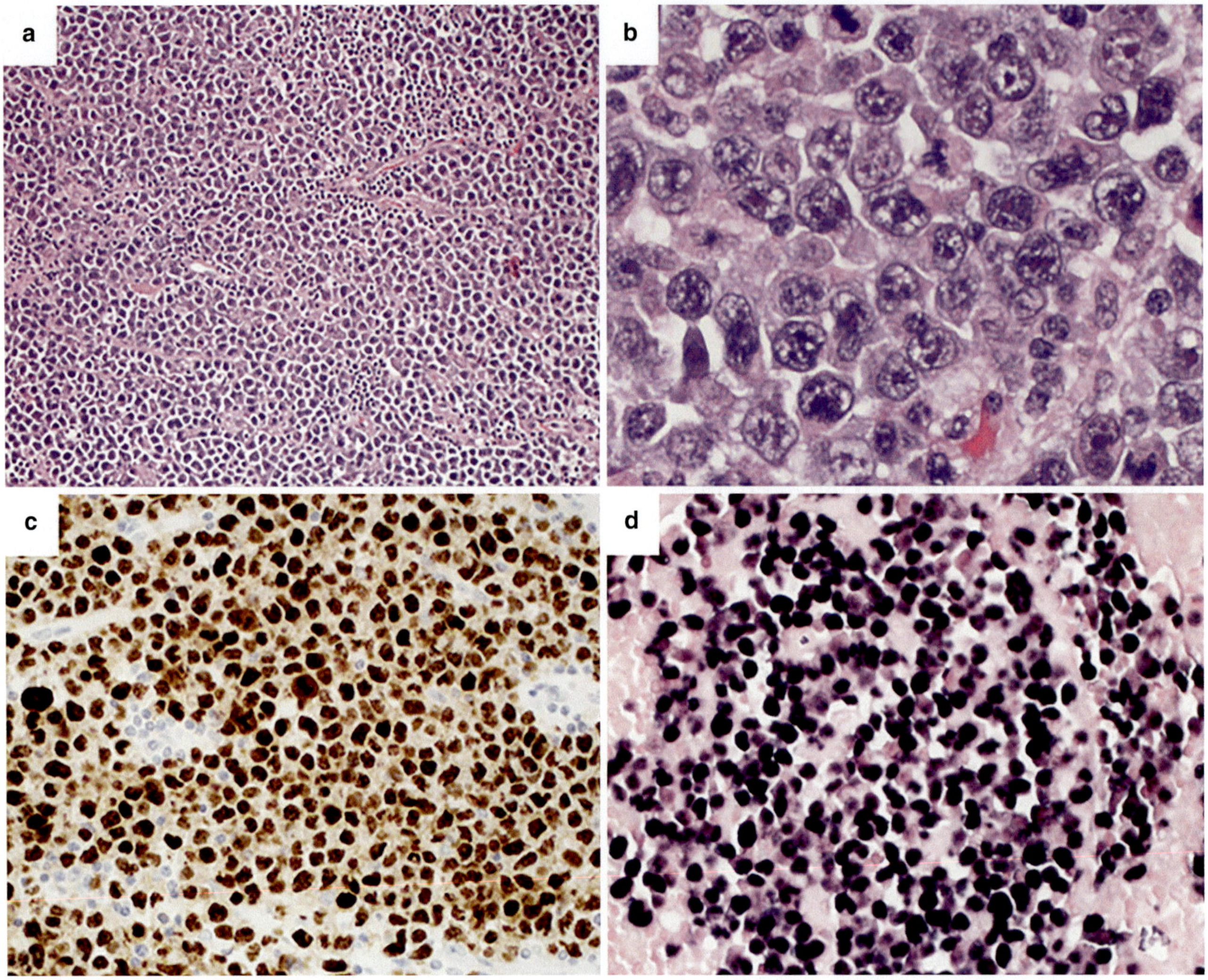

Fig. 19.4 A case of HHV8-positive, *EBV*-positive extracavitary PEL. The biopsy of large intestinal mass lesion shows a diffuse lymphoid proliferation (**a** H&E stain, 100×) composed of large cells with prominent central nucleoli (**b** H&E stain, 400×). Tumor cells are positive for HHV8 (**c** 200×) and EBER (**d** 200×)

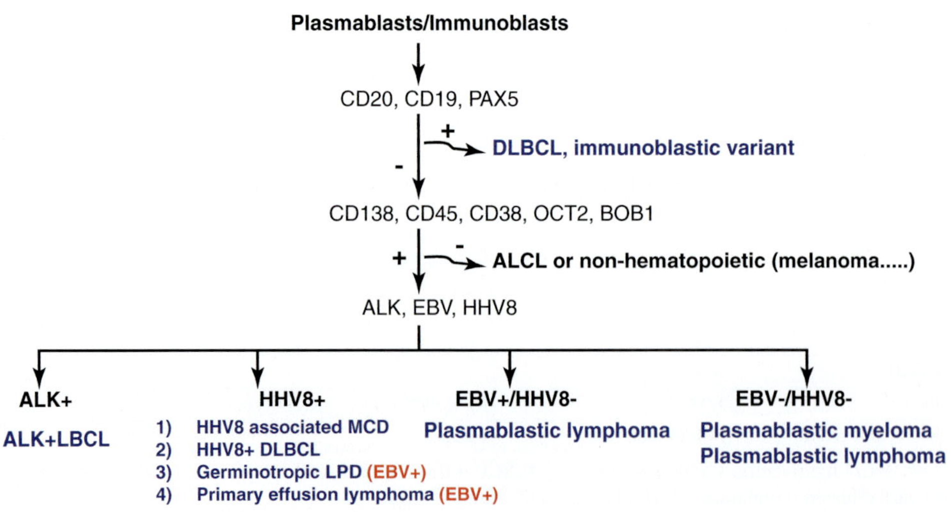

Fig. 19.5 The algorithm to distinguish lymphomas with immunoblastic/plasmablastic morphology

- In case of negative *EBV*, the differential diagnosis between plasmablastic lymphoma and plasmablastic myeloma can be challenging, but the absence of immunosuppression, the presence of bone involvement, and the presence of paraprotein favor myeloma over lymphoma.

8. When to perform a HHV8 immunostain?

- HHV8 immunostain is often not in the first batch of antibodies during a lymphoma workup. However, when the neoplastic cells show immunoblastic/plasmablastic morphology and are negative for common pan-B-cell markers, a HHV8 immunostain should be considered, as well as ALK1 and EBER.
- Of note, T-cell markers, especially CD3, have been reported to be positive in some cases of PEL and plasmablastic neoplasms [11, 12]. Thus, a positive CD3 should not stop one from performing a HHV8 stain. Morphology is the key.

9. What are the treatment options for patients with HHV8-associated LPDs?

Due to the rarity of most entities in this category, there is no standard therapy. However, for HHV8-positive MCD, IL-6 induced by HHV8 virus activates IL-6 receptor and plays a key role in the disease development. Accordingly, targeted therapy against IL-6 (siltuximab) and IL-6 receptor (tocilizumab) has improved patients' survival.

Case Presentations

Case 1 (Fig. 19.1)

Learning Objectives

1. To know the morphologic features and typical immunophenotype of HHV8-positive DLBCL, NOS
2. To know how to differentiate HHV8-positive DLBCL from other subtype of HHV8-positive LPD

Case History

A 63-year-old male with HIV presented with constitutional symptoms, generalized lymphadenopathy, and splenomegaly. PET scan revealed increased uptake in the neck, pelvis, and retroperitoneal lymph nodes. Left neck core biopsy was taken for evaluation.

Histologic Findings

- Core biopsy showed effacement of normal nodal architecture with proliferation of abnormal lymphoid cells. These abnormal cells displayed plasmablastic/immunoblastic morphology manifested as large cells with prominent central nucleoli.
- Occasional cells showed anaplastic morphology.
- Mitotic figures were frequently seen.

Morphologic Diagnosis

- Diffuse large cell lymphoma, immunoblastic variant
- Alternatively, plasmablastic lymphoma, extracavitary PEL, or HHV8-positive DLBCL

Flow Cytometry Analysis

- A large, CD38-positive, B-cell antigen-negative lymphoid population without definitive surface immunoglobulin light chains was detected

Immunohistochemical Stains

- Immunohistochemical stains showed the large cells are positive for MUM1, cytoplasmic IgM lambda light chain, and HHV8 LANA1.
- Negative for CD19, CD79a, CD138, and T-cell antigens except for focal CD3 staining.
- EBER in situ hybridization was negative.

IgH and TCR Gene Rearrangement

- Clonal *IGH* gene rearrangement was identified by PCR.
- No clonal *TCR* gene was detected.

Final Diagnosis

HHV8-positive diffuse large B-cell lymphoma, NOS

Take-Home Messages

1. HHV8-positive DLBCL, NOS tends to occur in HIV patients.
2. The morphology of HHV8-positive DLBCL often displays plasmablastic/immunoblastic features.
3. The neoplastic cells usually lack complete B-cell or plasma cell antigen profile.
4. HHV8 is positive, and *EBV* study is often negative.
5. B-cell clonality can be documented by lymphoid receptor gene rearrangement analysis.

Case 2 (Fig. 19.2)

Learning Objectives

1. To know the morphologic features and typical immunophenotype of HHV8-positive germinotropic lymphoproliferative disorder (GLPD)
2. To know how to differentiate HHV8-positive GLPD from other subtypes of HHV8-positive LPD

Case History

A 43-year-old male with unremarkable clinical history presented with left cervical lymphadenopathy. PET scan revealed increased uptake in the localized left neck lymph node. Left neck lymph node was excised for evaluation.

Histologic Findings

- The section of the biopsy showed altered nodal architecture with follicular hyperplasia. While some follicles demonstrated morphologic features suggestive of reactive follicular hyperplasia, other follicles contained abnormal germinal centers that were replaced by medium-sized to large lymphoid cells. These abnormal cells within germinal centers displayed plasmablastic/immunoblastic morphology.

Morphologic Diagnosis

- Follicular lymphoma, high grade, with partial involvement of the lymph node
- Reactive follicular hyperplasia
- HHV8-positive GLPD

Flow Cytometry Analysis

- Unremarkable or noncontributory

Immunohistochemical Stains

- Immunohistochemical stains showed the large cells are positive for MUM1, cytoplasmic kappa light chain restriction, and HHV8 LANA1.
- Negative for CD19, CD20, CD79a, CD138, and T-cell antigens.
- EBER in situ hybridization was positive.

IgH and TCR Gene Rearrangement Analysis with Microdissection of Abnormal Germinal Centers

- No clonal *IGH* gene rearrangement was identified by PCR.
- No clonal *TCR* gene was detected.

Final Diagnosis

HHV8-positive germinotropic lymphoproliferative disorder

Take-Home Messages

1. HHV8-positive GLPD tends to occur in immunocompetent patients.
2. The morphology of HHV8-positive GLPD often displays plasmablasts/immunoblasts replacing a fraction of germinal centers with otherwise follicular hyperplasia.
3. The plasmablasts/immunoblasts within germinal centers usually lack complete B-cell or plasma cell antigen profile.
4. Both HHV8 and *EBV* studies are positive.
5. B-cell clonality test often demonstrates either oligoclonal or polyclonal pattern of immunoglobulin gene rearrangements.

Case 3 (Fig. 19.3)

Learning Objectives

1. To know the morphologic features and typical immunophenotype of HHV8-positive multicentric Castleman disease
2. To know how to differentiate multicentric Castleman disease from other subtype of HHV8-positive LPD and reactive follicular hyperplasia

Case History

A 35-year-old male with HIV presented with constitutional symptoms, generalized lymphadenopathy, and splenomegaly. PET scan revealed increased uptake in the neck, pelvis, and retroperitoneal lymph nodes. Left neck lymph node was taken out for evaluation.

Histologic Findings

- Section of excisional biopsy showed lymphoid nodal architecture altered by follicles with expanded mantle zone cells that displayed concentric arrangement (onion skin-like appearance).
- Scattered hyperplastic follicles were present. Some germinal centers demonstrated atrophic changes with depleted lymphocytes and hyaline vascular penetration.
- Scattered plasmablasts/immunoblasts were noted within expanded mantle zone or in adjacent interfollicular areas.

Morphologic Diagnosis

- Multicentric Castleman disease
- Other HHV8-positive LPD
- Reactive follicular hyperplasia
- Mantle cell lymphoma

Flow Cytometry Analysis

- T-cells with inverted CD4:CD8 ratio; otherwise, no monoclonal B-cell population was detected.

Immunohistochemical Stains

- Immunohistochemical stains showed the scattered large cells are positive for MUM1, partial CD20, cytoplasmic IgM lambda light chain restriction, and HHV8 LANA1.
- Negative for CD19, CD79a, CD138, and T-cell antigens.
- EBER in situ hybridization was negative.

IgH/K Gene Rearrangement Analysis

- No clonal *IGH* gene rearrangement was identified by PCR.

Final Diagnosis

Multicentric Castleman disease, HHV8-positive

Take-Home Messages

1. Multicentric Castleman disease tends to occur in HIV patients.
2. The morphology of MCD often displays hyaline vascular germinal centers and expanded mantle zones with scattered plasmablasts/immunoblasts that are positive for HHV8.
3. The plasmablasts or immunoblasts usually lack complete B-cell or plasma cell antigen profile.
4. *EBV* study is negative.
5. B-cell clonality test shows no clonal *IGH/K* gene rearrangement.

Case 4 (Fig. 19.4)

Learning Objectives

1. To know the morphologic features and typical immunophenotype of extracavitary primary effusion lymphoma
2. To know how to differentiate extracavitary PEL from HHV8-positive DLBCL and other subtypes of HHV8-positive LPD

Case History

A 77-year-old female patient with unremarkable past medical history presented with constitutional symptoms and weight loss as well as symptom suggestive of bowel obstruction. Test for HIV was negative, and other causes for immunodeficiency were not noted. CT scan demonstrated a large mass lesion in large intestine. PET/CT scan revealed increased uptake in the mass lesion, but no significant lymphadenopathy or cavitary fluid collection. Endoscopic examination with biopsy of mass lesion was performed.

Histologic Findings

- The biopsy showed diffuse proliferation of abnormal lymphoid cells. These abnormal cells displayed plasmablastic/immunoblastic morphology manifested as large cells with prominent central nucleoli.

Morphologic Diagnosis

- Diffuse large cell lymphoma, possibly large B-cell lymphoma of ABC subtype
- Alternatively, plasmablastic lymphoma, extracavitary PEL or HHV8-positive DLBCL

Flow Cytometry Analysis

- A large, CD38-positive, B-cell antigen-negative lymphoid population without definitive surface immunoglobulin light chains was detected

Immunohistochemical Stains

- Immunohistochemical stains showed the large cells are positive for MUM1, CD138, cytoplasmic IgM lambda light chain restriction, and HHV8 LANA1.
- Negative for CD19, CD79a, CD20, and T-cell antigens except for focal CD3 staining.
- EBER in situ hybridization was positive.

IgH and TCR Gene Rearrangement Analysis

- Clonal *IGH* gene rearrangement was identified by PCR.
- No clonal *TCR* gene was detected.

Final Diagnosis

Extracavitary primary effusion lymphoma

Take-Home Messages

1. Primary effusion lymphoma including extracavitary variant tends to occur in HIV patients, but could occur in elderly patients with no identifiable immunodeficiency.
2. The morphology of extracavitary PEL often displays plasmablastic/immunoblastic features, as seen in other HHV8-positive LPD.
3. However, unlike other HHV8-positive DLBCL, the neoplastic cells of PEL demonstrate immunophenotypic profile suggestive of plasmacytic differentiation, including loss of pan-B-cell antigen and expression of bright CD38 and CD138.
4. Both HHV8 and *EBV* studies are positive.
5. B-cell clonality can be documented by lymphoid receptor gene rearrangement analysis.

References

1. Kim Y, Leventaki V, Bhaijee F, Jackson CC, Medeiros LJ, Vega F. Extracavitary/solid variant of primary effusion lymphoma. Ann Diagn Pathol. 2012;16(6):441–6.
2. Peker D, Alkan S, Zhang L, Martinez A. HIV-associated plasmablastic multicentric Castleman disease with microlymphoma coinfected with HHV8 and EBV. J Hematop. 2012;6(2):109–14.
3. Lee YM, Kim JM, Kim SY. Human herpes virus 8/Epstein-Barr virus-copositive, plasmablastic microlymphoma arising in multicentric Castleman's disease of an immunocompetent patient. J Pathol Transl Med. 2017;51(1):99–102.
4. Papoudou-Bai A, Hatzimichael E, Kyriazopoulou L, Briasoulis E, Kanavaros P. Rare variants in the spectrum of human herpesvirus 8/Epstein-Barr virus-copositive lymphoproliferations. Hum Pathol. 2015;46(10):1566–71.
5. Seliem RM, Griffith RC, Harris NL, Beheshti J, Schiffman FJ, Longtine J, Kutok J, et al. HHV-8+, EBV+ multicentric

plasmablastic microlymphoma in an HIV+ Man: the spectrum of HHV-8+ lymphoproliferative disorders expands. Am J Surg Pathol. 2007;31(9):1439–45.

6. Wang W, Kanagal-Shamanna R, Medeiros LJ. Lymphoproliferative disorders with concurrent HHV8 and EBV infection: beyond primary effusion lymphoma and germinotropic lymphoproliferative disorder. Histopathology. 2018;72(5):855–61.
7. Crane GM, Ambinder RF, Shirley CM, Fishman EK, Kasamon YL, Taube JM, et al. HHV-8-positive and EBV-positive intravascular lymphoma: an unusual presentation of extracavitary primary effusion lymphoma. Am J Surg Pathol. 2014;38(3):426–32.
8. Ferry JA, Sohani AR, Longtine JA, Schwartz RA, Harris NL. HHV8-positive, EBV-positive Hodgkin lymphoma-like large B-cell lymphoma and HHV8-positive intravascular large B-cell lymphoma. Mod Pathol. 2009;22(5):618–26.
9. Gonzalez-Farre B, Martinez D, Lopez-Guerra M, Xipell M, Monclus E, Rovira J, et al. HHV8-related lymphoid proliferations: a broad spectrum of lesions from reactive lymphoid hyperplasia to overt lymphoma. Mod Pathol. 2017;30(5):745–60.
10. Courville EL, Sohani AR, Hasserjian RP, Zukerberg LR, Harris NL, Ferry JA. Diverse clinicopathologic features in human herpesvirus 8-associated lymphomas lead to diagnostic problems. Am J Clin Pathol. 2014;142(6):816–29.
11. Pan ZG, et al. Extracavitary KSHV-associated large B-Cell lymphoma: a distinct entity or a subtype of primary effusion lymphoma? Study of 9 cases and review of an additional 43 cases. Am J Surg Pathol. 2012;36(8):1129–40.
12. Pan Z, Zhang QY, Lu ZB, Quinto T, Rozenvald IB, Liu LT, et al. CD3-positive plasmablastic B-cell neoplasms: a diagnostic pitfall. Mod Pathol. 2018;31:718.

Bone Marrow at Initial Diagnosis: Clinical Associations and Approach to Diagnosis

20

Anand Shreeram Lagoo and Nancy S. Rosenthal

List of Frequently Asked Questions

1. What is the relevance of morphological examination of bone marrow and the role of surgical pathologist in the era of molecular diagnostics?
2. What are the indications of bone marrow examination?
3. Are there specific indications in certain patient groups?
4. What are the contraindications for a bone marrow biopsy?
5. What is the optimal procedure for obtaining and processing bone marrow samples?
6. What is the role of imaging studies in bone marrow examination?
7. What clinical information is needed to adequately evaluate a bone marrow specimen and what does the information imply for underlying disease?
8. Which laboratory test results are needed to adequately evaluate most bone marrow specimens?
9. Which additional laboratory tests are needed for specific indications listed above?
10. What is the optimal specimen for cytological examination of the marrow?
11. How to judge the quality of aspirate smear?
12. What information is obtained from cytological examination of the marrow?
13. What is the role of the core biopsy?
14. What additional studies should be considered in the evaluation of a bone marrow?
15. Which findings are of immediate importance and should be reported to a clinician?
16. What is the optimal organization of the bone marrow report?
17. What are the mimics and what is the clinical relevance of misinterpretation between the true diagnosis and mimics with reference to mistreatment and/or prognosis?
18. Which morphological findings in the peripheral blood/BM aspirate/biopsy are reliably diagnostic? Which ones suggest the diagnosis? Which is (are) unreliable for diagnosis? Which findings rule out the diagnosis?
19. What should be the approach to provide maximum, but defensible information, from a limited specimen or work-up?
20. When is a diagnostic comment necessary and what should be discussed in the diagnostic comment?
21. When is it appropriate to seek external consultation for a bone marrow biopsy?

A. S. Lagoo (✉)
Department of Pathology, Duke University School of Medicine and Duke Health System, Durham, NC, USA
e-mail: anand.lagoo@duke.edu

N. S. Rosenthal
Department of Pathology, Wake Forest School of Medicine, Winston-Salem, NC, USA

1. What is the relevance of morphological examination of bone marrow and the role of a surgical pathologist in the era of molecular diagnostics?

Despite the emergence of many ancillary tests, morphological examination of the bone marrow remains the mainstay of diagnostic work-up for almost all neoplastic hematologic conditions and many non-neoplastic conditions as well, because:

- Availability: Bone marrow aspiration for pathological diagnosis dates back to 1903 [1], and the trephine biopsy taken from the posterior superior iliac crest has been an integral part of the diagnostic workup since the mid-1960s [2]. Morphological examination of bone marrow is now an established technique, requiring relatively simple equipment and reagents which are almost universally available.
- Objective and comprehensive morphological information: Morphology of individual cells and overall histology can be assessed, using the aspirate smear, clot section, and

E. Wang, A. S. Lagoo (eds.), *Practical Lymph Node and Bone Marrow Pathology*, Practical Anatomic Pathology,
https://doi.org/10.1007/978-3-030-32189-5_20

core biopsy. Objective, quantitative, and qualitative findings from each preparation can be recorded independently. Laboratory technologists can perform quantitative assessment such as bone marrow differential counts, providing an extra layer of unbiased observation.
- Correct classification of most neoplastic/clonal conditions according to the latest WHO guidelines still requires accurate morphologic identification and enumeration of abnormal cell types in the marrow [3]. Well-stained preparations which allow detailed cytological and histological examination and precise qualitative and quantitative assessment of each marrow component are critical for accurate diagnosis and to assess prognosis.
- Specimen triage decisions: The repertoire of ancillary studies has steadily grown in the past two decades. It is the responsibility of the pathologist to properly triage low volume specimens for competing demands of various ancillary techniques in a timely manner, someties based on limited clinical information and laboratory results. Thus, familiarity with requirements of tissue handling, amount of tissue required, and the relative advantages and disadvantages of different tests in the clinical context are needed.
- New Challenges: While combinations of clinical presentation with peripheral blood and laboratory findings are associated with a limited set of bone marrow morphological findings, newer therapies can produce unanticipated morphological changes and create new diagnostic pitfalls and challenges. Novel applications of older drugs (arsenic, thalidomide analogues), designer molecules targeting subcellular organelles (bortezomib) or precise molecular defects in individual hematological malignancies, as well as the various modalities of immunotherapy improve survival but can cause unexpected morphological changes in the bone marrow and can induce therapy-related secondary pathology.

2. What are the indications of bone marrow examination?

As the primary function of the bone marrow is production and maturation of cellular components of the blood, and to a lesser extent of lymphoid tissues, it is not surprising that most bone marrow biopsies are performed to evaluate quantitative or qualitative abnormalities of the blood. Indications for bone marrow examination and the key variables which may provide etiological clues are listed below.

- Abnormalities of the complete blood count and/or peripheral smear:
  - Evaluation of cytopenias – cells involved, duration
  - Evaluation of cytosis – cells involved, duration
  - Evaluation of circulating immature/abnormal cells – leukoerythroblastosis, acute leukemia, other tumor cells
- Evaluation of a monoclonal paraprotein, lytic bone lesions, and suspected amyloidosis
- Follow-up after therapy for a marrow-based malignancy
- Staging of lymphomas and non-hematolymphoid malignancies
- Work-up of a fever of unknown origin/infection
- Evaluation of a storage disease
- Evaluation of suspected hemophagocytic syndrome

Additional clues to possible etiologies in common indications are:

- Cytopenias: Copper deficiency can cause pancytopenia [4] and a myelopathy which may develop with zinc excess, after gastric bypass, and with total parenteral nutrition [5] (Fig. 20.1a). Evaluation of cytopenias in patients with a diagnosis of a systemic autoimmune disease may be particularly challenging, and bone marrow examination may reveal a specific cause such as MDS in about 20% of cases [6]. In one study, evaluation provided no new information and dysplasia often was reactive [7]. Patients may develop autoimmune myelofibrosis which must be distinguished from primary myelofibrosis [8]. Isolated immune-mediated thrombocytopenia does not produce consistent morphologic changes in the marrow [9], and bone marrow examination should be undertaken only when an alternate or additional pathological process is suspected. Detailed lists of possible etiologies of pancytopenia and suggestions for additional testing for definitive diagnosis are available [10, 11].
- Immature cells in blood: Presence of circulating blasts suggests a primary hematopoietic neoplasm, and circulating abnormal lymphoid cells suggest lymphoma. A leukoerythroblastic reaction can occur not only in hematopoietic neoplasms (primary myelofibrosis, etc.) but also in marrow involvement by metastases from non-hematolymphoid neoplasms [12] and some benign conditions [13–15].
- Staging bone marrow: In areas with high incidence of HIV/AIDS, a significant proportion of previously unsuspected lymphomas may be diagnosed on bone marrow examination [16]. The diagnostic yield for non-hematological neoplasms in unselected bone marrow specimens was found to be about 1% among the more than 10,000 bone marrows analyzed retrospectively [17]. Frequent clinical indications in these cases were microangiopathic hemolytic anemia, leukoerythroblastosis, or unexplained anemia [18]. About 50% of these metastases came from cancers of the lung, GI tract, and breast. Metastases are often associated with marrow fibrosis [12], which may be the reason why malignant cells cannot be

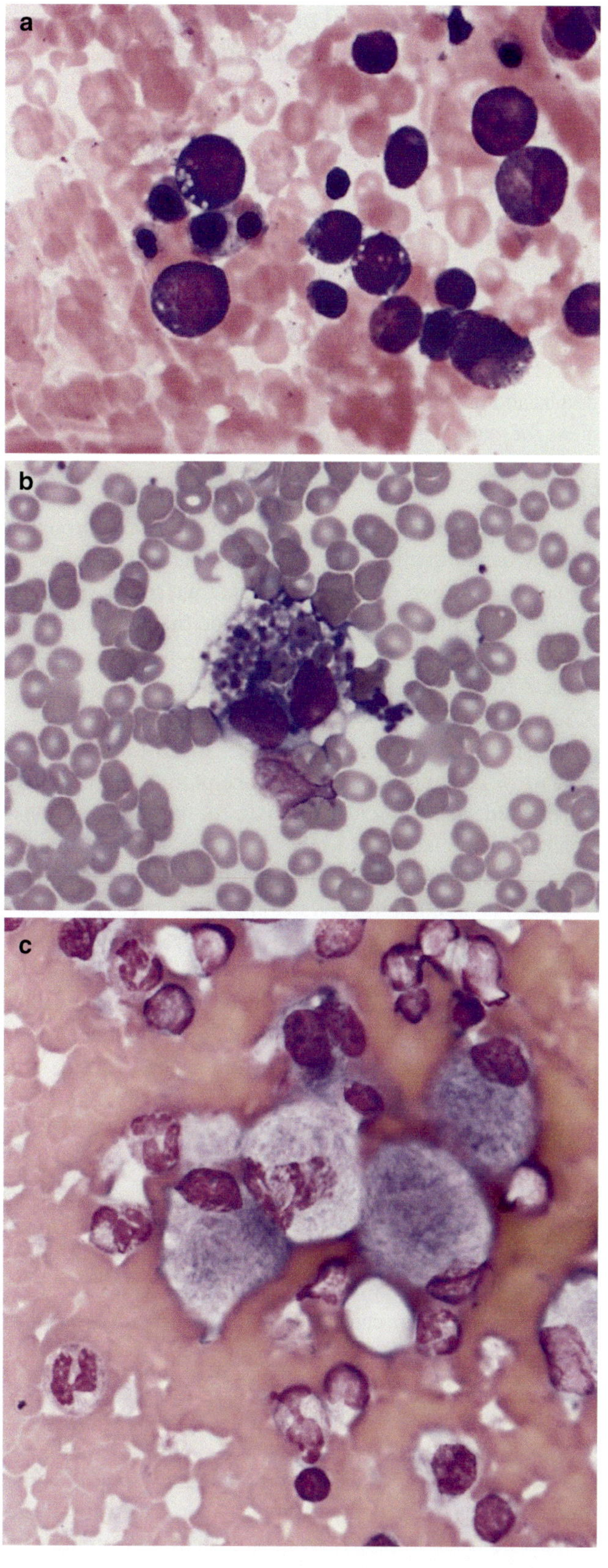

Fig. 20.1 Unusual bone marrow abnormalities in non-neoplastic bone marrow disorders (aspirate smears, Wright stain, 1000×). (**a**) Vacuolated red and white cell precursors in copper deficiency. (**b**) Hemophagocytic histiocytes in hemophagocytic lymphohistiocytosis. (**c**) Histiocytes with abundant "tissue paper" cytoplasm in Gaucher disease

identified in the aspirate smears from more than 25% of these cases.

- Suspected infections: The diagnostic yield for identification of infection is higher among immunosuppressed patients such as renal transplant recipients (about 10% compared to 1–2% in unselected bone marrows) [19, 20]. In contrast, bone marrow examination in liver transplant recipients did not detect specific infection or granulomata [21]. In HIV-AIDS patients, special stain for fungi on bone marrow biopsies appears to be as sensitive as blood and/or bone marrow culture, but only 30% bone marrows from patients with positive mycobacterial cultures demonstrate acid-fast organisms [22]. In immunocompetent patients with a fever of unknown origin, bone marrow examination is much more likely to show an underlying hematologic malignancy compared to an infectious etiology [23], and using a simple scoring system can increase the likelihood of a diagnostic bone marrow examination in such cases [24].
- Hemophagocytic syndrome: or hemophagocytic lymphohistiocytosis (HLH), often presents as fever of unknown origin (Fig. 20.1b). Hereditary abnormalities of cytotoxic molecules are responsible in a minority of cases, which generally present in children, while HLH in the vast majority of patients is triggered by infections or as paraneoplastic effect of a variety of malignancies, including lymphomas [25]. Rare nucleated red cells can be found inside macrophages in many bone marrow aspirates, without evidence of HLH, reducing the specificity of this finding in the diagnosis of HLH [26]. Conversely, the absence of microscopically demonstrable erythrophagocytosis in the marrow does not rule out the diagnosis [27]. Using "bone marrow index" incorporating laboratory values which reflect the functional status of the bone marrow is reported to be an independent predictor of HLH [28].

3. Are there specific indications in certain patient groups?

- Children and infants (Table 20.1): The indications in infants are evaluation of cytopenias and suspicion of storage disorders [29] (Fig. 20.1c). In one study, biopsies in infants constituted about 10% of pediatric bone marrow biopsies and yielded a satisfactory sample in over 95% biopsies, all of which were performed by pathologists. The commonest diagnoses were acute leukemia and storage disorders. In older children, cytopenias affecting more than one line account for over half the bone marrow examinations performed [30]. In these children, simultaneous occurrence of anemia and thrombocytopenia is the commonest finding, often accompanied by circulating blasts.
- In resource-limited settings, the indications are primarily pancytopenia, anemia, and suspected leukemia according

Table 20.1 Clinical indications for bone marrow evaluation in children [49]

Peripheral blood numerical abnormalities	Cytopenias (isolated or pancytopenia)
	With or without dysplastic features
	With or without circulating blasts
	Leukocytosis
	Blasts
	Neutrophilia and/or monocytosis with or without blasts
Systemic findings	Fever
	Lymphadenopathy and/or hepatosplenomegaly
	Bone pain
	Lytic bone lesions
	Masses suspicious for malignancy in anatomic sites that are difficult to sample; biopsy of bone marrow metastases may serve as the diagnostic sample
	Clinical manifestations of osteopetrosis

to a study from Sudan [31]. The diagnostic yield of such bone marrows was over 75%, with only a small minority of cases being normal. In a study of over 1100 bone marrows obtained over a 4-year period in Iran [20], about 10% of specimens were unsatisfactory. Sixty percent of the technically satisfactory specimens yielded a definite diagnosis. The likelihood of a definitive diagnosis varied according to the clinical indication for the bone marrow, being highest in suspected leukemia (54%), followed by plasma cell myeloma (30%), myeloproliferative neoplasms (25%), and lymphoma (16%). On the other hand, bone marrow examination rarely provided definite diagnosis in suspected storage disorders or infection (≤2%).

4. What are the contraindications for a bone marrow biopsy?

- Absolute contraindications: In adults, there are no absolute contraindications.
- Relative contraindications, particularly in children, are [32]:
  - A hemorrhagic disorder – correction of coagulation factor deficiency is advisable, but severe thrombocytopenia is not a contraindication if sufficiently prolonged pressure is applied post-biopsy. In obese patients, correction of severe thrombocytopenia is advisable.
  - Hereditary or acquired bone disorders such as osteogenesis imperfecta or osteomyelitis.
  - Skin infection or recent radiation to the biopsy site.

5. What is the optimal procedure for obtaining and processing bone marrow samples?

Guidelines for adult patients and pediatric patients differ to some extent:

Adults Instructional videos demonstrating the technique for obtaining the bone marrow sample are available (e.g., https://www.youtube.com/watch?v=EYd7OnCt7ug from the University of Oslo, https://www.youtube.com/watch?v=3hzVvCl8UkM by Dr. Alejandro Calvo), and various monographs and textbooks provide protocols for processing specimens for examination [33] or for harvesting stem cells [34].

- If needed, specimen quality can be improved through a systematic quality improvement initiative involving pathologists and relevant clinicians/ physician extenders [35]. The International Council for Standardization in Hematology has provided guidelines for a universal protocol for procurement and the contents of the pathology report [36].
- If aspirate smears are inadequate, touch imprints from marrow core biopsies are quite helpful. When correctly prepared, such "touch preps" have the advantage of transferring sufficient cells to the slide from fibrotic or otherwise inaspirable marrows and providing some architectural details in addition to good cytomorphology [37].
- A trephine core biopsy of the marrow provides information that is complimentary to the cytological preparations mentioned above. The biopsy can be done with a Jamshidi needle or a powered drill, which has been introduced relatively recently. The diagnoses from aspirate smears and core biopsies can be discordant in 20–30% cases [38]. The Hammersmith protocol, in which biopsy cores are fixed in acetic acid-zinc-formalin fixative and decalcified in 10% formic acid-5% formaldehyde, before processing for paraffin embedding, is widely adopted, as it allows sectioning at 1–2 micron thickness and renders excellent cytological and architectural details [39]. However, 10% buffered formalin can be used if other fixatives are not readily available.
- The precise site and order of the core biopsy with respect to the bone marrow aspiration are important determinants of the "aspiration artifact" in the core biopsy (Fig. 20.2a), which has the potential for limiting the usefulness of the core biopsy [40]. If the aspirate is performed first, care must be taken to biopsy from an area away from the site of the aspirate. Unilateral biopsy appears to be adequate for staging of non-Hodgkin lymphomas, provided the core is of sufficient length (≥26 mm according to one study) [16].

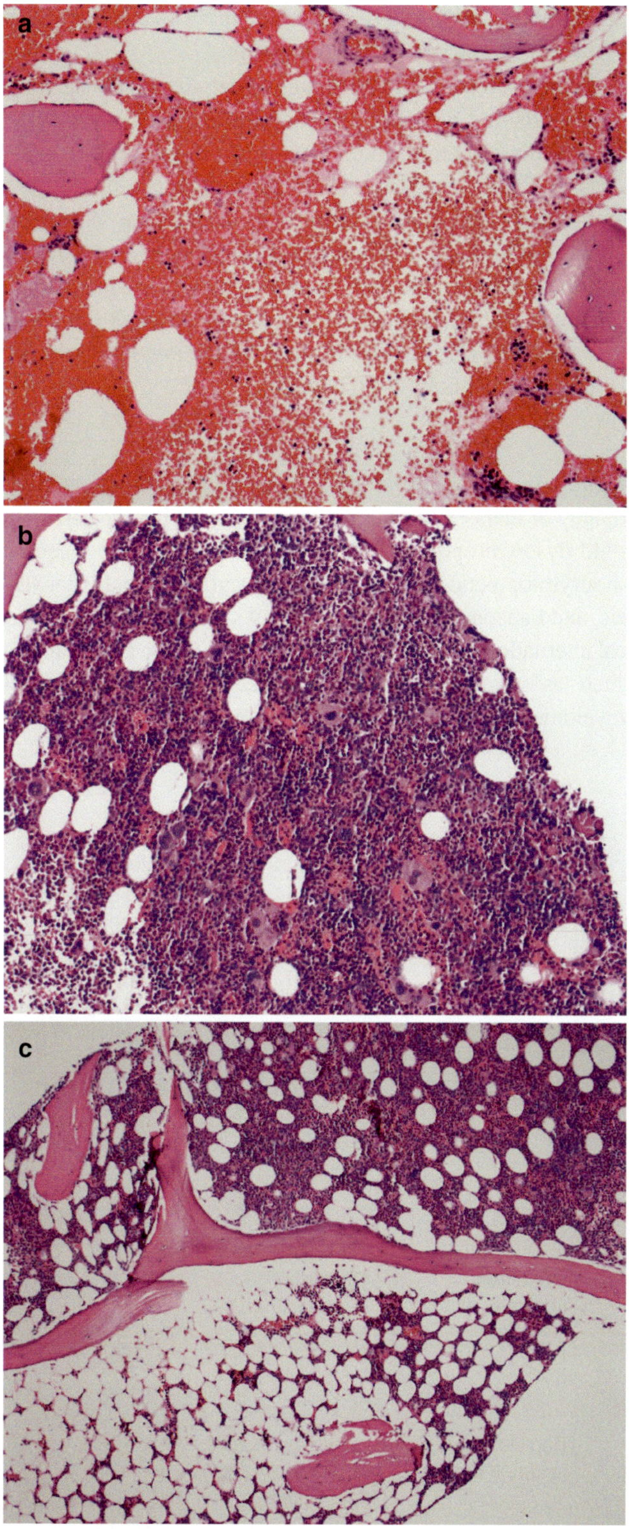

Fig. 20.2 Core biopsy, initial assessment (core biopsies, hematoxylin and eosin stain, 100×). (**a**) Aspiration artifact. The marrow contains hemorrhage and a paucity of hematopoietic cells as aspirate smear was obtained first and in the same location where the core biopsy was done. (**b**) Hypercellular marrow from an adult. (**c**) Variably cellular marrow from an adult

- While the unfixed cells obtained from an aspirate are essential for critical ancillary studies such as flow cytometry and cytogenetics, much of the same information can now be obtained from paraffin-embedded core biopsies. If decalcification and/or zinc-containing fixative preclude any type of testing, clot preparations prepared from residual aspirate material can be used. Most molecular tests for DNA and RNA as well as many fluorescent in situ hybridization (FISH) assays and immunohistochemistry can be performed on formalin-fixed, paraffin-embedded (FFPE) tissue. Alternatively, immunostaining protocols can be modified to work on decalcified and fixed bone marrow cores [41]. In resource-limited regions of the world, bone marrow aspiration by itself, when performed in patients with appropriate clinical presentations, can provide definitive diagnosis in a high proportion of cases [31].

Children Guidelines provided by Abla et al. [32] stress that the procedure should be performed only by well-trained professionals. Need for conscious sedation or anesthesia and performing the procedure in an operating room must be carefully assessed. A platelet count is recommended in all children prior to undergoing the procedure and basic coagulation tests (PT and aPTT) in those with history of coagulation defects or anticoagulant therapy. Posterior superior iliac crest is preferred in most patients, but the anterior superior iliac crest is more accessible in obese patients. Irrespective of the biopsy site (anterior or posterior iliac crest), it appears that biopsies shorter than 1.5 cm in length are more likely to produce inadequate samples [42], which suggests that the generally accepted lowest threshold of 0.5 cm [43] may be too short.

6. What is the role of imaging studies in bone marrow examination?

While not as crucial as in other areas of pathology (i.e., bone and soft tissue), evaluation of imaging studies can be helpful in interpretation of bone marrow specimens. For example, the presence of lytic lesions can lead to a diagnosis of plasma cell myeloma if the marrow shows clonal plasma cells, and the presence of lymphadenopathy or splenomegaly may help in evaluating lymphoid infiltrates. Positron emission tomography (PET) scans may be valuable in suspected benign and malignant conditions affecting the bone marrow [44]. In some cases, a positive PET scan can obviate the need for a staging marrow in lymphoma [45–47].

7. What clinical information is needed to adequately evaluate a bone marrow specimen and what does the information imply for underlying disease?

Age of the patient: This is critical in narrowing the differential diagnoses in several ways (Table 20.2):

- Is the observed cellularity normal, high, or low (Fig. 20.2b, c)? The first step in examination of bone marrow is to determine if the observed cellularity is hypocellular, normocellular, or hypercellular. The simple formula to find the normal expected cellularity for a patient is 100 minus age of the patient. However, the calculated value is too high in children [48] and too low in very old patients. Age-specific cellularity considered together with the peripheral blood findings is useful to guide further evaluation.
- Which conditions are likely to involve the marrow at this age? The common conditions seen at different age groups in Western countries are shown in Table 20.2. The incidence of these conditions varies in different parts of the world, and awareness of the local epidemiology of hematological conditions is very useful to increase the efficiency of bone marrow examination.
- Is the presence and percentage of certain cells normal for the patient's age? The percentage of mature lymphocytes, including hematogones (normal B-precursor cells) (Fig. 20.3b), decreases from infancy to adulthood [49], but may aberrantly increase in a regenerating marrow as well as unrelated conditions such as copper deficiency [50]. Plasma cells and mature lymphocytes increase in older adults [51]. Furthermore, the presence of lymphoid aggregates (Fig. 20.3b) in older adults is not necessarily pathological (see also Chap. 26).

Family history of hematologic conditions A hemoglobinopathy or thalassemia can produce erythroid hyperplasia with mild dyserythropoiesis, while rare conditions like congenital dyserythropoietic anemia, hemophagocytic lymphohistiocytosis, and Fanconi anemia are causes of significant morphological alternations in pediatric marrows [10]. Some malignancies such as chronic lymphocytic leukemia and plasma cell myeloma have a familial predisposition.

Table 20.2 Common bone marrow findings in different age groups

Age group		Infants (0–1 yr)	Children (1–10 yrs)	Adolescent/young adults (10–25 yrs)	Adult (25–65 yrs)	Elderly (65+ yrs)
Normal marrow cellularity		Can be lower than calculated by formula	Can be lower than calculated by formula	As calculated by formula	As calculated by formula	Can be higher than calculated by formula
Pathology	More likely at this age	Iron deficiency, congenital hemolytic anemia, +21 related MPN[a]	AA, ALL, BL, congenital anemia, nutritional deficiency, storage disorders	BL, cHL, CML, DLBCL	BL, cHL, CML, DLBCL, ET	AML, CLL, FL, MDS, myeloma, metastasis
	Possible at this age	ALL, AML, BL, DLBCL, infant leukemia, mastocytosis, metastases	AML, DLBCL, FL, MCL, PTCL, mastocytosis, metastases, pediatric MDS	AA, AITL, EATL, MCL, MZL, PTCL	AA, AITL, AML, EATL, FL, PMF, PTCL, PV, myeloma	AA, ALL, CML, PMF, PTCL, PV
	Rare at this age	AA, MDS, MPN	CML, PMF, PV	AA, CLL, mastocytosis, metastases, myeloma, storage disorders	Congenital anemia, metastases, storage disorders	Storage disorders
	Not seen at this age	CLL, myeloma	CLL, myeloma			Congenital anemias
Non-hematopoietic cells often present		Hematogones++, mature lymphs++, mast cells	Hematogones++, mature lymphs+++, mast cells	Hematogones+, mature lymphs++	Few plasma cells, rarely lymphoid aggregates	Interstitial lymphoid aggregates, plasma cells
Non-hematopoietic cells usually absent/rare		Lymphoid aggregates, plasma cells	Lymphoid aggregates, plasma cells	Lymphoid aggregates, plasma cells	Hematogones +/−	Hematogones −/+

[a]Abbreviations (in alphabetical order): *AA* aplastic anemia, *AITL* angioimmunoblastic T-cell lymphoma, *ALL* acute lymphoblastic leukemia, *AML* acute myeloid leukemia, *BL* Burkitt lymphoma, *cHL* classic Hodgkin lymphoma, *CLL* chronic lymphocytic leukemia, *CML* chronic myeloid leukemia, *DLBCL* diffuse large B-cell lymphoma, *EATL* enteropathy-associated T-cell lymphoma, *ET* essential thrombocythemia, *FL* follicular lymphoma, *MCL* mantle cell lymphoma, *MDS* myelodysplastic syndrome, *MPN* myeloproliferative neoplasm, *MZL* marginal zone lymphoma, *PMF* primary myelofibrosis, *PV* polycythemia vera, *PTCL* peripheral T-cell lymphoma, *NOS* not otherwise specified

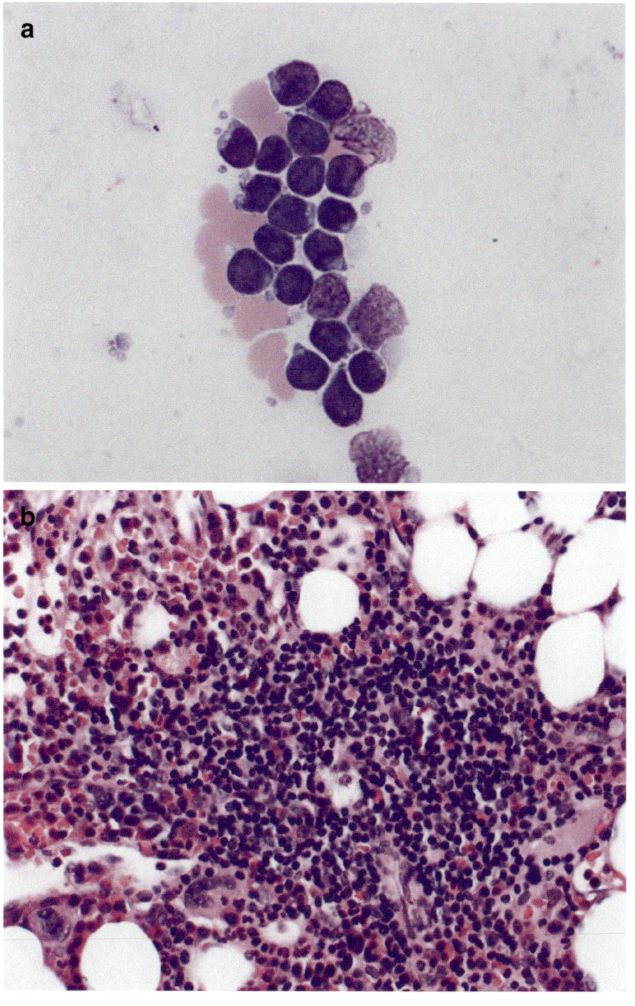

Fig. 20.3 Lymphoid cells in normal marrows. (**a**) Precursors of B lymphocytes (hematogones) in a marrow from a child undergoing evaluation for neuroblastoma; these cells with high nuclear/cytoplasmic ratios can be mistaken for blasts (aspirate smear, Wright stain, 1000×). (**b**) A well-circumscribed benign-appearing lymphoid aggregate. Lymphoid aggregates are seen with increased frequency in older patients (clot section, hematoxylin and eosin stain, 400×)

Prior malignancy and treatment Marrow recovery after chemotherapy and growth factor therapy can cause dyspoiesis and, in rare instances, increased blasts. History of prior cytotoxic drug or radiation therapy can lead to therapy-related myeloid neoplasms in a significant minority of patients [52]. Radiation field covering current biopsy site may lead to marrow suppression, fibrosis, and cellular atypia due to direct radiation effect. The effects of various immunotherapies, antibody based, stem cell based, or other, are not well documented but may mimic dysplasia or include left or right shift in maturation, hypoplasia, hyperplasia, and fibrosis.

Chronic diseases and medications Endocrinopathies including diabetes [53]and thyroid disease [54], chronic kidney disease [55], and chronic inflammatory conditions should be evaluated as there may be complex and unexpected interactive effects.

Immunodeficiency and autoimmune/rheumatic diseases These conditions can have variable functional and structural effects on the marrow. Patients with HIV-AIDS may have fungal and mycobacterial infections, lymphomas [16, 22], and pathological changes indistinguishable from MDS [56]. The pathology of immunodeficiency-associated lymphoid neoplasms is covered in detail in Chaps. 10 and 11. Autoimmune conditions may present with unexplained cytopenias [6], "primary" bone marrow fibrosis [57–59], and sometimes as combination of pancytopenia and myelofibrosis [60, 61].

Significant physical examination findings Splenomegaly and/or hepatomegaly can be a key finding to differentiate between myelodysplasia with fibrosis and a myeloproliferative neoplasm as well as some lymphomas. Lymphadenopathy is important in proper assessment of marrow lymphocytosis. Skin lesions may suggest a mast cell or Langerhans cell neoplasm as well as T-cell lymphomas such as adult T-cell leukemia/lymphoma and peripheral T-cell lymphoma NOS.

8. Which laboratory test results are needed to adequately evaluate most bone marrow specimens?

- Complete blood count (CBC) and evaluation of a well-spread and stained peripheral blood smear: Evaluation of the presence and degree of either cytopenias or cytosis may be helpful in determining a diagnosis. The MCV may be beneficial in determining the cause for an anemia (macrocytosis is often associated with myelodysplastic syndromes).
- A well-stained blood smear is important because features such as neutrophil granulation are prone to artifacts and may be misinterpreted as dysplasia. The WHO recommends a 200-cell WBC differential, excluding any nucleated red blood cells. Identification of blasts, blast equivalents, and other immature cells is critical for any case in which acute leukemia, myelodysplastic syndrome, or myeloproliferative neoplasm is suspected.

9. Which additional laboratory tests are needed for specific indications listed above?

- Tests performed to *rule out* a neoplastic/clonal hematologic process: Ideally, clinicians should rule out reactive, nutritional, or toxic causes of the peripheral blood changes before performing the bone marrow aspiration; however, knowledge of vitamin B12, folate, serum copper, and heavy metal (lead, mercury, and zinc) levels is important to avoid overdiagnosis of MDS. Iron studies, tests for hemoglobinopathies and other congenital red cell abnormalities, tests for immune hemolytic anemia, and tests for paroxysmal nocturnal hemoglobinuria may be helpful in microcytic and normocytic anemia.
- Tests performed to *confirm/classify* suspected hematologic neoplasms: Cytogenetic and/or molecular tests for suspected myeloproliferative neoplasms are often performed on blood. A suspected plasma cell neoplasm is further investigated with serum and/or urine protein electrophoresis, immunofixation electrophoresis, and serum light chain evaluation. Serum tryptase may be helpful in the evaluation of mast cell disorders.
- Laboratory tests in systemic diseases with hematological manifestations: Suspected autoimmune, metabolic, or infectious diseases are investigated with appropriate laboratory tests prior to bone marrow biopsy to clearly formulate a rationale for the procedure and to guide additional testing on the bone marrow specimen.

10. What is the optimal specimen for cytological examination of the marrow?

- Wedge "pull" smear versus crush film smear [62, 63]: In the authors' experience, both "crush" smears made by placing marrow particles directly from the aspirating syringe on coverslips (Fig. 20.4a) and well-made "pull" smears made at the bedside (Fig. 20.4b) can provide consistently high-quality cytomorphology and uniform staining.
- Smears prepared from EDTA anticoagulated marrow are not inferior to those prepared directly from the aspirated marrow [64], but the WHO recommendation is to prepare smears from fresh marrow whenever possible, and smears prepared from anticoagulated marrow beyond 2 hours from collection are not suitable for determination of dysplastic changes.
- If the aspirate does not contain particles, the touch preparation (Fig. 20.4c) provides an alternative for cytological examination. Touch preps may provide diagnostic material while aspirate smears do not in focal involvement of the marrow by conditions such as metastatic carcinoma and plasma cell myeloma and diseases frequently

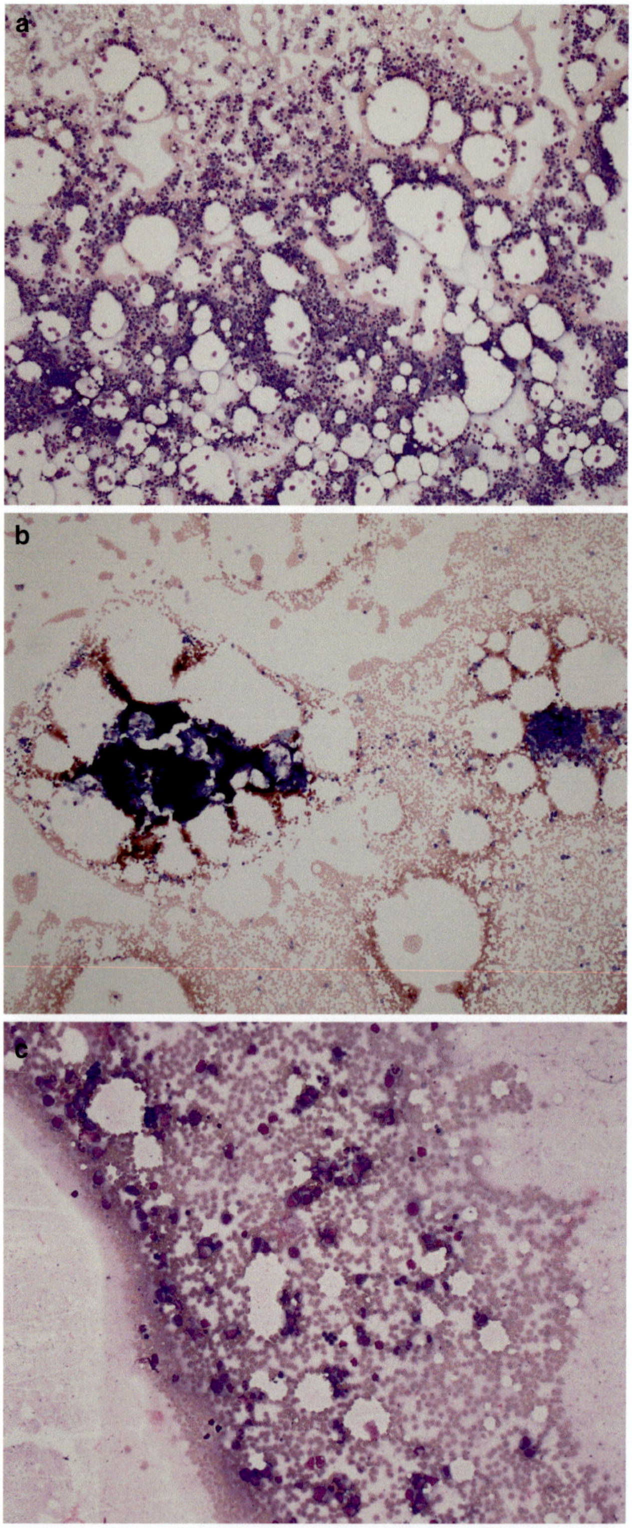

Fig. 20.4 Bone marrow aspirate preparations (aspirate smears, Wright stain, 100×). (**a**) Example of a crush preparation. (**b**) Example of a direct smear. (**c**) A touch preparation, made by touching the core biopsy on the glass slide. These can be helpful if the aspirate smear does not contain particles

associated with marrow fibrosis (various myeloproliferative neoplasms, MPNs, or MDS/PMN overlap).

11. How to judge the quality of aspirate smear?

- The presence of marrow particles (or spicules) in aspirate smears provides assurance that the findings are representative of the marrow. The proportion of various cell types expected in the marrow is best represented in the "tails" of smears following the marrow particles, where staining and cytologic details are optimal.
- Familiarity with the correct hues of basophilic, amphophilic, and eosinophilic staining at various stages of myeloid and erythroid precursors is essential to correctly assess dysplasia in these lineages. Avoid under-stained areas where blasts may be overestimated based on apparently fine chromatin.

12. What information is obtained from cytological examination of the marrow?

The aspirate smear (and/or the touch prep) is used for:

- Assessing proportion of erythroid and myeloid elements: A 500-cell differential of all nucleated cells is recommended, particularly when accurate and reproducible blast counts are critical for diagnosis or prognosis; however, in many cases, a 300-cell count suffices [61]. A differential count may be skipped if the total number of cells on the aspirate smear and touch preparation is limited as such counts are error-prone. The differential count includes myeloid (all three types of granulocytic and monocytic) and erythroid precursors as well as lymphocytes (mature and immature) and plasma cells (Fig. 20.5a). The megakaryocytes, mast cells, stromal cells, histiocytes, and any abnormal, non-hematopoietic cells, if present, are not included (Fig. 20.5b). The myeloid to erythroid ratio is calculated based on the differential count and should be normally 2–3:1. Ideally, the differential should be counted from several different slides.
- Assessing maturation of each line: Morphologic criteria for blasts and blast equivalents must be defined. Typical cells at various stages of myeloid and erythroid maturation are depicted in many standard texts, but it is important to recognize that maturation is a continuous process and each cell type spans a range of morphology. The laboratory should establish normal adult ranges for each cell type (Table 20.3). Widely accepted normal ranges for pediatric bone marrow are not available.
- Evaluating dysplasia: Despite the advances in molecular diagnostic methods, identification of cellular dysplasia is

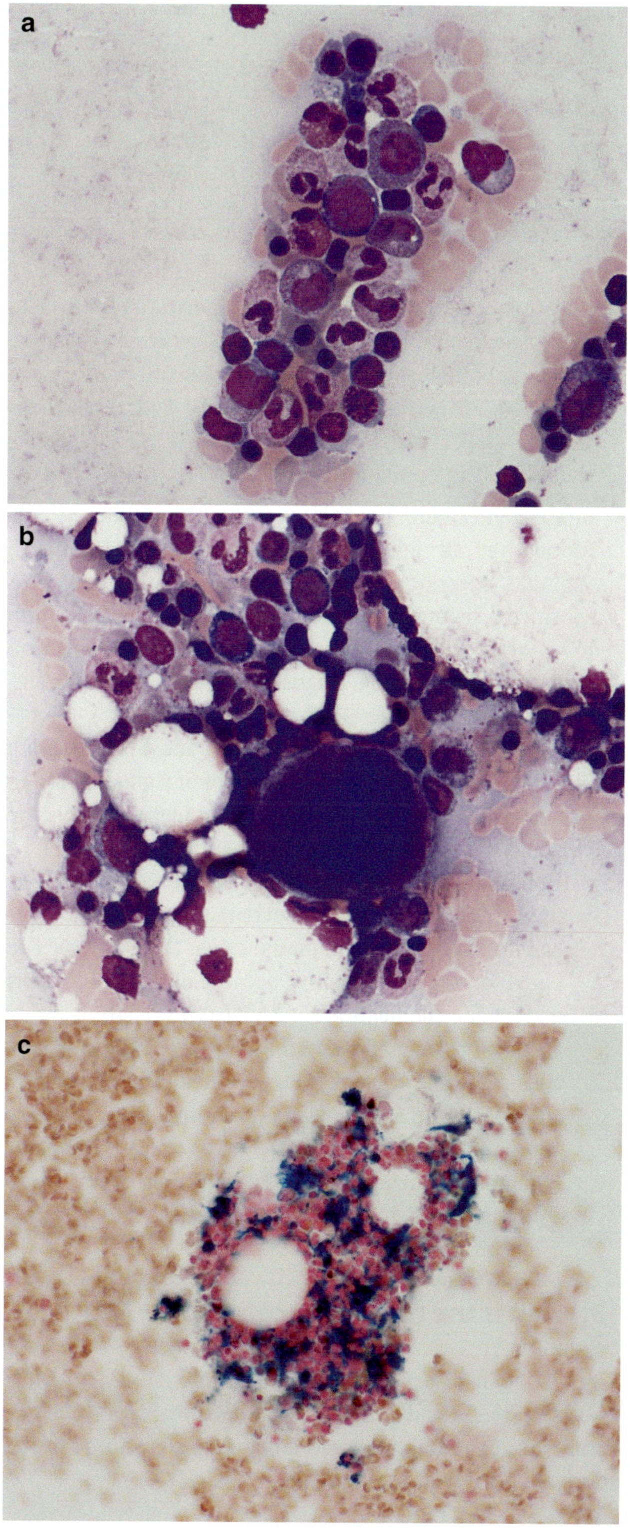

Fig. 20.5 Evaluation of bone marrow cells. (**a**) Normal myeloid and erythroid precursors. The myeloid to erythroid ratio should be approximately 2–3:1, and full maturation of both cell lines should be present (aspirate smear, Wright stain, 1000×). (**b**) Megakaryocytes are scattered on the smears (aspirate smear, Wright stain, 100×). (**c**) A Prussian blue for iron can be done on the aspirate smears or the clot sections (clot section Prussian blue stain, 40×)

Table 20.3 Reference ranges for bone marrow differential count in adults

Cell type	Reference range	Cell type	Reference range	Cell type	Reference range
Segs	(7–25)	Lymphocytes	(3–20)	Plasma cells	(0–3.5)
Bands	(6–36)	Atypical lymphocytes		RBC precursors	(10–30)
Metas	(9–25)	Lymphoblasts		Pronormoblasts	(0–3)
Myelos	(8–15)	Eosinophils	(0–4)	M:E ratio	
Promyelos	(1–6)	Basophils	(0–1)	Iron	(Scale 0–4+)
Myeloblasts	(0–3.5)	Monocytes	(0–2)		

a central pillar for diagnosis and categorization of myelodysplastic syndromes and some types of acute leukemia. The morphological findings of dysplasia are presented in Chap. 24. In addition to vitamin B12 and folate deficiency, copper deficiency as a cause of such changes should be kept in mind [65, 66].

- Storage and sideroblast iron: An iron stain should be performed on all initial adult bone marrow specimens. Aspirate smears containing particles are best suited for sensitive detection as well as quantification of storage iron [67]. We find a semi-quantitative, 4-point scale useful to grade iron stores; absent (grade 0 of 4) and trace of 4 stainable iron indicated reduced iron stores, grade 1–3 of 4 staining indicates normal stores, and grade 4 of 4 staining indicates increased stores. The amount of stainable iron in patients with normal iron stores varies widely, and only the two ends of the scale denote pathological finding.
  – Iron staining of clot section or core biopsy may be used if the aspirate does not contain particles and storage iron is not detected on the smear (Fig. 20.5c). The core biopsy is less sensitive because of tissue thickness and/or decalcification [68]. Iron-stained aspirate smears or touch preparations are required to assess ring sideroblasts which is important for classifying subtypes of myelodysplastic syndrome. Iron stains are less helpful in patients treated for a variety of hematologic malignancies as these patients often develop iron overload due to repeated transfusions.

13. What is the role of the core biopsy?

An H&E stained section (3–4uM) of a core biopsy, which is 1.5 cm in length and contains at least 10 marrow spaces, is optimal for examining the histological "architecture" of the marrow. This includes:

- Bone marrow cellularity: Cellularity is estimated in areas without significant aspiration or crush artifact. To estimate cellularity, it is useful to mentally estimate what percentage of the marrow space would be occupied if all the cells were together and all the fat was together. Highly fibrotic marrow may have very low proportion of fat, but also may contain few hematopoietic cells. A rare abnormality is gelatinous transformation or serous atrophy in which there is focal hypocellularity, accumulation of mucopolysaccharides, and normal fat replaced by a light pink granular material [69]. It occurs in a variety of clinical situations including anorexia nervosa, acute fever, HIV-AIDS, alcoholism, lymphoid and other malignancies, and chronic heart failure [70]. A similar change, called "marrow injury effect" or fibrinous necrosis (Fig. 20.6a) is often observed

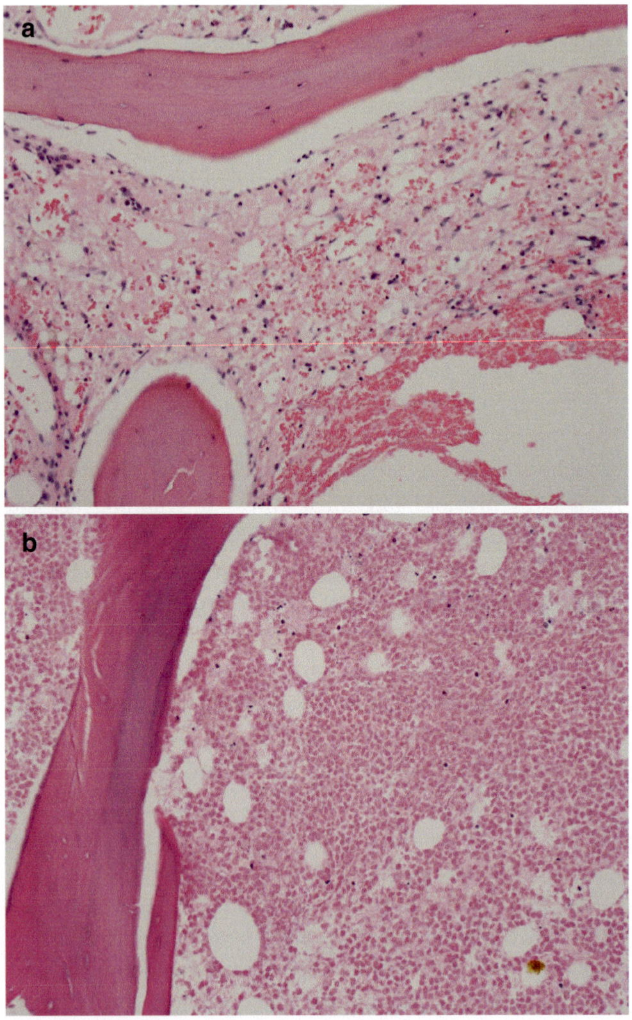

Fig. 20.6 Stromal abnormalities (core biopsies, hematoxylin and eosin stain, 100×). (**a**) Fibrinous necrosis. Stromal damage, hypocellularity, and focal hemorrhage due to recent chemotherapy. (**b**) Necrosis. Hypocellularity and necrotic tumor are seen in this example of marrow necrosis

after recent chemotherapy for a hematopoietic malignancy. It is more important to describe these abnormalities, rather than emphasizing a percentage cellularity. If the cellularity varies by more than 20%, the range should be mentioned and an average cellularity should be given. Subcortical marrow spaces can have lower cellularity than the rest of the marrow, and these should be avoided in calculating the average cellularity if possible.

- Appropriate distribution, proportion, and maturation of hematopoietic elements: Myeloid cells proliferate in paratrabecular areas (Fig. 20.7), and more mature myeloid elements are present in the interstitium. Erythroid cells are present as small colonies of cells at various stages of maturation in the interstitial areas. Megakaryocytes should be evenly distributed, away from bone. Adequacy of megakaryocytes is best assessed on the core biopsy as well as megakaryocyte dysplasia and clustering. The M:E ratio is assessed independently on the core biopsy and compared to that calculated on the aspirate smear. Left shift in maturation and collections of five or more immature precursors (myeloblasts and promyelocytes, proerythroblasts, monoblasts, and promonocytes) can be appreciated in the core biopsy, while it is generally not possible to verify minimal increase in immature cell types which are normally present in the marrow. An immunohistochemical stain for CD34 may be helpful in enumerating blasts.
- Marrow sinuses and vessels: The sinuses are inconspicuous unless they are dilated and/or filled with hematopoietic cells (as in primary myelofibrosis) (Fig. 20.8a) or abnormal infiltrating cells (as certain types of B- or T-cell lymphomas do). The normal marrow microvasculature is barely noticeable unless the vascularity is increased or the individual vessels have pathological changes. Small arteries are seen occasionally and when present are useful to assess amyloid deposition.
- Marrow fibrosis: A reticulin stain may be routinely or selectively performed depending on the institution but is essential in myeloproliferative neoplasms for accurate grading of the disease (Fig. 20.8b). It also can highlight early mastocytosis or minimal involvement by lymphoma. Fibrosis is rarely seen in conditions such as CLL/SLL, plasma cell neoplasms, and MDS. When present in these conditions, it may have prognostic significance [71]. A trichrome stain is required in selected cases of primary or secondary myelofibrosis for accurate grading.
- Infiltrative lesions: These may arise from neoplastic or inflammatory processes. The former may be hematolymphoid malignancies or other solid tumors metastasizing to the marrow (see also Chap. 27). Benign lymphoid aggre-

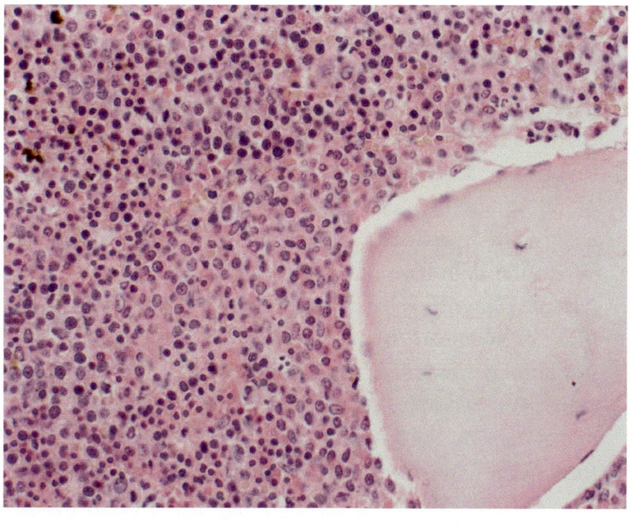

Fig. 20.7 Myeloid maturation (core biopsy, hematoxylin and eosin stain, 400×). Early myeloid precursors are seen in a paratrabecular location in this normal bone marrow

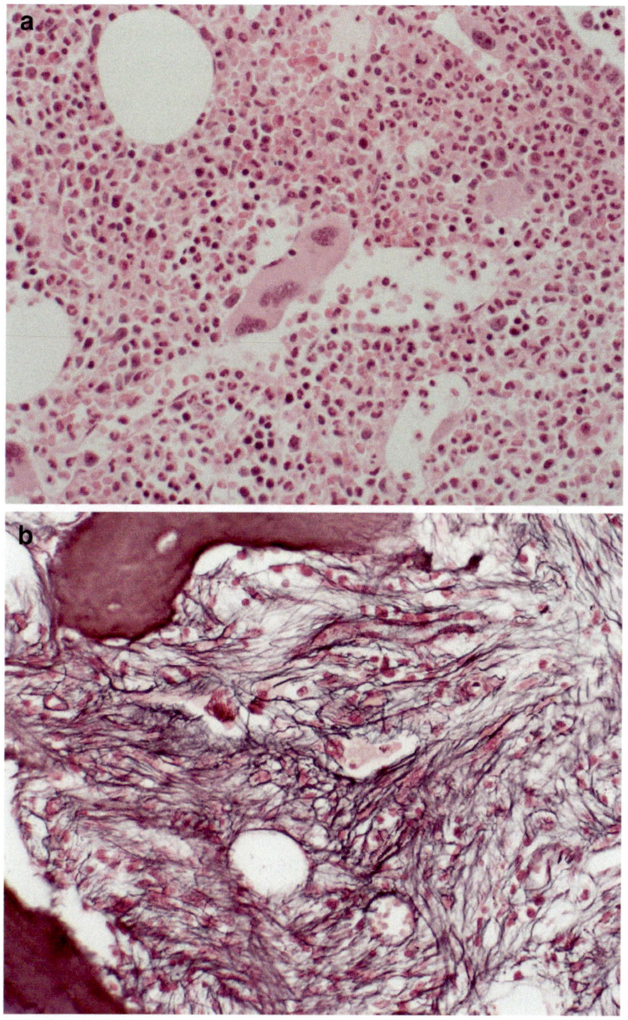

Fig. 20.8 Marrow sinusoids and fibrosis (core biopsies, hematoxylin and eosin stain, reticulin stain, 200×). (**a**) Dilated marrow sinusoids with intrasinusoidal hematopoiesis are present from a patient with primary myelofibrosis. (**b**) Increased reticulin fibrosis is present. Reticulin stains are essential in the evaluation of myeloproliferative disorders

gates may be seen with aging or a systemic chronic inflammatory condition. Other infiltrative/focal lesions most often are due to plasma cell neoplasms, systemic mastocytosis, Langerhans cell histiocytosis, and rarely histiocytic sarcomas. Granulomas are also seen in marrows and may be due to a variety of underlying causes [72].

- Necrosis: Diffuse necrosis of the bone marrow is seen in less than 1% bone marrows (Fig. 10.6b) and is almost always associated with metastatic or hematopoietic malignancy [73]. In some instances, extensive necrosis can make it difficult to determine the nature of the underlying malignancy.
- Changes in bone: While primary bone pathology is an infrequent finding in the bony trabeculae, evidence of hyperparathyroidism or Paget disease of bone may be present. Diffuse necrosis of bone marrow may be associated with karyolysis of osteocytes in the bony trabeculae and should be distinguished from true avascular necrosis of bone.
- Presence of unexpected "second" pathological process or disease: Particularly in older individuals, one can find evidence of a clinically unsuspected hematolymphoid process [74]. When both processes are relatively common, it is difficult to determine if they have any clonal or causal relationship or it is a chance occurrence [75]. (See Chap. 30 for more details).

14. What additional studies should be considered in the evaluation of a bone marrow?

Ancillary studies vary based on the indication for performing the bone marrow aspiration. The menu can be optimized by creating standard protocols [76, 77]. Some studies can be performed on routinely processed tissue, but some require additional specimen and decision to do these tests must be made at the time of collection. These studies include:

- Flow cytometry: A specimen should be collected in nearly every case. Two ml to 5 ml of marrow in a heparinized syringe is optimal. It is recommended that the first pull should be used for minimal residual disease (MRD) detection, especially for plasma cell myeloma [78]. In resource-poor settings, actual analysis can be safely delayed in almost all cases for 24–72 hours if the indication is not definitive.
- Karyotyping and FISH: Conventional cytogenetic analysis requires 2 ml or more of fresh (unfixed) heparinized marrow collected under aseptic conditions. FISH tests are often performed as a panel. FISH for *PML/RARA* translocation needs a rapid turnaround time if acute promyelocytic leukemia is suspected. These concerns must be communicated promptly to the performing laboratory so the test can be set up appropriately.
- Molecular tests: Most DNA-based tests can be performed on paraffin-embedded tissue, but decalcification can hamper some tests. However, DNA, and even more so RNA, promptly purified from fresh bone marrow collected in EDTA is more intact and provides more reliable results. Heparin may interfere in some PCR reactions. See Chap. 2 for additional precautions in collecting specimen for molecular tests.
- Bone marrow culture: When an infectious process is suspected, marrow should be submitted for culture, which can be more sensitive than morphological identification of mycobacteria (but not fungi) and blood culture [22].
- Additional unstained aspirate smears should be saved for performing cytochemical stains, including iron stain, as well as for FISH studies, particularly those involving numeric abnormalities.
- Ancillary tests which are performed on FFPE bone marrow biopsy and clot section include the following (see Chaps. 1 and 2 for more information about these tests):
  - Immunohistochemistry
  - Histochemical stains (Congo red, PAS, trichrome, etc.)
  - Paraffin FISH
  - Molecular tests (PCR-based amplification and sequencing, next-generation sequencing, RNA-based assays for gene expression)

15. Which findings are of immediate importance and should be reported to a clinician?

The following findings in the aspirate smear and/or touch preparation should be reported immediately to the clinician:

- Increased blasts (>20%) suggestive of acute leukemia, particularly if the morphology is suggestive of acute promyelocytic leukemia (see Chap. 21). Determining lymphoid versus myeloid leukemia may be difficult in the absence of Auer rods.
- When the definitive diagnosis from a set of limited differential diagnoses based on clinical or radiographic findings is obtained by morphological examination, the preliminary diagnosis should be conveyed to the clinicians; for example, metastasis versus plasma cell neoplasm causing lytic bone lesions.
- Presence of fungal or other organisms in the bone marrow – Histoplasma and candida may be detected in routinely stained aspirate smears. Prompt notification may help timely treatment and isolation of the patient.

16. What is the optimal organization of the bone marrow report?

- Bone marrow reports often include morphological descriptions. Pertinent parts of a concurrent CBC and microscopic findings in the peripheral blood and bone marrow aspirate (and/or touch preparation and clot section and core biopsy), including results of special stains, should be given. The choice of a narrative description versus a tabular reporting of findings varies from institution to institution. The College of American Pathologists has proposed synoptic report templates for hematologic neoplasms [79].
- In addition to morphology, flow cytometric, immunohistochemical, cytogenetic, FISH, and molecular results which are available at the time of completing the report may influence the specificity of the report.
- Bone marrow diagnoses can be broadly categorized based on degree of diagnostic certainty:
  - Definitive diagnosis of an entity: For neoplastic conditions, diagnosis according to WHO classification should be the goal [80]. Other clinically important findings or presence of a second pathological process should be mentioned as secondary diagnoses. In a comment, mention the key ancillary findings which support the diagnosis, such as positive FISH for *BCR/ABL* in a case of CML.
  - In case of a new malignant diagnosis, when all ancillary studies are completed, it is recommended that a comprehensive addendum diagnosis is issued which correlates the diagnostic, therapeutic, and prognostic impact of the additional results.
  - In follow-up marrows after therapy, the presence or absence of residual disease should be mentioned prominently so clinicians can easily find this information.
  - A descriptive diagnosis is appropriate when:
  - There are no pathological findings: The normal state of the marrow is conveyed by a phrase such as "Normocellular marrow with adequate trilineage hematopoiesis" along with status of iron stores.
- The pathological findings are not specific: The distinction between neoplastic and non-neoplastic conditions cannot be made with certainty, either because there is insufficient evidence of a clonal process (blast count is not high, flow cytometry is not diagnostic, etc.) or the morphological findings such as dysplasia, megakaryocytic abnormalities, or reticulin fibrosis are not well developed, or nutritional deficiencies, toxins, or infections can cause identical morphological change. In these situations, the key morphological findings, both normal and abnormal, are listed to provide a snapshot of the likely functional status of the marrow. Particularly in cases of cytopenias, the distinction between inability to produce enough cells or their destruction in the marrow or in the periphery is helpful. In these cases, the comment should include the likely differential diagnoses, the ancillary studies, and/or clinical/radiographic findings which can narrow the differential or provide a definitive diagnosis.

17. What are the mimics and what is the clinical relevance of misinterpretation between the true diagnosis and mimics with reference to mistreatment and/or wrong prognosis?

Caution should be exercised in interpreting following morphological findings, because they can be deceptively similar in the conditions listed below in the absence of ancillary studies:

- Small (8–9 uM diameter) blasts with high N:C ratio – hematogones (Fig. 20.3a), B-ALL (Fig. 20.9a), minimally differentiated AML

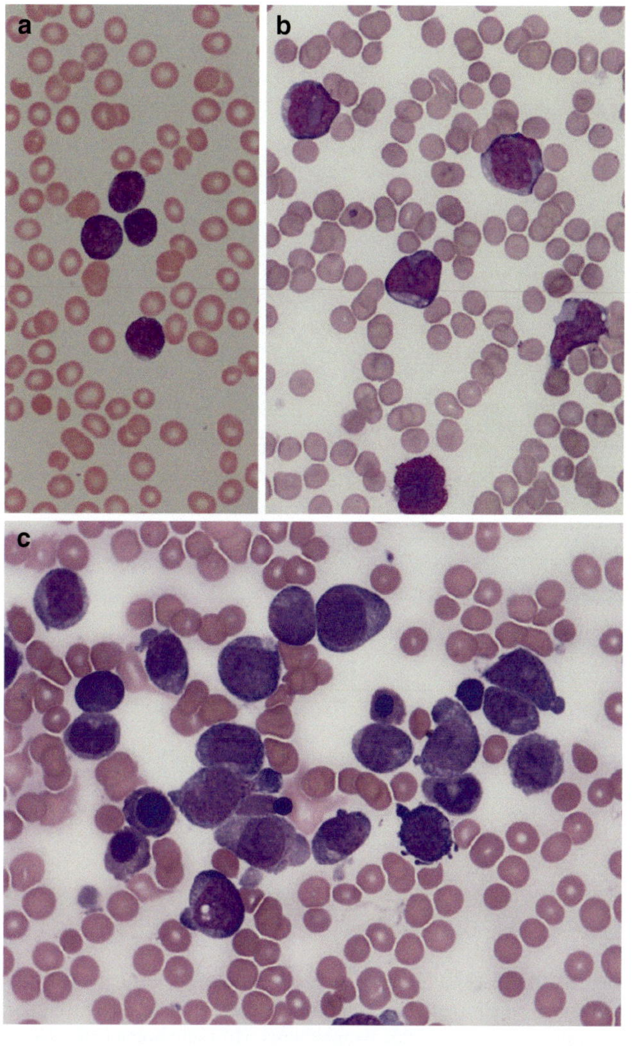

Fig. 20.9 Mimics (aspirate smears, Wright stain, 1000×). (**a**) Small blasts in B lymphoblastic leukemia should be differentiated from hematogones. Similarly, (**b**) hypogranular acute promyelocytic leukemia must not be mistaken for (**c**) Monocytic leukemia

- Large (12–18 uM diameter) immature cells with folded nuclei – hypogranular APL, monocytic acute leukemia (Fig. 20.9b,c)
- Blastoid cells – myeloblasts, plasmablasts, megaloblasts, metastases of small blue cell tumors (Fig. 20.10a), blastic plasmacytoid dendritic cell neoplasm, large cell lymphoma (Fig. 20.10b)
- Spindle cells, particularly in paratrabecular location – systemic mastocytosis (Fig. 20.11a), osteosclerotic myeloma, follicular lymphoma
- Giant cells – abnormal megakaryocytes, inflammatory giant cells (Fig. 20.11b), osteoclasts
- Abnormal granulocytes: toxic granules in infection and growth factor administration, hypolobate nuclei in benign Pelger-Huet anomaly or MDS

18. Which morphological findings in the peripheral blood/BM aspirate/biopsy are reliably diagnostic? Which ones suggest the diagnosis? Which is (are) unreliable for diagnosis? Which findings rule out the diagnosis?

Most morphological marrow findings must be interpreted in the context of clinical and other findings. Few are completely diagnostic or completely rule out a process.

- Pathognomonic findings: Auer rods (Fig. 20.12) are pathognomonic to distinguish abnormal myeloid from lymphoid blasts, but not acute leukemia from myelodysplasia. Amyloid identified by Congo red stain is consid-

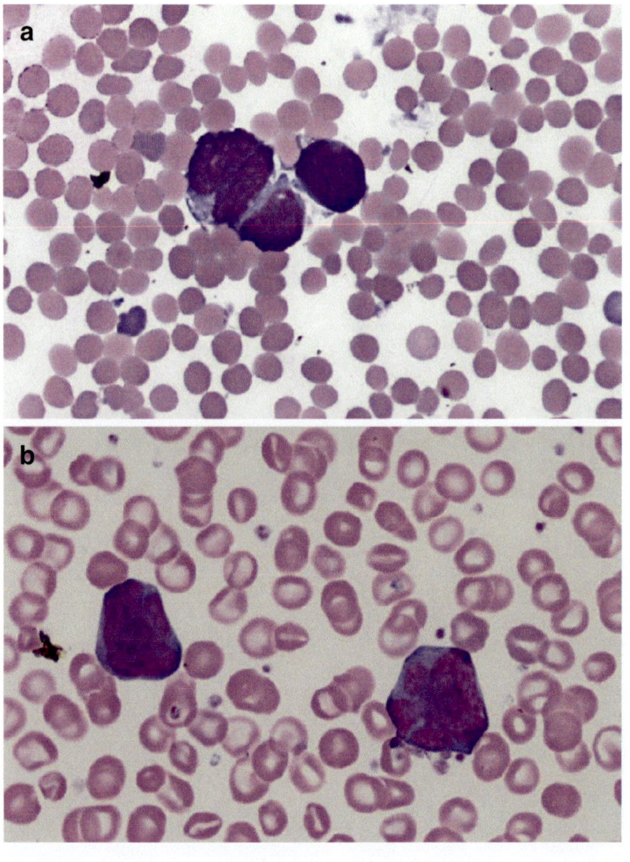

Fig. 20.10 Blastoid cells (aspirate smears, Wright stain, 1000×). (**a**) Metastatic small round blue cell tumor (neuroblastoma). These can be separate cells and resemble lymphoblasts. (**b**) Lymphoma cells. These cells may resemble blasts

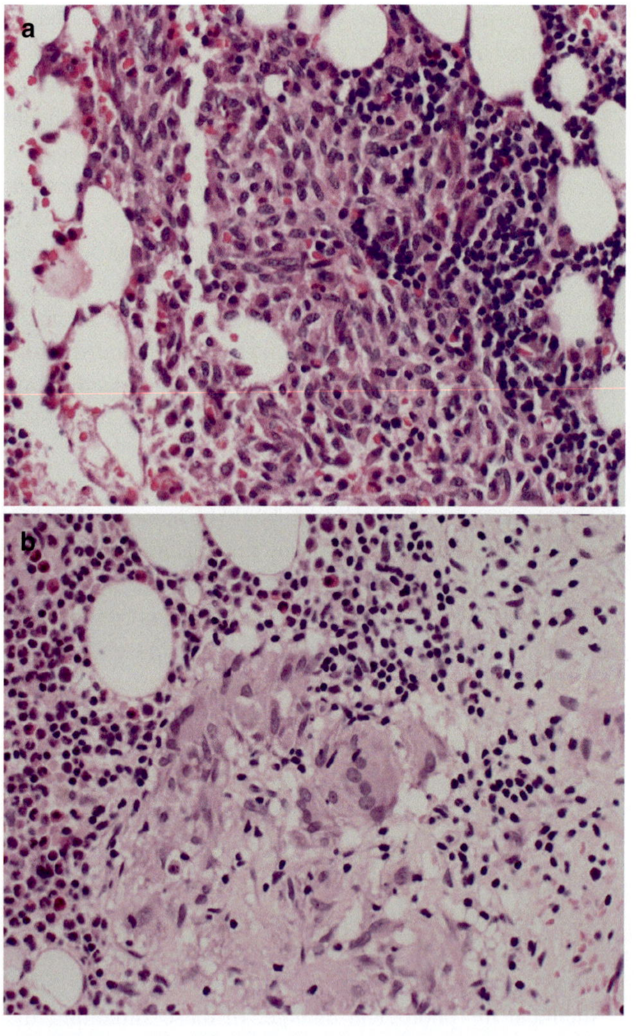

Fig. 20.11 Spindle cells and giant cells (core biopsy, hematoxylin and eosin stain, 400×). (**a**) Spindle cells in systemic mastocytosis shown here may be difficult to differentiate from fibroblasts. (**b**) Inflammatory giant cells need to be distinguished from megakaryocytes and osteoclasts

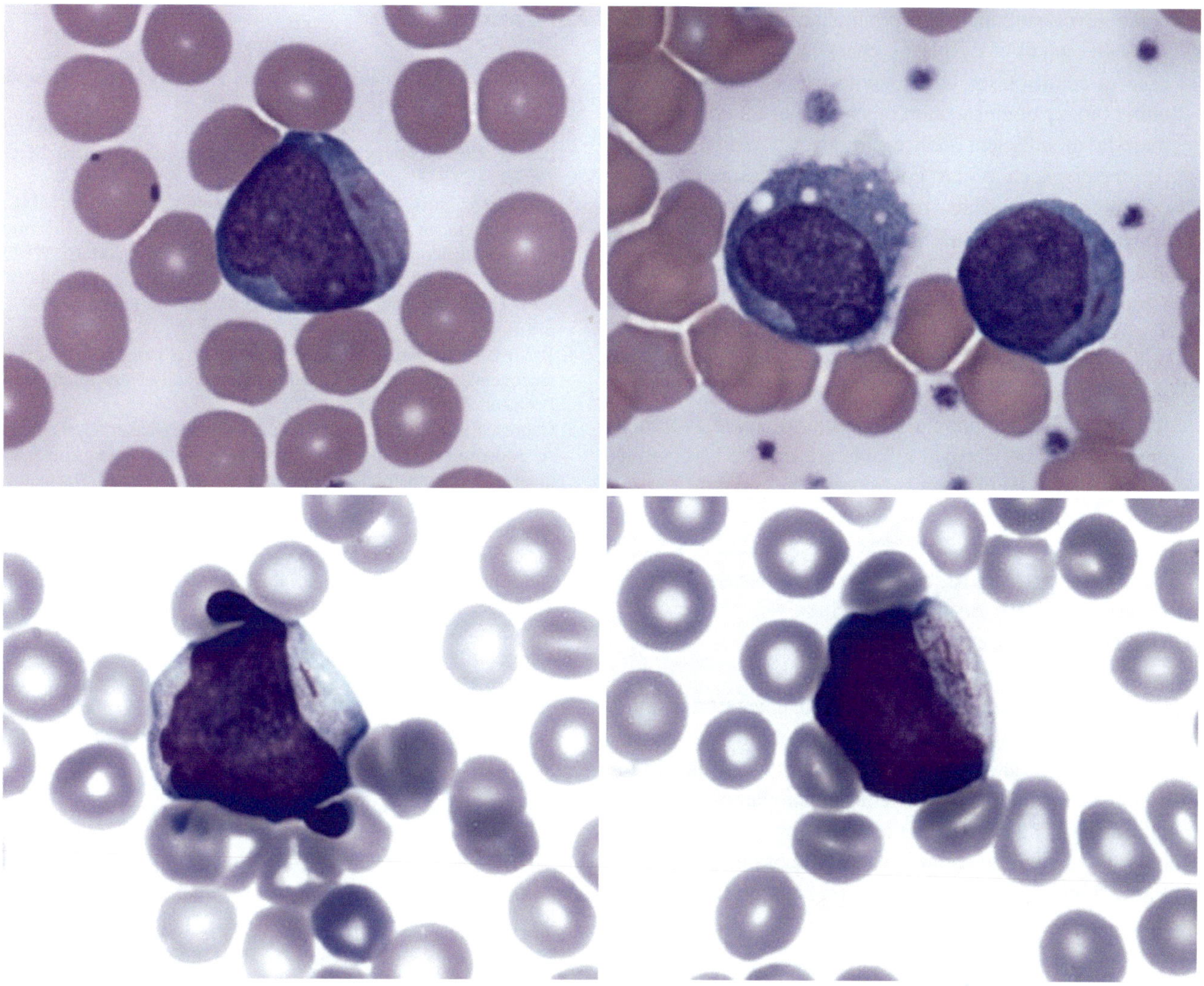

Fig. 20.12 Auer rods (Wright stain, 1000×). Auer rods are only seen in malignant myeloid blasts (upper panels) and abnormal promyelocytes (lower panels) and can be helpful in distinguishing lymphoid from myeloid blasts

ered specific; however; the determination of the underlying cause for the amyloid needs further study. Fungal and mycobacterial infections with appropriate special stains are considered sufficiently diagnostic even in the absence of additional proof by culture or molecular methods. A blast count above 20% of marrow cells based on morphological identification from a good quality aspirate smear is typically sufficient to diagnose acute leukemia, but exceptions occur such as infants with Down syndrome and patients receiving myeloid growth factor therapy.

- Suggestive of diagnosis: Dysplastic morphology is required for diagnosis in most MDS cases and is suggestive but is not sufficient for definitive diagnosis. Characteristic combinations of morphological findings are suggestive of the subtypes of MPNs, but diagnosis requires demonstration of specific mutations or ruling out reactive causes.
- Unreliable for diagnosis: See morphologic mimics above.
- Findings that rule out a diagnosis: Stainable storage iron rules out iron deficiency, but absence of stainable iron may be due to biological or technical reasons.

19. What should be the approach to provide maximum, but defensible information, from limited specimen or work-up?

- Following morphological findings tend to be unreliable in quantitatively limited specimens: proportion of various cells including M:E ratio and blast percentage in sparsely cellular aspirate smears, iron stores in aparticulate aspirate smears, marrow cellularity in subcortical marrow, and involvement by focal processes such as lymphoma, myeloma, metastases, etc., in small specimens (<5 mm long or <5 marrow spaces).

- Qualitatively suboptimal aspirate smears preclude accurate assessment of dysplastic changes and should not be used to count blasts. Often, some part of the specimen, either biopsy or clot section or aspirate or touch prep, has material of sufficient quality and quantity. Some of these parameters, such as blast count, can be measured by flow cytometry even when morphologically the specimen appears hopelessly inadequate with the caveat that blasts are often under-represented in flow cytometry specimens.
- The quality and quantity of the bone marrow core biopsy is less important in disorders like leukemia if there is a good aspirate smear compared to evaluation for infiltrative lesions like lymphoma or metastatic disease. Provided only the findings deemed reliable are reported, very few marrows are completely insufficient for diagnosis.

20. When is a diagnostic comment necessary and what should be discussed in the diagnostic comment?

A diagnostic comment is the rule rather an exception in bone marrow reports, because in many cases a definitive diagnosis of a well-defined entity is not possible. The report is part of an ongoing consultation between the hematopathologists and the clinicians. The content of the comment is dependent on whether the diagnosed entity is neoplastic or non-neoplastic and how definitive is the diagnosis (see the question about content of a bone marrow biopsy report).

21. When is it appropriate to seek external consultation for a bone marrow biopsy?

External consultation may be appropriate:

- If the clinical picture does not fit the pathological diagnosis. For example, the patient is clinically well and stable despite an apparent high-grade MDS.
- When there is a major discrepancy between the morphological diagnosis and the molecular/genetic results. For example, *BCR/ABL* translocation without any evidence of progressive leukocytosis, thrombocytosis, or acute leukemia.
- If certain pathological findings are not adequately explained by the overall diagnosis. Such findings may include reticulin fibrosis, histiocytic or lymphoid collections, deposition of acellular material of uncertain nature, etc.
- When the pathological findings are borderline or suggest a rare condition.
- In morphologically identical conditions with significant therapeutic differences.

References

1. Parapia LA. Trepanning or trephines: a history of bone marrow biopsy. Br J Haematol. 2007;139(1):14–9.
2. Ellis LD, Jensen WN, Westerman MP. Needle biopsy of bone and marrow; an experience with 1,445 biopsies. Arch Intern Med. 1964;114:213–21.
3. Arbor DA, Orazi A, Hasserjian RP, Brunning RD, Beau MML, Porwit A, et al. Introduction and overview of the classification of myeloid neoplasms. In: Swerdlow SH, et al., editors. WHO Classification of tumours of haematopoietic and lymphoid tissues. Lyon: International Agency for Research on Cancer; 2017. p. 16–27.
4. Wazir SM, Ghobrial I. Copper deficiency, a new triad: anemia, leucopenia, and myeloneuropathy. J Community Hosp Intern Med Perspect. 2017;7(4):265–8.
5. Gabreyes AA, Abbasi HN, Forbes KP, McQuaker G, Duncan A, Morrison I. et al. Hypocupremia associated cytopenia and myelopathy: a national retrospective review. Eur J Haematol. 2013;90(1):1–9.
6. Papageorgiou A, Ziakas PD, Tzioufas AG, Voulgarelis M. Indications for bone marrow examination in autoimmune disorders with concurrent haematologic alterations. Clin Exp Rheumatol. 2013;31(1):76–83.
7. Hunt KE, Salama ME, Sever CE, Foucar K. Bone marrow examination for unexplained cytopenias reveals nonspecific findings in patients with collagen vascular disease. Arch Pathol Lab Med. 2013;137(7):948–54.
8. Pullarkat V, Bass RD, Gong JZ, Feinstein DI, Brynes RK. Primary autoimmune myelofibrosis: definition of a distinct clinicopathologic syndrome. Am J Hematol. 2003;72(1):8–12.
9. Mahabir VK, Ross C, Popovic S, Sur ML, Bourgeois J, Lim W, et al. A blinded study of bone marrow examinations in patients with primary immune thrombocytopenia. Eur J Haematol. 2013;90(2):121–6.
10. Leguit RJ, van den Tweel JG. The pathology of bone marrow failure. Histopathology. 2010;57(5):655–70.
11. Weinzierl EP, Arber DA. The differential diagnosis and bone marrow evaluation of new-onset pancytopenia. Am J Clin Pathol. 2013;139(1):9–29.
12. Delsol G, Guiu-Godfrin B, Guiu M, Pris J, Corberand J, Fabre J. Leukoerythroblastosis and cancer frequency, prognosis, and physiopathologic significance. Cancer. 1979;44(3):1009–13.
13. Kakkar N, Mittal D, Das S, John JM, Rajamanickam T. Bone marrow involvement in systemic oxalosis: a rare cause of leukoerythroblastic anemia. Indian J Pathol Microbiol. 2011;54(3):659–60.
14. Simon D, Galambos JT. Leukoerythroblastosis with blasts in a patient with alcoholic hepatitis. J Clin Gastroenterol. 1987;9(2):217–8.
15. Tapia G, Navarro JT, Navarro M. Leukoerythroblastic anemia due to oxalosis with extensive bone marrow involvement. Am J Hematol. 2008;83(6):515–6.
16. Phillips L, Opie J. The utility of bone marrow sampling in the diagnosis and staging of lymphoma in South Africa. Int J Lab Hematol. 2018;40:276.
17. Xiao L, Luxi S, Ying T, Yizhi L, Lingyun W, Quan P. Diagnosis of unknown nonhematological tumors by bone marrow biopsy: a retrospective analysis of 10,112 samples. J Cancer Res Clin Oncol. 2009;135(5):687–93.
18. Ozkalemkas F, Ali R, Ozkocaman V, Ozcelik T, Ozan U, Ozturk H, et al. The bone marrow aspirate and biopsy in the diagnosis of unsuspected nonhematologic malignancy: a clinical study of 19 cases. BMC Cancer. 2005;5:144.
19. Garewal G, Ahluwalia J, Kumar V, Shukla R, Das R, Varma N, et al. The utility of bone marrow examination in renal transplanta-

tion: nine years of experience from north India. Transplantation. 2006;81(9):1354–6.
20. Mirzai AZ, Hosseini N, Sadeghipour A. Indications and diagnostic utility of bone marrow examination in different bone marrow disorders in Iran. Lab Hematol. 2009;15(4):38–44.
21. Borcek P, Ozdemir BH, Sercan C, Yilmaz Akcay E, Karakus S, Haberal M. Histologic changes in bone marrow biopsies from liver transplant patients. Exp Clin Transplant. 2016;14(Suppl 3):109–11.
22. Kilby JM, Marques MB, Jaye DL, Tabereaux PB, Reddy VB, Waites KB. The yield of bone marrow biopsy and culture compared with blood culture in the evaluation of HIV-infected patients for mycobacterial and fungal infections. Am J Med. 1998;104(2):123–8.
23. Hot A, Jaisson I, Girard C, French M, Durand DV, Rousset H, et al. Yield of bone marrow examination in diagnosing the source of fever of unknown origin. Arch Intern Med. 2009;169(21):2018–23.
24. Wang HY, Yang CF, Chiou TJ, Yang SH, Gau JP, Yu YB, et al. A "bone marrow score" for predicting hematological disease in immunocompetent patients with fevers of unknown origin. Medicine (Baltimore). 2014;93(27):e243.
25. Rosado FG, Kim AS. Hemophagocytic lymphohistiocytosis: an update on diagnosis and pathogenesis. Am J Clin Pathol. 2013;139(6):713–27.
26. Goel S, Polski JM, Imran H. Sensitivity and specificity of bone marrow hemophagocytosis in hemophagocytic lymphohistiocytosis. Ann Clin Lab Sci. 2012;42(1):21–5.
27. Gupta A, Tyrrell P, Valani R, Benseler S, Weitzman S, Abdelhaleem M. The role of the initial bone marrow aspirate in the diagnosis of hemophagocytic lymphohistiocytosis. Pediatr Blood Cancer. 2008;51(3):402–4.
28. Wang HY, Yang CF, Chiou TJ, Yang SH, Gau JP, Yu YB, et al. Risk of hemophagocytic lymphohistiocytosis in adults with fevers of unknown origin: the clinical utility of a new scoring system on early detection. Hematol Oncol. 2017;35(4):835–44.
29. Sreedharanunni S, Sachdeva MU, Kumar N, Sharma P, Naseem S, Ahluwalia J, et al. Spectrum of diseases diagnosed on bone marrow examination of 285 infants in a single tertiary care center. Hematology. 2015;20(3):175–81.
30. Naseem S, Varma N, Das R, Ahluwalia J, Sachdeva MU, Marwaha RK. Pediatric patients with bicytopenia/pancytopenia: review of etiologies and clinico-hematological profile at a tertiary center. Indian J Pathol Microbiol. 2011;54(1):75–80.
31. Elmadhoun WM, Noor SK, Bushara SO, Almobarak AO, Husain NE, Ahmed MH. Bone marrow aspiration in north Sudan: the procedure, indications and the diagnostic value. Int J Health Sci (Qassim). 2015;9(4):434–9.
32. Abla O, Friedman J, Doyle J. Performing bone marrow aspiration and biopsy in children: recommended guidelines. Paediatr Child Health. 2008;13(6):499–501.
33. Afkhami M, Vergara-Lluri M, Brynes RK, Siddiqi IN. Peripheral blood smears, bone marrow aspiration, trephine and clot biopsies: methods and protocols. Methods Mol Biol. 2014;1180:257–69.
34. Friedlis MF, Centeno CJ. Performing a better bone marrow aspiration. Phys Med Rehabil Clin N Am. 2016;27(4):919–39.
35. Yang RK, Nazeef M, Patel SS, Mattison R, Yang DT, Ranheim EA, et al. Improving bone marrow biopsy quality through peer discussion and data comparisons: a single institution experience. Int J Lab Hematol. 2018;40:419.
36. Lee SH, Erber WN, Porwit A, Tomonaga M, Peterson LC. ICSH guidelines for the standardization of bone marrow specimens and reports. Int J Lab Hematol. 2008;30(5):349–64.
37. Gong X, Lu X, Wu X, Xu R, Tang Q, Xu G, et al. Role of bone marrow imprints in haematological diagnosis: a detailed study of 3781 cases. Cytopathology. 2012;23(2):86–95.
38. Gilotra M, Gupta M, Singh S, Sen R. Comparison of bone marrow aspiration cytology with bone marrow trephine biopsy histopathology: an observational study. J Lab Physicians. 2017;9(3):182–9.
39. Naresh KN, Lampert I, Hasserjian R, Lykidis D, Elderfield K, Horncastle D, et al. Optimal processing of bone marrow trephine biopsy: the Hammersmith Protocol. J Clin Pathol. 2006;59(9):903–11.
40. Douglas DD, Risdall RJ. Bone marrow biopsy technic. Artifact induced by aspiration. Am J Clin Pathol. 1984;82(1):92–4.
41. Kremer M, Quintanilla-Martinez L, Nahrig J, von Schilling C, Fend F. Immunohistochemistry in bone marrow pathology: a useful adjunct for morphologic diagnosis. Virchows Arch. 2005;447(6):920–37.
42. Grant RC, Shaikh F, Abdelhaleem M, Alexander SW, Cada M. Risk factors for inadequate bone marrow biopsies in children. Am J Hematol. 2015;90(9):E187–9.
43. Reid MM, Roald B. Adequacy of bone marrow trephine biopsy specimens in children. J Clin Pathol. 1996;49(3):226–9.
44. van der Bruggen W, Glaudemans A, Vellenga E, Slart R. PET in benign bone marrow disorders. Semin Nucl Med. 2017;47(4):397–407.
45. El Karak F, Bou-Orm IR, Ghosn M, Kattan J, Farhat F, Ibrahim T, et al. PET/CT scanner and bone marrow biopsy in detection of bone marrow involvement in diffuse large B-cell lymphoma. PLoS One. 2017;12(1):e0170299.
46. Agbay R, Loghavi S, Zuo Z, Fayad L, Dabaja B, Medeiros LJ, et al. Bone marrow involvement in patients with nodular lymphocyte predominant Hodgkin lymphoma. Am J Surg Pathol. 2018;42(4):492–9.
47. Puccini B, Nassi L, Minoia C, Volpetti S, Ciancia R, Riccomagno PC, et al. Role of bone marrow biopsy in staging of patients with classical Hodgkin's lymphoma undergoing positron emission tomography/computed tomography. Ann Hematol. 2017;96(7):1147–53.
48. Friebert SE, Shepardson LB, Shurin SB, Rosenthal GE, Rosenthal NS. Pediatric bone marrow cellularity: are we expecting too much? J Pediatr Hematol Oncol. 1998;20(5):439–43.
49. Onciu M. Pediatric bone marrow interpretation. Surg Pathol Clin. 2010;3(4):1091–125.
50. Sutton L, Vusirikala M, Chen W. Hematogone hyperplasia in copper deficiency. Am J Clin Pathol. 2009;132(2):191–9; quiz 307.
51. Liang J, Malherbe JAJ, Fuller KA, Mirzai B, George C, Carter TL, et al. Automated enumeration of lymphoid and plasma cells in bone marrow to establish normal reference ranges. J Clin Pathol. 2018;71:916.
52. Ganser A, Heuser M. Therapy-related myeloid neoplasms. Curr Opin Hematol. 2017;24(2):152–8.
53. Fadini GP, Ciciliot S, Albiero M. Concise review: perspectives and clinical implications of bone marrow and circulating stem cell defects in diabetes. Stem Cells. 2017;35(1):106–16.
54. Soliman AT, De Sanctis V, Yassin M, Wagdy M, Soliman N. Chronic anemia and thyroid function. Acta Biomed. 2017;88(1):119–27.
55. Azevedo P, Cardoso PSR, Farah KP, de Melo FHC, Rezende SM. Complete reversal of bone marrow fibrosis after parathyroidectomy for secondary hyperparathyroidism. Br J Haematol. 2017;178(4):500.
56. Thiele J, Zirbes TK, Bertsch HP, Titius BR, Lorenzen J, Fischer R. AIDS-related bone marrow lesions--myelodysplastic features or predominant inflammatory-reactive changes (HIV-myelopathy)? A comparative morphometric study by immunohistochemistry with special emphasis on apoptosis and PCNA-labeling. Anal Cell Pathol. 1996;11(3):141–57.
57. Piatek CI, Vergara-Lluri ME, Pullarkat V, Siddiqi IN, O'Connell C, Brynes RK, et al. Autoimmune myelofibrosis: clinical features, course, and outcome. Acta Haematol. 2017;138(3):129–37.
58. Abaza Y, Yin CC, Bueso-Ramos CE, Wang SA, Verstovsek S. Primary autoimmune myelofibrosis: a case report and review of the literature. Int J Hematol. 2017;105(4):536–9.
59. Vergara-Lluri ME, Piatek CI, Pullarkat V, Siddiqi IN, O'Connell C, Feinstein DI, et al. Autoimmune myelofibrosis: an update on

morphologic features in 29 cases and review of the literature. Hum Pathol. 2014;45(11):2183–91.
60. Ungprasert P, Chowdhary VR, Davis MD, Makol A. Autoimmune myelofibrosis with pancytopenia as a presenting manifestation of systemic lupus erythematosus responsive to mycophenolate mofetil. Lupus. 2016;25(4):427–30.
61. Tang VK, Huh YO, Tayar JH, Rojas Hernandez CM. Primary autoimmune myelofibrosis as etiology of pancytopenia mimicking myelodysplastic syndrome. Leuk Lymphoma. 2016;57(3):731–4.
62. Lewandowski K, Complak A, Hellmann A. Microscopic examination of bone marrow aspirates in malignant disorders of haematopoiesis--a comparison of two slide preparation techniques. Ann Hematol. 2012;91(4):497–505.
63. Sharma P, Sachdeva MU, Varma N. Bone marrow aspirate smear preparation: morphological superiority of the timely wedge smear and the importance of imprints. Ann Hematol. 2014;93(6):1063–4.
64. Aleem A, Alsaleh K, Aljabry M, Aziz S, Iqbal Z, Almomen A. A comparison of two techniques of preparing bone marrow aspirate slides. J Pak Med Assoc. 2016;66(5):528–7.
65. Oo TH, Hu S. Copper deficiency-related bone marrow changes secondary to long-term total parenteral nutrition. Clin Case Rep. 2017;5(2):195–6.
66. Dalal N, Hooberman A, Mariani R, Sirota R, Lestingi T. Copper deficiency mimicking myelodysplastic syndrome. Clin Case Rep. 2015;3(5):325–7.
67. Beutler E. Clinical evaluation of iron stores. N Engl J Med. 1957;256(15):692–7.
68. Wallerstein RO. Marrow iron. JAMA. 1977;238(15):1661–2.
69. Das S, Mishra P, Kar R, Basu D. Gelatinous marrow transformation: a series of 11 cases from a tertiary care centre in South India. Turk J Haematol. 2014;31(2):175–9.
70. Bohm J. Gelatinous transformation of the bone marrow: the spectrum of underlying diseases. Am J Surg Pathol. 2000;24(1):56–65.
71. Tadmor T, Shvidel L, Aviv A, Ruchlemer R, Bairey O, Yuklea M, et al. Significance of bone marrow reticulin fibrosis in chronic lymphocytic leukemia at diagnosis: a study of 176 patients with prognostic implications. Cancer. 2013;119(10):1853–9.
72. Brackers de Hugo L, Ffrench M, Broussolle C, Seve P. Granulomatous lesions in bone marrow: clinicopathologic findings and significance in a study of 48 cases. Eur J Intern Med. 2013;24(5):468–73.
73. Wool GD, Deucher A. Bone marrow necrosis: ten-year retrospective review of bone marrow biopsy specimens. Am J Clin Pathol. 2015;143(2):201–13; quiz 306.
74. Himchak E, Marks E, Shi Y, Wang Y. Did I miss it? discovering hidden coexisting hematological neoplasms: a single institutional review of 100 collision tumors. Int J Surg Pathol. 2018;26(4):296–305.
75. Alley CL, Wang ED, Dunphy CH, Gong JZ, Lu CYM, Boswell EL, et al. Diagnostic and clinical considerations in concomitant bone marrow involvement by plasma cell myeloma and chronic lymphocytic leukemia/monoclonal B-cell lymphocytosis. Arch Pathol Lab Med. 2013;137(4):503–17.
76. Seegmiller AC, Kim AS, Mosse CA, Levy MA, Thompson MA, Kressin MK, et al. Optimizing personalized bone marrow testing using an evidence-based, interdisciplinary team approach. Am J Clin Pathol. 2013;140(5):643–50.
77. Seegmiller AC, Kim AS, Mosse CA, Shaver AC, Thompson MA, Li S, et al. Data-driven iterative refinement of bone marrow testing protocols leads to progressive improvement in cytogenetic and molecular test utilization. Am J Clin Pathol. 2016;146(5):585–93.
78. Arroz M, Came N, Lin P, Chen W, Yuan C, Lagoo A, et al. Consensus guidelines on plasma cell myeloma minimal residual disease analysis and reporting. Cytometry B Clin Cytom. 2016;90(1):31–9.
79. Sever C, Abbott CL, de Baca ME, Khoury JD, Perkins SL, Reichard KK, et al. Bone marrow synoptic reporting for hematologic neoplasms: guideline from the College of American Pathologists Pathology and Laboratory Quality Center. Arch Pathol Lab Med. 2016;140(9):932–49.
80. Swerdlow SH, Campo E, Harris NL, Jaffe ES, Pileri SA, Stein H, et al. WHO classification of tumours of haematopoietic and lymphoid tissues. In: Sosman FT, et al., editors. World Health Organization classification of tumours. Revised 4 ed. Lyon: International Agency for Research on Cancer; 2017. p. 585.

Acute Leukemias

21

Yang Shi, David D. Grier, and Jadee Neff

List of Frequently Asked Questions

1. What are the major types of acute leukemias?
2. What are the typical morphological findings in acute leukemias?
3. What are the mimics and what is the clinical relevance of misinterpretation between the true diagnosis and mimics with reference to mistreatment and/or wrong prognosis?
4. Which morphological findings in the peripheral blood/BM aspirate/biopsy are reliably diagnostic of acute leukemia? Which ones suggest the diagnosis? Which is (are) unreliable for diagnosis? Which findings rule out the diagnosis?
5. What is the minimal and optimal ancillary workup for diagnosis and subclassification of acute leukemias?
6. Which ancillary test results are diagnostic, suggestive of diagnosis, unreliable for diagnosis, or rule out the diagnosis?
7. What is the workup to provide prognostic and therapeutic target information? (Corollary – what treatments are available for this entity?)
8. Which subtypes of this entity are clinically relevant, and which are morphologically defined but have unproven/minimal clinical relevance?
9. What is an adequate specimen for this condition?
10. What information can be conveyed to the clinician during each stage of the workup?
11. What should be the approach to provide maximum, but defensible information, from limited specimen or workup? What is a descriptive diagnosis appropriate in such situations?
12. When is a diagnostic comment necessary, and what should be discussed in the diagnostic comment for this entity?
13. When it is appropriate to seek external consultation for this entity?

1. What are the major types of acute leukemias?

The classification of acute leukemias is complex and constantly evolving. The current classification system as defined by the 2017 WHO classification consists of three main categories [1]:

- Acute myeloid leukemias (AMLs)
- Acute lymphoblastic leukemias (ALL)
- Acute leukemias with ambiguous lineage

As shown in Table 21.1, the current WHO classification depends heavily on cytogenetic and molecular genetic findings as well as key clinical history such as prior radiation and/or chemotherapy. Morphological examination retains a central role in the diagnosis of acute leukemias for accurate identification and enumeration of blasts, to determine type of blasts in conjunction with flow cytometric immunophenotype, to document presence of myelodysplastic features, and to examine other hematopoietic elements. In particular, the classification of AML subtypes requires careful qualitative and quantitative assessment of marrow cells, clinical information, and integration of several ancillary test results. See Fig. 21.1 for an algorithmic approach to the diagnosis of AML.

Y. Shi
Department of Pathology, Montefiore Medical Center, Albert Einstein College of Medicine, Bronx, NY, USA
e-mail: yash@montefiore.org

D. D. Grier
Division of Pathology & Laboratory Medicine, Cincinnati Children's Hospital Medical Center, Cincinnati, OH, USA
e-mail: David.Grier@cchmc.org

J. Neff (✉)
Department of Pathology, Duke University School of Medicine, Durham, NC, USA
e-mail: jadee.neff@duke.edu

E. Wang, A. S. Lagoo (eds.), *Practical Lymph Node and Bone Marrow Pathology*, Practical Anatomic Pathology,
https://doi.org/10.1007/978-3-030-32189-5_21

Table 21.1 Classification system for acute leukemia (WHO 2017)

Myeloid leukemias	AML with recurrent genetic abnormalities
	AML with t(8;21)(q22;q22.1); *RUNX1-RUNX1T1*
	AML with inv(16)(p13.1q22) or t(16;16)(p13.1;q22) *CBFB-MYH11*
	Acute promyelocytic leukemia with *PML-RARA*
	AML with t(9;11)(p21.3;q23.3); *KMT2A-MLLT3*
	AML with t(6;9)(p23;q34.1); *DEK-NUP214*
	AML with inv(3)(q21.3q26.2) of t(3;3)(q21.3;q26.2); *GATA2, MECOM*
	AML (megakaryoblastic) with t(1;22)(p13.3;q13.1); *RBM15-MKL1*
	AML with *BCR-ABL1*
	AML with mutated *NPM1*
	AML with biallelic mutation of *CEBPA*
	AML with mutated *RUNX1*
	AML with myelodysplasia-related changes
	Therapy-related AML
	AML, NOS
	AML with minimal differentiation
	AML without maturation
	AML with maturation
	Acute myelomonocytic leukemia
	Acute monoblastic and monocytic leukemia
	Pure erythroid leukemia
	Acute megakaryoblastic leukemia
	Acute basophilic leukemia
	Acute panmyelosis with myelofibrosis
	Myeloid sarcoma
	Myeloid proliferations associated with Down syndrome
	Blastic plasmacytoid dendritic cell neoplasm (BPDCN)
Lymphoblastic leukemias	B-lymphoblastic leukemia/lymphoma (B-ALL/LBL)
	B-ALL/LBL, NOS
	B-ALL/LBL with t(9;22)(q34.1;q11.2); *BCR-ABL1*
	B-ALL/LBL with t(v;11q23.3); *KMT2A* rearranged
	B-ALL/LBL with t(12;21)(p13.2;q22.1); *ETV6-RUNX1*
	B-ALL/LBL with hyperdiploidy
	B-ALL/LBL with hypodiploidy
	B-ALL/LBL with t(5;14)(q31.1;q32.1); IGH/*IL3*
	B-ALL/LBL with t(1;19)(q23;p13.3); *TCF3-PBX1*
	B-ALL/LBL, *BCR-ABL1*-like
	B-ALL/LBL with iAMP21
	T-lymphoblastic leukemia/lymphoma
	Early T-cell precursor lymphoblastic leukemia
	NK-lymphoblastic leukemia/lymphoma
Leukemias of ambiguous lineage	Acute undifferentiated leukemia
	Mixed-phenotype acute leukemia (MPAL)
	MPAL with t(9;22)(q34.1;q11.2); *BCR-ABL1*
	MPAL with t(v;11q23.3); *KMT2A* rearranged
	MPAL, B/myeloid, NOS
	MPAL, T/myeloid, NOS
	MPAL, NOS, rare types
	Acute leukemia of ambiguous lineage, NOS

2. What are the typical morphological findings in acute leukemias?

The diagnosis of acute leukemia is frequently based on clinical findings, morphology, cytogenetics, and molecular studies. Despite new diagnostic modalities, recognizing acute leukemia by morphology is critical for the diagnosis and cannot be over emphasized. In order to diagnose acute leukemia, the blast percentage in peripheral blood and/or bone marrow must reach at least 20% with several exceptions [1]. On the peripheral blood smear and/or bone marrow aspirate smears, blasts might show different morphology in different subtypes.

They usually share some common features:

- Increased nucleus/cytoplasm ratio
- Fine chromatin
- Prominent/distinct nucleoli

Acute Myeloid Leukemia vs Acute Lymphoblastic Leukemia

According to the lineage of the blasts, acute leukemias are subclassified into acute myeloid leukemia (AML), acute lymphoblastic leukemia (ALL), and acute leukemia of ambiguous lineage. AML originates from myeloid precursors and ALL from lymphoid precursors. The classification is mostly based on immunophenotypic findings by flow cytometry. Morphologic features of the blasts can frequently provide some clues before the flow cytometry results are available [2].

- On peripheral blood smear/bone marrow aspirate smears, myeloblasts usually have the following features:
  - Medium to large size (2–4 times the diameter of RBC).
  - Round, oval, or indented nuclei with invaginated nuclear membrane.
  - Moderate to abundant cytoplasm.

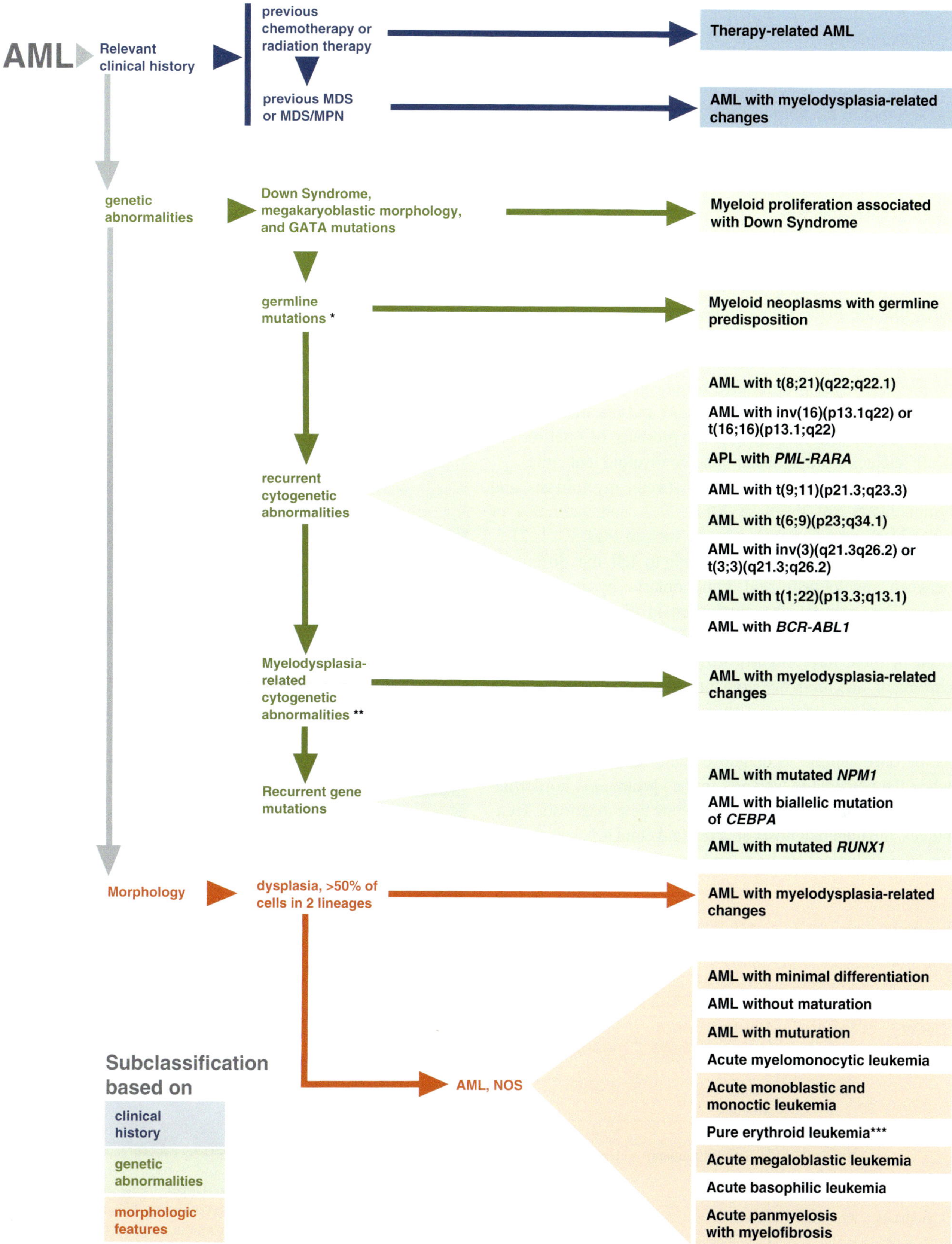

Fig. 21.1 Flow chart 22.1: AML classification (WHO 2017). ∗Germline alterations such as mutations in *CEBPA*, *DDX41*, *RUNX1*, *ANKRD26*, *ETV6*, or *GATA2*, bone marrow failure syndromes, and telomere biology disorders. ∗∗See Table 21.5 for a complete list. ∗∗∗Pure erythroid leukemias (PEL) typically have complex cytogenetic abnormalities including −5/del(5q) and/or −7/del(7q) [13]. Per the current WHO guidelines, these should NOT be diagnosed as AML-MRC if they meet the morphologic criteria of PEL (see Fig. 21.5) [1]

 - Absent, rare, to numerous azurophilic granules in the cytoplasm.
 - Auer rods might be present.
- Lymphoblasts usually have the following features:
 - Small to medium in size (1.5–3 times the diameter of RBC)
 - Round to oval nuclear contour without obvious invagination or irregularity
 - Scant cytoplasm
 - Agranular cytoplasm (almost always).

Auer rods are azurophilic long, thin, needle-shaped structures that are made of crystallized granules. Auer rods are almost exclusively seen in myeloid neoplasms, most frequently in AML, and sometimes in myelodysplastic syndromes and myeloproliferative neoplasms. The presence of Auer rod-like structures in lymphoid and plasma cell neoplasms is extremely rare [3, 4]. The presence of Auer rods in acute leukemia is diagnostic of acute myeloid leukemia.

The morphologic differences between myeloblasts and lymphoblasts are listed in Table 21.2, and examples of myeloblasts and lymphoblasts are seen in Figs. 21.2, 21.3, and 21.4. Frequently, it is difficult to tell the difference between myeloblasts and lymphoblasts by morphology alone. For example, the myeloblast in Fig. 21.4a and the lymphoblast in Fig. 21.4e share very similar morphology. Both of them have slightly irregular nuclear contour, fine chromatin, and moderate amount of agranular cytoplasm. In these situations, additional studies, especially flow cytometry, are very helpful. Flow cytometry should not be counted as the only method to diagnose acute leukemia, especially when the percentage of blasts in the specimen is borderline (approaching 20% of all cells). Despite new diagnostic techniques, the final diagnosis of acute leukemia is based on both the morphological findings and the flow cytometry result, especially when it is an erythroid predominant bone marrow specimen (Fig. 21.5) and in acute myeloid leukemia with monocytic differentiation (please refer to the later section of this question for details).

Table 21.2 Morphologic differences between myeloblasts and lymphoblasts

		Myeloblasts	Lymphoblasts
Nuclei	Size	Mostly medium to large, occasionally small	Small to medium, occasionally large
	Shape	Round, oval, irregular	Round to oval
	Chromatin	Fine	Fine
	Nucleoli	Usually prominent/distinct	Usually distinct, can be indistinct or absent
Cytoplasm	Amount	Moderate to abundant	Usually scant
	Granules	Various in number, usually present	Agranular
	Auer rod	Can be present	Absent

Acute Myeloid Leukemia

There are several types of acute myeloid leukemia that have distinct morphologic, immunophenotypic, and genetic features.

Acute Promyelocytic Leukemia

These cases represent true medical emergencies, and prompt and correct diagnosis is crucial for appropriate treatment and life-saving supportive measures.

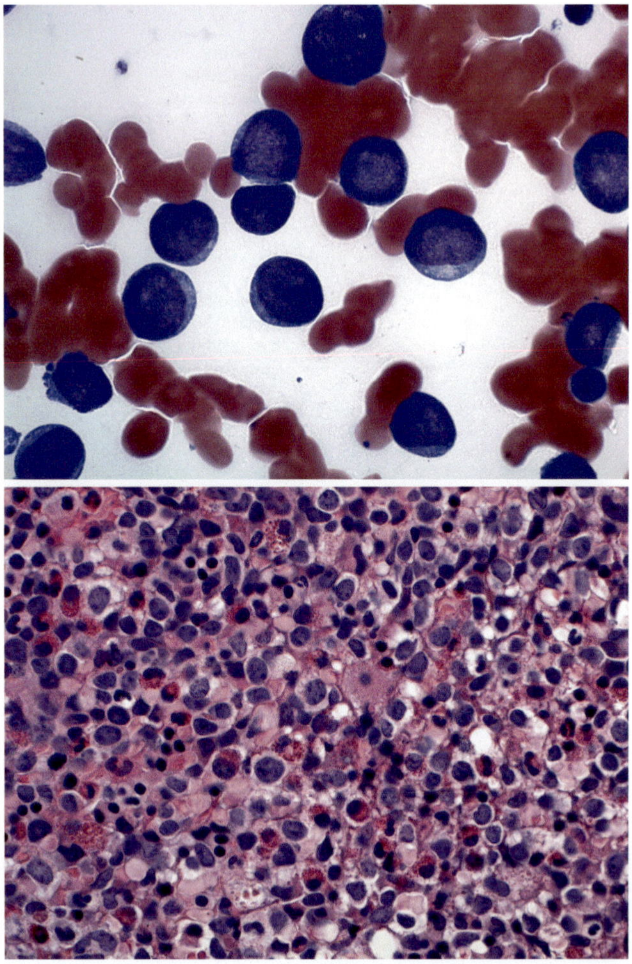

Fig. 21.2 Acute myeloid leukemia. Upper: bone marrow aspirate smear shows marked increase in myeloblasts. The myeloblasts are medium to large in size, with fine chromatin, slightly irregular nuclear contour, and moderate amount of cytoplasm (original magnification 1000×). Lower: core biopsy reveals sheets of myeloblasts. The myeloblasts have open chromatin and distinct nucleoli (original magnification 400×)

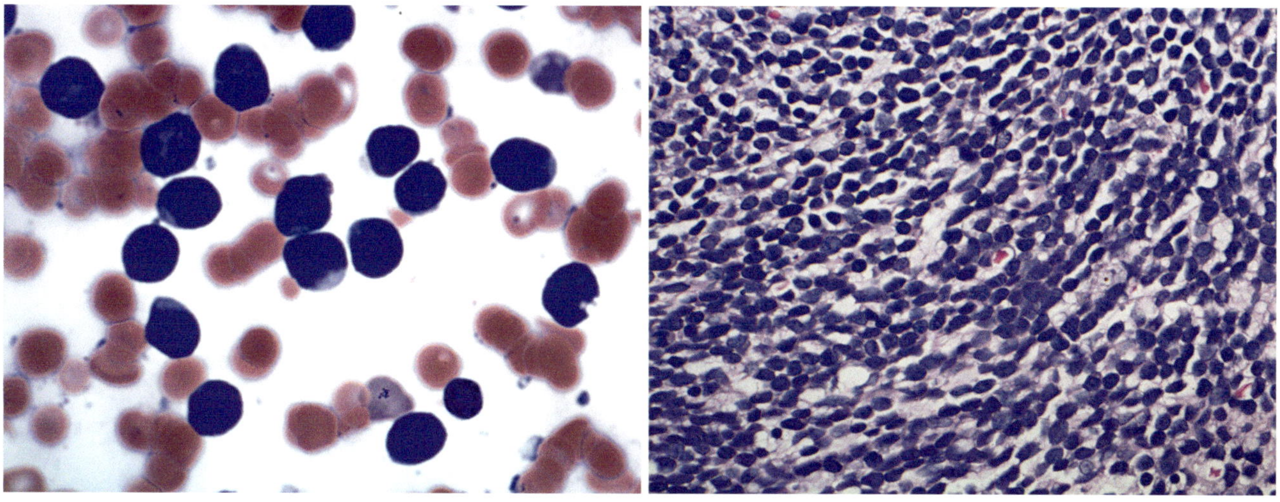

Fig. 21.3 Acute lymphoblastic leukemia. *Left*: bone marrow aspirate smear shows that the lymphoblasts are small to medium in size, with round to oval nuclear contour, slightly condensed chromatin, and scant cytoplasm (original magnification 1000×). *Right*: core biopsy shows sheets of lymphoblasts. The lymphoblasts are small to medium in size. They have round to oval nuclei, slightly condensed nuclei, and very scant cytoplasm. The nucleoli are absent (original magnification 400×)

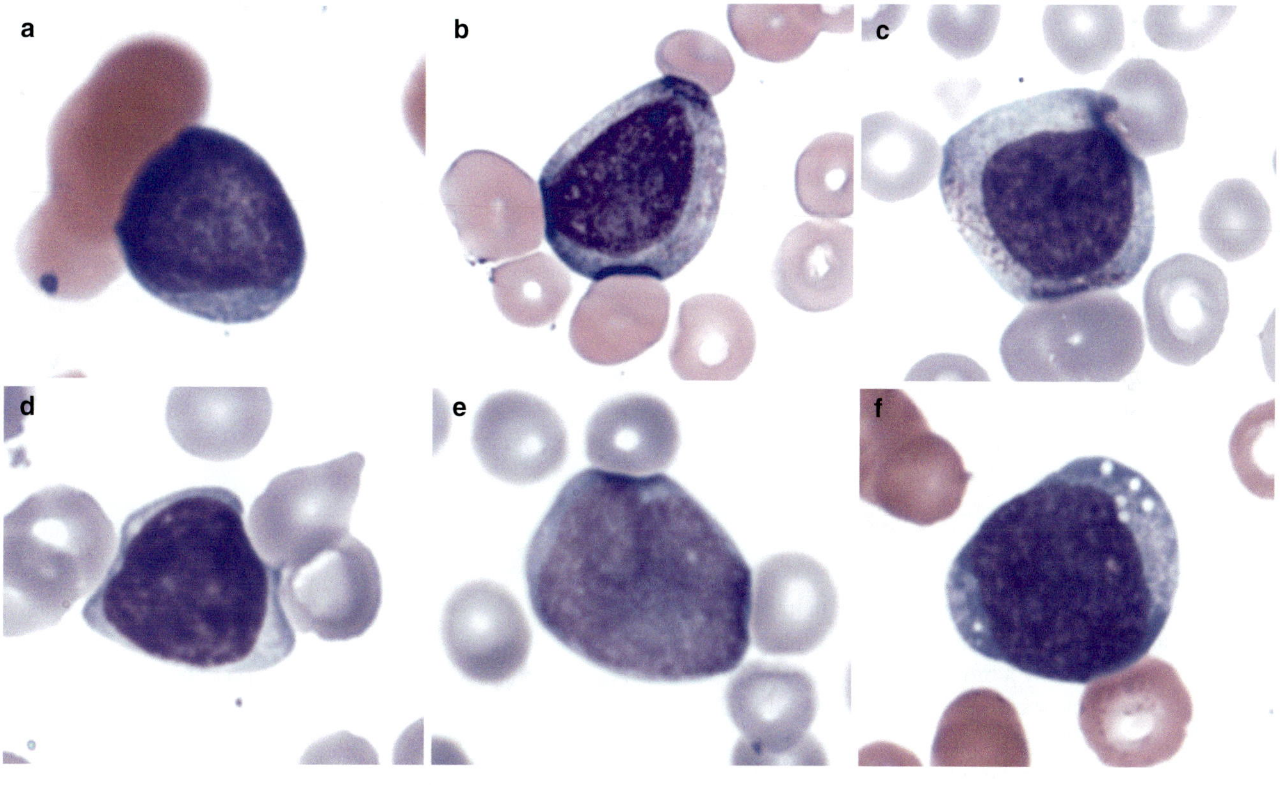

Fig. 21.4 Myeloblasts vs lymphoblasts. Upper panels: myeloblasts; Lower panels: lymphoblasts. (**a**) This myeloblast (M0) is small to medium in size, with slightly condensed chromatin and scant agranular cytoplasm. (**b**) This myeloblast (M1) is medium to large in size, with distinct nucleoli and some granules in the cytoplasm. (**c**) This myeloblast (M2) is medium to large in size, with azurophilic granules and Auer rods in the cytoplasm. (**d**) This lymphoblast (L1) is small to medium in size, with round to oval nuclear contour, slightly condensed chromatin, and scant cytoplasm. (**e**) This lymphoblast (L2) is medium to large in size, slightly irregular nuclear contour, fine chromatin, and agranular cytoplasm. (**f**) This lymphoblast (L3) shows slightly clumped chromatin and several vacuoles in the cytoplasm (original magnification 1000×)

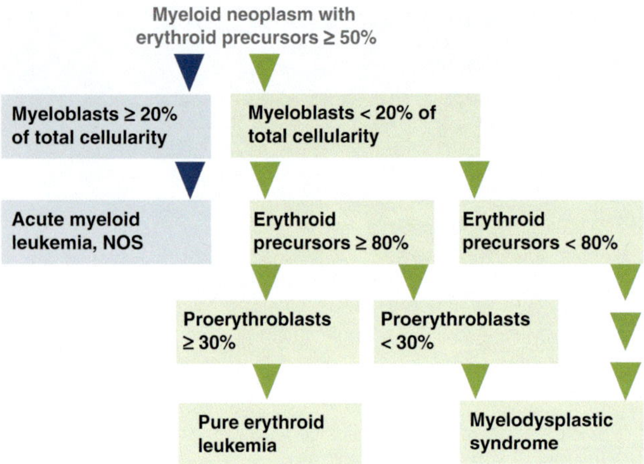

Fig. 21.5 Working strategy for erythroid predominant myeloid neoplasm

- Acute promyelocytic leukemia (APL) with *PML-RARA* (referred to as M3 by the French-American-British (FAB) classification) comprises approximately 10% of AML [5, 6].
- APL is characterized by myeloid maturation arrest at the promyelocyte stage. Promyelocytes are medium to large (2–4 times the diameter of RBC) blasts or blastoid cells and have bilobed, kidney-shaped, or butterfly-like nuclei. Nuclear chromatin varies from fine to unevenly condensed, and nucleoli are variably distinct. The nucleus/cytoplasm ratio usually is not very high (Fig. 21.6a).
- There are two morphologic variants of APL: hypergranular and microgranular/hypogranular variant.
- The hypergranular variant is characterized by:
  - Bilobed/butterfly/kidney-shaped nuclei
  - Many large Auer rods
  - Abundant densely packed azurophilic granules in the cytoplasm
  - Occasional blasts may contain clusters of Auer rods resembling bundles of sticks
- The microgranular/hypogranular variant is characterized by the following:
  - Very fine or even lack of granules in the cytoplasm.
  - The shape of nuclei is as same as that in hypergranular variant, but in bilobed nuclei, the two lobes are typically connected by a broad but fine "vail-like" nuclear material. Nuclear chromatin is usually uniformly fine and nucleoli are present.
  - Rare Auer rods can be seen in a small subset of blasts in many cases.

The differences between the two variants of acute promyelocytic leukemia can be seen in Table 21.3 and Fig. 21.6. In most cases, morphologic and flow cytometric findings can give us a strong clue for APL, but only documentation of the t(15;17) cytogenetic abnormality or other rare variant abnormalities involving the *RARA* gene can confirm the diagnosis.

Table 21.3 Morphologic differences between hypergranular and hypogranular acute promyelocytic leukemia

		Hypergranular	Hypogranular
Nuclei		Bilobed, butterfly, kidney-shaped	Bilobed, butterfly, kidney-shaped
Cytoplasm	Granules	Many, densely packed, sometimes cover the nuclei	A few, rarely absolutely absent
	Auer rod	Large in size, frequent	Usually present in a few blasts, rarely absolutely absent

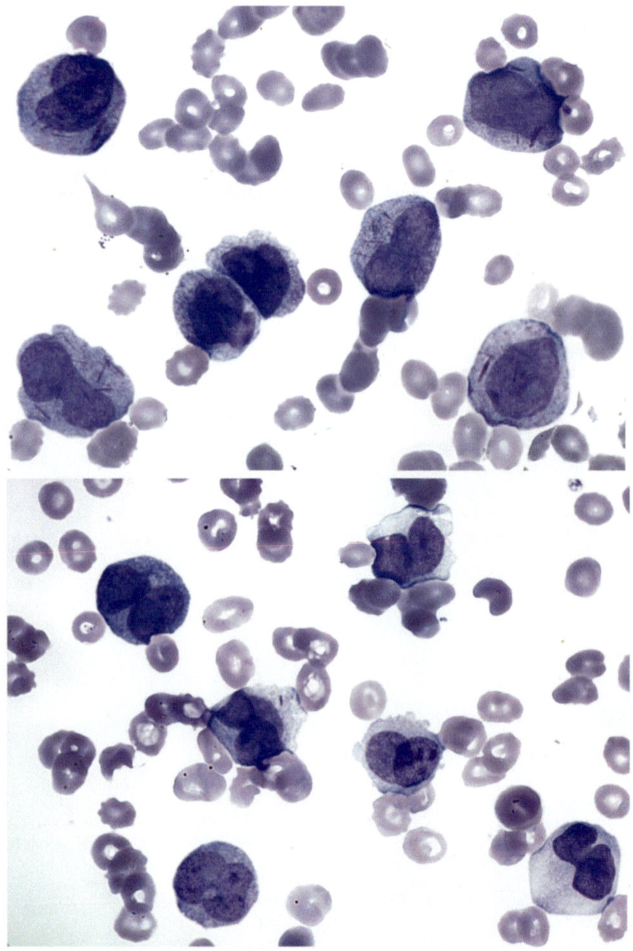

Fig. 21.6 Acute promyelocytic leukemia (M3). Upper: hypergranular variant, bilobed nuclei with many azurophilic coarse granules, and Auer rods in the cytoplasm; lower: microgranular variant, bilobed or butterfly-like nuclei with few granules, and rare Auer rods in the cytoplasm (original magnification 1000×)

Of note, patients with hypergranular APL often present with pancytopenia, with only 10–30% of patients presenting with leukocytosis. For those patients with severe pancytopenia, it is very important for pathologists to review the peripheral blood smear carefully and identify the blasts suspicious for APL. Blast percentage ≥ 20% is not required for the diagnosis of APL; thus, the diagnosis of APL can be rendered even when the blast percentage is less than 20% if *PML-RARA* fusion can be confirmed by conventional cytogenetics, FISH, or polymerase chain reaction (PCR) [7, 8].

Acute Myeloid Leukemia with Monocytic Differentiation

This category includes the following:

- Acute myelomonocytic leukemia
- Acute monoblastic leukemia
- Acute monocytic leukemia
- Monoblasts are morphologically characterized by the following:
  - Large size (3–4 times the diameter of RBC)
  - Round, oval, or irregular nuclei
  - Delicate lacy chromatin
  - Prominent nucleoli
  - Abundant basophilic cytoplasm that might contain several fine azurophilic granules and vacuoles
- Promonocytes are blast equivalents and are morphologically characterized by the following:
  - Irregular or delicately convoluted nuclear contour
  - Small indistinct nucleoli
  - Abundant cytoplasm which might contain several large azurophilic granules and/or vacuoles

The morphologic differences between monocytes, promonocytes, and abnormal monocytes are shown in Table 21.4 and Fig. 21.7.

Table 21.4 Morphologic comparison of monoblasts, promonocytes, and abnormal monocytes

		Monoblasts	Promonocytes	Abnormal monocytes
N/C ratio		High	Moderate	Low
Nuclei	Contour	Round to oval	Delicately convoluted, indented, grooved	More irregular, indented, folded
	Chromatin	Delicate fine/lace-like chromatin	Finely dispersed chromatin	More clumped chromatin
	Nucleoli	One or more prominent nucleoli	Small indistinct nucleoli	Absent
Cytoplasm	Amount	Relatively less	Moderate	Abundant
	Color	Moderately to intensely basophilic	Less basophilic	Gray, pale
	Granules	Sparse fine azurophilic granules	More obviously granulated, with occasional large azurophilic granules	More abundant granules
	Vacuoles	Maybe present	Maybe present	Maybe present

Acute Myelomonocytic Leukemia

- Defined as proliferation of both neutrophilic and monocytic lineages and the combination of myeloblasts and monoblasts/promonocytes is ≥20%.
- Usually, there are at least 20% monocytes and monocytic precursors and greater than 20% granulocytes and granulocytic precursors.

Acute Monoblastic Leukemia and Acute Monocytic Leukemia.

- At least 80% cells of monocytic lineage and the monoblasts/promonocytes are ≥20%.
- In acute monoblastic leukemia, ≥80% of the monocytic lineage cells are monoblasts.
- In acute monocytic leukemia, the majority of monocytic cells are promonocytes and abnormal monocytes (Fig. 21.8) [1].
- It can be difficult to differentiate promonocytes from abnormal monocytes on bone marrow aspirate smears. High-quality peripheral blood smears prepared from fresh blood are often helpful. Monocytes on peripheral blood smears tend to be more mature than those on the bone marrow aspirate smears.

Acute Myeloid Leukemia with t(8;21)(q22;q22.1); *RUNX1-RUNX1T1*

- Most blasts are large in size with abundant basophilic cytoplasm and perinuclear clearing (hof). Azurophilic granules and Auer rods, characteristically thin, needle-like, can be seen in cytoplasm (Fig. 21.9).

Acute Myeloid Leukemia with inv(16)(p13.1q22) or t(16;16)(p13.1;q22); *CBFB-MYH11*

- The blasts usually have monocytic differentiation with increased number of abnormal eosinophils.
- The eosinophils are at different stages of maturation.
- The granules in the eosinophils can be larger and coarser than those in normal eosinophils [9] (Fig. 21.10). Note that the granules in eosinophilic myelocytes and early metamyelocytes are often basophilic. The granules in the abnormal eosinophils stain positive for chloroacetate esterase ("specific" esterase) similar to neutrophil granules (but unlike normal eosinophils).

Pure Erythroid Leukemia

- Defined as acute leukemia in which erythroid precursors consist of more than 80% of the total bone marrow cellularity and proerythroblasts are ≥30% [1].

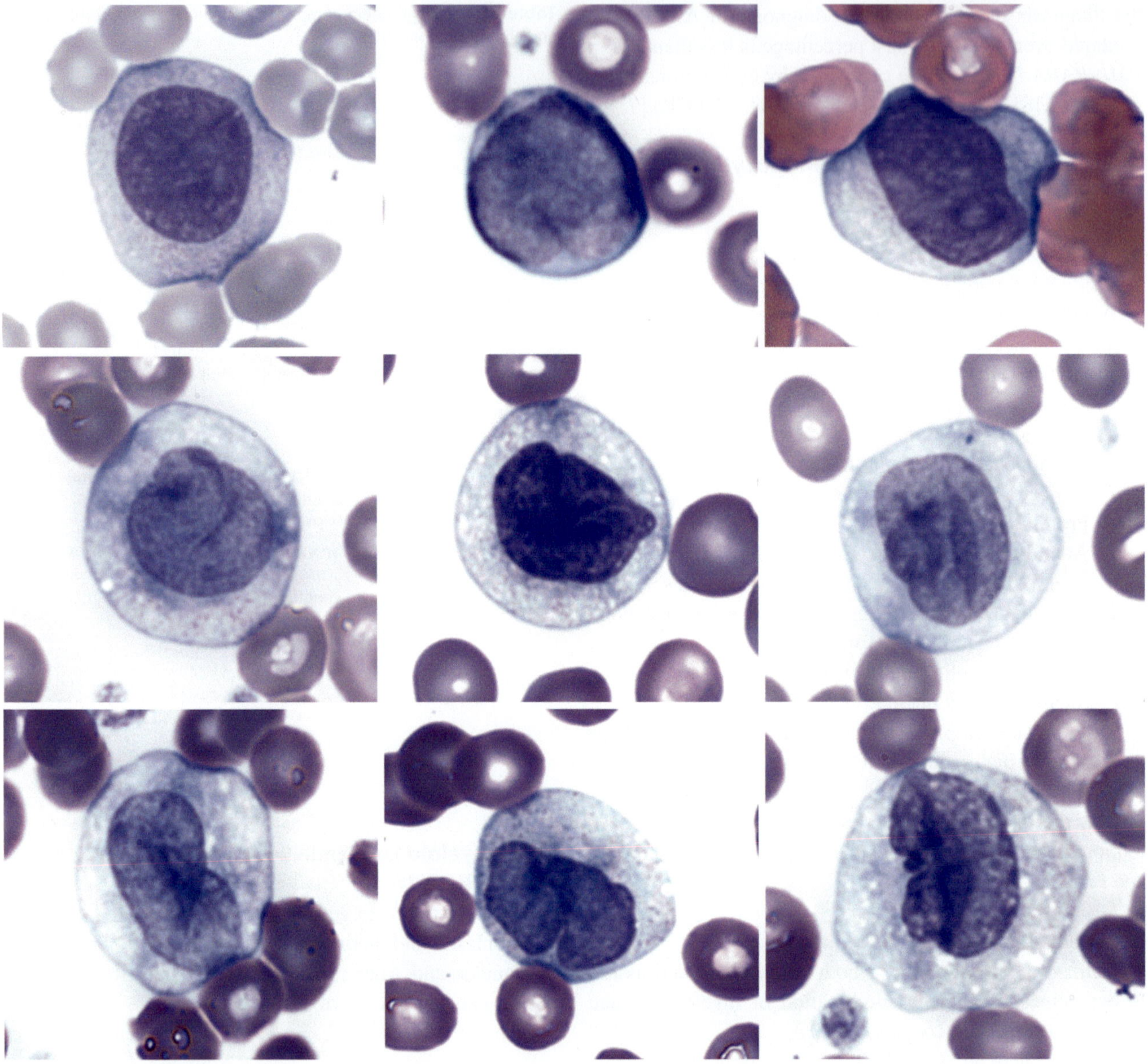

Fig. 21.7 Monoblasts, promonocytes, and abnormal monocytes. Upper: monoblasts show relatively high nucleus/cytoplasm ratio, slightly irregular nuclear contour, fine chromatin, distinct nucleoli, and moderate amount of cytoplasm. Middle: promonocytes have moderate nucleus/cytoplasm ratio, folded nuclei, relatively fine chromatin, and more cytoplasm. Lower: abnormal monocytes have low nucleus/cytoplasm ratio, deeply folded nuclei, condensed chromatin, and large amount of cytoplasm (original magnification 1000×)

- Proerythroblasts are characterized by:
  - Medium- to large-sized blasts
  - Round nuclei
  - Fine chromatin
  - Distinct nucleoli
  - Deep basophilic agranular cytoplasm with occasional vacuoles
- On the core biopsy or blood clots, marrow shows marked left-shifted erythroid hyperplasia (Fig. 21.11) [10–13].

Acute Myeloid Leukemia with Myelodysplasia-Related Changes

- Acute myeloid leukemia with myelodysplasia-related changes (AML-MRC) is a subtype of acute myeloid leukemia with myelodysplastic features, or the patient has a previous history of myelodysplastic syndrome/myeloproliferative neoplasm, or with MDS-related cytogenetic abnormalities, and no AML-related recurrent genetic abnormalities or any previous history of cytotoxic/radiation therapy.
- Besides ≥20% myeloblasts, both of the following diagnosis criteria are required [1]:

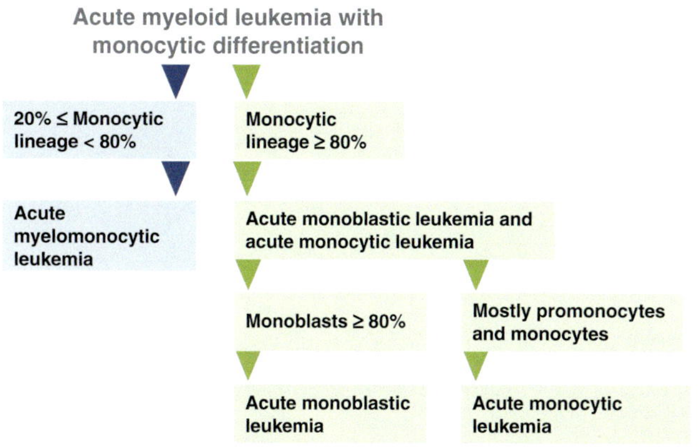

Fig. 21.8 Working strategy for acute myeloid leukemia with monocytic differentiation

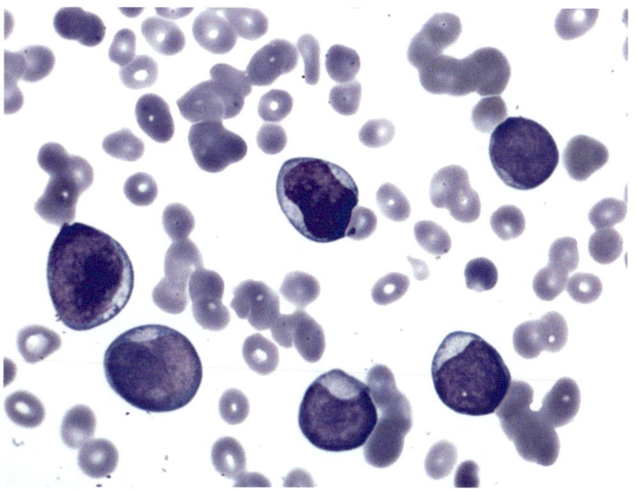

Fig. 21.9 Acute myeloid leukemia with t(8;21)(q22;q22.1); *RUNX1-RUNX1T1*. Bone marrow aspirate smear shows the myeloblasts are medium to large in size, fine chromatin, and perinuclear clearing (original magnification 1000×)

1. One or more of the following three conditions must be met:
   - History of MDS or MDS/MPN
   - MDS-related cytogenetic abnormality (see Table 21.5)
   - Multilineage dysplasia (see Table 21.6)
2. Absence of both:
   - Prior cytotoxic or radiation therapy for unrelated disease
   - AML with recurrent genetic abnormalities

- Of note, in order to diagnose AML-MRC by morphology, dysplasia must be present in *≥50% of the cells in at least two hematopoietic lineages*. AML-MRC usually show complex cytogenetic changes and carry dismal prognosis [14].

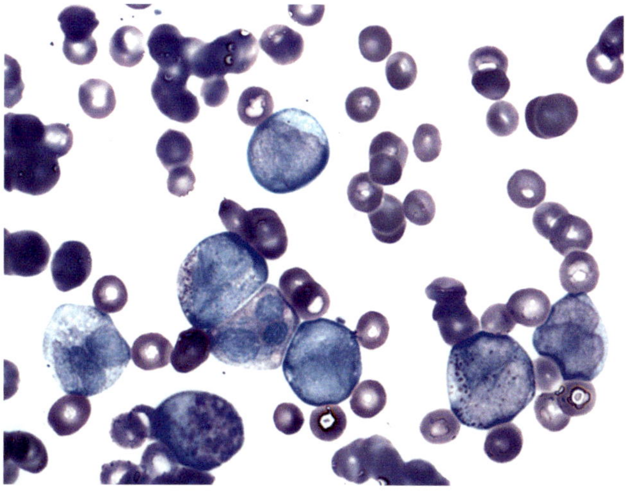

Fig. 21.10 Acute myeloid leukemia with inv(16)(p13.1q22). Bone marrow aspirate smears show increased blasts with monocytic differentiation and a variable number of abnormal eosinophils at different stages of maturation. The eosinophils show large coarse eosinophilic and basophilic granules. The granules obscure the nucleus of the cell in the left lower corner (original magnification 1000×)

Acute Lymphoblastic Leukemia

The morphologic features of the lymphoblasts are summarized in earlier section in this question (Fig. 21.3). Based on the differentiation of the lymphoblasts, there are two types of acute lymphoblastic leukemia: B-lymphoblastic leukemia and T-lymphoblastic leukemia. Morphologically, they resemble each other. According to the FAB classification, B-acute lymphoblastic leukemia (B-ALL) can be subclassified into types L1, L2, and L3 by morphology (Fig. 21.4 lower panel) [15].

- L1 is the most common subtype. They are characterized by:
  - Monotonous, intermediate-sized blasts (1.5–2.5 times the diameter of RBC)
  - Round to oval nuclear contour
  - Slightly condensed chromatin
  - Indistinct or no nucleoli
  - Scant cytoplasm
- L2 blasts are characterized by:
  - Heterogeneous blast size (2–4 times the diameter of RBC)
  - Fine chromatin
  - Prominent nucleoli
  - Moderate amount of cytoplasm
- L3 refers to the leukemic phase of Burkitt lymphoma. They show:
  - Very homogeneous, medium-sized atypical cells (2–3 times the diameter of RBC)

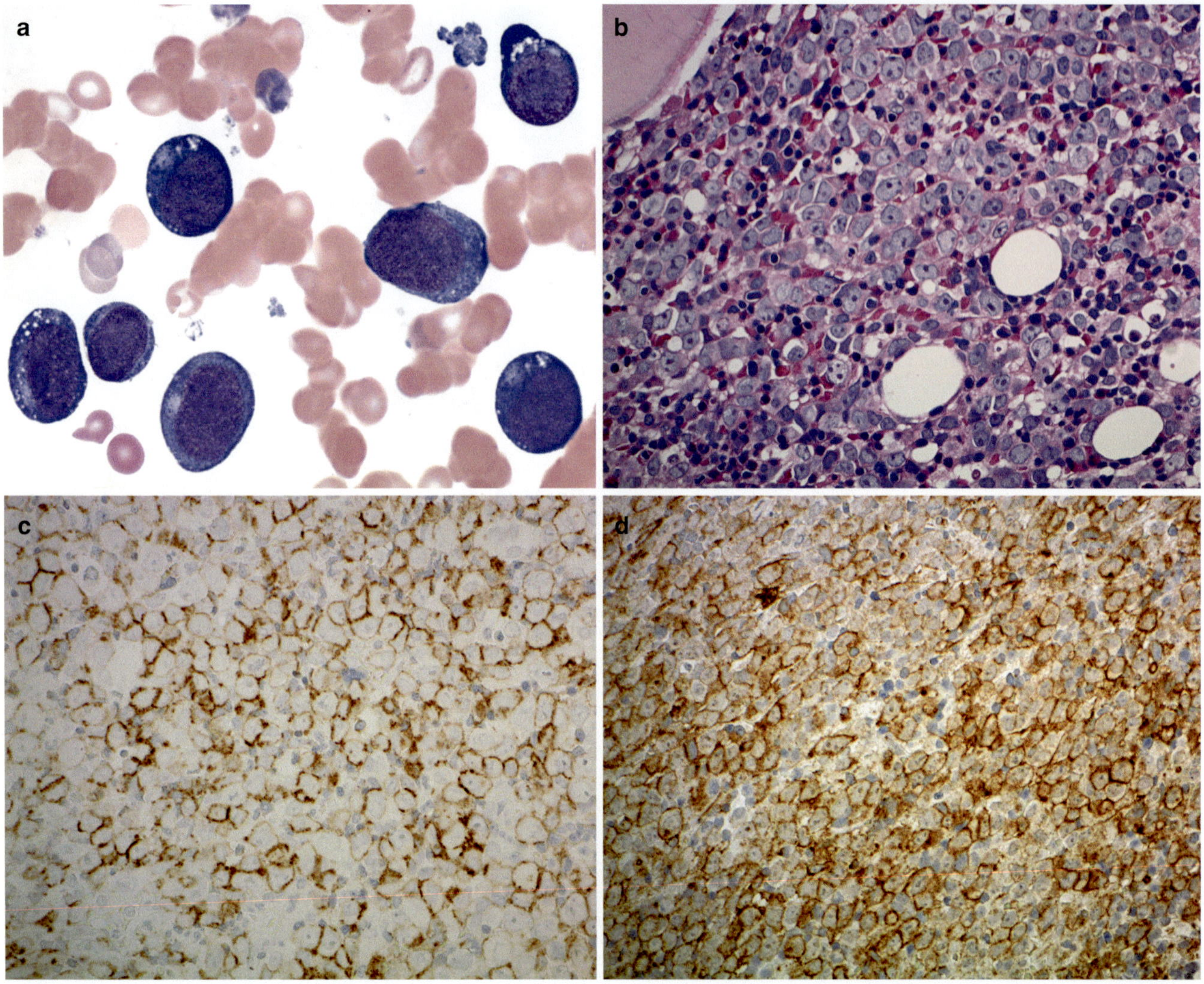

Fig. 21.11 Pure erythroid leukemia. (**a**) Bone marrow aspirate shows that the erythroid precursors consist of ≥80% of the total population and proerythroblasts consist of ≥30% of the total cellularity (original magnification 1000×). (**b**) Bone marrow core biopsy reveals marked left-shifted erythroid hyperplasia consisting of mainly early erythroid precursors (original magnification 400×). (**c**) Most of the cells are positive for E-cadherin (original magnification 400×). (**d**) Most of the cells are positive for CD117 (original magnification 400×)

Table 21.5 Cytogenetic abnormalities diagnostic of AML-MRC

Unbalanced abnormalities
−7/del(7q)
del(5q)/t(5q)
i17q/t(17p)
−13/del(13q)
del(11q)
del(12p)/t(12p)
idic(X)(q13)
Balanced translocations
t(11;16)(q23.3;p13.3)
t(3;21)(q26.2;q22.1)
t(1;3)(p36.3;q21.2)
t(2;11)(p21;q23.3)
t(5;12)(q32;p13.2)
t(5;7)(q32;q11.2)
t(5;17)(q32;p13.2)
t(5;10)(q32;q21)
t(3;5)(q25.3;q35.1)
≥3 cytogenetic abnormalities involving at least 1 of the above

Table 21.6 Morphologic features of dysplasia in hematopoietic cells*

Cell lines	Dysplastic features
Dyserythropoiesis	1. Megaloblastoid changes 2. Karyorrhexis 3. Nuclear irregularity 4. Nuclear fragmentation 5. Multinucleation 6. Ring sideroblasts 7. Cytoplasmic vacuoles 8. Periodic acid-Schiff (PAS) positivity
Dysgranulopoiesis	1. Neutrophils with hypogranular cytoplasm 2. Neutrophils with hyposegmented nuclei (pseudo-Pelger-Huet anomaly) 3. Bizarrely segmented nuclei
Dysmegakaryopoiesis	1. Micromegakaryocytes 2. Normal-sized or large megakaryocytes with monolobated or multiple nuclei

* See Chapter 24, Table 24.2 and Figures 24.2, 24.3, and 24.4 for representative microphotographs depicting these abnormalities

- Round nuclear contour
- Mildly clumped chromatin
- Several distinct nucleoli
- Moderate amount of basophilic cytoplasm
- Cytoplasmic vacuoles

The morphologic subtypes of L1 and L2 do not correlate with the cytogenetic findings or prognosis; however, the larger blasts with L2 morphology can mimic myeloblasts. L3 morphology is usually, but not invariably, seen in Burkitt lymphoma. While Burkitt lymphoma is a mature B-cell lymphoma (and by definition does not belong to the B-ALL category), it should be emphasized that rare cases of B-ALL do have the L3 morphology. Therefore, this morphological classification mainly serves as a reminder to avoid misdiagnosis and for the description of the blast morphology for future reference.

Acute Leukemia with Ambiguous Lineage

Acute leukemias with ambiguous lineage are defined as leukemias that show no definite differentiation toward any single lineage.

- They include acute undifferentiated leukemia and mixed-phenotype acute leukemia. Acute undifferentiated leukemias show no definite lineage-differentiation markers. There are two types of mixed-phenotype acute leukemias:
  - Acute leukemia with at least two different populations of blasts and each population shows different lineage differentiation, such as acute myeloid leukemia and B-lymphoblastic leukemia.
  - Acute leukemia with one population of blasts that express multiple antigens with different lineage differentiation.
- Morphologically, the blasts can be similar to both AML and ALL.
- The lineage definition markers are summarized in Table 21.7. Acute leukemia with ambiguous lineage consists of less than 5% of all acute leukemia cases and in general shows worse prognosis than acute myeloid leukemia or acute lymphoblastic leukemia. Due to its rarity, there is no definite guideline for therapy, but usually, the patients are treated with ALL-like protocol followed by consolidation chemotherapy and stem cell transplant [16].

3. What are the mimics and what is the clinical relevance of misinterpretation between the true diagnosis and mimics with reference to mistreatment and/or wrong prognosis?

Distinction between the following entities which can resemble each other closely is critical to avoid inappropriate treatment.

Table 21.7 Required phenotype for lineage assignment in mixed-phenotype acute leukemia

AML (granulocytic differentiation)	MPO (by flow cytometry, cytochemistry, or immunohistochemistry)
AML (monocytic differentiation)	CD11c, CD14, CD64, lysozyme, nonspecific esterase (need ≥ 2)
B-ALL	CD19 (strong) *and* CD10, CD79a, cytoplasmic CD22, PAX5 (≥1) *-or-* CD19 (weak) *and* CD10, CD79a, cytoplasmic CD22, PAX5 (≥2)
T-ALL	Cytoplasmic CD3 or surface CD3 (by flow cytometry)

Note: the above immunophenotypic criteria should ONLY be used when considering a diagnosis of MPAL. For example, in the absence of T-lineage or B-lineage differentiation, blasts with morphologic and immunophenotypic features of myeloid differentiation but no MPO would be classified as AML with minimal differentiation

Acute Promyelocytic Leukemia vs Acute Myeloid Leukemia with Monocytic Differentiation or Acute Myeloid Leukemia, NOS

- Blasts in some cases of hypogranular APL might show folded/bilobed nuclei and agranular cytoplasm that mimics monoblasts, promonocytes, or myeloblasts.
- In such cases, one important clue is that increased abnormal monocytes are frequently seen, particularly in peripheral blood, in AML with monocytic differentiation, but not in APL.
- Cytochemical stains and flow cytometry are very helpful in such cases [17]. These differences are summarized in Table 21.8.
  - APL blasts are usually strongly positive for myeloperoxidase (MPO).
  - AML with monocytic differentiation is strongly positive for nonspecific esterase (NSE). Approximately 25% of APL blasts may be weakly positive for NSE and should not be confused with AML with monocytic differentiation [18].
  - By flow cytometry, APL is positive for CD117 (usually, but not invariably), CD33 (strong, uniform), CD13 (heterogeneous) and MPO (strong) and usually but not invariably negative or very weakly positive for CD34 and HLA-DR. AML with monocytic differentiation are positive for one or more monocytic markers such as CD4, CD11b, CD11c, CD14 and CD64 and usually express HLA-DR.
- Sometimes it is difficult to differentiate APL from AML, NOS. Not all APL blasts show eosinophilic cytoplasmic granules, Auer rods, and characteristic nuclear contours. They may be irregular, but may not show characteristic bilobed or butterfly-shaped nuclei. In these cases, flow cytometry may be helpful.
- If there is any suspicion for APL either by morphology or by flow cytometry, demonstration of *PML-RARA* fusion is necessary to ensure the correct treatment (ATRA and/or arsenic

Table 21.8 Hypogranular acute promyelocytic leukemia vs acute myeloid leukemia with monocytic differentiation

	Hypogranular APL	AML with monocytic differentiation
Nuclei	Bilobed/kidney-shaped/butterfly-like; fine chromatin	Convoluted, indented, grooved; delicate fine/lace-like or finely dispersed chromatin
Cytoplasm	Agranular/rare granules with rare Auer rods	Agranular
Monocytes	No definite increase in monocytes	Might be accompanied by marked increase in abnormal monocytes
Cytochemistry	Strongly positive for MPO	Strongly positive for NSE
Flow cytometry	Positive for CD117, CD13 (heterogeneous), CD33 (homogeneous bright). Usually negative for CD34, HLA-DR, CD15, CD65, and monocytic markers.	Monoblasts and promonocytes are usually positive for CD13 and CD33 but frequently negative for CD34 and CD117. They usually show monocytic markers such as CD14, CD4, CD11b, CD11c, CD64, CD68, CD36, and lysozyme. Most cases are positive for HLA-DR. MPO is sometime expressed in acute monocytic leukemia but usually not in acute monoblastic leukemia
Cytogenetics	t(15;17)(q24.1;q21.2) – most frequent t(11;17)(q23.2;q21.2) – rare t(5;17)(q35.1;q21.2) – rare	Nonspecific; sometimes t(8;16)(p11.2;p13.3)

APL acute promyelocytic leukemia, *AML* acute myeloid leukemia, *MPO* myeloperoxidase, *NSE* nonspecific esterase

trioxide) is administered. *PML-RARA* can be detected by FISH, conventional cytogenetics, or RT-PCR. FISH is usually the fastest, most convenient way to identify the translocation for initial diagnosis. RT-PCR is usually used for following up for residual disease [19–21].

Acute Promyelocytic Leukemia vs Growth Factor Effect

- Administration of human recombinant granulocyte colony-stimulating growth factor (G-CSF) and granulocyte-macrophage colony-stimulating factor (GM-CSF) in patients with severely hypoplastic or aplastic marrow may result in the bone marrow containing predominantly promyelocytes and myelocytes.
- This may mimic APL [22]; however, the myeloid cells may contain toxic granules, Döhle bodies, and occasionally vacuoles in the cytoplasm. Prominent perinuclear hofs can also be seen. Auer rods are almost never seen in growth factor administration, unless there is an underlying hypocellular myelodysplasia or treated acute leukemia.
- Flow cytometry studies usually are very helpful. The "blasts" in APL are positive for CD117, but negative for CD34 and are usually greater than 20%. Although the myeloid maturation is left-shifted in bone marrow with growth factor effect, the blast percentage is usually less than 5%, except in very rare instances [23].
- In bone marrow biopsy with growth factor changes, both myeloid and erythroid precursors show left-shifted maturation in parallel with each other. However, in APL cases, the erythroid precursors are hypoplastic and the erythroid cells present show full progressive maturation.

Acute Myelomonocytic/Monocytic Leukemia vs Chronic Myelomonocytic Leukemia/Juvenile Myelomonocytic Leukemia

- In some cases, the distinction between acute myelomonocytic/monocytic leukemia and chronic myelomonocytic leukemia (CMML)/juvenile myelomonocytic leukemia (JMML) may be extremely difficult. (See Chap. 25 for primary description of CMML and JMML.)
- AML with monocytic differentiation is characterized by at least 20% myeloblasts/monoblasts/promonocytes, while in CMML and JMML, most atypical cells are abnormal monocytes and dysplastic myeloid cells with the myeloblasts/monoblasts/promonocytes less than 20%.
- Since monoblasts and promonocytes are usually negative for both CD34 and CD117 by flow cytometry and immunohistochemistry stains, morphologic evaluation is almost the only way to differentiate AML with monocytic differentiation from CMML/JMML.
- High-quality bone marrow aspirate smears and peripheral blood smears are critical for the diagnosis.
- Promonocytes usually show slightly higher nucleus/cytoplasm ratio; delicately convoluted, indented, or grooved nuclei; and small indistinct nucleoli.
- Abnormal monocytes usually have relatively low nucleus/cytoplasm ratio, more obviously folded nuclei, and no nucleoli.
- These morphologic differences between monocytes, promonocytes, and abnormal monocytes are summarized in Table 21.4 and Fig. 21.7.
- It is equally important to distinguish AML with monocytic differentiation arising from transformation of CMML/JMML, because prognosis and treatment options vary significantly [24].

Pure Erythroid Leukemia vs Acute Myeloid Leukemia, Not Otherwise Specified, Erythroid Predominant Myelodysplastic Syndrome and Reactive Erythroid Hyperplasia

- Pure erythroid leukemia (PEL) is very rare and usually has an aggressive course. In the 2017 WHO classification, pure erythroid leukemia is defined as >80% erythroid precursors and ≥30% proerythroblasts in the bone marrow [1]. (Note that the category of erythroleukemia, myeloid/erythroid, defined in prior editions of the WHO classification, is eliminated.) The following morphological characteristics are helpful:
  - Proerythroblasts are large in size (2–3 times the diameter of RBC) and have fine nuclear chromatin, one or more nucleoli, an indistinct perinuclear clear Golgi area, deep basophilic agranular cytoplasm, and occasional small vacuoles in the cytoplasm.
  - Basophilic erythroblasts (early normoblasts) are medium in size, have more chromatin clumping, and have deep basophilic cytoplasm.
  - Polychromatic erythroblasts (intermediate normoblasts) are medium-sized and more condensed, with light basophilic cytoplasm, lower nucleus/cytoplasm ratio, and focally clumped chromatin.
  - Orthochromatic erythroblasts (late normoblasts) are small in size, have prominent chromatin clumping culminating in "ink dot" nucleus in which chromatin details are imperceptible, and have very low nucleus/cytoplasm ratio, and cytoplasm approaches a polychromatophilic red blood cell.
- If there are ≥50% erythroid precursors and myeloblasts are ≥20% of the total cellularity, it is classified as acute myeloid leukemia, not otherwise specified according to the 2017 WHO classification.
- If there are myelodysplastic changes, the erythroid precursors are ≥50% of the total cellularity, the proerythroblasts are <30% of the total cellularity and the myeloblasts are <20% of the total cellularity, then it is classified as myelodysplastic syndrome (MDS) by the WHO 2017 classification [1, 25, 26]. The algorithmic approach to diagnosis of erythroid predominant myeloid neoplasms is shown in Fig. 21.5.
- Pure erythroid leukemia shows almost pure erythroid lineage proliferation with maturation arrest characterized by proerythroblasts ≥30%, while acute myeloid leukemia NOS is defined as myeloblasts ≥20%. Erythroid predominant myeloid proliferations with myeloblasts between 5% and 19% and/or prominent dyserythropoiesis are classified as myelodysplastic syndrome.
- Pure erythroid leukemia must also be differentiated from reactive erythroid hyperplasia including:
  - Vitamin B12 or folate deficiency
  - Heavy metal poisoning
  - Congenital dyserythropoiesis
  - Excess production of erythropoietin or paraneoplastic effect of substances synthesized by certain tumors or exogenous erythropoietin usage
- These mimickers can be recognized by the following features:
  - Patients with vitamin B12 or folate deficiency have a long history of anemia, and bone marrow biopsy shows trilineage proliferation with prominent erythroid hyperplasia and dyserythropoiesis. Both myeloid and erythroid lineages usually show full maturation without maturation arrest, and the myeloid lineage can show features like megaloblastoid changes and hypersegmented neutrophils (Fig. 21.12).
  - In heavy metal poisoning, the erythroid precursors might show prominent vacuoles in the cytoplasm. There is no maturation arrest, and myeloblasts are less than 20%.
  - Congenital dyserythropoietic anemia is usually, but not invariably, seen in pediatric patients with a history of anemia since early age while patients with pure erythroid leukemia usually present with a sudden onset of pancytopenia with no previous history of anemia.
  - Erythropoietin administration can lead to a transient left-shifted erythroid hyperplasia. In this scenario, a repeat bone marrow biopsy after discontinuing the usage of erythropoietin is usually helpful.
- In summary, it is always very important to check the clinical history of patients including nutritional deficiency and medications before the diagnosis of pure erythroid leukemia is rendered [10, 13].

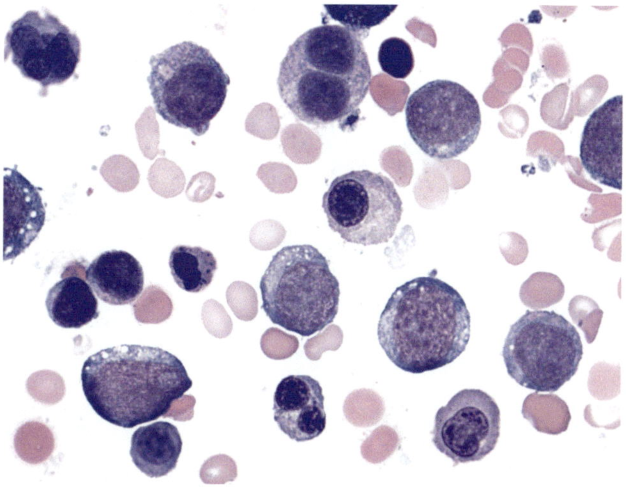

Fig. 21.12 Acute myeloid leukemia with myelodysplasia-related changes. The erythroid precursors show megaloblastoid changes, multinucleation, binucleation, irregular nucleation, irregular nuclear contour, and cytoplasmic vacuoles. A myeloid cell shows binucleation (original magnification 1000×)

Transient Abnormal Myelopoiesis Associated with Down Syndrome vs Acute Megakaryoblastic Leukemia

- Transient abnormal myelopoiesis (TAM) associated with Down syndrome is seen in approximately 10% of newborns with Down syndrome between the 3rd and 7th postnatal day. Some patients are asymptomatic, and routine complete blood count (CBC) shows thrombocytopenia. Some patients present with prominent leukocytosis and hepatosplenomegaly [27]. Peripheral blood smear shows circulating megakaryoblasts with high nucleus/cytoplasm ratio, fine chromatin, basophilic cytoplasm, and cytoplasmic blebbing (Fig. 21.13).
- The blasts usually show megakaryocytic differentiation by flow cytometry:
  - Positive for CD34, CD117, CD13, CD33, CD41, CD42, CD61, CD71, and HLA-DR
  - Negative for MPO, CD11, CD14, CD15, and glycophorin A
- Most cases demonstrated *GATA1* mutation in addition to trisomy 21. Bone marrow biopsy shows increased megakaryoblasts but usually less than those seen in peripheral blood. The blasts are positive for megakaryocytic markers such as CD41, CD42b, and CD61 as well as immature markers including CD34 and CD117.
- The majority of patients spontaneously recover within 3 months though rare cases of hydrops fetalis or progressive hepatic fibrosis have been reported. 20–30% of patients might acquire further molecular mutations and develop true acute myeloid leukemia within 1–3 years [28, 29].

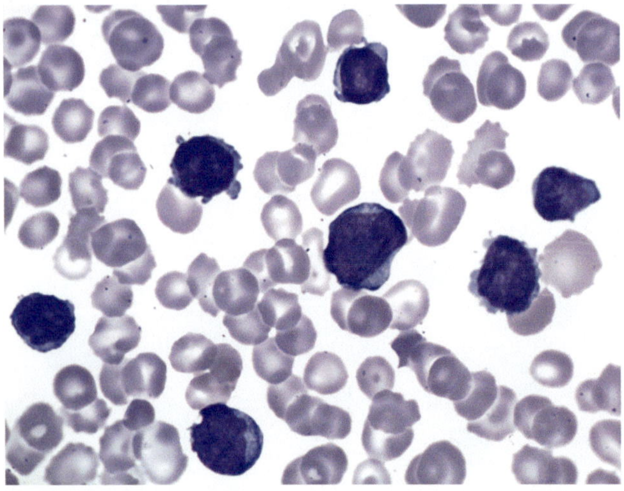

Fig. 21.13 Transient abnormal myelopoiesis associated with Down syndrome. Bone marrow aspirate smear shows marked increase in megakaryoblasts. The blasts are large in size, with round nuclear contour, slightly condensed chromatin, and deep basophilic cytoplasm with blebbing (original magnification 1000×)

- It is difficult to differentiate TAM vs true acute megakaryoblastic leukemia by morphology or immunophenotyping. Although TAM has been reported in non-Down syndrome newborns, this is very rare.
- An asymptomatic newborn with physical features suggestive of Down syndrome and relatively normal CBC except for thrombocytopenia is the classical presentation of TAM, while a very sick baby with marked leukocytosis, severe anemia, and thrombocytopenia is more typical for patients with AML.
- TAM might show a *GATA1* mutation, while acute megakaryocytic leukemia might show complex cytogenetic and molecular changes [12, 30, 31].

Mimics of Acute Leukemia

Acute leukemia cells are characterized by high nucleus/cytoplasm ratio, fine chromatin, and distinct nucleoli in peripheral blood/bone marrow. Other cells can have similar morphology and mimic blasts. Careful observation and thorough immunophenotyping are needed to differentiate them and avoid misinterpretation.

B-cell Prolymphocytic Leukemia Mimicking Acute Leukemia

- B-cell prolymphocytic leukemia (B-PLL) is a mature B-cell neoplasm characterized by B-prolymphocytes involving peripheral blood, bone marrow, and spleen.
- Prolymphocytes are characterized by:
  - Medium-sized.
  - Round nuclear contour.
  - Moderately condensed chromatin.
  - Prominent central nucleolus.
  - Moderate amount of agranular cytoplasm.
- B-PLL is diagnosed when more than 55% of the circulating cells are prolymphocytes.
- The prominent nucleoli might resemble acute leukemia. The chromatin in B-PLL is usually more condense than that in acute leukemia.
- Flow cytometry shows that B-PLL cells express B-cell markers including CD19, CD20, CD22, CD79a, CD79b, and FMC7. CD5 and CD23 are positive in approximately 20% of the cases. They express surface immunoglobulin light chain kappa or lambda and are negative for immature markers such as CD34 and TdT. On the contrary, B-ALL, being a precursor B-cell neoplasm, lacks surface immunoglobulin light chains and expresses immature markers CD34, CD123, and/or TdT.

T-cell Prolymphocytic Leukemia and HTLV1+ Adult T-Cell Leukemia Lymphoma (ATLL) Mimicking Acute Leukemia

- T-cell prolymphocytic leukemia (T-PLL) is an aggressive mature T-cell leukemia characterized by small- to medium-sized lymphocytes involving peripheral blood, bone marrow, lymph nodes, liver, spleen, and skin. ATLL has more variable clinical presentation, but some cases may closely mimic an acute leukemia.
- T-PLL cells have round, oval, or irregular nuclear contour, distinct nucleoli, and abundant agranular cytoplasm [32]. Although the chromatin is relatively denser than that in acute leukemia, the prolymphocytes can mimic leukemia cells morphologically.
- ATLL cells can have irregular nuclear contour and relatively condensed chromatin, resembling "flower cells."
- Flow cytometry can help to differentiate these two entities but also may be confusing because about 40% of T-PLL show a CD4+/CD8+ "double-positive" phenotype generally associated with immature T cells.
  - T-PLL can show dimmer expression of CD3, but they lack immature markers such as CD34, TdT, or CD1a and express CD52 brightly. The comparison of T-lymphoblastic leukemia (T-ALL) and T-PLL can be seen in Table 21.9 (Fig. 21.14).
  - ATLL typically shows CD4+ T cells and loss of CD7 while retaining CD2 and CD5. Occasionally, they can show dimmer expression of CD3 or even loss of CD3 expression. Rarely, they can express both CD4 and CD8 or lack both CD4 and CD8, mimicking T-acute lymphoblastic leukemia. Typically, ATLL express CD25. However, they lack expression of immature markers such as CD34, TdT, or CD1a.

Table 21.9 Comparison of T-acute lymphoblastic leukemia (T-ALL) vs T-cell prolymphocytic leukemia (T-PLL)

	Age	Morphology	Flow cytometry
T-ALL	Both pediatric and adults	Relatively fine chromatin, inconspicuous nucleoli, scant agranular cytoplasm	Surface CD3 is usually negative, cytoplasmic CD3 is usually positive; variably express CD2, CD5, CD7; usually CD4+/CD8+ or CD4-/CD8-, can be CD4+ or CD8+; maybe positive for one or more immature markers such as CD34, TdT, and CD1a
T-PLL	Median age: 65 (30–94), extremely rare in pediatric patients	Relatively condensed chromatin, prominent nucleoli, abundant agranular cytoplasm	CD2+, surface CD3 might be weak, CD5+, CD7+, CD4+/CD8- (60%); CD4+/CD8+ (25%); CD4-/CD8+ (15%), negative for CD34, TdT, and CD1a

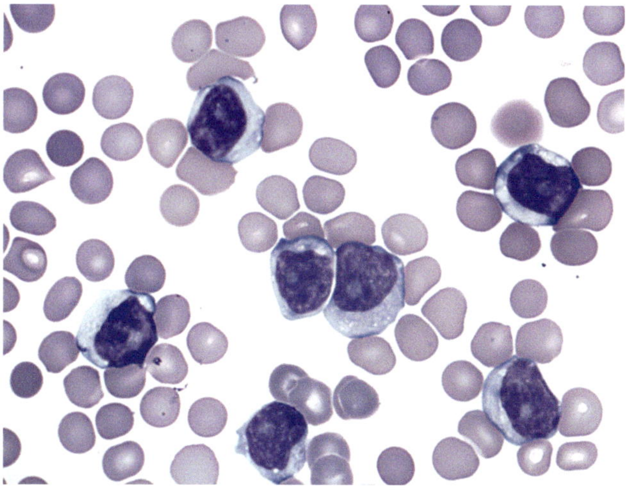

Fig. 21.14 T-cell prolymphocytic leukemia mimicking acute leukemia. Peripheral blood smear shows marked increase in atypical cells with distinct nucleoli (original magnification 1000×)

Aggressive B-Cell Lymphoma Involving Peripheral Blood and/or Bone Marrow Mimicking Acute Leukemia

- Aggressive B-cell lymphoma, including diffuse large B-cell lymphoma (DLBCL), high-grade B-cell lymphoma with *MYC* and *BCL2* and/or *BCL6* rearrangements (the so called "double-hit or triple-hit lymphoma"), and blastoid mantle cell lymphoma, usually do not involve peripheral blood or bone marrow.
- When there is diffuse involvement in bone marrow and/or peripheral blood, DLBCL might mimic acute leukemia because they are large cells with prominent nucleoli [33–35]. Usually, the aggressive B-cell lymphomas show more condensed chromatin, and the cells are more pleomorphic.
- They are positive for B-cell markers such as CD19, CD20, CD22, and CD79a and are monoclonal for surface immunoglobulin light chain kappa or lambda. They are usually negative for immature markers CD34 or TdT. High-grade B-cell lymphoma with *MYC* and *BCL2* and/or *BCL6* rearrangement (the so-called double-hit or triple-hit lymphoma) can show more monotonous blastoid morphology and relatively fine chromatin [36]. The cells occasionally express dim CD45 and TdT, lack CD20 (especially after rituximab therapy), and lack surface immunoglobulin light chain by flow cytometry [37, 38].
- When aggressive lymphoma has a leukemic presentation, a careful clinical history including the patient's previous rituximab treatment and full workup including evaluation of cell morphology, flow cytometry, and cytogenetic study including FISH is needed for a definite diagnosis.

Atypical Chronic Lymphocytic Leukemia Mimicking Acute Leukemia

- Circulating lymphocytes with condensed chromatin usually rule out the diagnosis of acute leukemia, especially chronic lymphocytic leukemia (CLL). Atypical CLL might show less condensed chromatin and distinct nucleoli and might cause confusion with acute leukemia.
- CLL is usually positive for CD5, CD19, CD20, CD23, and CD79a. CD20 expression might be dim/heterogeneous, and the surface immunoglobulin expression might be negative. They are negative for markers of immaturity including CD34 and TdT.

4. Which morphological findings in the peripheral blood/BM aspirate/biopsy are reliably diagnostic of acute leukemia? Which ones suggest the diagnosis? Which is (are) unreliable for diagnosis? Which findings rule out the diagnosis?

In most cases, at least 20% blasts on peripheral blood smears and/or bone marrow aspirate smears are diagnostic of acute leukemia. The blasts are identified by their morphological features, but flow cytometry and/or immunohistochemistry for CD34 or CD117 may be used to identify and quantify myeloid blasts, while CD19, CD79a, CD10, and TdT may be used for B-ALL, and CD3, CD7, and TdT may be used for T-ALL blasts. There are two scenarios in which acute leukemia may be diagnosed by morphology alone:-

Acute Myeloid Leukemia with the Presence of Auer Rods in Blasts

- Myeloblasts show various amount of azurophilic granules in the cytoplasm. The presence of abundant azurophilic granules is highly suggestive for myeloblasts, while identification of Auer rods in the cytoplasm of blasts is diagnostic of acute myeloid leukemia. Flow cytometry is usually performed to confirm the diagnosis of acute myeloid leukemia and rule out mixed-phenotype acute leukemia.

Acute Myeloid Leukemia with Monocytic Differentiation

- Monoblasts/promonocytes are typically negative for CD34 and CD117 by flow cytometry. Morphologic evaluation of the peripheral blood smear/bone marrow aspirate smears is usually the only way to diagnose acute myeloid leukemia with monocytic differentiation. (See discussion in Q3 and Fig. 21.4 and Table 21.4.)

Acute Leukemia with <20% Blasts

- In most cases, at least 20% blasts are required for the diagnosis of acute leukemia (and 30% proerythroblasts are required for diagnosis of erythroleukemia). A blast percentage of 20% is not required in the following three types of AML:
  - Acute myeloid leukemia with t(8;21)(q22;q22.1); *RUNX1-RUNX1T1*
  - Acute myeloid leukemia with inv(16)(p13.1q22) or t(16;16)(p13.1;q22); *CBFB-MYH11*
  - Acute promyelocytic leukemia (APL) with *PML-RARA*

Aleukemic Acute Leukemia

- Aleukemic acute leukemia is generally an early phase of developing acute leukemia in some cases when blasts are absent in the blood. A bone marrow biopsy is required for these patients.

Cases with Hypercellularity, Fibrosis, or Dysplasia

- The bone marrow spaces in patients with acute leukemia are often, but not invariably, hypercellular (usually >90%). The marrow can be fibrotic, and the remaining hematopoietic cells can show dysplasia, especially the erythroid precursors. These features might suggest, but are not diagnostic of acute leukemia. Careful observation and necessary immunophenotyping are very helpful to rule out the possibility of acute leukemia.

Hematogone Hyperplasia

- Hematogone hyperplasia can be a mimicker for B-lymphoblastic leukemia (B-ALL).
- Hematogones are the B-lymphocyte precursors in the bone marrow. They share very similar morphologic and immunophenotypic findings with B-lymphoblasts. They have very high nucleus/cytoplasm ratio, relatively fine homogenous chromatin, round nuclei, and scant cytoplasm. Usually, they do not have discernable nucleoli.
- They are positive for CD19, CD10, CD34 (dim, heterogenous), and CD20 (heterogenous) by flow cytometry. They do not have aberrant myeloid markers such as CD13 and CD33 and show a normal maturation pattern by flow cytometry. More mature hematogones express surface immunoglobulin light chains. B-lymphoblasts rarely express surface immunoglobulin light chains [39, 40].
- Hematogones are usually <5% in adults but can be much higher in pediatric patients especially during viral infection and regeneration after chemotherapy and bone marrow transplant. By morphology alone, it is difficult to differentiate hematogones from residual lymphoblasts in patients with a history of B-ALL.

5. What is the minimal and optimal ancillary workup for diagnosis and subclassification of acute leukemias?

The proper classification of acute leukemia is of vital importance due to the differences in treatment regimens and prognosis. Acute leukemias can be roughly divided into three lineage categories: myeloid, lymphoblastic, and leukemias of ambiguous lineage. This basic subdivision, with a few notable exceptions, drives initial therapy.

A minimal workup in every new case of suspected acute leukemia should include the following [41]:

- Peripheral blood smear and complete blood count.
- Bone marrow aspirate with good-quality smears stained with Romanowsky stain.
- An adequate H&E-stained core biopsy and/or clot section (preferably both).
- Additional stains for aspirate smears – iron and myeloperoxidase.
- Flow cytometry with analysis of stem cell, myeloid, monocytic, lymphoid (B, T, and NK-cell specific), erythroid, and megakaryocytic antigens. The antibody repertoire selected must have sufficient redundancy to accommodate loss of antigen and/or aberrant expression of antigens to define the lineage of the leukemic cells clearly. A larger antibody panel is more likely to provide a leukemia-associated immunophenotype (LAIP), which may be crucial in identifying minimal residual disease after treatment. Immunophenotyping should almost always be performed by flow cytometry. Lineage determination can be done by immunohistochemistry, but only if an aspirate sample for flow cytometry is not available.
- Karyotyping by conventional cytogenetics.

Depending on the morphological and flow cytometry findings, appropriate FISH panels are performed:

- AML FISH panel for the following abnormities (probe target/gene or sequence) [42]:
  - t(8;21)(q22;q22)/*RUNX1T1-RUNX1*
  - inv(16)/(p13.3q22)/*CBFB-MYH11*
  - inv(3) or t(3;3)/*RPN1-MECOM*
  - 11q23/*KMT2A*
  - del(5)(q31)/*EGR1*
  - del(7)(q31)/D7S486
- Stat FISH for t(15;17) if APL is suspected.
- ALL FISH for the following abnormities (probe target/gene) [43]:
  - 11q23/*KMT2A*
  - t(12;21)(p13;q22)/*ETV6-RUNX*
  - t(1;19)(q23;p13.3)/*TCF3-PBX1*
  - Enumeration probes for chromosomes 4, 10, and 17
  - t(5;13)(q31.1;q32.1) *IGH/IL3*
  - t(9;22)(q34;q11.2)/*BCR-ABL1*
- Molecular and myeloid NGS panel [42].
  - Testing is based on finding most common genomic alterations, as well as actionable mutations.
  - A minimal analysis for AML subclassification would include *NPM1, CEBPA,* and *RUNX1* analysis.
  - A minimal analysis for actionable alterations includes *FLT3* (both for internal tandem duplications [ITDs] and mutant-to-wild-type allelic ratio) and *IDH1/IDH2* analysis.
  - *KIT* mutation testing should be performed for patients with t(8;21)(q22;q22)/*RUNX1T1-RUNX1* or inv(16)/(p13.3q22)/*CBFB-MYH11*.
  - Although not done in every case of AML, next-generation sequencing panel (NGS) highlights the most common and prognostic genetic alterations including *TP53*, *ETV6*, *EZH2*, and *ASXL1*. Panels will vary from institution and vendor.

Comments: The above workup should be abbreviated only if the material received for pathological examination is insufficient. For example, if there is no aspirate smear due to fibrosis, then flow cytometry and cytogenetics may not be options. In such cases, flow cytometry may be performed on peripheral blood if sufficient circulating blasts are present to determine lineage.

While the diagnosis can sometimes be established on peripheral blood alone (>20% circulating blasts), a bone marrow biopsy and aspirate for morphologic assessment are recommended. Recent studies have shown that in pediatric leukemias, flow cytometry is reliable in most cases with the exception of early T-cell precursor ALL, mixed-phenotype acute leukemia, and acute megakaryoblastic leukemia [44].

6. Which ancillary test results are diagnostic, suggestive of diagnosis, unreliable for diagnosis, or rule out the diagnosis?

Immunophenotyping (Flow Cytometry and/or Immunohistochemistry)

- If a smear is suboptimal or unavailable, CD34, CD117, and/or TdT expression by immunohistochemistry or flow cytometry may be used to identify and quantify blasts.
  - When possible, immunohistochemistry or flow cytometry should not replace cytomorphologic examination, which is the gold standard for blast identification and quantification [1, 45].
  - Note: Rarely, some cases of progressed or aggressive mature B-cell lymphomas can show weak or patchy TdT expression [46], but they otherwise lack morphologic or other phenotypic features of blasts and should

not be diagnosed as lymphoblastic leukemia/ lymphoma.

- CD34, CD117, and/or TdT are not reliable for blast identification in following situations:
  – Monoblasts, megakaryoblasts, and erythroblasts are negative for TdT and can also be negative for both CD34 and CD117. In these instances, blasts must be identified and quantified by morphology.
- Surface immunoglobulin light chain can rule out B-acute lymphoblastic leukemia.
  – Surface immunoglobulin light chain expression typically excludes a diagnosis of B-acute lymphoblastic leukemia.
  – Note: B-lymphoblastic leukemia can very rarely express surface immunoglobulin light chain [47–52], but in these rare cases, blasts are confirmed by strong CD34 or TdT expression.
- Thorough immunophenotyping is required for broad lineage subclassification:
  – AML – Show features of granulocytic, monocytic, megakaryocytic, or erythroid differentiation. See Table 21.10 for a list of commonly used antigens to define or support myeloid blast lineage.
  – B-ALL/B-LBL – See Table 21.10 for a list of commonly used antigens to define or support B-lineage blasts.

Table 21.10 Phenotype supportive of lineage determination

	AML myeloid	AML monocytic	AML erythroid	AML Mk	BPDCN	B-ALL	T-ALL
CD34	++	+/−	−/+	+/−	−/+	++	+
CD117	+/−	−/+	+	−	−/+	−	−/+
HLA-DR	++	+	−	−	+	+	+
CD123	+/−	+/−	−	−	++	+/−	/−+
MPO	++	−	−	−	×	−	−
CD13	+	+	−	−	×	−/+	−/+
CD33	+	+	−	−	+	−/+	−/+
CD11c	−	+	−	−	−	−	−
CD64	−	+	−	−	−	−	−
CD14	−	+	−	−	−	−	−
CD4	−	+	−	−	+	−	+/−
Lysozyme	++	++	−	−	×	−	−
NSE	−	+	−	−	−	−	−
E-cadherin	−	−	++	−	−	−	−
Glycophorin A	−	−	+	−	−	−	−
CD71	−/+	−/+	++	−/+	−/+	−	−
Hemoglobin	−	−	−/+	−	−	−	−
CD41	−	−	−	++	−	−	−
CD42b	−	−	−	++	−	−	−
CD61	−	−	−	++	−	−	−
CD56	−/+	−/+	−	−	+	−	−
TCL1a	−	−	−	−	++	−	−
TdT	−/+	−	−	−	−/+	++	++
CD19	−/+	−	−	−	×	++	−
CD10	−	−	−	−	−	+/−	+/−
CD79a	−	−	−	−	−/+	+	−/+
cCD22	−	−	−	−	−	+	−
PAX5	−/+	−	−	−	−	+	−
cCD3	−	−	−	−	×	−	++
CD2	−	−	−	−	−/+	−	+
CD5	−	−	−	−	−/+	−	+
CD7	−/+	−	−	−	+	−	+
CD8	−	−	−	−	−	−	+/−
CD1a	−	−	−	−	−	−	+
CD99	−	−	−	−	−	−	+

Mk megakaryocyte, *BPDCN* blastic plasmacytoid dendritic cell neoplasm, *B-ALL* B-lymphoblastic leukemia/lymphoma, *T-ALL* T-lymphoblastic leukemia/lymphoma. Symbols in bold font indicate the antigen is either specific for blast lineage assignment (**+**) or rules out blast lineage assignment (**×**). The phenotypes listed above are typical but are not absolute unless otherwise noted

- T-ALL/T-LBL – See Table 21.10 for a list of commonly used antigens to define or support T-lineage blasts.
- Mixed-phenotype acute leukemia (MPAL) – Immunophenotypic evidence for more than one lineage is present (see Table 21.7 for immunophenotypic requirements to diagnose MPAL). This category includes acute leukemias with two different blast populations that are of different lineages as well as acute leukemias with a single blast population that expresses antigens from different lineages [1, 53].
- BPDCN – Blastic plasmacytoid dendritic cell neoplasm is also defined by a blast morphology and a unique immunophenotype (see Table 21.10 for additional details).
  - Note: expression of other lineage-defining antigens such as MPO, lysozyme, CD3, CD16, CD19, or CD20 rules out a diagnosis of BPDCN [1].
- Acute undifferentiated leukemia – This is a diagnosis of exclusion; thorough immunophenotyping must be performed to exclude any myeloid or lymphoid differentiation. These typically only express CD34, HLA-DR, and/or CD38. TdT or CD7 may be expressed and does not exclude this diagnosis [1].

- Some antigens are strongly associated with one lineage but lack fidelity so are unreliable for lineage assignment.
  - CD13, CD33 – Usually myeloid but can be seen in ALL and BPDCN
  - PAX5 – Usually B-lineage but can be seen in AML
  - TdT – Usually lymphoid but can be seen in AML and BPDCN
  - CD7 – usually strongly associated with T-lineage but can be seen in AML or BPDCN

Cytogenetic Studies (Karyotype and/or FISH)

- Abnormalities that are diagnostic of AML regardless of blast count:
  - t(8;21)(q22;q22)/*RUNX1T1-RUNX1*
  - inv(16)/(p13.3q22) or t(16;16)(p13.1;q22)/*CBFB-MYH11*
  - *PML-RARA*
- Cytogenetic studies are required for subclassification of AML, MPAL, and B-ALL/B-LBL.
  - AML – Required for AML with recurrent cytogenetic abnormalities (see Table 21.1 and Fig. 21.1) versus normal karyotype AML
  - MPAL – Required for MPAL with *BCR-ABL1* or MPAL with *KMT2A* rearrangements
  - B-ALL/B-LBL – Required for B-ALL/B-LBL with recurrent cytogenetic abnormalities (see Table 21.1)
- Cytogenetic abnormalities do not define the acute leukemia outside of the context of blast lineage.
  - Example 1:
  - A hypodiploid karyotype has no relevance in subclassifying AML or T-ALL/T-LBL.
  - Example 2:
  - *BCR-ABL1* fusion and *KMT2A* rearrangements can be seen in AML, MPAL, and B-ALL/B-LBL and should first be categorized by lineage and then by the cytogenetic abnormality.
- *JAK2-PCM1* fusion or *PDGFRA*, *PDGFRB*, or *FGFR1* rearrangements exclude a diagnosis of AML or ALL.

Special note should be made of any acute leukemia with eosinophilia or other myeloproliferative neoplasm (MPN)-like background (i.e., myeloid-predominant hypercellularity, often with eosinophilia) without a known preexisting MPN diagnosis. In some instances, the MPN-like background may not become apparent until after induction therapy, and the blast count is reduced to around 10% or lower. In these instances, FISH studies should be performed for *BCR-ABL1* fusion (if not already performed for subclassification), *JAK2-PCM1* fusion, and rearrangements in *PDGFRA*, *PDGFRB*, and *FGFR1*. If a *BCR-ABL1* fusion is detected, then a diagnosis of blast phase chronic myeloid leukemia (CML) must be considered. If rearrangements in *PDGFRA*, *PDGFRB*, or *FGFR1* are detected or a *JAK2-PCM1* fusion is detected, then a diagnosis of AML or ALL/LBL would be excluded and instead a diagnosis of myeloid/lymphoid neoplasm with eosinophilia and gene rearrangement in blast phase would instead be given.

Molecular Studies

- *NPM1*, *CEBPA*, and *RUNX1* mutation analyses are required for subclassification of normal karyotype AML (see Table 21.1 and Fig. 21.1).
- Gene expression arrays or NGS panels for rearrangements and mutations in genes involved in the JAK-STAT pathway are often used in the diagnosis of *BCR-ABL1*-like B-ALL/B-LBL. It should be noted that this testing is complex and not widely performed at this time.

7. What is the workup to provide prognostic and therapeutic target information? (Corollary – what treatments are available for this entity?)

See Table 21.11 for the prognostic and therapeutic implications of the more commonly informative phenotypic, cytogenetic, and molecular findings in acute leukemia [54–56].

Table 21.11 Prognostic and therapeutic implications of immunophenotypic, cytogenetic, and molecular findings

	Method of detection				Prognosis	Specific therapy[a]
	FC/IHC	FISH	Chr.	Mol.		
Acute myeloid leukemia						
CD33	X					**Y**
TdT	X				Good[b]	
−7/del(7q)		X	X		Worst	**Y**
del(5q)/t(5q)		X	X		Worst	**Y**
i17q/t(17p)		X	X		Worst	**Y**
−13/del(13q)		X	X		Poor	**Y**
del(11q)		X	X		Poor	**Y**
del(12p)/t(12p)		X	X		Poor	**Y**
idic(X)(q13)			X		Poor	**Y**
t(11;16)(q23.3;p13.3)			X		Poor	**Y**
t(3;21)(q26.2;q22.1)			X		Poor	**Y**
t(1;3)(p36.3;q21.2)			X		Poor	**Y**
t(2;11)(p21;q23.3)			X		Poor	**Y**
t(5;12)(q32;p13.2)			X		Poor	**Y**
t(5;7)(q32;q11.2)			X		Poor	**Y**
t(5;17)(q32;p13.2)			X		Poor	**Y**
t(5;10)(q32;q21)			X		Poor	**Y**
t(3;5)(q25.3;q35.1)			X		Poor	**Y**
≥3 cytogenetic abnormalities			X		Worst	**Y**
t(8;21)(q22;q22.1); *RUNX1-RUNX1T1*		X	X		Best	Y
inv(16)(p13.1q22) or t(16;16)(p13.1;q22) *CBFB-MYH11*		X	X		Best	Y
PML-RARA fusion		X			Best	**Y**
t(9;11)(p21.3;q23.3); *KMT2A-MLLT3*		X	X		Intermed	
KMT2A rearranged (other than *KMT2A-MLLT3*)		X			Poor	
t(6;9)(p23;q34.1); *DEK-NUP214*		X	X		Poor	
inv(3)(q21.3q26.2) of t(3;3)(q21.3;q26.2); *GATA2, MECOM*		X	X		Poor	
t(1;22)(p13.3;q13.1); *RBM15-MKL1*		X	X		Poor	
BCR-ABL1 fusion		X			Poor	Y
NPM1				X	Best[c]	Y
Biallelic *CEBPA*				X	Best	Y
RUNX1				X	Poor	
KIT				X	Poor[d]	**Y**
IDH1				X	Mixed	Y
IDH2				X	Mixed	**Y**
FLT3				X	Poor	**Y**
TP53				X	Worst	**Y**
ASXL1				X	Poor	
SRSF2				X	Poor[e]	
SF3B1				X	Poor[e]	
U2AF1				X	Poor[e]	
ZRSR2				X	Poor[e]	
B-lymphoblastic leukemia/lymphoma						
CD19	X					**Y**
CD20	X					Y
CD22	X					**Y**
CD52	X					Y
t(9;22)(q34.1;q11.2); *BCR-ABL1*		X	X		Poor	Y
t(v;11q23.3); *KMT2A* rearranged		X			Worst	
t(12;21)(p13.2;q22.1); *ETV6-RUNX1*		X	X		Best	
Hyperdiploidy			X		Best	
Hypodiploidy			X		Poor	
t(5;14)(q31.1;q32.1); IGH/*IL3*		X	X			
t(1;19)(q23;p13.3); *TCF3-PBX1*		X	X		Poor	
BCR-ABL1-like		X		X	Poor	Y
iAMP21		X			Poor	
ERG				X	Good	
IKZF1				X	Poor	
TP53				X	Poor	

(continued)

Table 21.11 (continued)

	Method of detection				Prognosis	Specific therapy[a]
	FC/IHC	FISH	Chr.	Mol.		
CREBBP				X	Poor	
FLT3				X		Y
BPDCN						
CD123	X					Y

FC/IHC flow cytometry/immunohistochemistry, *FISH* fluorescence in situ hybridization, *Chr.* chromosome analysis (karyotype), *Mol.* molecular, *BPDCN* blastic plasmacytoid dendritic cell neoplasm

[a]Specific therapies include targeted monoclonal antibodies, CAR-T cells, small molecular inhibitors, and specific chemotherapeutic regimens for that alteration. Therapies in **bold** are FDA approved specifically for acute leukemia. Some therapies in preclinical studies or very early-phase clinical studies may not be represented. Specific drugs or therapeutic regimens are beyond the scope of this chapter.

[b]TdT expression is a good prognostic indicator only for AML with minimal differentiation

[c]*NPM1* mutation has an excellent prognosis only for normal karyotype AML and wild-type *FLT3*

[d]*KIT* mutations confer a poor prognosis in AML with *RUNX1-RUNX1T1* or *CBFB-MYH11*

[e]Spliceosome gene mutations (*SRSF2, SF3B1, U2AF1*, and *ZRSR2*) have a poor prognosis when co-mutated with chromatin-modifying genes (*ASXL1, STAG2, BCOR, KMT2A, EZH2*, and *PHF6*)

Reticulin Stain on Core Biopsy

- For AML not otherwise specified (see flowchart 22.1), the presence of significant marrow fibrosis would be compatible with acute panmyelosis with myelofibrosis, which has an extremely poor prognosis [57, 58].

Immunophenotyping (Flow Cytometry)

- All acute leukemias should be thoroughly immunophenotyped.
- Distinction between myeloid and lymphoid lineage guides immediate therapy.
- Identification of MPAL has a very poor prognosis.
- TdT expression in AML with minimal differentiation has been associated with a favorable prognosis [59].
- Targeted therapies are available [54–56]:
  - AML – CD33
  - B-ALL/B-LBL – CD19, CD20, CD22, or CD52
  - BPDCN – CD123

Chromosome Analysis and FISH

- All AML and B-ALL/B-LBL should be cytogenetically characterized.
- AML with *RUNX1-RUNX1T1, CBFB-MYH11,* or APL with *PML-RARA* has a very good prognosis and can be treated with less aggressive therapies [54].
- Cases of APL with *PML-RARA* are urgently treated with ATRA [21].
- Complex cytogenetic abnormalities and myelodysplasia-related abnormalities have a poor prognosis and are eligible for the newly FDA-approved therapy CPX-351 (Vyxeos®) [54].
- In B-ALL/B-LBL, hyperdiploidy and *ETV6-RUNX1* fusions have the best prognosis, while *KMT2A* rearrangements, *BCR-ABL1* fusions, and hypodiploidy have a poor prognosis [56].
- B-ALL/B-LBL with *BCR-ABL1* fusions and *BCR-ABL1*-like B-ALL/B-LBL are eligible for tyrosine kinase inhibitor therapy. Commonly rearranged genes that fall under the classification of *BCR-ABL1*-like B-ALL/B-LBL include *CRLF2, JAK2, EPOR, ABL2, PDGFRB, NTRK3, TYK2*, and *CSF1R* [56].

Molecular Studies

- B-ALL/B-LBL: *ERG* mutations have a favorable prognosis [56, 60], while *IKZF1* and *TP53* mutations have a poor prognosis [56, 61–66]. *CREBBP* deletions and mutations are associated with increased risk of relapse, even in otherwise favorable prognosis B-ALL/B-LBL [56, 67, 68].
- *ABL1* and *JAK1/2/3* mutations are common in *BCR-ABL1*-like B-ALL/B-LBL and are eligible for tyrosine kinase inhibitor therapy [56].
- *FLT3* mutations can occur in *KMT2A*-rearranged B-ALL/B-LBL and are eligible for *FLT3* inhibitor therapy [55, 69, 70].
- *NOTCH1* mutations are common in T-ALL/T-LBL and are therefore promising therapeutic targets currently being investigated in preclinical and early clinical trials [55, 71, 72].
- *NPM1* and biallelic *CEBPA* mutations are favorably prognostic in normal karyotype AML and can be treated with less aggressive therapies [54].
- *KIT* D816 mutations confer a poor prognosis in the otherwise favorable AML with *RUNX1-RUNX1T1* and AML with *CBFB-MYH11*; these are eligible for KIT-targeted therapies [54, 73, 74].
- *FLT3* mutations are prognostically unfavorable and are eligible for FDA-approved FLT3 inhibitors [54].
- *TP53* mutations have a very poor prognosis and are eligible for the newly FDA-approved therapy CPX-351 (Vyxeos) [54].
- *IDH1* or *IDH2* mutations are eligible for IDH1/2 inhibitor therapies [54].
- Splicing factor mutations (*ASXL1, SRSF2, SF3B1, USAF1*, and *ZRSR2*) confer a poor prognosis in AML and are highly suggestive of secondary AML (i.e., AML-MRC) [75, 76]. Though the presence of these mutations

in AML is not yet sufficient for the diagnosis of AML-MRC, the strong association may allow for future use of CPX-351 (Vyxeos) in these cases.

8. Which subtypes of this entity are clinically relevant, and which are morphologically defined but have unproven/minimal clinical relevance?

- *Acute promyelocytic leukemia (APL, M3) needs special treatment*
- Patients with acute promyelocytic leukemia (APL, M3) carry high risk of hypercoagulation and are treated with ATRA and sometimes arsenic trioxide. These therapies lead to complete remission in 90–100% cases and an overall survival of 86–97% [1, 77]. Chemotherapy is only limited to those patients with high risk [78]. It is critical to differentiate APL from the other subtypes of acute myeloid leukemia. The morphologic features of APL and how to differentiate it from AML with monocytic differentiation can be found in Questions 2 and 3.
- *Acute myeloid leukemia with myelodysplasia-related changes carries poor prognosis*
- Acute myeloid leukemia with myelodysplasia-related changes (AML-MRC) carries a poor prognosis except for some cases with a prior history of MDS and 20–29% blasts in the bone marrow biopsy [79]. In order to make a diagnosis of AML-MRC, the pathologist has to answer the following questions:
  - The patient's history: Does the patient have any previous history of MDS/MPN? Did the patient have previous history of radiation or chemotherapy unrelated to the disease?
  - Cytogenetic changes: Any MDS-related abnormalities? Any recurrent abnormalities described in AML with recurrent cytogenetic abnormalities?
  - Morphologic dysplasia: Does the patient have any dysplasia, how many lineages, and what percentage?

The diagnostic criteria of AML-MRC can be found in Question 2. The morphologic features of dysplasia are listed in Table 21.6. The cytogenetic features are listed in Table 21.5.

AML with Minimal Differentiation, AML Without Maturation, and AML with Maturation are Morphologically Distinct but Similar in Prognosis

- AML with minimal differentiation (FAB classification M0)
  - The blasts do not have morphologic or cytochemical evidence of myeloid differentiation by definition. The main clinical significance is to distinguish these from acute lymphoblastic leukemias. The blasts are usually characterized by:
    - Medium-sized.
    - Round to slightly irregular nuclear contour.
    - One or two nucleoli.
  - They may resemble lymphoblasts and have small nuclei, relatively more condensed chromatin, inconspicuous nucleoli, and scant cytoplasm.
  - The blasts show no cytoplasmic granules, no Auer rods.
  - Less than 3% blasts are positive for myeloperoxidase, Sudan Black B, and nonspecific esterase by cytochemistry stains.
  - Myeloid differentiation can be seen by CD13, CD33, and CD117 (KIT) expressions. They do not show monocytic markers including CD11b, CD14, and CD64.
  - Although MPO is negative by cytochemistry, MPO can be positive by flow cytometry and/or immunohistochemistry (Fig. 21.4a).
- AML without maturation (FAB classification M1)
  - Some blasts may show azurophilic granules and/or Auer rods. Some may have agranular cytoplasm.
  - MPO and Sudan Black B are positive in ≥3% of the blasts by cytochemistry stains.
  - The maturing granulocytic cells, including promyelocytes, myelocytes, metamyelocytes, and neutrophils, consist of <10% of the total nucleated bone marrow cells.
  - The immunophenotype of the blasts might resemble those seen in AML with minimal differentiation except that some blasts might express CD11b (Fig. 21.4b).
- AML with maturation (FAB classification M2)
  - The blasts may or may not have azurophilic granules in the cytoplasm.
  - Auer rods are typically more frequently seen than in other leukemias.
  - The maturing granulocytes consist of ≥10% of the total nucleated bone marrow cells.
  - The blasts might show more mature granulocytic markers such as CD15 and CD65 by immunophenotyping. CD11b expression is more frequent. They usually lack monocytic markers such as CD14 and CD64 (Fig. 21.4c).

The morphologic and immunophenotypic differences between the above entities are listed in Table 21.12 [80]. If the dysplastic cells are ≤50% in two lineages, and there is no previous related chemotherapy/radiation therapy, the AML can be classified into these categories based on morphologic and immunophenotypic findings before the cytogenetic and molecular results are available. If the case fits into any of the recurrent genetic abnormalities listed in 2017 WHO classification such as t(8;21), inv(16)(p13.1q22), and t(16; 16)

Table 21.12 Morphologic and immunophenotypic differences of AML with minimal differentiation, AML without maturation, and AML with maturation

	Morphology	Cytochemistry	Immunophenotype
AML with minimal differentiation	No cytoplasmic granules; no Auer rods	Negative for MPO, Sudan Black, and ACE (<3%)	Positive for CD13, CD33, CD34, CD117, HLA-DR, MPO Negative for CD11b, CD14, CD15, CD64, CD65
AML without maturation	Azurophilic granules and/or Auer rods are present; maturing granulocytic cells consisting of <10% of the total nucleated bone marrow cells	Positive for MPO, Sudan Black (≥3%)	Positive for CD11b (subset), CD13, CD33, CD34, CD117, HLA-DR, MPO Negative for CD14, CD15, CD64, CD65
AML with maturation	Azurophilic granules may be present; Auer rods are more frequent; maturing granulocytic cells consisting of ≥10% of the total nucleated bone marrow cells	Positive for MPO, Sudan Black (≥3%)	Positive for CD11b, CD13, CD15, CD33, CD34, CD65, CD117, HLA-DR, MPO Negative for CD14, CD64

MPO myeloperoxidase, *NSE* nonspecific esterase, *ACE* naphthol AS-D chloroacetate esterase

(p13.1;q22), the case should be reclassified as AML with recurrent genetic abnormalities. If cases with *NPM1* and *CEBPA* mutations are excluded, the morphologic differences between AML with minimal differentiation (M0), AML without maturation (M1), and AML with maturation (M2) do not provide any clinical or prognostic information [81].

Of note, one AML case might qualify for several entities, but usually only one entity is assigned. AML can be classified according to the following order (see Fig. 21.1):

- Therapy-related MDS/AML
- AML with classic recurrent genetic abnormalities
- AML-MRC (AML with myelodysplasia-related changes) (characteristic cytogenetic abnormalities [Table 21.5] or originating from preexisting myeloid neoplasm)
- AML with mutated *NPM1*, biallelic *CEBPA*, *RUNX1*
- AML-MRC defined by morphologic dysplasia
- AML, NOS

According to the FAB classification, B-acute lymphoblastic leukemia (B-ALL) can be subclassified into types L1, L2, and L3 by morphology [15]. The description of the morphologic features of B-ALL can be found in Question 2 section B. The cytomorphologic types of L1 and L2 do not correspond to the cytogenetics/molecular features or the prognosis of B-ALL. Therefore, the L1 and L2 subtypes of B-ALL have unproven/minimal clinical relevance. It is very important to recognize the L3 morphology, because the treatment for Burkitt lymphoma, being a mature B-cell lymphoma, is different from acute lymphoblastic leukemia. Additional auxiliary studies such as flow cytometry, immunohistochemistry, and cytogenetic study are very helpful. L1 and L2 usually show immature markers such as CD34 and TdT, while L3 demonstrates mature B-cell markers such as CD20 and surface immunoglobulin light chain restriction. L3 usually shows translocation involving c*MYC* gene. t(8;14)(q24;q32) involving *IGH* is the most common one, accounting for 85% of the cases, while t(2;8)(p12;q24) involving kappa light chain and t(8;22)(q24;q11) involving lambda light chain are relatively rare. A three-way translocation, involving t(8;14;18), has also been reported [82].

9. What is an adequate specimen for this condition?

Bone Marrow Aspirate

- The most important specimen for the diagnosis and classification of acute leukemia is the bone marrow aspirate.
- Ideally, 10–15 mL should be collected in total, with the first pull (about 5 mL) used for preparation of aspirate smears and flow cytometry. Subsequent pulls, which are more hemodiluted, should be collected for chromosome analysis, FISH, and molecular studies [41].
- An adequate aspirate smear should consist of 2–3 slides containing a total of 4–5 cellular marrow particles such that 500 nucleated cells can easily be counted near the particles. Multiple slides should be examined to minimize the effects of uneven blast distribution [1].
- A formalin-fixed, paraffin-embedded (FFPE) clot section should also be prepared if possible. Some immunohistochemical studies do not perform well in decalcified tissue and can thus be performed on the clot section, which is not decalcified. In addition, the clot section may be able to be used for FISH or molecular studies if sufficient material was not obtained at the time of biopsy.

Bone Marrow Core Biopsy

- An adequate bone marrow core biopsy should be 1.5 cm in length, taken perpendicular to the cortical bone, and should contain ≥10 intertrabecular marrow spaces for examination [1].
- Touch preparation slides should also be performed when a core biopsy is obtained in case the aspirate smears are too hemodiluted for accurate blast quantification. The cores should be handled carefully so as not to crush the cells or the delicate bony trabeculae.

Peripheral Blood

- A peripheral blood smear should be examined and correlated with a peripheral blood count [1, 41].
- An adequate peripheral blood smear should contain at least 200 nucleated cells for accurate blast quantification.
- If there is insufficient bone marrow aspirate and if the peripheral blood blast count is sufficiently high, then additional blood may be sent for flow cytometry, chromosome analysis, FISH, and molecular studies.

10. What information can be conveyed to the clinician during each stage of the workup?

- *Peripheral blood smear, aspirate smear, and touch preparations*
- Depending on workflow, the smears and touch preparations can be ready for review as early as 1–2 hours after bone marrow collection. At this stage, the percent blasts can be relayed to the clinician. If Auer rods are identified or a myeloperoxidase cytochemical stain is positive, then a diagnosis of acute myeloid leukemia can be confidently rendered. For cases with a history of myelodysplasia or cytotoxic therapy, a final diagnosis of acute myeloid leukemia with myelodysplasia-related changes (AML-MRC) or therapy-related acute myeloid leukemia (t-AML) can also be reported.
- *Flow cytometry and/or immunohistochemistry*
- If available onsite, flow cytometry is typically faster and can be ready for review within 4–6 hours after bone marrow collection depending on workflow and whether the case is prioritized. If not available onsite, then immunohistochemistry may be available first and would typically be available 24–48 hours after bone marrow collection. At this stage, broad classification may be conveyed (acute myeloid leukemia (AML), B-lymphoblastic leukemia/lymphoma (B-ALL/B-LBL), T-lymphoblastic leukemia/lymphoma (T-ALL/T-LBL), blastic plasmacytoid dendritic cell neoplasm (BPDCN), or mixed-phenotype leukemias (MPAL)). For T-ALL/LBL, this is sufficient for definitive subclassification. For all other acute leukemias, the case is typically given a preliminary diagnosis at this stage so that clinicians can begin treatment, with final subclassification to occur after cytogenetic and molecular studies are complete.
- *Chromosome analysis and FISH*
- Some FISH tests, like FISH for *PML-RARA* fusion, have been optimized to result in ≤24 hours. Most FISH panels and chromosome analysis can be completed within 1–2 weeks. If a recurrent cytogenetic abnormality is identified, then a final subclassification with the specific cytogenetic abnormality may be given at this stage. Also, for B-ALL/LBL, MPAL, and BPDCN, a final subclassification may be given even if no cytogenetic abnormalities are identified.
- *Molecular studies in AML*
- Molecular mutation analysis of *NPM1*, *CEBPA*, and *RUNX1* can typically be resulted as quickly as 3 days after ordering if offered as separate stand-alone tests but may take 2–3 weeks if performed as part of a next-generation sequencing (NGS) panel. A diagnostic subclassification of AML can only be based on the presence of a molecular mutation if all cytogenetic studies are normal.
- AML samples are also frequently tested for *FLT3*, *IDH1/2*, and *TP53* mutations, which would have a similar turnaround time depending on the testing methodology. These mutations are not informative for diagnostic subclassification but do provide important therapeutic information (see Question 7 and Table 21.11).

11. What should be the approach to provide maximum, but defensible information, from limited specimen or workup? What is a descriptive diagnosis appropriate in such situations?

- *Limited aspirate*
  - If there is insufficient aspirate for all ancillary studies, then the sample should be prioritized in following order:
  - Smears for morphology
  - Flow cytometry for phenotyping (if available onsite)∗
  - Conventional karyotyping∗∗
  - Molecular studies
  - FISH
  - Flow cytometry for phenotyping (if not available onsite)∗

    ∗If flow cytometry is available onsite, then it should be prioritized just below smears for morphology since it will be able to provide blast lineage in the most time efficient manner. If flow cytometry is not available onsite, then it should be prioritized last since adequate immunophenotyping for blast lineage can typically be performed by immunohistochemistry on the core biopsy.

**Conventional karyotyping is prioritized above molecular studies and FISH because peripheral blood blasts typically do not grow well in culture. In contrast, both molecular studies and interphase FISH can be performed on the peripheral blood if necessary as long as there are sufficient circulating blasts.

- *Inadequate aspirate*
  - If the aspirate is inadequate or not obtained, a complete workup should be attempted on a peripheral blood specimen if there are adequate circulating blasts. If there are too few circulating blasts, then touch preparation slides should be created for morphology and FISH testing, and a portion of the core may be sent for a limited flow cytometry panel focusing on blast identification and basic phenotyping (e.g., CD45, CD34, CD117, CD19, CD10, CD13, CD33, CD7). Additional phenotyping should be performed by immunohistochemistry as necessary to establish blast lineage (AML, B-ALL/LBL, T-ALL/LBL, MPAL, BPDCN). FISH studies may be performed on touch preparations to rule out critical translocations like *PML-RARA* fusions, but these can also be performed on peripheral blood if the blast count is sufficiently high.
- *Suboptimal/inadequate aspirate and inadequate core*
  - In some instances, both the aspirate and the core are suboptimal or inadequate, and a descriptive diagnosis must be given. For example, if ≥20% blasts are seen by morphology but cannot be immunophenotyped, then a diagnosis of "acute leukemia" can be reported with a recommendation for repeat biopsy. Another example would be if there appears to be ≥20% immature blast-like cells on the core biopsy, but they are negative for CD34 and CD117, and the aspirate smear is too hemodiluted or otherwise inadequate to verify true blast count or morphology. In this case, a descriptive diagnosis can be given with a comment raising the suspicion for acute leukemia and recommending repeat biopsy.

12. When is a diagnostic comment necessary, and what should be discussed in the diagnostic comment for this entity?

A diagnostic comment and morphologic description are almost always required in the diagnosis of acute leukemia for several reasons: Since it is impossible to diagnose an acute leukemia by morphology alone, ancillary techniques (e.g., flow cytometry, immunohistochemistry, special stains, etc.) are required, and the results must be integrated into the report. Morphologic findings are also critical, especially in the case of myelodysplasia-related leukemias or the presence unusual findings (e.g., Auer rods). Overall, the purpose of a diagnostic comment is to integrate all the parts of a biopsy (i.e., morphology, clinical history and findings, ancillary studies), to include relevant information that is not a diagnosis, and to communicate uncertainty [83, 84].

13. When it is appropriate to seek external consultation for this entity?

Like any field of medicine, external consultation should be obtained if the provider is unfamiliar or uncomfortable with the diagnosis. Since there are several ancillary techniques involved with the diagnosis of acute leukemia, outside performance of the test and interpretation may be required if the technique and expertise are not available in-house.

Case Presentations

Case 1 (Fig. 21.15)

Learning Objectives

1. To generate the differential diagnoses in cases of circulating abnormal/immature monocytic cells
2. To become familiar with the diagnostic criteria for relevant entities
3. Understand how to differentiate AML from chronic myeloid leukemia blast phase

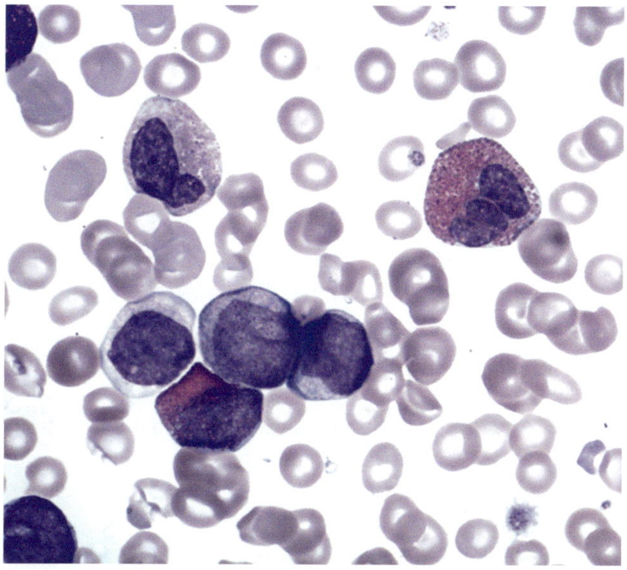

Fig. 21.15 Case 1: Acute myeloid leukemia, *BCR-ABL1*. There is marked increase in blasts, resembling monoblasts and promonocytes (original magnification 1000×)

Case History

A 69-year-old female presented to the emergency room with complaints of shortness of breath and body aches for 3 weeks. CBC: WBC 90.3 $\times 10^9$/L; Hgb 9.0 g/dl; Plt 95 $\times 10^9$/L. The patient has no previous history of leukocytosis.

Histologic Findings

- Peripheral blood smear: Marked leukocytosis with many monoblasts/promonocytes

Differential Diagnosis

- Acute monocytic leukemia
- Chronic myelomonocytic leukemia 2
- Chronic myeloid leukemia, accelerated phase
- Chronic myeloid leukemia, blast phase

Ancillary Studies

- Flow cytometry: Some atypical cells are positive for CD11b, CD11c (small subset), CD33, and CD45. They are negative for CD10, CD19, CD34, CD117, and other B or T or myeloid markers.
- Cytogenetics: 46, XX, t(9;22)(q34;q11.2)
- Next-generation sequencing: *NPM1* mutation

Final Diagnosis

Acute myeloid leukemia with *BCR-ABL1*

Take-Home Messages

1. Extremely rare <1% all acute myeloid leukemia
2. Compared to blast transformation of chronic myeloid leukemia, AML with *BCR-ABL1* shows:
   (a) Less frequent splenomegaly.
   (b) Less frequent dwarf megakaryocytes.
   (c) Relatively normal M:E ratio in non-blast cells.
   (d) *NPM1* and *FLT3*-ITD are seen in AML with *BCR-ABL1* but not in CML blast phase.
   References: [85–87]

Case 2 (Fig. 21.16)

Learning Objectives

1. To generate the differential diagnoses for circulating lymphoblasts
2. To become familiar with the diagnostic criteria for the relevant entities
3. Understand how to differentiate the relevant entity from T-acute lymphoblastic leukemia, NOS

Case History

A 25-year-old male presented with cough and chest pain. X-ray showed mediastinal mass. CBC: WBC 37 $\times 10^9$/L; Hgb 7.3 g/dl; Plt 251 $\times 10^9$/L.

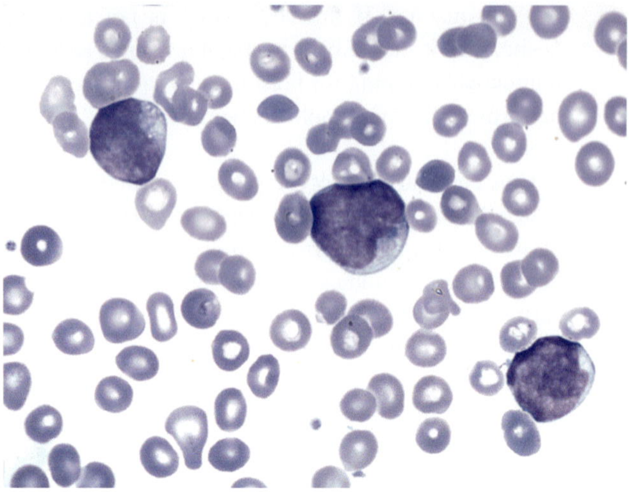

Fig. 21.16 Case 2: Early T-cell precursor lymphoblastic leukemia. The blasts are medium to large in size, with fine chromatin, slightly irregular nuclear contour, and moderate amount of agranular cytoplasm (original magnification 1000×)

Histologic Findings

- Peripheral blood smear: Marked increase in blasts. The blasts are medium to large in size, with fine chromatin, slightly irregular nuclear contour, and moderate amount of agranular cytoplasm.

Differential Diagnosis

- T-acute lymphoblastic leukemia
- B-acute lymphoblastic leukemia
- Acute myeloid leukemia

Ancillary Studies

- Flow cytometry: 62.2% blasts
- They are positive for cCD3, CD7, CD33 (dim, subset), CD34, CD45, and CD56
- They are negative for CD1a, CD2, CD3, CD4, CD5, CD8, CD9, CD10, MPO, TdT, and other B or myeloid markers

Final Diagnosis

Early T-cell precursor lymphoblastic leukemia

Take-Home Messages

1. Immunophenotype:
   (a) Positive for cytoplasmic CD3.
   (b) May express CD2, CD4, and/or CD7.
   (c) Usually negative for CD1a, CD5, and CD8. When CD5 is positive, it is dim and present on <75% of the blast population.
   (d) Positive for CD34 and one or more of the myeloid/markers CD117, CD13, CD33, HLA-DR, CD11b, and CD65.
   (e) Negative for myeloperoxidase (MPO).

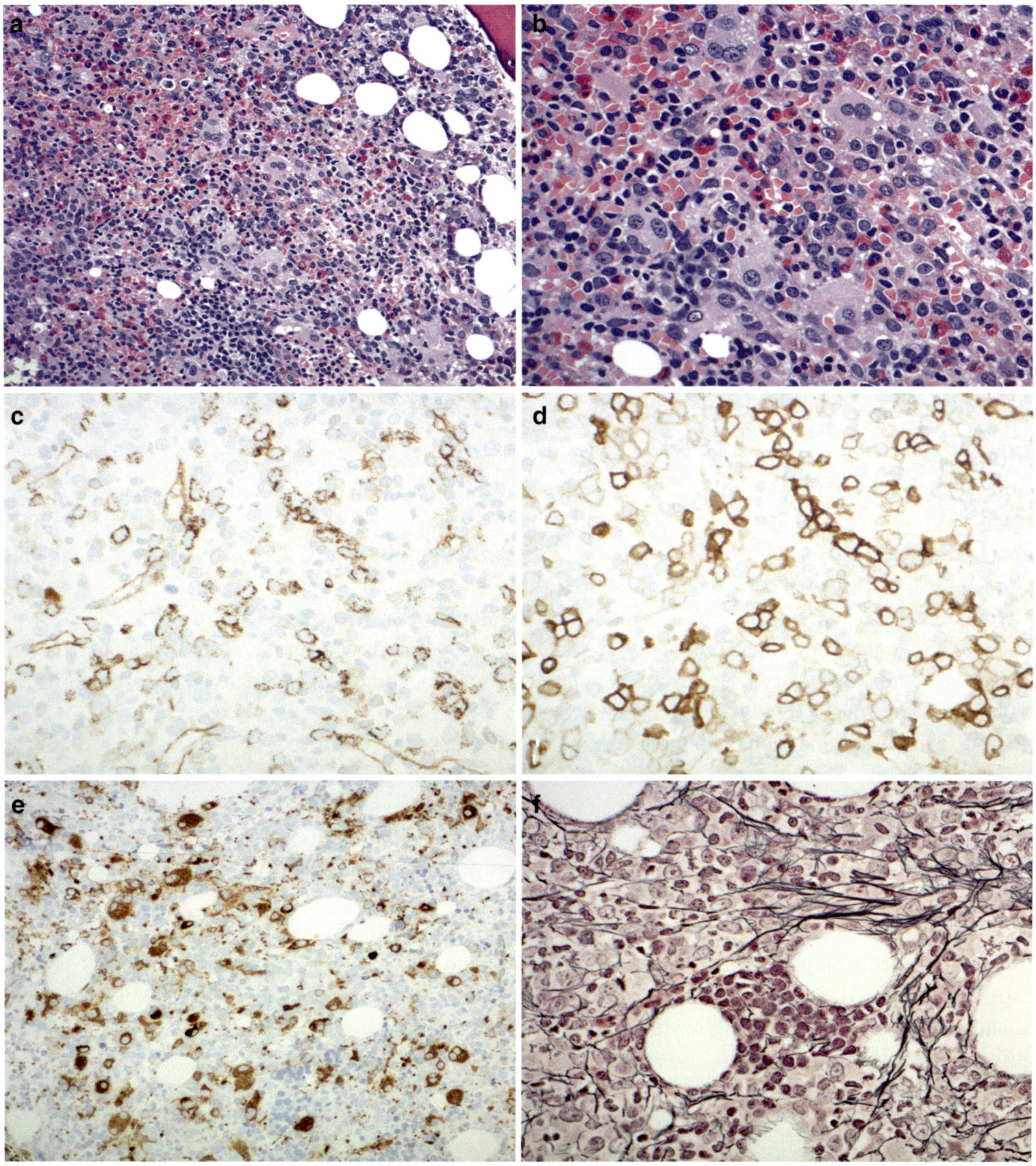

Fig. 21.17 Case 3: Therapy-related acute myeloid leukemia. Upper panel: Bone marrow core biopsy shows hypercellular marrow (>90%) with increased atypical megakaryocytes and mononuclear cells resembling blasts; (**a**) original magnification 200×; (**b**) original magnification 400×. Middle panel: increased blasts (20%) by CD34; (**c**) original magnification 400×; and CD117 immunohistochemistry stains (**d**) original magnification 400×. Lower panel: markedly increased megakaryocytes of various sizes by CD61; (**e**) original magnification 200×; and reticulin stain showing severe myelofibrosis; (**f**) original magnification 400×

2. Prognosis may be worse than T-ALL, NOS but this is controversial.
   References: [88–91]

Case 3 (Fig. 21.17)

Learning Objectives

1. To become familiar with the diagnostic criteria for certain subtypes of acute leukemia
2. To generate the differential diagnoses
3. Understand how to differentiate acute panmyelosis with myelofibrosis, therapy-related acute myeloid leukemia, and acute megakaryoblastic leukemia

Case History

A 64-year-old male with past medical history of stage IV prostate cancer with metastatic disease to the bone, status post chemotherapy, presented with pancytopenia. CBC: WBC 3.1 $\times 10^9$/L; Hgb 8.6 g/dl; Plt 123 $\times 10^9$/L.

Histologic Findings

- Bone marrow core biopsy: Hypercellular marrow (>90%) with myelofibrosis, markedly increased atypical megakaryocytes and increased mononuclear cells, resembling blasts. Some megakaryocytes are small and hypolobated. Some megakaryocytes have widely separated lobes.

Ancillary Studies

- Immunohistochemistry stains: The blasts are positive for CD34 and/or CD117, consisting of 20% of the total cellularity. CD61 highlights markedly increased megakaryocytes, many in small mononuclear forms. Diffuse 3+/3 reticulin fibrosis.

Final Diagnosis

Therapy-related acute myeloid leukemia

Take-Home Messages

1. Therapy-related acute myeloid leukemia is defined as acute myeloid leukemia after cytotoxic chemotherapy and/or radiation therapy. They frequently show morphologic dysplasia with megakaryocytes showing nonlobated or hypolobated nuclei or widely separated nuclear lobes. Reticulin fibrosis is common. While these features are often present, neither is required for the diagnosis.
2. Acute panmyelosis with myelofibrosis is defined as acute panmyeloid proliferation with ≥20% blasts and myelofibrosis. The cases do not fulfill the criteria of AML with recurrent genetic abnormalities, AML with myelodysplasia-related changes, or therapy-related AML. Bone marrow core biopsies usually show hypercellular marrow with marked trilineage proliferation, myelofibrosis, and increased blasts. Megakaryocytes frequently show different degrees of dysplasia.
3. Acute megakaryoblastic leukemia is characterized by a proliferation of predominantly megakaryoblasts without definite proliferation of myeloid or erythroid lineages. Various degrees of myelofibrosis might be present.
   References: [12, 57, 92]

Case 4 (Fig. 21.18)

Learning Objectives

1. To recognize morphologic features suggestive of acute leukemia with recurrent cytogenetic abnormality
2. To generate the differential diagnoses

Case History

A 30-year-old female presented to her primary care physician with fatigue for 2–3 weeks and recent gingival bleeding after brushing. CBC: WBC 83.4 $\times 10^9$/L; Hgb 9.2 g/dl; Plt 11 $\times 10^9$/L.

Histologic Findings

- Bone marrow aspirate: Increased numbers of blasts with monocytic features and atypical eosinophilic precursors.

Differential Diagnosis

- Acute myeloid leukemia with inv(16)
- Acute myelomonocytic leukemia
- Acute monoblastic leukemia
- Chronic myeloid leukemia, blast phase

Ancillary Studies

- Flow cytometry: There was a blast population that expressed CD34, CD117, CD13, CD33, myeloperoxidase, and dim CD64
- Cytogenetics: 46, XX, inv(16)(p13.1 q22)

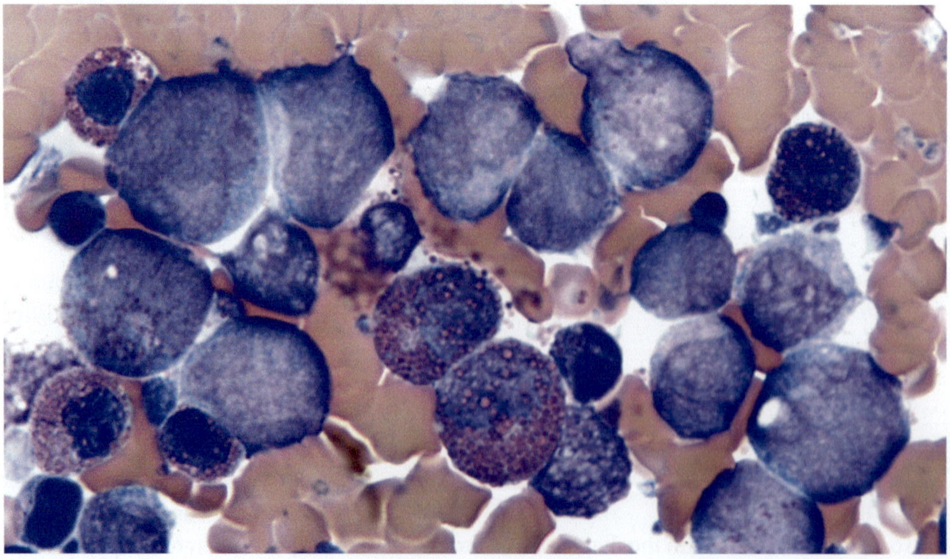

Fig. 21.18 Case 4: Acute myeloid leukemia with inv(16). The blasts are large with monocytic features (large size, agranular or sparsely granular cytoplasm, indented/bean-shaped nuclei with fine chromatin). There are atypical immature eosinophilic precursors with coarse granules (original magnification 1000×)

Final Diagnosis

Acute myeloid leukemia with inv(16)

Take-Home Messages

1. An acute leukemia with monocytic differentiation and atypical eosinophilic precursors.
2. The eosinophilic precursors have immature granules and can be purple-violet in color.
3. Eosinophils are usually not increased in acute myelomonocytic leukemia.
4. Even if blasts are <20%, cases with inv(16) should be classified as acute myeloid leukemia.
5. The atypical eosinophilic granules should raise suspicion for this entity, and FISH for inv(16) should be ordered; however, inv(16) can be seen on conventional karyotyping.
   References: [1]

Case 5 (Fig. 21.19)

Learning Objectives

1. To become familiar with diagnostic algorithm for circulating blasts with limited bone marrow specimen
2. To generate the differential diagnoses and guide further workup
3. Understand how to differentiate a CD20 positive B-lymphoblastic leukemia from an aggressive B-cell non-Hodgkin lymphoma

Case History

A 21-year-old female presented to an outside hospital with fatigue and rare circulating blasts. A bone marrow was performed, but was not diagnostic. She was transferred and second marrow was performed, but an aspirate could not be obtained. CBC: WBC 1.3 $\times 10^9$/L; Hgb 7.2 g/dl; Plt 26 $\times 10^9$/L.

Histologic Findings

- Bone marrow core biopsy: The marrow was almost completely replaced with small atypical lymphoid cells. There was extensive necrosis.

Differential Diagnosis

- B-acute lymphoblastic leukemia
- T-acute lymphoblastic leukemia
- Burkitt lymphoma
- Aggressive "double-hit" non-Hodgkin lymphoma

Ancillary Studies

- By immunohistochemistry, the blasts expressed CD19, CD10, CD79a, BCL2, TdT, and CD20. They were negative for CD3, CD34, CD45, CD30, and myeloperoxidase.
- FISH studies for 11q23 revealed a rearrangement.

Final Diagnosis

B-lymphoblastic leukemia with 11q23.3 rearrangement

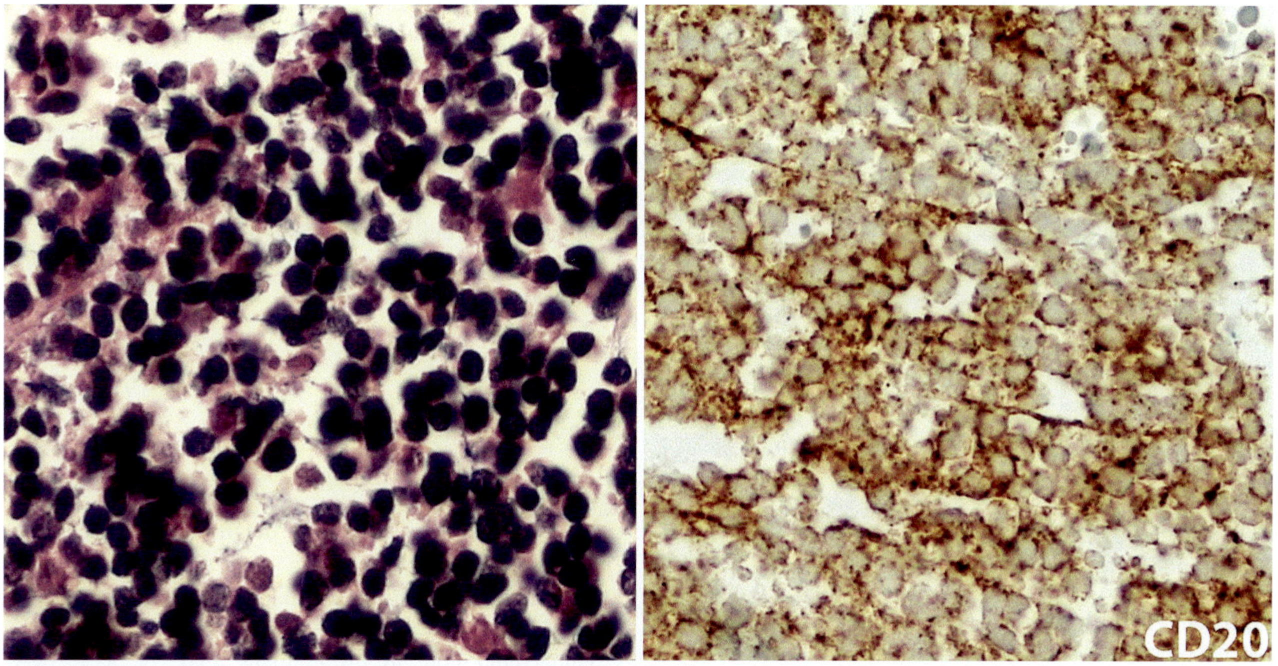

Fig. 21.19 Case 5: B-lymphoblastic leukemia with CD20 expression. The left panel shows a hypercellular marrow that has been replaced by lymphoblasts. The right panel shows the CD20 expression in the lymphoblast population (original magnification 400×)

Take-Home Messages

1. CD20 expression ranges from 40% to 50% in B-lymphoblastic leukemia.
2. CD20 expression in adult B-lymphoblastic leukemia appears to be associated with a poor prognosis.
3. Distinguishing between B-lymphoblastic leukemia and a mature lymphoma can be done by looking for markers of immaturity such as CD34 and TdT.

References: [93]

Case 6 (Fig. 21.20)

Learning Objectives

1. To generate the differential diagnoses for marked erythroid predominance and left shift
2. To become familiar with the diagnostic criteria of the relevant diagnosis
3. Understand how to differentiate erythroid predominant MDS from pure erythroid leukemia and AML-MRC

Case History

A 51-year-old male presented with 2 weeks of progressive fatigue, weakness, decreased appetite, hip pain, and subjective fevers. CBC: WBC 14.8 $\times 10^9$/L; Hgb 5.1 g/dl; Plt 4 $\times 10^9$/L.

Histologic Findings

- Bone marrow aspirate smear: 71% blasts with large nuclei, dispersed chromatin, very prominent nucleoli, deeply basophilic cytoplasm, and occasional cytoplasmic vacuoles. Marked dyspoiesis in maturing erythroid precursors. Numerous ring sideroblasts (approximately 30%).

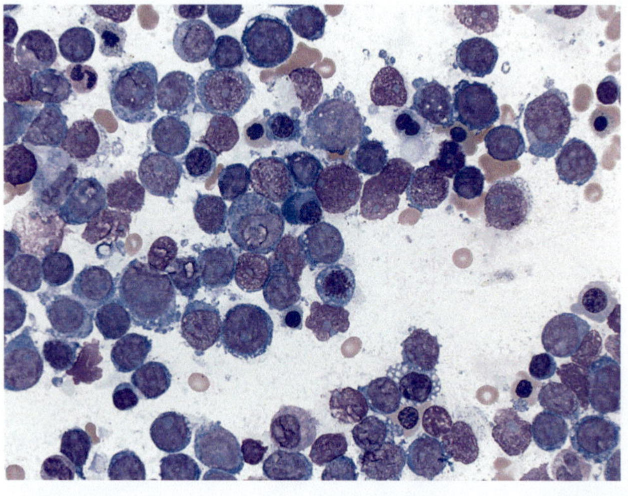

Fig. 21.20 Case 6: Pure erythroid leukemia. Blasts have a pronormoblast morphology with fine chromatin, large prominent nucleoli, deeply basophilic cytoplasm, and cytoplasmic vacuoles. Maturing erythroid precursors are dysplastic with nuclear to cytoplasmic dyssynchrony and nuclear blebs (original magnification 500×)

Differential Diagnosis

- Pure erythroid leukemia
- Erythroid predominant myelodysplastic syndrome
- Acute myeloid leukemia with myelodysplasia-related changes

Ancillary Studies

- Immunohistochemistry and special stains: The blasts were positive for PAS (granular, partial) and E-cadherin (partial). They were negative for CD68 and lysozyme.
- Flow cytometry: The blasts were positive for CD71 (strong), CD117 (dim), CD13 (dim), CD33, and CD7 (partial). They were negative for CD11c, CD14, CD19, CD34, CD61, and CD63, and MPO was not significant.
- Chromosome analysis: 40,XY,del(5)(q12q35),-14,-15,-16,der(17)t(14;17)(q11.2;p12),-18,-19,-20,-21,-22,+2mar[3]/49~53,X,-Y,+1,+2,-3,del(5)(q12q35),der(6)t(6;14)(q21;q11.2),+8,add(9)(p24),+del(11)(q21q23),-13,-14,der(16)t(?8;16)(q22;q22),+18,+add(18)(q23),add(19)(q13.3),idic(21)(p11.2),+add(21)(p11.2),-22,+1~6mar[cp15]/46,XY[2].
- Next-generation sequencing: *TP53* mutation.

Final Diagnosis

Pure erythroid leukemia

Take-Home Messages

1. Pure erythroid leukemia (PEL) is a morphologic diagnosis that requires ≥80% erythroid precursors and ≥ 30% pronormoblasts.
2. PEL may arise de novo or may progress from a preceding myelodysplastic syndrome.
3. PEL nearly always has complex cytogenetics, typically including −5/del(5q) or −7/del(7q).
4. PEL frequently has *TP53* mutations.
5. PEL has a dismal prognosis.

References: [1, 10, 12, 13, 25]

Case 7 (Fig. 21.21)

Learning Objectives

1. To generate the differential diagnoses for circulating blasts and eosinophils
2. To become familiar with the diagnostic criteria for the relevant entities
3. Understand how to differentiate AML or ALL from myeloid/lymphoid neoplasms with eosinophilia and recurrent genetic abnormality

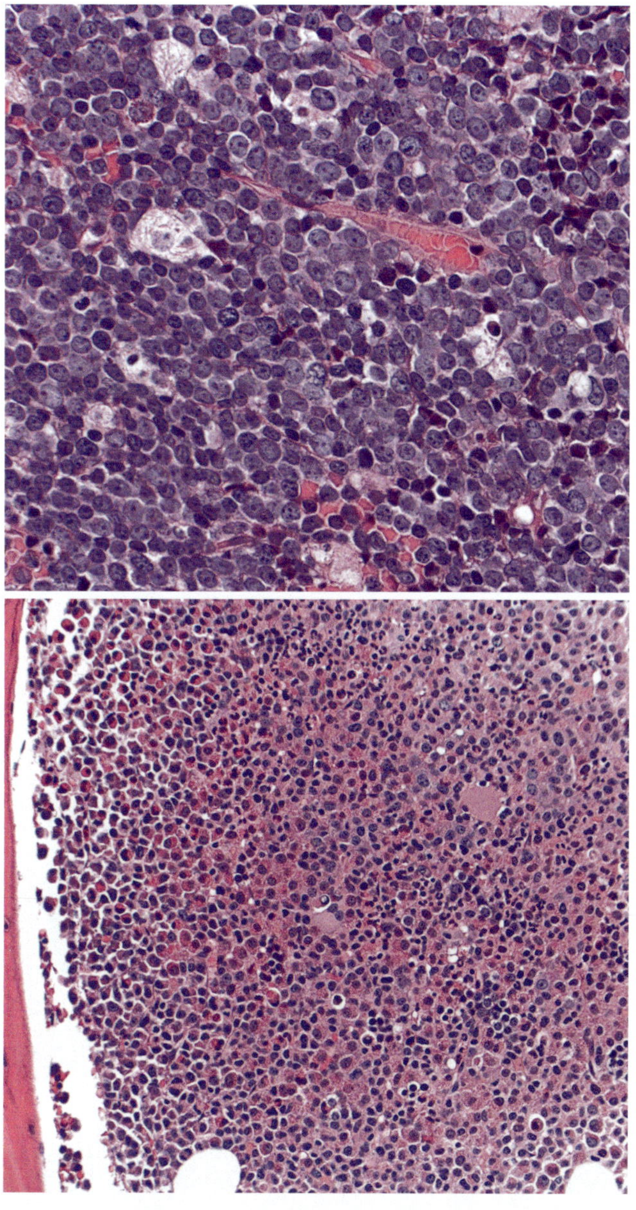

Fig. 21.21 Case 7: Myeloid/lymphoid neoplasm with eosinophilia and *PDGFRA* rearrangement. Upper panel: C3 biopsy shows sheets of blasts with open chromatin, small nucleoli, and scant cytoplasm (original magnification 400×). Lower panel: bone marrow biopsy shows markedly hypercellular marrow with eosinophilia but no increase in blasts (original magnification 200×)

Case History

A 56-year-old male presented to an outside hospital with acutely worsening neck/back pain in a history of chronic pain issues. MRI revealed an area concerning for abscess vs mass in the area of C3 with extension into the epidural space. One week after the C3 biopsy, the patient transferred to our institution for bone marrow biopsy. CBC: WBC 24.2 $\times 10^9$/L; Hgb 12.6 g/dl; Plt 310 $\times 10^9$/L.

Histologic Findings

- C3 biopsy: Sheets of small- to medium-sized blasts with open chromatin, small nucleoli, and scant cytoplasm (Fig. 21.21 top).
- Peripheral blood smear: Leukoerythroblastosis and eosinophilia.
- Bone marrow aspirate smear: Myeloid predominance with eosinophilia and left-shift.
- Bone marrow core biopsy: Markedly hypercellular marrow with myeloid predominance, eosinophilia, and mild fibrosis. Blasts were not increased (2%) (Fig. 21.21 bottom).

Differential Diagnosis

- Blast phase chronic myeloid leukemia
- B-lymphoblastic lymphoma and reactive/leukemoid reaction
- Myeloid/lymphoid neoplasm with eosinophilia and gene rearrangement

Ancillary Studies

- Immunohistochemical studies on the C3 biopsy: Blasts were positive for TdT (strong), CD20 (partial), CD79a (partial), BCL2, and CD45 (slightly dim). They were negative for CD3, CD10, BCL6, and cytokeratins.
- Bone marrow flow cytometry: Eosinophilia without phenotypic abnormalities. Negative for B-lymphoblasts (limit of detection 0.01%), and no phenotypically abnormal populations or increase in blasts.
- Chromosome analysis: 46,XY[20].
- FISH studies: Positive for *PDGFRA* rearrangement. Negative for *BCR-ABL1* fusion and negative for rearrangements in *ABL1*, *ABL2*, *PDGFRB*, *JAK2*, and *FGFR1*.

Final Diagnosis

Myeloid/lymphoid neoplasm with eosinophilia and *PDGFRA* rearrangement

Take-Home Messages

1. Myeloid/lymphoid neoplasms with eosinophilia and *PDGFRA*, *PDGFRB*, *FGFR1* rearrangement or *PCM1-JAK2* fusion can present in a variety of ways including as a chronic myeloproliferative neoplasm, chronic myelodysplastic/myeloproliferative neoplasm, acute myeloid leukemia, T-lymphoblastic leukemia/lymphoma, or B-lymphoblastic leukemia/lymphoma. They typically show some degree of eosinophilia.
2. An underlying chronic myeloid neoplasm should be considered in all cases of lymphoblastic leukemia with

accompanying eosinophilia or myeloproliferative picture in the bone marrow. In some cases, the eosinophilia or myeloproliferative picture may not become apparent until after chemotherapy.

3. An appropriate FISH panel would include probes for *BCR-ABL1* fusion, *PCM1-JAK2* fusion, and rearrangements in *PDGFRA*, *PDGFRB*, and *FGFR1*.
4. Cases with rearrangements in *PDGFRA* or *PDGFRB* are sensitive to tyrosine kinase inhibitors like imatinib, so identification is important for prompt initiation of appropriate therapy.

References: [1, 94, 95]

Case 8 (Fig. 21.22)

Learning Objectives

1. To generate the differential diagnoses for patients presenting with circulating blasts and skin lesions
2. To become familiar with the diagnostic criteria of the relevant entity
3. Understand how to differentiate AML with mutated *NPM1* from AML-MRC
4. Understand how to differentiate BPDCN from AML with monocytic features

Case History

A 75-year-old male presented with 6 weeks of rashes on his back and abdomen. The rashes were small, raised, red, non-painful, non-pruritic lesions. He noticed some fatigue but no other symptoms. Outside biopsy of the rash was diagnosed as blastic plasmacytoid dendritic cell neoplasm. He then presented to our institution for further workup. CBC: WBC 24.0 $\times 10^9$/L; Hgb 7.5 g/dl; Plt 30 $\times 10^9$/L.

Histologic Findings

- Bone marrow aspirate smear: 40% blasts with monocytoid features and erythroid and megakaryocyte dysplasia in >50% of cells in each lineage. Numerous ring sideroblasts (approximately 40%) (Fig. 21.22a, b)
- Bone marrow clot section: markedly hypercellular marrow with increased blasts and dysplastic megakaryocytes (Fig. 21.22c)

Differential Diagnosis

- Blastic plasmacytoid dendritic cell neoplasm
- Acute myeloid leukemia with myelodysplasia-related changes
- Acute monocytic/monoblastic leukemia
- Acute myelomonocytic leukemia
- Acute myeloid leukemia with mutated *NPM1*

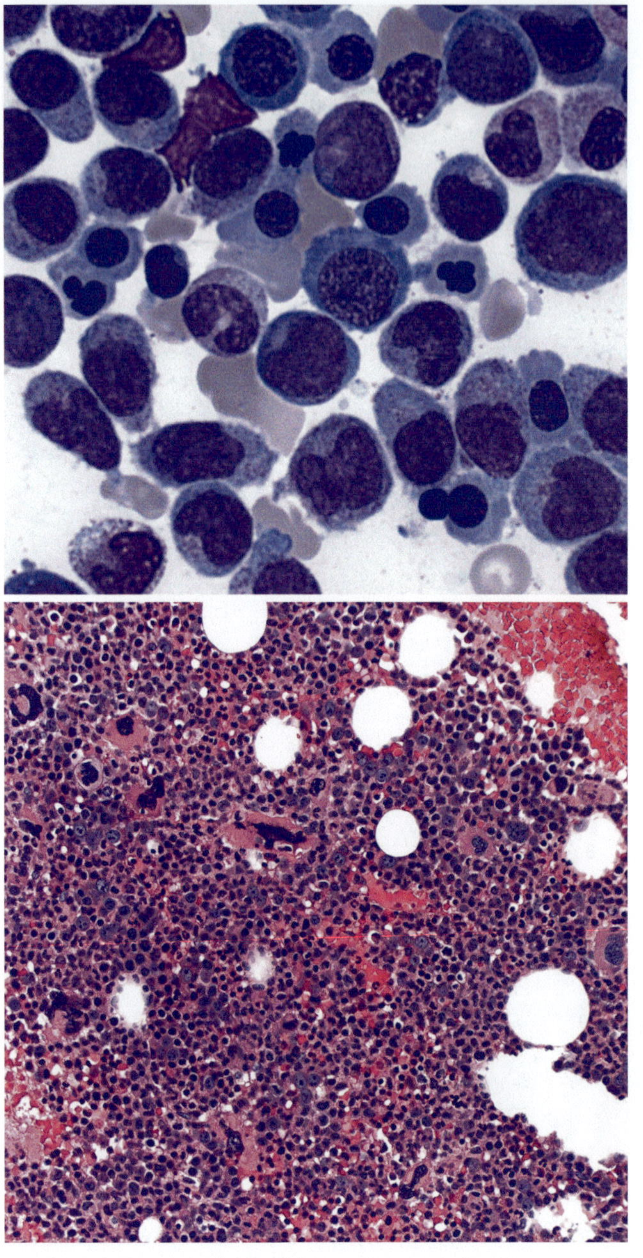

Fig. 21.22 Case 8: AML with NPM1. Upper panel: Blasts have monocytoid features with open chromatin, prominent nucleoli, nuclear indentations, and delicate nuclear folds. Erythroid precursors are dysplastic (original magnification 500×). Lower panel: bone marrow clot section shows increased blasts and increased dysplastic megakaryocytes (original magnification 200×)

Ancillary Studies

- Immunohistochemistry: Blasts were positive for CD4 (weak), CD56, CD68 (weak), MPO (partial), and lysozyme (strong). They were negative for CD123, CD34, CD117, TdT, and CD3. CD61 highlighted the dysplastic megakaryocytes.

- Flow cytometry: Blasts expressed CD11c (bright), CD14 (partial), CD33 (bright), CD56, CD64, and HLA-DR. CD123 was very dim in a minor subset of the blasts. They did not express CD4, CD34, or CD117.
- Chromosome analysis: 46,XY[20].
- FISH: Negative for abnormalities in chromosomes 5, 7, 8, *MLL*, *CBFB*, *PML/RARA*, and *RUNX1/RUNX1T1*.
- Next-generation sequencing: Mutations in *NPM1*, *NF1*, and *SF3B1*.

Final Diagnosis

AML with mutated *NPM1*

Take-Home Messages

1. Acute myeloid leukemia with mutated *NPM1* must be cytogenetically normal and have mutated *NPM1*.
2. These cases often show morphologic dysplasia and/or monocytic differentiation in the blasts.
3. AML with mutated *NPM1* has a favorable prognosis, especially if *FLT3* is not mutated. These may be treated with a less aggressive therapeutic regimen.
4. Blasts with monocytic features can be easily misdiagnosed as blastic plasmacytoid dendritic cell neoplasm (BPDCN) because monocytoid blasts can express CD123, CD4, and CD56.
5. BPDCN must be negative for lysozyme, MPO, CD34, CD3, CD19, and CD20 in order for the diagnosis to be made.
   References: [1, 54, 96–99]

References

1. Swerdlow SH, Campo E, Harris NL, Jaffe ES, Pileri SA, Stein H, et al. WHO classification of tumours of haematopoietic and lymphoid tissues. Revised 4th ed. Lyon: The International Agency for Research on Cancer (IARC); 2017.
2. Palmer L, Briggs C, McFadden S, Zini G, Burthem J, Rozenberg G, et al. ICSH recommendations for the standardization of nomenclature and grading of peripheral blood cell morphological features. Int J Lab Hematol. 2015;37(3):287–303.
3. Sylvia MT, Jacob SE, Basu D. Multiple myeloma with crystalline and Auer rod-like inclusions. Br J Haematol. 2017;179(1):8.
4. Oberley MJ, Yang DT. Lymphoproliferative disorder with Auer rod-like inclusions. Blood. 2014;124(16):2607.
5. Pulsoni A, Stazi A, Cotichini R, Allione B, Cerri R, Di Bona E, et al. Acute promyelocytic leukaemia: epidemiology and risk factors. A report of the GIMEMA Italian archive of adult acute leukaemia. GIMEMA Cooperative Group. Eur J Haematol. 1998;61(5):327–32.
6. Dores GM, Devesa SS, Curtis RE, Linet MS, Morton LM. Acute leukemia incidence and patient survival among children and adults in the United States, 2001-2007. Blood. 2012;119(1):34–43.
7. Golomb HM, Rowley JD, Vardiman JW, Testa JR, Butler A. "Microgranular" acute promyelocytic leukemia: a distinct clinical, ultrastructural, and cytogenetic entity. Blood. 1980;55(2):253–9.
8. McKenna RW, Parkin J, Bloomfield CD, Sundberg RD, Brunning RD. Acute promyelocytic leukaemia: a study of 39 cases with identification of a hyperbasophilic microgranular variant. Br J Haematol. 1982;50(2):201–14.
9. Mrozek K, Prior TW, Edwards C, Marcucci G, Carroll AJ, Snyder PJ, et al. Comparison of cytogenetic and molecular genetic detection of t(8;21) and inv(16) in a prospective series of adults with de novo acute myeloid leukemia: a Cancer and Leukemia Group B Study. J Clin Oncol. 2001;19(9):2482–92.
10. Liu W, Hasserjian RP, Hu Y, Zhang L, Miranda RN, Medeiros LJ, et al. Pure erythroid leukemia: a reassessment of the entity using the 2008 World Health Organization classification. Mod Pathol. 2011;24(3):375–83.
11. Kowal-Vern A, Cotelingam J, Schumacher HR. The prognostic significance of proerythroblasts in acute erythroleukemia. Am J Clin Pathol. 1992;98(1):34–40.
12. Wang SA, Hasserjian RP. Acute erythroleukemias, acute megakaryoblastic leukemias, and reactive mimics: a guide to a number of perplexing entities. Am J Clin Pathol. 2015;144(1):44–60.
13. Reinig EF, Greipp PT, Chiu A, Howard MT, Reichard KK. De novo pure erythroid leukemia: refining the clinicopathologic and cytogenetic characteristics of a rare entity. Mod Pathol. 2018;31(5):705–17.
14. Arber DA, Stein AS, Carter NH, Ikle D, Forman SJ, Slovak ML. Prognostic impact of acute myeloid leukemia classification. Importance of detection of recurring cytogenetic abnormalities and multilineage dysplasia on survival. Am J Clin Pathol. 2003;119(5):672–80.
15. Khalidi HS, Chang KL, Medeiros LJ, Brynes RK, Slovak ML, Murata-Collins JL, et al. Acute lymphoblastic leukemia. Survey of immunophenotype, French-American-British classification, frequency of myeloid antigen expression, and karyotypic abnormalities in 210 pediatric and adult cases. Am J Clin Pathol. 1999;111(4):467–76.
16. Khan M, Siddiqi R, Naqvi K. An update on classification, genetics, and clinical approach to mixed phenotype acute leukemia (MPAL). Ann Hematol. 2018;97(6):945–53.
17. Tavassoli M, Shaklai M, Crosby WH. Cytochemical diagnosis of acute myelomonocytic leukemia. Am J Clin Pathol. 1979;72(1):59–62.
18. Matsuo T, Jain NC, Bennett JM. Nonspecific esterase of acute promyelocytic leukemia (M3). Am J Hematol. 1988;29(3):148–51.
19. Dash A, Gilliland DG. Molecular genetics of acute myeloid leukaemia. Best Pract Res Clin Haematol. 2001;14(1):49–64.
20. Ravandi F, Stone R. Acute promyelocytic leukemia: a perspective. Clin Lymphoma Myeloma Leuk. 2017;17(9):543–4.
21. Sanz MA, Fenaux P, Tallman MS, Estey EH, Lowenberg B, Naoe T, et al. Management of acute promyelocytic leukemia: updated recommendations from an expert panel of the European LeukemiaNet. Blood. 2019;133(15):1630–43.
22. Harris AC, Todd WM, Hackney MH, Ben-Ezra J. Bone marrow changes associated with recombinant granulocyte-macrophage and granulocyte colony-stimulating factors. Discrimination of granulocytic regeneration. Arch Pathol Lab Med. 1994;118(6):624–9.
23. Meyerson HJ, Farhi DC, Rosenthal NS. Transient increase in blasts mimicking acute leukemia and progressing myelodysplasia in patients receiving growth factor. Am J Clin Pathol. 1998;109(6):675–81.
24. Patnaik MM, Tefferi A. Chronic myelomonocytic leukemia: 2018 update on diagnosis, risk stratification and management. Am J Hematol. 2018;93(6):824–40.
25. Wang W, Wang SA, Medeiros LJ, Khoury JD. Pure erythroid leukemia. Am J Hematol. 2017;92(3):292–6.
26. Greenberg PL, Stone RM, Al-Kali A, Barta SK, Bejar R, Bennett JM, et al. Myelodysplastic syndromes, version 2.2017, NCCN clinical practice guidelines in oncology. J Natl Compr Cancer Netw. 2017;15(1):60–87.
27. Zipursky A, Brown EJ, Christensen H, Doyle J. Transient myeloproliferative disorder (transient leukemia) and hematologic manifestations of Down syndrome. Clin Lab Med. 1999;19(1):157–67, vii.

28. Litz CE, Davies S, Brunning RD, Kueck B, Parkin JL, Gajl Peczalska K, et al. Acute leukemia and the transient myeloproliferative disorder associated with Down syndrome: morphologic, immunophenotypic and cytogenetic manifestations. Leukemia. 1995;9(9):1432–9.
29. Brink DS. Transient leukemia (transient myeloproliferative disorder, transient abnormal myelopoiesis) of Down syndrome. Adv Anat Pathol. 2006;13(5):256–62.
30. Yoshida K, Toki T, Okuno Y, Kanezaki R, Shiraishi Y, Sato-Otsubo A, et al. The landscape of somatic mutations in Down syndrome-related myeloid disorders. Nat Genet. 2013;45(11):1293–9.
31. Rozen L, Huybrechts S, Dedeken L, Heijmans C, Dessars B, Heimann P, et al. Transient leukemia in a newborn without Down syndrome: case report and review of the literature. Eur J Pediatr. 2014;173(12):1643–7.
32. Foucar K. Mature T-cell leukemias including T-prolymphocytic leukemia, adult T-cell leukemia/lymphoma, and Sezary syndrome. Am J Clin Pathol. 2007;127(4):496–510.
33. Chen Z, Hu S. MYC/BCL2 double-hit lymphoma/leukemia mimicking acute leukemia at initial presentation. Blood. 2016;127(8):1072.
34. Molina TJ, Delmer A, Cymbalista F, Le Tourneau A, Perrot JY, Ramond S, et al. Mantle cell lymphoma, in leukaemic phase with prominent splenomegaly. A report of eight cases with similar clinical presentation and aggressive outcome. Virchows Arch. 2000;437(6):591–8.
35. Matutes E, Parry-Jones N, Brito-Babapulle V, Wotherspoon A, Morilla R, Atkinson S, et al. The leukemic presentation of mantle-cell lymphoma: disease features and prognostic factors in 58 patients. Leuk Lymphoma. 2004;45(10):2007–15.
36. Ott G. Aggressive B-cell lymphomas in the update of the 4th edition of the World Health Organization classification of haematopoietic and lymphatic tissues: refinements of the classification, new entities and genetic findings. Br J Haematol. 2017;178(6):871–87.
37. Moench L, Sachs Z, Aasen G, Dolan M, Dayton V, Courville EL. Double- and triple-hit lymphomas can present with features suggestive of immaturity, including TdT expression, and create diagnostic challenges. Leuk Lymphoma. 2016;57(11):2626–35.
38. Rashidi A, Fisher SI. Double-hit lymphoma mimicking acute lymphoblastic leukemia at presentation. Eur J Haematol. 2015;94(4):374–6.
39. Sedek L, Bulsa J, Sonsala A, Twardoch M, Wieczorek M, Malinowska I, et al. The immunophenotypes of blast cells in B-cell precursor acute lymphoblastic leukemia: how different are they from their normal counterparts? Cytometry B Clin Cytom. 2014;86(5):329–39.
40. Rimsza LM, Larson RS, Winter SS, Foucar K, Chong YY, Garner KW, et al. Benign hematogone-rich lymphoid proliferations can be distinguished from B-lineage acute lymphoblastic leukemia by integration of morphology, immunophenotype, adhesion molecule expression, and architectural features. Am J Clin Pathol. 2000;114(1):66–75.
41. Arber DA, Borowitz MJ, Cessna M, Etzell J, Foucar K, Hasserjian RP, et al. Initial diagnostic workup of acute leukemia: guideline from the College of American Pathologists and the American Society of Hematology. Arch Pathol Lab Med. 2017;141(10):1342–93.
42. Dohner H, Estey E, Grimwade D, Amadori S, Appelbaum FR, Buchner T, et al. Diagnosis and management of AML in adults: 2017 ELN recommendations from an international expert panel. Blood. 2017;129(4):424–47.
43. Hoelzer D, Bassan R, Dombret H, Fielding A, Ribera JM, Buske C, et al. Acute lymphoblastic leukaemia in adult patients: ESMO Clinical Practice Guidelines for diagnosis, treatment and follow-up. Ann Oncol. 2016;27(suppl 5):v69–82.
44. Cheng J, Klairmont MM, Choi JK. Peripheral blood flow cytometry for the diagnosis of pediatric acute leukemia: highly reliable with rare exceptions. Pediatr Blood Cancer. 2019;66(1):e27453.
45. Wongprajun S, Auewarakul CU. A method comparison study of flow cytometry and cytomorphology to determine the percentages of blasts in patients with acute leukemia after induction and consolidation chemotherapy. J Med Assoc Thail. 2010;93(Suppl 1):S157–64.
46. Ok CY, Medeiros LJ, Thakral B, Tang G, Jain N, Jabbour E, et al. High-grade B-cell lymphomas with TdT expression: a diagnostic and classification dilemma. Mod Pathol. 2019;32(1):48–58.
47. Vasef MA, Brynes RK, Murata-Collins JL, Arber DA, Medeiros LJ. Surface immunoglobulin light chain-positive acute lymphoblastic leukemia of FAB L1 or L2 type: a report of 6 cases in adults. Am J Clin Pathol. 1998;110(2):143–9.
48. Tsao L, Draoua HY, Osunkwo I, Nandula SV, Murty VV, Mansukhani M, et al. Mature B-cell acute lymphoblastic leukemia with t(9;11) translocation: a distinct subset of B-cell acute lymphoblastic leukemia. Mod Pathol. 2004;17(7):832–9.
49. Rabade N, Bibi A, Ghodke K, Patkar N, Tembhare P, Amare P, et al. Lymphoblastic leukemia with surface light chain restriction: a diagnostic dilemma. Indian J Pathol Microbiol. 2016;59(3):410–2.
50. Kim B, Lee ST, Kim HJ, Lee SH, Yoo KH, Koo HH, et al. Acute lymphoblastic leukemia with mature B-cell phenotype and t(9;11;11)(p22;q23;p11.2): a case study and literature review. Ann Lab Med. 2014;34(2):166–9.
51. Kansal R, Deeb G, Barcos M, Wetzler M, Brecher ML, Block AW, et al. Precursor B lymphoblastic leukemia with surface light chain immunoglobulin restriction: a report of 15 patients. Am J Clin Pathol. 2004;121(4):512–25.
52. Hirzel AC, Cotrell A, Gasparini R, Sriganeshan V. Precursor B-cell acute lymphoblastic leukemia/lymphoma with L3 morphology, Philadelphia chromosome, MYC gene translocation, and coexpression of TdT and surface light chains: a case report. Case Rep Pathol. 2013;2013:679892.
53. Charles NJ, Boyer DF. Mixed-phenotype acute leukemia: diagnostic criteria and pitfalls. Arch Pathol Lab Med. 2017;141(11):1462–8.
54. Perl AE. The role of targeted therapy in the management of patients with AML. Blood Adv. 2017;1(24):2281–94.
55. Portell CA, Advani AS. Novel targeted therapies in acute lymphoblastic leukemia. Leuk Lymphoma. 2014;55(4):737–48.
56. Zhang X, Rastogi P, Shah B, Zhang L. B lymphoblastic leukemia/lymphoma: new insights into genetics, molecular aberrations, subclassification and targeted therapy. Oncotarget. 2017;8(39):66728–41.
57. Orazi A, O'Malley DP, Jiang J, Vance GH, Thomas J, Czader M, et al. Acute panmyelosis with myelofibrosis: an entity distinct from acute megakaryoblastic leukemia. Mod Pathol. 2005;18(5):603–14.
58. Suvajdzic N, Marisavljevic D, Kraguljac N, Pantic M, Djordjevic V, Jankovic G, et al. Acute panmyelosis with myelofibrosis: clinical, immunophenotypic and cytogenetic study of twelve cases. Leuk Lymphoma. 2004;45(9):1873–9.
59. Patel KP, Khokhar FA, Muzzafar T, James You M, Bueso-Ramos CE, Ravandi F, et al. TdT expression in acute myeloid leukemia with minimal differentiation is associated with distinctive clinicopathological features and better overall survival following stem cell transplantation. Mod Pathol. 2013;26(2):195–203.
60. Clappier E, Auclerc MF, Rapion J, Bakkus M, Caye A, Khemiri A, et al. An intragenic ERG deletion is a marker of an oncogenic subtype of B-cell precursor acute lymphoblastic leukemia with a favorable outcome despite frequent IKZF1 deletions. Leukemia. 2014;28(1):70–7.
61. Boer JM, van der Veer A, Rizopoulos D, Fiocco M, Sonneveld E, de Groot-Kruseman HA, et al. Prognostic value of rare IKZF1 deletion in childhood B-cell precursor acute lymphoblastic leukemia: an international collaborative study. Leukemia. 2016;30(1):32–8.
62. Clappier E, Grardel N, Bakkus M, Rapion J, De Moerloose B, Kastner P, et al. IKZF1 deletion is an independent prognostic marker in childhood B-cell precursor acute lymphoblastic leukemia, and distinguishes patients benefiting from pulses during maintenance therapy: results of the EORTC Children's Leukemia Group study 58951. Leukemia. 2015;29(11):2154–61.
63. Martinelli G, Iacobucci I, Storlazzi CT, Vignetti M, Paoloni F, Cilloni D, et al. IKZF1 (Ikaros) deletions in BCR-ABL1-positive

acute lymphoblastic leukemia are associated with short disease-free survival and high rate of cumulative incidence of relapse: a GIMEMA AL WP report. J Clin Oncol. 2009;27(31):5202–7.
64. Yao QM, Liu KY, Gale RP, Jiang B, Liu YR, Jiang Q, et al. Prognostic impact of IKZF1 deletion in adults with common B-cell acute lymphoblastic leukemia. BMC Cancer. 2016;16:269.
65. Hof J, Krentz S, van Schewick C, Korner G, Shalapour S, Rhein P, et al. Mutations and deletions of the TP53 gene predict nonresponse to treatment and poor outcome in first relapse of childhood acute lymphoblastic leukemia. J Clin Oncol. 2011;29(23):3185–93.
66. Salmoiraghi S, Montalvo ML, Ubiali G, Tosi M, Peruta B, Zanghi P, et al. Mutations of TP53 gene in adult acute lymphoblastic leukemia at diagnosis do not affect the achievement of hematologic response but correlate with early relapse and very poor survival. Haematologica. 2016;101(6):e245–8.
67. Inthal A, Zeitlhofer P, Zeginigg M, Morak M, Grausenburger R, Fronkova E, et al. CREBBP HAT domain mutations prevail in relapse cases of high hyperdiploid childhood acute lymphoblastic leukemia. Leukemia. 2012;26(8):1797–803.
68. Mullighan CG, Zhang J, Kasper LH, Lerach S, Payne-Turner D, Phillips LA, et al. CREBBP mutations in relapsed acute lymphoblastic leukaemia. Nature. 2011;471(7337):235–9.
69. Armstrong SA, Mabon ME, Silverman LB, Li A, Gribben JG, Fox EA, et al. FLT3 mutations in childhood acute lymphoblastic leukemia. Blood. 2004;103(9):3544–6.
70. Chillon MC, Gomez-Casares MT, Lopez-Jorge CE, Rodriguez-Medina C, Molines A, Sarasquete ME, et al. Prognostic significance of FLT3 mutational status and expression levels in MLL-AF4+ and MLL-germline acute lymphoblastic leukemia. Leukemia. 2012;26(11):2360–6.
71. Girardi T, Vicente C, Cools J, De Keersmaecker K. The genetics and molecular biology of T-ALL. Blood. 2017;129(9):1113–23.
72. Weng AP, Ferrando AA, Lee W, Morris JPt, Silverman LB, Sanchez-Irizarry C, et al. Activating mutations of NOTCH1 in human T cell acute lymphoblastic leukemia. Science. 2004;306(5694):269–71.
73. Ayatollahi H, Shajiei A, Sadeghian MH, Sheikhi M, Yazdandoust E, Ghazanfarpour M, et al. Prognostic importance of C-KIT mutations in core binding factor acute myeloid leukemia: a systematic review. Hematol Oncol Stem Cell Ther. 2017;10(1):1–7.
74. Yui S, Kurosawa S, Yamaguchi H, Kanamori H, Ueki T, Uoshima N, et al. D816 mutation of the KIT gene in core binding factor acute myeloid leukemia is associated with poorer prognosis than other KIT gene mutations. Ann Hematol. 2017;96(10):1641–52.
75. Lindsley RC, Mar BG, Mazzola E, Grauman PV, Shareef S, Allen SL, et al. Acute myeloid leukemia ontogeny is defined by distinct somatic mutations. Blood. 2015;125(9):1367–76.
76. Sperling AS, Gibson CJ, Ebert BL. The genetics of myelodysplastic syndrome: from clonal haematopoiesis to secondary leukaemia. Nat Rev Cancer. 2017;17(1):5–19.
77. Lo-Coco F, Di Donato L, Gimema, Schlenk RF, German-Austrian Acute Myeloid Leukemia Study G, Study Alliance L. Targeted therapy alone for acute promyelocytic leukemia. N Engl J Med. 2016;374(12):1197–8.
78. Sanz MA, Montesinos P, Rayon C, Holowiecka A, de la Serna J, Milone G, et al. Risk-adapted treatment of acute promyelocytic leukemia based on all-trans retinoic acid and anthracycline with addition of cytarabine in consolidation therapy for high-risk patients: further improvements in treatment outcome. Blood. 2010;115(25):5137–46.
79. Hasserjian RP, Campigotto F, Klepeis V, Fu B, Wang SA, Bueso-Ramos C, et al. De novo acute myeloid leukemia with 20-29% blasts is less aggressive than acute myeloid leukemia with >/=30% blasts in older adults: a Bone Marrow Pathology Group study. Am J Hematol. 2014;89(11):E193–9.
80. Bennett JM, Catovsky D, Daniel MT, Flandrin G, Galton DA, Gralnick HR, et al. Proposals for the classification of the acute leukaemias. French-American-British (FAB) co-operative group. Br J Haematol. 1976;33(4):451–8.
81. Walter RB, Othus M, Burnett AK, Lowenberg B, Kantarjian HM, Ossenkoppele GJ, et al. Significance of FAB subclassification of "acute myeloid leukemia, NOS" in the 2008 WHO classification: analysis of 5848 newly diagnosed patients. Blood. 2013;121(13):2424–31.
82. Knuutila S, Elonen E, Heinonen K, Borgstrom GH, Lakkala-Paranko T, Perkkio M, et al. Chromosome abnormalities in 16 Finnish patients with Burkitt's lymphoma or L3 acute lymphocytic leukemia. Cancer Genet Cytogenet. 1984;13(2):139–51.
83. Smith SM, Yearsley M. Constructing comments in a pathology report: advice for the pathology resident. Arch Pathol Lab Med. 2016;140(10):1023–4.
84. Lindley SW, Gillies EM, Hassell LA. Communicating diagnostic uncertainty in surgical pathology reports: disparities between sender and receiver. Pathol Res Pract. 2014;210(10):628–33.
85. Konoplev S, Yin CC, Kornblau SM, Kantarjian HM, Konopleva M, Andreeff M, et al. Molecular characterization of de novo Philadelphia chromosome-positive acute myeloid leukemia. Leuk Lymphoma. 2013;54(1):138–44.
86. Nacheva EP, Grace CD, Brazma D, Gancheva K, Howard-Reeves J, Rai L, et al. Does BCR/ABL1 positive acute myeloid leukaemia exist? Br J Haematol. 2013;161(4):541–50.
87. Soupir CP, Vergilio JA, Dal Cin P, Muzikansky A, Kantarjian H, Jones D, et al. Philadelphia chromosome-positive acute myeloid leukemia: a rare aggressive leukemia with clinicopathologic features distinct from chronic myeloid leukemia in myeloid blast crisis. Am J Clin Pathol. 2007;127(4):642–50.
88. Coustan-Smith E, Mullighan CG, Onciu M, Behm FG, Raimondi SC, Pei D, et al. Early T-cell precursor leukaemia: a subtype of very high-risk acute lymphoblastic leukaemia. Lancet Oncol. 2009;10(2):147–56.
89. Zhang J, Ding L, Holmfeldt L, Wu G, Heatley SL, Payne-Turner D, et al. The genetic basis of early T-cell precursor acute lymphoblastic leukaemia. Nature. 2012;481(7380):157–63.
90. Jain N, Lamb AV, O'Brien S, Ravandi F, Konopleva M, Jabbour E, et al. Early T-cell precursor acute lymphoblastic leukemia/lymphoma (ETP-ALL/LBL) in adolescents and adults: a high-risk subtype. Blood. 2016;127(15):1863–9.
91. Chopra A, Bakhshi S, Pramanik SK, Pandey RM, Singh S, Gajendra S, et al. Immunophenotypic analysis of T-acute lymphoblastic leukemia. A CD5-based ETP-ALL perspective of non-ETP T-ALL. Eur J Haematol. 2014;92(3):211–8.
92. Bueso-Ramos CE, Kanagal-Shamanna R, Routbort MJ, Hanson CA. Therapy-related myeloid neoplasms. Am J Clin Pathol. 2015;144(2):207–18.
93. Thomas DA, O'Brien S, Jorgensen JL, Cortes J, Faderl S, Garcia-Manero G, et al. Prognostic significance of CD20 expression in adults with de novo precursor B-lineage acute lymphoblastic leukemia. Blood. 2009;113(25):6330–7.
94. Baer C, Muehlbacher V, Kern W, Haferlach C, Haferlach T. Molecular genetic characterization of myeloid/lymphoid neoplasms associated with eosinophilia and rearrangement of PDGFRA, PDGFRB, FGFR1 or PCM1-JAK2. Haematologica. 2018;103(8):e348–50.
95. Reiter A, Gotlib J. Myeloid neoplasms with eosinophilia. Blood. 2017;129(6):704–14.
96. Dohner K, Schlenk RF, Habdank M, Scholl C, Rucker FG, Corbacioglu A, et al. Mutant nucleophosmin (NPM1) predicts favorable prognosis in younger adults with acute myeloid leukemia and normal cytogenetics: interaction with other gene mutations. Blood. 2005;106(12):3740–6.
97. Lee JM, Kim IS, Lee JN, Park SH, Kim HH, Chang CL, et al. Acute myeloid leukemia with MLL rearrangement and CD4+/CD56+ expression can be misdiagnosed as blastic plasmacytoid dendritic cell neoplasm: two case reports. Ann Lab Med. 2016;36(5):494–7.
98. Pagano L, Valentini CG, Grammatico S, Pulsoni A. Blastic plasmacytoid dendritic cell neoplasm: diagnostic criteria and therapeutical approaches. Br J Haematol. 2016;174(2):188–202.
99. Reichard KK. Blastic plasmacytoid dendritic cell neoplasm: how do you distinguish it from acute myeloid leukemia? Surg Pathol Clin. 2013;6(4):743–65.

Chronic Myeloid Leukemia

22

Ting Zhou and Shimin Hu

List of Frequently Asked Questions

1. How is chronic myeloid leukemia defined? What is its presentation and natural course?
2. What are the morphological features of CML in CP, AP, and BP?
3. What are the diagnostic criteria for CML-CP?
4. What are the diagnostic criteria for CML-AP?
5. What are the diagnostic criteria for CML-BP?
6. What are the diagnostic and prognostic work-ups for CML?
7. What is the differential diagnosis for CML?
8. How is CML treated?
9. How is CML treatment response monitored?
10. What are the mechanisms of TKI resistance?
11. What is the significance of *BCR-ABL1* transcript subtypes?
12. What is the significance of variant Ph?
13. What is the significance of additional chromosomal abnormalities in Ph+ cells?
14. What is the significance of chromosomal abnormalities in Ph-negative cells?
15. What other types of de novo leukemia are Ph+?
16. What is the significance of Ph acquired during therapy of MDS and acute leukemia?
17. What is the significance of Ph acquired during therapy of Ph-negative MPN?

T. Zhou
Pathology & Immunology, Baylor College of Medicine, Houston, TX, USA

S. Hu (✉)
Department of Hematopathology, The University of Texas MD Anderson Cancer Center, Houston, TX, USA
e-mail: SHu1@mdanderson.org

1. How is chronic myeloid leukemia defined? What is its presentation and natural course?

- Chronic myeloid leukemia (CML) is a myeloproliferative neoplasm (MPN) characterized by *BCR-ABL1* fusion gene resulting from the Philadelphia chromosome (Ph)/der(22)t(9;22)(q34;q11.2), its variant translocations, or rarely, cytogenetically cryptic chromosomal rearrangements.
  - While this genetic abnormality is required for the diagnosis of CML, it is not sufficient for diagnosis because it can occur in other conditions as well (see Questions 15–17).
  - CML must be separated from other MPNs primarily because it has a uniquely successful and specific treatment in the form of tyrosine kinase inhibitors (TKIs) which target the fusion gene product of the Ph chromosome.
- It is characterized by a biphasic or triphasic natural history: an indolent chronic phase (CP) followed by an accelerated phase (AP), an aggressive blast phase (BP), or both.
  - About 95% of CML patients are diagnosed in CP, and nearly half of them are asymptomatic and diagnosed incidentally in a routine complete blood count (CBC) work-up.
  - In the symptomatic patients, the common findings include fatigue, weight loss, night sweats, and hepatosplenomegaly.
- Without treatment or even in a small fraction of patients receiving TKI therapy, the disease will eventually progress to BP within 3–5 years after initial diagnosis of CP.
  - The progression is characterized by gradual but persistent deterioration in clinical status and hematological parameters, and associated with accumulation of cytogenetic and molecular genetic alterations. The clinical and pathological characteristics of the BP resemble those of acute leukemia.

E. Wang, A. S. Lagoo (eds.), *Practical Lymph Node and Bone Marrow Pathology*, Practical Anatomic Pathology,
https://doi.org/10.1007/978-3-030-32189-5_22

2. What are the morphological features of CML in CP, AP, and BP?

- Most cases of CML show rather characteristic morphological findings in various phases of the disease (Table 22.1). However, the diagnosis of CML and of various phases of the disease is based on well-defined numeric criteria for blood and marrow components, cytogenetic and molecular genetic abnormalities, and response to TKI therapy.
- Broadly speaking, the morphological features of CML reflect the underlying myeloid hyperplasia with retained capacity to differentiate into different granulocytic stages (Figs. 22.1 and 22.2).
  - In chronic phase of CML, left shift in myeloid maturation is observed with blasts typically <2% in the peripheral blood.
  - While erythroid precursors are relatively decreased, variable increases in basophils, eosinophils, monocytes, and megakaryocytes, as well as reticulin fibrosis, are seen in most cases.
  - Dysplasia of erythroid or myeloid precursors is typically absent in CML-CP.
  - Although not a defining feature of CML-AP, marked fibrosis in bone marrow accompanied by dysplastic megakaryopoiesis also reflects disease progression.
  - Persistent leukocytosis, thrombocytosis, or thrombocytopenia also indicate disease progression. Morphologically, CML-BP resembles acute leukemia.
- The morphological features in these stages of the disease are listed in Table 22.1, and the detailed diagnostic criteria for each phase of the disease are given below (Questions 3–5).

Table 22.1 Comparison of morphological and cytogenetic features of CML-CP, AP, and BP

	Chronic phase	Accelerated phase	Blast phase
Peripheral blood	Blasts usually <2% of WBCs Leukocytosis Predominantly neutrophilic lineage in different stages of maturation Characteristic "myelocyte bulge" Absolute basophilia invariably present; eosinophilia common Thrombocytosis Anemia	10–19% blasts ≥20% basophils Persistent leukocytosis Persistent thrombocytosis or thrombocytopenia	>20% blasts Myeloid origin in 70% of cases B-cell origin in 30% of cases Rarely, T-cell origin
Bone marrow	Blasts usually <5%, always <10% Hypercellularity with increased myeloid-to-erythroid ratio Widening of paratrabecular cuff of immature granulocytes Spectrum of maturing granulocytes with "myelocyte bulge" Basophils and eosinophils conspicuous Megakaryocytes usually normal or increased in number, with "dwarf" morphology No significant dysplasia in granulocytes and erythroid precursors Pseudo-Gaucher or "Sea blue" histiocytes present Reticulin fibers normal to moderately increased	10–19% blasts ≥20% basophils Dysplastic features in any myeloid lineages Sizable clusters of megakaryocytes, including micro-megakaryocytes similar to those in MDS Significant reticulin or collagen fibrosis	>20% blasts Myeloid origin in 70% of cases B-cell origin in 30% of cases Rarely, T-cell origin
Extramedullary tissue	Infiltrate in spleen, liver, and occasionally lymph nodes Mixture of immature and mature granulocytes		Any extramedullary tissue can be infiltrated, but most commonly spleen, liver, lymph nodes, and soft tissue
Cytogenetics	Clonal ACAs in 5–10% of cases	Clonal ACAs in 30% of cases [35, 54]. Any clonal ACAs acquired during therapy Major-route ACAs, complex karyotype, or 3q26.2 abnormalities at initial diagnosis	Clonal ACAs in 70–80% of cases [35, 54].

Abbreviations: *CP* chronic phase, *AP* accelerated phase, *BP* blast phase, *WBC* white blood cells, *MDS* myelodysplastic syndrome, *ACA* additional chromosomal abnormality

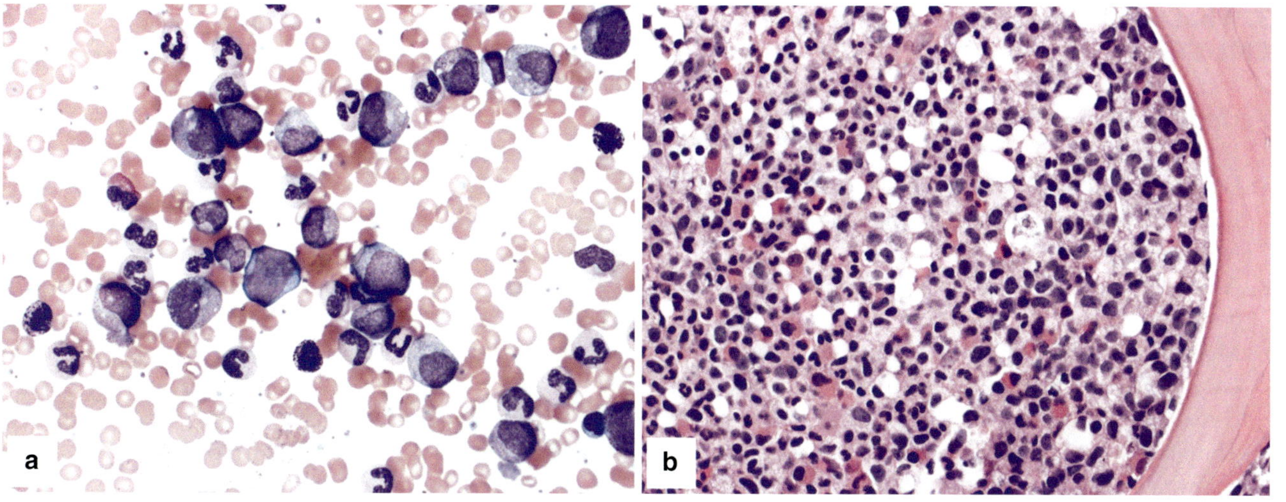

Fig. 22.1 Typical morphological features of CML-CP. (**a**) Peripheral blood shows left-shifted neutrophilia with myelocyte bulge, basophilia, eosinophilia, and occasional circulating blasts. (**b**) Bone marrow is hypercellular with myeloid hyperplasia, widening of paratrabecular cuff of immature myeloid cells, increased eosinophils, and decreased erythroid precursors

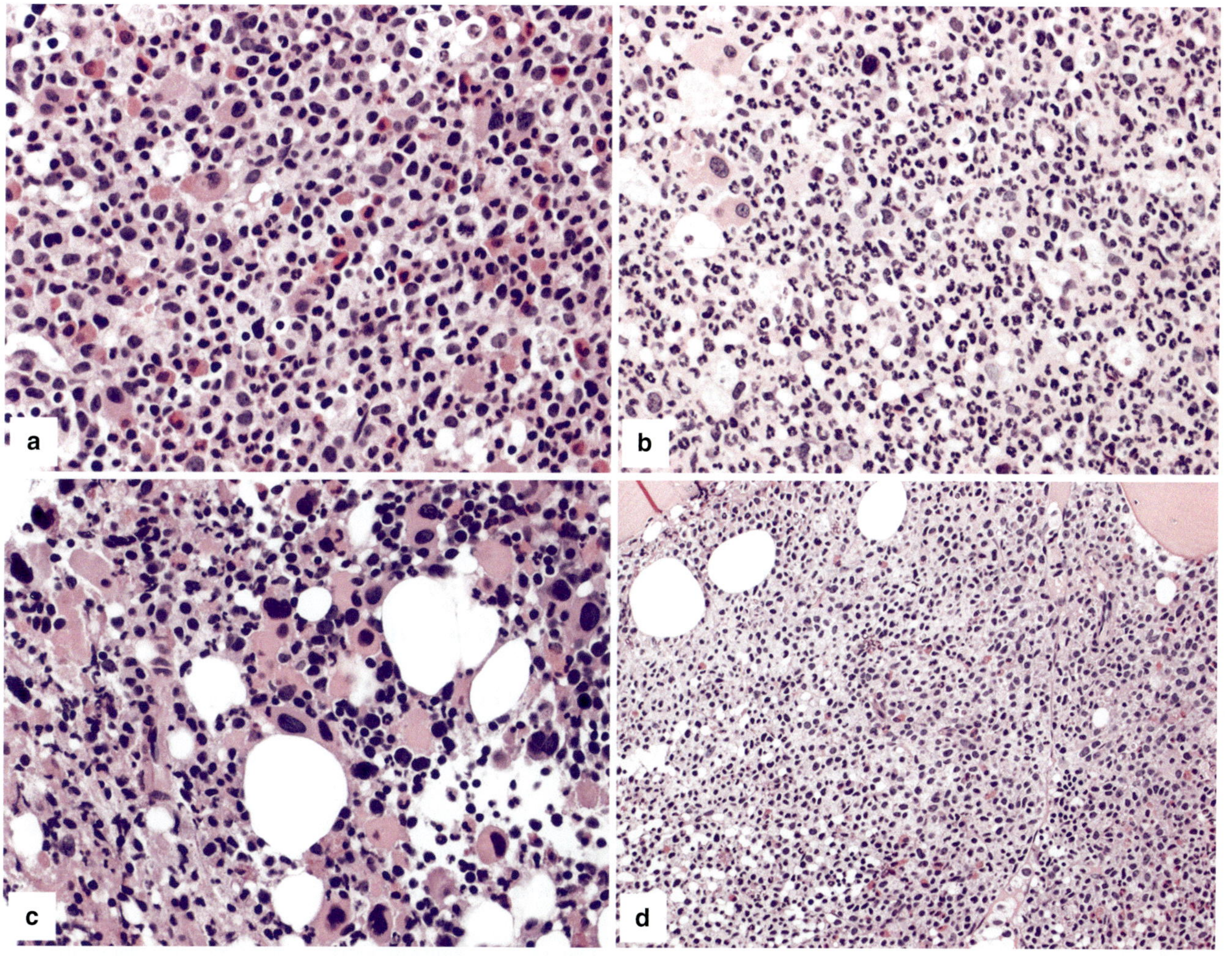

Fig. 22.2 Morphological spectrum of CML-CP. (**a**) Bone marrow shows left-shifted myeloid hyperplasia. Most myeloid cells are immature. Eosinophils are frequently seen. (**b**) Bone marrow shows right-shifted myeloid hyperplasia. Most myeloid cells are mature neutrophils. Eosinophils are rarely seen. (**c**) Bone marrow shows markedly increased dwarf megakaryocytes (megakaryocyte rich). (**d**) Bone marrow shows markedly decreased megakaryocytes (megakaryocyte poor/null). In rare cases, megakaryocytes may be mostly morphologically unremarkable

3. What are the diagnostic criteria for CML-CP?

Peripheral Blood (Fig. 22.1a)

- Leukocytosis composed of predominantly neutrophilic lineage in different stages of maturation with a characteristic myelocyte bulge
- Absolute basophilia invariably present and eosinophilia common
- Monocytosis, usually <3%, except in rare cases, particularly in those with P190 BCR-ABL1, which may mimic chronic myelomonocytic leukemia
- Thrombocytosis; cases of isolated thrombocytosis present, which may mimic essential thrombocythemia
- Blasts usually <2%
- Anemia
- No significant dysplasia in granulocytes and erythroid precursors

Bone Marrow (Figs. 22.1b and 22.2)

- Hypercellularity with myeloid hyperplasia and elevated myeloid-to-erythroid ratio
- Spectrum of maturing myeloid cells with myelocyte bulge; basophils and eosinophils conspicuous
- Widening of paratrabecular cuff of immature myeloid cells
- Megakaryocytes may be decreased but usually normal or increased in number, with "dwarf" morphology
- Pseudo-Gaucher or "sea blue" histiocytes present
- Blasts usually <2%
- No significant dysplasia in granulocytes and erythroid precursors

4. What are the diagnostic criteria for CML-AP?

CML-AP is defined by the presence of one or more of the following hematological, cytogenetic, or provisional criteria [1].

Hematological Criteria

- Persistent or increasing leukocytosis (>10 × 10^9/L), unresponsive to therapy
- Persistent or increasing splenomegaly, unresponsive to therapy
- Persistent thrombocytosis, unresponsive to therapy
- Persistent thrombocytopenia, unrelated to therapy
- ≥20% basophils in peripheral blood
- 10–19% blasts in peripheral blood and/or bone marrow

Cytogenetic Criteria

- Any clonal additional chromosomal abnormalities (ACAs) in Ph+ cells acquired during therapy
- Clonal ACAs in Ph+ cells at diagnosis, including major-route ACAs (+8, i(17q), +19, +Ph), complex karyotype, and abnormalities of 3q26.2

Provisional Response-to-TKI Criteria

- Hematological resistance (lack of complete hematological remission) to the first TKI
- Any hematological, cytogenetic, and molecular indications of resistance to two sequential TKIs
- Occurrence of two or more mutations in the *BCR-ABL1* during TKI therapy

Presumptive Evidence of AP

- Large clusters or sheets of small dwarf megakaryocytes associated with marked reticulin or collagen fibrosis in biopsy specimens

5. What are the diagnostic criteria for CML-BP?

CML-BP is defined by [1]:

- ≥20% blasts in peripheral blood and/or bone marrow
- Presence of an extramedullary proliferation of blasts

Presumptive Evidence of BP

- Sheets of blasts occupy focal but substantial areas of the bone marrow (an entire intertrabecular space or more) in biopsy specimens

6. What are the diagnostic and prognostic work-ups for CML?

The goal of diagnostic work-ups for CML is to detect the two essential diagnostic features, namely characteristic peripheral blood findings and the presence of Ph chromosome or

BCR-ABL1. Additional tests can be done to assess the phase of the disease and provide valuable prognostic and predictive information. Accordingly, the National Comprehensive Cancer Network practice guidelines recommend that in addition to a thorough clinical history and physical examination, the work-ups of CML should include [2]:

- CBC with leukocyte differential and chemistry profile
- Bone marrow aspiration: mandatory to obtain materials for chromosomal analysis to detect the Ph chromosome and ACAs, as well as for morphological evaluation to assess the phase of the disease
- Bone marrow core biopsy: not mandatory, unless the peripheral blood findings are atypical or a marrow aspirate cannot be obtained
- Fluorescence in situ hybridization (FISH) studies: needed to identify cryptic *BCR-ABL1* rearrangement
- Quantitative real-time reverse-transcriptase polymerase chain reaction (qRT-PCR): necessary to identify the fusion transcript subtype and quantify the baseline level of *BCR-ABL1* transcripts for monitoring treatment response
- Flow cytometry and immunohistochemistry: traditionally limited to analysis of blasts, including blast enumeration and lineage assignment, to help identify advanced-stage disease

7. What is the differential diagnosis of CML?

- The differential diagnosis for CML-CP and AP includes chronic neutrophilic leukemia (particularly in cases with P230 BCR-ABL1) [3], essential thrombocythemia (particularly in cases with P230) [4, 5], Ph-negative MPN with eosinophilia, atypical CML, chronic myelomonocytic leukemia (particularly in cases with P190) [6], juvenile myelomonocytic leukemia, and extreme leukemoid reaction. The fundamental key for the diagnosis of CML lies in the presence of *BCR-ABL1*. Hematological and morphological features, including characteristic myelocyte bulge and basophilia particularly, also provide valuable clues.
- The *BCR-ABL1* fusion gene can be found in several types of de novo acute leukemia, including acute lymphoblastic leukemia (ALL), acute myeloid leukemia (AML), and mixed phenotype acute leukemia (MPAL). In the absence of a history of pre-existing CML, the differentiation between CML presenting initially in BP and de novo Ph+ acute leukemia can be very challenging and sometimes impossible. Presence of the following clinical, morphological, and genetic features may favor CML-BP over Ph+ de novo acute leukemia [7].
  - Evidence of an antecedent blood disorder, such as leukocytosis and splenomegaly, points to CML-BP. Presence of background CML-related morphological features can be helpful in diagnosing CML-BP, including granulocytes with a left shift, "myelocyte bulge," and basophilia or dwarf megakaryocytes.
  - Evidence of CP or AP after induction chemotherapy, such as persistent t(9;22)(q34;q11.2), supports the diagnosis of CML.
  - P190 (e1a2) is very rare in CML (1–2%) [8, 9]. The presence of P190 strongly favors the diagnosis of de novo Ph+ acute leukemia although a diagnosis of CML carrying P190 cannot be completely excluded.

8. How is CML treated?

- First-line treatment: According to the current European LeukemiaNet (ELN) recommendations [10], any of the three TKIs approved for CML (imatinib, dasatinib, and nilotinib) can be used as the first-line treatment for CML-CP. The choice can be made based on the characteristics of the disease (high-risk ACAs), individual comorbidities, and the side effect profile of the drugs, as well as the presence of certain mutations that confer resistance to a particular TKI. When intolerance occurs, the other two first-line TKIs should be considered.
- Second-line treatment: For patients who fail the first-line treatment, second-line treatments include switching to the other first-line TKIs or transitioning to ponatinib or bosutinib. Following second-line treatment failure, any one of the remaining TKIs or allogeneic hematopoietic stem cell transplant (allo-HSCT) should be considered. In the situation of T315I mutation, the choices are limited to ponatinib and allo-HSCT.
- For CML-AP, the optimal therapeutic approaches differ dependent on whether the patient is TKI-naïve or has evolved from CML-CP following TKI failure. Patients with de novo CML-AP have a good outcome with frontline TKI therapy, particularly if treated with a second-generation TKI. These patients can be treated following the same guidelines as those for CML-CP and continue TKI therapy as their long-term treatment after they achieve a complete cytogenetic remission; allo-HSCT is considered only upon treatment failure with two TKIs. Patients who progress to AP from CP while on TKI therapy have a much worse prognosis and may be best treated more aggressively with a second-generation TKI followed by allo-HSCT [11, 12].
- The aim of treatment for CML-BP is to obtain reversion to CP, followed promptly by allo-HSCT. Patients are treated with a standard ALL or AML induction chemotherapy with or without the addition of TKIs, and allo-HSCT is performed as soon as the patient is back to

CP. Posttransplant TKI maintenance may also be considered. For those who are not candidates for transplant, TKI monotherapy or in combination with chemotherapy remains a good option [11, 12].

9. How is CML treatment response monitored?

- Ongoing assessment is required for early identification of patients who are not responding optimally so that alternative treatment strategies can be considered. Based on the time taken to reach various levels of responses, treatment responses can be categorized into three groups: optimal, failure, and warning (Table 22.2) [10, 13].
  - Optimal response is associated with the best long-term outcome, and the patients are expected to live a similar life span to that of the general population. Continuing the current therapy plan is appropriate in this group.
  - "Failure" means that a different treatment should be initiated to limit the risk of progression and death.
  - "Warning" implies that although the current treatment may still be beneficial, the long-term outcome of treatment is less likely to be favorable. More frequent monitoring is required to permit timely changes in therapy in case of treatment failure.
- Per ELN recommendations, responses can be assessed with either cytogenetic analysis or qRT-PCR alone; when local laboratory facilities permit, both cytogenetic and molecular tests are recommended until a complete cytogenetic remission is achieved [10]. Following these landmarks, molecular tests alone may be sufficient (Table 22.3).
  - In case of suspicion of warning, failure, or progression, cytogenetic analysis is mandated. In addition, mutation analysis is recommended in certain situations, as following imatinib failure, up to 48% of cases with primary resistance and 68% of cases with secondary resistance show mutations in the *BCR-ABL1* kinase domain [14].
  - A single measurement of the *BCR-ABL1* transcript level is not sufficient to define failure. Two tests at 3 and 6 months and supplementary tests in-between should be performed before a decision is made to change the treatment. Furthermore, failures must be distinguished as either primary (lack of initial response) or secondary (loss of an established response).

Table 22.2 Definition of responses to TKIs as first-line treatment

	Optimal	Warning	Failure
Baseline/ diagnosis	N/A	High-risk or major-route ACAs	N/A
3 months	*BCR-ABL1* ≤10% and/or Ph+ ≤35%	*BCR-ABL1* >10% and/or Ph+ 36–95%	Non-CHR and/ or Ph+ >95%
6 months	*BCR-ABL1* <1% and/or Ph+ 0%	*BCR-ABL1* 1–10% and/or Ph+ 1–35%	*BCR-ABL1* >10% and/or Ph+ >35%
12 months	*BCR-ABL1* ≤0.1% (MMR)	*BCR-ABL1* >0.1–1%	*BCR-ABL1* >1% and/or Ph+ >0%
After 12 months	*BCR-ABL1* ≤0.1%	Cytogenetic changes in Ph-negative cells (−7 or 7q-)	Loss of CCyR Confirmed loss of MMR Mutations ACA in Ph+ cells

Data adapted from the ELN recommendations [10] and Cancer Cytogenetics [13]

Abbreviations: *ACAs* additional chromosomal abnormalities, *CHR* complete hematologic remission (WBC <10 × 10^9/L, platelet count <450 × 10^9/L, no immature granulocytes in differential, and spleen nonpalpable), *CCyR* complete cytogenetic remission (no Ph+ metaphase), *MMR* major molecular response (*BCR-ABL1* expression of ≤0.1%), *N/A* not applicable, *TKI* tyrosine kinase inhibitor

10. What are the mechanisms of TKI resistance?

TKIs act as competitive inhibitors for ATPs and freeze BCR-ABL1 kinase in the inactive non-ATP-binding conformation. This blocks the tyrosine kinase activity and prevents BCR-ABL1-mediated autophosphorylation, and in turn, substrate phosphorylation, thereby switching off the downstream signaling pathways [15].

Table 22.3 Recommendations for cytogenetic and molecular monitoring of CML

At diagnosis	CBA of bone marrow metaphases FISH in case of Ph negativity to identify variant translocations or cryptic *BCR-ABL1* rearrangement qRT-PCR to identify the fusion transcript type and quantify the baseline level of *BCR-ABL1* expression on the international scale
During treatment	qRT-PCR of *BCR-ABL1* on the international scale Every 3 months until MMR achieved After MMR: every 3–6 months CBA of bone marrow metaphases At 3, 6, and 12 months until CCyR achieved After CCyR: every 12 months[a] FISH on blood cells After CCyR achieved
Failure, progression	qRT-PCR, mutation analysis, and CBA of bone marrow metaphases Immunophenotyping in BP
Warning	Molecular and cytogenetic analyses performed more frequently CBA of bone marrow cells in case of myelodysplasia or clonal cytogenetic changes in Ph-negative cells with chromosome 7 abnormalities

Data adapted from the ELN recommendations [10] and Cancer Cytogenetics [13]

Abbreviations: *CBA* chromosome banding analysis, *CCyR* complete cytogenetic remission, *MMR* major molecular remission, *qRT-PCR* quantitative real-time reverse-transcription polymerase chain reaction

[a]After CCyR is achieved, if adequate qRT-PCR can be ensured, cytogenetic analysis can be omitted

- TKI resistance (~13% of patients) [16] can develop from a number of mechanisms involving both BCR-ABL1-dependent and BCR-ABL1-independent pathways. The BCR-ABL1-dependent pathways include mutations [17–19] and amplification of *BCR-ABL1* [20]; the BCR-ABL1-independent pathways include inherent resistance of CML stem cells to TKIs [21, 22], clonal evolution [23, 24], activation of other tyrosine kinases [25, 26], pharmacokinetic variability, and drug transport mechanisms [27].
  - More than 100 mutations in *BCR-ABL1* have been identified to confer TKI resistance [28]. The frequency of mutation increases as the disease progresses, with mutations detected in 27%, 52%, and 75% of patients with CP, AP, and myeloid BP, respectively [29]. Additionally, they are more common in acquired resistance than primary resistance [12, 30].

11. What is the significance of *BCR-ABL1* transcript subtypes?

- The breakpoints in *ABL1* gene are distributed over a large region in the intron between exons 1b and 1a or the intron between exons 1a and 2 [31]. Depending on the location of breakpoints in *BCR* gene, different types of fusion genes can be formed. In *BCR*, three breakpoint cluster regions are characterized: minor (*m-BCR*), major (*M-BCR*), and micro (*μ-BCR*) breakpoint clusters.
  - The *m-BCR* is located in the 3' half of the first *BCR* intron, the *M-BCR* region encompasses exons 12–15, and the *μ-BCR* is located further downstream between exons 19 and 21, corresponding to three fusion transcript subtypes e1a2, e13a2/e14a2 (or b2a2/b3a2), and e19a2 that encode P190, P210, and P230, respectively [32].
  - The rare *BCR-ABL1* transcript variants include fusion transcripts lacking exon 2 of *ABL1* (ela3, e13a3, and e14a3), e2a2, e6a2, e12a1, or "bizarre" insertions or breakpoints within exons [33, 34].
- There is a clear association of different forms of the *BCR-ABL1* transcript subtypes with different disease phenotypes (Table 22.4).
  - The e13a2/e14a2 (P210) *BCR-ABL1* is reported in ~98% of CML. In contrast, the e1a2 (P190) *BCR-ABL1* is present in ~80% of Ph+ B-ALL but only rarely observed in CML patients (1–2%).
  - CML patients with the e1a2 (P190) fusion transcript tend to be older, present with monocytosis, and have a higher frequency of BP at initial presentation [9]. Those who are not in BP initially have a higher risk of subsequent blastic transformation.
  - The rare e19a2 (P230) has been described in a small fraction of CML patients who often present with prominent neutrophilic maturation or thrombocytosis [3]. Because of the low frequency, the significance of other rare atypical transcripts is unclear.

Table 22.4 *BCR-ABL1* fusion subtype genotype and phenotype correlation

P190	P210	P230
CML (1–2%) [8, 9]	CML (~98%) [9]	CML (<1%)
B-ALL (~14%) [55] 68–83% of Ph+ ALL in adults [55–57] 78.8% of Ph+ ALL in children [55]	B-ALL (~3%) [55] 17–28% of Ph+ ALL in adults [55–57] 13.4% of Ph+ ALL in children [55]	
B/M MPAL (~20%) [58] 61.9% of Ph+ MPAL	B/M MPAL (~10%) [58] 28.6% of Ph+ MPAL	
AML (<1%) 17–41% of Ph+ AML [7, 59, 60]	AML (<1%) 59–83% of Ph+ AML [7, 59, 60]	

Abbreviations: *CML* chronic myeloid leukemia, *ALL* acute lymphoblastic leukemia, *B/M MPAL* B/myeloid mixed phenotype acute leukemia, *AML* acute myeloid leukemia, *Ph* Philadelphia chromosome

12. What is the significance of variant Ph?

- In about 6% of CML patients, *BCR-ABL1* are generated from variant rearrangements involving one or more additional chromosomes besides chromosomes 9 and 22. All chromosomes, including chromosome Y, have been demonstrated to participate in the variant rearrangements. The most commonly involved chromosomes include chromosomes 11, 14, 12, 1 and 7, with a frequency of at least 8% of all variant rearrangements [35, 36].
- Variant Ph translocations were considered an adverse prognostic factor in the pre-TKI era. Studies in the TKI era suggest variant translocations confer a similar prognosis to the standard Ph. However, a recent large study indicates a role of complexity of variant rearrangements in CML. Although variant translocations as a whole appear prognostically similar to the stand Ph, patients with variant translocations involving four or more breakpoints have a lower rate of molecular response to TKI therapy, a higher frequency of blastic transformation, and an inferior overall survival than those with variant translocations involving only three breakpoints [36].

13. What is the significance of additional chromosomal abnormalities in Ph+ cells?

- In the 2017 update of WHO Classification of Tumors of Hematopoietic and Lymphoid Tissue, major-route ACAs (+8, i(17q), +19, +Ph), complex karyotype, and 3q26.2

abnormalities at initial diagnosis as well as any ACAs emerging during therapy are considered defining criteria for AP [1]. Per ELN recommendations [10], only major-route ACAs emerging during therapy, but not minor-route ACAs emerging during TKI therapy nor any ACAs detected at initial diagnosis, define TKI failure and mandate the change of treatment.

- Most recent studies [37, 38] establish a four-tier risk stratification model based on the presence or absence of ACAs and the types of ACAs. These four different groups confer different risk of blastic transformation and survival:
  - High risk: 3q26.2 rearrangement, −7/7q-, or i(17q), either as a single ACA or as a component of a complex karyotype
  - Intermediate risk 2: complex karyotypes without any of the three high-risk components
  - Intermediate risk 1: any single ACAs other than the three high-risk ACAs
  - Standard risk: no ACAs

This four-tier stratification remains somewhat valid for ACAs, particularly the high-risk ACAs, detected at initial diagnosis of CML. When all patients are included, the 5-year cumulative probability of blastic transformation from initial diagnosis of CML for these four groups is 67.4%, 41.7%, 28.0%, and 9.8%, respectively. TKI therapy does not alter the natural course of CML with the high-risk ACAs. The pre-BP disease course in patients with high-risk ACAs and treated in the TKI era highly resembles that observed in patients treated with busulfan or hydroxyurea in the pre-TKI era. These patients may benefit from early hematopoietic stem cell transplantation to prevent the onset of blastic transformation. Regardless of the risk of ACAs in pre-BP disease course, the prognostic impact of the type of ACAs is minimized once the disease progresses to BP [24, 38].

14. What is the significance of chromosomal abnormalities in Ph-negative cells?

- About 5–10% of patients who receive imatinib develop clonal chromosomal abnormalities in Ph-negative cells, most commonly, −7, +8, and −Y [39–41]. However, only a small subset of these patients (2–10%) develops clinically evident myelodysplastic syndrome (MDS) or AML [42].
- In the absence of dysplasia, the presence of chromosomal abnormalities in Ph-negative cells does not adversely affect the outcome, with the exception of −7 and del(7q). About 30% of patients with −7 develop MDS or AML, frequently within the first 6 months after the detection of −7. According to the ELN recommendations [10], −7 and del(7q) detected during TKI treatment is a "warning" sign and requires more frequent cytogenetic and molecular genetic monitoring and long-term follow-up.
- Other clonal chromosomal abnormalities in Ph-negative cells do not necessitate immediate therapeutic intervention or more frequent monitoring. Bone marrow examination is reserved for cases with cytopenia or dysplasia.

15. What other types of de novo leukemia are Ph+?

- B-ALL: The Ph is the most commonly detected cytogenetic abnormality in B-ALL patients. The frequency of Ph positivity in B-ALL increases with age: ~3% of pediatric patients, ~25% of adult patients, and may reach up to 50% of patients older than 50 years [43]. The e1a2 (P190) *BCR-ABL1* is documented in ~80% of Ph+ B-ALL cases. Patients with Ph+ B-ALL tend to have a high WBC count and a high incidence of central nervous system involvement. Microscopically, Ph+ B-ALL is similar to Ph-negative B-ALL. Ph+ B-ALL frequently expresses myeloid-associated antigens including CD13 and CD33, and highly characteristically CD25 [44]. Very rare cases of Ph+ T-ALL have also been reported [45].
- MPAL: As is the case in ALL, the Ph is the most common recurrent cytogenetic abnormality in MPAL and is found in ~30% of cases. The e1a2 (P190) *BCR-ABL1* is detected in ~60% of Ph+ MPAL cases. Patients with Ph+ MPAL present with a high WBC count and are otherwise clinically similar to patients with Ph-negative MPAL. The vast majority of cases have a B/myeloid phenotype, with few cases reported to show T/myeloid phenotype.
- Ph+ AML: In the 2017 update of WHO Classification, Ph+ AML is included as a new provisional entity. It is rare and comprises <1% of all cases of AML. The majority of Ph+ AML cases express the e13a2/e14a2 (P210) transcript (Table 22.4). It occurs primarily in adults and shows distinct hematological, morphological, and genetic characteristics from CML-BP, such as the absence of basophilia, a slightly lower bone marrow cellularity, a lower myeloid-to-erythroid ratio, a more prominent dysplasia with lack of significant myeloid maturation, and a significantly lower frequency of major-route ACAs [7].
- De novo Ph+ MDS is exceedingly rare [46, 47]. In some cases of Ph+ MDS reported in literature, the Ph was acquired secondarily during therapy, while other cases may represent CML in preleukemic phase [46, 48]. CML following treatment for primary neoplasms or other medical conditions has a clinical presentation, pathologic features, and cytogenetic profile similar to those of de novo CML [49].

16. What is the significance of Ph acquired during therapy of MDS and acute leukemia?

The Ph acquired secondarily during chemotherapy of myeloid or lymphoid neoplasms is rare and has been reported in patients with AML, MDS, B-ALL, and T-ALL [48].

- The emergence of secondary Ph is almost always associated with the advanced stage of disease: during relapse or in refractory stage of de novo AML or ALL or after acute transformation from MDS. The *BCR-ABL1* transcript subtype is overwhelmingly of the e1a2 (P190). The diseases before and after the emergence of Ph+ clones are clonally related by karyotyping or molecular analyses in the vast majority of patients, and usually show similar morphological or immunophenotypic features.
- Features of CML after the emergence of Ph+ clones are rare regardless of the size of Ph+ clones. The emergence of secondary Ph is not essential for maintenance of the leukemic process. Incorporating TKIs into treatment may eradicate the Ph+ clones and could potentially change the disease prognosis in a small subset of patients. However, most patients have persistent or refractory disease despite the eradication of the Ph+ clones.

17. What is the significance of Ph acquired during therapy of Ph-negative MPN?

An increasing number of cases of patients with both CML and Ph-negative MPN have been described, either simultaneously or sequentially (CML after Ph-negative MPN or Ph-negative MPN after CML). Herein, we only discuss the Ph arising in patients with a previous history of Ph-negative MPN.

- To date, <40 cases have been reported in the literature, predominantly in patients with a history of polycythemia vera (~70%), followed by essential thrombocythemia and primary myelofibrosis [50–53]. However, the karyotype and mutational status of *JAK2*, *MPL*, and CALR were unknown in some reported cases of Ph-negative MPN, and therefore, it is uncertain whether some of these cases represented genuine Ph-negative MPN.
- The Ph acquired after Ph-negative MPN is often the e13a2/e14a2 (P210) subtype (~70%) [51]. Additionally, the disease in most patients, if not all, is bona fide CML. These two features are in sharp contrast to the Ph acquired during therapy in MDS and acute leukemia, where the transcript subtype is of overwhelmingly the e1a2 (P190) subtype and features of CML are rare.

Case Presentations

Case 1

Learning Objectives

1. To become familiar with the typical CBC profile of CML
2. To become familiar with the age spectrum of patients with CML

Case History

A 2-year-old boy presented with a 1-month history of progressive pallor and several days of fever, and was thought to have an infection.

Morphologic Findings

- WBC 48.7, Hgb 9.6, MCV 100, PLT 386.
- Differential (%): neutrophils 44, metamyelocytes 6, blasts 1, lymphocytes 42, monocytes 1, eosinophils 4, basophils 2.
- Bone marrow was 100% cellular. Megakaryocytes were not increased and occasional dwarf forms were seen.
- Bone marrow differential (%): blasts 2, promyelocytes 3, myelocytes 15, metamyelocytes 11, granulocytes 35, eosinophils 4, basophils 1, lymphocytes 15, monocytes 4, erythroid precursors 10.

Differential Diagnosis

- Infection
- CML
- JMML

Ancillary Studies Performed on the Bone Marrow

- Karyotype: 46,XY,t(9;22)(q34;q11.2)[20]
- FISH: positive for *BCR-ABL1* rearrangement in 188/200 interphases
- qRT-PCR: b2a2 *BCR-ABL1* fusion transcript detected, *BCR-ABL1* to *ABL1* ratio >100%

Final Diagnosis

Chronic myeloid leukemia, *BCR-ABL1* positive, chronic phase

Take-Home Messages

1. This patient is very young (2 years old). Usually, pediatric patients with CML are older than 10 years.
2. CML is rare in pediatric patients and may be misdiagnosed as infection.

Case 2

Learning Objectives

1. To become familiar with the atypical CBC profile of CML

2. To become familiar with the concept of preleukemic phase of CML

Case History

A 66-year-old man who had a history of polycythemia secondary to testosterone usage and treated with phlebotomies was found to have *BCR-ABL1* at 0.04, which gradually increased over the next 18 months. He was referred to us for further evaluation.

Morphologic Findings

- WBC 8.4, Hgb 12.7, MCV 81, PLT 395.
- Differential (%): neutrophils 61, lymphocytes 29, monocytes 6, eosinophils 4.
- Bone marrow was normocellular with occasional dwarf megakaryocytes.
- Bone marrow differential (%): blasts 0, promyelocytes 0, myelocytes 10, metamyelocytes 12, granulocytes 30, eosinophils 4, basophils 1, lymphocytes 17, plasma cells 1, monocytes 3, erythroid precursors 22.

Differential Diagnosis

- Reactive changes with low level of *BCR-ABL1*
- Preleukemic phase of CML

Ancillary Studies Performed on the Bone Marrow and Peripheral Blood

- Karyotype: 46,XY,t(9;22)(q34;q11.2)[3]/46,XY[17] (on bone marrow)
- FISH: positive for *BCR-ABL1* rearrangement in 7/200 interphases (on bone marrow)
- qRT-PCR: b3a2 *BCR-ABL1* fusion transcript detected, *BCR-ABL1* to *ABL1* ratio 2.24% (on peripheral blood)

Final Diagnosis

Chronic myeloid leukemia, *BCR-ABL1* positive, preleukemic phase

Take-Home Message

Patients with preleukemic phase of CML may have near normal CBC and bone marrow findings. Basophilia is not always a feature of preleukemic phase of CML.

Case 3

Learning Objectives

1. To become familiar with the unusual presentations of CML
2. To become familiar with the discordant manifestations in the extramedullary site, peripheral blood, and bone marrow
3. To become familiar with the morphologic spectrum of megakaryocytes in CML

Case History

A 72-year-old man presented with a 2-year history of back pain that was getting worse for the last 2 months. MRI revealed a 15.8 × 10.8 × 8.3 cm right paraspinal mass.

Morphologic Findings

- A biopsy of the mass revealed myeloid sarcoma (Fig. 22.3).
- WBC 8.0, Hgb 12.9, MCV 95, PLT 183.
- Differential (%): neutrophils 63, lymphocytes 21, monocytes 10, eosinophils 3, basophils 3.
- Bone marrow was 50% cellular with myeloid hyperplasia. Megakaryocytes were unremarkable in number and in morphology.

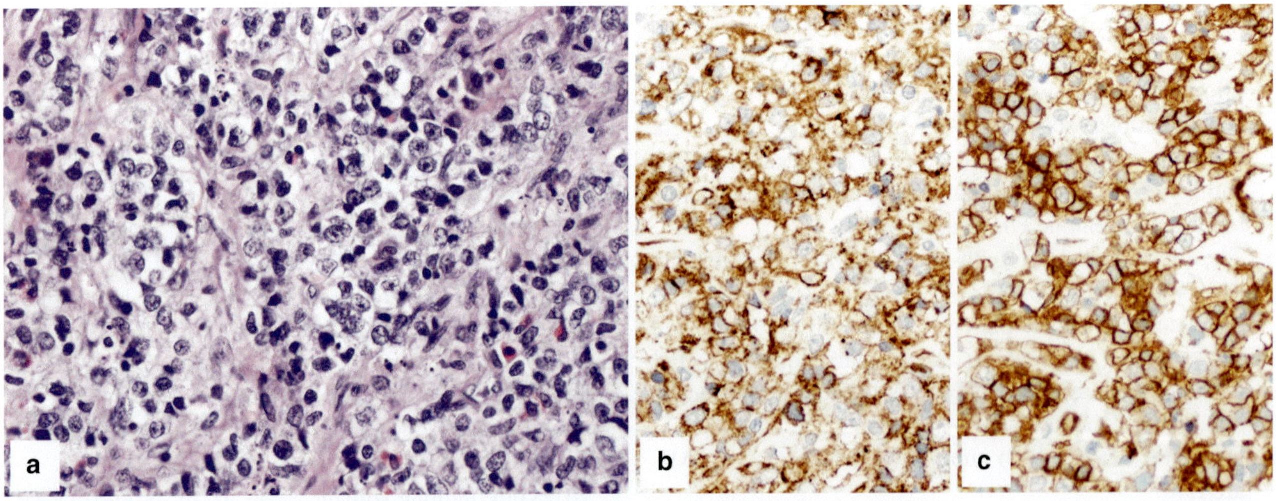

Fig. 22.3 Myeloid sarcoma as the initial presentation of CML. A paraspinal mass biopsy revealed myeloid sarcoma (**a**: H&E, **b**: CD34, **c**: CD117) in a patient with CML-CP in the bone marrow and a normal CBC

- Bone marrow differential (%): blasts 1, promyelocytes 2, myelocytes 14, metamyelocytes 25, granulocytes 39, eosinophils 3, basophils 0, lymphocytes 5, plasma cells 1, monocytes 3, erythroid precursors 7.

Differential Diagnosis

- De novo myeloid sarcoma
- CML, extramedullary BP

Ancillary Studies performed on the bone marrow:
- Karyotype: 46,XY,t(9;22)(q34;q11.2)[15]/48,idem,+8,+21[3]/46,XY[2]
- FISH: positive for *BCR-ABL1* rearrangement in 69/200 interphases
- qRT-PCR: b2a2 *BCR-ABL1* fusion transcript detected, *BCR-ABL1* to *ABL1* ratio 38.84%

Final Diagnosis

Chronic myeloid leukemia, *BCR-ABL1* positive, extramedullary myeloid blast phase

Take-Home Messages

1. The patient had CML in three different phases: extramedullary BP (myeloid sarcoma), CP in the bone marrow, and preleukemic phase in peripheral blood.
2. Normal morphology of megakaryocytes does not exclude the diagnosis of CML.

Case 4

Learning Objectives

To learn how to distinguish CML, lymphoid BP vs de novo ALL/LBL

Case History

A 23-year-old man was found to have anemia, thrombocytopenia, and leukocytosis with 4% circulating blasts in a routine work-up in an outside hospital. A hemodiluted bone marrow aspirate showed 5% blasts. Karyotyping on the bone marrow revealed t(9;22)(q34;q11.2) in 19/20 cells. He also had splenomegaly. The patient was treated with hydrea, allopurinol, and dasatinib. Four months later, he was referred to us for fever.

Morphologic Findings

- WBC 5.9, HGB 13.0, MCV 87, PLT 63.
- Differential (%): neutrophils 35, metamyelocytes 3, blasts 25, lymphocytes 33, monocytes 3, basophils 1.
- Bone marrow was nearly entirely replaced by sheets of blasts. Megakaryocytes were not seen.
- Bone marrow differential (%): blasts 90, promyelocytes 0, myelocytes 2, metamyelocytes 1, granulocytes 0, eosinophils 2, basophils 0, lymphocytes 3, monocytes 0, erythroid precursors 2.

Ancillary Studies Performed on the Bone Marrow
- Karyotype: 45,XY,der(7;9)(q10;q10),t(9;22)(q34;q11.2),del(17)(p11.2)[5]/46,XY[15]
- FISH: positive for *BCR-ABL1* rearrangement in 174/200 interphases and *CRLF2* rearrangement in 185/200 interphases
- qRT-PCR: b2a2 *BCR-ABL1* fusion transcript detected, *BCR-ABL1* to *ABL1* ratio >100%
- Flow cytometry: blasts positive for CD10 (bright), CD19, CD20, CD22, CD34 (small subset), CD79a, and TDT, and negative for MPO

Differential Diagnosis

Given the lack of CML features in the current bone marrow, a differential diagnosis of B-ALL/LBL vs CML, lymphoid BP was raised. However, a further review of the initial peripheral blood revealed left-shifted granulocytosis. WBC 38.23, HGB 9.7, MCV 97.2, PLT 88. Differential (%): neutrophils 70, immature granulocytes 23, lymphocytes 2, monocytes 1, blasts 4.

Final Diagnosis

Chronic myeloid leukemia, *BCR-ABL1* positive, lymphoid blast phase

Take-Home Message

1. Evidence of an antecedent left-shifted neutrophilia and splenomegaly point to CML-BP.
2. Detection of t(9;22) in non-blast cells confirms the diagnosis of CML-BP. In the initial outside bone marrow, there were only 5% blasts but t(9;22) was detected in 19/20 cells.
3. *CRLF2* rearrangement can be observed in CML.

Case 5

Learning Objectives

To learn how to distinguish CML, initial myeloid BP vs de novo AML

Case History

A 67-year-old woman was referred for newly diagnosed untreated acute leukemia.

Morphologic Findings

- WBC 18.0, HGB 9.3, MCV 101, PLT 151.
- Differential (%): neutrophils 50, metamyelocytes 1, blast 28, lymphocytes 12, monocytes 2, basophils 7.
- Bone marrow was 100% cellular with markedly increased immature myeloid cells. Megakaryocytes and erythroid were rare (Fig. 22.4).

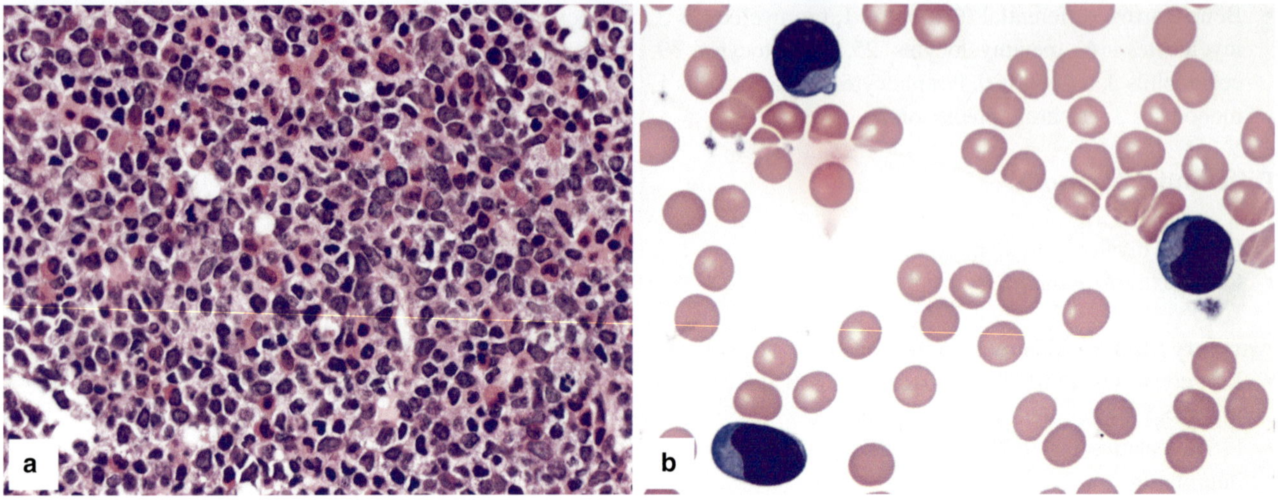

Fig. 22.4 CML, initial myeloid BP, with NPM1 mutation. Bone marrow core biopsy (**a**) and smear (**b**) from a patient with CML-BP and NPM1 mutation at initial presentation. The blasts show cup-like morphology

- Aparticulate bone marrow differential (%): blasts 25, promyelocytes 2, myelocytes 16, metamyelocytes 16, granulocytes 24, eosinophils 1, basophils 1, lymphocytes 11, monocytes 2, erythroid precursors 2.

Differential Diagnosis

- De novo acute leukemia
- CML-BP

Ancillary Studies Performed on the Bone Marrow

- Karyotype: 46,XX,t(9;22)(q34;q11.2)[17]/47,idem,+8[3]
- FISH: positive for *BCR-ABL1* rearrangement in 190/200 interphases
- qRT-PCR: b3a2 *BCR-ABL1* fusion transcript detected, *BCR-ABL1* to *ABL1* ratio 84.68%
- Mutation screen: positive for *NPM1* (p.W288fs), *RUNX1* and *WT1* mutations
- Flow cytometry: blasts positive for CD4 (partial), CD13, CD33 (bright), CD34 (partial), CD38, CD117 (partial), CD123, HLA-DR (partial) and MPO (partial)

Final Diagnosis

Chronic myeloid leukemia, *BCR-ABL1* positive, myeloid blast phase, with *NPM1* mutation

Treatment

The patient was treated with decitabine and dasatinib. In multiple follow-up bone marrow specimens, t(9;22)(q34;q11.2) and *NPM1* mutation were persistent despite only very low level of residual AML detected by flow cytometry.

Take-Home Messages

1. Reversion to CP after chemotherapy points to CML-BP.
2. Detection of t(9;22) in non-blast cells confirms the diagnosis of CML-BP. There was only 25% blasts by differential, but t(9;22) was detected in 20/20 cells by karyotyping and *BCR-ABL1* in 190/200 interphases by FISH, and *BCR-ABL1* level was high by qRT-PCR.
3. *NPM1* mutation is not only observed in de novo AML but also in CML, even in CP.

Case 6

Learning Objectives

1. To become familiar with the atypical CBC profile of CML
2. To learn how to distinguish CML, preleukemic phase vs MDS

Case History

A 44-year-old woman who had a long-standing history of chronic back pain, status post multiple lumbar spine surgeries presented to an outside hospital with jaundice. WBC 2.8, Hgb 11.1, MCV 91.4, PLT 267. A bone marrow revealed 46,XX,t(9;22)(q34;q11.2)[4]/46,XX[16]. With an outside provisional diagnosis of MDS, she was referred to us for further evaluation.

Morphologic Findings

- WBC 3.6, HGB 11.4, MCV 94, PLT 225.
- Differential (%): neutrophils 49, immature granulocytes 0, lymphocytes 39, monocytes 10, eosinophils 0, basophils 2.
- Bone marrow was 70–80% cellular with erythroid hyperplasia. Megakaryocytes were mildly increased in number with occasional dwarf forms.

- Bone marrow differential (%): blasts 3, promyelocytes 2, myelocytes 8, metamyelocytes 7, granulocytes 18, lymphocytes 5, monocytes 3, erythroid precursors 54. No dysplasia in granulocytes and erythroid lineage.

Differential Diagnosis

- MDS
- CML, preleukemic phase
- Nonneoplastic etiology

Ancillary Studies Performed on the Bone Marrow
- Karyotype: 46,XX,t(9;22)(q34;q11.2)[7]/46,XX[13]
- FISH: positive for *BCR-ABL1* rearrangement in 20/200 interphases
- qRT-PCR: b2a2 *BCR-ABL1* fusion transcript detected, *BCR-ABL1* to *ABL1* ratio 32.61%

Final Diagnosis
Chronic myeloid leukemia, *BCR-ABL1*, preleukemic phase

Treatment
The patient was started on dasatinib and then switched to imatinib due to adverse effects. Eight months later, she developed B-lymphoid BP involving cerebrospinal fluid (54% by differential). At this time, WBC 4.1, HGB 10.2, MCV 90, and PLT 310. The blast count was 0% in peripheral blood and 2% in bone marrow. Myeloid-to-erythroid ratio in the bone marrow was normalized.

Take-Home Message
1. CML patients may present cytopenia, possibly due to other etiology.
2. CML, preleukemic phase can progress, in this patient, to isolated lymphoid BP involving cerebrospinal fluid.

Case 7

Learning Objectives
1. To learn how to distinguish CML, initial lymphoid BP vs de novo ALL/LBL

Case History
A 35-year-old man presented with progressive bone pain, fatigue, nausea, vomiting, and swollen lymph nodes.

Morphologic Findings

- WBC 46.8, HGB 9.6, MCV 93, PLT 16.
- Differential (%): neutrophils 2, metamyelocytes 1, lymphocytes 15, blasts 82.
- Bone marrow was 90% cellular. Megakaryocytes were too few.
- Bone marrow differential (%): blasts 82, granulocytes 1, lymphocytes 12, monocytes 5.

Differential Diagnosis

- De novo acute leukemia
- CML, initial BP

Ancillary Studies Performed on the Bone Marrow
- Karyotype: 46,XY,t(9;22)(q34;q11.2)[9]/47,idem,+der(22)t(9;22)[2]/46,XY[9]
- FISH: positive for *BCR-ABL1* in 179/200 of interphase
- qRT-PCR: b3a2 *BCR-ABL1* fusion transcript detected, *BCR-ABL1* to *ABL1* ratio >100%
- Flow cytometry: blasts positive for CD10, CD19, CD20, CD22, CD34, CD38, CD45 dim, CD66c (partial), cytoCD79a, CD123 (partial), HLA-DR, and TdT; negative for MPO and other myeloid and T-cell markers

Diagnosis
The patient was diagnosed with **B-ALL/LBL, *BCR-ABL1 positive***, treated with hyper-CVAD plus dasatinib, and achieved complete remission. Six months after the initial diagnosis, the patient had a relapse.

Morphologic Findings

- WBC 68.7, HGB 16.3, MCV 93, PLT 446.
- Differential (%): neutrophils 43, metamyelocytes 17, lymphocytes 5, monocytes 4, basophils 1, blasts 30.
- Bone marrow was 100% cellular. Megakaryocytes were increased and "dysplastic."
- Bone marrow differential (%): blasts 78, myelocytes 2, metamyelocytes 4, granulocytes 11, eosinophils 2, lymphocytes 1, normoblasts 2.

Differential Diagnosis

- Relapsed B-ALL/LBL
- CML, lymphoid BP

Ancillary Studies Performed on the Bone Marrow
- Karyotype: 46,XY,t(9;22)(q34;q11.2)[8]/47,idem,+der(22)t(9;22)[12]
- FISH: positive for *BCR-ABL1* in 196/200 of interphase
- qRT-PCR: b3a2 *BCR-ABL1* fusion transcript detected, *BCR-ABL1* to *ABL1* ratio >100%
- Flow cytometry: blasts with a phenotype similar to that at initial diagnosis

Diagnosis
The patient was diagnosed with **relapsed B-ALL/LBL, *BCR-ABL1 positive***, treated with hyper-CVAD plus dasat-

inib, and achieved complete remission. Fourteen months after the initial diagnosis, the patient had a second relapse.

Morphologic Findings

- WBC 226.1, HGB 12.5, MCV 96, PLT 719.
- Differential (%): neutrophils 62, metamyelocytes 15, promyelocytes 2, lymphocytes 4, monocytes 4, basophils 4, eosinophils 2, blasts 7.
- Bone marrow was 100% cellular. Megakaryocytes were increased and mostly of dwarf forms.
- Bone marrow differential (%): blasts 6, promyelocytes 3, myelocytes 15, metamyelocytes 24, granulocytes 41, eosinophils 5, basophils 2, lymphocytes 1, monocytes 1, normoblasts 2.

Differential Diagnosis

- Leukemoid reaction
- CML, second CP
- De novo CML

Ancillary Studies Performed on the Bone Marrow
- Karyotype: 46,XY,t(9;22)(q34;q11.2)[20]
- FISH: positive for *BCR-ABL1* in 189/200 of interphase
- qRT-PCR: b3a2 *BCR-ABL1* fusion transcript detected, *BCR-ABL1* to *ABL1* ratio >100%
- Flow cytometry: 0.01% B-lymphoblasts and 3.1% aberrant myeloblasts

Final Diagnosis
Chronic myeloid leukemia, *BCR-ABL1*, chronic phase. Retrospectively, the disease at initial presentation represented CML, initial lymphoid BP.

Take-Home Messages
1. It is quite challenging and sometimes may be impossible to distinguish CML, initial lymphoid BP from de novo Ph+ B-ALL/LBL.
2. Retrospectively, reversion to CP supports the diagnosis of CML, initial lymphoid BP.

References

1. Swerdlow SH, Campo E, Harris NL, Jaffe ES, Pileri SA, Stein H, et al. WHO classification of tumours of haematopoietic and lymphoid tissues. 4th ed. Switzerland: WHO Press; 2017.
2. O'Brien S, Radich JP, Abboud CN, Akhtari M, Altman JK, Berman E, et al. Chronic myelogenous leukemia, version 1.2015. J Natl Compr Cancer Netw. 2014;12(11):1590–610.
3. Pane F, Frigeri F, Sindona M, Luciano L, Ferrara F, Cimino R, et al. Neutrophilic-chronic myeloid leukemia: a distinct disease with a specific molecular marker (BCR/ABL with C3/A2 junction). Blood. 1996;88(7):2410–4.
4. Cervantes F, Urbano-Ispizua A, Villamor N, Feliu E, Milla F, Lopez-Guillermo A, et al. Ph-positive chronic myeloid leukemia mimicking essential thrombocythemia and terminating into megakaryoblastic blast crisis: report of two cases with molecular studies. Leukemia. 1993;7(2):327–30.
5. Parilla M, Venkataraman G. The thin line between CML and CMML. Blood. 2017;129(17):2456.
6. Asinari MB, Zeballos M, Alicia S, Ricchi BN, Basquiera AL. A case of chronic myeloid leukemia with the m-bcr (p190) molecular rearrangement identified during treatment. Rev Bras Hematol Hemoter. 2015;37(1):55–7.
7. Soupir CP, Muzikansky A, Kantarjian H, Jones D, et al. Philadelphia chromosome-positive acute myeloid leukemia: a rare aggressive leukemia with clinicopathologic features distinct from chronic myeloid leukemia in myeloid blast crisis. Am J Clin Pathol. 2007;127(4):642–50.
8. Verma D, Kantarjian HM, Jones D, Luthra R, Borthakur G, Verstovsek S, et al. Chronic myeloid leukemia (CML) with P190 BCR-ABL: analysis of characteristics, outcomes, and prognostic significance. Blood. 2009;114(11):2232–5.
9. Gong Z, Medeiros LJ, Cortes JE, Zheng L, Khoury JD, Wang W, et al. Clinical and prognostic significance of e1a2 BCR-ABL1 transcript subtype in chronic myeloid leukemia. Blood Cancer J. 2017;7(7):e583.
10. Baccarani M, Deininger MW, Rosti G, Hochhaus A, Soverini S, Apperley JF, et al. European LeukemiaNet recommendations for the management of chronic myeloid leukemia: 2013. Blood. 2013;122(6):872–84.
11. Thompson PA, Kantarjian HM, Cortes JE. Diagnosis and treatment of chronic myeloid leukemia in 2015. Mayo Clin Proc. 2015;90(10):1440–54.
12. Jabbour E, Kantarjian H. Chronic myeloid leukemia: 2016 update on diagnosis, therapy, and monitoring. Am J Hematol. 2016;91(2):252–65.
13. Fioretos T. Chronic myeloid leukemia, In: Heim S, Mitelman F, editors. Cancer Cytogenetics: Wiley & Sons, Ltd Hoboken, NJ, USA; 2016. p. 153–74.
14. Soverini S, et al. Implications of BCR-ABL1 kinase domain-mediated resistance in chronic myeloid leukemia. Leuk Res. 2014;38(1):10–20.
15. Takimoto CH, Calvo E. Principles of oncological pharmacotherapy. In: Pazdur R, et al., editors. Cancer management: a multidisciplinary approach; UBM Medica, Norwalk, CT, USA. 2008.
16. Chaitanya PK, Kumar KA, Stalin B, Sadashivudu G, Srinivas ML. The role of mutation testing in patients with chronic myeloid leukemia in chronic phase after imatinib failure and their outcomes after treatment modification: single-institutional experience over 13 years. Indian J Med Paediatr Oncol. 2017;38(3):328–33.
17. Apperley JF. Part I: mechanisms of resistance to imatinib in chronic myeloid leukaemia. Lancet Oncol. 2007;8(11):1018–29.
18. Sherbenou DW, Hantschel O, Kaupe I, Willis S, Bumm T, Turaga LP, et al. BCR-ABL SH3-SH2 domain mutations in chronic myeloid leukemia patients on imatinib. Blood. 2010; 116(17):3278–85.
19. O'Hare T, Zabriskie MS, Eiring AM, Deininger MW. Pushing the limits of targeted therapy in chronic myeloid leukaemia. Nat Rev Cancer. 2012;12(8):513–26.
20. Barnes DJ, Palaiologou D, Panousopoulou E, Schultheis B, Yong AS, Wong A, et al. Bcr-Abl expression levels determine the rate of development of resistance to imatinib mesylate in chronic myeloid leukemia. Cancer Res. 2005;65(19):8912–9.
21. Thomas J, Wang L, Clark RE, Pirmohamed M. Active transport of imatinib into and out of cells: implications for drug resistance. Blood. 2004;104(12):3739–45.

22. Jiang X, Smith C, Eaves A, Eaves C. The challenges of targeting chronic myeloid leukemia stem cells. Clin Lymphoma Myeloma. 2007;7(Suppl 2):S71–80.
23. Wang W, Cortes JE, Lin P, Beaty MW, Ai D, Amin HM, et al. Clinical and prognostic significance of 3q26.2 and other chromosome 3 abnormalities in CML in the era of tyrosine kinase inhibitors. Blood. 2015;126(14):1699–706.
24. Chen Z, Shao C, Wang W, Zuo Z, Mou X, Hu SJ, et al. Cytogenetic landscape and impact in blast phase of chronic myeloid leukemia in the era of tyrosine kinase inhibitor therapy. Leukemia. 2017;31(3):585–92.
25. Wu J, Meng F, Kong LY, Peng Z, Ying Y, Bornmann WG, et al. Association between imatinib-resistant BCR-ABL mutation-negative leukemia and persistent activation of LYN kinase. J Natl Cancer Inst. 2008;100(13):926–39.
26. Quentmeier H, Eberth S, Romani J, Zaborski M, Drexler HG. BCR-ABL1-independent PI3Kinase activation causing imatinib-resistance. J Hematol Oncol. 2011;4:6.
27. Milojkovic D, Apperley J. Mechanisms of resistance to imatinib and second-generation tyrosine inhibitors in chronic myeloid leukemia. Clin Cancer Res. 2009;15(24):7519–27.
28. Quintas-Cardama A, Kantarjian HM, Cortes JE. Mechanisms of primary and secondary resistance to imatinib in chronic myeloid leukemia. Cancer Control. 2009;16(2):122–31.
29. Comert M, Baran Y, Saydam G. Changes in molecular biology of chronic myeloid leukemia in tyrosine kinase inhibitor era. Am J Blood Res. 2013;3(3):191–200.
30. Soverini S, et al. Contribution of ABL kinase domain mutations to imatinib resistance in different subsets of Philadelphia-positive patients: by the GIMEMA Working Party on Chronic Myeloid Leukemia. Clin Cancer Res. 2006;12(24):7374–9.
31. Ross DM, O'Hely M, Bartley PA, Dang P, Score J, Goyne JM, et al. Distribution of genomic breakpoints in chronic myeloid leukemia: analysis of 308 patients. Leukemia. 2013;27(10):2105–7.
32. Melo JV. The diversity of BCR-ABL fusion proteins and their relationship to leukemia phenotype. Blood. 1996;88(7):2375–84.
33. Barnes DJ, Melo JV. Cytogenetic and molecular genetic aspects of chronic myeloid leukaemia. Acta Haematol. 2002;108(4):180–202.
34. Burmeister T, Reinhardt R. A multiplex PCR for improved detection of typical and atypical BCR-ABL fusion transcripts. Leuk Res. 2008;32(4):579–85.
35. Johansson B, Fioretos T, Mitelman F. Cytogenetic and molecular genetic evolution of chronic myeloid leukemia. Acta Haematol. 2002;107(2):76–94.
36. Gong Z, Zheng L, Tang Z, Chen Z, Wang W, Bai S, et al. Role of complexity of variant Philadelphia chromosome in chronic myeloid leukemia in the era of tyrosine kinase inhibitor therapy. Ann Hematol. 2017;96(3):501–4.
37. Chen Z, Wang W, Cortes JE, Liu E, Miranda RN, Zhao C, et al. Differential clinical and prognostic impact of myeloid sarcoma vs medullary myeloid blast phase of chronic myelogenous leukemia in the era of tyrosine kinase inhibitor therapy. Blood Cancer J. 2016;6:e418.
38. Gong Z, Medeiros LJ, Cortes JE, Chen Z, Zheng L, Li Y, et al. Cytogenetics-based risk prediction of blastic transformation of chronic myeloid leukemia in the era of TKI therapy. Blood Adv. 2017;1(26):2541–52.
39. Medina J, Kantarjian H, Talpaz M, O'Brien S, Garcia-Manero G, Giles F, et al. Chromosomal abnormalities in Philadelphia chromosome-negative metaphases appearing during imatinib mesylate therapy in patients with Philadelphia chromosome-positive chronic myelogenous leukemia in chronic phase. Cancer. 2003;98(9):1905–11.
40. O'Dwyer ME, Gatter KM, Loriaux M, Druker BJ, Olson SB, Magenis RE, et al. Demonstration of Philadelphia chromosome negative abnormal clones in patients with chronic myelogenous leukemia during major cytogenetic responses induced by imatinib mesylate. Leukemia. 2003;17(3):481–7.
41. Jabbour E, Kantarjian HM, Abruzzo LV, O'Brien S, Garcia-Manero G, Verstovsek S, et al. Chromosomal abnormalities in Philadelphia chromosome negative metaphases appearing during imatinib mesylate therapy in patients with newly diagnosed chronic myeloid leukemia in chronic phase. Blood. 2007;110(8):2991–5.
42. Kovitz C, Kantarjian H, Garcia-Manero G, Abruzzo LV, Cortes J. Myelodysplastic syndromes and acute leukemia developing after imatinib mesylate therapy for chronic myeloid leukemia. Blood. 2006;108(8):2811–3.
43. de Franca Azevedo I, da Silva Júnior RM, de Vasconcelos AV, das Neves WB, de Barros Correia Melo FC, Melo RA. Frequency of p190 and p210 BCR-ABL rearrangements and survival in Brazilian adult patients with acute lymphoblastic leukemia. Rev Bras Hematol Hemoter. 2014;36(5):351–5.
44. Jaso J, Thomas DA, Cunningham K, Jorgensen JL, Kantarjian HM, Medeiros LJ, et al. Prognostic significance of immunophenotypic and karyotypic features of Philadelphia positive B-lymphoblastic leukemia in the era of tyrosine kinase inhibitors. Cancer. 2011;117(17):4009–17.
45. Verrma SP, Dutta TK, Vinod KV, Dubashi B, Ariga KK. Philadelphia chromosome positive pre-T cell acute lymphoblastic leukemia: a rare case report and short review. Indian J Hematol Blood Transfus. 2014;30(Suppl 1):177–9.
46. Armas A, Chen C, Mims M, Rivero G. Uncovering clinical features of De Novo Philadelphia positive myelodysplasia. Case Rep Hematol. 2017;2017:5404131.
47. Gale RP, Hlatky L, Sachs RK, Radivoyevitch T. Why is there so much therapy-related AML and MDS and so little therapy-related CML? Leuk Res. 2014;38(10):1162–4.
48. Kurt H, Zheng L, Kantarjian HM, Tang G, Ravandi-Kashani F, Garcia-Manero G, et al. Secondary Philadelphia chromosome acquired during therapy of acute leukemia and myelodysplastic syndrome. Mod Pathol. 2018;31:1141–54.
49. Yang LH, Su P, Luedke C, Lu CM, Louissaint A, McCall CM, et al. Chronic myeloid leukemia following treatment for primary neoplasms or other medical conditions: a report of 21 cases and review of the literature. Am J Clin Pathol. 2018;150(3):246–58.
50. Chen Z, Wang W, Verstovsek S, Cortes JE, Medeiros LJ, Hu S. Chronic myelogenous leukemia in patients with MPL or JAK2 mutation-positive myeloproliferative neoplasm. Int J Lab Hematol. 2015;37(6):e150–2.
51. Soderquist CR, Ewalt MD, Czuchlewski DR, Geyer JT, Rogers HJ, Hsi ED, et al. Myeloproliferative neoplasms with concurrent BCR-ABL1 translocation and JAK2 V617F mutation: a multi-institutional study from the bone marrow pathology group. Mod Pathol. 2018;31(5):690–704.
52. Pingali SR, Mathiason MA, Lovrich SD, Go RS. Emergence of chronic myelogenous leukemia from a background of myeloproliferative disorder: JAK2V617F as a potential risk factor for BCR-ABL translocation. Clin Lymphoma Myeloma. 2009;9(5):E25–9.
53. Mirza I, Frantz C, Clarke G, Voth AJ, Turner R. Transformation of polycythemia vera to chronic myelogenous leukemia. Arch Pathol Lab Med. 2007;131(11):1719–24.
54. Mu Q, Ma Q, Wang Y, Chen Z, Tong X, Chen FF, et al. Cytogenetic profile of 1,863 Ph/BCR-ABL-positive chronic myelogenous leukemia patients from the Chinese population. Ann Hematol. 2012;91(7):1065–72.
55. Arana-Trejo RM, Ignatio G, Amador-Sanchez R, Cruz-Rico J, Hernandez M, Salvidar I, et al. Frequency of p190 and p210 BCR-ABL fusions genes in acute lymphoblastic leukemia in a long group of adults and childhood. Blood. 2016;128(22):1.
56. Gleissner B, Gökbuget N, Bartram CR, Janssen B, Rieder H, Janssen JW, Fonatsch C, et al. Leading prognostic relevance of the BCR-ABL translocation in adult acute B-lineage lymphoblas-

tic leukemia: a prospective study of the German Multicenter Trial Group and confirmed polymerase chain reaction analysis. Blood. 2002;99(5):1536–43.
57. Dombret H, Gabert J, Boiron JM, Rigal-Huguet F, Blaise D, Thomas X, et al. Outcome of treatment in adults with Philadelphia chromosome-positive acute lymphoblastic leukemia--results of the prospective multicenter LALA-94 trial. Blood. 2002;100(7):2357–66.
58. Wang Y, Gu M, Mi Y, Qiu L, Bian S, Wang J. Clinical characteristics and outcomes of mixed phenotype acute leukemia with Philadelphia chromosome positive and/or bcr-abl positive in adult. Int J Hematol. 2011;94(6):552–5.
59. Konopleva M, Cardama AQ, Kantarjian H, Cortes J. Molecular Biology and Cytogenetics of Chronic Myeloid Leukemia, in: Wiemik PH, Dutcher JP, Gertz MA, editors. Neoplastic disease of the blood: 6th ed, Springer Cham, Switzerland. pp 29–47, 2018.
60. Reboursiere E, Chantepie S, Gac AC, Reman O. Rare but authentic Philadelphia-positive acute myeloblastic leukemia: two case reports and a literature review of characteristics, treatment and outcome. Hematol Oncol Stem Cell Ther. 2015;8(1):28–33.

Chronic Myeloproliferative Neoplasms (Other Than Chronic Myeloid Leukemia)

23

Matthew E. Keeney and Sharathkumar Bhagavathi

List of Frequently Asked Questions

1. What are the major subtypes of myeloproliferative neoplasms?
2. What are the typical morphological findings in MPNs?
3. What are mimics of MPNs, and what are the clinical implications of misinterpretation of the true diagnosis and mimics with regard to mistreatment and/or prognosis?
4. Which morphological findings in the peripheral blood/BM aspirate/biopsy are reliably diagnostic? Which ones suggest the diagnosis? Which is (are) unreliable for diagnosis? Which findings rule out the diagnosis?
5. What is the minimal and optimal ancillary workup for diagnosis and subclassification of MPNs?
6. Which ancillary test results are diagnostic, suggestive of diagnosis, unreliable for diagnosis, or rule out the diagnosis?
7. What is the workup to provide prognostic and therapeutic target information? What treatments are available for MPNs?
8. Which subtypes of MPNs are clinically relevant and which are morphologically defined but have unproven or minimal clinical relevance?
9. What is an adequate specimen for MPNs?
10. What information can be conveyed to the clinician during each stage of the workup?
11. What should be the approach to provide maximum, but defensible, information from limited specimen or workup? What is an appropriate descriptive diagnosis in such situations?
12. When is a diagnostic comment necessary and what should be discussed in the diagnostic comment for MPNs?
13. When is it appropriate to seek external consultation for this entity?

M. E. Keeney (✉)
Pathology, University of Iowa Hospitals and Clinics, Iowa City, IA, USA
e-mail: mekeeney@llu.edu

S. Bhagavathi
Pathology and Laboratory Medicine, University of Iowa Carver College of Medicine, Iowa City, IA, USA
e-mail: Sharathkumar-bhagavathi@uiowa.edu

1. What are the major subtypes of myeloproliferative neoplasms (MPNs)?

- Major subtypes of myeloproliferative neoplasms according to the 2017 World Health Organization Classification of Tumors of Hematopoietic and Lymphoid Tissues [1] include:
  - Chronic myeloid leukemia, *BCR-ABL1* positive (CML)
  - Chronic neutrophilic leukemia (CNL)
  - Polycythemia vera (PV)
  - Primary myelofibrosis (PMF) including both pre-fibrotic/early primary myelofibrosis and overt primary myelofibrosis
  - Essential thrombocythemia (ET)
  - Chronic eosinophilic leukemia, not otherwise specified (CEL, NOS)
  - Myeloproliferative neoplasm, unclassifiable (MPN-U)
- Mastocytosis and myeloid/lymphoid neoplasms with eosinophilia and gene rearrangement are separate chapters of the 2017 WHO, but they are included here for convenience.
- CML is the most common subtype of MPN but is considered separately in Chap. 22 because its overall biology, diagnosis, treatment, and clinical behavior are uniquely connected to the presence of the *BCR/ABL* translocation.
- A pluripotent hematopoietic stem cell is the postulated cell of origin for MPNs. Most MPNs have mutated tyrosine kinases or mutations/rearrangements involving

E. Wang, A. S. Lagoo (eds.), *Practical Lymph Node and Bone Marrow Pathology*, Practical Anatomic Pathology,
https://doi.org/10.1007/978-3-030-32189-5_23

downstream kinases resulting in the overactivation of transcriptionally active proteins. Just as these entities have similar and sometimes identical molecular drivers, so too they have similar morphologic and clinical presentations. MPNs are subclassified based on clinical, morphological, and laboratory (histochemical, cytogenetic, molecular) findings.

- MPNs typically have insidious onsets and are often detected incidentally. Many MPNs are discovered early in their disease course on routine blood work. Unexplained itching, tingling, or burning sensation of skin, characteristically induced by contact with water (aquagenic pruritus) is a frequent early symptom in PV and less often in ET. PMF tends to have the greatest symptom burden (constitutional symptoms including weight loss and cachexia) but presents asymptomatically in nearly a third of cases.

2. What are the typical morphological findings in MPNs?

The clonal myeloid proliferations in MPNs are productive in contrast to myelodysplastic syndrome. Hence, MPN should be suspected in the setting of prolonged leukocytosis, increased hemoglobin/hematocrit, thrombocytosis, or a combination of these. Early MPNs show marrow hypercellularity. Hepatosplenomegaly is commonly seen. All MPNs have the potential to progress to acute leukemia, myelofibrosis, and/or myelodysplasia. Depending on the timing of the biopsy in the natural course of the disease, morphological findings can vary significantly within the same patient.

CNL

- Peripheral blood neutrophilia with ≥80% mature neutrophils and bands, only rare blasts, and <10% early neutrophil precursors is characteristic of CNL. Patients tend to have splenomegaly often with accompanying hepatomegaly. The bone marrow tends to be hypercellular with an elevated M:E ratio. Blasts are not increased above 5% and dyspoiesis is absent. Proliferation of megakaryocytes and erythrocytes may be seen, but a neutrophilic predominance is essential.
- CNL is extremely rare, and a reactive leukemoid reaction will show significant laboratory and morphological overlap. A recently discovered mutation in *CSF3R* gene can assist in diagnosis.
- Diagnostic criteria per WHO [1]:
  1. Blood WBC count >25 × 10^9/L.
     Segmented and band neutrophils compose more than 80%.
     Neutrophil precursors compose less than 10%.
     Blasts are rare.
     Monocyte count <1 × 10^9/L.
     No dysgranulopoiesis.
  2. Bone marrow hypercellularity.
     Neutrophils increased in number and percentages.
     Normal maturation of neutrophils.
     Myeloblasts comprise less than 5%.
  3. Not meeting criteria for chronic myeloid leukemia, polycythemia vera, essential thrombocythemia, or primary myelofibrosis.
  4. No rearrangement of *PDGFRA*, *PDGFRB*, *FGFR1*, or *PCM1-JAK2* fusion.
  5. *CSF3R* T618I or another activating *CSF3R* mutation.
     Or
     Persistent neutrophilia (>3 months), splenomegaly, and no identifiable cause of reactive neutrophilia including absence of a plasma cell neoplasm or, if a plasma cell neoplasm is present, demonstration of clonality of myeloid cells by cytogenetic or molecular studies.

PV

- Erythrocytosis and marrow hypercellularity with panmyelosis must be seen to consider PV. In addition, *either* the presence of a *JAK2* V617F or *JAK2* exon 12 mutation *or* a subnormal serum erythropoietin level is required for the diagnosis. Circulating blasts are rare or absent. A prominent increase in erythroid and megakaryocytic precursors is commonly seen in the marrow. The megakaryocytes lack significant atypia, but they may show hyperlobated nuclei and morphologic overlap with the megakaryocytes of ET. Those of PV should show pleomorphism with a mixture of normally lobated and normally folded nuclei. The finding of at least moderate fibrosis may indicate post–polycythemia vera myelofibrosis.
- Diagnostic criteria per WHO [1]:
  - Diagnosis of PV requires three major criteria or the first two major criteria and the minor criterion.
  - Major criteria:
    1. Elevated Hb (>16.5 g/dL in men; >16 g/dL in women) or HCT (>49% in men; >48% in women) or RBC mass (>25% above mean normal)
    2. Bone marrow hypercellularity with panmyelosis
    3. Presence of *JAK2* V617F or *JAK2* exon 12 mutation
  - Minor criterion:
    Subnormal serum erythropoietin level

PMF

- The classic "book picture" of PMF is a hypocellular, fibrotic bone marrow (grade 2–3 out of 3) with megakaryocyte atypia, and subsequent peripheral blood leukoerythroblastosis with tear drop cells. However, these findings are characteristic of PMF in later stages of its natural course and are not seen in early or pre-fibrotic PMF.

- A diagnosis of pre-fibrotic PMF requires megakaryocyte proliferation and atypia and increased marrow cellularity with grade ≤1 fibrosis. Note that pre-fibrotic PMF may be diagnosed without any marrow fibrosis provided that there is megakaryocyte proliferation and atypia, a characteristic mutation (*JAK2, MPL, CALR,* or other; see Question 5), and the fulfillment of at least one minor criterion (anemia, leukocytosis, splenomegaly, elevated lactate dehydrogenase, leukoerythroblastosis). These same criteria in a marrow with grade 2–3 fibrosis would be sufficient for a diagnosis of PMF (fibrotic phase).
- The megakaryocytes of pre-fibrotic PMF are the most atypical megakaryocytes of all MPNs. They are large with cloud-like or hyperchromatic balloon-shaped nuclei. They tend to form clusters, particularly near trabeculae and vascular sinuses. Naked megakaryocyte nuclei are frequently seen. These morphologic features help to make the clinically important distinction between pre-fibrotic PMF with thrombocytosis and ET. Unfortunately, these pathological findings may not be sufficiently characteristic in every case, and the final classification of the MPN may have to be deferred to clinical findings and/or a future biopsy.
- Diagnostic criteria [1]:
  - PMF (pre-fibrotic stage) diagnosis requires three major criteria and at least one minor criterion.
  - Major criteria:
    1. Megakaryocytic hyperplasia and atypia with reticulin fibrosis less than 1, granulocytic hyperplasia, and often erythroid hypoplasia
    2. Not meeting criteria for CML, PV, ET, MDS, or other myeloid neoplasm
    3. *JAK2*, *CALR*, or *MPL* mutation
       Or
       Presence of another clonal marker
       Or
       Absence of minor reactive bone marrow reticulin fibrosis
  - Minor criteria:
    Presence of at least one, confirmed in two consecutive samples:
    Anemia not due to comorbid condition
    Leukocytosis > 11 × 10^9/L
    Palpable splenomegaly
    Increased LDH level
- Diagnostic criteria:
  - PMF (fibrotic stage) diagnosis requires three major criteria and at least one minor criterion.
  - Major criteria:
    1. Megakaryocytic hyperplasia and dysplasia with more than grade 1 reticulin and or collagen fibrosis.
    2. Not meeting criteria for ET, PV, CML, MDS, or other myeloid disorder.
    3. *JAK2*, *CALR*, or *MPL* mutation
       Or
       Presence of another clonal marker
       Or
       Absence of reactive myelofibrosis
  - Minor criteria:
    Presence of at least one, confirmed in two consecutive samples:
    - Anemia not due to comorbid condition
    - Leukocytosis > 11 × 10^9/L
    - Palpable splenomegaly
    - Increased LDH
    - Leukoerythroblastosis

ET

- Peripheral blood thrombocytosis and megakaryocyte proliferation with atypia are characteristic of ET. Platelets vary significantly in size and shape and may show occasional dysplastic forms (hypogranular platelets with bizarre shapes). The bone marrow cellularity is typically normal or slightly increased with proliferation of the megakaryocyte lineage. Megakaryocyte atypia of ET differs substantially from that of PMF.
- Megakaryocytes of ET are large with abundant cytoplasm and multilobated, staghorn-like nuclei. Unlike the megakaryocytes of PMF, ET megakaryocytes rarely form clusters. ET should have no, or only minimal, fibrosis. ET can eventually progress, and the finding of at least moderate fibrosis may indicate post-essential thrombocythemia myelofibrosis.
- Diagnostic criteria [1]:
  - Requires all major or three major criteria plus one minor criterion.
  - Major criteria:
    1. Platelet count > 450 × 10^9/L.
    2. Bone marrow showing predominantly megakaryocytic hyperplasia with mature enlarged hyperlobated nuclei. No significant erythroid and myeloid hyperplasia or left shift. Reticulin fibrosis should be equal or less than grade 1.
    3. WHO criteria for CML, PV, PMF, or other myeloid disorders not met.
    4. *JAK2*, *CALR*, or *MPL* mutation.
  - Minor criteria:
    Presence of a clonal marker or absence of evidence of reactive thrombocytosis

CEL, NOS

- Peripheral blood eosinophilia is required for the diagnosis of CEL, NOS. In addition, diagnostic criteria for other MPNs must not be met. If peripheral blood or bone marrow blasts are <2% or <5%, respectively, a clonal cytogenetic or molecular marker must be present (but not *PDGFRA, PDGFRB, FGFR1, PCM1-JAK2, ETV6-JAK2,* or *BCR-JAK2* fusions as these would categorize the process as a myeloid/lymphoid neoplasm with eosinophilia and gene rearrangement). Bone marrow is typically hypercellular with increased eosinophilic precursors. Increased blasts and dysplastic eosinophilic maturation favor a diagnosis of CEL, NOS over reactive eosinophilia.

- Diagnostic criteria [1]:
  1. Eosinophilia (eosinophil count $\geq 1.5 \times 10^9/L$).
  2. WHO criteria for CML, PV, ET, PMF, CNL, CMML, and atypical CML are not met.
  3. No rearrangement of *PDGFRA*, *PDGFRB*, or *FGFR1* or no *PCM1-JAK2*, *ETV6-JAK2*, or *BCR-JAK2* fusion.
  4. Blast cells constitute <20% of the cells (blood or bone marrow) and inv (16)(p13.1q22), t(16;16)(p13.1;q22), t(8;21)(q22;q22.1), and other diagnostic features of acute myeloid leukemia are absent.
  5. There is a clonal cytogenetic or molecular abnormality.[a]
     Or
     Blast cells account for ≥2% of cells in the peripheral blood or ≥5% in the bone marrow.
     ([a]Mutations of *TET2*, *ASXL1*, and *DNMT3A* genes can occur in elderly as aging process, and all reactive conditions for eosinophilia should be excluded).

MPN-U

- The types of cases that fall within this diagnostic category can be thought of as too early, too late, or too confounded. The "too early" cases are those which have features of an MPN, but have yet to fully manifest the characteristic findings. "Too late" cases are those that have reached a final common pathway of MPNs and show severe myelofibrosis, increased blasts, or dysplastic changes that mask the underlying disorder. The "too confounded" cases are those in which an MPN is suspected, but a concurrent inflammatory condition or neoplasm disguise diagnostic laboratory or pathological features.
- Diagnostic criteria [1]:
  1. Features of myeloproliferative neoplasms are met.
  2. WHO criteria for other MPNs, MDS,[a] and MDS/MPN are not met.
  3. *JAK2*, *CALR*, or *MPL* mutations associated with MPN.
     Or
     Presence of another clonal marker[b]
     Or
     Absence of a cause of reactive fibrosis[c]

[a]History of any treatment, comorbidity, and natural progression of the disease process must be excluded.
[b]If *JAK2*, *CALR*, and *MPL* mutations are absent, mutations of *ASXL1*, *EZH2*, *TET2*, *IDH1*, *IDH2*, *SRSF2*, and *SF3B1* may be of help to confirm clonal myeloid process.
[c]Marrow fibrosis secondary to infection, inflammatory, autoimmune, myeloid, and nonmyeloid malignancy.

Mastocytosis

- Mastocytosis is a clinically heterogeneous disease ranging from mild skin involvement to organ failure and death. This rare neoplasm is divided clinically into rarer subcategories depending on the extent and sites of involvement. Fortunately, for the pathologist evaluating bone marrow biopsies, mastocytosis is relatively straightforward, requiring the identification of an abnormal mast cell infiltrate in the marrow defined as: more than one aggregate of at least 15 mast cells with
  - Cytologic atypia: >25% of mast cells are spindled or immature in appearance.
  - Abnormal phenotype: expression of CD25.
  - Serum tryptase level persistently above 20 ng/mL.
  - Presence of an activating mutation in the *KIT* gene at codon 816.
- In the presence of bone marrow aggregates of mast cells, only one atypical feature is required for the diagnosis of systemic mastocytosis. Three atypical features are required for the diagnosis in the absence of bone marrow mast cell aggregates.
- If these features are seen in addition to a hematological neoplasm, such as AML, MDS, or other nonmast cell MPN, a diagnosis of systemic mastocytosis with an associated hematological neoplasm is appropriate.
- Diagnostic criteria [1]:
  - Cutaneous mastocytosis
    Typical skin lesions of urticaria pigmentosa/maculopapular cutaneous mastocytosis/diffuse cutaneous mastocytosis or solitary mastocytoma with typical histological infiltrates (diffuse or multifocal) of mast cells in skin biopsy.
  - Systemic mastocytosis
    - Require either major criteriaon (multifocal dense infiltrates of mast cells detected in bone marrow or other extracutaneous organs) plus one minor criterion or at least three minor criteria are met.
    - Minor criteria:
      1. In biopsy sections
         >25% of the mast cells in the infiltrate are spindle-shaped or have atypical morphology
         or

>25% of all mast cells in bone marrow aspirate smears are immature or atypical.
2. Activating mutation at codon 816 of *KIT* (blood or bone marrow or extracutaneous organ).
3. Mast cells express CD25 with or without CD2 in addition to other mast cell markers.
4. Serum total tryptase is persistently >20 ng/mL, unless there is an associated myeloid neoplasm, in which case this parameter is void.

Myeloid/Lymphoid Neoplasms with Eosinophilia and Gene Rearrangement

- When eosinophilia is seen in conjunction with a myeloid or lymphoid neoplasm, the presence of a disease defining translocation should be investigated. Although eosinophilia is typically present and used within the name, it is not always seen in this diagnostic category.
- The morphologic features vary depending on the myeloid/lymphoid neoplasm and range from myeloid sarcoma to T-lymphoblastic leukemia. Peripheral blood eosinophilia and bone marrow hypercellularity with increased eosinophils are characteristic findings. Eosinophils showing dysplastic (smaller and sparse granulation, hypolobation, cytoplasmic vacuoles) maturation favor a neoplastic process over a reactive process.
- The translocations seen in myeloid/lymphoid neoplasms with eosinophilia and gene rearrangement involve the *PDGFRA, PDGFRB,* and *FGFR1* genes. A provisional category is included in the current WHO for myeloid/lymphoid neoplasms with eosinophilia and *PCM1-JAK2* translocation. Reported cases with this translocation show highly variable survival.

3. What are mimics of MPNs, and what are the clinical implications of misinterpretation of the true diagnosis and mimics with regard to mistreatment and/or prognosis?

Not too long ago, MPN was considered a diagnosis of exclusion, as reactive conditions are notorious mimics. However, with recent discovery of molecular events and advent of cost effective molecular testing, the diagnosis is increasingly based on molecular tests. The mimics are broadly based on blood and bone marrow findings.

- Mimics based on complete blood count and morphology: Reactive neutrophilia secondary to infection or malignancy may mimic chronic neutrophilic leukemia. Polycythemia vera has a number of mimics which include both primary (congenital) and secondary (physiologic or compensatory) causes of erythrocytosis. There are many causes of eosinophilia (mnemonic NAACP: neoplasm, allergic, adrenal insufficiency, collagen vascular disease, parasites). The use of ancillary cytogenetic and molecular studies and correlation with the clinical presentation, bone marrow, and laboratory data are crucial for the accurate diagnosis of MPNs.
- Mimics based on bone marrow hypercellularity: Any process causing marrow hypercellularity may mimic an early MPN. Mimics of pre-fibrotic PMF include other MPNs and reactive inflammatory conditions. Similarly, overt PMF will have an appearance that may closely resemble post-PV or post-ET myelofibrosis. Distinguishing between an MPN and a reactive condition by marrow biopsy alone is challenging. Definitive exclusion of an infection or alternative malignancy as the cause of a leukemoid reaction requires clinical and radiographic information often not available to the pathologist evaluating the bone marrow biopsy. In such cases, and in the absence of ancillary molecular data, a descriptive comment suggesting alternate explanations of the observed pathology is prudent.
- A frequently encountered problem is the distinction of one MPN from another. The distinction of pre-fibrotic PMF from ET is particularly problematic as both will have peripheral blood thrombocytosis. Cases of early PV with thrombocytosis can be confused with ET as well. While prognosis differs significantly, the therapeutic consequences of a misdiagnosis between MPNs are often mitigated by the fact that they each have similar management depending on the patient's clinical presentation and risk as assessed by several scoring systems including the International prognostic scoring system (IPSS) and the Dynamic International Prognostic Scoring System (DIPSS). See Question 7 regarding the prognosis and treatments for myeloproliferative neoplasms.

4. Which morphological findings in the peripheral blood/BM aspirate/ biopsy are reliably diagnostic? Which ones suggest the diagnosis? Which is (are) unreliable for diagnosis? Which findings rule out the diagnosis?

- Peripheral blood findings in MPNs show significant overlap. Prolonged leukocytosis, thrombocytosis, and/or erythrocytosis without clinically identifiable etiology should raise the suspicion of an MPN. Marked thrombocytosis with variably sized platelets may suggest MPN, but there are no morphologic findings on the peripheral blood smear that are pathognomonic for an MPN. Eosinophilia may be seen in several MPNs and reactive states, but marked eosinophilia with atypical forms is more suggestive of a neoplastic process and should clue the pathologist into the differential diagnosis of CEL-NOS or myeloid/lymphoid neoplasms with eosinophilia and gene rearrangement. Leukoerythroblastosis with dacrocytes is nonspecific, but it suggests a diagnosis of PMF.

- Dysplastic findings in a majority of peripheral blood granulocytes and platelets should *not* be seen and would instead suggest a diagnosis of MDS or an overlap of MDS/MPN.
- Bone marrow morphology also shows overlap among the MPNs with most early disease showing age-adjusted marrow hypercellularity and expansion of one or more lineages.
- Dysplastic changes (refer to MDS chapter for specific microscopic findings) should be rare to absent. Attention should be focused on the megakaryocyte distribution and morphology as these can provide clues to the specific MPN.
- Classic megakaryocyte findings in MPNs are summarized in Table 23.1. The megakaryocyte morphologies are not entirely specific to each corresponding MPN and should be interpreted in the context of the clinical and laboratory presentation.

Table 23.1 Characteristic of megakaryocyte findings in MPNs

	Morphology	Example
CML	Small, hypolobate Dispersed throughout marrow	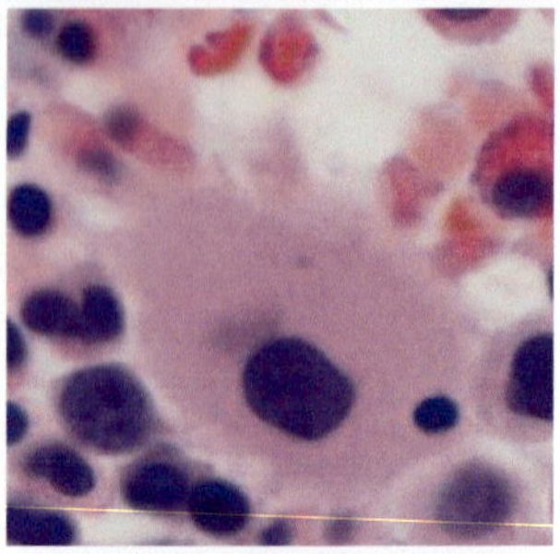
PV	Variably sized, increased in number, frequent hypersegmented nuclei Loose clusters	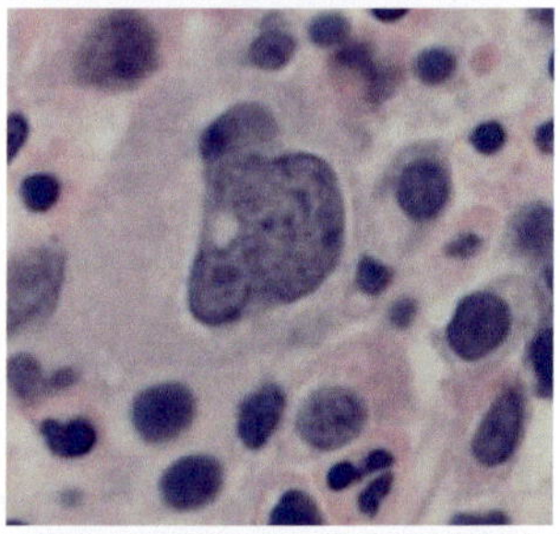
PMF	Enlarged with hyperchromatic bizarre, bulbous, balloon-like nuclei Dense clusters of megakaryocytes near sinuses and trabeculae	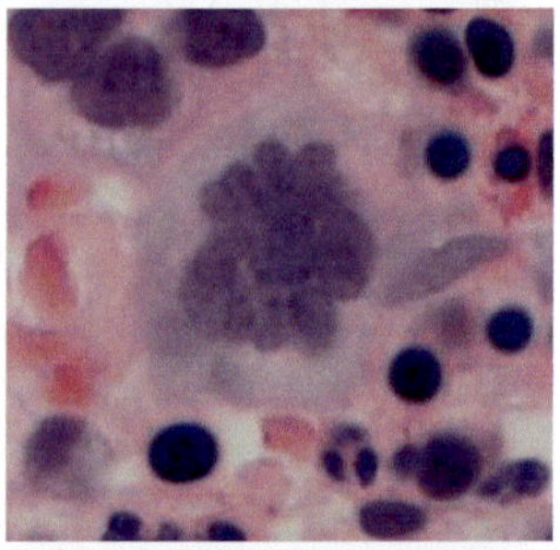
ET	Large with abundant cytoplasm and hypersegmented, staghorn-like nuclei Dispersed or loose clusters	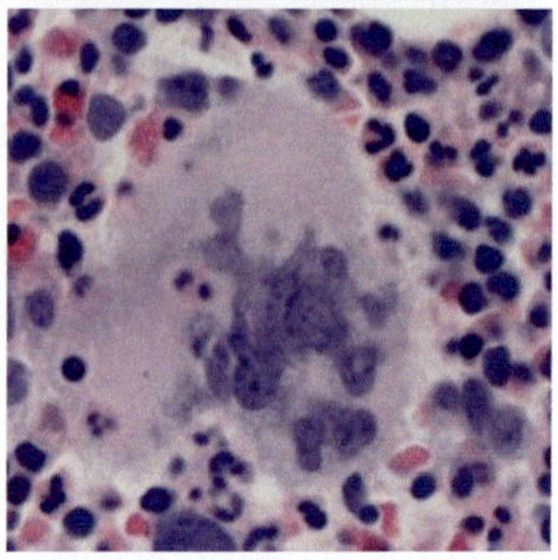

5. What is the minimal and optimal ancillary workup for diagnosis and subclassification of MPNs?

- Morphologic evaluation of peripheral blood with a complete blood count and differential, assessment of bone marrow aspirate smears with iron stain, and a core biopsy with reticulin and trichrome are the minimum requirements to suggest the diagnosis of a myeloid neoplasm.
- The minimum molecular or cytogenetic workup at the time of diagnosis is the evaluation of peripheral blood or bone marrow aspirate for the *BCR-ABL* translocation as the exclusion of *BCR-ABL1*-positive CML is a required major criterion for CNL, PMF, ET, and CEL-NOS.
- The addition of molecular studies to detect *JAK2* V617F, *JAK2* exon 12, *CALR*, and *MPL* mutations would assist in the diagnosis of the vast majority PV, PMF, and ET cases [2].
- A minority of PMF and ET cases (roughly 15%) will not be detected with this panel. For such cases, the addition of *ASXL1, EZH2, TET2, SRSF2,* and *SF3B1* could be considered. For the rare diagnosis of CNL, testing for mutations in *CSF3R* is recommended [3, 4].
- The optimal ancillary workup for marrow involvement by mastocytosis (spindled mast cells with a background of eosinophils and lymphocytes) would include flow cytometry or immunohistochemical staining for CD2 and CD25 and molecular testing for *KIT* codon 816 mutations.
- The required ancillary workup for myeloid/lymphoid neoplasms with eosinophilia and gene rearrangement would include fluorescence in situ hybridization (FISH) to detect rearrangements of *PDGFRA, PDGFRB,* and *FGFR1*. Of note, the common *FIP1L1-PDGFRA* fusion gene is cryptic (not detected with a karyotype) as it results from a deletion of a portion of the long arm of chromosome 4. This results in the deletion of the *CHIC2* gene in

patients with this fusion. While RT-PCR can be used to detect this translocation, a FISH probe for the *CHIC2* gene can be used as a surrogate.

6. Which ancillary test results are diagnostic, suggestive of diagnosis, unreliable for diagnosis, or rule out the diagnosis?

- The vast majority of MPNs will contain a well-characterized mutation or translocation. As a major criterion for each respective diagnosis, these mutations or translocations essentially seal the diagnosis when found in a case meeting the quantitative requirements and morphologic appearance of a suspected diagnosis. Note that the *JAK2* mutations are seen in PV, while *JAK2, CALR,* and *MPL* mutations are seen in ET and PMF. Because of this molecular overlap, no one mutation is pathognomonic for one MPN and instead must be used in context of the morphologic and laboratory findings.
- The characteristic molecular findings of MPNs are summarized in Fig. 23.1. The presence of the *BCR-ABL1* translocation rules out the diagnosis of CNL, PMF, ET, and CEL-NOS. The morphological finding with clonality (translocations, point mutations, amplification, etc.) detection by cytogenetics, FISH, NGS, or molecular assay will be diagnostic. Peripheral blood can be sent for clonality testing in most cases. It is important to note that *JAK2* and *BCR-ABL1* mutations can occur at very low copy number in healthy people, especially in elderly population [5, 6].

7. What is the workup to provide prognostic and therapeutic target information? What treatments are available for MPNs?

- Fortunately, the ancillary studies that aid in the diagnosis of an MPN also provide prognostic and therapeutic information. Ruxolitinib, a JAK inhibitor, is used in the treatment of PV, ET, and PMF even in the absence of *JAK2* mutations [7]. Other JAK inhibitors are in different stages of development [8]. Table 23.2 summarizes current therapies for PV, ET, and PMF.

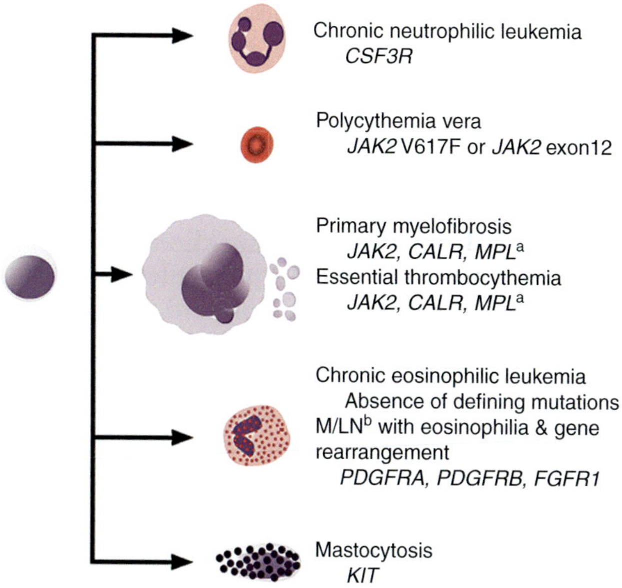

Fig. 23.1 A schematic displaying the characteristic mutations of MPNs. [a]Most commonly mutated genes other than *JAK2, CALR,* and *MPL*: *ASLX1, EZH2, TET2, SRSF2, SF3B1*. [b]M/LN, myeloid/lymphoid neoplasm. Figure credit: Clare L Keeney

Table 23.2 Summary of clinical information regarding PV, ET, and PMF

	Clinical concerns	Prognosis	Treatment	
			Low risk	High risk
PV	Risk of thrombosis, hemorrhage, evolution to MF, AML, MDS	Median survival 10.9 years	Aspirin, phlebotomy	Hydroxyurea, pegylated interferon, anagrelide, ruxolitinib[a]
ET	Risk of thrombosis, hemorrhage, evolution to MF, AML, MDS	Low-risk ET patients have mortality ratio approaching 1	Aspirin	Hydroxyurea, pegylated interferon, anegralide, ruxolitinib[a]
PMF	High symptom burden: constitutional symptoms, cachexia, low quality of life, splenomegaly, anemia	With overt fibrosis, median survival 5.7 years[b] (pre-fibrotic is decades)	Supportive therapy: hydroxyurea, splenectomy,[c] corticosteroids, erythropoietin, danazol	Ruxolitinib[a] or experimental TKIs Stem cell transplant in <10% of patients

[a]Patients who fail hydroxyurea
[b]Highly dependent on IPSS Plus score
[c]In select patients

- The defining translocations of myeloid/lymphoid neoplasms with eosinophilia and gene rearrangement involve the *PDGFRA, PDGFRB,* and *FGFR1* genes. It is essential to recognize these entities as patients with rearrangements of *PDGFRA* or *PDGFRB* can be treated with imatinib, drastically improving survival [9, 10], while those with *FGFR1* rearrangement have a poor prognosis and stem cell transplantation may be used. Imatinib can also be used in the treatment of systemic mastocytosis in patients with *KIT* mutations [11].
- Prognosis of MPNs is largely dependent on clinical parameters which are integrated into scoring systems such as the IPSS and DIPSS plus. However, myelofibrosis, karyotype, and commonly identified mutations (which can be detected by sequencing gene panels) continue to show potential prognostic value [12]. Higher grade of fibrosis, complex karyotype, and p53 mutations are associated with worse prognosis.

8. Which subtypes of MPNs are clinically relevant and which are morphologically defined but have unproven or minimal clinical relevance?

- The MPNs discussed in this chapter are all clinically relevant due to either specific treatment or prognosis. Myeloid and lymphoid neoplasms with *PCM1-JAK2* are defined and contained within the WHO as a provisional entity. Variants of this neoplasm result from translocations involving *JAK2* and one of two alternative partners, *BCR* or *ETV6* [13]. Like the other MPNs, a chronic phase may precede a blast phase which can be myeloid or lymphoid. Survival is highly variable and depends on the phase at diagnosis.
- Of note, pre-fibrotic PMF has been defined relatively recently and was typically categorized as ET previously. As such, contemporary survival data may differ substantially from earlier studies of ET and PMF.

9. What is an adequate specimen for MPNs?

- A peripheral blood smear, bone marrow aspirate smears, and bone marrow core biopsy are required for the diagnosis of a non-CML MPN. Classification of MPNs relies heavily on bone marrow core biopsy morphology. In cases with a dry tap, biopsy touch preparation can be utilized for morphological examination. The recommended bone marrow biopsy length is 1.5 cm taken perpendicularly to the cortical bone. The first milliliter of marrow aspirate should be dedicated to slides to be stained with Wright-Giemsa or May-Grünwald-Giemsa stain for morphologic evaluation. Additional marrow aspirate should be collected for ancillary studies: approximately 3 mL in a sodium heparin tube for chromosome analysis, 1–2 mL in a sodium heparin tube for FISH, and 2 mL in an EDTA tube for molecular studies (gene sequencing). Flow cytometry is not required for the diagnosis of an MPN; however, 2–4 mL of marrow aspirate is typically saved at the time of collection in an ACD, Na-heparin, or EDTA tube.
- Once a *BCR-ABL1* translocation is excluded, molecular analysis inclusion of *JAK2, CALR,* and *MPL* genes will detect a large majority of MPNs. An extended panel should include the next most commonly mutated genes in MPNs: *ASXL1, EZH2, TET2, SRSF2,* and *SF3B1* [14].
- For cases with suspected mastocytosis, sequencing of the *KIT* gene for mutations in codon 816 should be performed as this has both diagnostic and therapeutic implications [15].
- If eosinophilia is present, FISH for *PDGFRA, PDGFRB,* and *FGFR1* rearrangements should be performed [16]. A probe for *CHIC2* (which will be deleted in *FIP1L1-PDGFRA* rearranged neoplasms) and break-apart probes for *PDGFRB* and *FGFR1* are available from commercial mail-out laboratories. Keep in mind that FISH will not detect the translocation partner, but this is not required for the diagnosis. If above tests are negative, to differentiate reactive from clonal process, NGS myeloid panel testing can be performed [17].

10. What information can be conveyed to the clinician during each stage of the workup?

- The WHO criteria for the diagnosis MPNs contain CBC values or laboratory parameters already available to the clinician. The pathologist can provide additional information once the morphology of the aspirate smears is reviewed. The absence of myelodysplasia and no increase in blasts is helpful information that further supports an MPN. While definitive characterization should be deferred to the evaluation of the bone marrow core biopsy, megakaryocyte morphology can be described on aspirate smears. A hemodilute marrow aspirate may indicate a suboptimal biopsy or the presence of significant marrow fibrosis.
- With appropriate laboratory data, a final diagnosis can often be provided once the core biopsy has been examined. If not, the presence/absence of marrow fibrosis and the status of (and reasoning for) ancillary studies provide additional helpful information. The results of ancillary studies should be added to the original bone marrow report with a confirmed or modified diagnosis if applicable.

11. What should be the approach to provide maximum, but defensible, information from limited specimen or workup? What is an appropriate descriptive diagnosis in such situations?

- The most important sample for a suspected MPN is the bone marrow core biopsy. Molecular and cytogenetic diagnostics can be performed on peripheral blood as the neoplastic cells are circulating in the patient. Thus, if triaging of the marrow aspirate is required, priority should be given to morphologic evaluation for the exclusion of myelodysplasia and blast enumeration.
- A subcortical, fragmented, or small bone marrow core biopsy can make the diagnosis of an MPN challenging and the quantification of fibrosis impossible. In such situations, a comment explaining the nature of the specimen and the need for repeat biopsy should be provided.

12. When is a diagnostic comment necessary and what should be discussed in the diagnostic comment for MPNs?

Descriptive comments for MPNs are often warranted given their significant morphologic, clinical, and molecular overlap with each other and benign reactive states.

- As mentioned previously, excluding secondary causes of high blood counts or panmyelosis may require information unavailable to the pathologist. In the setting of a negative or absent molecular and cytogenetic workup, a diagnostic comment should be used to suggest these secondary causes.
- When biopsy material is limited or contains morphologic characteristics of multiple MPNs, a diagnosis of "*JAK2*-positive myeloproliferative neoplasm, see comment" may be appropriate. The diagnostic comment should discuss the differential diagnosis and address the interpretive challenges specific to the case.
- A repeat biopsy should be recommended only with a suboptimal sample and a clinical diagnosis as ambiguous as the pathology. An example would include a case in which clustering megakaryocytes with large, bulky, hyperchromatic nuclei are seen in addition to an occasional megakaryocyte with large, irregular "staghorn" nuclear lobes on a small core biopsy with minimal clinical and laboratory data. The presence of a *JAK2*, *CALR*, or *MPL* mutation would not differentiate ET from pre-fibrotic PMF. Instead, close correlation with the clinical presentation and laboratory data would better aid in the definitive characterization of the disease.

13. When is it appropriate to seek external consultation for this entity?

- External consultation should be sought in three settings:
  - The ancillary studies available to the pathologist are limited and fail to identify a clonal process. There is often an insistence that no secondary cause of the peripheral blood findings can be found. It is appropriate to seek external consultation and/or send available specimen to a reference laboratory with a broader panel of molecular and cytogenetic tests.
  - When the morphologic and ancillary studies show significant overlap and a descriptive comment does not provide the information needed to treat the patient. The inability to distinguish pre-fibrotic PMF from ET may not result in a change to patient management. However, in a setting of a myeloid neoplasm with eosinophilia, a descriptive comment will not suffice given the marked difference in treatment and survival among patients with *PDGFRA* or *PDGFRB* rearrangements compared to those with *FGFR1* rearrangements.
  - When the responsible pathologist is unsure of a diagnosis and is struggling with a decision that would drastically alter the patient's management.

Case Presentations

Case 1

Learning Objectives

1. Identify pertinent CBC findings in the workup of a myeloproliferative neoplasm
2. Generate a differential diagnosis given CBC and bone marrow biopsy findings
3. Identify the appropriate ancillary studies to order for a suspected MPN

Case History

A 75-year-old woman with history of beta thalassemia minor was found to have thrombocytosis (1133 K/mL) and a mild leukocytosis (13 K/mL) on routine follow-up. The patient had symptoms of fatigue, and a bone marrow biopsy was performed.

Histologic Findings

- Hypercellular bone marrow.
- Focal grade 1 of 3 fibrosis.
- Loosely clustered megakaryocytes with hyperchromatic nuclei (Fig. 23.2). Some megakaryocytes have bulky nuclei, while others appear hyperlobated.

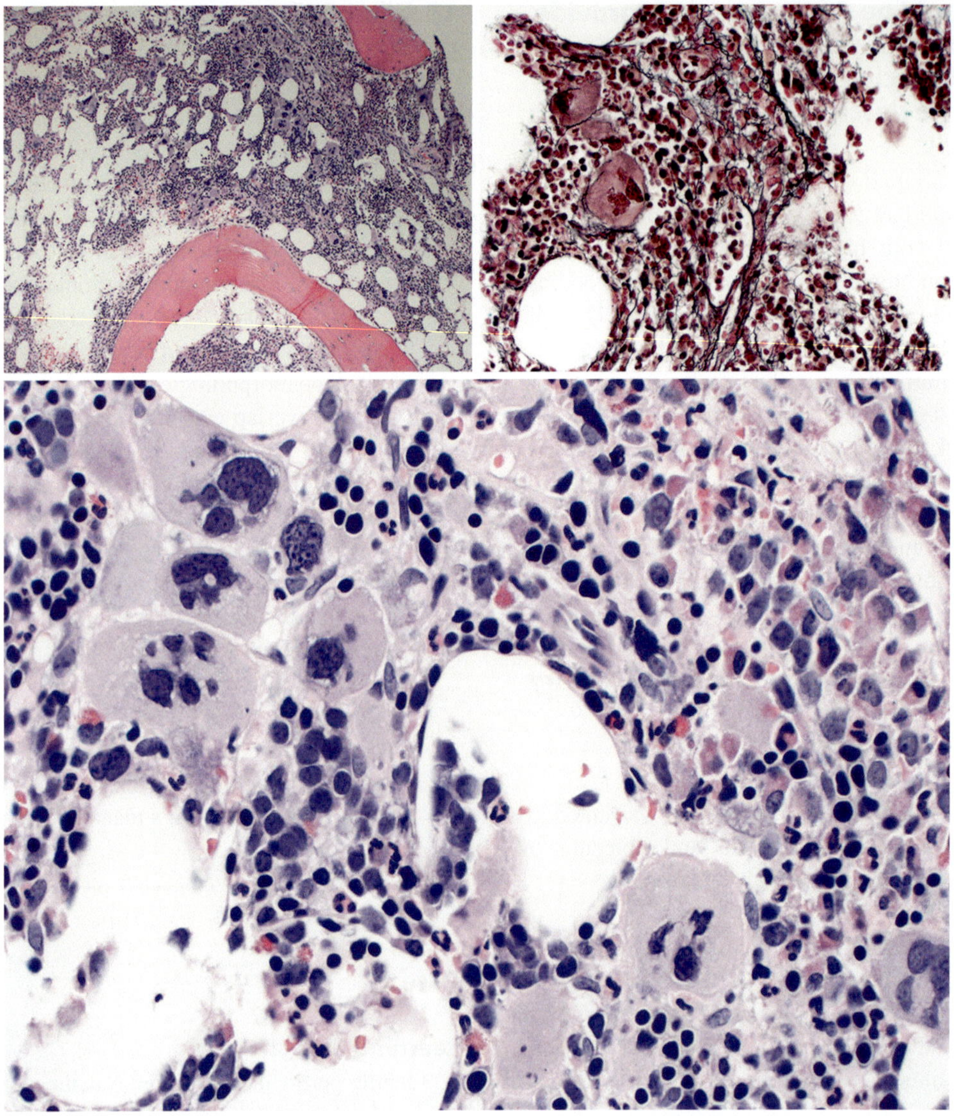

Fig. 23.2 Top left: bone marrow core biopsy at 100× magnification showing marrow hypercellularity. Top right: reticulin stain showing focal grade 1 of 3 marrow fibrosis. Bottom: core biopsy at 500× showing clustered megakaryocytes with atypical, hyperchromatic nuclei. While some contain "cloud-like" nuclei, others appear hypersegmented

Ancillary Studies

- Massive parallel sequencing (myeloid mutation panel) detected a c.1544G>T mutation in the *MPL* gene.

Final Diagnosis

Myeloproliferative neoplasm in a hypercellular bone marrow with increased megakaryocytes showing clustering and hyperchromasia, grade 1 fibrosis, and 1% blasts

Diagnostic Comment

A *MPL* mutation is identified. The differential diagnosis includes essential thrombocythemia and pre-fibrotic primary myelofibrosis. The marrow hypercellularity and clustering of megakaryocytes are most compatible with a diagnosis of pre-fibrotic primary myelofibrosis.

Take-Home Messages

1. Mutations in *JAK2, CALR,* and *MPL* are not specific to a single myeloproliferative neoplasm.
2. A spectrum of atypical megakaryocytes is often seen in each case of MPN. The predominant morphology is not always apparent.
3. A descriptive comment is often required. In this case, a diagnosis of ET is not excluded, as marrow hypercellularity could be the result of erythroid hyperplasia given the patient's beta thalassemia and a decreased M:E ratio. This patient also had thrombocytosis with some megakaryocytes showing hypersegmented, branching nuclei. For these reasons, a descriptive comment was added that ultimately favored one diagnosis over the other.

Case 2

Learning Objectives

1. Identify pertinent CBC findings in a patient with suspected MPN
2. Know when to suspect neutrophilic leukemia
3. Be aware of confounding factors and mimics of MPNs

Case History

A 70-year-old woman with a 3-week history of diarrhea was found to have a markedly elevated WBC (181 K/mL) with 89% neutrophils and 3% band forms. The patient was referred to a hematologist who performed a bone marrow biopsy.

Histologic Findings (Fig. 23.3)

- Peripheral blood with toxic neutrophilia consisting of mature forms
- Markedly hypercellular bone marrow without fibrosis
- Markedly increased M:E ratio with left-shifted granulocytes

Ancillary Studies

- Massive parallel sequencing (myeloid mutation panel) detected a c.566C>A mutation of the *CEBPA* gene with an allele frequency of 8%.
- Cytogenetics showed a karyotype of 46,XX.

Final Diagnosis

Hypercellular bone marrow with increased M:E ratio, toxic and left-shifted granulopoiesis, no fibrosis, and no increase in blasts

Diagnostic Comment

The *CEBPA* mutation detected by massive parallel sequencing is of undetermined significance. The differential diagnosis includes a leukemoid reaction.

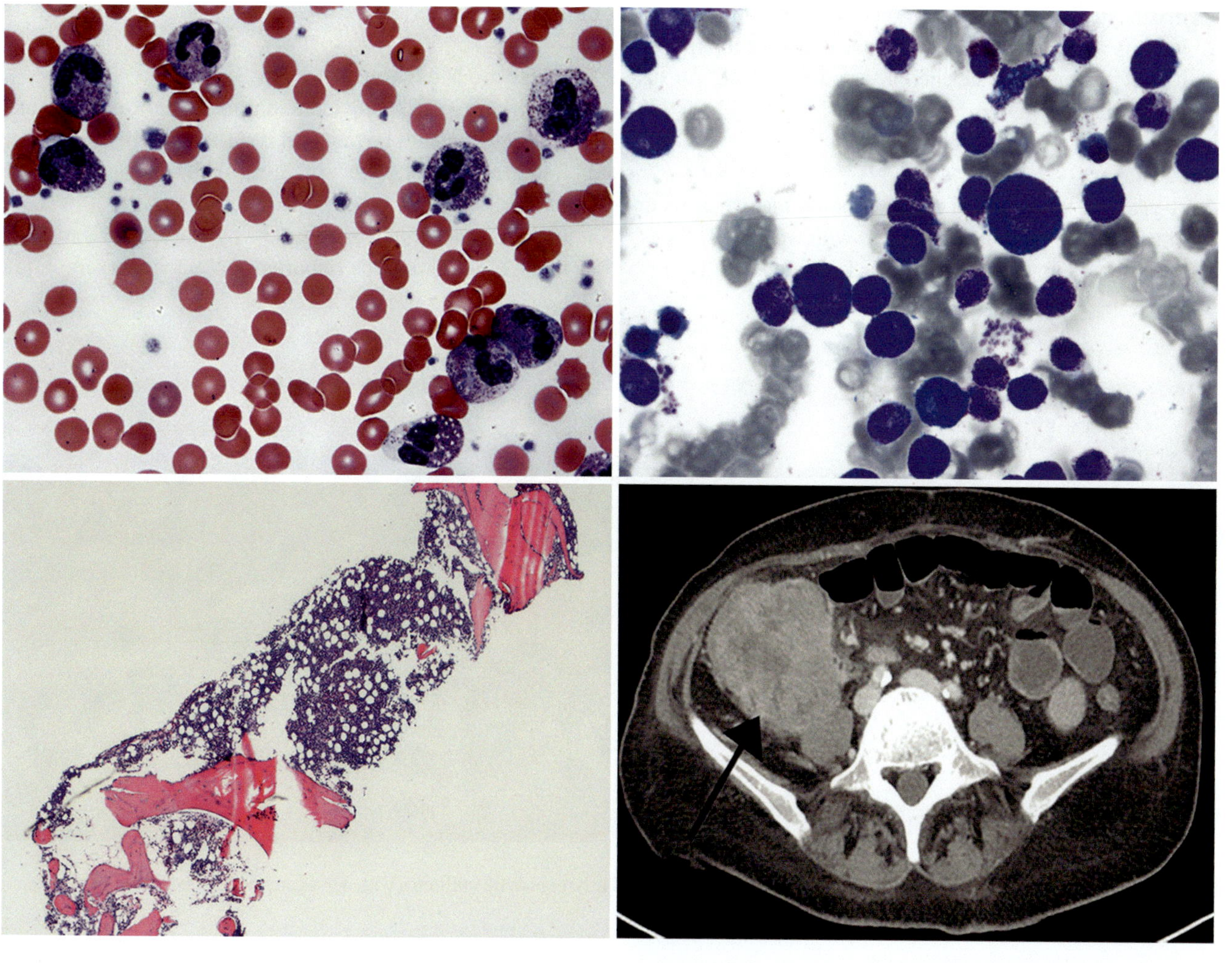

Fig. 23.3 Top left: peripheral blood smear showing toxic neutrophilia and mild thrombocytosis. Top right: bone marrow aspirate showing left-shifted granulocytes with an increased M:E ratio. Bottom left: bone marrow core biopsy showing a marked age-adjusted hypercellularity. Bottom right: additional workup included a CT of the abdomen and pelvis which showed a large sigmoid colon mass

Additional Workup

An abdominal CT scan showed a large mass involving the sigmoid colon. Surgical resection revealed an undifferentiated carcinoma. The patient's WBC decreased to 42 K/mL 1 day after surgical resection.

Take-Home Messages

1. Somatic mutations of undetermined clinical significance may be found in elderly individuals and do not equate to a diagnosis of neoplasia.
2. CNL is characterized by mutations in *CSF3R*.
3. Secondary causes of a leukemoid reaction must be excluded before extensive work-up of CNL which is very rare.

Case 3

Learning Objectives

1. Identify pertinent clinical findings that suggest mastocytosis
2. Identify atypical mast cells on bone marrow biopsy
3. Identify the appropriate ancillary studies to order for suspected mastocytosis

Case History

A 61-year-old woman with a longstanding history of recurrent rash of the extremities presented with worsened "flares" and progression to the thighs and back. A biopsy of the rash was diagnosed as urticaria pigmentosa. The patient was found to have an elevated tryptase level, and a bone marrow biopsy was performed to evaluate for systemic mastocytosis.

Histologic Findings (Fig. 23.4)

- Slightly hypercellular bone marrow.
- Atypical mast cells with spindled morphology are seen on aspirate smear.
- Focal lymphoid aggregates surrounded by a mast cell infiltrate. Overall, the mast cells accounted for approximately 10% of the marrow cellularity.

Ancillary Studies

- Sequencing of the *KIT* gene identified the D816V mutation.

Final Diagnosis

Systemic mastocytosis involving a hypercellular bone marrow with approximately 10% mast cells with spindle morphology

Take-Home Messages

1. Mutations in *KIT* provide additional diagnostic support, although may not be required if sufficient criteria are met.
2. Spindled morphology of mast cells is an atypical finding.
3. Involvement of the bone marrow by mastocytosis may be focal, highlighting the importance of adequate sampling.

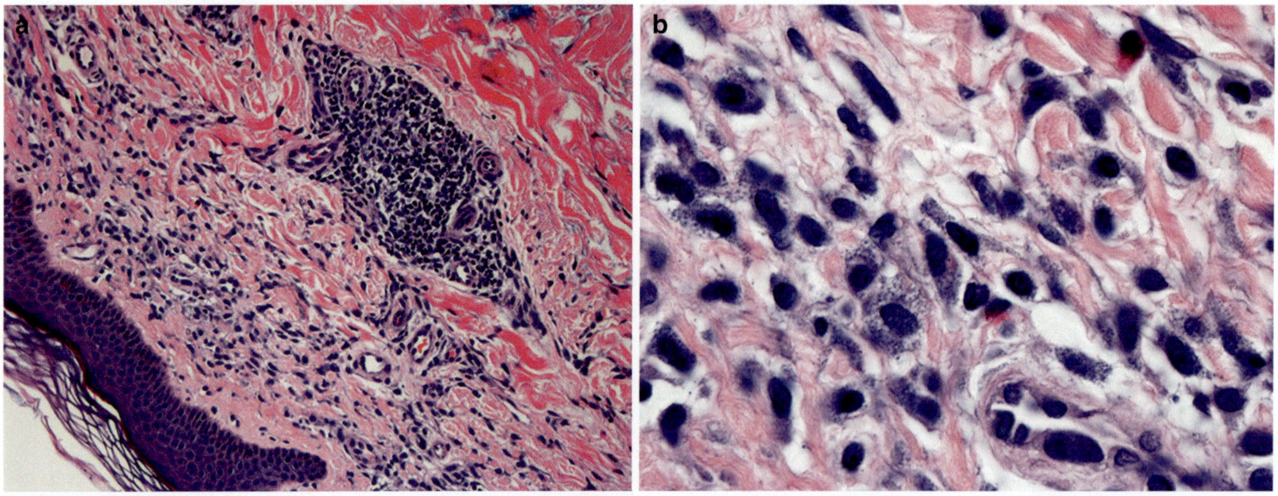

Fig. 23.4 (**a**, **b**) Representative sections of skin rash showing perivascular lymphocytic infiltrates with aggregates of mast cells within the superficial dermis.

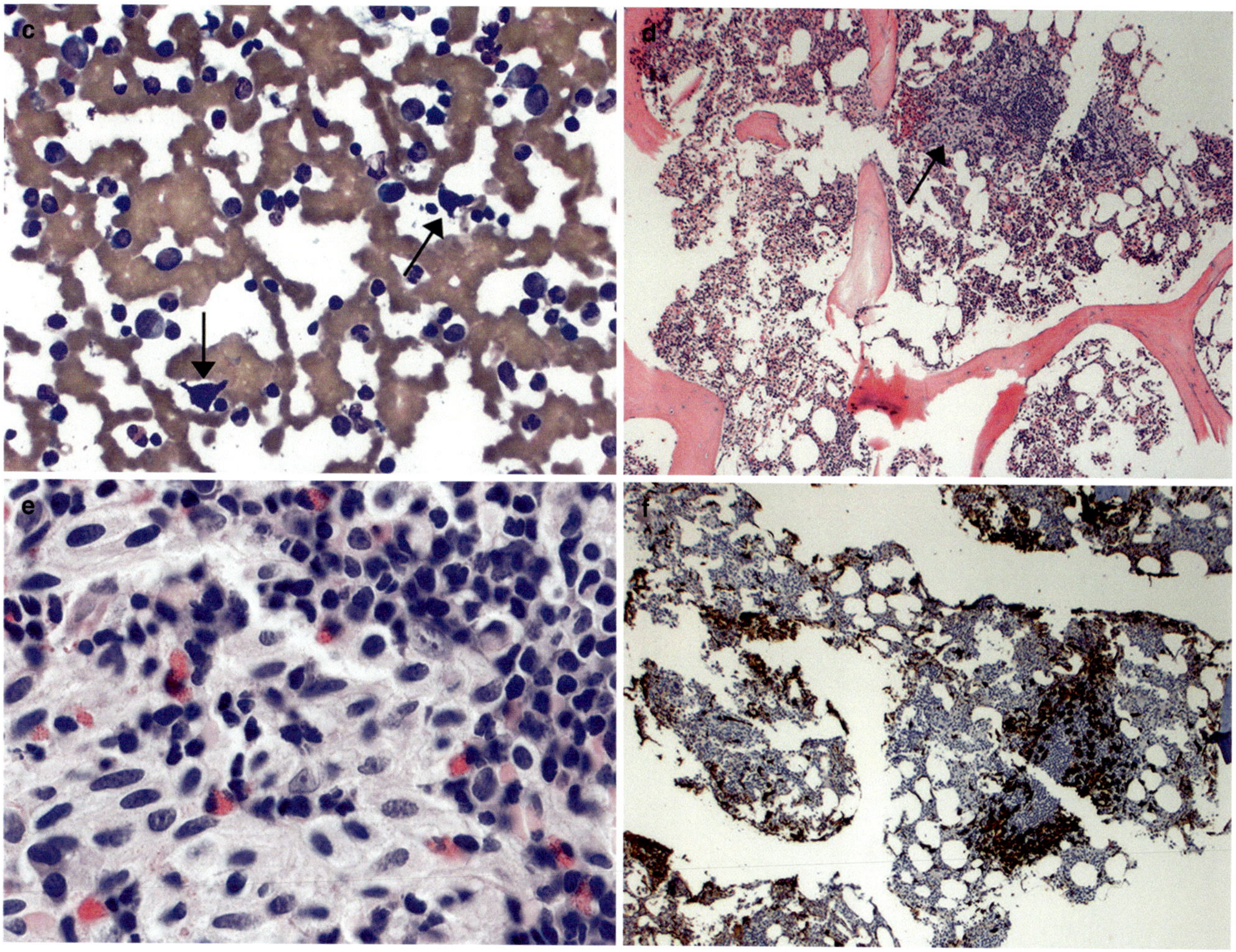

Fig. 23.4 (continued) (**c**) Bone marrow aspirate showing occasional spindled mast cells (*arrows*). (**d**, **e**) Bone marrow core biopsy showing a small lymphoid aggregate surrounded by spindled mast cells. (**f**) Tryptase immunostain highlighting mast cells which also stained positively for CD117

References

1. Swerdlow SH, Campo E, Harris NL, Jaffe E, Pileri S, Stein H, et al. WHO classification of tumours of haematopoietic and lymphoid tissues. (revised 4th edition). Lyon: IARC; 2017.
2. Tefferi A. Novel mutations and their functional and clinical relevance in myeloproliferative neoplasms. JAK2, MPL, TET2, ASXL1, CBL, IDH and IKZF1. Leukemia. 2010;24:1128–38.
3. Maxson JE, Gotlib J, Pollyea DA, Fleischman AG, Agarwal A, Eide CA, et al. Oncogenic CSF3R mutations in chronic neutrophilic leukemia and atypical CML. N Engl J Med. 2013;368:1381–90.
4. Tefferi A, Elliott M, Pardanani A. Chronic neutrophilic leukemia: novel mutations and their impact on clinical practice. Curr Opin Hematol. 2015;22:171–6.
5. Ismail SI, Naffa RG, Yousef AF, Ghanim MT. Incidence of bcr-abl fusion transcripts in healthy individuals. Mol Med Rep. 2014;9(4):1271–76
6. Nielsen C, Bojesen SE, Nordestgaard BG, Kofoed KF, Birgens HS. JAK2V617F somatic mutation in the general population: myeloproliferative neoplasm development and progression rate. Haematol. 2014;99(9):1448–55.
7. Vannucchi AM, Harrison CN. Emerging treatments for classical myeloproliferative neoplasms. Blood. 2017;129(6):693–703.
8. Stahl M, Zeidan AM. Management of myelofibrosis: JAK inhibition and beyond. Expert Rev Hematol. 2017;10(5):459–77.
9. Cools J, DeAngelo DJ, Gotlib J, Stover EH, Legare RD, Cortes J, et al. A tyrosine kinase created by fusion of the PDGFRA and FIP1L1 genes as a therapeutic target of imatinib in idiopathic hypereosinophilic syndrome. N Engl J Med. 2003;348(13):1201–14.
10. Cheah CY, Burbury K, Apperley JF, Huguet F, Pitini V, Gardembas M, et al. Patients with myeloid malignancies bearing PDGFRB fusion genes achieve durable long-term remissions with imatinib. Blood. 2014;123(23):3574–7.
11. Alvarez-Twose I, Matito A, Morgado JM, Sánchez-Muñoz L, Jara-Acevedo M, García-Montero A, et al. Imatinib in systemic mastocytosis: a phase IV clinical trial in patients lacking exon 17. Oncotarget. 2017;8(40):68950–63.
12. Zhou A, Afzal A, Oh ST. Prognostication in Philadelphia chromosome negative myeloproliferative neoplasms: a review of the recent literature. Curr Hematol Malig Rep. 2017;12(5):397–405.
13. Reiter A, Gotlib A. Myeloid neoplasms with eosinophilia. Blood. 2017;129:704–14.

14. Tefferi A, Lasho TL, Finke CM, Knudson RA, Ketterling R, Hanson CH, et al. CALR vs JAK2 vs MPL-mutated or triple-negative myelofibrosis. Clinical, cytogenetic and molecular comparisons. Leukemia. 2014;28:1472–7.
15. Valent P, Akin C, Arock M, Brockow K, Butterfield JH, Carter MC, et al. Definitions, criteria, and global classification of mast cell disorders with special reference to mast cell activation syndromes: a consensus proposal. Int Arch Allergy Immunol. 2012;157:215–25.
16. Boyer DF. Blood and bone marrow evaluation for eosinophilia. Arch Pathol Lab Med. 2016;140:1060–7.
17. Wang SA, Tam W, Tsai AG, Arber DA, Hasserjian RP, Geyer JT, et al. Targeted next-generation sequencing identifies a subset of idiopathic hypereosinophilic syndromes with features similar to chronic eosinophilic syndrome, not otherwise specified. Mod Pathol. 2016;29:854–64.

Myelodysplastic Syndromes

24

Jason X. Cheng and James W. Vardiman

Frequently Asked Questions

1. What are the major subtypes of myelodysplastic syndromes (MDS)?
2. What are the 2017 WHO criteria for myelodysplasia, cytopenia, and ring sideroblasts?
3. What are the major changes in the 2017 WHO classification?
4. What are the typical clinical, laboratory and morphological findings of MDS?
5. What are the MDS mimics and what is the clinical impact of misdiagnosis?
6. What germline predispositions and inherited syndromes are relevant to MDS and its differential diagnosis?
7. What other pre-MDS conditions are relevant to MDS differential diagnosis?
8. What are the practical guidelines for diagnosis of MDS? What are the findings suggestive of MDS and the findings that rule out MDS?
9. What is the minimal and optimal ancillary work up for MDS and subclassification of MDS?
10. What additional ancillary tests are helpful for the diagnosis of MDS?
11. What is the workup to provide prognostic information?
12. What workup provides therapeutic target information for MDS?
13. What is an appropriate practical approach for diagnosis of MDS? When is a diagnostic comment necessary and what should be discussed in the diagnostic comment for this entity? When is it appropriate to seek external consultation for this entity?
14. Which features set MDS apart from closely related hematologic neoplasms?

1. What are the major subtypes of myelodysplastic syndromes (MDS)?

- Myelodysplastic syndromes (MDS) are a heterogeneous group of clonal hematopoietic stem cell disorders characterized by morphologic dysplasia and ineffective hematopoiesis affecting one or more of the myeloid lineages that usually result in peripheral blood cytopenia(s) in the face of a hypercellular bone marrow [1–4].
- The 2017 WHO classification recognizes 7 major subtypes of MDS based on (1) the lineages affected; (2) the percentages of blasts in the peripheral blood (PB) and bone marrow (BM); (3) the number of ring sideroblasts in the BM; (4) the presence of the specific chromosome abnormality, isolated del 5q; and (6) the age of the patient [1] (Table 24.1):
  1. MDS with single-lineage dysplasia (MDS-SLD)
  2. MDS with multilineage dysplasia (MDS-MLD)
  3. MDS with ring sideroblasts (MDS-RS)
  4. MDS with isolated del(5q)
  5. MDS with excess blasts (MDS-EB)
  6. MDS, unclassifiable (MDS-U)
  7. Refractory cytopenia of childhood
- Of note, pancytopenia can be seen in MDS-MLD, but not in MDS-SLD. MDS-SLD, MDS-MLD, MDS-RS, and MDS-del(5q) should have no increase in blasts and no Auer rods at the time of diagnosis.
  - MDS-EB is characterized by 2–19% blasts in the blood or 5–19% in the bone marrow but can be further subdivided into MDS-EB-1 with 2–4% blasts in the blood and/or 5–9% in the bone marrow or MDS-EB-2, with 5–19% blasts in the peripheral blood or 10–19% blasts in the bone marrow.

J. X. Cheng (✉) · J. W. Vardiman
Department of Pathology, University of Chicago, Chicago, IL, USA
e-mail: Jason.Cheng@uchospitals.edu; james.vardiman@uchospitals.edu

E. Wang, A. S. Lagoo (eds.), *Practical Lymph Node and Bone Marrow Pathology*, Practical Anatomic Pathology, https://doi.org/10.1007/978-3-030-32189-5_24

Table 24.1 The 2017 WHO Classification of myelodysplastic syndromes (MDS)

Entity	Dysplastic lineage(s)[a]	Peripheral blood (PB)	Bone marrow (BM)	Ring sideroblasts%[b]	Cytogenetics by conventional karyotyping
MDS with single-lineage dysplasia (MDS-SLD)	1	Unicytopenia[c] or bicytopenia <1% blasts No Auer rods No monocytosis	Unilineage dysplasia < 5% blasts No Auer rods	<15% or <5% if *SF3B1* mutation is present	Any, unless fulfills all criteria for MDS with isolated del(5q)
MDS with multilineage dysplasia (MDS-MLD)	2–3	Bicytopenia or pancytopenia <1% blasts No Auer rod No monocytosis	Multilineage dysplasia <5% blasts No Auer rods	<15% <5% if *SF3B1* mutation is present	Any, unless fulfills all criteria for MDS with isolated del(5q)
MDS with ring sideroblasts (MDS-RS) MDS-RS-SLD MDS-RS-MLD	 1 2–3	<1% blasts No Auer rod No monocytosis Uni–/bicytopenia Uni-,bi- or pan-cytopenia	<5% blasts No Auer rods Unilineage dysplasia Multilineage dysplasia	≥15% or ≥5% with *SF3B1* mutation	Any, unless fulfills all criteria for MDS with isolated del(5q)
MDS with excess blasts (MDS-EB) MDS-EB-1 MDS-EB-2	1–3	Any cytopenia(s) No monocytosis Blasts: 2–4% No Auer rods Blast: 5–19% or 2–4% blasts with Auer rods	Any dysplasia Blasts: 5–9% No Auer rods Blasts: 10–19% with or without Auer rods	None or any None or any	Any Any
MDS associated with isolated del(5q)	1–3	Uni-, bi- or pan-cytopenia <1% blasts No monocytosis No Auer rods	< 5% blasts No Auer rods	None or any	del(5q) alone or with 1 additional abnormality, except −7 or del(7)
Myelodysplastic syndrome, unclassifiable with 1% blasts in PB with SLD and pancytopenia with MDS-defining cytogenetics	 1–3 1 None	No Auer rods 1% blasts on ≥2 occasions Pancytopenia <1% blasts Any cytopenia <1% blasts	No Auer rods < 5% blasts Any dysplasia Uni-lineage dysplasia No dysplasia	None or any <15% or < 5% if *SF3B1* mutation is present	Any Any MDS-defining abnormality
Refractory cytopenia of Childhood	1–3	Cytopenia(s) <2% blasts	< 5% blasts, no Auer rods	None or any	Any

Adapted and modified from the Table 6.01 of the book, *WHO Classification of Tumours of Haematopoietic and Lymphoid Tissues. Lyon, France: IARC; 2017*

[a]Dysplasia is defined as ≥10% dysplastic cells in the same lineage cells

[b]Percentage (%) of ring sideroblasts is defined as % ring sideroblasts of the BM erythroid elements

[c]Cytopenias defined as <10 g/dL, platelet count <100 x 10^9/L, and absolute neutrophil count <1.8 x 10^9/L

- The finding of Auer rods in a case of MDS is sufficient to designate the case as MDS-EB-2 as long as the blast count in the blood and marrow is less than 20%. However, in cases of MDS-EB-2 with Auer rods, it is important to exclude the rare instances of AML with t(8;21)(q22;q22.1); *RUNX1-RUNX1T1,* which may rarely present with <20% blasts.

2. What are the WHO criteria for myelodysplasia, cytopenia and ring sideroblasts?

- Myelodysplasia is characterized by morphologic abnormalities that reflect the ineffective and clonal hematopoiesis in one or more myeloid cell lineages. The presence of ≥10% dysplastic cells in a cell lineage currently is used as a practical marker to consider a lineage as being dysplastic.
- The cytopenias are defined as anemia, hemoglobin <10 g/dL; thrombocytopenia, platelet count <100 x 10^9/L; and neutropenia, absolute neutrophil count <1.8 x 10^9/L.
- An increase in blasts is defined as blasts ≥1% in the peripheral blood (PB) or ≥ 5% in the bone marrow (BM).
- Ring sideroblasts (RS) are erythroid precursors with a minimum of 5 siderotic granules detected by Prussian blue staining that surround at least one-third of the nuclear circumference. They are considered as increased when they account for ≥15% of the BM erythroid precursors or ≥ 5% in the presence of an *SF3B1* mutation. Assessment

of RS requires cellular bone marrow aspirate smears or touch preparations; iron stains on bone marrow core biopsy specimens are unreliable for this purpose.

3. What are the major changes in the 2017 WHO classification?

- Nomenclature: Identification of some entities according to specific cytopenias, such as "refractory anemia," which often failed to correlate with the specific cytopenia of concern or the numbers of lineages affected and did not fully emphasize the significance of the blast percentage, is no longer used. The updated nomenclature first identifies the disorder as a "myelodysplastic syndrome" and then further specifies the number of lineages involved, whether blasts are increased in percentage, the presence of specific morphologic abnormalities of clinical importance such as ring sideroblasts and the specific cytogenetic abnormality, isolated del(5q).
- Myeloid neoplasms with ≥50% erythroid precursors: Previously, in such cases, if the percentage of blasts was 20% or more of the nonerythroid marrow cell component, the diagnosis of acute erythroleukemia was made, even if the percentage of nonerythroid cells was very small. Now, for all cases – including those in which erythroid precursors account for more than 50% of the marrow cells – the bone marrow blast percentage is expressed as a percentage of all nucleated bone marrow cells, including erythroid and nonerythroid components. Thus, many cases previously diagnosed as acute erythroleukemia will now be diagnosed as MDS, most likely MDS with excess of blasts (MDS-EB). However, for those rare cases in which 80% or more of the marrow cells are immature erythroid precursors, with more than 30% proerythroblasts, the diagnosis of pure erythroid leukemia is justified (AML, NOS, pure erythroid leukemia).
- Definition of MDS, unclassifiable (MDS-U): MDS-U is now defined by the presence of any of the following three conditions (see Table 24.1):
  - 1% blasts in the PB on at least 2 separate occasions, associated with findings that would otherwise suggest MDS with single-lineage dysplasia, MDS with multilineage dysplasia, MDS with ring sideroblasts and single or multilineage dysplasia, or MDS with isolated del(5q), with <5% BM blasts and no Auer rods.
  - Unilineage dysplasia, with pancytopenia, but no increase in blasts in the PB or BM and no Auer rods.
  - MDS-defining cytogenetic abnormality, with no dysplasia in any of the major myeloid lineages and no increase in blasts in the PB or BM and no Auer rods.

4. What are the typical clinical, laboratory, and morphological findings of MDS?

- Clinical findings of MDS:
  - Earliest stage: most patients have no symptoms but may come to the physician's attention because of anemia, neutropenia, and/or thrombocytopenia discovered on routine blood counts.
  - Later, patients often develop fatigue, dyspnea, easy bruisability, bleeding, and infections. Physical findings in MDS are nonspecific, but importantly, hepatomegaly, splenomegaly, and lymphadenopathy are uncommon [5, 6].
- Anemia and dyserythropoiesis: Anemia is the most common hematologic finding in MDS. Approximately 60% of MDS patients have normocytic (MCV of 80–100 fL) or macrocytic anemia (MCV > 100 FL [7–9], and anisocytosis of RBCs with macro-ovalocytes is commonly observed on the peripheral blood smear (Fig. 24.1 and Table 24.2) [10]. Less commonly, a dimorphic pattern with coexisting macrocytic and normocytic or even microcytic cell populations are seen, particularly in MDS-RS (Fig. 24.1a).
  - Abnormalities such as elliptocytes, schistocytes, acanthocytes, and spherocytes can be seen due to abnormalities of the RBC cytoskeletal proteins [11–15]. Teardrop-shaped RBCs are occasionally seen in MDS with reticulin fibrosis in the marrow and have been reported to be associated with a worse outcome [16].
  - Hypochromia and microcytosis are unusual, but a subpopulation of patients has hypochromic, microcytic red cells with anisocytosis, with or without ring sideroblasts in the BM [17, 18].
  - Occasional MDS patients develop acquired hemoglobinopathy/acquired α-thalassemia with microcytic red blood cells (RBCs) and hemoglobin H inclusions consisting of beta-globin tetramers. This latter finding may be caused by deletion of cis-elements of the *α-globin* gene cluster or more commonly by somatic mutations of *ATRX* that result in trans-inactivation of *α-globin* genes [19].
  - The morphologic features of erythroid dysplasia in the BM include asynchrony of nuclear and cytoplasmic maturation (Fig. 24.2), i.e., megaloblastoid maturation (Fig. 24.2a), nuclear irregularities (Fig. 24.2b), apoptotic or fragmented nuclei (Fig. 24.2c), multinucleation (Fig. 24.2d), nuclear budding, internuclear bridging, and small gaps in the nuclear membrane [1, 20]. Cytoplasmic vacuolization (Fig. 24.2e), periodic acid-Schiff (PAS)-positive granules and/ or ring sideroblasts (Fig. 24.2f) are also common [21–25].
- Neutropenia and dysgranulopoiesis: Neutropenia, granulocytic dysplasia, and dysfunctional neutrophils are common in MDS. Neutropenia occurs in 15–20% of patients with

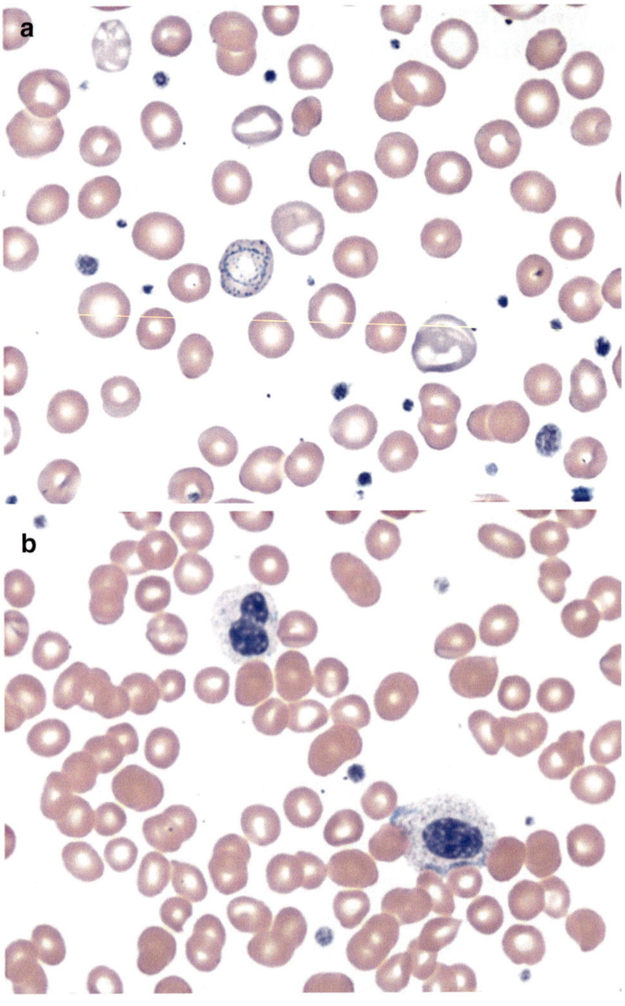

Fig. 24.1 The peripheral blood (PB) smears from patients with myelodysplastic syndrome with multilineage dysplasia (MDS-MLD). (**a**) Marked macrocytic anemia with RBC anisocytosis, dimorphic RBCs, and rare Cabot rings. (**b**) Granulocytic dysplasia with hyposegmented nuclei, abnormal chromatin patterns, and hypogranulated cytoplasm

lower-risk MDS but 70–80% of patients with higher-risk MDS [26, 27] (see Fig. 24.3 and Table 24.2).

- Eosinophilia (absolute eosinophils >450/μL) and basophilia (basophils >200/μL) are typical features of myeloproliferative neoplasms but may also be present in patients with MDS, in which case, they reportedly have a negative impact on prognosis [28–31].
- Granulocytic dysplasia is characterized by nuclear and/or cytoplasmic abnormalities [1, 4, 27, 32, 33]. Dysplastic granulocytes often show hypogranular cytoplasm (Fig. 24.3a), but rarely, giant azurophilic granules resembling those seen in the neutrophils of Chediak-Higashi syndrome (Fig. 24.3b) may be seen [34]. The nuclear abnormalities of dysplastic neutrophils include abnormal nuclear size and segmentation (Fig. 24.3c) including bi-lobed or nonsegmented nuclei (pseudo-Pelger-Huët abnormality) (Fig. 24.3d), nuclear hypersegmentation (6 or more nuclear lobes), and abnormal nuclear chromatin patterns with hypercondensed chromatin, nuclear excrescences, and nuclear sticks. Ring-shaped nuclei may also be seen [35].
- Hypercellularity with left-shifted myelopoiesis (Fig. 24.3e) is seen in a majority of the BM specimens from patients with MDS. Granulocytic dysplasia is usually more prominent in the BM aspirate smears than the PB smears, but the morphologic features are similar (Fig. 24.3f).

• Thrombocytopenia and dysmegakaryopoiesis: Thrombocytopenia (platelet count <100,000/μL) is found in 40–65% of patients with MDS [36] (Table 24.2).

- The platelet morphology, platelet mass, and platelet count have been reported to correlate with platelet function and to have a significant impact on prognosis in patients with MDS [37]. Hypogranular platelets

Table 24.2 The morphologic features of myelodysplasia in MDS

Lineage	Morphologic features of peripheral blood (PB) and bone marrow (BM)		
	Cell number and size	Nuclei	Cytoplasm
Erythroid dysplasia	Macrocytic or normocytic anemia, microcytic anemia (uncommon), anisopoikilocytosis including ovalocytes, elliptocytes, acanthocytes, echinocytes, teardrop cells	Asynchrony of nuclear/cytoplasmic maturation, megaloblastoid changes, nuclear irregularities or budding, internuclear bridging, karyorrhexis, bi- or multinucleation	Basophilic stippling, cytoplasmic vacuolization, periodic acid-Schiff positive inclusions, ring sideroblasts, polychromasia, incomplete hemoglobinization, Howell-Jolly bodies, Cabot ring (rare)
Granulocytic dysplasia	Neutropenia, increased immature granulocytic precursors or myeloblasts in PB or BM, dysfunctional neutrophils	Abnormal nuclear size and segmentation, bi-lobed or nonsegmented nuclei (pseudo-Pelger-Huët abnormality), nuclear hypersegmentation (6 or more nuclear lobes), abnormal hypercondensed chromatin, nuclear excrescences, nuclear sticks, and rare ring-shaped nuclei	Hypogranulation, abnormal granulation, including giant azurophilic granules (pseudo-Chediak-Higashi granules), Döhle bodies, Auer rods
Megakaryocytic dysplasia	*Platelets:* Large/giant platelets, small platelets, platelet anisocytosis, "balloon-like" platelets *Megakaryocytes:* Small or micro-megakaryocytes, giant bizarre-shaped megakaryocytes	Hypolobated or monolobated megakaryocytes, widely separate nuclear lobes, "pawn ball-like" nuclei, hyperchromatic nuclei (uncommon)	Dissociation between cytoplasmic and nuclear maturation, cytoplasmic hypogranulation, cytoplasmic vacuolation

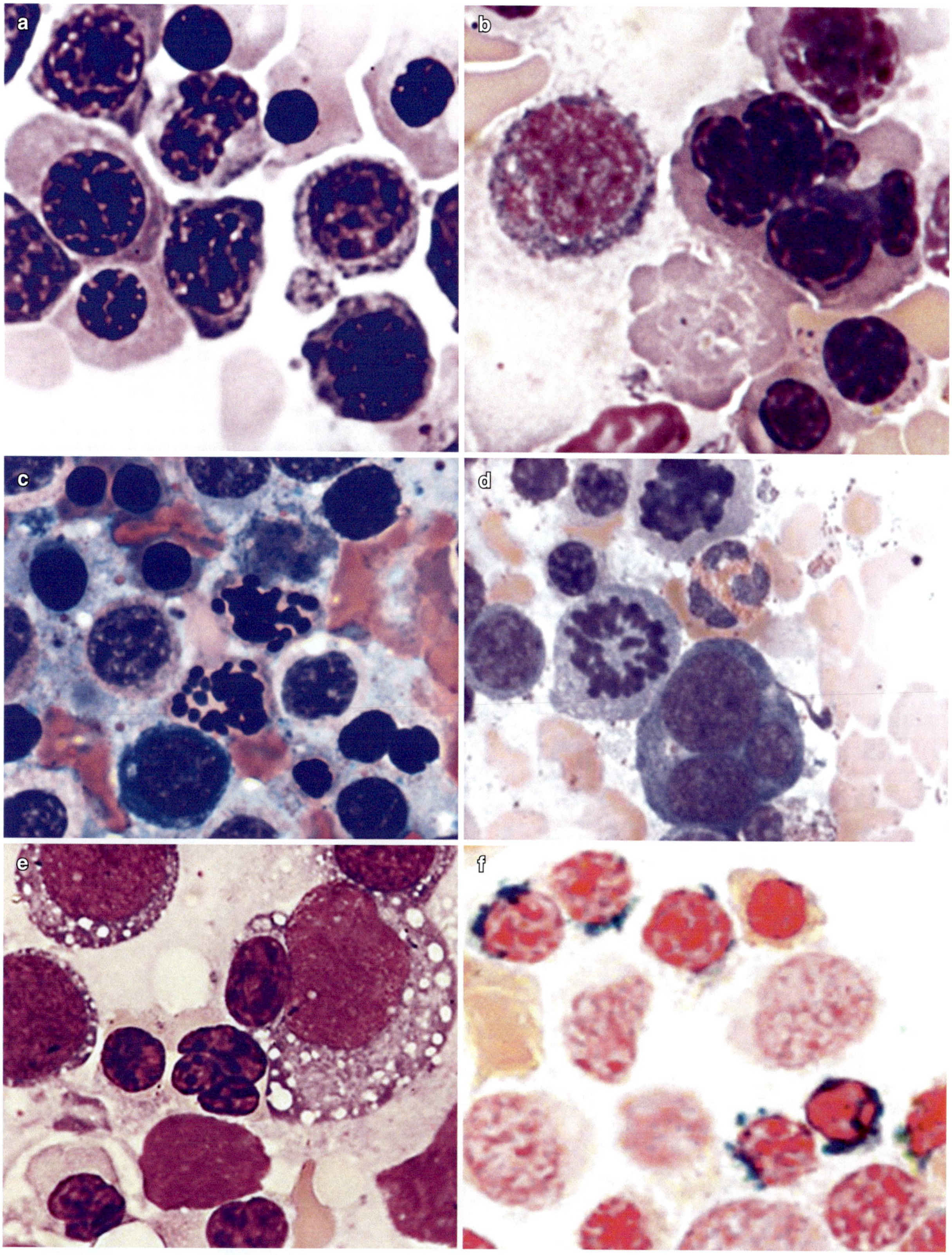

Fig. 24.2 The morphologic features of dyserythropoiesis in the bone marrow (BM) of patients with myelodysplastic syndromes (MDS). (**a**) Marked erythroid hyperplasia and erythroid precursors with megaloblastoid changes and asynchrony of nuclear/cytoplasmic maturation. (**b**) Dysplastic erythroid precursors with nuclear irregularities and abnormal chromatin patterns. (**c**) Dysplastic erythroid precursors with nuclear fragmentation (apoptotic changes). (**d**) Dysplastic erythroid precursors with multinucleation and increased mitoses and apoptosis. (**e**) Dysplastic erythroid precursors with cytoplasmic vacuolation and dysplastic megakaryocyte with widely separate nuclear lobes. (**f**) Markedly increased ring sideroblasts

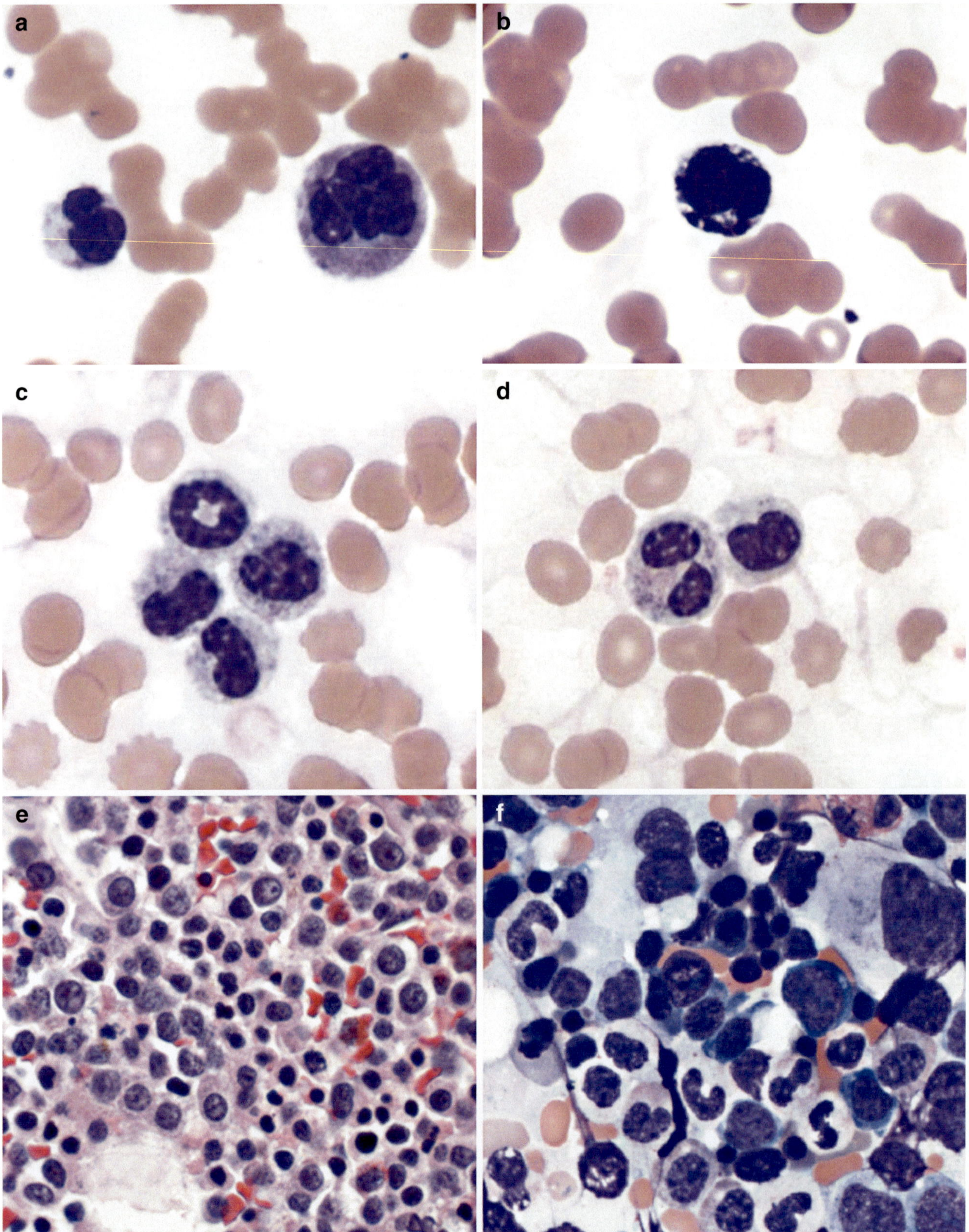

Fig. 24.3 The morphologic features of granulocytic dysplasia in the peripheral blood (PB) and bone marrow aspirate smears of patients with myelodysplastic syndromes (MDS). (**a**) A dysplastic granulocyte with cytoplasmic hypogranulation (left); and a dysplastic giant granulocyte (right) in the PB. (**b**) A dysplastic granulocyte with pseudo-Chediak-Higashi granules in the PB. (**c**) Dysplastic granulocytes with abnormal nuclear shapes/segmentation and chromatin patterns in the PB. (**d**) Dysplastic neutrophils with pseudo-Pelger-Huët anomaly or monolobated nuclei in the PB. (**e**) Hypercellular BM with marked left-shifted myelopoiesis. (**f**) BM cells show marked granulocytic dysplasia with cytoplasmic hypogranulation and abnormal nuclear segmentation and chromatin patterns in the BM

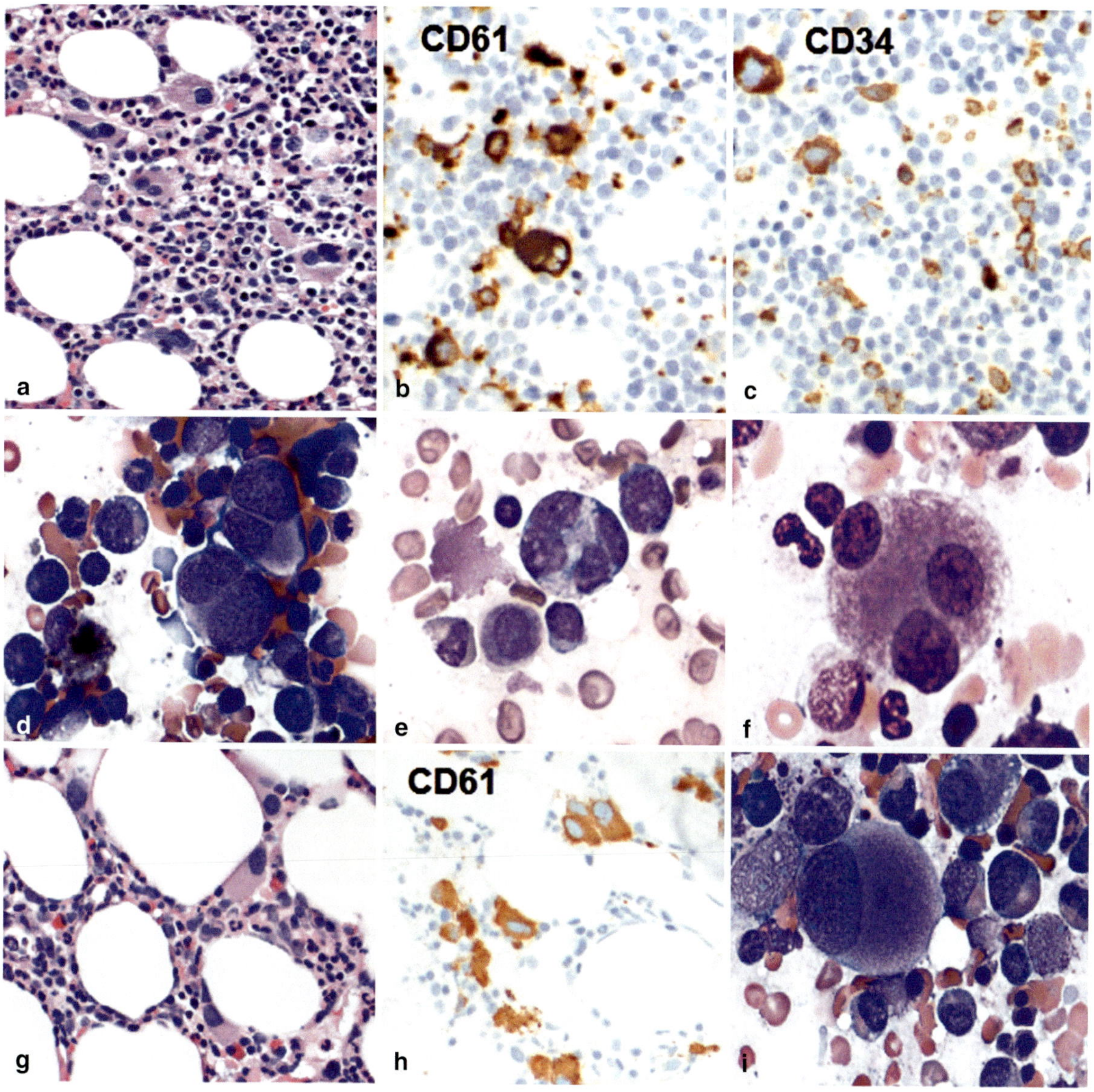

Fig. 24.4 The morphologic features of megakaryocytic dysplasia in the bone marrow (BM) of patients with myelodysplastic syndromes (MDS). (**a**) Dysplastic megakaryocytes with hypolobated and abnormally shaped nuclei in the BM core. (**b**) CD61 immunostain highlights dysplastic megakaryocytes in the BM core; there are many small hypolobated forms. (**c**) CD34 immunostains show increased CD34+ blasts in the BM core; the dysplastic megakaryocytes are abnormally positive for CD34. (**d**) Dysplastic small megakaryocytes with abnormal hypolobation in the BM aspirate smears. (**e**) Micromegakaryocytes and large hypolobated megakaryocytes in the BM aspirate smears. (**f**) Dysplastic large megakaryocytes with widely separate nuclear lobes in the BM aspirate smears. (**g**) Dysplastic monolobated megakaryocytes in the BM core from a patient with MDS associated with isolated del(5q). (**h**) CD61 immunostain highlights dysplastic monolobated small megakaryocytes in the BM core of the de(5q) MDS patient. (**i**) Dysplastic monolobated small megakaryocytes in the BM aspirate smear of the de(5q) MDS patient

and/or large "balloon-like" platelets are commonly observed [38].

- The morphologic features of dysmegakaryopoiesis include micro-megakaryocytes, small or large mononuclear forms, megakaryocytes with abnormal nuclear shape, nuclear hypolobation, multiple dispersed nuclear lobes ("pawn ball" changes), and small mature megakaryocytes with pale cytoplasm and defective platelet formation (Fig. 24.4a–f, Table 24.2) [1, 4, 39]. Mononuclear megakaryocytes may be identified, particularly in association with the 5q- syndrome (Fig. 24.4g–h) [40–43]. Whenever possible, evaluation of at least 30 megakaryocytes is strongly recommended to document the percentage of dysplastic megakaryocytes. This is best done using well-prepared aspirate smears, although biopsy specimens are also informative [44].

- Blasts and Auer rods (Fig. 24.5): According to the WHO classification [1, 4], the myeloblast percentage in the PB and BM of patients with MDS may be normal or increased, but is always less than 20% in blood and in bone marrow specimens.
  - An International Working Group on Morphology of Myelodysplastic Syndrome (IWGM-MDS) has recommended criteria for defining a myeloblast. These criteria include a high nuclear/cytoplasmic ratio, easily visible nucleoli, and usually, but not invariably, finely distributed nuclear chromatin. They have variably basophilic cytoplasm with or without a few granules, but no Golgi zone is detected [22].
  - Auer rods are needle- or rod-shaped azurophilic cytoplasmic inclusions first described in 1905 by Thomas McCrae, a Canadian physician at Johns Hopkins Hospital [45]. One year later, John Auer, a US physiologist, described the same structure [46]. Usually, in MDS, Auer rods are associated with increased blast counts, but they have also been reported in MDS cases with less than 5% blasts in the BM (Fig. 24.5a). Although most reports indicate Auer rods are associated with rapid disease progression [47, 48], some authors dispute their prognostic significance [49–54]. However, if a diagnosis of MDS is contemplated when Auer rods are present, correlation with cytogenetic findings is essential. Acute myeloid leukemia (AML) with t(8;21)(q22;q22.1); *RUNX-RUNX1T1* (Fig. 24.5b), AML with inv(16)(p13.1q22) or t(16;16)(p13.1;q22); *CBFB-MYH11*, and acute promyelocytic leukemia (APL) with t(15;17)(q22;q11–12); *PML-RARA* (Fig. 24.5c) do occasionally present with less than 20% blasts or abnormal promyelocytes in the blood and/or marrow, and the diagnosis in such cases is AML or APL, not MDS.
- Abnormalities of BM cellularity, cellular composition, and cellular distribution: The BM specimens in MDS are often hypercellular with increased proliferation, but premature apoptosis (Fig. 24.6a, b) which results in the classic paradox of a hypercellular BM associated with peripheral cytopenia(s) [55–57].
  - Some cases of MDS, particularly in pediatric patients, may have decreased BM cellularity (Fig. 24.6c, d) that can mimic aplastic anemia [58, 59]. Reduced marrow cellularity, often associated with reticulin fibrosis, is also common in therapy-related myeloid neoplasms (t-MN) [41, 60–62].
  - Abnormal distribution of hematopoietic cells, including abnormal localization of immature precursors (ALIP) and/or the displacement of erythroid precur-

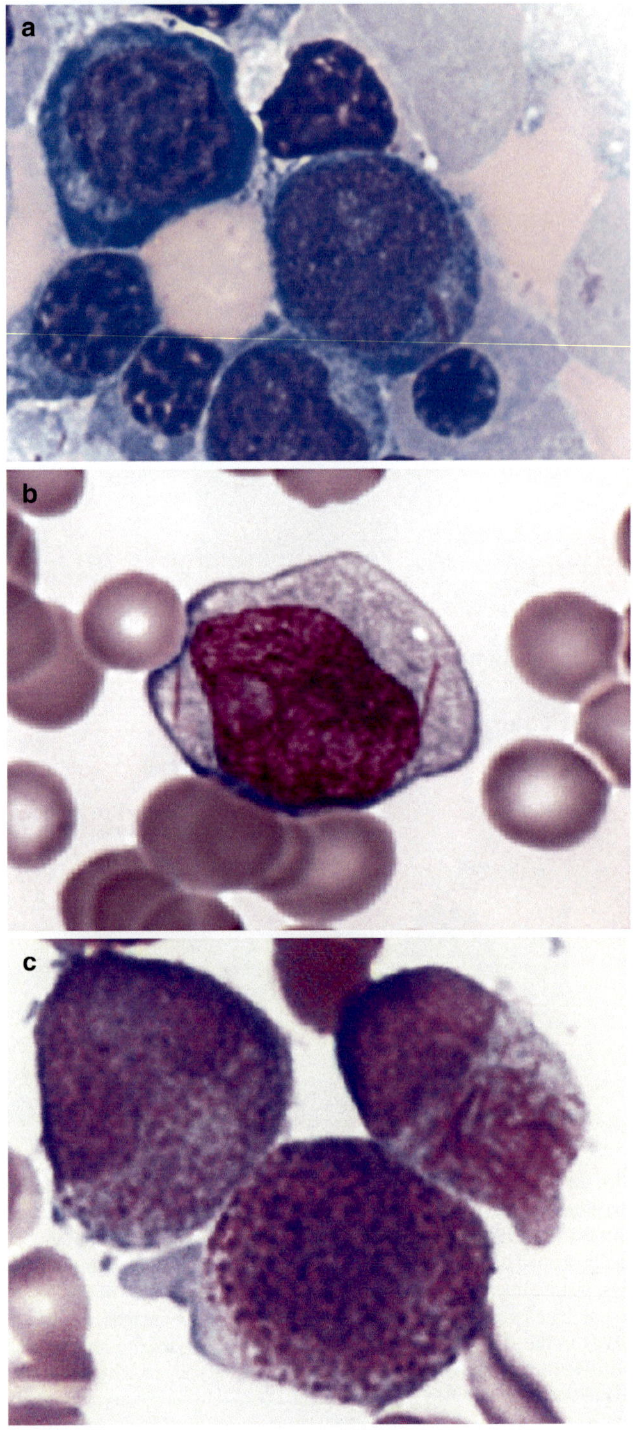

Fig. 24.5 Different types of blasts with Auer rods in patients with myelodysplastic syndromes (MDS), acute myeloid leukemia (AML), and acute promyelocytic leukemia (APL). (**a**) A blast with Auer rods in the BM aspirate smear of a patient with MDS with 4% blasts, classified as MDS-EB-1. (**b**) A blast with a long thin Auer rods in the PB smear of a patients with AML with t(8;21)(q22;q22.1) *RUNX-RUNX1T1*. (**c**) Blasts with bundles of Auer rods in the PB smear of a patients with APL with t(15;17)((q22;q11–12) *PML-RARA*

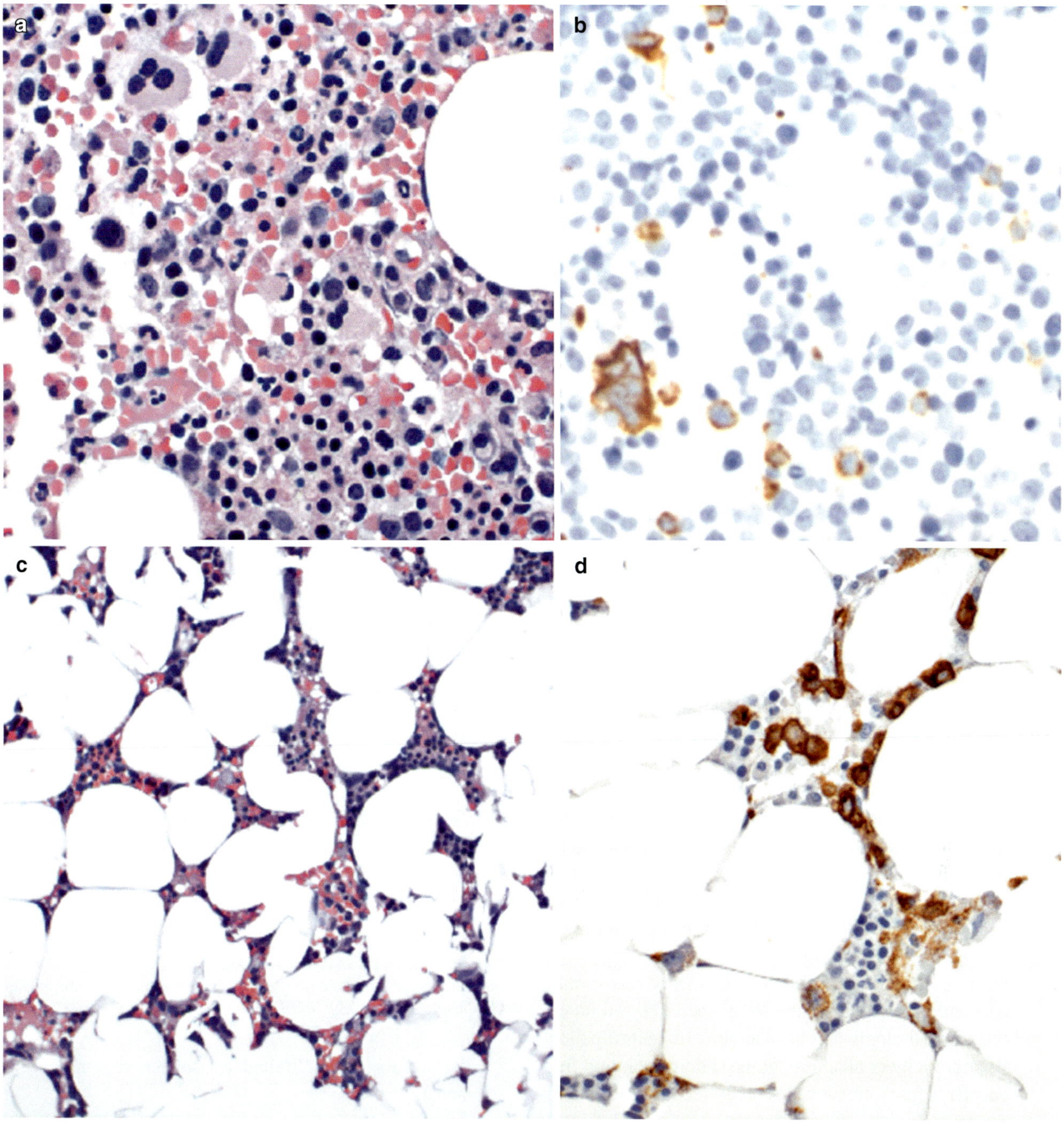

Fig. 24.6 Hypercellular vs. hypoplastic myelodysplastic syndromes (MDS). (**a**) Hypercellular BM of a patient with MDS-EB-1. (**b**) Increased CD34+ blasts in the hypercellular BM. (**c**) Hypocellular BM of a patient with MDS-EB-1. (**d**) Increased CD34+ blasts in the hypocellular BM

sors from their normal, intertrabecular location to paratrabecular regions, is common in MDS and can generally be appreciated in BM biopsies. BM core biopsies also provide material for immunohistochemical studies. In particular, CD34 is often expressed by MDS blasts, and can be very helpful in providing a more accurate assessment of the number of blasts.

5. What are the MDS mimics and what is the clinical impact of misdiagnosis?

It is very important, but often challenging, to distinguish MDS from MDS mimics that range from laboratory artifacts, to cytopenia and myelodysplasia induced by nutritional deficiencies, chronic inflammatory diseases, drugs/medications,

Table 24.3 MDS mimics and diagnostic approaches

MDS Mimics	Diagnostic approaches
Laboratory/staining artifacts	Re-stain slides by using an appropriate staining solution and protocol as well as well-prepared slides; avoid using stored specimens if possible
Idiopathic dysplasia of unknown significance (IDUS)	If there is significant dysplasia, thorough hematologic workup and cytogenetic/molecular studies are highly recommended
Nutritional deficiencies	Perform laboratory tests for iron, vitamin B_{12} and folic acid deficiency or copper deficiencies
Infections	Perform laboratory tests for parvovirus B19, HIV, *EBV*, CMV, leishmaniasis, or tuberculosis (TB)
Autoimmune diseases	Perform flow cytometric analysis to detect PNH clones and to assess the clonality of B cells and the immunophenotypes of B cells, T cells and NK cells, lymphoid cells and/or the laboratory tests for lupus and other autoimmune diseases
Alcohol, toxins, drugs, and organ (liver or renal) failure	Perform laboratory tests folate and thiamine, lead, and other toxins/drugs accordingly

and other toxins, to other hematologic and non-hematologic malignancies [63–65]. Table 24.3 lists common MDS mimics and practical approaches to their recognition.

- Laboratory/staining artifacts: A precise morphologic assessment for any hematologic disorder requires well-prepared PB and cellular BM aspirate smears, and one of the most common pitfalls, particularly in the evaluation of suspected cases of MDS, is trying to assess dysplasia on poorly prepared PB and BM smears.
  - For morphologic evaluation of PB smears, one should concentrate on areas of the slide where the red blood cells appear singly and have an area of central pallor. Hypertonicity or alkalinity of the staining solution frequently causes crenated red cells (echinocytes), and stomatocytes may form when the staining solution is too acidic [66].
  - Refrigerated storage and excessive EDTA can induce morphologic changes in PB and BM smears that mimic dysplastic features including erythroid nuclear irregularities, hypolobated neutrophils, small neutrophils, and micromegakaryocytes [67, 68].
  - A useful clue to distinguish genuine dysplasia from artifactual dysplastic changes is that MDS usually demonstrates at least some mixture of dysplastic, variably dysplastic and even nondysplastic cells, whereas MDS-like artifacts induced by improper staining or storage tend to be homogenous and affect all cells in the smears or are limited to isolated regions of the smear.
  - Although assessment of cytoplasmic hypogranularity of neutrophils is often problematic in poorly stained slides, usually, in MDS, the dysplastic neutrophils have additional abnormal features, such as abnormal nuclear segmentation and nuclear contours (Fig. 24.7).
- Nutritional deficiencies: Deficiencies of some essential nutrients can cause cytopenia(s) and dysplasia that mimic MDS. These deficiencies include iron, vitamin B_{12}, and folic acid, as well as essential mineral deficiencies, such as zinc-induced copper deficiency.
  - Vitamin B_{12} and folic acid deficiencies often cause marked erythroid proliferation, megaloblastoid

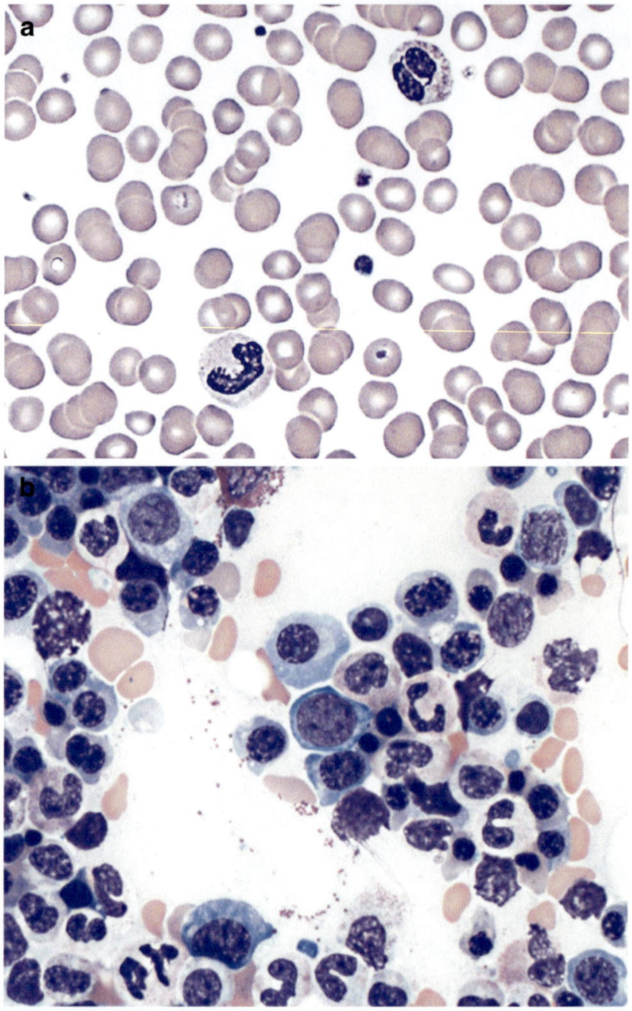

Fig. 24.7 Mixed populations of normally granulated and hypogranulated neutrophils in myelodysplastic syndromes (MDS). (**a**) Dysplastic granulocyte with cytoplasmic hypogranulation and nuclear abnormalities, including nuclear membrane projections (left) or hyposegmented nuclei (right) in the PB smears of a MDS patient. (**b**) Mixed populations of normally granulated granulocytes and hypogranulated neutrophils in the BM aspirate smear of a MDS patient

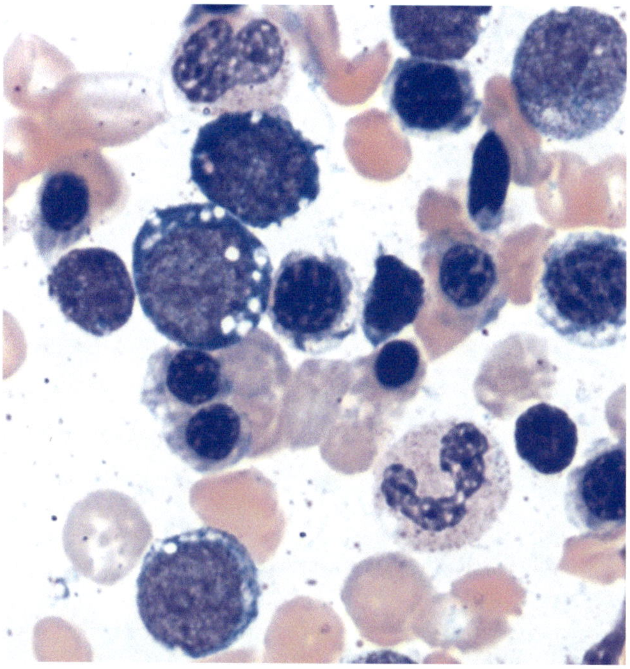

Fig. 24.8 Erythroid precursors with vacuolated cytoplasm in a patient of zinc-induced copper deficiency

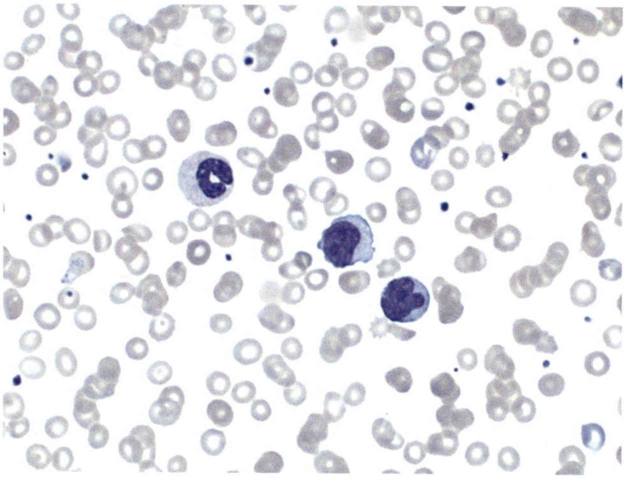

Fig. 24.9 A hypogranulated neutrophil and malignant lymphoma cells in the peripheral blood smear of a HIV patient

changes, nuclear/cytoplasmic maturation asynchrony and neutrophilic nuclear hypersegmentation and giant bands [69], and assessment of B_{12} and folic acid is recommended in the evaluation of all suspected MDS cases.

- Copper deficiency is characteristically associated with cytoplasmic vacuoles in erythroid and myeloid precursors (Fig. 24.8), is often related to zinc toxicity, and should be considered when patients present with cytopenia, erythroid, and myeloid dysplasia with vacuolization in erythroid and myeloid precursors. Neuropathy is often clinically present in such cases of copper deficiency as well [70, 71]. Pathologists should suggest appropriate chemical laboratory tests when the morphologic findings are suggestive of copper deficiency.

- Infections: Infections, such as Parvovirus B19, HIV, *EBV*, CMV, leishmaniasis, and tuberculosis (TB), can cause cytopenia(s) and morphologic abnormalities of the hematopoietic cells that mimic those seen in MDS. HIV infection may be associated with significant cytopenias and myelodysplasia (Fig. 24.9) [72–75]. Acute parvovirus B19 infection can cause a transient maturation arrest of erythroid precursors, and abnormal, giant proerythroblasts in the BM with marked anemia in the PB (Fig. 24.10). Chronic parvovirus B19 infections can cause significant marrow damage and impairment of multilineage hematopoiesis, leading to pancytopenia and multilineage dysplasia [76, 77].
- Autoimmune diseases: Various autoimmune conditions can cause marrow damage. Rheumatoid arthritis, systemic lupus erythematosus (Fig. 24.11), sarcoidosis (Fig. 24.12), and other autoimmune disorders often present with various degrees of cytopenias [78], and some patients may show some morphologic features in their PB and BM cells that resemble the changes of MDS.
  - Note that approximately 10% of MDS patients have concurrent autoimmune disorders [79, 80], and those cases may pose a challenge in clinical diagnosis as shown in Fig. 24.13, which illustrates a BM biopsy from a patient with the morphologic features of autoimmune myelofibrosis but was associated with del(7)(q22q36) plus a *JAK2V617F* mutation.
  - Paroxysmal nocturnal hemoglobinuria (PNH) can also mimic MDS, and clones of PNH cells of varying sizes are frequently associated with aplastic anemia [81, 82]. Flow cytometry provides a sensitive and definitive tool for diagnosis of PNH and should be performed when PNH is suspected.
- Alcohol, toxins, drugs/medications, and organ (liver or renal) failure:
  - Excessive alcohol consumption is one of the most common causes of cytopenia(s) and marrow damage as well as of dysplastic features [83]. Excessive alcohol consumption causes nutritional deficiencies, especially folate and thiamine deficiencies, leading to impaired hematopoiesis [83].
  - Numerous cytotoxic drugs, such as methotrexate, azathioprine, mechlorethamine (nitrogen mustard), procarbazine, chlorambucil, cyclophosphamide, ifosfamide, etoposide, teniposide, doxorubicin, arsenic compounds and tacrolimus, can also cause cytopenia(s) and dysplastic morphology [84, 85].

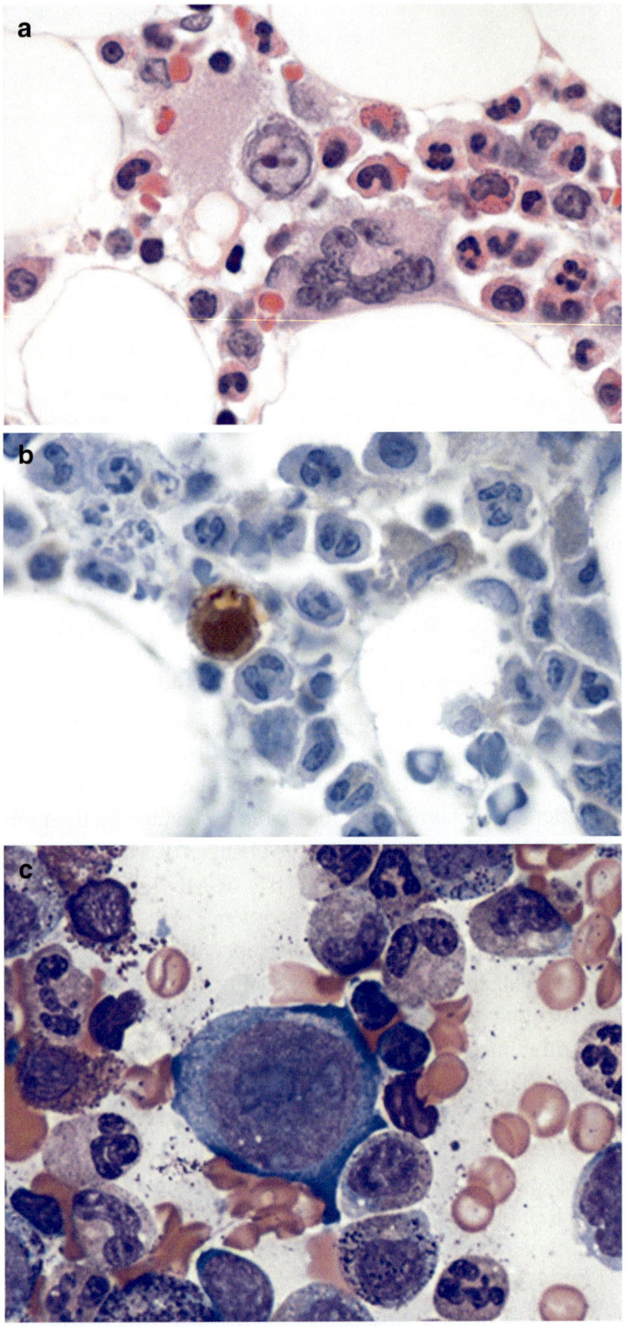

Fig. 24.10 Morphologic features of erythroid precursors in the bone marrow of a patient with parvovirus B19 infection. (**a**) A large atypical erythroid precursor with an intranuclear inclusion in the BM core. (**b**) The intranuclear inclusion is strongly positive for anti-parvovirus antibody in the BM core. (**c**) A giant pronormoblast with large intranuclear inclusions in the BM aspirate

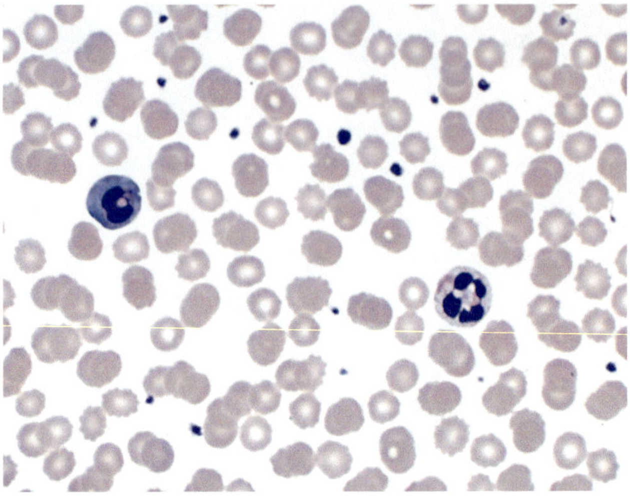

Fig. 24.11 Abnormal neutrophils in the peripheral blood smear of a patient with systemic lupus erythematous

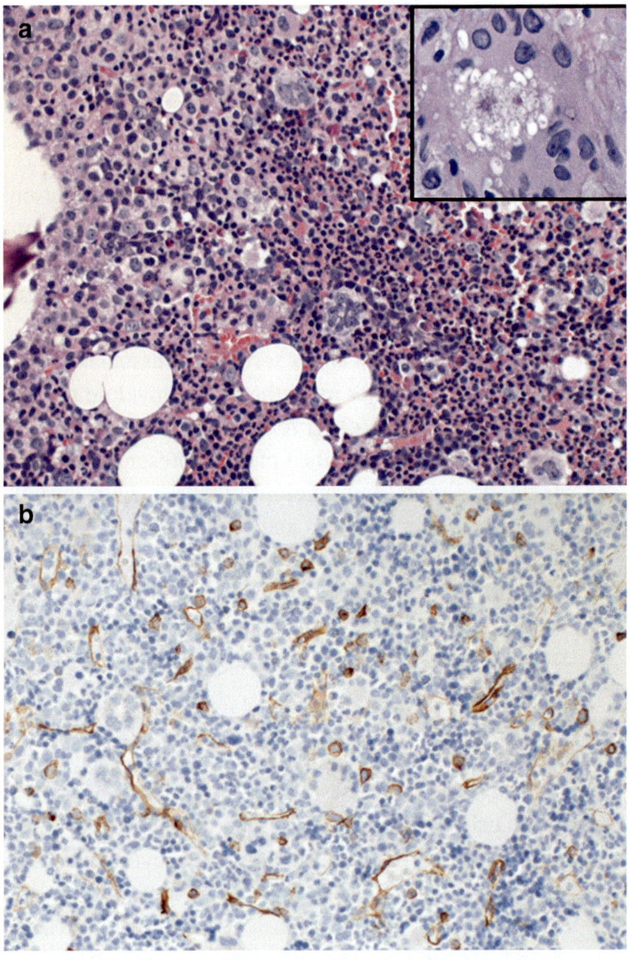

Fig. 24.12 Abnormal neutrophils in the peripheral blood smear of a patient with systemic lupus erythematous. (**a**) Markedly increased cellularity and immature myeloid cells in the BM core of a patient with sarcoidosis. The figure inset shows granuloma with an asteroid body. (**b**) Immunohistochemistry shows Increased CD34+ myeloid precursors/blasts in the BM core

– Tacrolimus and mycophenolate mofetil are immunosuppressive drugs commonly used after allogeneic organ transplantation, and these drugs can cause significant neutrophilic dysplasia (Fig. 24.14a), with pseudo-Pelger-Huët anomaly [86, 87]. Differing from drug (tacrolimus and mycophenolate)-induced cases,

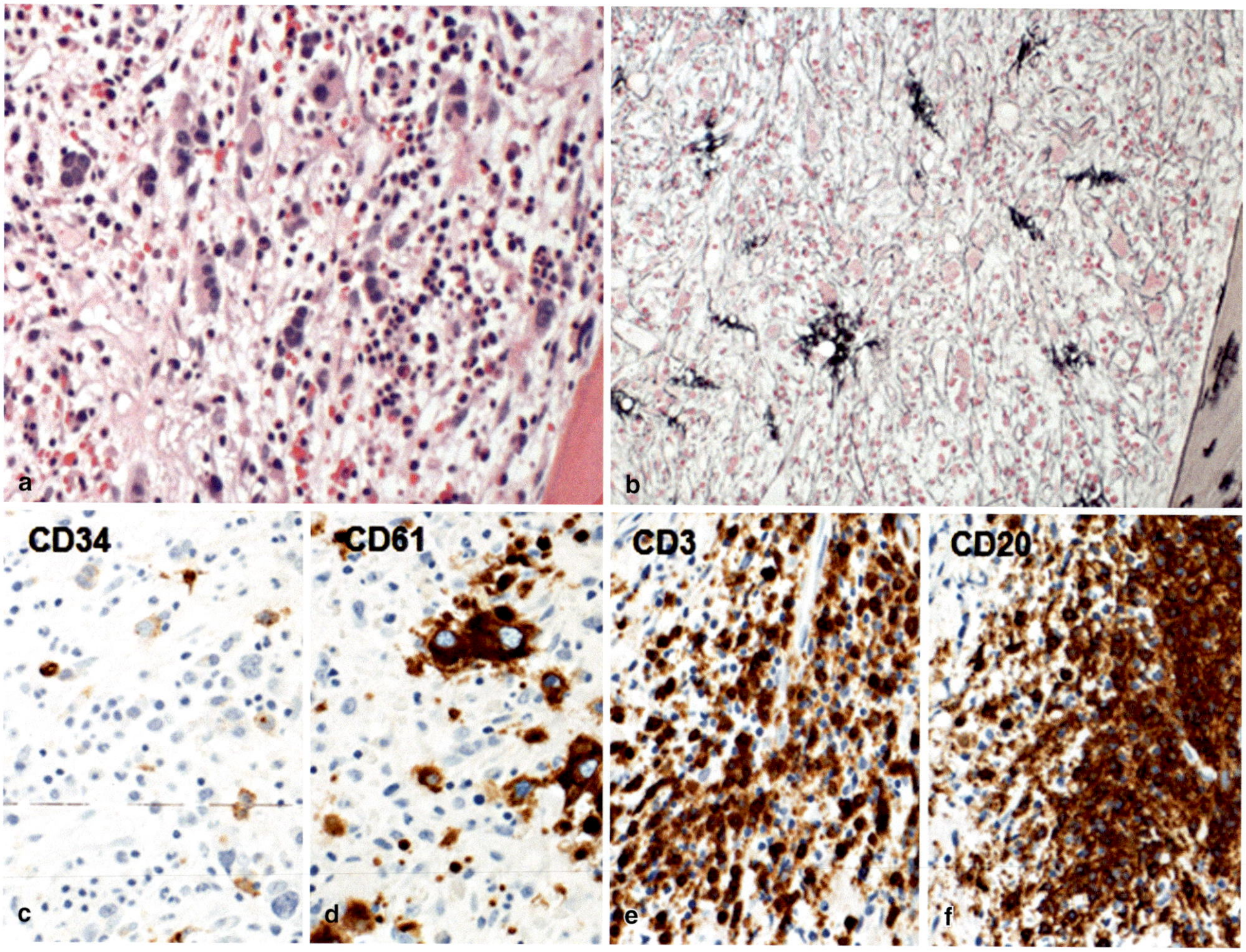

Fig. 24.13 Concurrence of myelodysplastic syndrome (MDS) and autoimmune myelofibrosis. (**a**) Hypocellular BM with markedly reduced myelopoiesis, relatively megakaryocytic hyperproliferation, stromal serous atrophy and lymphoplasmacytic infiltrate. (**b**) Reticulin stain shows markedly increased myelofibrosis. (**c–f**) Immunohistochemical studies for CD34, CD61, CD3 and CD20, respectively

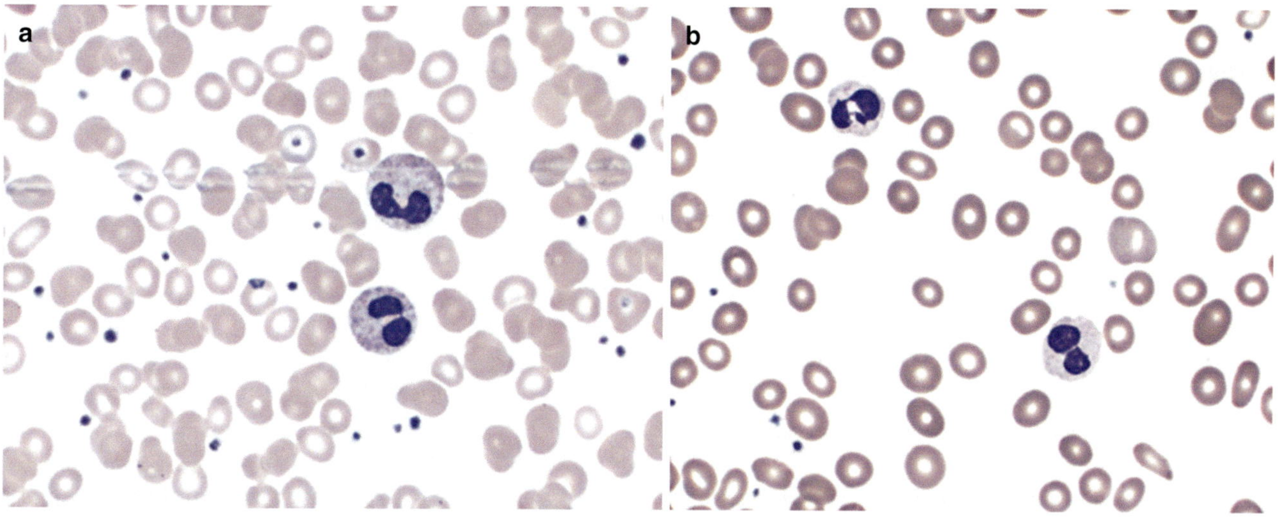

Fig. 24.14 Drug (tacrolimus)-induced pseudo-Pelger-Huët abnormality vs. pseudo-Pelger-Huët abnormality in myelodysplastic syndromes (MDS). (**a**) Neutrophils with pseudo-Pelger-Huët abnormality in the peripheral blood smear of a patient on tacrolimus treatment. (**b**) Dysplastic neutrophils with hypogranulation, abnormal nuclear membrane projections and chromatin patterns as well as pseudo-Pelger-Huët abnormality in the peripheral blood smear of a patient with MDS

MDS with pseudo-Pelger-Huët anomaly is often associated with other nuclear and cytoplasmic abnormalities in neutrophils and other lineage cells (Fig. 24.14b).
– Recombinant granulocyte (G-CSF) or granulocyte macrophage colony-stimulating growth factor (GM-CSF) can cause a transient left shift in myelopoiesis with increased blasts and myelodysplasia in the PB and BM that resembles MDS [88, 89].

6. What germline predispositions and inherited syndromes are relevant to MDS and its differential diagnosis?

See also Chap. 28 for a full discussion of myeloid neoplasms with germline predispositions and inherited syndromes. The following paragraphs briefly summarize the overlapping clinical and laboratory findings and morphological similarities with MDS.

- Germline predispositions to myeloid neoplasms: Several germline gene mutations, including *CEBPA*, *DDX41*, *RUNX1*, *ANKRD26*, *ETV6*, *GATA2,* and *SRP72*, confer an increased inherited risk for myeloid or lymphoid neoplasms, including MDS and AML. Myeloid neoplasms with germline predisposition are now recognized by the 2017 WHO classification (Table 24.4) and subdivided into three categories (and multiple subtypes in each category) depending on the gene involved and presence or absence of preexisting conditions and/ or organ dysfunction [1, 63]. Though rare, the presence of cytopenias and/ or dysplastic morphology of hematopoietic cells in many of these conditions makes them important differential considerations.
- Inherited bone marrow failure syndromes (IBMFs): IBMFs often present with peripheral blood cytopenias and hypocellular BM specimens with variable dysplastic changes and carry an increased risk for MDS and AML. They may have a number of systemic non-hematologic abnormalities as well, such as short stature, skeletal and facial abnormalities, skin and nail deformities, and organ dysfunction [64]. Classical IBMFs include the following 4 syndromes (Table 24.5):
  1. Fanconi Anemia (FA) caused by DNA repair gene mutations in the *FA/BRCA* pathway.
  2. Dyskeratosis Congenita (DC) caused by aberrations in key telomere biology genes.
  3. Diamond Blackfan Anemia (DBA) caused by ribosomal biology defects [65].
  4. Shwachman Diamond Syndrome (SDS) caused by *SBDS* gene mutations.

Table 24.4 The 2017 WHO classification of myeloid neoplasms with germline predisposition[1]

Classification	Subclassification
Myeloid neoplasms with germline predisposition without a preexisting disorder or organ dysfunction	Acute myeloid leukemia with germline *CEBPA* mutation Myeloid neoplasms with germline *DDX41* mutation[2]
Myeloid neoplasms with germline predisposition and preexisting platelet disorder	Myeloid neoplasms with germline *RUNX1* mutation[2] Myeloid neoplasms with germline *ANKRD26* mutation[2] Myeloid neoplasms with germline *ETV6* mutation[2]
Myeloid neoplasms with germline predisposition and organ dysfunction	Myeloid neoplasms with germline *GATA2* mutation Myeloid neoplasms with germline BM failure syndrome Myeloid neoplasms with germline BM telomere syndrome Juvenile myelomonocytic leukemia with neurofibromatosis, Noonan syndrome or Noonan syndrome-like disorders Myeloid neoplasms with Down syndrome

[1]Adapted from the book, WHO Classification of Tumours of Haematopoietic and Lymphoid Tissues. Lyon, France: IARC; 2017
[2]Lymphoid neoplasms are also reported to be associated with these mutations

- Three other inherited conditions leading to bone marrow failure are discussed below. For discussion of other, rarer subtypes of these syndromes, see Chap. 28.
  – Congenital neutropenia (CN): It is caused by a spectrum of mutations (Table 24.6) associated with variable clinical courses [90, 91].
    To date, over 100 mutations have been identified based on data from the Severe Chronic Neutropenia International Registry. However, in approximately 30–40 percent of the cases of CN, the genetic basis remains unknown [92].
    Kostmann syndrome is a group of disorders that affect early myelopoiesis and cause severe congenital neutropenia (SCN) usually without other physical malformations [93, 94]. The most common form, SCN1, is caused by autosomal dominant *ELANE* (*ELA2*) mutations and accounts for 60–80% of SCN cases. *ELANE* (*ELA2*) gene encodes a neutrophil elastase, and cyclic neutropenia is also caused by autosomal dominantly inherited mutations in *ELANE* (*ELA2*) [95]. SCN2 is caused by heterozygous autosomal dominant) mutation in *GFI1* [93]. Kostmann disease (SCN3) was initially described in 1956 Kostmann [96]. About one-third of patients with Kostmann disease (SCN3) also

Table 24.5 Inherited bone marrow failure syndromes and telomere biology disorders

Disorders	Hematologic and physical features	BM findings	Gene mutations	Diagnostic tests
Fanconi anemia (FA)	Thrombocytopenia, macrocytic anemia, or macrocytosis of RBC, then progressing to pancytopenia later; BM failure (~90%) or hematologic malignancies (MDS/AML) or solid tumors by age 40; Short stature; Abnormalities of skin, arms, head, renal, gonadal, CNS, GI, or cardiopulmonary systems	Progressively reducing BM cellularity, with erythroid hyperplasia and megaloblastoid changes, to aplastic BM in ~90% by age 40 Erythroid dysplasia is common	[1]AR: *FANCA* [2]XLR: *FANCB, FANCC, FANCD1 (BRCA2), FANCD2, FANCE, FANCF, FANCG, FNACI, FANCJ (BRIP1), FANCL, FANCM, FANCN (PALB2), RAD51C, SLX4 (BTBD12)*	Screening: Chromosomal breakage or cell-cycle arrest induced by mitomycin C or Diepoxybutane Gene sequencing for relevant mutations
Dyskeratosis congenita (DC) and telomere biology disorders	Cytopenia, progressing to pancytopenia Triad: Lacey reticular skin pigmentation, nail dystrophy, and oral leukoplakia	Progressive BM failure, similar to FA, initially normocellular BM to aplastic BM (~40%) by age 40	XLR: *DKC1* [3]AD: *TERT, TERC, TINF2, RTEL1* AR: *NOP10, NHP2, WARAP53, RTEL1, TERT, CTC1*	Telomere length measurement by flow-FISH; Gene sequencing for the relevant mutations
Shwachman-Diamond syndrome (SDS)	Neutropenia in majority, intermittent in 2/3 or chronic in 1/3; normocytic or macrocytic anemia in 1/2, and thrombocytopenia in 1/3 Exocrine pancreatic dysfunction/steatorrhea; Skeletal abnormalities: Short stature, asphyxiating thoracic dystrophy (Jeune syndrome), metaphyseal dysostosis	Progressively reducing BM cellularity Prominent granulocytic hypoplasia and left-shifted myelopoiesis Note: Granulocytic dysplasia may be present	AR: *SBDS* Common deleterious mutations including 258 T > C and 183–4 TA > CT Note: 10% patients lack *SBDS* mutations	Screening: Low serum trypsinogen (age < 3 yo), low pancreatic isoamylase (age > 3 yo) Gene sequencing for *SBDS* mutations
Diamond-Blackfan anemia (DBA)	Macrocytic anemia, typically 2–3 months of age, ~25% presented at birth Thumb anomalies; craniofacial dysmorphologies (Pierre Robin syndrome); cardiac and genitourinary anomalies; short stature	Marked erythroid hypoplasia with defected maturation Frequently normocellular BM, Normal granulopoiesis and megakaryopoiesis	AR: *RPS19, RPS17, RPS24, RPS7, RPS10, RPS26, RPL35A, RPL5, RPL11* XLR: *GATA1*	Screening: Hemoglobin F; elevated erythrocyte adenosine deaminase; Gene sequencing

[1]AR: Autosomal recessivea
[2]XLR: X-lined recessive
[3]AD: Autosomal dominant

have neurological changes including seizures, learning disabilities, or developmental delay. This type (SCN3) has an autosomal recessive form and is caused homozygous mutations in the *HAX1* gene [97]. Other gene mutations involved in SCN include the Wiskott-Aldrich syndrome gene *WASP*, *CSF3R*, *G6PC3*, *SBDS*, and *JAGN1* [97–101].

Mild CN has benign intermittent neutropenia usually detected later in life and is associated with the mutations in *CHD2* or *HUWE1* genes [90], which encode a chromodomain/helicase-containing chromatin modifier and an E3 ubiquitin-protein ligase, respectively, and are involved in neurodevelopment [102, 103].

Patients with moderate to severe CN and intellectual disability is associated with dominant mutations in *KAT6A* [90], so-called KAT6A syndrome [104–106]. *KAT6A (MOZ)* encodes a lysine (K) acetyltransferase, a member of the MYST family of proteins, that is essential for the maintenance of adult hematopoietic stem cells [107], and the chromosomal translocation of t(8;16)(p11;p13) involving *KAT6A/CREBBP* gene fusion causes AML with unique cytomorphological, cytogenetic, and prognostic features [108].

- Congenital dyserythropoietic anemias (CDA): Congenital dyserythropoietic anemias (CDA) are characterized by distinct morphologic abnormalities of erythroid precursors and caused by gene mutations in the major CDA subgroups, including I-*CDAN1*, II-*SEC23B*, and III-*KIF23* [109, 110]. CDA variants with mutations in erythroid transcription factor genes (*KLF1* and *GATA1*) have been recently identified as well [109]. Table 24.6 lists the hematologic features, gene mutations, and diagnostic approaches of the four most common types of CDA, but even these are extremely rare.
- Monocytopenia and mycobacterial infection (MonoMAC) syndrome: MonoMAC syndrome is caused by heterozygous mutations in *GATA2*, which result in the developmental defects of dendritic cell (DC), monocyte, B and natural killer (NK) lymphoid cell lineages [111–114]. The clinical features associated with germline *GATA2* mutations are quite variable, and may be manifest initially by infection, MDS or AML, or

Table 24.6 Congenital neutropenia (CN), congenital dyserythropoietic anemias (CDA), and monocytopenia and mycobacterial infection (MonoMAC) syndrome

Disorders/subtypes	Hematologic and physical features	Gene mutations	Diagnostic tests
Severe CN and Kostmann syndrome	Isolated neutropenia with an ANC <500/uL; normo- or hypocellularity with a myeloid arrest at an early stage, nuclear atypia, and cytoplasmic vacuolization 2 Frequent upper respiratory infections, often due to staphylococci and streptococci	[a]AD: *ELANE, CSF3R, GFI1* [b]AR: *HAX1, G6PC3* [c]XLR: *WAS* Unknown ~40%	Gene sequencing
Mild CN with gene mutations implicated in neurodevelopmental disorders	Benign nonsymptomatic intermittent neutropenia (1000–1500/uL) Neurodevelopmental disorders	AD: *CHD2* XLR: *HUWE1*	Gene sequencing
Moderate to severe CN with KAT6A syndrome	Moderate to severe intermittent neutropenia (<1000/uL) KAT6A syndrome/intellectual disability and neurodevelopment defects	AR: *KAT6A*	Gene sequencing
CDA type I (CDA-I)	Macrocytic anemia, with extramedullary hematopoiesis Hypocellular BM with nuclear chromatin bridges between erythroblasts and marked dyserythropoiesis	AR: *CDAN1*	Gene sequencing
CDA type II (CDA-II)	Normocytic anemia, with extramedullary hematopoiesis Hypercellular BM with a large number of bi-nucleated, rarely multinuclear erythroblasts	AR: *SEC23B*	Electrophoresis (SDS-PAGE) Gene sequencing
CDA type III (CDA-III)	Intravascular hemolysis Hypercellular BM with erythroid hyperplasia and dyserythropoiesis with large multinucleated erythroblasts	AD: *KIF23*	↑LDH, ↓Hepatoglobin Gene sequencing
CDA type IV (CDA-IV)	Normocytic anemia and/or hemolysis Hypercellular BM with erythroid hyperplasia and various dyserythropoiesis	AD: *KLF1*	↑HbF Gene sequencing
MonoMAC syndrome	Profoundly decreased or absent circulating monocytes, DCs, NK cells, and B cells Severe infections with *M. avium* complex (MAC) Hypocellular BM, often with myelofibrosis and multilineage dysplasia	AD: *GATA2* No cytogenetic abnormalities No mutations in *TERT* or *KRAS*	Negative for chromosomal fragility studies DNA sequencing for *GATA2* mutations

[a]*AD* autosomal dominant; [b]*AR* autosomal recessive; [c]*XLR* X-lined recessive

lymphedema (Table 24.6). The majority of patients with MonoMAC syndrome have hypocellular marrows with reticulin fibrosis and multilineage dysplasia [115], which are often difficult to distinguish from hypoplastic MDS.

- Clinical Implications: Patients with germline mutations and inherited/congenital syndromes have a spectrum of clinical presentations and variable outcomes. In general, it is difficult to predict their clinical courses or to make a diagnosis of MDS at the right time in those patients. Genetic evaluation and genetic counseling should be recommended for patients with germline predispositions and inherited syndromes, and periodic BM examinations may be considered for assessing disease progression. Importantly, these abnormalities should be particularly considered and assessed in family members who are being considered as possible donors for patients requiring bone marrow transplantation for any hematologic neoplasm.

7. What other pre-MDS conditions are relevant to MDS differential diagnosis?

- Idiopathic dysplasia of unknown significance (IDUS) and idiopathic cytopenia of undetermined significance (ICUS). Previous studies have shown that dysmyelopoiesis and even multilineage dysplasia can be seen in a small yet significant proportion of the BM specimens from healthy unrelated BM donors [116–119]. The terms IDUS and/or ICUS are used to describe those situations in which there is dysplasia in 10% or more of any hematopoietic lineage and/or persistent (>4 months duration) cytopenia(s) after exclusion of secondary causes of dyspoiesis as well as exclusion of MDS-related cytogenetic abnormalities [118, 120].
  - In ICUS, cytopenia is present, but the dysplasia is not sufficient to fulfill the WHO criteria for MDS.
  - In IDUS, the dysplasia is prominent but cytopenia is not present, or if detectable, is very mild.
  - Both conditions may progress to an overt myelodysplastic syndrome (MDS), but progression to other

Table 24.7 Recurrent gene mutations in myelodysplastic syndromes (MDS)

Pathways/genes	Gene locus	Frequency	Prognostic impact
Epigenetic regulation			
TET2	4q24	~25%	Unclear
ASXL1	20q11	15–20%	Adverse
DNMT3A	2p23	~10%	Adverse
EZH2	7q35-q36	5–10%	Adverse
IDH1/2	2q33.3/15q26.1	~5%	Unclear
UTX	Xp11.2	~1%	Unclear
SETBP1	18q21.1	~1%	Adverse
RNA splicing/processing			
SF3B1	2q33.1	~25%	Favorable
U2AF1	21q22.3	5–10%	Adverse
SRSF2	17q25.1	5–10%	Adverse
ZRSR2	Xp22.1	5–10%	Unclear
PRPF8	17p13.3	1–3%	Unclear
Transcription factors and cofactors			
RUNX1	21q22.3	~10%	Adverse
TP53	17p13.1	~5–10%	Adverse
BCOR/BCORL1	Xp11.4/Xq25-q26.1	~5%	Adverse
Signal transduction pathway			
JAK2	9p24	5–10%	Unclear
CBL	11q23.3	~5%	Adverse
N/K-RAS	1p13.2/12p12.1	~5%	Adverse
Cohesion complex			
STAG2	Xq25	5–7%	Adverse
RAD21	8p24	~2%	Adverse
SMC3	10q25	~2%	Adverse
SMC1A	Xp11.22-p11.21	<1%	Adverse

myeloid neoplasms is also possible. For both of these ill-defined entities, a thorough hematologic work and follow-up is recommended [121].

- Clonal hematopoiesis of indeterminate potential (CHIP) and clonal cytopenia of unknown significance (CCUS): The advent of next-generation DNA sequencing has allowed for identification of many somatic mutations in MDS (Table 24.7). Clonal hematopoiesis is defined as the expansion of a clonal population of blood cells with one or more somatic mutations [122, 123]. The term "CHIP" was coined to describe individuals with a somatic mutation identified in their blood and/or marrow that has been reported to be associated with a hematologic neoplasm, but who lack other diagnostic criteria for a hematologic malignancy [124].
  - However, individuals with CHIP may have an increased risk of acquiring a hematologic malignancy, including therapy-related myeloid neoplasms [125]. CHIP does signify age-related clonal hematopoiesis and has a striking association with an increased risk for cardiovascular diseases [126].
  - The term "CHIP" should only be used for individuals who have a normal blood count. CCUS should be reserved for rare patients with cytopenia who have clonal abnormalities but no dysplasia.
- It should be emphasized that ICUS, IDUS, CHIP, and CCUS are not synonymous with low-grade MDS, and patients with these conditions may or may not develop MDS or may develop other types of neoplasms or nonneoplastic disorders [1, 57]. Individuals with clonal hematopoiesis have an estimated risk of progression to a frank neoplasm of 0.5–1% per year but also have a much higher risk of cardiovascular diseases [127–129]. In addition, clonal hematopoiesis is common in healthy elderly individuals and may be a part of the aging process. When dealing with patients with recurrent MDS/AML-associated gene mutation, one should adhere to the 2017 WHO diagnostic criteria for MDS.

8. What are the practical guidelines for diagnosis of MDS? What are the findings suggestive of MDS and the findings that rule out MDS?

- Findings serving as presumptive evidence of MDS:
  - The presence of MDS-related cytogenetic abnormalities (Table 24.8) by conventional cytogenetic studies, except for +8, del(20q) and −Y, can serve as

Table 24.8 Recurring chromosomal abnormalities in the myelodysplastic syndromes (MDS)

Chromosome abnormality	Genes involved	Frequency	IPSS-R risk category
Unbalanced			
Gain of chromosome 8[a]	Unknown	5–7%	intermediate
Loss of chromosome 7 or del(7q)	*EZH2, MLL3, CUX1*	10%	Poor
del(5q)	*CSNK1A1, RPS14, EGR1, APC, DDX41, HSPA9, NPM1, TIFAB, DIAPH1, miR-145, miR-146a*	10%	Good
del(20q)[a]	*MYBL2, TP53RK, TP53TG5*	5–8%	Good
Loss of Y chromosome (-Y)[a]	Unknown	5%	Very good
Isochromsome 17q i(17q) or t(17p)	*TP53*	3%	Intermediate
Loss of chromosome 13 or del(13q)	Unknown	3%	Intermediate
del(11q)	Unknown	3%	Good
del(12p) or t(12p)	Unknown	3%	Good
del(9q)	Unknown	1–2%	Intermediate
idic(X)(q13)	Unknown	1–2%	Intermediate
Balanced			
t(11;16)(q23.3;p13.3)	*KMT2A/CREBBP*	3%	Intermediate
t(3;21)(q26.2;q22.1)	*MECOM/RUNX1*	2%	Intermediate
t(1:3)(p36.3;q21.2)	*PRDM16/RPN1*	1%	Intermediate
t(2;11)(p21;q23.3)	Unknown, without *MLL* gene rearrangement.	1%	Intermediate
inv(3)(q21.3q26.2)/t(3;3)(q21.3;q26.2)	*MECOM (EVI1)/RPN1*	1%	Poor
Complex karyotype (≥3 abnormalities)		5–6%	Very poor

[a]Not MDS-defining cytogenetic abnormalities

presumptive evidence of MDS, if the blasts are <20% in PB or BM.
  - Persistent excess of blasts (2–19% in PB and 5–19% in BM) with or without Auer rods, in an appropriate setting, e.g., persistent cytopenia, an inappropriate level of response to EPO, and no recent chemotherapy, infections or G-CSF treatment, can serve as presumptive evidence of MDS. The presence of Auer rods warrants diagnosis of a higher grade MDS if the blasts are within the MDS range.
  - A diagnosis of MDS-RS can be made if there are >15% ring sideroblasts in the BM aspirate smears with or without *SF3B1* mutation or if there are >5% ring sideroblasts in the BM aspirate smears with *SF3B1* mutation.
- Findings suggestive of MDS:
  - Significant dysplasia, especially granulocytic dysplasia that accompanies cytopenia(s) with or without erythroid and/or megakaryocytic dysplasia, is most suggestive of MDS.
  - The presence of a significant population of small megakaryocytes or micromegakaryocytes with hypo- or mono-lobated nuclei in BM core biopsies or aspirate smears, in the presence of cytopenia(s), is highly suggestive of MDS.
- Findings to be considered cautiously in making a definite diagnosis of MDS:
  - If only single-lineage dysplasia is present – especially only erythroid dysplasia – a definitive diagnosis of MDS should be deferred until there is additional substantiating evidence for MDS, such as definitive genetic abnormalities or evidence of further evolution. Nonneoplastic causes of cytopenia or erythroid dysplasia are particularly common in the elderly [130].
  - The presence of demonstrable clonal hematopoiesis by molecular studies (Table 24.7), without significant myelodysplasia and/or cytopenia(s), does not warrant a diagnosis of early or low-grade MDS. Clonal hematopoiesis can be a part of aging-related hematologic changes [131, 132].
  - The presence of an autoimmune condition does not exclude the diagnosis of MDS. An autoimmune disease can be concurrent with MDS or perhaps contribute to MDS pathogenesis [133]. In the cases of concurrent myelodysplasia and autoimmune disease (Fig. 24.13), careful assessment of the degree of myelodysplasia and information regarding cytogenetics – including the response to immunomodulating therapies – may provide important clues to the correct diagnoses.
  - In rare MDS cases, such as those with *GATA2* mutation or *MECOM (EVI1)* rearrangements, patients may have myelodysplasia and/or increased blasts or thrombocytosis, but no cytopenia. In patients with significant myelodysplasia, but no cytopenia(s), exclusion of myelodysplasia mimics and myeloproliferative/myelodysplastic neoplasms is necessary.
  - In rare cases, clonal cytogenetic abnormalities of undetermined significance (CCAUS) as well as some chromosomal abnormalities identified by FISH or PCR may not be necessarily associated with an underlying myelodysplastic syndrome [134]. Still, such CCAUS cases are rare in our experience and extra caution should be exerted. Close follow-up is highly recommended in such cases.
- Findings ruling out the diagnosis of MDS:

- The blast count in the PB or BM of MDS patients should always be <20%. If the blast count is ≥20% in the PB or BM, the diagnosis is acute leukemia, but not MDS.
- The diagnosis of MDS should not be made in cases in which cytogenetic abnormalities are found that define subtypes of AML, e.g., t(8;21)(q22;q22), inv(16)(p13q22)/t(16;16)(p13;q22), and t(15;17)(q22;q21).
- MDS does not have myeloproliferative neoplasm-defined molecular or cytogenetic abnormalities, i.e., *BCR-ABL1, PCM1-JAK2* fusions or *PDGFRA*, *PDGFRB,* and *FGFR1* gene rearrangements, which identify other specific hematologic neoplasms.
- A patient with a history of previous chemo- or radiation therapy should be classified as a therapy-related myeloid neoplasm (t-MN); if blasts are <20% in the PB or BM and myelodysplastic features are present, the case may be classified as therapy-related neoplasm with myelodysplastic features, but further subclassification according to the guidelines used to subclassify de novo MDS may be misleading for prediction of prognosis [61].
- MDS is not associated with a marked increase in peripheral blood monocytes or neutrophils, which is often seen in myelodysplastic/myeloproliferative neoplasms (MDS/MPN).
- Thrombocytopenia is common in MDS, but some MDS cases with inv(3) or t(3;3) may have significant thrombocytosis.
- A definite diagnoses and classification of MDS should be deferred in patients who are undergoing or just finished chemotherapy, G-CSF or other growth factor therapy, or stem cell mobilizing procedures.

9. What is the minimal and optimal ancillary workup for MDS and subclassification of MDS?

- Patient history and physical examination: The history should include detailed information regarding any hematologic diseases in the family as well as the patient's exposure to any previous chemotherapy or radiation therapy, exposure to toxins such as benzene, and a detailed catalogue of previous medication including "alternative medication," alcohol intake, smoking, bleeding/bruising, and infection. A complete physical examination that includes determination of the size of the spleen and the liver should be performed.
- Blood tests and morphologic examination: A complete blood cell count (CBC) and leukocyte differential with assessment of the morphology of red cells, white cells, and platelets is mandatory. Morphologic evaluation should be performed on optimally prepared PB smears, with a required differential count of at least 200 WBC when possible. Other blood tests to further exclude MDS mimics (see the following section) may be performed based on the patient history, clinical and physical findings, and the results of the initial basic blood tests and morphologic evaluation.
- Morphologic evaluation of bone marrow specimens: Generally, this is a mandatory step in the diagnostic workup for MDS and should include the evaluation of BM core biopsies and aspirate smears, as well as reticulin and/or trichrome stains of the BM core biopsies, and iron stains of the BM aspirate smears. See Chap. 20 for characteristics of an adequate bone marrow specimen.
- Conventional cytogenetic analysis of bone marrow aspirate: A conventional cytogenetic analysis is required for all initial suspected MDS cases. Cytogenetic studies or fluorescence in situ hybridization (FISH) with a MDS panel of probes on peripheral blood may be performed in case of inadequate BM aspirates or dry taps, but should not considered as an adequate replacement for a complete karyotype.

10. What additional ancillary tests are helpful for the diagnosis of MDS?

- Fluorescence in situ hybridization (FISH): When an accurate assessment of the karyotype is not possible due to no cell growth or insufficient metaphases, FISH should be performed in order to determine whether specific cytogenetic abnormalities are present. Probes for FISH analysis should cover abnormalities in at least the following chromosomal regions: 5q31, cep7, 7q31, 20q, cep8, cepY, and p53 [118, 135]. However, FISH should not be routinely considered in lieu of a complete karyotype. The cytogenetic findings at diagnosis may not only provide important diagnostic information but also provide one of the most important prognostic indicators in MDS; and evidence of clonal cytogenetic evolution suggests a poor outcome [1, 20, 136].
- Immunohistochemical staining (IHC): The immunostains for CD34 and CD61 are recommended to assist in assessing the numbers and distribution patterns of blasts and megakaryocytes, respectively, in BM core biopsies [137]. These stains are particularly useful if the marrow aspirate is hypocellular or hemodilute, or the marrow is fibrotic. However, CD34 IHC highlights not only myeloblasts but also hematogones, lymphoid blasts, and endothelial cells. Importantly, monoblasts usually do not express CD34, and erythroid and megakaryocytic blasts are usually nonreactive for CD34 as well, although it may be aberrantly expressed in dysplastic megakaryocytes [138, 139]. Therefore, although of considerable value when good aspirate smears cannot be obtained, CD34 staining by IHC does have some limitations.

- Flow cytometry: Multi-parameter flow cytometry (MFC) of PB and/or BM aspirate specimens may detect abnormal populations of cells with aberrantly expressed differentiation and/or lineage-associated antigens in cases of MDS.
  - Coexpression of CD34 with antigens usually expressed on more mature cells, such as CD15, CD11b, and/or CD56, diminished CD10 expression in mature granulocytes, or coexpression of lymphoid-related antigens, such as CD7, CD2, and CD19, on myeloid cells, are examples of antigenic changes that, in the appropriate setting, may be suggestive of MDS [140–142].
  - To date, however, there is no generally accepted or standardized MFC protocol for MDS. Therefore, MFC is generally considered as providing supportive but not entirely diagnostic evidence for the diagnosis of MDS. Several flow cytometry-based prognostic scoring systems have been reported to have both diagnostic and prognostic value in MDS [143–147].
  - Certain antigenic aberrancies may have a value to assist in prognostication of MDS; for example, the increased expression of CD117 in myeloid progenitors was reported to be associated with a poorer prognosis, and on the other hand, patients with decreased CD13 expression in mature monocytes had a better prognosis [141, 146, 148].
- DNA sequencing: MDS-related gene mutations are clustered in 5 major groups of genes as listed in Table 24.7:
  - Epigenetic regulator genes
  - RNA processing/splicing factor genes
  - Transcription factor and cofactor genes
  - Signal transduction pathway factor genes
  - Cohesion complex component genes

    DNA sequencing technologies are increasingly used to identify MDS-related recurrent mutations or germline mutations that predispose to myeloid neoplasms or other cancers [149–151]. Not uncommonly, however, the findings are gene mutations of uncertain significance, and these results have led to an increasing number of patient referrals to hematology centers for further evaluations. However, it should be emphasized that those gene mutations listed in Table 24.7 are not specific for MDS, and they can be seen in normal aging hematopoiesis and other types of hematologic or non-hematologic malignancies.

11. What is the workup to provide prognostic information?

- Prognostic scoring systems: Prognosis of MDS can be estimated using a number of scoring systems, but the Revised International Prognostic Scoring System (IPSS-R) is the most accepted and widely used system [152]. The IPSS-R and other scoring systems are based on the following five major parameters.
  - Hemoglobin (g/dL)
  - Absolute neutrophil count (x10^9/L)
  - Platelet count (x10^9/L)
  - Blast count in BM (%), and
  - Cytogenetic categories (very good, good, intermediate, poor, and very poor)

    The IPSS-R system includes 16 cytogenetic abnormalities that are the most important factor in determining MDS prognosis [153]. Tables 24.9 and 24.10a, b, summarize the IPSS-R cytogenetic prognostic subgroups and the scores and risk values. Further information regarding the IPSS-R score calculation can be found at https://www.mds-foundation.org/calculator/advanced/.
  - Other features that have been reported to have a prognostic significance in MDS include age (> 60 years), LDH (high vs normal), ferritin (>350 ng/mL), beta-2 microglobulin (>2 g/mL), and BM fibrosis, as those conditions are associated with shorter overall survival in patients with MDS [152, 153].
- Gene mutation-based prognostic value: Many recurrent somatic mutations are identified in MDS (Table 24.7).

Table 24.9 IPSS-R Cytogenetic risk groups

Cytogenetic prognostic subgroups	Cytogenetic abnormalities
Very good	−Y, del(11q)
Good	Normal, del(5q), del(12p), del(20q), double including del(5q)
Intermediate	del(7q), +8, +19, i(17q), any other single or double independent clones
Poor	−7, inv(3)/t(3q)/del(3q), double including −7/del(7q), Complex: 3 abnormalities
Very poor	Complex: >3 abnormalities

Table 24.10a IPSS-R Prognostic Score Values

Prognostic variable	0	0.5	1	1.5	2	3	4
Cytogenetics	Very good		Good		Intermediate	Poor	Very poor
BM blast %	≤2		2–4%		5–10%	>10%	
Hemoglobin	≥10		≥8 to <10	<8			
Platelets	≥100	≥50 to <100	<50				
ANC	≥0.8	<0.8					

Table 24.10b IPSS-R Prognostic Risk Categories/Scores

Risk category	Risk score
Very low	≤1.5
Low	>1.5–3
Intermediate	>3–4.5
High	>4.5–6
Very high	>6

- Mutations in *TP53, EZH2, ETV6, RUNX1, ASXL1, DNMT3A, IDH1/2, BCOR, SRSF2, NRAS, CBL*, and *STAG2* have been reported to be associated with shortened survival [150, 151].
- *SF3B1* mutation is associated with favorable outcome.
- Among these mutations, *TP53*, *TET2*, *DNMT3A*, and *SRSF2* are most frequently mutated in therapy-related myeloid neoplasms (t-MN)/t-MDS, and *TP53* mutations have the most negative prognostic impact in both t-MN and MDS [154, 155]. The presence of *ASXL1*, *EZH2*, or *TP53* mutations shows additional adverse prognosis in patients with lower-risk MDS [156], and *TP53*, *TET2*, or *DNMT3A* mutations identified at pretransplantation indicate an inferior posttransplant survival [157].

12. What workup provides therapeutic target information for MDS?

- Gene mutations: As shown in Table 24.7, there are five major groups of recurrent somatic mutations in MDS, and some of them may provide therapeutic targets for MDS.
  - Hypomethylating agents (HMA), such as azacitidine and decitabine, have been widely used to treat MDS, and mutations in *TET2* and *DNMT3A* may predict for an increased likelihood of response to HMA [158, 159]. Ongoing clinical trials for MDS include the use of new agents/drugs, such as histone deacetylase inhibitors [160], HMA with improved pharmacokinetic properties such as SGI110 [161], and HMA combined with other drugs, such as venetoclax, a BCL2 inhibitor [162].
  - A recent study demonstrated that patients with AML and MDS with cytogenetic abnormalities often associated with unfavorable risk, *TP53* mutations, or both, had favorable clinical responses and robust (but incomplete) mutation clearance after receiving decitabine [163].
- Cytogenetic abnormalities – MDS with isolated del(5q) and lenalidomide: Lenalidomide is one of three FDA-approved agents for the treatment of MDS, specifically for the WHO-defined MDS with isolated del(5q) subtype [164–166]. A recent study demonstrated that the action mechanism of lenalidomide in MDS is through binding cereblon and ubiquitinating CSK1A1 serine/threonine kinase [167].
- Hypoplastic MDS and immunosuppressive therapy (IST): Hypoplastic MDS is defined as bone marrow cellularity of less than 30% in patients younger than 70 years or less than 20% in those older than 70 years. Hypoplastic MDS and MDS associated with paroxysmal nocturnal hemoglobinuria (PNH) clone or autoimmune-associated class II alleles including HLA-DRB1–15 are characterized by significant immune deregulation. These MDS cases are associated with a high responsive rate to antithymocyte globulin (ATG) and cyclosporine [168–170].

13. What is an appropriate practical approach for diagnosis of MDS? When is a diagnostic comment necessary and what should be discussed in the diagnostic comment for this entity? When is it appropriate to seek external consultation for this entity?

- A recommended algorithm and the mandatory steps for diagnosis of MDS: In the era of molecular testing, it is challenging for hematopathologists to select appropriate cost-effective diagnostic tests and to make accurate diagnosis and prognosis of MDS in day-to-day clinical practice. We recommend an integrated approach based on clinical information and morphology to select appropriate ancillary tests for diagnosis of MDS as schematically illustrated in Fig. 24.15. We emphasize the importance of a comprehensive clinical and family history and careful examination of the parameters and morphology of the PB and BM cells in the initial diagnostic workup for MDS.
- Diagnostic comments: We recommend following the diagnostic algorithm for MDS (Fig. 24.15). If there are difficulties in diagnosis of MDS, such as inadequate clinical information, missing any of the mandatory diagnostic tests or poor-quality specimens, the pathologist should discuss the diagnostic difficulties with the treating physician. A diagnostic comment should be added to document the diagnostic difficulties and to suggest further studies that might enable a final, unequivocal diagnosis.
- Appropriate timing to seek for external consultation: The following are common issues in the diagnosis of MDS, and external consultation may be considered in such situations:
  - Unable to obtain good-quality BM aspirates stains or necessary cytogenetic studies.
  - Discrepancies between morphologic findings and molecular or cytogenetic findings.

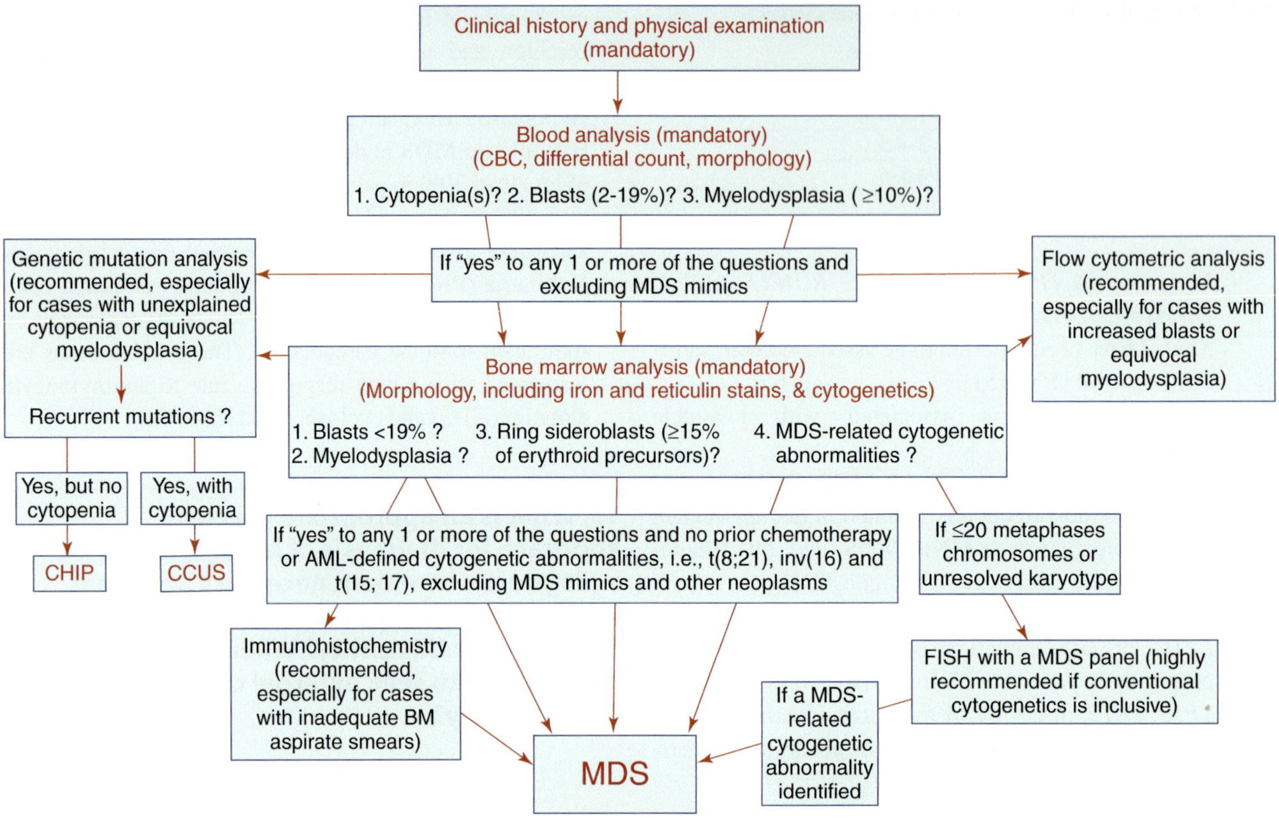

Fig. 24.15 A morphology/clinical data-based integrated diagnostic algorithm for myelodysplastic syndromes (MDS). The text in red indicates the mandatory tests/procedures for diagnosis/differential diagnosis of MDS, CHIP and CCUS

  - Concurrence of myelodysplasia with other reactive conditions or other malignancies, which may cause a diagnostic difficulty.
  - Pediatric MDS. MDS is rare in children, and a thorough study should be performed to exclude a secondary cause for cytopenia and/or dysplasia. If there is any uncertainty regarding the diagnosis, external review may be helpful.
  - Patients with germline predispositions or inherited syndromes. These patients often present with myelodysplasia and their disease courses are often unpredictable. Therefore, it is very difficult to make the diagnosis of MDS and initiate MDS treatment at right timing. An external consultation may be helpful.

14. Which features set MDS apart from closely related hematologic neoplasms?

Even though MDS, myeloproliferative neoplasms (MPN) and acute myeloid leukemia (AML) have some overlapping features, and indeed the mixed category of MDS/MPN is well recognized, it is critical to identify the differences in the morphology and immunophenotype of each category and classify them correctly because each category has a unique biology and clinical course as summarized below.

- Biology and clinical course: MDS is comprised of a group of myeloid neoplasms characterized by ineffective myelopoiesis and dysplastic morphology; although there is a tendency for the disease to evolve to a blastic, acute leukemia-like phase, more patients will die of complications of their cytopenia rather than acute leukemia. Thus, it is not appropriate to consider MDS as merely "preleukemia." In contrast to the myeloproliferative neoplasms (MPN), the hematopoietic proliferation in MDS is ineffective, and thus associated with one or more cytopenias, in contrast to the effective proliferation of the MPNs [171, 172].
- The differences in the morphology and immunophenotype: Besides ineffective and clonal myelopoiesis, MDS has abnormal differentiation and lineage specification of myeloid cells, which is caused by underlying epigenetic and/or genetic alterations. In contrast, acute myeloid leukemia (AML, including acute promyelocytic leukemia, APL) are characterized by markedly increased proliferation of myeloid progenitors/blasts or promyelocytes with a defect in maturation and chronic myeloproliferative neoplasms are caused by increased proliferation of myeloid components without a significant maturation defect. In the latter, myeloid cells can reach the terminal differentiation stage in a markedly increased quantity, i.e., effective hematopoiesis,

with normal or NON-dysplastic morphology. Most acute leukemias also do not have significant dysplasia or aberrancies in cell lineage specification, except AML-MRC and t-MN/AML.

- In practice, an increase in myeloid blast count in the ranges of 2–19% and 5–19% in the PB and BM, respectively, with myelodysplasia, is consistent with the diagnosis of MDS. Significant dysplasia in one or more myeloid lineages is typically seen in MDS or MDS-related processes, but not in other chronic myeloid neoplasms. However, it is not uncommon to find some myelodysplasia at the time of progression or acceleration of a myeloproliferative neoplasm to a more advanced stage, and the morphologic boundary between MPN with disease progression, MDS and MDS/MPN may be obscure, particularly if there is no clinical history of a preceding hematologic neoplasm at the time of diagnosis. The finding of the MDS-defining cytogenetic abnormalities (Table 24.8) with or without increased blast count supports the diagnosis of MDS or MDS-related processes in such cases.

• Myelodysplastic/myeloproliferative neoplasms (MDS/MPN): MDS/MPN is an important, often challenging, entity that needs to be distinguished from MDS and is discussed in Chap. 25. The MDS/MPN category includes myeloid disorders that have both dysplastic and proliferative features at the time of initial presentation [172–174].
  - Practically, if there is a significant myelodysplasia and persistent absolute monocytosis ($\geq$ 1 x 10^9/L in the PB) or leukocytosis ($\geq$ 13 x 10^9/L in the PB) with increased neutrophils and their precursors ($\geq$ 10% of the leukocytes) or persistent thrombocytosis with platelet count $\geq$450 x 10^9/L in the PB and $\geq$ 15% ring sideroblasts, the correct diagnosis is one of the MDS/MPN, and not MDS.
  - Unfortunately, cytogenetic abnormalities and gene mutations overlap between MDS and MDS/MPN, and have a limited value in distinguishing these two entities. Careful evaluation of differential counts and morphology of patients' PB and BM is a key to differentiate MDS from other types of hematologic malignancies.

Case Presentations

See Chap. 25 for combined Case Presentations.

References

1. Arber DA, Orazi A, Hasserjian R, Thiele J, Borowitz MJ, Le Beau MM, et al. The 2016 revision to the World Health Organization classification of myeloid neoplasms and acute leukemia. Blood. 2016;127(20):2391–405.
2. Vardiman J. The classification of MDS: from FAB to WHO and beyond. Leuk Res. 2012;36(12):1453–8.
3. Vardiman JW. The World Health Organization (WHO) classification of tumors of the hematopoietic and lymphoid tissues: an overview with emphasis on the myeloid neoplasms. Chem Biol Interact. 2010;184(1–2):16–20.
4. Vardiman JW, Harris NL, Brunning RD. The World Health Organization (WHO) classification of the myeloid neoplasms. Blood. 2002;100(7):2292–302.
5. Koeffler HP, Golde DW. Human preleukemia. Ann Intern Med. 1980;93(2):347–53.
6. Kraus MD, Bartlett NL, Fleming MD, Dorfman DM. Splenic pathology in myelodysplasia: a report of 13 cases with clinical correlation. Am J Surg Pathol. 1998;22(10):1255–66.
7. Foucar K, Langdon RM 2nd, Armitage JO, Olson DB, Carroll TJ Jr. Myelodysplastic syndromes. A clinical and pathologic analysis of 109 cases. Cancer. 1985;56(3):553–61.
8. Goldberg SL, Chen E, Corral M, Guo A, Mody-Patel N, Pecora AL, et al. Incidence and clinical complications of myelodysplastic syndromes among United States Medicare beneficiaries. J Clin Oncol. 2010;28(17):2847–52.
9. Guralnik JM, Eisenstaedt RS, Ferrucci L, Klein HG, Woodman RC. Prevalence of anemia in persons 65 years and older in the United States: evidence for a high rate of unexplained anemia. Blood. 2004;104(8):2263–8.
10. Linman JW, Bagby C Jr. The preleukemic syndrome: clinical and laboratory features, natural course, and management. Nouv Rev Fr Hematol Blood Cells. 1976;17(1–2):11–31.
11. Rummens JL, Verfaillie C, Criel A, Hidajat M, Vanhoof A, Van den Berghe H, et al. Elliptocytosis and schistocytosis in myelodysplasia: report of two cases. Acta Haematol. 1986;75(3):174–7.
12. Doll DC, List AF, Dayhoff DA, Loy TS, Ringenberg QS, Yarbro JW. Acanthocytosis associated with myelodysplasia. J Clin Oncol. 1989;7(10):1569–72.
13. de Cataldo F, Cairoli R, Baudo F, Pezzetti L, Lo Cunsolo CL, Perutelli P, et al. Abnormalities of cytoskeletal proteins of the red blood cells in myelodysplastic syndromes. Int J Hematol. 1994;59(3):227–9.
14. Hertenstein B, Kurrle E, Redenbacher M, Arnold R, Heimpel H. Pseudoreticulocytosis in a patient with myelodysplasia. Ann Hematol. 1993;67(3):127–8.
15. Aleem A, Murray JA. Spherocytosis preceding the development of myelodysplasia. Clin Lab Haematol. 2001;23(4):249–51.
16. Lambertenghi-Deliliers G, Orazi A, Luksch R, Annaloro C, Soligo D. Myelodysplastic syndrome with increased marrow fibrosis: a distinct clinico-pathological entity. Br J Haematol. 1991;78(2):161–6.
17. Tulliez M, Testa U, Rochant H, Henri A, Vainchenker W, Touboul J, et al. Reticulocytosis, hypochromia, and microcytosis: an unusual presentation of the preleukemic syndrome. Blood. 1982;59(2):293–9.
18. Tefferi A, Dingli D, Li CY, Mesa RA. Microcytosis in agnogenic myeloid metaplasia: prevalence and clinical correlates. Leuk Res. 2006;30(6):677–80.
19. Steensma DP, Gibbons RJ, Higgs DR. Acquired alpha-thalassemia in association with myelodysplastic syndrome and other hematologic malignancies. Blood. 2005;105(2):443–52.
20. Vardiman JW, Thiele J, Arber DA, Brunning RD, Borowitz MJ, Porwit A, et al. The 2008 revision of the World Health Organization (WHO) classification of myeloid neoplasms and acute leukemia: rationale and important changes. Blood. 2009;114(5):937–51.
21. Head DR, Kopecky K, Bennett JM, Grenier K, Morrison FS, Miller KB, et al. Pathogenetic implications of internuclear bridging in myelodysplastic syndrome. An Eastern Cooperative Oncology Group/Southwest Oncology Group Cooperative Study. Cancer. 1989;64(11):2199–202.

22. Mufti GJ, Bennett JM, Goasguen J, Bain BJ, Baumann I, Brunning R, et al. Diagnosis and classification of myelodysplastic syndrome: International Working Group on Morphology of myelodysplastic syndrome (IWGM-MDS) consensus proposals for the definition and enumeration of myeloblasts and ring sideroblasts. Haematologica. 2008;93(11):1712–7.
23. Montalban-Bravo G, Garcia-Manero G. Myelodysplastic syndromes: 2018 update on diagnosis, risk-stratification and management. Am J Hematol. 2018;93(1):129–47.
24. Wang SA, Tang G, Fadare O, Hao S, Raza A, Woda BA, et al. Erythroid-predominant myelodysplastic syndromes: enumeration of blasts from nonerythroid rather than total marrow cells provides superior risk stratification. Mod Pathol. 2008;21(11):1394–402.
25. Calvo X, Arenillas L, Luno E, Senent L, Arnan M, Ramos F, et al. Enumerating bone marrow blasts from nonerythroid cellularity improves outcome prediction in myelodysplastic syndromes and permits a better definition of the intermediate risk category of the Revised International Prognostic Scoring System (IPSS-R). Am J Hematol. 2017;92(7):614–21.
26. Toma A, Fenaux P, Dreyfus F, Cordonnier C. Infections in myelodysplastic syndromes. Haematologica. 2012;97(10):1459–70.
27. Boogaerts MA, Nelissen V, Roelant C, Goossens W. Blood neutrophil function in primary myelodysplastic syndromes. Br J Haematol. 1983;55(2):217–27.
28. Matsushima T, Handa H, Yokohama A, Nagasaki J, Koiso H, Kin Y, et al. Prevalence and clinical characteristics of myelodysplastic syndrome with bone marrow eosinophilia or basophilia. Blood. 2003;101(9):3386–90.
29. Fureder W, Schernthaner GH, Ghannadan M, Hauswirth A, Sperr WR, Semper H, et al. Quantitative, phenotypic, and functional evaluation of basophils in myelodysplastic syndromes. Eur J Clin Investig. 2001;31(10):894–901.
30. Shibata K, Watanabe M, Yano H, Matsuzaki M, Funai N, Sano M. Importance of basophilia in haematopoietic disorders. Haematologia (Budap). 1998;29(3):241–53.
31. Wimazal F, Baumgartner C, Sonneck K, Zauner C, Geissler P, Schur S, et al. Mixed-lineage eosinophil/basophil crisis in MDS: a rare form of progression. Eur J Clin Investig. 2008;38(6):447–55.
32. Goasguen JE, Bennett JM, Bain BJ, Brunning R, Vallespi MT, Tomonaga M, et al. Proposal for refining the definition of dysgranulopoiesis in acute myeloid leukemia and myelodysplastic syndromes. Leuk Res. 2014;38(4):447–53.
33. Strupp C, Nachtkamp K, Hildebrandt B, Giagounidis A, Haas R, Gattermann N, et al. New proposals of the WHO working group (2016) for the diagnosis of myelodysplastic syndromes (MDS): characteristics of refined MDS types. Leuk Res. 2017;57:78–84.
34. Gallardo R, Kranwinkel RN. Pseudo-Chediak-Higashi anomaly. Am J Clin Pathol. 1985;83(1):127–9.
35. Langenhuijsen MM. Neutrophils with ring-shaped nuclei in myeloproliferative disease. Br J Haematol. 1984;58(2):227–30.
36. Kantarjian H, Giles F, List A, Lyons R, Sekeres MA, Pierce S, et al. The incidence and impact of thrombocytopenia in myelodysplastic syndromes. Cancer. 2007;109(9):1705–14.
37. Germing U, Platzbecker U, Giagounidis A, Aul C. Platelet morphology, platelet mass, platelet count and prognosis in patients with myelodysplastic syndromes. Br J Haematol. 2007;138(3):399–400.
38. Widell S, Hast R. Balloon-like platelets in myelodysplastic syndromes – a feature of dysmegakaryopoiesis? Leuk Res. 1987;11(8):747–52.
39. Bennett JM, Brunning RD, Vardiman JW. Myelodysplastic syndromes: from French-American-British to World Health Organization: a commentary. Blood. 2002;99(8):3074–5.
40. Van den Berghe H, Vermaelen K, Mecucci C, Barbieri D, Tricot G. The 5q-anomaly. Cancer Genet Cytogenet. 1985;17(3):189–255.
41. Le Beau MM, Albain KS, Larson RA, Vardiman JW, Davis EM, Blough RR, et al. Clinical and cytogenetic correlations in 63 patients with therapy-related myelodysplastic syndromes and acute nonlymphocytic leukemia: further evidence for characteristic abnormalities of chromosomes no. 5 and 7. J Clin Oncol. 1986;4(3):325–45.
42. Thiede T, Engquist L, Billstrom R. Application of megakaryocytic morphology in diagnosing 5q- syndrome. Eur J Haematol. 1988;41(5):434–7.
43. Podolak-Dawidziak M, Geddes D, Bowen D. Megakaryocytopoiesis in patients with myelodysplastic syndromes (MDS) with and without del(5q). Eur J Haematol. 1990;45(2):115–6.
44. Goasguen JE, Bennett JM, Bain BJ, Brunning RD, Vallespi MT, Tomonaga M, et al. Quality control initiative on the evaluation of the dysmegakaryopoiesis in myeloid neoplasms: difficulties in the assessment of dysplasia. Leuk Res. 2016;45:75–81.
45. McCrae T. Acute lymphatic leukaemia, with the report of five cases. Br Med J. 1905;1(2304):404–8.
46. Freeman JA. Origin of Auer bodies. Blood. 1966;27(4):499–510.
47. Seymour JF, Estey EH. The contribution of Auer rods to the classification and prognosis of myelodysplastic syndromes. Leuk Lymphoma. 1995;17(1–2):79–85.
48. Willis MS, McKenna RW, Peterson LC, Coad JE, Kroft SH. Low blast count myeloid disorders with Auer rods: a clinicopathologic analysis of 9 cases. Am J Clin Pathol. 2005;124(2):191–8.
49. Yoshida Y, Oguma S, Ohno H. John Auer and Auer rods; controversies revisited. Leuk Res. 2009;33(5):614–6.
50. Strupp C, Gattermann N, Giagounidis A, Aul C, Hildebrandt B, Haas R, et al. Refractory anemia with excess of blasts in transformation: analysis of reclassification according to the WHO proposals. Leuk Res. 2003;27(5):397–404.
51. Seymour JF, Estey EH. The prognostic significance of Auer rods in myelodysplasia. Br J Haematol. 1993;85(1):67–76.
52. Seigneurin D, Audhuy B. Auer rods in refractory anemia with excess of blasts: presence and significance. Am J Clin Pathol. 1983;80(3):359–62.
53. Weisdorf DJ, Oken MM, Johnson GJ, Rydell RE. Auer rod positive dysmyelopoietic syndrome. Am J Hematol. 1981;11(4):397–402.
54. Mertelsmann R, Tzvi Thaler H, To L, Gee TS, McKenzie S, Schauer P, et al. Morphological classification, response to therapy, and survival in 263 adult patients with acute nonlymphoblastic leukemia. Blood. 1980;56(5):773–81.
55. Raza A, Gezer S, Mundle S, Gao XZ, Alvi S, Borok R, et al. Apoptosis in bone marrow biopsy samples involving stromal and hematopoietic cells in 50 patients with myelodysplastic syndromes. Blood. 1995;86(1):268–76.
56. Shetty V, Hussaini S, Broady-Robinson L, Allampallam K, Mundle S, Borok R, et al. Intramedullary apoptosis of hematopoietic cells in myelodysplastic syndrome patients can be massive: apoptotic cells recovered from high-density fraction of bone marrow aspirates. Blood. 2000;96(4):1388–92.
57. Della Porta MG, Travaglino E, Boveri E, Ponzoni M, Malcovati L, Papaemmanuil E, et al. Minimal morphological criteria for defining bone marrow dysplasia: a basis for clinical implementation of WHO classification of myelodysplastic syndromes. Leukemia. 2015;29(1):66–75.
58. Niemeyer CM, Baumann I. Classification of childhood aplastic anemia and myelodysplastic syndrome. Hematology Am Soc Hematol Educ Program. 2011;2011:84–9.
59. Tuzuner N, Cox C, Rowe JM, Watrous D, Bennett JM. Hypocellular myelodysplastic syndromes (MDS): new proposals. Br J Haematol. 1995;91(3):612–7.
60. Larson RA, LeBeau MM, Vardiman JW, Rowley JD. Myeloid leukemia after hematotoxins. Environ Health Perspect. 1996;104(Suppl 6):1303–7.
61. Singh ZN, Huo D, Anastasi J, Smith SM, Karrison T, Le Beau MM, et al. Therapy-related myelodysplastic syndrome: morphologic subclassification may not be clinically relevant. Am J Clin Pathol. 2007;127(2):197–205.

62. Fu B, Ok CY, Goswami M, Xei W, Jaso JM, Muzzafar T, et al. The clinical importance of moderate/severe bone marrow fibrosis in patients with therapy-related myelodysplastic syndromes. Ann Hematol. 2013;92(10):1335–43.
63. Furutani E, Shimamura A. Germline genetic predisposition to hematologic malignancy. J Clin Oncol. 2017;35(9):1018–28.
64. Savage SA, Dufour C. Classical inherited bone marrow failure syndromes with high risk for myelodysplastic syndrome and acute myelogenous leukemia. Semin Hematol. 2017;54(2):105–14.
65. Schaefer EJ, Lindsley RC. Significance of clonal mutations in bone marrow failure and inherited myelodysplastic syndrome/acute myeloid leukemia predisposition syndromes. Hematol Oncol Clin North Am. 2018;32(4):643–55.
66. Bessis M. Red cell shapes. An illustrated classification and its rationale. Nouv Rev Fr Hematol. 1972;12(6):721–45.
67. Wang LJ, Glasser L. Spurious dyserythropoiesis. Am J Clin Pathol. 2002;117(1):57–9.
68. Lee SH, van der Weyden C, Mayson E, Desai S. Excessive EDTA induces morphologic changes in bone marrow smears that mimic specific features of dysplasia. Int J Lab Hematol. 2013;35(2):163–9.
69. Yang DT, Cook RJ. Spurious elevations of vitamin B12 with pernicious anemia. N Engl J Med. 2012;366(18):1742–3.
70. Kumar N, Elliott MA, Hoyer JD, Harper CM Jr, Ahlskog JE, Phyliky RL. "Myelodysplasia," myeloneuropathy, and copper deficiency. Mayo Clin Proc. 2005;80(7):943–6.
71. Haddad AS, Subbiah V, Lichtin AE, Theil KS, Maciejewski JP. Hypocupremia and bone marrow failure. Haematologica. 2008;93(1):e1–5.
72. Thiele J, Titius BR, Quitmann H, Fischer R, Salzberger B, Dienemann D, et al. Megakaryocytopoiesis in bone marrow biopsies of patients with acquired immunodeficiency syndrome (AIDS). An immunohistochemical and morphometric evaluation with special emphasis on myelodysplastic features and precursor cells. Pathol Res Pract. 1992;188(6):722–8.
73. Dhurve SA, Dhurve AS. Bone marrow abnormalities in HIV disease. Mediterr J Hematol Infect Dis. 2013;5(1):e2013033.
74. Ryu T, Ikeda M, Okazaki Y, Tokuda H, Yoshino N, Honda M, et al. Myelodysplasia associated with acquired immunodeficiency syndrome. Intern Med. 2001;40(8):795–801.
75. Delacretaz F, Perey L, Schmidt PM, Chave JP, Costa J. Histopathology of bone marrow in human immunodeficiency virus infection. Virchows Arch A Pathol Anat Histopathol. 1987;411(6):543–51.
76. Baurmann H, Schwarz TF, Oertel J, Serke S, Roggendorf M, Huhn D. Acute parvovirus B19 infection mimicking myelodysplastic syndrome of the bone marrow. Ann Hematol. 1992;64(1):43–5.
77. Kerr JR. A review of blood diseases and cytopenias associated with human parvovirus B19 infection. Rev Med Virol. 2015;25(4):224–40.
78. Giannouli S, Kanellopoulou T, Voulgarelis M. Myelodysplasia and autoimmunity. Curr Opin Rheumatol. 2012;24(1):97–102.
79. Voulgarelis M, Giannouli S, Ritis K, Tzioufas AG. Myelodysplasia-associated autoimmunity: clinical and pathophysiologic concepts. Eur J Clin Investig. 2004;34(10):690–700.
80. Valent P. Low blood counts: immune mediated, idiopathic, or myelodysplasia. Hematology Am Soc Hematol Educ Program. 2012;2012:485–91.
81. DeZern AE, Sekeres MA. The challenging world of cytopenias: distinguishing myelodysplastic syndromes from other disorders of marrow failure. Oncologist. 2014;19(7):735–45.
82. Devalet B, Mullier F, Chatelain B, Dogne JM, Chatelain C. Pathophysiology, diagnosis, and treatment of paroxysmal nocturnal hemoglobinuria: a review. Eur J Haematol. 2015;95(3):190–8.
83. Ballard HS. The hematological complications of alcoholism. Alcohol Health Res World. 1997;21(1):42–52.
84. Yoon JH, Kwak WS, Ahn YS. A brief review of relationship between occupational benzene exposure and hematopoietic cancer. Ann Occup Environ Med. 2018;30:33.
85. Rezuke WN, Anderson C, Pastuszak WT, Conway SR, Firshein SI. Arsenic intoxication presenting as a myelodysplastic syndrome: a case report. Am J Hematol. 1991;36(4):291–3.
86. Banerjee R, Halil O, Bain BJ, Cummins D, Banner NR. Neutrophil dysplasia caused by mycophenolate mofetil. Transplantation. 2000;70(11):1608–10.
87. Wang E, Boswell E, Siddiqi I, Lu CM, Sebastian S, Rehder C, et al. Pseudo-Pelger-Huet anomaly induced by medications: a clinicopathologic study in comparison with myelodysplastic syndrome-related pseudo-Pelger-Huet anomaly. Am J Clin Pathol. 2011;135(2):291–303.
88. Meyerson HJ, Farhi DC, Rosenthal NS. Transient increase in blasts mimicking acute leukemia and progressing myelodysplasia in patients receiving growth factor. Am J Clin Pathol. 1998;109(6):675–81.
89. Schmitz LL, Litz CE, Brunning RD. Morphologic and quantitative alterations in hematopoietic cells associated with growth factor therapy: review of the literature. Hematol Pathol. 1994;8(3):55–73.
90. Gauthier-Vasserot A, Thauvin-Robinet C, Bruel AL, Duffourd Y, St-Onge J, Jouan T, et al. Application of whole-exome sequencing to unravel the molecular basis of undiagnosed syndromic congenital neutropenia with intellectual disability. Am J Med Genet A. 2017;173(1):62–71.
91. Donadieu J, Beaupain B, Fenneteau O, Bellanne-Chantelot C. Congenital neutropenia in the era of genomics: classification, diagnosis, and natural history. Br J Haematol. 2017;179(4):557–74.
92. Kutler DI, Singh B, Satagopan J, Batish SD, Berwick M, Giampietro PF, et al. A 20-year perspective on the International Fanconi Anemia Registry (IFAR). Blood. 2003;101(4):1249–56.
93. Klein C. Genetic defects in severe congenital neutropenia: emerging insights into life and death of human neutrophil granulocytes. Annu Rev Immunol. 2011;29:399–413.
94. Zeidler C, Welte K. Kostmann syndrome and severe congenital neutropenia. Semin Hematol. 2002;39(2):82–8.
95. Sera Y, Kawaguchi H, Nakamura K, Sato T, Habara M, Okada S, et al. A comparison of the defective granulopoiesis in childhood cyclic neutropenia and in severe congenital neutropenia. Haematologica. 2005;90(8):1032–41.
96. Kostmann R. Infantile genetic agranulocytosis; agranulocytosis infantilis hereditaria. Acta Paediatr Suppl. 1956;45(Suppl 105):1–78.
97. Klein C, Grudzien M, Appaswamy G, Germeshausen M, Sandrock I, Schaffer AA, et al. HAX1 deficiency causes autosomal recessive severe congenital neutropenia (Kostmann disease). Nat Genet. 2007;39(1):86–92.
98. Boxer LA, Newburger PE. A molecular classification of congenital neutropenia syndromes. Pediatr Blood Cancer. 2007;49(5):609–14.
99. Xia J, Bolyard AA, Rodger E, Stein S, Aprikyan AA, Dale DC, et al. Prevalence of mutations in ELANE, GFI1, HAX1, SBDS, WAS and G6PC3 in patients with severe congenital neutropenia. Br J Haematol. 2009;147(4):535–42.
100. McDermott DH, De Ravin SS, Jun HS, Liu Q, Priel DA, Noel P, et al. Severe congenital neutropenia resulting from G6PC3 deficiency with increased neutrophil CXCR4 expression and myelokathexis. Blood. 2010;116(15):2793–802.
101. Boztug K, Jarvinen PM, Salzer E, Racek T, Monch S, Garncarz W, et al. JAGN1 deficiency causes aberrant myeloid cell homeostasis and congenital neutropenia. Nat Genet. 2014;46(9):1021–7.
102. Liu JC, Ferreira CG, Yusufzai T. Human CHD2 is a chromatin assembly ATPase regulated by its chromo- and DNA-binding domains. J Biol Chem. 2015;290(1):25–34.

103. Kao SH, Wu HT. Wu KJ. Ubiquitination by HUWE1 in tumorigenesis and beyond. J Biomed Sci. 2018;25(1):67.
104. Tham E, Lindstrand A, Santani A, Malmgren H, Nesbitt A, Dubbs HA, et al. Dominant mutations in KAT6A cause intellectual disability with recognizable syndromic features. Am J Hum Genet. 2015;96(3):507–13.
105. Arboleda VA, Lee H, Dorrani N, Zadeh N, Willis M, Macmurdo CF, et al. De novo nonsense mutations in KAT6A, a lysine acetyl-transferase gene, cause a syndrome including microcephaly and global developmental delay. Am J Hum Genet. 2015;96(3):498–506.
106. Millan F, Cho MT, Retterer K, Monaghan KG, Bai R, Vitazka P, et al. Whole exome sequencing reveals de novo pathogenic variants in KAT6A as a cause of a neurodevelopmental disorder. Am J Med Genet A. 2016;170(7):1791–8.
107. Sheikh BN, Yang Y, Schreuder J, Nilsson SK, Bilardi R, Carotta S, et al. MOZ (KAT6A) is essential for the maintenance of classically defined adult hematopoietic stem cells. Blood. 2016;128(19):2307–18.
108. Haferlach T, Kohlmann A, Klein HU, Ruckert C, Dugas M, Williams PM, et al. AML with translocation t(8;16)(p11;p13) demonstrates unique cytomorphological, cytogenetic, molecular and prognostic features. Leukemia. 2009;23(5):934–43.
109. Gambale A, Iolascon A, Andolfo I, Russo R. Diagnosis and management of congenital dyserythropoietic anemias. Expert Rev Hematol. 2016;9(3):283–96.
110. Iolascon A, Heimpel H, Wahlin A, Tamary H. Congenital dyserythropoietic anemias: molecular insights and diagnostic approach. Blood. 2013;122(13):2162–6.
111. Vinh DC, Patel SY, Uzel G, Anderson VL, Freeman AF, Olivier KN, et al. Autosomal dominant and sporadic monocytopenia with susceptibility to mycobacteria, fungi, papillomaviruses, and myelodysplasia. Blood. 2010;115(8):1519–29.
112. Hsu AP, Sampaio EP, Khan J, Calvo KR, Lemieux JE, Patel SY, et al. Mutations in GATA2 are associated with the autosomal dominant and sporadic monocytopenia and mycobacterial infection (MonoMAC) syndrome. Blood. 2011;118(10):2653–5.
113. Crispino JD, Horwitz MS. GATA factor mutations in hematologic disease. Blood. 2017;129(15):2103–10.
114. Hirabayashi S, Wlodarski MW, Kozyra E, Niemeyer CM. Heterogeneity of GATA2-related myeloid neoplasms. Int J Hematol. 2017;106(2):175–82.
115. Calvo KR, Vinh DC, Maric I, Wang W, Noel P, Stetler-Stevenson M, et al. Myelodysplasia in autosomal dominant and sporadic monocytopenia immunodeficiency syndrome: diagnostic features and clinical implications. Haematologica. 2011;96(8):1221–5.
116. Bain BJ. The bone marrow aspirate of healthy subjects. Br J Haematol. 1996;94(1):206–9.
117. Valent P, Jager E, Mitterbauer-Hohendanner G, Mullauer L, Schwarzinger I, Sperr WR, et al. Idiopathic bone marrow dysplasia of unknown significance (IDUS): definition, pathogenesis, follow up, and prognosis. Am J Cancer Res. 2011;1(4):531–41.
118. Valent P, Orazi A, Steensma DP, Ebert BL, Haase D, Malcovati L, et al. Proposed minimal diagnostic criteria for myelodysplastic syndromes (MDS) and potential pre-MDS conditions. Oncotarget. 2017;8(43):73483–500.
119. Parmentier S, Schetelig J, Lorenz K, Kramer M, Ireland R, Schuler U, et al. Assessment of dysplastic hematopoiesis: lessons from healthy bone marrow donors. Haematologica. 2012;97(5):723–30.
120. Valent P, Bain BJ, Bennett JM, Wimazal F, Sperr WR, Mufti G, et al. Idiopathic cytopenia of undetermined significance (ICUS) and idiopathic dysplasia of uncertain significance (IDUS), and their distinction from low risk MDS. Leuk Res. 2012;36(1):1–5.
121. Valent P. ICUS, IDUS, CHIP and CCUS: Diagnostic Criteria, Separation from MDS and Clinical Implications. Pathobiology. 2019;86(1):30–38.
122. Bowman RL, Busque L, Levine RL. Clonal hematopoiesis and evolution to hematopoietic malignancies. Cell Stem Cell. 2018;22(2):157–70.
123. Jan M, Ebert BL, Jaiswal S. Clonal hematopoiesis. Semin Hematol. 2017;54(1):43–50.
124. Steensma DP, Bejar R, Jaiswal S, Lindsley RC, Sekeres MA, Hasserjian RP, et al. Clonal hematopoiesis of indeterminate potential and its distinction from myelodysplastic syndromes. Blood. 2015;126(1):9–16.
125. Gillis NK, Ball M, Zhang Q, Ma Z, Zhao Y, Yoder SJ, et al. Clonal haemopoiesis and therapy-related myeloid malignancies in elderly patients: a proof-of-concept, case-control study. Lancet Oncol. 2017;18(1):112–21.
126. Jaiswal S, Natarajan P, Silver AJ, Gibson CJ, Bick AG, Shvartz E, et al. Clonal hematopoiesis and risk of atherosclerotic cardiovascular disease. N Engl J Med. 2017;377(2):111–21.
127. Steensma DP. Clinical implications of clonal hematopoiesis. Mayo Clin Proc. 2018;93(8):1122–30.
128. Sperling AS, Gibson CJ, Ebert BL. The genetics of myelodysplastic syndrome: from clonal haematopoiesis to secondary leukaemia. Nat Rev Cancer. 2017;17(1):5–19.
129. Chung SS, Park CY. Aging, hematopoiesis, and the myelodysplastic syndromes. Blood Adv. 2017;1(26):2572–8.
130. Stauder R, Valent P, Theurl I. Anemia at older age: etiologies, clinical implications, and management. Blood. 2018;131(5):505–14.
131. Malcovati L, Cazzola M. The shadowlands of MDS: idiopathic cytopenias of undetermined significance (ICUS) and clonal hematopoiesis of indeterminate potential (CHIP). Hematology Am Soc Hematol Educ Program. 2015;2015:299–307.
132. Jain M, Tripathi A. ICUS/CCUS/CHIP: basics & beyond. Expert Rev Hematol. 2017;10(10):915–20.
133. Barcellini W. The relationship between idiopathic cytopenias/dysplasias of uncertain significance (ICUS/IDUS) and autoimmunity. Expert Rev Hematol. 2017;10(7):649–57.
134. Tang G, Medeiros LJ, Wang SA. How I investigate clonal cytogenetic abnormalities of undetermined significance. Int J Lab Hematol. 2018;40(4):385–91.
135. Braulke F, Platzbecker U, Muller-Thomas C, Gotze K, Germing U, Brummendorf TH, et al. Validation of cytogenetic risk groups according to international prognostic scoring systems by peripheral blood CD34+FISH: results from a German diagnostic study in comparison with an international control group. Haematologica. 2015;100(2):205–13.
136. Schanz J, Tuchler H, Sole F, Mallo M, Luno E, Cervera J, et al. New comprehensive cytogenetic scoring system for primary myelodysplastic syndromes (MDS) and oligoblastic acute myeloid leukemia after MDS derived from an international database merge. J Clin Oncol. 2012;30(8):820–9.
137. Valent P, Orazi A, Busche G, Schmitt-Graff A, George TI, Sotlar K, et al. Standards and impact of hematopathology in myelodysplastic syndromes (MDS). Oncotarget. 2010;1(7):483–96.
138. Pellegrini W, Facchetti F, Marocolo D, Pelizzari AM, Capucci A, Rossi G. Expression of CD34 by megakaryocytes in myelodysplastic syndromes. Haematologica. 2000;85(10):1117–8.
139. Tang G, Wang SA, Menon M, Dresser K, Woda BA, Hao S. High-level CD34 expression on megakaryocytes independently predicts an adverse outcome in patients with myelodysplastic syndromes. Leuk Res. 2011;35(6):766–70.
140. Porwit A, van de Loosdrecht AA, Bettelheim P, Brodersen LE, Burbury K, Cremers E, et al. Revisiting guidelines for integration of flow cytometry results in the WHO classification of myelodysplastic syndromes-proposal from the International/European LeukemiaNet Working Group for Flow Cytometry in MDS. Leukemia. 2014;28(9):1793–8.
141. Bento LC, Correia RP, Pitangueiras Mangueira CL, De Souza Barroso R, Rocha FA, Bacal NS, et al. The use of flow cytometry in myelodysplastic syndromes: a review. Front Oncol. 2017;7:270.

142. Cremers EM, Westers TM, Alhan C, Cali C, Visser-Wisselaar HA, Chitu DA, et al. Implementation of erythroid lineage analysis by flow cytometry in diagnostic models for myelodysplastic syndromes. Haematologica. 2017;102(2):320–6.
143. Wells DA, Benesch M, Loken MR, Vallejo C, Myerson D, Leisenring WM, et al. Myeloid and monocytic dyspoiesis as determined by flow cytometric scoring in myelodysplastic syndrome correlates with the IPSS and with outcome after hematopoietic stem cell transplantation. Blood. 2003;102(1):394–403.
144. Westers TM, Cremers EM, Oelschlaegel U, Johansson U, Bettelheim P, Matarraz S, et al. Immunophenotypic analysis of erythroid dysplasia in myelodysplastic syndromes. A report from the IMDSFlow working group. Haematologica. 2017;102(2): 308–19.
145. Scott BL, Wells DA, Loken MR, Myerson D, Leisenring WM, Deeg HJ. Validation of a flow cytometric scoring system as a prognostic indicator for posttransplantation outcome in patients with myelodysplastic syndrome. Blood. 2008;112(7):2681–6.
146. Alhan C, Westers TM, Cremers EM, Cali C, Witte BI, Ossenkoppele GJ, et al. The myelodysplastic syndromes flow cytometric score: a three-parameter prognostic flow cytometric scoring system. Leukemia. 2016;30(3):658–65.
147. Alhan C, Westers TM, Cremers EM, Cali C, Witte BI, Ossenkoppele GJ, et al. High flow cytometric scores identify adverse prognostic subgroups within the revised international prognostic scoring system for myelodysplastic syndromes. Br J Haematol. 2014;167(1):100–9.
148. Kern W, Bacher U, Haferlach C, Alpermann T, Schnittger S, Haferlach T. Multiparameter flow cytometry provides independent prognostic information in patients with suspected myelodysplastic syndromes: a study on 804 patients. Cytometry B Clin Cytom. 2015;88(3):154–64.
149. Papaemmanuil E, Gerstung M, Malcovati L, Tauro S, Gundem G, Van Loo P, et al. Clinical and biological implications of driver mutations in myelodysplastic syndromes. Blood. 2013;122(22): 3616–27; quiz 99.
150. Haferlach T, Nagata Y, Grossmann V, Okuno Y, Bacher U, Nagae G, et al. Landscape of genetic lesions in 944 patients with myelodysplastic syndromes. Leukemia. 2014;28(2):241–7.
151. Bejar R, Greenberg PL. The impact of somatic and germline mutations in myelodysplastic syndromes and related disorders. J Natl Compr Cancer Netw. 2017;15(1):131–5.
152. Greenberg PL, Tuechler H, Schanz J, Sanz G, Garcia-Manero G, Sole F, et al. Revised international prognostic scoring system for myelodysplastic syndromes. Blood. 2012;120(12):2454–65.
153. Jonas BA, Greenberg PL. MDS prognostic scoring systems - past, present, and future. Best Pract Res Clin Haematol. 2015;28(1):3–13.
154. Walter MJ, Shen D, Shao J, Ding L, White BS, Kandoth C, et al. Clonal diversity of recurrently mutated genes in myelodysplastic syndromes. Leukemia. 2013;27(6):1275–82.
155. Shih AH, Chung SS, Dolezal EK, Zhang SJ, Abdel-Wahab OI, Park CY, et al. Mutational analysis of therapy-related myelodysplastic syndromes and acute myelogenous leukemia. Haematologica. 2013;98(6):908–12.
156. Bejar R, Stevenson KE, Caughey BA, Abdel-Wahab O, Steensma DP, Galili N, et al. Validation of a prognostic model and the impact of mutations in patients with lower-risk myelodysplastic syndromes. J Clin Oncol. 2012;30(27):3376–82.
157. Bejar R, Stevenson KE, Caughey B, Lindsley RC, Mar BG, Stojanov P, et al. Somatic mutations predict poor outcome in patients with myelodysplastic syndrome after hematopoietic stem-cell transplantation. J Clin Oncol. 2014;32(25):2691–8.
158. Itzykson R, Kosmider O, Cluzeau T, Mansat-De Mas V, Dreyfus F, Beyne-Rauzy O, et al. Impact of TET2 mutations on response rate to azacitidine in myelodysplastic syndromes and low blast count acute myeloid leukemias. Leukemia. 2011;25(7):1147–52.
159. Traina F, Visconte V, Elson P, Tabarroki A, Jankowska AM, Hasrouni E, et al. Impact of molecular mutations on treatment response to DNMT inhibitors in myelodysplasia and related neoplasms. Leukemia. 2014;28(1):78–87.
160. Ornstein MC, Mukherjee S, Sekeres MA. More is better: combination therapies for myelodysplastic syndromes. Best Pract Res Clin Haematol. 2015;28(1):22–31.
161. Issa JJ, Roboz G, Rizzieri D, Jabbour E, Stock W, O'Connell C, et al. Safety and tolerability of guadecitabine (SGI-110) in patients with myelodysplastic syndrome and acute myeloid leukaemia: a multicentre, randomised, dose-escalation phase 1 study. Lancet Oncol. 2015;16(9):1099–110.
162. DiNardo CD, Daver N, Jabbour E, Kadia T, Borthakur G, Konopleva M, et al. Sequential azacitidine and lenalidomide in patients with high-risk myelodysplastic syndromes and acute myeloid leukaemia: a single-arm, phase 1/2 study. Lancet Haematol. 2015;2(1):e12–20.
163. Welch JS, Petti AA, Miller CA, Fronick CC, O'Laughlin M, Fulton RS, et al. TP53 and decitabine in acute myeloid leukemia and myelodysplastic syndromes. N Engl J Med. 2016;375(21):2023–36.
164. List A, Dewald G, Bennett J, Giagounidis A, Raza A, Feldman E, et al. Lenalidomide in the myelodysplastic syndrome with chromosome 5q deletion. N Engl J Med. 2006;355(14):1456–65.
165. Defina M, Rondoni M, Gozzetti A, Aprile L, Chitarrelli I, Fabbri A, et al. Lenalidomide on alternative days is effective in myelodysplastic syndrome with 5q- deletion. Br J Haematol. 2010;148(3):483–4.
166. Garcia-Manero G. Myelodysplastic syndromes: 2015 update on diagnosis, risk-stratification and management. Am J Hematol. 2015;90(9):831–41.
167. Kronke J, Fink EC, Hollenbach PW, MacBeth KJ, Hurst SN, Udeshi ND, et al. Lenalidomide induces ubiquitination and degradation of CK1alpha in del(5q) MDS. Nature. 2015;523(7559):183–8.
168. Sloand EM, Wu CO, Greenberg P, Young N, Barrett J. Factors affecting response and survival in patients with myelodysplasia treated with immunosuppressive therapy. J Clin Oncol. 2008;26(15):2505–11.
169. Passweg JR, Giagounidis AA, Simcock M, Aul C, Dobbelstein C, Stadler M, et al. Immunosuppressive therapy for patients with myelodysplastic syndrome: a prospective randomized multicenter phase III trial comparing antithymocyte globulin plus cyclosporine with best supportive care--SAKK 33/99. J Clin Oncol. 2011;29(3):303–9.
170. Aalbers AM, van der Velden VH, Yoshimi A, Fischer A, Noellke P, Zwaan CM, et al. The clinical relevance of minor paroxysmal nocturnal hemoglobinuria clones in refractory cytopenia of childhood: a prospective study by EWOG-MDS. Leukemia. 2014;28(1):189–92.
171. Vardiman JW. Myelodysplastic syndromes, chronic myeloproliferative diseases, and myelodysplastic/myeloproliferative diseases. Semin Diagn Pathol. 2003;20(3):154–79.
172. Vardiman JW. Hematopathological concepts and controversies in the diagnosis and classification of myelodysplastic syndromes. Hematology Am Soc Hematol Educ Program. 2006:199–204.
173. Vardiman JW. Myelodysplastic/myeloproliferative diseases. Cancer Treat Res. 2004;121:13–43.
174. Hyjek E, Vardiman JW. Myelodysplastic/myeloproliferative neoplasms. Semin Diagn Pathol. 2011;28(4):283–97.

25 Myelodysplastic/Myeloproliferative Neoplasms

Jason X. Cheng and James W. Vardiman

Frequently Asked Questions

1. What are myelodysplastic and myeloproliferative neoplasms (MDS/MPN), and what are the major subtypes of MDS/MPN?
2. What are the laboratory and morphologic findings of CMML?
3. What are the mimics and differential diagnostic considerations for CMML?
4. What work-up provides prognostic information for CMML?
5. What work-up provides information regarding therapeutic targets and clinical management information for CMML?
6. What are the laboratory and morphologic findings of aCML?
7. What are the mimics and differential diagnostic considerations for aCML?
8. What work-up provides prognostic information for aCML?
9. What work-up provides therapeutic targets and clinical management information for aCML?
10. What are the laboratory and morphologic findings of JMML?
11. What are the mimics and differential diagnostic considerations for JMML?
12. What work-up provides prognostic information for JMML?
13. What work-up provides therapeutic targets and clinical management information for JMML?
14. What are the laboratory and morphologic findings of MDS/MPN-RS-T?
15. What are the mimics and differential considerations for MDS/MPN-RS-T?
16. What work-up provides prognostic information for MDS/MPN-RS-T?
17. What work-up provides therapeutic targets and clinical management information for MDS/MPN-RS-T?
18. What are the laboratory and morphologic findings of MDS/MPN-U?
19. What work-up provides therapeutic targets and clinical management information for MDS/MPN-U?
20. Which morphological and laboratory findings in the PB/BM aspirate/biopsy are reliably diagnostic for MDS/MPN? Which ones suggest the diagnosis? Which is (are) unreliable for diagnosis? Which findings rule out the diagnosis?
21. What is the minimal and optimal ancillary work-up for diagnosis and subclassification of the different categories of MDS/MPN?
22. What is an appropriate practical approach for diagnosis of MDS/MPN? When is a diagnostic comment necessary, and what should be discussed in the diagnostic comment for this entity? When is it appropriate to seek external consultation for this entity?

J. X. Cheng (✉) · J. W. Vardiman
Department of Pathology, University of Chicago, Chicago, IL, USA
e-mail: Jason.Cheng@uchospitals.edu

1. What are myelodysplastic and myeloproliferative neoplasms (MDS/MPN), and what are the major subtypes of MDS/MPN?

The MDS/MPN category is comprised of a group of clonal myeloid neoplasms that at the time of diagnosis have some clinical, laboratory, and/or morphologic features that support the diagnosis of MDS, whereas other features suggest the

E. Wang, A. S. Lagoo (eds.), *Practical Lymph Node and Bone Marrow Pathology*, Practical Anatomic Pathology,
https://doi.org/10.1007/978-3-030-32189-5_25

diagnosis of an MPN [1–4]. Due to the overlapping morphological and laboratory findings, the diagnosis of these entities is often challenging. Please also see Chaps. 22 and 23 for features of various MPN entities and Chap. 24 for features of MDS.

The 2017 WHO classification of myeloid neoplasms recognizes five subtypes of MDS/MPN [4]:

1. Chronic myelomonocytic leukemia (CMML) (see section "Chronic Myelomonocytic Leukemia (CMML)")
2. Atypical chronic myeloid leukemia, *BCR-ABL1*-negative (aCML, *BCR-ABL1*-) (see section "Atypical Chronic Myeloid Leukemia, *BCR-ABL1*-negative (aCML, *BCR-ABL1*-)")
3. Juvenile myelomonocytic leukemia (JMML) (see section "Juvenile Myelomonocytic Leukemia (JMML)")
4. MDS/MPN with ring sideroblasts and thrombocytosis (MDS/MPN-RS-T) (see section "MDS/MPN With Ring Sideroblasts and Thrombocytosis (MDS/MPN-RS-T)")
5. MDS/MPN, unclassifiable (MDS/MPN-U) (see section "Myelodysplastic/Myeloproliferative Neoplasms, Unclassifiable (MDS/MPN-U)")

In the next five sections, we discuss each entity in detail by answering the following four questions:

- What are the laboratory and morphologic findings in this entity?
- What are the mimics and differential diagnostic considerations for this entity?
- What work-up provides prognostic information for this entity?
- What work-up provides information regarding therapeutic targets and clinical management in this entity?

After discussing individual conditions, we provide answers to the following general questions applicable to all entities discussed:

- Which morphological and laboratory findings in the PB/BM aspirate/biopsy are reliably diagnostic for MDS/MPN? Which ones suggest the diagnosis? Which is (are) unreliable for diagnosis? Which findings rule out the diagnosis (Question 20)?
- What is the minimal and optimal ancillary work-up for MDS/MPN and subclassification of this category of conditions (Question 21)?
- What is an appropriate practical approach for diagnosis of MDS/MPN? When is a diagnostic comment necessary, and what should be discussed in the diagnostic comment for this entity? When is it appropriate to seek external consultation for this entity (Question 22)?

Chronic Myelomonocytic Leukemia (CMML)

Chronic myelomonocytic leukemia was originally considered as a myelodysplastic syndrome in the French-American-British (FAB) classification of leukemia [5], but after fierce debate it was acknowledged that CMML has both myeloproliferative and myelodysplastic features and became the first myeloid neoplasm to be accepted as a "hybrid" MDS/MPN disorder and the model for the MDS/MPN category that was introduced in the 3rd edition of the World Health Organization Classification of Hematopoietic Neoplasms [6–8].

2. What are the laboratory and morphologic findings of CMML?

- Peripheral blood findings. The 2017 WHO diagnostic criteria for CMML [4] are listed in Table 25.1. Persistent monocytosis is a key defining feature of CMML, and in all cases increased numbers of monocytes ($\geq 1 \times 10^9$/L) must be present, and they account for $\geq$10% of the WBCs. However, only in about 50% of CMML cases is the total WBC count increased, and normal or decreased WBC counts also occur. Although monocytes may range from 1 to >200 × 10^9/L, they are less than 5 × 10^9/L in the majority of cases.
  - The monocyte morphology is variable; often they are mature with fairly normal morphology, but some may be atypical, with unusually folded nuclei, abnormally dense chromatin, or abnormal granulation (Fig. 25.1a).
  - Neutrophils are usually normal or moderately increased in number, but can vary from <0.5 to nearly 200 × 10^9/L, and demonstrate variable degrees of dysplasia. Immature neutrophils (promyelocytes and myelocytes) typically account for fewer than 10% of the WBCs in the blood at diagnosis [9]. Blasts plus promonocytes are always less than 20% of the WBCs. There are usually fewer than 2% basophils.
  - Eosinophils are often normal or mildly increased, but if they are persistently >1.5 × 10^9/L, the diagnosis of CMML with eosinophilia can be made, assuming that myeloid neoplasms associated with eosinophilia and specific genetic abnormalities are excluded (Table 25.1) [2, 4].
  - Mild thrombocytopenia and anemia are common, but thrombocytosis may also be seen [2, 10, 11]. Often the anemia is normocytic, but macrocytosis can be seen as well.
- Myelodysplasia. Dysplasia involving one or more myeloid lineages is a major diagnostic criterion for CMML. Careful morphologic evaluation of the PB and BM cells in well-prepared smears is the gold standard for

Table 25.1 The 2017 WHO diagnostic criteria for chronic myelomonocytic leukemia (CMML)

Diagnostic criteria
1. Persistent peripheral blood monocytosis ($\geq 1 \times 10^9$ /L) with monocytes accounting for ≥10% of the leukocyte count
2. WHO criteria for *BCR-ABL1*-positive chronic myeloid leukemia, primary myelofibrosis, polycythemia vera, and essential thrombocythemia[a] are not met
3. No rearrangements of *PDGFRA*, *PDGFRB*, or *FGFR1* and no *PCM1-JAK2* fusion (which should be specifically excluded in cases with eosinophilia)
4. Blasts[b] constitute <20% of the cells in the PB and BM
5. Dysplasia involving one or more myeloid lineages or If myelodysplasia is absent or minimal, criteria 1–4 are met and: An acquired, clonal cytogenetic or molecular genetic abnormality is present in hematopoietic cells[c] or The monocytosis has persisted for ≥3 months, and all other causes of monocytosis (e.g., malignancy, infection, and inflammation) have been excluded

[a]Myeloproliferative neoplasms (MPN) can be associated with monocytosis or it can develop during the course of the diseases; such cases can mimic CMML. In these rare instances, a documented history of MPN excludes CMML, whereas the presence of MPN features in the BM and/or MPN-associated mutations (in *JAK2*, *CALR*, or *MPL*) tends to support MPN with monocytosis rather than CMML
[b]Blasts and blast equivalents include myeloblasts, monoblasts, and promonocytes
[c]In the appropriate clinical context, mutations in genes often associated with CMML (e.g., *TET2*, *SRSF2*, *ASXL1*, and *SETBP1*) support the diagnosis. However, some of these mutations can be age-related or present in other neoplasms; therefore, these genetic findings must be interpreted with caution

assessing abnormalities in the various hematopoietic lineages (see also Chap. 24) [1, 7]. Neutrophils often show mild to moderate dysplasia (abnormal nuclear segmentation, hypogranular cytoplasm, etc.) in the PB smears (Fig. 25.1a) and BM aspirate smears (Fig. 25.1b) of CMML, but the degree of granulocytic dysplasia varies greatly.

- Cytochemical stains for naphthol AS-D chloroacetate esterase (CAE) and naphthyl butyrate or acetate esterase are sensitive and specific means to distinguish atypical, dysplastic neutrophils and their precursors (CAE positive, naphthyl butyrate/acetate esterase negative or weak) from immature and dyspoietic monocytes (CAE negative or weak, naphthyl butyrate/acetate esterase positive) (Fig. 25.1c).
- Dyserythropoiesis including megaloblastoid changes, abnormal nuclear features, or ring sideroblasts may be seen in the BM aspirate smears of CMML, but these features are often mild, and the number of erythroid precursors may vary from markedly decreased to normal or even increased [10, 11].
- Megakaryocytes may be increased, normal, or decreased in quantity, but markedly increased numbers of megakaryocytes with clustering is unusual [1]. However, up to 75% of CMML patients have variable numbers of small, dysplastic megakaryocytes, which can be more easily recognized with CD61 immunostains on BM core biopsies [12, 13].

• Blasts and promonocytes in CMML. A number of difficulties can be encountered in making the diagnosis of CMML, particularly in distinguishing between normal monocytes, neoplastic monocytes, promonocytes, and monoblasts in the PB and BM.

- Promonocytes are considered as “blast equivalents” in the WHO classification and thus tallied in the blast count [1–4]. Monoblasts have large, round to irregular nuclei with fine chromatin, prominent nucleoli, and blue-gray cytoplasm (Fig. 25.2a). Promonocytes are morphologically characterized by delicately convoluted, folded, or grooved nuclei with finely dispersed delicate/lacelike chromatin, variably prominent nucleoli, and slight cytoplasmic granulation (Fig. 25.2b) [7, 14–16]. In CMML, the monocytes in the peripheral blood may exhibit abnormal granulation and/or nuclear lobation, but their chromatin patterns may vary greatly (Fig. 25.2c). According to the 2017 WHO diagnostic criteria, CMML is further divided into three subtypes according to the blast plus promonocyte counts (Table 25.2).
- The 2017 WHO classification also recommends distinction between “proliferative” and “dysplastic” subtypes of CMML [4] according to the total leukocyte count (Table 25.2).

• Bone marrow cellularity and other findings. The BM is hypercellular in most cases of CMML (Fig. 25.3a) but may be normocellular or even hypocellular [11–13].

- The marrow biopsy often shows prominent granulocytic proliferation with a significant increase in the myeloid-to-erythroid (M:E) ratio. Monocytic proliferation is invariably increased but can be difficult to recognize in BM biopsy sections. Immunohistochemistry (IHC) of the BM core for CD14 and CD68 on BM biopsies may help identify monocytes, although they often tend to underestimate monocytes (Fig. 25.3c).
  • Cytochemical stains for nonspecific esterase on the PB or BM aspirate smears are more reliable than

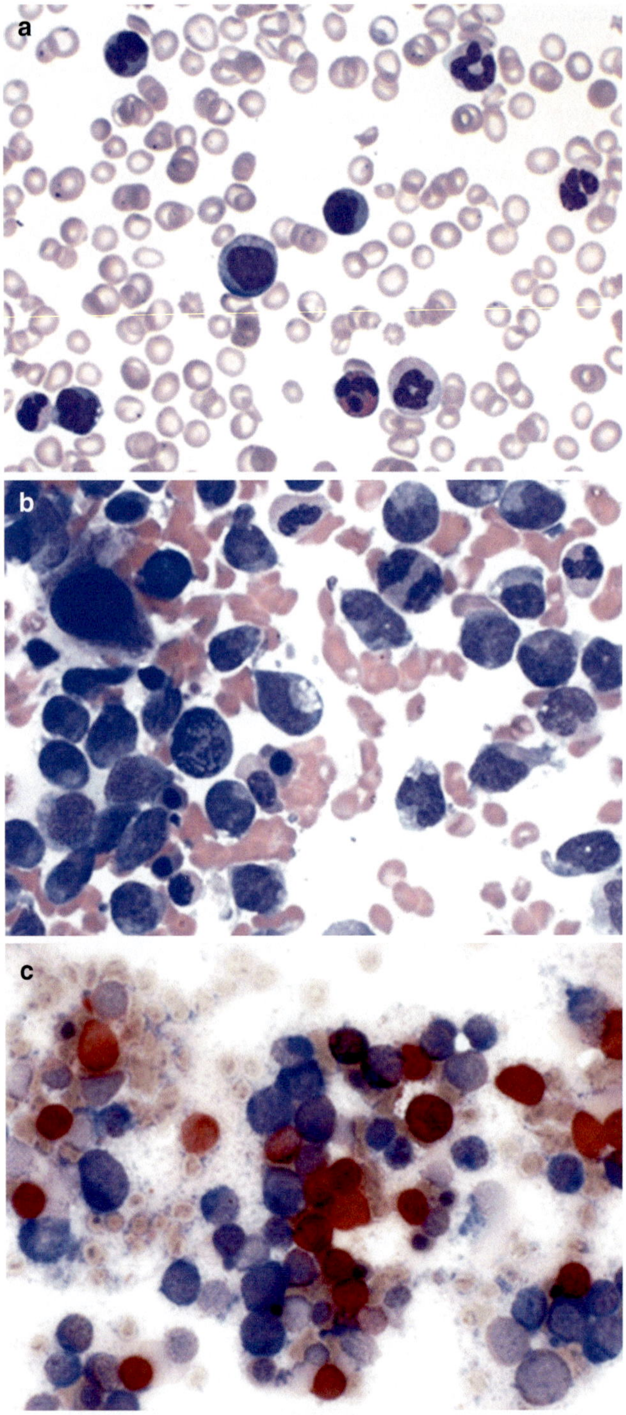

Fig. 25.1 The PB smear and the BM aspirate smear and combined esterase stain of CMML. (**a**) The PB smear demonstrates monocytosis with rare circulating blasts/promonocytes and occasional dysplastic granulocytes. (**b**) The BM aspirate smear demonstrates monocytosis, mildly increased monoblasts and promonocytes, myelodysplasia, and micromegakaryocytes. (**c**) The combined esterase stain that is to combine naphthol ASD chloroacetate esterase (CAE) reaction (neutrophils are blue) with naphthyl butyrate esterase (monocytes are brown)

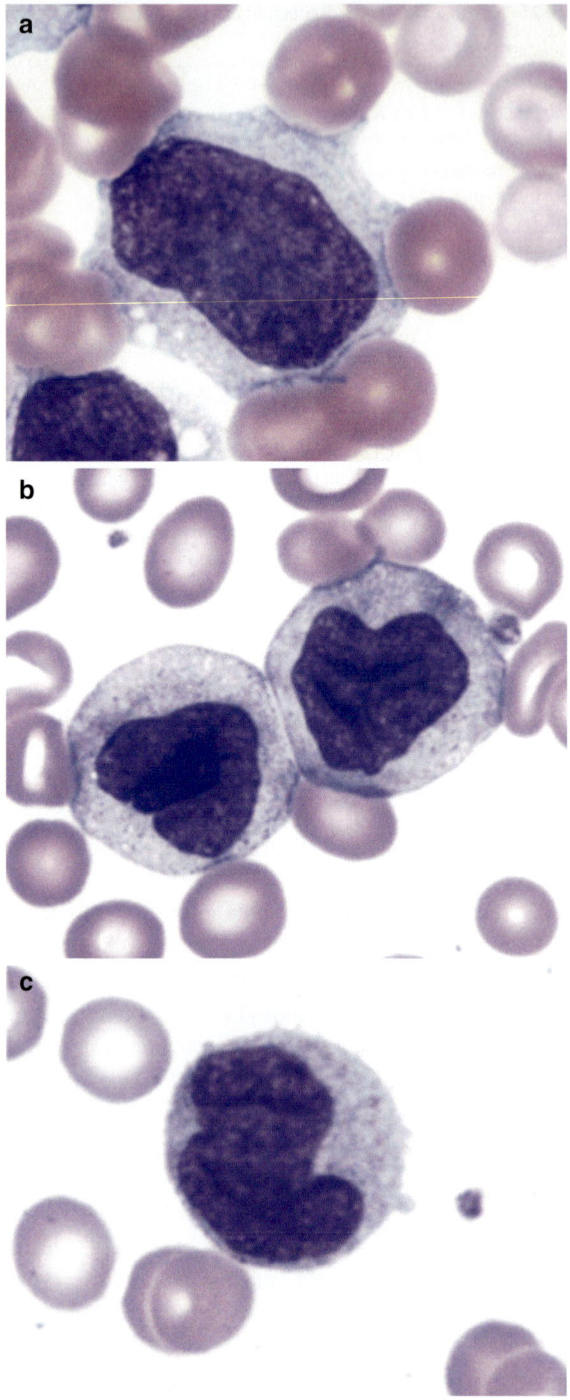

Fig. 25.2 The morphologic features of monoblasts, promonocytes, and abnormal monocytes. (**a**) Monoblasts are large, with round to oval nuclei that may be slightly irregular, lacy chromatin, one or more variably prominent nucleoli, and moderate to abundant cytoplasm that may contain a few vacuoles and fine granules. (**b**) Promonocytes have slightly more irregular and slightly folded nuclei with fine chromatin, indistinct nucleoli, and moderate to abundant finely granulated cytoplasm that may contain a few vacuoles. (**c**) The abnormal monocytes in CMML may appear slightly immature; however, they have condensed chromatin, abnormally shaped, irregular, or folded nuclei, and abundant grayish cytoplasmic granules and often may contain cytoplasmic vacuoles

Table 25.2 The subtypes of chronic myelomonocytic leukemia (CMML)

Categories	Criteria
CMML-0	Blasts including promonocytes account for <2% in the PB and <5% in the BM; no Auer rods
CMML-1	Blasts including promonocytes account for 2–4% in the PB or 5–9% in the BM; <5% blasts in the PB, <10% in the BM, and no Auer rods
CMML-2	Blasts including promonocytes account for 5–19% in the PB and 10–19% in the BM, or Auer rods are present
Proliferative subtype	WBC $\geq 13 \times 10^9$/L in the PB
Dysplastic subtype	WBC $<13 \times 10^9$/L in the PB

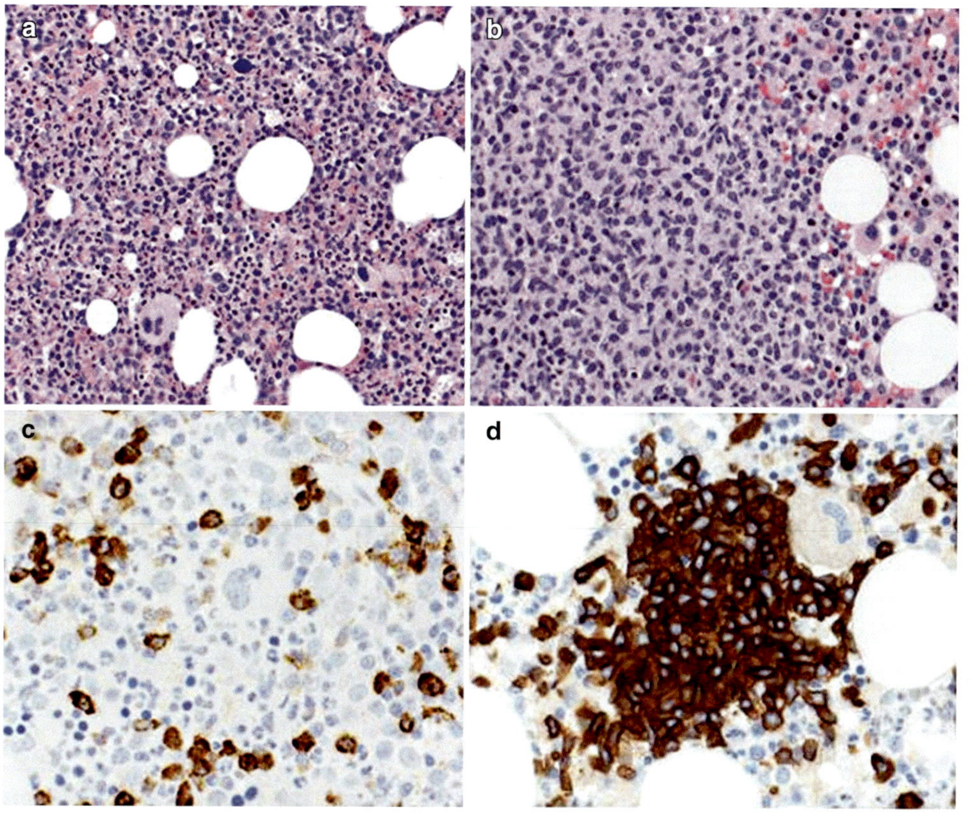

Fig. 25.3 The morphologic features in the BM core biopsy of CMML. (**a**) Bone marrow biopsy is hypercellular with prominent granulocytic and monocytic cells and variably sized megakaryocytes. (**b**) A nodule of plasmacytoid dendritic cells in the bone marrow. (**c**) An immunostain for CD14 demonstrates increased monocytes. (**d**) An immunostain for CD123 highlights the plasmacytoid dendritic cells in the nodule

IHC for identifying monocytes and are strongly recommended to aid in establishing the diagnosis of CMML [1, 12, 13].

- Of note, the percentage of monocytes in the BM required for the diagnosis of CMML has never been established, as the minimal percentages of BM monocytes in CMML reported in the literature vary widely.
- Importantly, monoblasts and promonocytes usually do not express CD34; thus immunohistochemical staining of the bone marrow biopsy for CD34 (and for CD117) is likely to be misleading in regard to the numbers of these immature cells.

- Plasmacytoid dendritic cell nodules in the BM and myelofibrosis. In up to 20% of CMML-1 cases and in even more CMML-2 cases, variably sized nodules of plasmacytoid dendritic cells can be identified in the BM core biopsy (Fig. 25.3b). These aggregates can be highlighted with CD123 IHC (Fig. 25.3d) [1, 3, 17]. A mild increase in reticulin fibers has been reported in most cases of CMML, particularly those with CMML-2 [18], but prominent myelofibrosis in CMML is associated with increased megakaryopoiesis, splenomegaly, and a shorter median time to disease progression [19, 20].
- Extramedullary involvement in CMML. The spleen, liver, skin, and lymph nodes are the most frequent sites of extramedullary involvement by CMML.
  - Splenic enlargement is caused by leukemic infiltration, primarily in the red pulp [1, 3, 10].

Table 25.3 Recurrent mutations in myelodysplastic/myeloproliferative neoplasms (MDS/MPN)

Gene mutation	CMML (%)	aCML (%)	JMML (%)	MDS/MPN-RS-T (%)
Epigenetic regulators:				
TET2	50–60%	~40%	–	~25%
ASXL1	30–40%	~25%	~4%	~20%
DNMT3A	4–5%	<1%	<1%	~15%
IDH1/2	<1%	–	–	–
UTX	~10%	–	–	–
EZH2	~10%	–	–	~25%
SETBP1	~5%	~30%	~7%	~10%
RNA splicing/processing factors:				
SF3B1	5–10%	–	–	~85%
U2AF1	~5%	–	–	–
SRSF2	~50%	~40%	–	–
Cell signaling components:				
NRAS	~20%	~20%	~10%	–
KRAS	5–10%	~10%	~10%	–
PTPN11	~5%	–	~40%	–
CBL	~10%	~5–10%	~15%	–
NF1	1%	–	–	–
FLT3	~4%	<5%	–	–
CSF3R	~10%	5–10%	–	–
JAK2	5–10%	–	–	~50%
CALR	–	–	–	10–15%
MPL	–	–	–	10%
Transcription factors and others:				
NPM1	~5–10%	–	–	–
TP53	~1%	–	–	–
RUNX1	~20%	~5%	–	–

  - Lymph node enlargement is seen in a minority of CMML patients and often represents nodular proliferation of plasmacytoid dendritic cells in the paracortical regions of the involved nodes [17, 21–24]. The tumoral proliferation of plasmacytoid dendritic cells in the nodal and extranodal tissue shares the same clonal, neoplastic nature as the associated CMML cells in the BM specimens [23]. Nevertheless, biopsy of an enlarged lymph node or any other mass lesion is strongly recommended in any patient with CMML, as it may indicate extramedullary transformation to acute leukemia, i.e., "myeloid sarcoma" [1].
- Cytogenetic abnormalities and gene mutations in CMML. Cytogenetic abnormalities are detected in ~40–50% of cases, the most frequent of which are +8, −Y, −7, del(7q), +21, and del(20q) [25]. Some patients with i(17q) may have the features of CMML, and such cases were reported to have an aggressive clinical course with rapid progression toward acute myeloid leukemia [26–30]. The abnormalities of chromosome 11q23 are uncommon in CMML and should raise concern for an acute leukemia [31–33]. Gene mutations are frequently detected in CMML as well. The most common mutations involve four major groups of genes that include (1) epigenetic regulators and chromatin modifiers (*TET2* ~50–60% of all CMML cases, *ASXL1* ~30–40%), (2) spliceosome components (*SRSF2* ~50%), (3) transcription factors (*RUNX1* ~15–20%), and (4) signal pathways (*RAS* ~20–30%, *CBL* ~10%) [25, 34] (Table 25.3). Of note, these gene mutations are not specific for CMML and can be seen in other hematologic malignancies and aging-related processes.

3. What are the mimics and differential diagnostic considerations for CMML?

The major differential considerations for CMML with suggested approaches to their recognition and differentiation from CMML are listed in Table 25.4 and discussed below:

- Reactive monocytosis. Infections, including viral, fungal, protozoal, rickettsial, and mycobacterial infections, are commonly associated with monocytosis, as are autoimmune diseases and other chronic inflammatory disorders. Monocytosis is also often seen in regenerative bone marrows after various infections and biological or chemical insults (Fig. 25.4).
  - CMML can also coexist with reactive or other neoplastic diseases that are commonly associated with monocytosis, such as autoimmune diseases. Careful review and analysis of the morphology of the PB and BM cells, examination of the history and clinical findings, such as splenomegaly, as well as the genetic studies will enable distinction of reactive monocytosis from CMML in most cases [1–3, 13, 35].

Table 25.4 The major differential considerations and diagnostic approaches for CMML, JMML, and aCML

MDS/MPN	Differential	Diagnostic approaches
CMML JMML	Reactive monocytosis	Rule out (1) infections including viruses, fungi, protozoa, rickettsia, and mycobacteria; (2) autoimmune; and (3) other neoplasms
	AML with monocytic differentiation	PB and BM for morphologic, immunophenotypic, and cytogenetic studies
	CML, *BCR-ABL1*⁺, particularly p190 CML	Molecular and cytogenetic for t(9;22)(q34;q11) *BCR-ABL1*
	Myeloid neoplasms with eosinophilia and *PDGFRB*, *PDGFRA*, or *FGFR1* rearrangement or *PCM1-JAK2* fusion	Cytogenetic/FISH/molecular studies
	BCR-ABL1-negative MPN associated with monocytosis	PB and BM for morphologic, immunophenotypic, and cytogenetic studies
	MDS	PB and BM for morphologic, immunophenotypic, and cytogenetic studies
	Lymphomas, Langerhans cell, histiocytic or melanocytic or dendritic neoplasms	Biopsy of tumoral lesions for morphologic, immunophenotypic, and cytogenetic studies
	Transient JMML-like myeloproliferative disorder with Noonan syndrome (TMD-NS)	Genetic sequencing for germline *PTPN11*, *KRAS*, or *NRAS* mutations
	CBL germline mutation and "CBL syndrome"	Genetic sequencing for germline *PTPN11*, *KRAS*, or *NRAS* mutations
	Transient myeloproliferative disorder of Down syndrome (TMD-DS)	Cytogenetic analysis for trisomy 21 and molecular studies for *GATA1* mutation
	Wiskott-Aldrich syndrome (WAS)	Screening: Flow cytometry to measure WASP Diagnosis: Genetic sequencing for *WASP* mutations
	Malignant infantile osteopetrosis (MIOP)	Skeletal findings in radiography
aCML	CML, *BCR-ABL1*⁺	Molecular and cytogenetic to exclude t(9;22)(q34;q11) *BCR-ABL1*
	BCR-ABL1-negative MPN, especially CNL	PB and BM for morphologic and molecular/cytogenetic studies, especially for *CSF3R* mutation
	Other types of MDS/MPN	PB and BM for morphologic and molecular/cytogenetic studies
	Myeloid neoplasms with eosinophilia and *PDGFRB*, *PDGFRA*, or *FGFR1* rearrangement or *PCM1-JAK2* fusion	Cytogenetic/FISH/molecular studies

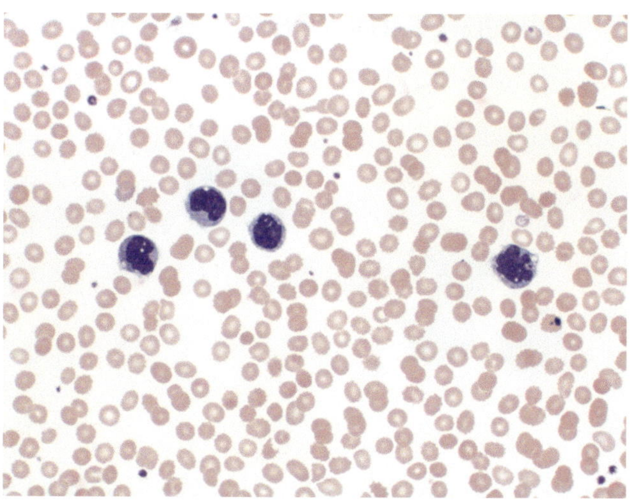

Fig. 25.4 Reactive monocytosis from a patient status post bone marrow transplant with *EBV* infection

- CML, *BCR-ABL1*⁺, particularly "p190 CML." The distinction between CML, *BCR-ABL1*⁺, and CMML is made on the basis of morphology combined with cytogenetics and molecular/genetic studies that show the *BCR-ABL1* fusion in CML, but not in CMML. The rare cases of CML with p190 BCR/ABL1 is characteristically associated with increased monocytes (see also Chap. 21) and thus may closely mimic the findings in CMML [1, 36]. Therefore, cytogenetic and genetic testing for the *BCR-ABL1* fusion is strongly recommended whenever the diagnosis of CMML is considered.
- *BCR-ABL1*-negative MPN associated with monocytosis. Monocytosis has been described in up to 15% of patients with *BCR-ABL1*-negative MPN, such as primary myelofibrosis (PMF), in which cases the monocytosis is reportedly an independent adverse predictive factor, particularly in younger patients [37, 38].
  - CMML may be associated with prominent reticulin fibrosis [39]. In such cases its distinction from PMF may be very difficult, but the finding of clusters of pleomorphic, bizarre megakaryocytes in the BM favors PMF rather than CMML [1].
- Myelodysplastic syndrome (MDS). CMML cases, particularly those with normal or low WBC counts and prominent dysplasia, i.e., "dysplastic-type CMML," may be difficult to distinguish from MDS. If the WHO criteria

are carefully applied, the finding of monocytosis ($\geq 1 \times 10^9$/L) with significant myelodysplasia is sufficient for the diagnosis of CMML rather than MDS.

  - In rare cases, early CMML may present with marked monocytosis in the BM, but not in the PB [40]. In such cases, follow-up repeats of the peripheral CBC and differential count after suitable intervals may provide evidence for a diagnosis of CMML.

- Acute myeloid leukemia (AML). AML with or without *NPM1* or *FLT3* mutation must be considered in the differential diagnosis of all CMML cases, and well-prepared BM aspirate smears and core biopsies are crucial in distinguishing between these entities, along with mutational analysis. *NPM1* or *FLT3* mutations are very rarely, if ever, found in CMML, and if present, a diagnosis of AML rather than CMML should be considered first. The finding of "cuplike" myeloblasts in such cases (Fig. 25.5) is suggestive of the presence of *NPM1* or *FLT3* mutation and provides a useful clue for the diagnosis of AML [41–44].
- Myeloid/lymphoid neoplasms associated with eosinophilia and *PDGFRB*, *PDGFRA*, or *FGFR1* rearrangements or *PCM1-JAK2* fusion. This group of myeloid neoplasms is characteristically associated with eosinophilia [45–47]. In addition to eosinophilia and leukocytosis, monocytosis is common in myeloid neoplasms with eosinophilia and *PDGFRB* rearrangement and is occasionally seen in the myeloid neoplasms with rearranged *PDGFRA* or *FGFR1* and with *PCM1-JAK2* fusion. In all suspected CMML cases with eosinophilia, cytogenetic, FISH, and molecular studies should be performed [1].
- Other hematopoietic neoplasms and lymphomas. Hodgkin and non-Hodgkin lymphoma, NK-cell neoplasms, plasma cell myeloma, and blastic plasmacytoid dendritic neoplasms may produce cytokines that stimulate myeloid and monocytic cell proliferation and lead to leukocytosis and monocytosis in the PB. Furthermore, the morphology of circulating or infiltrating neoplastic cells may sometimes resemble the abnormal (neoplastic) monocytes seen in CMML.
  - Figure 25.6 shows circulating peripheral T-cell lymphoma cells with large multilobated nuclei and monocytoid morphology. Rare plasma cell myeloma cases can have monocytoid morphology (Fig. 25.7), and such myeloma cases often have an aggressive clinical course [48]. Langerhans cell, histiocytic, melanocytic, or dendritic neoplasms can resemble extramedullary involvement by CMML, resulting in diagnostic difficulties [49–51].
  - CMML often involves extramedullary organs/tissues, such as the liver, spleen, skin, lymph nodes, and other organs/tissues. Figure 25.8 shows that CMML involves gastrointestinal walls.
  - Conversely, many benign and neoplastic soft-tissue diseases, such as Langerhans cell, histiocytic, dendritic, and melanocytic lineages, can be associated with marked monocytosis in the PB and BM and pose a diagnostic challenge. Figure 25.9 shows a BM core biopsy of Rosai-Dorfman disease cases with markedly increased monocytes and histiocytes in the BM and with monocytosis in the PB, which closely mimics CMML. In such cases, a panel of immunohistochemical markers, including CD45, CD3, CD20, CD30,

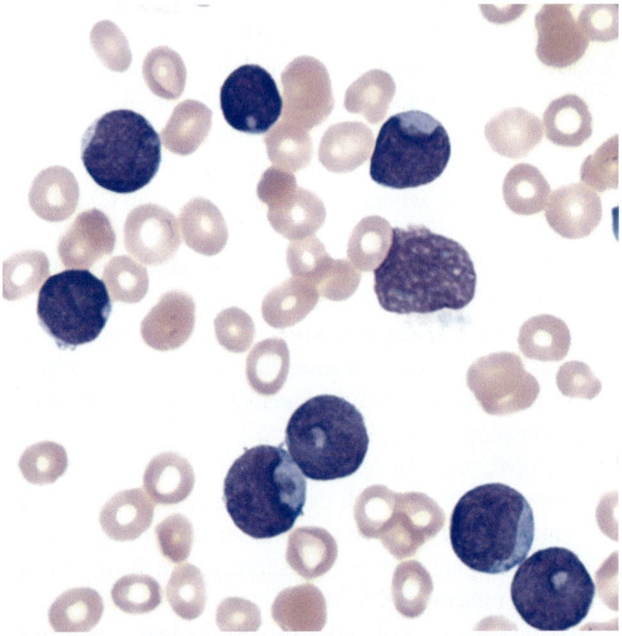

Fig. 25.5 Myeloblasts with "cuplike" monocytoid morphology from a patient with acute myeloid leukemia (AML) with mutated *NPM1*

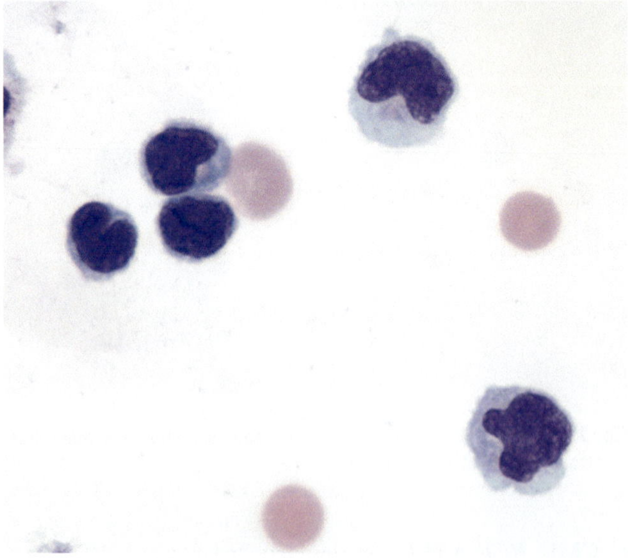

Fig. 25.6 Circulating peripheral T-cell lymphoma cells with large multilobated nuclei and monocytoid morphology

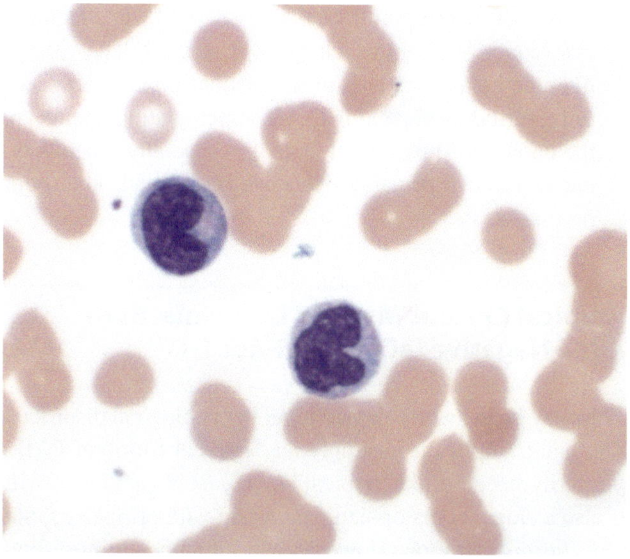

Fig. 25.7 Circulating myeloma cells with large irregular cleaved nuclei and monocytoid morphology. These cells were shown to be monoclonal plasma cells by flow cytometry

CD34, CD68, CD1a, S100, Langerin, TCL1, and CD123, may be useful to distinguish CMML from Hodgkin and non-Hodgkin lymphomas and Langerhans cell, histiocytic, melanocytic, or dendritic neoplasms [51]. Flow-cytometry studies can also provide useful information for differential diagnosis.

4. What work-up provides prognostic information for CMML?

- Prognostic scoring systems. The clinical course of CMML is highly variable, the overall survival times ranging from 1 to 100 months [52, 53]. Several prognostic scoring systems, including the MD Anderson prognostic scoring system (MDAPS), the Dusseldorf system, the Global MDAPS, the CMML-specific prognostic scoring system (CPSS), and the Mayo CMML prognostic model, have been developed to estimate CMML prognosis [34, 54–67]. Genetic abnormalities – including gene mutations – have also been reported to affect the outcome of CMML [67, 68]. See Table 25.5 for the detailed information about the score calculation and risk stratification of the Mayo CMML prognostic model [69], MDAPS [60], and CPSS [54].

5. What work-up provides information regarding therapeutic targets and clinical management information for CMML?

- Gene mutations and targeted therapy: Table 25.3 lists the common recurrent mutations in CMML, some of which may provide promising therapeutic targets. Currently, many new gene/protein or pathway targeting therapies are in active clinical trials (Table 25.6).

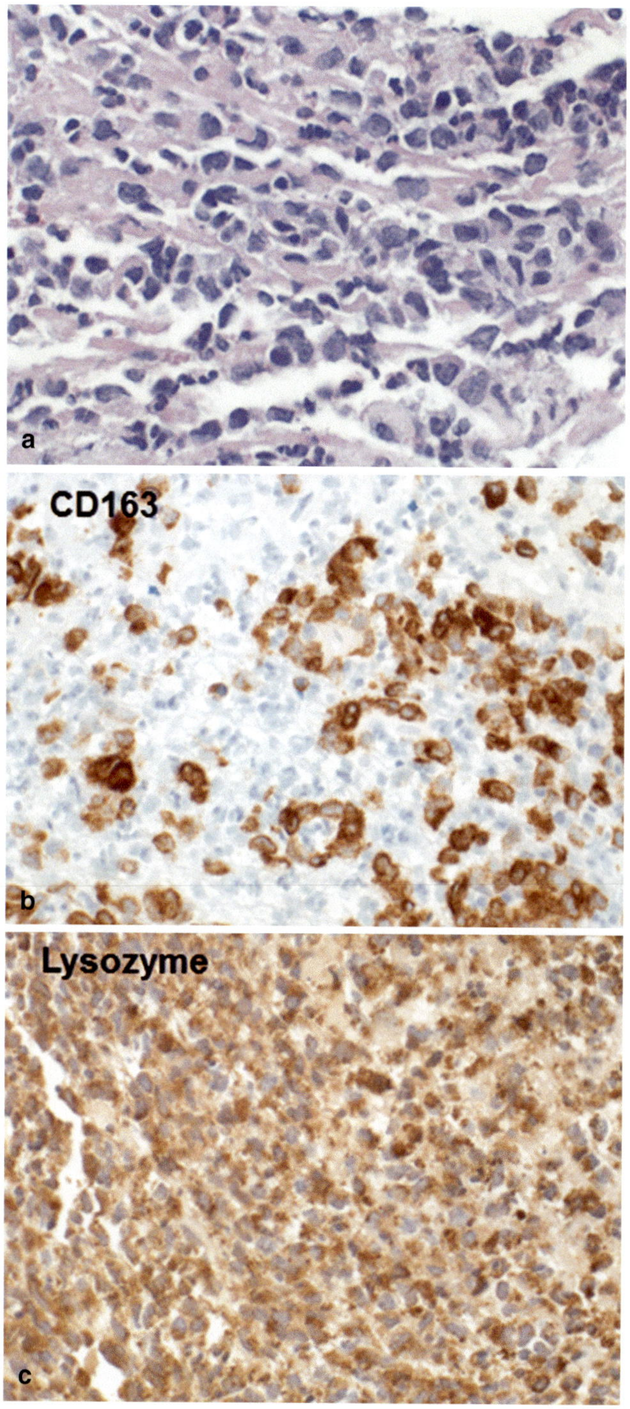

Fig. 25.8 A GI biopsy shows involvement by monocytic leukemia cells in a patient with CMML. (**a**) The GI biopsy shows sheets of neoplastic cells with large irregular nuclei, conspicuous nucleoli, and ample amount of amphophilic cytoplasm. (**b**) CD163 IHC highlights more mature monocytes/histiocytes. (**c**) Lysozyme IHC highlights both mature and immature monocytes as well as myelomonocytes

- Clinical management in CMML: Currently, the only curative option for CMML is allogeneic stem cell transplantation (ASCT). If transplantation is not a suitable choice, a personalized strategy guided by cytopenia-induced vs.

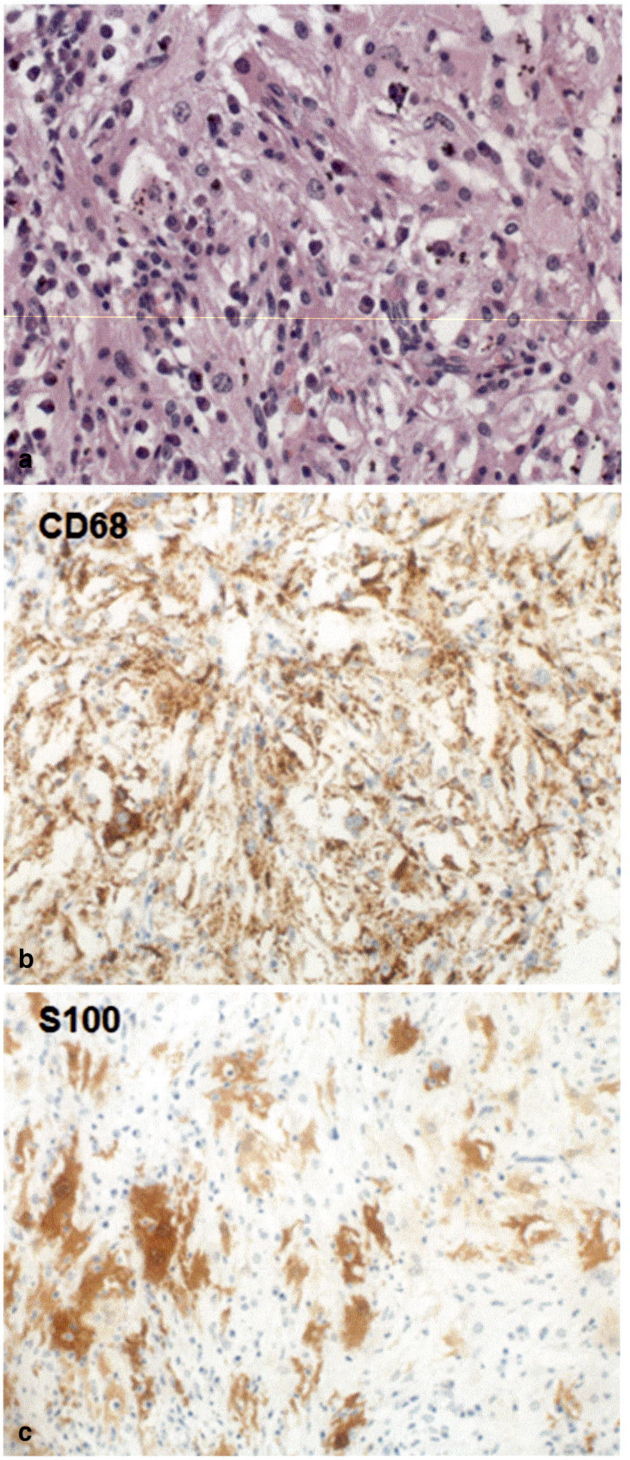

Fig. 25.9 Bone marrow involvement by Rosai-Dorfman disease morphologically resembling CMML with myelofibrosis. (**a**) The BM shows marked histiocytic and dendritic cell proliferation with plasmacytosis. (**b**) CD68 IHC highlights numerous histiocytes. (**c**) S100 is expressed in the histiocytic/dendritic cells

proliferation-associated symptoms is recommended [67]. The management of myelodysplastic-type CMML includes erythropoiesis-stimulating agents for management of severe anemia and supportive care. The management of myeloproliferative-type CMML includes cytoreductive agents such as hydroxyurea. The role of hypomethylating agents in this patient population needs to be further evaluated [67]. Hypomethylating agents are the choice for progressed CMML, especially when there are severe cytopenia(s), excessive blasts, and other poor prognostic factors.

Atypical Chronic Myeloid Leukemia, *BCR-ABL1*-Negative (aCML, *BCR-ABL1*-)

This may be the worst-named of all hematological disorders! The name implies it is simply an "atypical form" of CML, primarily because like "typical" CML, *BCR-ABL1*+, aCML is also a clonal hematopoietic neoplasm with primarily granulocytic proliferation. However, the granulocytic proliferation in aCML is dysplastic, and the patients with aCML do not respond to imatinib therapy (because they lack the *BCR-ABL1* fusion) and have a very poor prognosis [1, 9, 70–72].

6. What are the laboratory and morphologic findings of aCML?

- Dysplastic neutrophilic leukocytosis. The hallmarks of aCML are persistent leukocytosis ($\geq 13 \times 10^9$/L) due to increased numbers of neutrophils, with neutrophilic precursors accounting for ≥10% of the peripheral blood WBCs (Table 25.7) [1, 7, 9], and prominent granulocytic dysplasia, including neutrophils with hypogranular cytoplasm, and abnormal nuclear segmentation and chromatin patterns, including pseudo-Pelger-Huët-like nuclei (Fig. 25.10a) [73].
  - Blasts are usually <5% and always less than 20%, but promyelocytes, myelocytes, and metamyelocytes account for 10% or more of the WBCs.
  - A variant of aCML is characterized by markedly abnormal condensation and clumping of the neutrophil nuclear chromatin ("syndrome of abnormal chromatin clumping"), but the clinical course of these patients is similar to that of other patients with aCML [74].
- No or minimal basophilia or monocytosis. Basophils and monocytes should constitute <2% and <10% of the peripheral blood leukocytes, respectively, although in rare cases, monocytes may exceed 1000/μL (Table 25.7).
- Anemia and thrombocytopenia. Moderate normocytic anemia and thrombocytopenia are common in aCML, but the degree of anemia and thrombocytopenia and the morphology of RBCs and platelets may vary from case to case.
- Hypercellular BM with granulocytic proliferation. In aCML, the BM biopsies and aspirate smears are hypercellular due to

Table 25.5 Three prognostic scoring systems for CMML

	Parameters and prognostic scores	Risk stratification
Mayo CMML prognostic model	1. Absolute monocytes: ≤10,000/mL → 0 point; > 10,000/mL → 1 point 2. Circulating immature cells, i.e., myeloblasts, myelocytes, metamyelocytes, and/or promyelocytes: no → 0 point; yes → 1 point 3. Anemia: HGB ≤10 g/dL → 0 point; HGB <10 g/dL → 1 point 4. Thrombocytopenia: platelets >100 × 10^9/L → 0 point; platelets ≤100 × 10^9/L → 1 point	0 point: Low risk with 32-month median survival 1 point: Intermediate risk with 18.5-month median survival 2–4 points: High risk with 10-month median survival
MD Anderson prognostic scoring system (MDAPS)	1. Age: <60 yo → 0 point; 60–64 yo → 1 point; ≥ 65 yo → 2 points 2. History of prior transfusion: no → 0 point; yes → 1 point 3. Performance status: 2 or higher status → 2 points 4. Leukocytosis: WBC >20 × 10^9/L → 2 points 5. Anemia: HGB <10 g/dL → 2 points 6. Thrombocytopenia: platelets ≥200 × 10^9/L → 0 point; platelets >50–199 × 10^9/L → 1 point; 30–49 × 10^9/L → 2 points; <30 × 10^9/L → 2 points. 7. Blasts in the BM: <5% → 0 point; 5–10% → 1 point; >10% → 2 points 8. Karyotype: chromosome 7 abnormality or complex ≥3 abnormalities → 3 points	0–4 points: The median survival of 54 months; 63% at 3 years and 38% at 6 years 5–6 points: The median survival of 25 months; 34% at 3 years and 13% at 6 years 7–8 points: The median survival of 14 months; 16% at 3 years and 6% at 6 years 9–17 points: The median survival of 6 months; 4% at 3 years and 0.4% at 6 years
CMML-specific prognostic scoring system (CPSS)	1. Leukocytosis: WBC <13 × 10^9/L → 0 point; WBC ≥13 × 10^9/L → 1 point. 2. RBC transfusion dependency: no → 0 point; yes → 1 point 3. BM blasts: <5% → 0 point; ≥5% → 1 point 4. Cytogenetics: low risk (normal and isolated –Y) → 0 point; intermediate risk (other abnormalities) → 1 point; and high risk (trisomy 8, complex karyotype, i.e., ≥3 abnormalities) and abnormalities of chromosome 7 → 2 points 5. Gene mutations: Low risk (no mutations in *ASXL1*, *NRAS*, *RUNX1*, and *SEPBP1*) → 0 point; intermediate risk (no mutations in *ASXL1*, *NRAS*, or *SEPBP1*, but not *RUNX1*) → 1 point; high risk (no *RUNX1*) → 2 points	0 point: Low risk with unreached (at least >70 months) median survival 1 point: Intermediate risk-1 with 68-month median survival 1 point: Intermediate risk-2 with 30-month median survival 2–4 points: High risk with 17-month median survival

Table 25.6 Gene/pathway targeting therapeutic agents in clinical usages and trials for hematologic malignancies

Targets	Drugs/inhibitors
Epigenetics:	
Hypomethylating agents	Decitabine, azacitidine, guadecitabine (SGI-110), ASTX727
HDAC	Mocetinostat, pracinostat, vorinostat, entinostat
BRD4/BET	ABBV-075
IDH1, IDH2	Ivosidenib, enasidenib
Signal transduction pathway:	
RAS/MEK/PI3K/AKT pathway	Binimetinib (MEK162), rigosertib
FLT3	Quizartinib, crenolanib, gilteritinib
Pim kinase/PLK-1	LGH447, volasertib
Janus kinase (JAK) pathway	Ruxolitinib and baricitinib (JAK1/JAK2 inhibitors) Oclacitinib (JAK1 inhibitor) Tofacitinib (JAK3 inhibitor)
Hedgehog pathway	Sonidegib (erismodegib)
CK1α degradation	Lenalidomide
TGF-β superfamily ligands	Luspatercept, sotatercept
Spliceosomes and RNA-binding factors:	
Modulator of SF3B complex	H3B-8800
Apoptosis	
TP53 and MDMX/MDM2 complex	ALRN-6924
BCL2	Venetoclax
N/K-RAS	
DNA repair and telomerase dysfunction:	
Poly(ADP-ribose) polymerase (PARP)	Olaparib, talazoparib, veliparib, temozolomide
Telomerase	Imetelstat
Immunomodulating complex:	
CTLA-4	Ipilimumab
PD1/PD-L1	Atezolizumab, durvalumab, pembrolizumab
Erythropoiesis	
Erythropoietin	Epoetin alfa or darbepoetin alfa

Table 25.7 The 2017 WHO diagnostic criteria for atypical chronic myeloid leukemia *BCR-ABL1*⁻ (aCML)

Diagnostic criteria
1. Peripheral blood leukocytosis ≥13 × 10^9 /L, due to increased numbers of neutrophils and their precursors (i.e., promyelocytes, myelocytes, and metamyelocytes), with neutrophil precursors ≥10% of the leukocytes
2. Dysgranulopoiesis, which may include abnormal chromatin clumping
3. No or minimal absolute basophilia; basophils constitute <2% of the peripheral blood leukocytes
4. No or minimal absolute monocytosis; monocytes constitute <10% of the peripheral leukocytes
5. Hypercellular bone marrow with granulocytic proliferation and granulocytic dysplasia, with or without erythroid and megakaryocytic dysplasia
6. <20% blasts in the blood and bone marrow
7. No rearrangements of *PDGFRA*, *PDGFRB*, or *FGFR1* or *PCM1-JAK2* fusion (which should be specifically excluded in cases with eosinophilia)
8. WHO criteria for *BCR-ABL1*⁺ chronic myeloid leukemia, primary myelofibrosis, polycythemia vera, or essential thrombocythemia are not met[a]

[a]MPN, in particular those in accelerated phase and/or in post-polycythemia vera or post-essential thrombocythemia myelofibrosis, may simulate aCML. A history of MPN, the presence of MPN features in the bone marrow, and/or MPN-associated mutations (in *JAK2*, *CALR*, or *MPL*) tend to exclude the diagnosis of aCML; conversely, the diagnosis of aCML is supported by the presence of *SETBP1* and/or *ETNK1* mutations. *CSF3R* mutation is uncommon and, if detected, should prompt careful morphological review to exclude an alternative diagnosis of chronic neutrophilic leukemia or another myeloid neoplasm

prominent granulocytic proliferation and expansion, with an increased M:E ratio, often >10:1 (Fig. 25.10b).

- Myelodysplasia. Dysgranulopoiesis is always present and often best appreciated in the BM aspirate smears, with dysplastic changes similar to those described in the PB [73, 75]. Dyserythropoiesis is present in about 40% of aCML cases. Megakaryocytes are usually normal or increased in number but often show dysplastic changes, including micromegakaryocytes, small megakaryocytes with hypolobated nuclei, and/or large megakaryocytes with widely separate nuclear lobes [76–78].
- Extramedullary leukemic involvement. Splenic and hepatic involvement is very common in aCML. The liver and spleen are enlarged due to infiltration of atypical neoplastic granulocytes and their precursors, which may cause organ failure [9, 73, 79].
- Cytogenetic abnormalities and gene mutations in aCML. By definition, there is no cytogenetic or molecular genetic evidence of *BCR-ABL1* fusion in aCML. Cytogenetic abnormalities and gene mutations are common, seen in 50–65% cases of aCML overall [72, 77, 80–82] (Table 25.3).
  - The most common cytogenetic abnormalities include +8 and del(20q), but monosomy 7; del(12p); deletions of 5q, 13q, 17p, 12q, and 11q; and t(6;8)(p23;q22) are seen as well [76, 77].
  - aCML is reported to have a relatively high frequency of mutations in *SETBP1*, *ASXL1*, *N/K-RAS*, *SRSF2*, and *TET2* (>20% of the all reported aCML cases) and relatively low frequency of mutations (<10%) in *CBL*, *CSF3R*, *JAK2*, and *ETNK1* [70, 80].
    - *SETBP1* mutations have been reported to be associated with an aggressive clinical course [83, 84]. *SETBP1* mutations have also been shown to be associated with −7 and i(17)(q10) cytogenetic abnormalities and with *ASXL1* and *CBL* mutations, but not with *TET2* or *JAK2* gene mutations [83, 84].

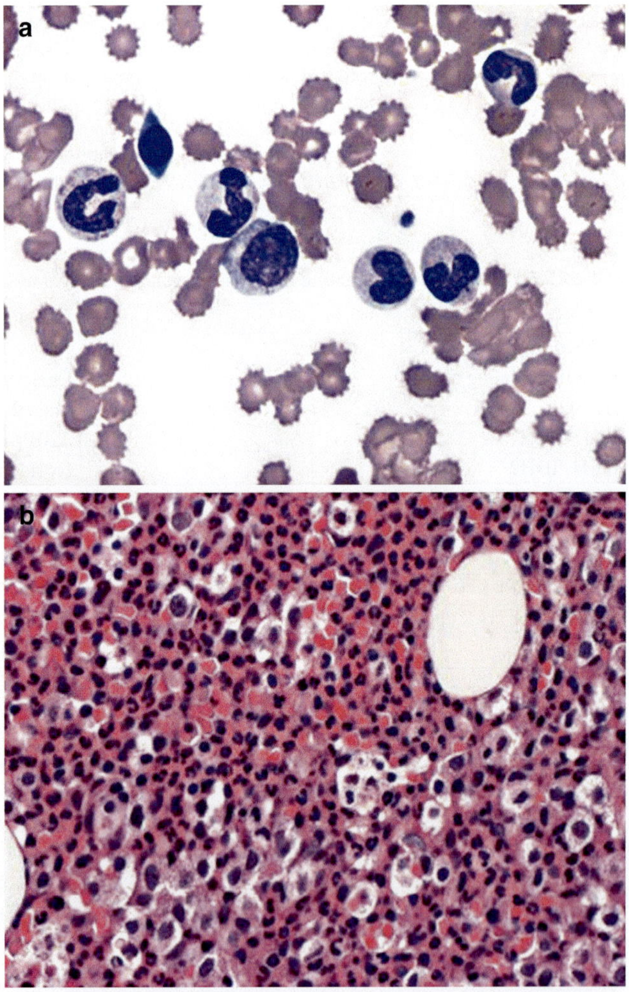

Fig. 25.10 The PB smear and the BM core biopsy of a patient with atypical CML, *BCR-ABL1*⁻ (aCML). (**a**) The PB smear shows neutrophilia with marked granulocytic dysplasia. The granulocytes display abnormally segmented nuclei, abnormally clumped chromatin, and hypogranular cytoplasm. (**b**) The BM core biopsy from a patient with aCML shows a hypercellular bone marrow with granulocytic proliferation, with hyper-condensed nuclear chromatin, left-shifted myelopoiesis, and a markedly increased M:E ratio

7. What are the mimics and differential diagnostic considerations for aCML?

The following are the major differential diagnostic considerations for aCML, and approaches to their recognition are listed in Table 25.4:

- Reactive granulocytic hyperplasia/leukemoid reactions. aCML is usually easily distinguished from reactive granulocytosis based on the dysplasia of the granulocytes in aCML. However, it is prudent to verify that the patient is not receiving G-CSF or other medications that may cause granulocytic dysplasia or pelgeroid neutrophils (see Chap. 31).
- *BCR-ABL1*-positive CML. One of the prerequisites for the diagnosis of aCML is to exclude *BCR-ABL1*-positive CML by cytogenetic and/or molecular analysis that excludes the presence of the t(9;22)(q34.1;q11.2) *BCR-ABL1* fusion gene [85, 86]. It is important to note that in *BCR-ABL1*-positive CML, dysplasia may be prominent in the accelerated phase, and thus exclusion of this diagnosis is mandatory by genetic testing. Conversely, rare cases of CML with e19a2 *BCR-ABL1* fusion that results in a p230 product may not be detected in routine molecular testing.
- Chronic neutrophilic leukemia (CNL). Both aCML and CNL present with marked neutrophilia in the PB and granulocytic expansion in the BM, as well as hepatosplenomegaly. The morphologic distinction between these two neoplasms includes the percentage of immature neutrophils in the blood (≥10% in aCML and <10% in CNL) and the presence of significant granulocytic dysplasia in aCML but not in CNL. Mutations in the colony-stimulating factor 3 receptor gene (*CSF3R*) are found in a majority (~80%) of CNL patients but also reported in a small number (~10%) of patients with aCML [58, 70, 85, 87, 88].
- Other types of MDS/MPN:
  - Proliferative-type CMML can present with marked leukocytosis and increased numbers of neutrophils but always has 10% or more monocytes in the peripheral blood and absolute monocytosis. Rarely, mild absolute monocytosis is present in aCML, but in contrast to CMML, the monocyte percentage in the blood is always less than 10% in aCML.
  - MDS/MPN-U cases can also have a WBC $\geq 13 \times 10^9$/L and granulocytic dysplasia, but the granulocyte counts are generally lower than in aCML, and granulocytic dysplasia is less severe. When compared to MDS/MPN-U, aCML shows inferior overall survival [72, 89].
  - Recently, some molecular markers have been reported to be helpful in the differential diagnosis of these entities. *ASXL1*, *SRSF2*, and *TET2* are more frequently mutated in CMML, whereas *SETBP1* is more frequently mutated in aCML, but also often coexistent with *ASXL1* and/or *CBL* mutations. *SETBP1* mutations are strongly associated with *ASXL1* and *CBL* mutations and mutually exclusive of *JAK2* and *TET2* mutations [84].
- Myeloid/lymphoid neoplasms associated with eosinophilia and *PDGFRA*, *PDGFRB*, or *FGFR1* rearrangement or *PCM1-JAK2* fusion [45, 47]. These myeloid neoplasms may present with leukocytosis and granulocytic dysplasia, in addition to eosinophilia. However, rearrangements of *PDGFRA*, *PDGFRB*, *FGFR1*, or *PCM1-JAK2* fusion exclude the diagnosis of aCML.

8. What work-up provides prognostic information for aCML?

The prognosis of aCML is poor, with reported median survival times of 12–25 months [73]. Approximately 30–40% of patients evolve to AML, and most of the remaining patients die of BM failure [72, 76, 77, 79, 80]. The following are reported independent, adverse prognostic factors that affect the overall survival (OS) and leukemia-free survival (LFS) of aCML [77, 80, 81, 90]:

- Marked leukocytosis (WBC counts $>50 \times 10^9$/L).
- Increased percentage of peripheral blood granulocytic precursors.
- Anemia (Hb < 10 g/dL), red cell transfusion dependence and erythroid dysplasia [77].
- Female sex.
- Older age (>65 years old).
- Mutational status; *SETBP1* mutations are associated with a higher leukocyte count, lower hemoglobin and platelet counts, and a worse overall survival in aCML [83]. *TET2*, *NRAS*, *PTPN11* mutations and the presence of ≥3 gene mutations were also reported to have a negative impact on prognosis [82].

9. What work-up provides therapeutic targets and clinical management information for aCML?

- Gene mutations and targeted therapy: The common recurrent mutations in aCML are listed in Table 25.3. Clinical trials that target specific genes or molecular pathways are listed in Table 25.6. Imatinib has not been shown to be efficacious in aCML due to absence of BCR-ABL1 fusion protein, but other specific targeted therapies are emerging based on genetic studies, particularly in cases with *CSF3R*, *NRAS*, or *KRAS* mutations [89]. However, no clear molecularly driven therapy for *SETBP1* mutation is currently available [89].

- Clinical management of aCML: Currently, no standard treatment protocols, consensus recommendations, or risk-based treatment algorithms have been established to help guide therapy in aCML or decide for a watch-and-wait approach vs. initiation of therapy in clinical settings [80]. Hematopoietic stem cell transplantation (HSCT) for eligible patients with a suitable donor should be considered, and hypomethylating agents, such as azacitidine or decitabine, are recommended as a bridging therapy for those who are eligible for HSCT or as stand-alone treatment of patients who are not eligible for HSCT or clinical trial [80].

Juvenile Myelomonocytic Leukemia (JMML)

JMML is a rare disorder that occurs primarily in children less than 3 years of age, although it may be seen in teenagers as well. There is a predilection for young boys, for infants with Noonan syndrome-like disorders, and for children with neurofibromatosis type 1. Mutations involving genes in the RAS pathway are most frequently involved. The presentation of JMML often mimics an infection, but hepatosplenomegaly is prominent in most cases from the onset.

10. What are the laboratory and morphologic findings of JMML?

- Leukocytosis with monocytosis, anemia, and thrombocytopenia. The 2017 WHO diagnostic criteria for JMML are listed in Table 25.8. Leukocytosis with absolute monocytosis ($\geq 1 \times 10^9$/L) is always present (Fig. 25.11a) [4, 91]. In one large cohort of JMML patients [9], the reported median WBC count was 33×10^9/L (ranging from 5 to 259 WBCs $\times 10^9$/L). Patients with monosomy 7, however, tend to have lower WBC counts than other JMML patients [92]. Anemia and thrombocytopenia are common. Nucleated RBCs and macrocytosis are frequently seen. Blasts (including promonocytes) are always less than 20% of the WBCs in the peripheral blood, and Auer rods are not seen.
- Myelodysplasia. Dysplastic granulocytes and atypical monocytes may be seen in the PB, but granulocytic dysplasia is usually not prominent (Fig. 25.11a). Dysgranulopoiesis with cytoplasmic hypogranulation and pseudo-Pelger-Huët changes can also be seen in the BM aspirate smears of JMML cases, but marked dysplasia is unusual in any of the myeloid lineages. Macrocytosis of the RBCs is commonly observed and reflects underlying megaloblastic erythropoiesis in the marrow, which, in JMML, is a manifestation of a shift toward fetal erythropoiesis [92–94]. Dysgranulopoiesis with cytoplasmic hypogranulation and pseudo-Pelger-Huët changes can be seen in the BM aspirate smears of JMML cases as well, but marked dysplasia is unusual in any of the myeloid lineages. Although megakaryocytes are often reduced in number, they are usually not markedly dysplastic.
- Increased fetal hemoglobin (HbF) and fetal erythropoiesis. JMML cases, especially those with a normal karyotype, characteristically show increased levels of fetal hemoglobin (HbF), which is due to the shift toward fetal-type erythropoiesis (Fig. 25.11a) [95].
- Cellular bone marrow (BM) with granulocytic and monocytic proliferation and myelodysplasia. The bone marrow findings in JMML are not, by themselves, entirely diagnostic. The BM core biopsy and aspirate smears are usually highly cellular with marked granulocytic proliferation (Fig. 25.11b), although occasionally there is very prominent erythroid proliferation. Megakaryocytes are often reduced in number. Monocytes in the BM are usually less prominent than in the PB. Blasts plus promonocytes are always <20% of all nucleated bone marrow cells, and Auer rods are not present [4, 91]. Mild dysplasia can be seen in one or more of the marrow lineages.
- Extramedullary involvement. Splenomegaly is a requirement for the diagnosis of JMML (Table 25.8). More than 90% of JMML patients initially present with splenomegaly, but virtually all patients develop splenomegaly within several weeks to months of the initial presentation [93]. The splenomegaly is due to leukemic infiltration, which also affects the liver, and hepatomegaly is not uncommon in JMML patients.
- Genetic abnormalities and gene mutations. Genetic and molecular findings are important for the diagnosis of JMML.
  - Cytogenetic abnormalities in bone marrow cells have been reported in 30–40% of patients with JMML; about 26% exhibit monosomy 7 [92].
  - Mutations in *NF1*, *NRAS*, *KRAS*, *PTPN11*, or *CBL*, which encode proteins important in activation of the RAS pathway, occur in 85% of JMML patients, and recurrent mutations are often seen in the genes involved in signal transduction, RNA splicing, the polycomb repressive complex 2 (PRC2), and transcriptional regulation [96, 97] (Table 25.3).
    - Importantly, one of the major diagnostic criteria for JMML includes the presence of one of the genetic/molecular findings of (1) somatic mutation in *PTPN11*, *KRAS*, or *NRAS*, (2) clinical diagnosis of neurofibromatosis type 1 or *NF1* mutation, or (3) germline *CBL* mutation and loss of heterozygosity (Table 25.8).

Table 25.8 The 2017 WHO diagnostic criteria for juvenile myelomonocytic leukemia (JMML)

Diagnostic criteria
Clinical and hematologic criteria (all four criteria are required):
Persistent PB monocytosis ($\geq 1 \times 10^9$ /L)
Blasts: <20% in the PB and BM
Splenomegaly
No Philadelphia (Ph) chromosome or *BCR-ABL1* fusion
Genetic criteria (any one criterion is sufficient):
Somatic mutation in *PTPN11*, *KRAS*, or *NRAS*[a]
Clinical diagnosis of neurofibromatosis type 1 or *NF1* mutation
Germline *CBL* mutation[b] and loss of heterozygosity[c]
Other criteria (cases that do not meet any of the genetic criteria above must meet the following criteria in addition to the clinical and hematologic criteria above):
Monosomy 7 or any other chromosomal abnormalities
or
≥2 of the following:
1. Increased hemoglobin F
2. Myeloid or erythroid precursors on the PB smears
3. Granulocyte-macrophage colony-stimulating factor (GM-CSF) hypersensitivity in colony assay
4. Hyperphosphorylation of STAT5

[a]If a mutation is found in *PTPN11*, *KRAS*, or *NRAS*, it is essential to consider that it might be a germline mutation and the diagnosis of transient abnormal myelopoiesis of Noonan syndrome must be considered
[b]A spontaneous remission is seen in some of the germline *CBL* mutation cases
[c]Occasional cases have heterozygous splice-site mutations

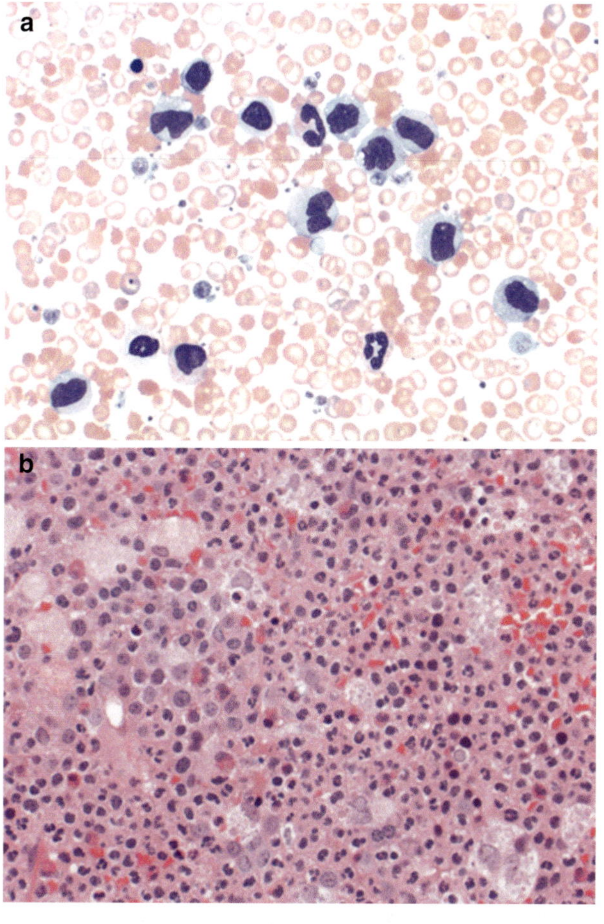

Fig. 25.11 The PB smear and the BM core biopsy of a patient with JMML. (**a**) The PB smear demonstrates rare circulating blasts/promonocytes, monocytosis, circulating nucleated erythrocytes, and dysplastic granulocytes. (**b**) The BM core biopsy shows a cellular bone marrow with marked granulocytic and monocytic proliferation. Occasional small megakaryocytes with hypolobated nuclei are seen

11. What are the mimics and differential diagnostic considerations for JMML?

The major differential considerations for JMML and the approaches to their recognition are outlined in Table 25.4 and discussed briefly below:

- Viral infections. Viral infections are commonly seen in the age group affected by JMML and may have clinical features and laboratory findings (marked monocytosis, anemia, and splenomegaly) similar to JMML.
  - Patients with viral infections may show an increased response to granulocyte-macrophage colony-stimulating factor (GM-CSF) or STAT5 in their *in vitro* colony-forming assays or hyperphosphorylation of STAT5 by flow cytometry, which is similar to that observed in JMML [98–101]. These features often pose a diagnostic challenge [93, 102, 103]. Furthermore, JMML may coexist with a viral infection [104], further contributing to the diagnostic difficulty.
  - The most common viral infections in the differential diagnosis of JMML include Epstein-Barr virus (*EBV*) (Fig. 25.12), cytomegalovirus (CMV), and human herpesvirus 6 (HHV-6) [105].
  - Approximately 85–90% of JMML cases have cytogenetic and/or molecular abnormalities, which are useful in differentiating JMML from viral infections as well as from other types of neoplasms. Identification of a congenital syndrome (e.g., neurofibromatosis-1, Noonan syndrome) or a JMML-associated cytogenetic and molecular abnormality is extremely helpful in differential diagnosis of such cases. A panel of molecular/

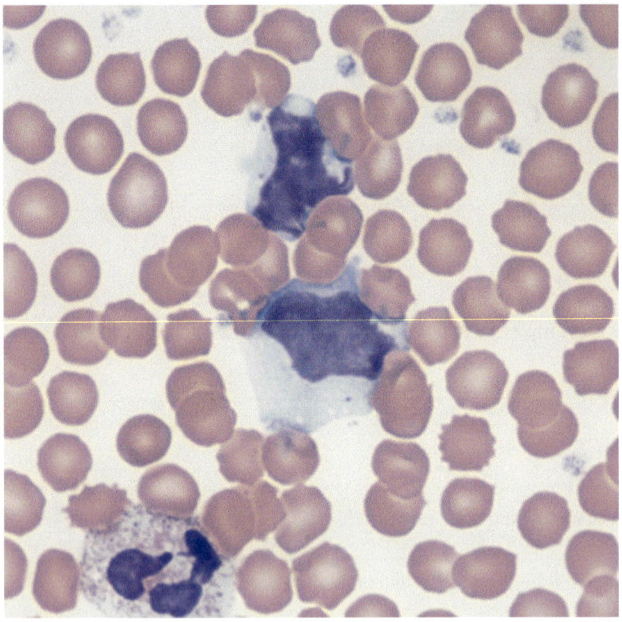

Fig. 25.12 Circulating reactive monocytoid T-lymphocytes in a patient with infectious mononucleosis

genetic tests has been proposed as a part of the mandatory work-up for diagnosis of JMML by an international consensus on the diagnostic criteria for JMML [103].

- Chronic myeloid leukemia (CML), *BCR-ABL1*-positive, and acute myeloid leukemia (AML). Although rare, CML, *BCR-ABL1+*, does occur in children, with clinical presentations similar to JMML, although often with much higher WBC counts. The demonstration of t(9;22)(q34;q11.2) and/or *BCR-ABL1* fusion by cytogenetic, FISH, or RT-PCR studies is sufficient to exclude JMML in such cases. A careful examination of the number of blasts and promonocytes is the key to differentiate JMML from AML. If blasts plus promonocytes are ≥20% in the PB or BM, the diagnosis is AML, not JMML. Cytochemical studies (for nonspecific esterase), immunohistochemistry, and flow cytometry may be useful in characterizing the immature cells in such cases.
- Transient JMML-like myeloproliferative disorder with Noonan syndrome (TMD-NS). Noonan syndrome (NS) is an autosomal dominant congenital disorder caused by genetic alterations that abnormally activate the RAS-MAPK signaling pathway. Infants with Noonan syndrome (NS) may have a transient JMML-like myeloproliferative disorder (TMD-NS) with spontaneous regression [106, 107]. Germline *PTPN11* mutations are identified in 50% of patients with NS, and somatic *PTPN11* mutations occur in 35% of the cases. Importantly, in the majority of patients with germline *PTPN11* mutations, the JMML-like hematologic abnormalities gradually resolve, but this process may take several years [108–110]. (See also Chap. 28, Case 14.)
- Transient myeloproliferative disorder of Down syndrome (TMD-DS). TMD-DS is seen in patients with Down syndrome, usually in the first several weeks of life. Patients with TMD-MDS usually present with leukocytosis, circulating blasts with megakaryocytic features, and hepatosplenomegaly. Cytogenetic analysis for trisomy 21 and molecular studies for *GATA1* mutation are extremely helpful in distinguishing JMML from TMD-DS, although overall, TMD-DS is more likely to be misdiagnosed as acute leukemia rather than JMML. (See also Chap. 28, Case 11.)
- *CBL* germline mutation and "CBL syndrome." The *CBL* gene encodes a member of the CBL family of proteins, which functions as an E3 ubiquitin ligase. A heterozygous germline *CBL* p.Y371H substitution is found in ~15% of JMML cases [111] (Table 25.3). These children have germline *CBL* mutations and develop JMML because they are at increased risk of developing loss of heterozygosity (LOH) for the *CBL* locus in hematopoietic stem/progenitor cells.
  - All children with JMML and *CBL* mutations reportedly have germline CBL missense mutation on one allele and acquired LOH on the other allele in leukemic cells [103]. These patients may display a variable combination of dysmorphic features, hyperpigmented skin lesions, and microcephaly, i.e., so-called CBL syndrome; patients with "CBL syndrome" have a predisposition to JMML [111–113].
  - Compared with *CBL* wild-type JMML, JMML patients with the germline *CBL* mutation show earlier presentation and lower hemoglobin F levels and may have spontaneous remission [114–116].
- Wiskott-Aldrich syndrome (WAS). WAS is a rare, recessive X-linked disease that is caused by mutations in WASP gene at chromosome Xp11.23. Clinically, WAS is characterized by the triad of recurrent bacterial sinopulmonary infections, eczema, and a bleeding diathesis caused by thrombocytopenia and platelet dysfunction [117]. Children with WAS exhibit thrombocytopenia, leukocytosis, monocytosis in the PB, and hypercellular BM with dysplasia as well as hypersensitivity to G/M CSF by in vitro culture, which is similar to JMML [118].
  - No splenomegaly or mutations in the *PTPN11*, *RAS*, and *CBL* genes or clinical features of neurofibromatosis type 1 are detected in patients with WAS [119]. Flow-cytometry analysis of WASP protein expression is a useful screening tool in all cases of suspected WAS. For the definite diagnosis of WAS, sequencing of the *WASP* gene is required. (See also Chap. 28, Case 9.)

- Malignant infantile osteopetrosis (MIOP). MIOP is a rare infantile autosomal recessive (AR) severe disorder of osteoclast development and/or function. Children with MIOP present with severe symptoms soon after birth or within the first years of life, including abnormal bone remodeling with a characteristic macrocephaly with frontal bossing, exophthalmus, bone fractures, and failure to thrive. Patients with MIOP have hematologic abnormalities with bone marrow failure and extramedullary hematopoiesis. Clinical and laboratory manifestations of MIOP include anemia, thrombocytopenia, leukocytosis, hepatosplenomegaly, and hypersensitivity to G/M CSF [105, 120].
  - In contrast to JMML, MIOP has characteristic bony lesions, elevation of alkaline phosphatase, and hypogammaglobulinemia. Skeletal findings in radiography are essentially diagnostic for MIOP. Morphologic evaluation of the bone core biopsies and marrow aspirate smears from suspected patients and genetic sequencing for mutations in *TCIRG1*, *OSTM1*, *ClCN7*, and *TNFRSF11A* genes are helpful in the diagnosis [121].
- Histiocytic and Langerhans cell disorders. Langerhans cell histiocytosis (LCH), Rosai-Dorfman disease (RDD), juvenile xanthogranuloma (JXG), and Erdheim-Chester disease (ECD) are not uncommon in children, and they can involve multiple organs [122].
  - Langerhans cell histiocytosis (LCH) can exhibit leukocytosis, monocytosis, anemia, and hepatosplenomegaly [123]. Germline *NF1* and *NF2* mutations associated with JMML have been reported in children with JXG [124–126].
  - ECD is histopathologically characterized by an infiltration of predominantly lipid-laden histiocytes/macrophages, multinucleated giant cells, and some lymphocytes in the BM as well as a generalized sclerosis of the long bones. Patients with ECD characteristically have symmetrical long bone involvement, cardiovascular infiltration, kidney and/or liver failure, and retroperitoneal fibrosis [127]. More than one-half of ECD patients carry the *BRAF-V600E* mutation or recurrent mutations in the genes involving the MAP kinase and PI3K pathways [122, 128].
  - A careful morphologic evaluation, along with carefully designed panels of immunohistochemical stains, such as CD34, NPM1, CD68, CD1a, S100, Langerin, and CD163, is the key to distinguish JMML from such disorders. Cytogenetic and molecular studies for gene mutations, particularly *BRAF-V600E*, *NRAS*, and *NPM1* mutations, may also aid in differentiating those disorders from JMML.
- Lymphoblastic leukemia, lymphoma, and hemophagocytic lymphohistiocytosis (HLH). In addition to JMML, Noonan syndrome (NS) or RASopathy is associated with other malignancies including B- and T-cell lymphoblastic leukemia, Hodgkin lymphoma, and neuroblastoma [129–132]. JMML can be concurrently present with a B-cell lymphoblastic leukemia [133–137] or a T-cell lymphoblastic leukemia [138, 139]. Lymphoblastic leukemia can be a manifestation of a lymphoid blast crisis of JMML or develop after complete remission of JMML [140]. Hemophagocytic lymphohistiocytosis (HLH) [141] and Hodgkin lymphoma [142] have also been reported concurrently with JMML.

12. What work-up provides prognostic information for JMML?

Both the clinical and molecular characteristics of JMML contribute to the prognosis of a patient with JMML [102]. The following factors have been reported to have a negative impact on the OS or LFS of JMML [92, 112, 114, 143–145]: (1) blast count (> 5% in the BM); (2) older age >2 years; (3) increased fetal hemoglobin (HbF) $\geq$10%; (4) platelet count (<33 × 10^9 /L at diagnosis); (5) female sex; and (6) *SETBP1* and *JAK3* mutations were reported to be associated with poor clinical outcomes [146, 147].

13. What work-up provides therapeutic targets and clinical management information for JMML?

- Gene mutations and targeted therapy: The common recurrent mutations in JMML are listed in Table 25.3. Clinical trials that target specific genes or molecular pathways are listed in Table 25.6. These genetic alterations may provide useful prognostic indicators and therapeutic targets for JMML [148, 149]. However, a recent clinical trial with the farnesyl transferase inhibitor (RAS pathway inhibitor) tipifarnib as pre-transplant therapy in patients with JMML showed no overall survival benefit in those patients who received tipifarnib [150].
- Clinical management of JMML: Immediate allogeneic HSCT is recommended for most of children with JMML, especially those associated with *NF1* mutation and somatic *PTPN11* and *KRAS* mutations, and for most children with somatic *NRAS* mutations. Close observation without immediate allogeneic HSCT is warranted for JMML patients who also have (i) germline *CBL* mutation;

(ii) Noonan syndrome; and (iii) acquired *RAS* mutations, with normal hemoglobin F and higher platelet counts [103, 145]. These JMML patients may have a long-term remission without HSCT. A high platelet count and low HbF in these patients predict a more indolent course in such patients, warranting close observation without immediate HSCT.

MDS/MPN with Ring Sideroblasts and Thrombocytosis (MDS/MPN-RS-T)

This disorder is characterized by the concomitant presence of myelodysplasia in the erythroid lineage, characterized by ring sideroblasts, and by megakaryocytes that not only have myeloproliferative morphology but also are effective in producing platelets. There is a strong association with mutated *SF3B1*, which may be concurrent with mutated *JAK2*, *CALR*, or *MPL* W515 mutations. Although in general, a history of a previous MPN or MDS (except MDS with ring sideroblasts) excludes the diagnosis of MDS/MPN-RS-T, the possibility that the disorder began as an MPN but then acquired an *SF3B1* mutation and ring sideroblasts may not always be easily excluded.

14. What are the laboratory and morphologic findings of MDS/MPN-RS-T?

- Persistent thrombocytosis. The 2017 WHO diagnostic criteria for MDS/MPN-RS-T are listed in Table 25.9. Thrombocytosis (platelet count ≥450/μL) is the major diagnostic criterion and always present in MDS/MPN-RS-T cases (Fig. 25.13a).
- Anemia. Normocytic anemia is typically present in the PB, and the WBC is usually normal or mildly elevated (Fig. 25.13a) [151].
- No increased blasts in the PB or BM. A major diagnostic criteria is <1% blasts in the PB and <5% blasts in the BM (Table 25.9).
- Hypercellular BM with increased erythropoiesis and megakaryopoiesis. A decreased or reversed M:E ratio is usually seen due to increased (but ineffective) erythropoiesis. Megakaryocyte proliferation is present in all cases, with focal clustering. Megakaryocytes are variable in size and morphology but are often large with hypersegmented nuclear lobes (Fig. 25.13b).
- Dyserythropoiesis with increased ring sideroblasts. Dyserythropoiesis is similar to that of MDS with ring sideroblasts (MDS-RS), and multilineage dysplasia may be seen as well. Iron stains on the BM aspirate smears show ≥15% RS of the erythroid precursors (Fig. 25.13c). It is important to realize that ring sideroblasts are difficult to visualize in iron stains performed on biopsy sections. Furthermore, decalcification procedures generally remove iron from the biopsy, further complicating interpretation of iron stains in routinely processed biopsies.
- Cytogenetic abnormalities and gene mutations. Cytogenetic abnormalities are uncommon (~10%) in MDS/MPN-RS-T [151, 152]. However, cases of MDS/MPN-RS-T frequently have gene mutations in *SF3B1* (~85%) and *JAK2* V617F (~50%) and less frequently in other genes, such as *CALR* and *MPL* (Table 25.3). An *SF3B1* mutation together with a *JAK2 V617F*, *CALR*, or *MPL* mutation strongly supports the diagnosis.

15. What are the mimics and differential considerations for MDS/MPN-RS-T?

Both MDS/MPN-RS-T and MDS-RS have RS ≥15% of the erythroid precursors, but MDS/MPN-RS-T additionally has thrombocytosis (platelets ≥ 450/μL). MDS/MPN-RS-T and MDS-RS also need to be distinguished from non-clonal conditions associated with RS, which include

Table 25.9 The 2017 WHO diagnostic criteria for myelodysplastic/myeloproliferative neoplasm with ring sideroblasts and thrombocytosis (MDS/MPN-RS-T)

Diagnostic criteria
1. Anemia associated with dyserythropoiesis, with or without multilineage dysplasia; ≥15% ring sideroblasts[a]
2. Persistent thrombocytosis with platelet count ≥450 × 10^9/L
3. <1% blasts in the PB and <5% blasts in the BM
4. *SF3B1* mutation or, in the absence of *SF3B1* mutation, no history of recent cytotoxic or growth factor therapy that could explain the MDS/MPN features[b]
5. No *BCR-ABL1* or *PCM1-JAK2* fusions; no rearrangements of *PDGFRA*, *PDGFRB*, or *FGFR1*; and no t(3;3)(q21;q26), inv(3)(q21q26), or del(5q)[c]
6. No history of MPN, MDS (except MDS with ring sideroblasts), or other MDS/MPN

[a]≥15% ring sideroblasts is a required criterion even if *SF3B1* mutation is detected
[b]The diagnosis of MDS/MPN-RS-T is strongly supported by the presence of *SF3B1* mutation together with a *JAK2 V617F*, *CALR*, or *MPL* mutation
[c]In a case that otherwise meets the diagnostic criteria for MDS with isolated del(5q)

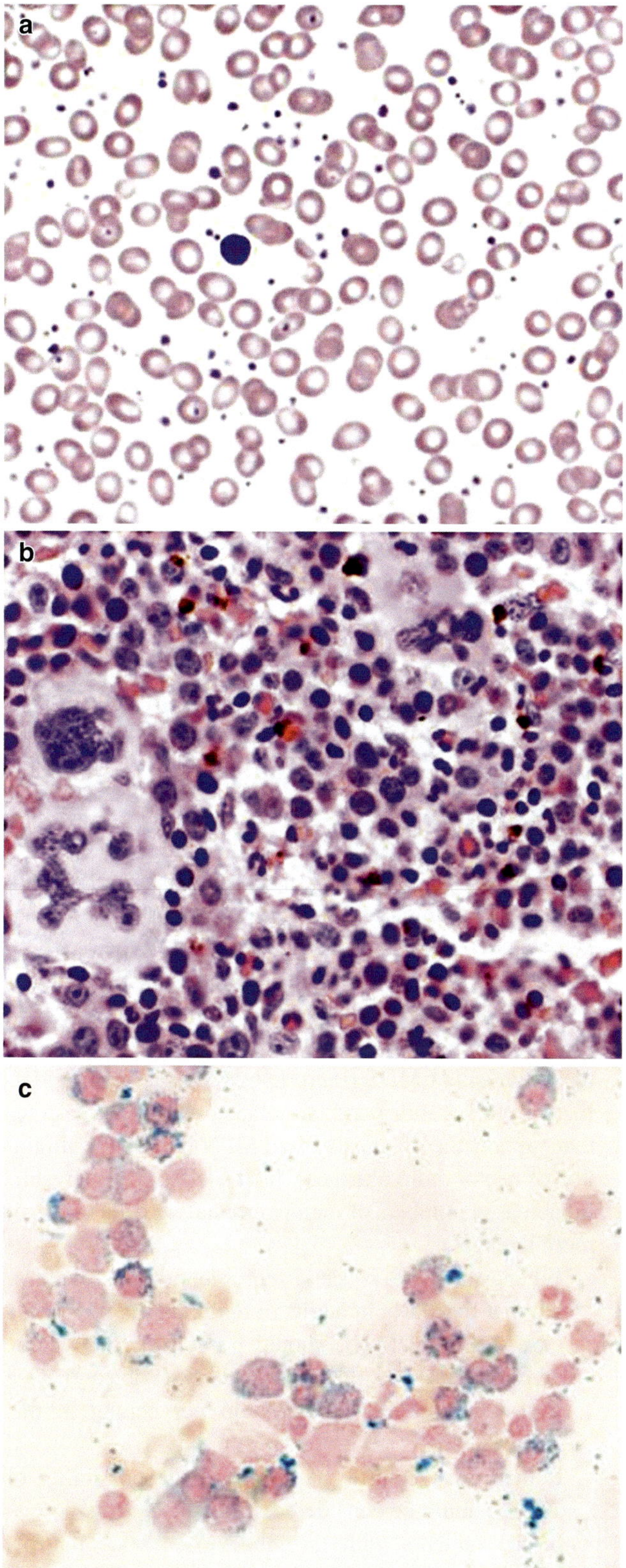

Fig. 25.13 The PB smear and the BM core biopsy of a patient with MDS/MPN-RS-T. (**a**) The PB shows macrocytic anemia with hypochromic red blood cells and marked increase in platelets with platelet anisocytosis. (**b**) The BM core shows a hypercellular bone marrow with marked megakaryocytic and erythroid proliferation, and dyserythropoiesis. (**c**) An iron stain demonstrates numerous ring sideroblasts

excess alcohol use, lead toxicity, copper or pyridoxine deficiency, isoniazid therapy, and congenital sideroblastic anemias (CSA).

16. What work-up provides prognostic information for MDS/MPN-RS-T?

Patients with MDS/MPN-RS-T have a median overall survival (OS) of 76 months, and the median OS for MDS-RS-SLD and ET is 63 months and 117 months, respectively [153]. The following factors have been reported to have an adverse effect on the prognosis of MDS/MPN-RS-T [151, 154]:

- Anemia (Hb < 10 g/dL).
- Abnormal karyotype.
- Mutational status. Mutations in *SETBP1* or *ASXL1* are independently prognostic for inferior survival.

17. What work-up provides therapeutic targets and clinical management information for MDS/MPN-RS-T?

- Gene mutations and targeted therapy. The common recurrent mutations in MDS/MPN-RS-T are listed in Table 25.3. Clinical trials that target specific genes or molecular pathways are listed in Table 25.6. The high frequency of mutations in the genes involving tyrosine kinase pathway provides promising therapeutic interventions using tyrosine kinase inhibitors, such as ruxolitinib, in patients with MDS/MPN-RS-T.
- Clinical management of MDS/MPN-RS-T. No formal guidelines have been established for the management of MDS/MPN-RS-T [151]. Patients with MDS/MPN-RS-T have a higher incidence of thrombosis and often require antiplatelet and/or cytoreductive therapy. However, cytoreductive therapy may exacerbate anemia, which is the most frequent disease manifestation of MDS/MPN-RS-T [151]. Hydroxyurea, lenalidomide, interferon alpha, and busulfan have been reported to be effective in some patients with MDS/MPN-RS-T [151, 155–157].

Myelodysplastic/Myeloproliferative Neoplasms, Unclassifiable (MDS/MPN-U)

Patients who fall into this category have, at the time of initial presentation, some clinical, morphologic, and laboratory features that are most consistent with MDS and others that are more consistent with an MPN, yet do not meet the criteria for any of the other MDS/MPN categories. The following cases should NOT be included in this category:

Table 25.10 The 2017 WHO diagnostic criteria for myelodysplastic/myeloproliferative neoplasm, unclassifiable (MDS/MPN-U)

Myeloid neoplasms with mixed features of MPN and MDS at onset, not meeting the following WHO criteria for any other MDS/MPN, MDS, or MPN
1. <20% blasts in the PB and BM
2. Clinical and morphologic features of one of the categories of MDS[a]
3. Clinical and morphological MPN features manifested as a platelet count of ≥450 × 10^9/L associated with megakaryocytic proliferation in the BM and/or a WBC ≥13 × 10^9/L in the PB
4. No recent cytotoxic or growth factor therapy that could explain the MDS/MPN features
5. No *BCR-ABL1* or *PCM1-JAK2* fusions, no rearrangements of *PDGFRA*, *PDGFRB*, or *FGFR1*

[a]Cases that meet criteria for MDS with isolated de(5q) are excluded irrespective of the presence of thrombocytosis or leukocytosis

- Patients with a previously documented MPN, who later develop MDS-like features.
- Cases with features of MDS/MPN who have history of prior chemo- and/or radiation therapy should be classified in the therapy-related myeloid neoplasm category [1–4].

18. What are the laboratory and morphologic findings of MDS/MPN-U?

- Laboratory and morphologic features. The 2017 WHO diagnostic criteria for MDS/MPN-U are listed in Table 25.10. MDS/MPN-U cases have, at the time of initial presentation, some clinical and morphologic features of one of the categories of MDS but also manifest some clinical and morphological MPN features, such as thrombocytosis (platelet count of ≥450 × 10^9/L) and/or a WBC ≥13 × 10^9/L in the PB. MDS/MPN-U may have MPN-like megakaryocytic proliferation in the BM, but does not meet the criteria for any of the other MDS/MPN categories described above.
- Cytogenetic abnormalities and gene mutations. A recent study showed no statistically significant difference in cytogenetics (karyotyping) findings between aCML and MDS/MPN-U. However, MDS/MPN-U appeared to have more *JAK2* p.V617F (7% vs. 19%) and less *RAS* (35% vs. 14%) than aCML [72]. *SETBP1* mutations were reported to be present more frequently in aCML than MDS/MPN-U (30% vs. 95%) and tend to be associated with monosomy 7, i(17)(q10), *ASXL1*, and *CBL* mutations in aCML cases [84].

19. What work-up provides therapeutic targets and clinical management information for MDS/MPN-U?

- Gene mutations and targeted therapy. There are no specific cytogenetic or molecular abnormalities for MDS/MPN-U [84]. Currently, little information is available about clinical trials for patients with MDS/MPN-U [151, 155–157].
- Clinical management of MDS/MPN-U. No formal guidelines have been established for the management of patients with MDS/MPN-U. The paucity of clinical treatment available secondary to unclear pathogenesis and rarity of these diseases makes the management of these entities clinically challenging [151].

20. Which morphological and laboratory findings in the PB/BM aspirate/biopsy are reliably diagnostic for MDS/MPN? Which ones suggest the diagnosis? Which is (are) unreliable for diagnosis? Which findings rule out the diagnosis?

- Findings diagnostic or suggestive of MDS/MPN: Table 25.11 summarizes the clinical, morphological, and cytogenetic/molecular features of each subtype of MDS/MPN. As noted in the introductory paragraphs, the diagnosis of MDS/MPN is suggested whenever there are, at the time of initial diagnosis, some features that support the diagnosis of MDS (morphologic dysplasia with ineffective proliferation) and, simultaneously, other features that support the diagnosis of an MPN (marked proliferation of one or more lineages which is effective and results in increased numbers of mature circulating cells in one or more lineages).
  - Whenever there is persistent monocytosis with or without dysplasia in adults or children, the possibility of CMML or JMML should be considered. On the other hand, cases that have clearly evolved from a well-defined MDS or MPN do not belong in this category.
  - If there is dysplastic neutrophilia, the possibility of aCML should be considered.
  - In the patients with thrombocytosis, bone marrow biopsies and iron stains should be performed to evaluate the possible diagnosis of MDS/MPN-RS-T. See the above sections and the summary Table 25.11 as well as Tables 25.1, 25.7, 25.8, 25.9, and 25.10 for the 2017 WHO diagnostic criteria for CMML, aCML, JMML, MDS/MPN-RS-T, and MDS/MPN-U, respectively.

Table 25.11 Summary of the clinical, morphological, and cytogenetic/molecular features of MDS/MPN

	Clinical Findings	Findings excluding MDS/MPN	Disease entities	Findings in the peripheral blood (PB)		Findings in the bone marrow (BM)		Cytogenetic/ Molecular findings
MDS/ MPN	Symptoms (fatigue, weakness, short of breath) related to anemia.		CMML	Persistent monocytosis (≥1 × 10^9/L; monocytes ≥10% of the leukocytes)	Dysplasia in 1 or more myeloid lineages	Hypercellular BM with prominent granulocytic proliferation (↑M:E). ↑ monocyte count	Dysplasia in 1 or more myeloid lineages	Cytogenetic abnormalities in ~40–50% of cases, most frequently +8, −Y, −7, del(7q), +21, and del(20q). Gene mutations in ~60% of cases, most frequently *TET2, SRSF2, ASXL1* and *SETBP1.*
	Infections related to abnormal WBC counts and/or function. Easy bruising or bleeding related to abnormal platelet counts or platelet function.	Exclusive findings: ≥20% blasts in the PB or BM.	aCML	Neutrophilic leukocytosis (≥13 × 10^9/L; neutrophilic precursors ≥10% of the leukocytes); No or minimal absolute basophilia or monocytosis (basophils and monocytes constitute <2% and <10% of the leukocytes, respectively).	Granulocytic dysplasia-major diagnostic criterion	Hypercellular BM with prominent granulocytic proliferation (↑ M:E ratio)	Marked granulocytic dysplasia with or without erythroid and megakaryocytic dysplasia	Cyto genetic abnormalities in ~50–65% of cases, most frequently +8 and del(20q), but monosomy 7, del(12p), deletions of 5q, 13q, 17p, 12q, and 11q, and t(6;8)(p23;q22) are seen as well. Gene mutations in ~50–65% of cases include high frequency (>20%) mutations in *SETBP1, ASXL1, N/K-RAS, SRSF2,* and *TET2* and low frequency (<10%) mutations in *CBL, CSF3R, JAK2,* and *ETNK1.*
	Splenomegaly and/or hepatosplenomegaly is common	Presence of *BCR-ABL1 or PCM1- JAK2* fusions. Presence of rearrangements of *PDGFRA, PDGFRB,* or *FGFR1.*	JMML	Persistent PB monocytosis (≥1 × 10^9 /L)-major diagnostic criterion; Increased hemoglobin F and circulating myeloid or erythroid precursors	GM-CSF hypersensitivity; Hyperphosphorylation of STAT5; Granulocytic dysplasia	Cellular BM with granulocytic and monocytic proliferation.	Dysplasia in 1 or more myeloid lineages (usually mild)	Cytogenetic abnormalities in ~30–40% of cases, Most frequently monosomy 7. Mutations in *NF1, NRAS, KRAS, PTPN1 1* or *CBL,* in 85% of all cases
	Splenomegaly is a required diagnostic criterion for JMML.		MDS/ MPN-RS-T	Anemia (Hb < 10 g/dL). MDS/M Persistent thrombocytosis (≥450 × 10^9/L). <1% circulating blasts.		Hypercellular BM with increased erythropoiesis and megakaryopoiesis; <5% blasts in the BM	Dyserythropoiesis, with or without multilineage dysplasia; ≥15% ring sideroblasts	Cytogenetic abnormalities are uncommon (~10%); Mutational analysis (recommended): Frequent gene mutations in *SF3B1* (~85%) and *JAK2 V617F* (~50%), and less frequent mutations in other genes, such as *CALR* and *MPL.*
	Clinical diagnosis of neurofibromatosis type 1 is an additional diagnostic criterion for JMML.		MDS/ MPN-U	Having some clinical and morphologic findings of one of the categories of MDS, but also manifest some clinical and morphological MPN features. However, these findings do not meet the criteria for any of the other MDS/MPN categories described above. May have thrombocytosis (platelet count of ≥450 × 10^9/L) and/or a WBC ≥13 × 10^9/L,at the time of initial diagnosis May have a hypercellular BM with MPN-like megakaryocytic proliferation				Cytogenetic abnormalities similar to those in aCML, but have have more *JAK2p.V617F* (7% vs 19%) and less *RAS* (35% vs 14%) than aCML

- Findings which warrant extra caution before making a definite diagnosis of MDS/MPN:
  - Monocytosis in patients with previously diagnosed MPN or MDS. Monocytosis has been reported in up to 15% of patients with PMF [37]. The presence of morphological features of MPN in the BM and/or MPN-associated mutations in *JAK2*, *CALR*, or *MPL* tends to support MPN with monocytosis rather than CMML in such cases. On the other hand, patients with MDS may develop monocytosis after chemotherapy or other treatments, and in such cases, a diagnosis of CMML should also be avoided.
  - Recent chemotherapy or G-CSF treatment, infections or autoimmune diseases.
  - Cases with peripheral blood and/or bone marrow monocytosis, but no definite myelodysplasia. In such cases, ancillary studies such as cytogenetic studies may support a diagnosis of CMML, but if there is no convincing evidence for a neoplastic process, a diagnosis of CMML should be deferred, and the patients observed for a period of time (>3 months) to exclude reactive monocytosis.
  - Rare cases with prominent dysplasia and monocytosis in the BM, but no peripheral monocytosis (monocyte count $<1 \times 10^9$/L) in the PB. Such cases have been reported to share clinical and molecular characteristics with CMML [40]. Repeating CBC and differential counts is warranted before making a definite diagnosis of MDS or CMML in such patients.
- Morphological and laboratory findings which exclude diagnosis of MDS/MPN:
  - Blasts constitute ≥20% of the cells in the PB or BM.
  - Molecular/cytogenetic studies that demonstrate the presence of *BCR-ABL1* or *PCM1-JAK2* fusion genes or rearrangements of *PDGFRA*, *PDGFRB*, and *FGFR1*.

21. What is the minimal and optimal ancillary work-up for diagnosis and subclassification of the different categories of MDS/MPN?

The diagnostic steps for CMML, aCML, and MDS/MPN-RS-T are schematically illustrated in Fig. 25.14. Steps 1 through 4 are mandatory for the initial diagnosis of all MDS/MPN cases, and steps 5–6 are highly recommended in all adult MDS/MPN cases. Of note, genetic analysis of somatic and germline mutations plays a critical role in diagnosis and prognosis of JMML and constitutes a mandatory diagnostic procedure (Fig. 25.15).

22. What is an appropriate practical approach for diagnosis of MDS/MPN? When is a diagnostic comment necessary, and what should be discussed in the diagnostic comment for this entity? When is it appropriate to seek external consultation for this entity?

- Diagnostic approach for MDS/MPN: We recommend an integrated approach based on clinical information and morphology as schematically illustrated in Figs. 25.14 and 25.15. The importance of comprehensive clinical history and careful examination of the hematologic parameters and the morphology of the PB and marrow cells in the initial diagnostic work-up for MDS/MPN cannot be overemphasized. It is also important to follow the 2017 WHO diagnostic guidelines [4] carefully for the diagnosis and classification of suspected MDS/MPN cases at the first encounter, as these findings can change with time and/ or prior treatment.
- Diagnostic comments and external consultation: In the following situations, a definite diagnosis and classification of MDS/MPN may be deferred, and external consultation is recommended.
  - Unable to perform or obtain good-quality BM aspirates, informative stains, or necessary cytogenetic/molecular studies.
  - Uncertain about the definite diagnosis or classification of MDS/MPN cases, especially suspected JMML cases. JMML often has a more rapid clinical course compared to CMML. Moreover, numerous conditions, including viral infections, congenital syndromes/disorders, and other malignancies, can mimic JMML. Consequently, it is often challenging to diagnose JMML at early stage in clinical settings. We recommend seeking an external consultation whenever there is difficulty in making a diagnosis of JMML or any other MDS/MPN, particularly, for those cases that lack genetic and molecular abnormalities or evidence of neurofibromatosis. Furthermore, the diagnostic report should carefully define the characteristics of the disease, the reasons that a definitive diagnosis cannot be made, and the steps for further evaluation of the patient.

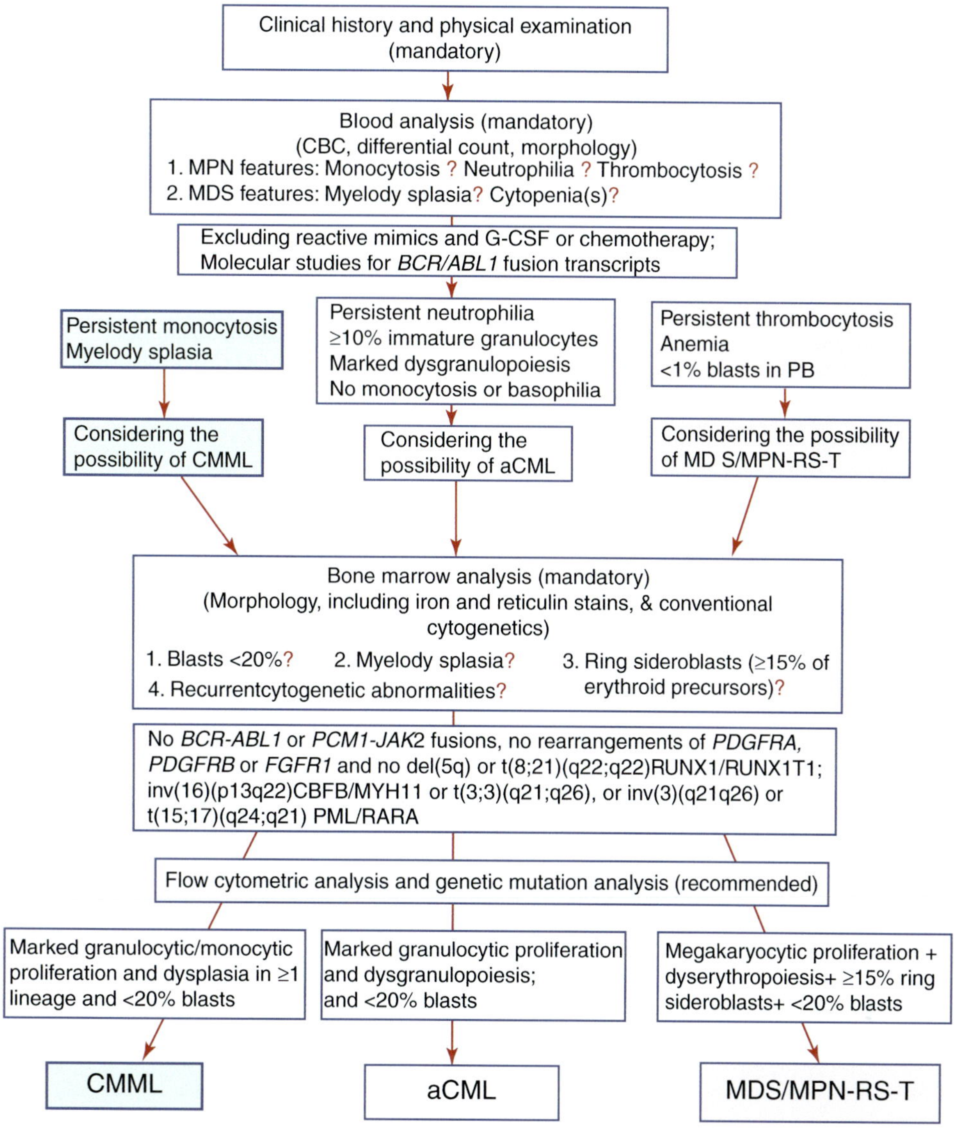

Fig. 25.14 A morphology and clinical data-based integrated diagnostic algorithm for myelodysplastic/myeloproliferative neoplasms (MDS/MPN)

- Discrepancies between morphologic findings and molecular or cytogenetic findings.
- Concurrence with reactive conditions, congenital syndromes/disorders, or other malignancies.

Case Presentations

We will use three clinical cases to illustrate some challenges in diagnosis of MDS and MDS/MPN in the era of molecular testing and a practical approach to the correct diagnosis and classification of MDS/MPN.

Case 1

Learning Objectives

1. Illustrate the clinical challenges and considerations in differential diagnosis of reactive (secondary) monocytosis, MDS, CMML (dysplastic type), and other hematologic malignancies.
2. Introduce an integrative and practical approach to (evolving) CMML or undetermined monocytosis.
3. Emphasize on the importance of morphologic evaluation and integration of immunohistochemical, flow cytometric, and cytogenetic/molecular studies, as well as clinical information.

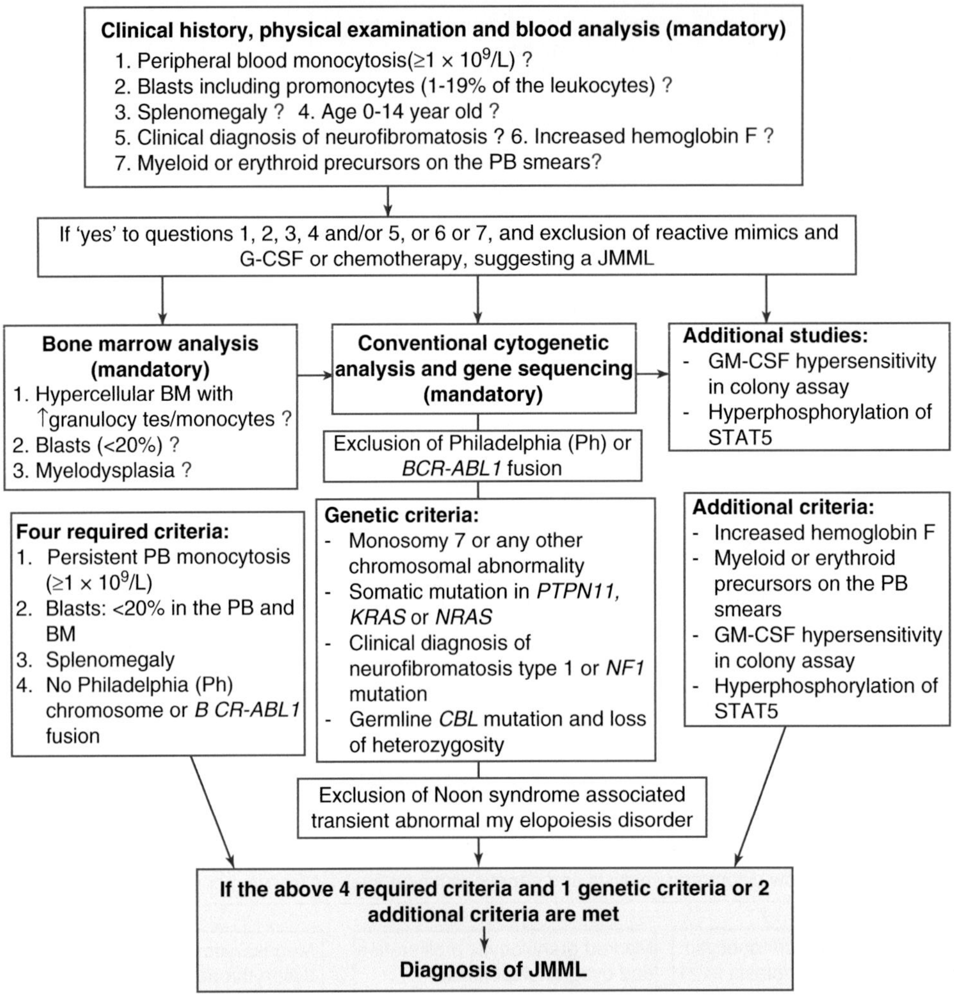

Fig. 25.15 An integrated diagnostic algorithm for juvenile myelomonocytic leukemia (JMML)

Case History

A 60-year-old man with pancytopenia underwent a bone marrow biopsy. His iron and B12 levels were within the normal range. The patient had a history of ulcerative granulomatous lymphoid infiltrate with monoclonal *TCR* gene rearrangements in his GI biopsy. His physical examination was normal. No palpable lymphadenopathy or hepatosplenomegaly was appreciated.

Histologic Findings

- His complete blood cell count (CBC) showed white blood cell (WBC) count 2.6×10^9/L, hemoglobin (HGB) 11.0 g/dL, MCV 103 fL, and platelet count (PLT) 160×10^9/L.
- The differential count of the PB showed 18% neutrophils, 1% eosinophils, 45% lymphocytes, and 36% monocytes. His PB smear showed no blasts, and there was relative, but not absolute, monocytosis (36%, 0.94×10^9/L) (Fig. 25.16a). The neutrophils showed significant dysplasia with cytoplasmic hypogranularity, aberrant nuclear segmentation, and abnormal chromatin patterns (Fig. 25.16b).
- His BM core biopsy showed hypercellular (~60%) BM with myelomonocytic expansion, and no atypical lymphoid aggregates or infiltrate was seen (Fig. 25.17a).
- The BM aspirate smears showed moderate dyserythropoiesis and dysmegakaryopoiesis and mild dysgranulopoiesis (Fig. 25.17b).
- The differential count of the BM aspirate smears showed 1.8% blasts, 1.7% promyelocytes, 33.4% myelocytes, 11.8% bands, 9.4% segmented neutrophils, 1.4% eosinophils, 0.2% basophils, 7.4% lymphocytes, 2.4% plasma cells, 12% monocytes, and 18.5% erythroid precursors.

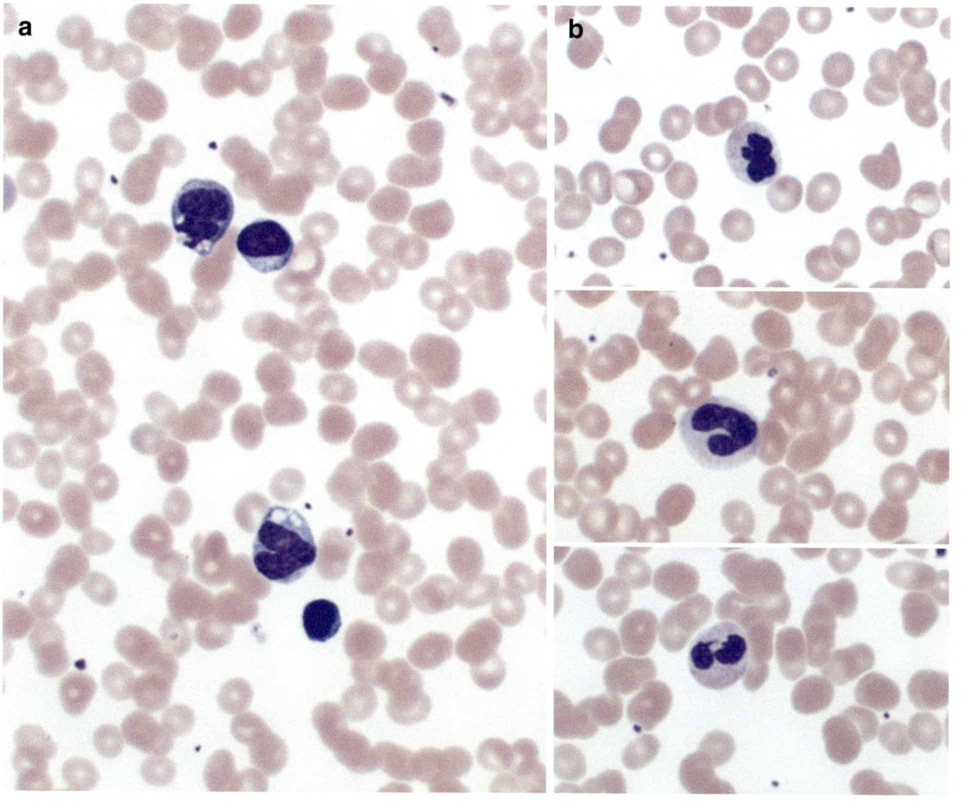

Fig. 25.16 Case presentation #1, peripheral blood (PB) smear. (**a**) The PB shows anemia and relative monocytosis. (**b**) Dysplastic neutrophils in the PB smear

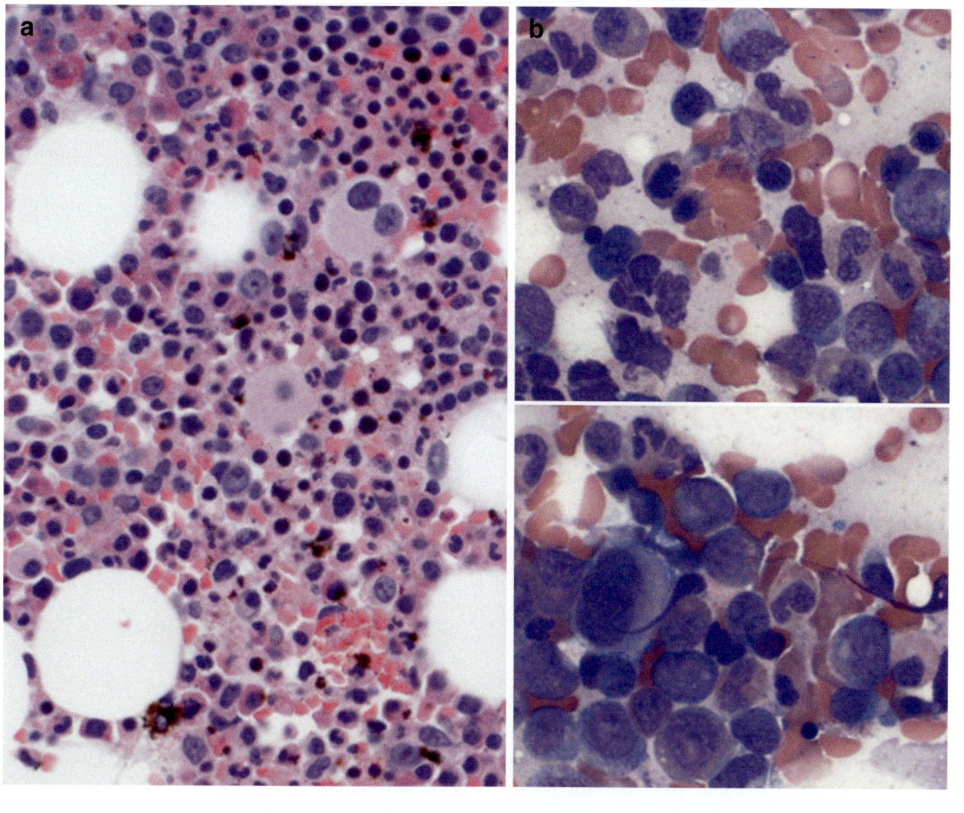

Fig. 25.17 Case presentation #1, bone marrow (BM) core biopsy and aspirate smears. (**a**) The BM biopsy shows a hypercellular BM with granulocytic proliferation and increased M:E ratio. (**b**) The BM aspirate smear shows multilineage dysplasia and increased granulocytes and monocytes

Other Ancillary Studies

- The immunohistochemical studies on the BM core showed ~2% CD34+ cells (Fig. 25.18a). CD61 stain highlighted occasional small hypolobated (dysplastic) megakaryocytes (Fig. 25.18b). CD3 and CD20 stains showed scattered T-cells and B-cells, respectively (Fig. 25.18c, d).
- Flow cytometric analysis of the BM aspirate showed no increase in blasts. No monoclonal B-cells or T-cells with an aberrant phenotype were detected.
- Cytogenetic studies revealed a normal karyotype.
- FISH studies with a MDS panel (for abnormalities/deletions of 5, 7, 5q or 7q, +8, 20q-, or 11q23) were negative.

Differential Diagnosis

Based on the clinical history and the morphologic findings in the PB and the BM, the diagnostic considerations include:

- Bone marrow involvement by the previously diagnosed T-cell lymphoproliferative disorder
- MDS with multilineage dysplasia (MDS-MLD)
- (Evolving) CMML

The morphology of the bone marrow biopsy and the negative immunohistochemical and flow cytometric findings could help quickly exclude the possibility of bone

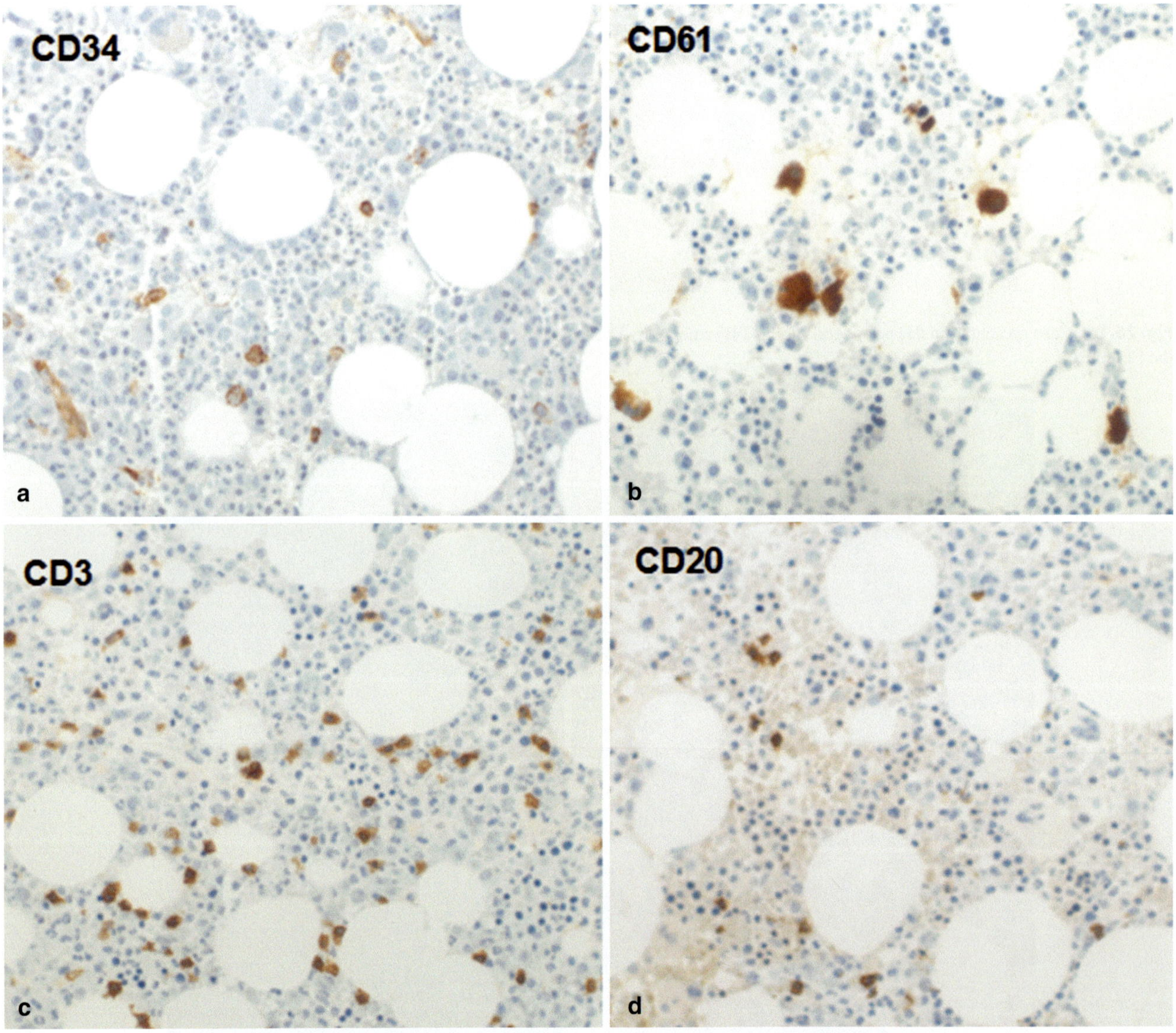

Fig. 25.18 Case presentation #1, immunohistochemical stains performed on the bone marrow (BM) core biopsy. (**a**) CD34 immunostain shows no increase in CD34+ blasts. (**b**) CD61 immunostain shows small hypolobated (dysplastic) megakaryocytes. (**c**) CD3 immunostain shows occasional scattered T-cells. (**d**) CD20 immunostain shows rare scattered B-cells

marrow involvement by a T-cell proliferative disorder. Although the morphologic findings would fulfill the WHO diagnostic criteria [4] for MDS-MLD, the levels of monocytes in the PB and the BM caused a concern for (evolving) CMML. However, the minimal level of the monocytes in the BM to confirm the diagnosis of CMML has never been established [1, 7]. The peripheral monocyte count did not meet the minimal requirement (≥1000/uL) for CMML. We thought that it was prudent to defer a definite diagnosis and to follow up for CBC and differential count for a period of time.

Final Diagnosis

In the following month, the absolute monocyte count was increased to 1200/uL, and a definite diagnosis of CMML was made. Meanwhile next-generation sequencing (NGS) reported a *TET2* mutation (c.1924C > T, p.Q642).

Take-Home Messages

1. Carefully following the WHO 2017 diagnostic guidelines and the integrative approach (Fig. 25.14) to make a diagnosis of CMML or other MDS and MDS/MPN.
2. Morphology remains a cornerstone in the diagnosis of MDS and MDS/MPN.
3. In the cases of possible evolving CMML or having difficulties to differentiate CMML from reactive monocytosis, it is prudent to defer a definite diagnosis and to follow up for CBC and differentiate count and morphological evaluation for a period of time.
4. *TET2* mutation is seen in about one half of CMML cases with a normal karyotype. However, it is also seen in MDS and normal aging process, and hence cannot be used as a diagnostic criterion of CMML per se.

Case 2

Learning Objectives

1. Illustrate the diagnostic challenges in diagnosis of aCML and the key features for differentiating aCML from CNL and other MDS/MPN.
2. Discuss the value and limitation of molecular (sequencing) studies in the diagnosis of CNL, aCML, and other MDS/MPN.
3. Demonstrate the possible impact of diagnosis of aCML vs. CNL on the treatment choices of hypomethylating agents vs. ruxolitinib.

Case History

A 73-year-old female presented with fatigue, easy bruising, and 10 lb weight loss over the past 1–2 months. She had no history of previously diagnosed malignancies or chemotherapies. Her physical examination showed non-tender splenomegaly (~6 cm below the left costal margin) and no hepatomegaly. The skin examination showed ecchymoses on her arms and legs.

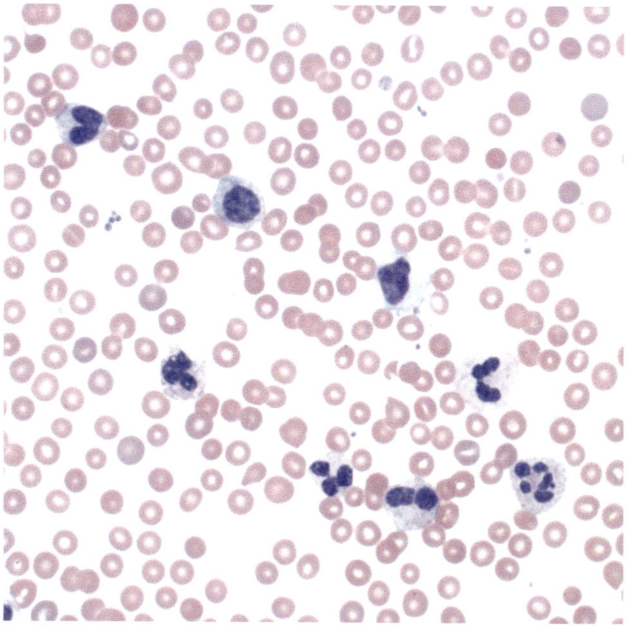

Fig. 25.19 Case presentation #2, peripheral blood (PB) smear

Histologic Findings

- CBC showed WBC 84.7 × 10^9/L, HGB 10.1 g/dL, MCV 92.3 fL, and PLT 102 × 10^9/L.
- The PB smear showed predominantly dysplastic neutrophils (Fig. 25.19). The differential count of the PB showed 2% blasts, 83% neutrophils, 3% metamyelocytes, 6% myelocytes, 1% monocytes, 4% lymphocytes, and 2% nucleated RBCs.
- Her BM core biopsy showed markedly hypercellular (~100%) BM with granulocytic expansion with a left shift in maturation and some small hypolobated megakaryocytes, i.e., moderate dysmegakaryopoiesis (Fig. 25.20a).
- The differential count of the BM aspirate smears showed markedly increased granulopoiesis with dysplasia, mild dyserythropoiesis, and no significant increase in blasts (Fig. 25.20b).

Other Ancillary Studies

- Cytogenetics showed a normal female karyotype.
- FISH for *BCR-ABL1* translocation was negative. FISH studies performed on the BM aspirate with the MDS panel were negative as well.
- Molecular studies later reported to be negative for *BCR-ABL1* fusions and *JAK2* p.V617F mutation.
- The results of NGS on the BM aspirate are pending.

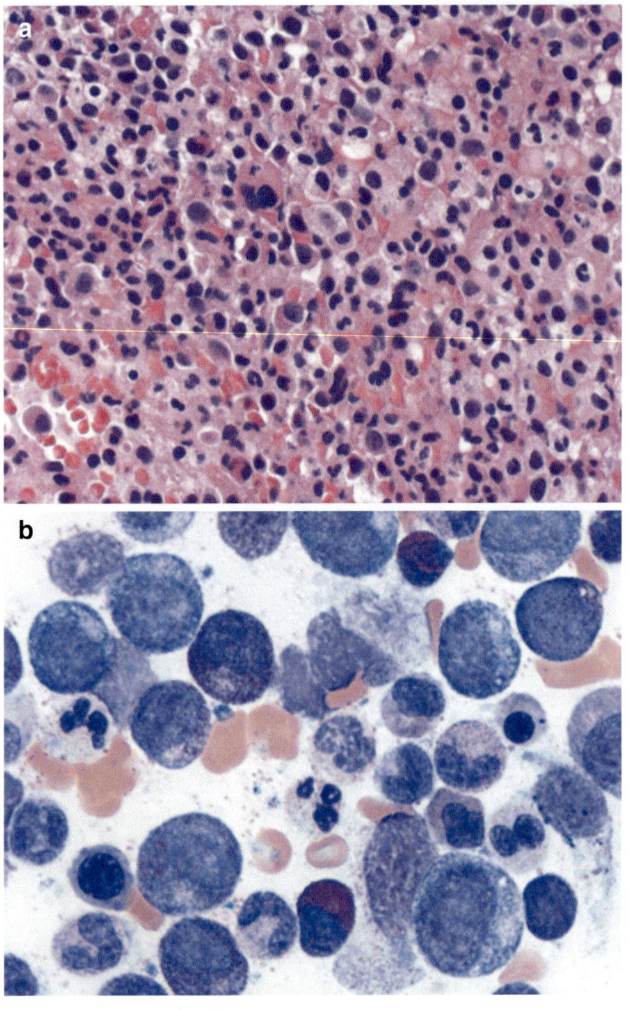

Fig. 25.20 Case presentation #2, bone marrow (BM) core biopsy and aspirate smear. (**a**) The bone core biopsy shows a hypercellular BM with marked granulocytic proliferation, left-shifted myelopoiesis, and increased M:E ratio. (**b**) The BM aspirate smear shows markedly increased granulocytes and granulocytic dysplasia

Differential Diagnosis

- The major differential diagnosis in this case is between a MPN and a MPN/MDS.
- The specific differential diagnoses include:
  - *Ph+* chronic myeloid leukemia (CML)
  - Chronic neutrophilic leukemia (CNL)
  - *BCR-ABL1*- atypical CML

A diagnosis of CMML was excluded due to the lack of absolute monocytosis. Importantly, the diagnosis of CML was unlikely due to the lack of basophilia and was definitely excluded by the negative FISH and PCR studies for *BCR-ABL1* fusions. Given her marked neutrophilia ($\geq 25 \times 10^9$ /L with >80% neutrophils), CNL was included in our initial differential diagnosis. However, the findings of circulating blasts and increased myeloid precursors ($\geq$10%) as well as significant myelodysplasia spoke against the diagnosis of CNL [1, 4].

Final Diagnosis and Follow Up

A final diagnosis of aCML was made on this case, and the patient was immediately treated with a hypomethylating agent, decitabine. Her leukocytosis dramatically reduced on decitabine. However, the NGS results came in about 3–4 weeks later and reported a *CSF3R* T618I mutation. Oncogenic *CSF3R* mutations were reported to be characteristically recurrent mutations for chronic neutrophilic leukemia and atypical CML [81, 88]. Some reports claimed that *CSF3R* T618I mutation is highly specific for CNL [158]. As a matter of fact, although *CSF3R* T618I is prevalent in CNL, this finding can also be seen in CMML and aCML. This patient finished four rounds of decitabine treatment, and her leukocytes were markedly reduced (to 0.8/uL), and HGB and platelet count gradually improved to 11.1 g/dL and 131/uL, respectively. No ruxolitinib was given to this patient because of a very good response to decitabine alone.

Take-Home Messages

1. Morphology remains a cornerstone in the diagnosis of aCML, and careful evaluation of the differential count and granulocytic dysplasia is the key for differential diagnosis of aCML vs. CNL or CMML.
2. *CSF3R* p.T618I mutation is highly prevalent in CNL, but is not specific or diagnostic for CNL. It can be seen in a small subset (~10%) of aCML and CMML cases.
3. Some aCML patients even with *CSF3R* p.T618I mutation may respond to hypomethylating agents, such as azacitidine and decitabine.

Case 3

Learning Objectives

1. Illustrating the diagnostic challenges in dealing with fibrotic bone marrow specimens
2. Discussing the differential diagnoses for CMML with marked myelofibrosis and the usefulness and limitation of ancillary diagnostic studies, including cytochemical stain of combined esterase (CO-ES), CD34, and other immunostains
3. Discussing the impact of morphology and myelofibrosis as well as *CSF3R* and *ASXL1* mutations on the diagnosis and prognosis of CMML

Case History

A 62-year-old man with a long history of rheumatoid osteoarthritis, who was recently found to have abnormal blood counts. His physical examination was unremarkable. No lymphadenopathy or hepatosplenomegaly was detected.

Histologic Findings

- CBC showed WBC 23.2 × 10^9/L, HGB 7.8 g/dL, MCV 100.8 fL, and platelet count 100 × 10^9/L.
- The PB smear showed many myelocytes and predominantly neutrophils with mild granulocytic dysplasia (Fig. 25.21a). Differential count of the PB showed 2% blasts, 1% promyelocytes, 20% myelocytes, 7% metamyelocytes, 8% bands, 48% neutrophils, 1% eosinophils, 7% lymphocytes, 14% monocytes, and occasional nucleated RBCs. There was absolute monocytosis (3200/μL) confirmed by combined esterase (CO-ES) stain (Fig. 25.21b).
- His BM core biopsy showed a markedly hypercellular (~95%) BM with marked myelomonocytic proliferation, increased immature myeloid precursors, and occasional small hypolobated (dysplastic) megakaryocytes (Fig. 25.22a).
- Reticulin stain showed marked myelofibrosis (MF-3, WHO 2017) (Fig. 25.22b).
- No BM aspirate smears were obtained due to a dry tap.
- A touch imprint from the BM core showed ~5.7% blasts, but the quality of the touch imprint was inadequate for a precise assessment of the differential count and myelodysplasia.

Other Ancillary Studies

- The immunohistochemical studies performed on the BM core showed no increase in CD34+ blasts (Fig. 25.23a).
- CD33 and glycophorin C stains showed markedly increased granulocytic and monocytic elements and reduced erythroid precursors (Fig. 25.23b, c).
- CD138 showed occasional plasma cells (Fig. 25.23d).
- CD3 and CD20 showed markedly increased T- and B-cells, respectively, in focal areas of the BM core (Fig. 25.23e, f).
- FISH studies performed on the PB with the MDS panel were negative.

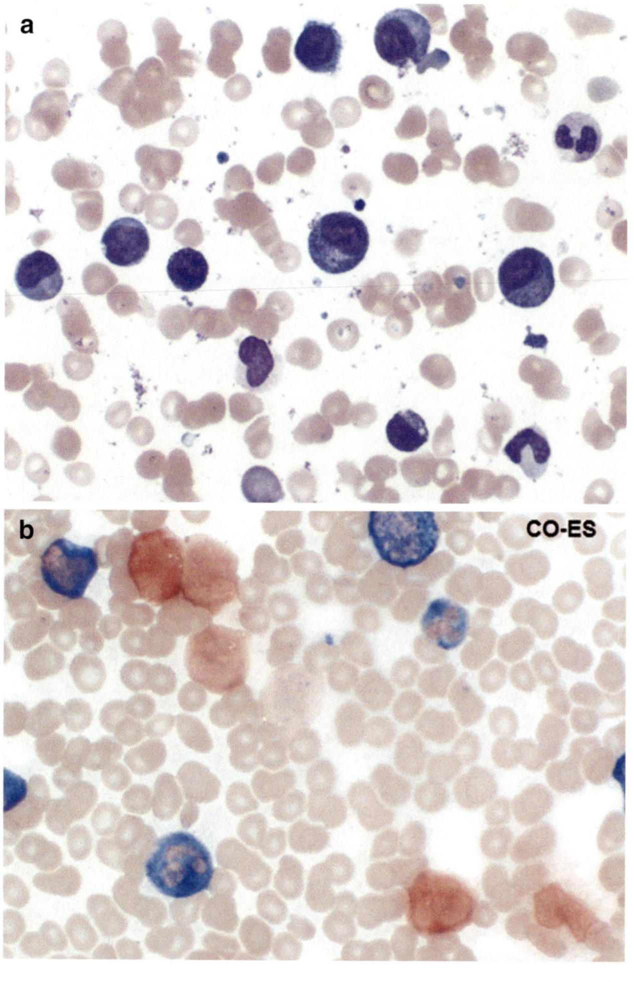

Fig. 25.21 Case presentation #3, peripheral blood (PB) smear. (**a**) The PB smear shows anemia and marked monocytosis. (**b**) The combined esterase stain, chloroacetate esterase (CAE) and alpha-naphthyl butyrate esterase (ANBE) double stain, shows granulocytes in blue and monocytes and their precursors in brown

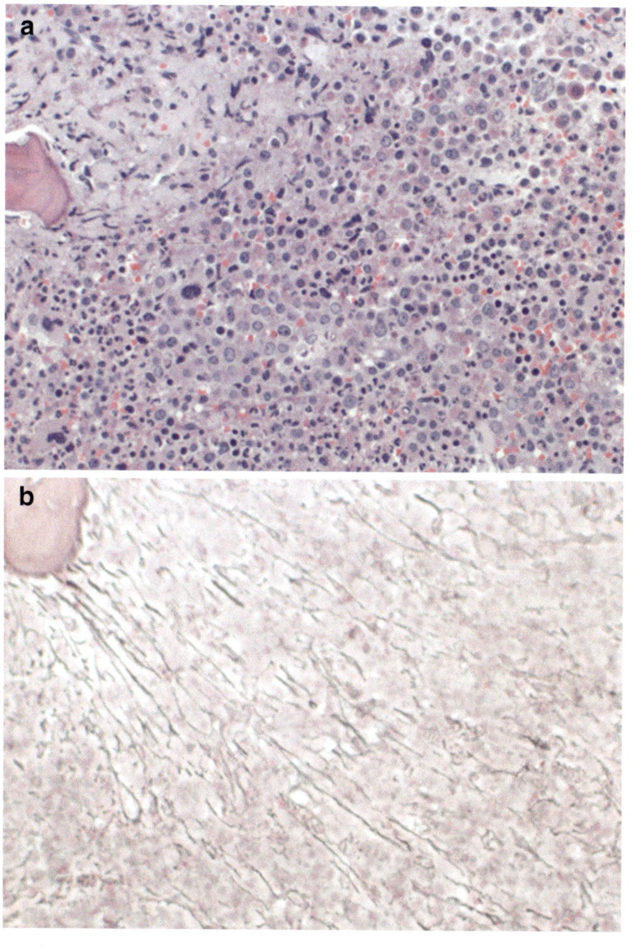

Fig. 25.22 Case presentation #3, bone marrow (BM) core biopsy and aspirate smear. (**a**) The bone core biopsy shows a hypercellular BM with left-shifted myelopoiesis, marked granulocytic/monocytic proliferation, and increased M:E ratio. (**b**) The reticulin stains show moderate to marked myelofibrosis, MF-2-3 WHO 2017

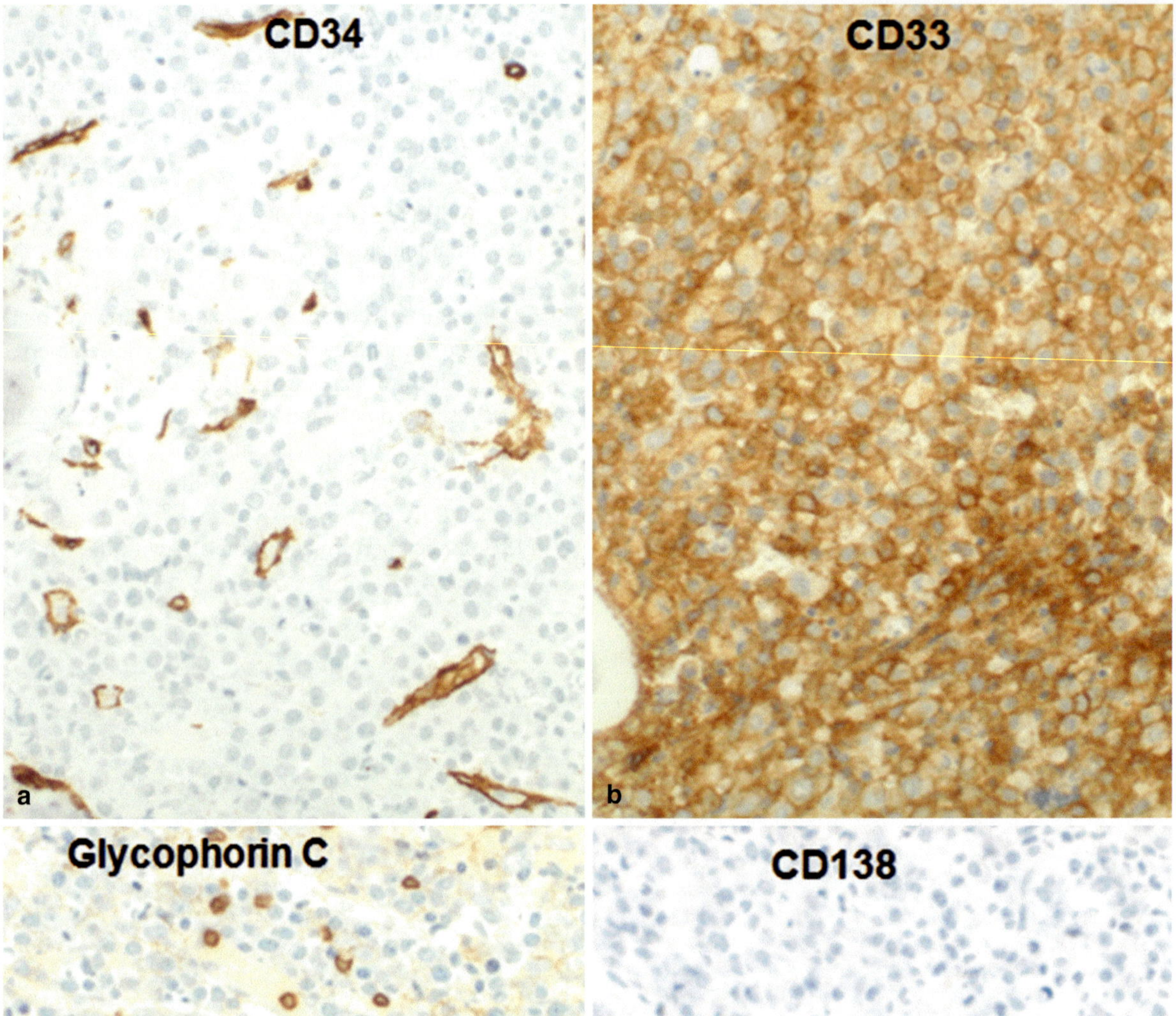

Fig. 25.23 Case presentation #3, immunohistochemical stains performed on the bone marrow (BM) core biopsy. (**a**) CD34 immunostain shows no increase in CD34+ blasts. (**b**) CD33 immunostain shows marked myeloid expansion. (**c**) Glycophorin C immunostain shows markedly reduced erythroid precursors. (**d**) CD138 immunostain shows a few plasma cells. (**e**, **f**) CD3 and CD20 immunostains show markedly increased T- and B-cells, respectively, in focal areas of the BM core

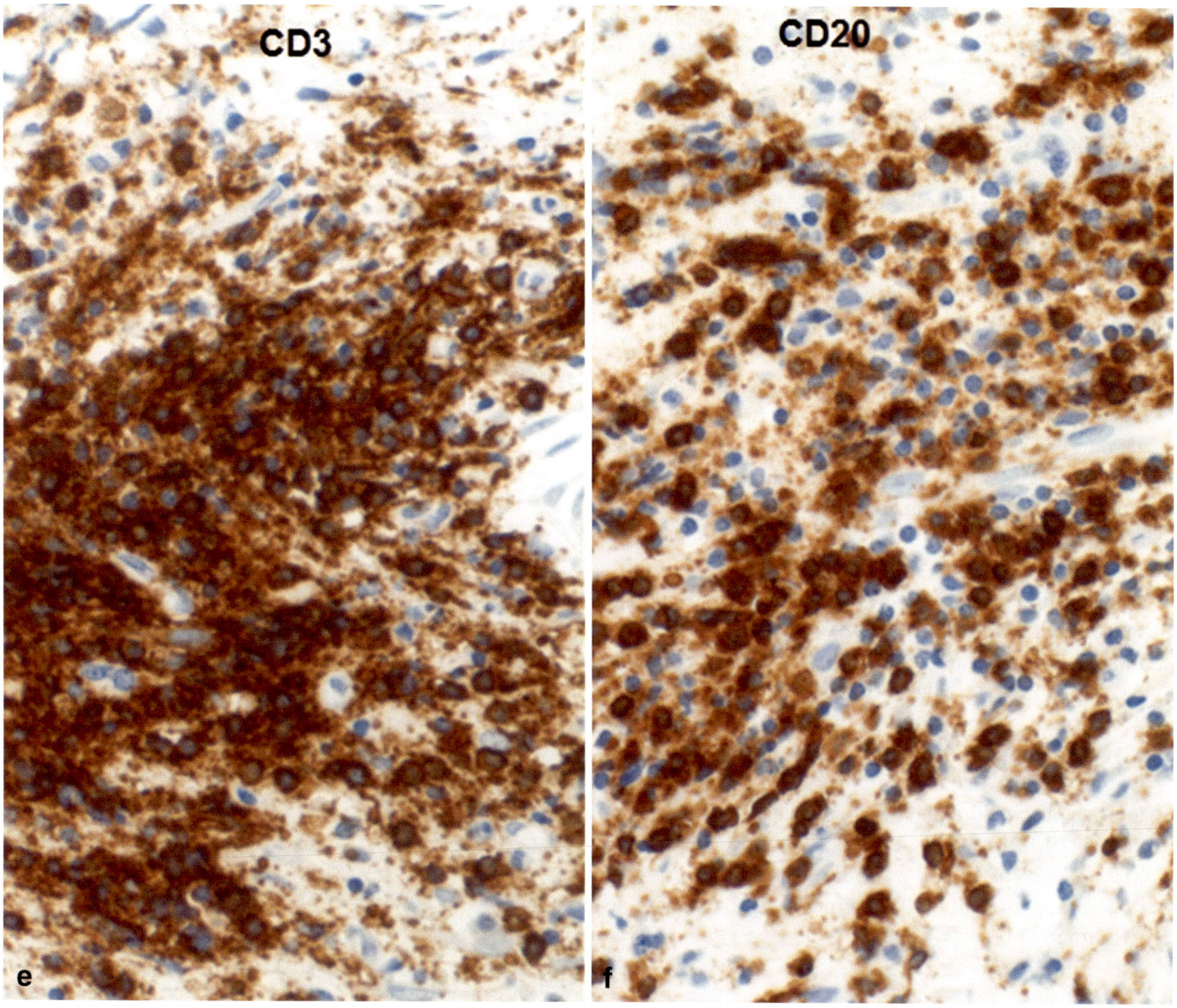

Fig. 25.23 (continued)

- Molecular studies performed on the PB were negative for *BCR-ABL1* fusions and *JAK2* p.V617F mutation.
- The results of NGS on the BM aspirate are pending.

Differential Diagnosis

Given a history of autoimmune disease (rheumatoid osteoarthritis) and the findings of neutrophilia and monocytosis in the PB and granulocytic proliferation and marked fibrosis, the differential diagnosis of this case could be very broad, ranging from:

- Reactive/autoimmune myelofibrosis
- MPN including CNL, CML, and PMF
- MDS/MPN, such as:
  - CMML
  - aCML

The diagnosis of CML was quickly ruled out based on the morphologic findings of presence of significant monocytosis and absent basophilia in the PB and the negative molecular studies for *BCR-ABL1* fusions. The diagnosis of PMF was also excluded based on the morphology of the megakaryocytes and the absence of *JAK2* p.V617F mutation. Of note, NGS indeed detected mutations in *CSF3R* (p.Q766 and T6181I) and *ASXL1* genes in this case. Although *CSF3R* (p.Q766 and T6181I) mutation was reported to be prevalent in CNL [81, 88], the findings of circulating blasts and increased myeloid precursors (≥10%) excluded CNL in this case. The diagnosis of aCML was not favored because of the relatively mild granulocytic dysplasia and absolute monocytosis. This exclusive diagnostic approach led to a major differential diagnosis between autoimmune myelofibrosis and CMML in this case, which is often challenging because autoimmune diseases can be seen in ~10% of patients with MDS and CMML and may play a role in the pathogenesis of MDS and CMML [159–163].

Final Diagnosis and Follow Up

A final diagnosis of CMML was made largely based on the morphologic features. However, it was impossible to precisely determine the blast count and the myelodysplasia of the BM cells due to the combination of a lack of aspirate smears and the negative CD34 stain in monoblasts. The patient was treated with ruxolitinib, and unfortunately, the patient did not respond to the treatment, and his CMML progressed to AML with 38% circulating blasts 3 months later. It is worth noting that *CSF3R* T618I mutation and *ASXL1* mutation were reported to be associated with a poor prognosis in CMML [68, 164], but others disputed the prognostic value of *CSF3R* p.T618I mutation in CMML and CNL [165].

Take-Home Messages

1. Extra caution should be exercised to differentiate autoimmune myelofibrosis from CMML with myelofibrosis, and the presence of autoimmune disorder does not exclude the diagnosis of MDS, CMML, or other myeloid neoplasms.
2. Myelofibrosis is associated with a poor prognosis in CMML. The *ASXL1* and *CSF3R* as well as *SETBP1* mutations are also reported to be associated with a poor prognosis in CMML.
3. The presence of *CSF3R* p.T618I mutation does not warrant a diagnosis of CNL nor therapeutic response to ruxolitinib.

References

1. Hyjek E, Vardiman JW. Myelodysplastic/myeloproliferative neoplasms. Semin Diagn Pathol. 2011;28(4):283–97.
2. Vardiman JW, Thiele J, Arber DA, Brunning RD, Borowitz MJ, Porwit A, et al. The 2008 revision of the World Health Organization (WHO) classification of myeloid neoplasms and acute leukemia: rationale and important changes. Blood. 2009;114(5):937–51.
3. Orazi A, Germing U. The myelodysplastic/myeloproliferative neoplasms: myeloproliferative diseases with dysplastic features. Leukemia. 2008;22(7):1308–19.
4. Arber DA, Orazi A, Hasserjian R, Thiele J, Borowitz MJ, Le Beau MM, et al. The 2016 revision to the World Health Organization classification of myeloid neoplasms and acute leukemia. Blood. 2016;127(20):2391–405.
5. Bennett JM, Brunning RD, Vardiman JW. Myelodysplastic syndromes: from French-American-British to World Health Organization: a commentary. Blood. 2002;99(8):3074–5.
6. Vardiman JW. The new World Health Organization classification of myeloid neoplasms: Q&A with James W. Vardiman, MD. Clin Adv Hematol Oncol. 2003;1(1):18–21.
7. Vardiman JW. Myelodysplastic/myeloproliferative diseases. Cancer Treat Res. 2004;121:13–43.
8. Vardiman JW, Harris NL, Brunning RD. The World Health Organization (WHO) classification of the myeloid neoplasms. Blood. 2002;100(7):2292–302.
9. Bennett JM, Catovsky D, Daniel MT, Flandrin G, Galton DA, Gralnick H, et al. The chronic myeloid leukaemias: guidelines for distinguishing chronic granulocytic, atypical chronic myeloid, and chronic myelomonocytic leukaemia. Proposals by the French-American-British Cooperative Leukaemia Group. Br J Haematol. 1994;87(4):746–54.
10. Germing U, Gattermann N, Minning H, Heyll A, Aul C. Problems in the classification of CMML--dysplastic versus proliferative type. Leuk Res. 1998;22(10):871–8.
11. Michaux JL, Martiat P. Chronic myelomonocytic leukaemia (CMML)--a myelodysplastic or myeloproliferative syndrome? Leuk Lymphoma. 1993;9(1–2):35–41.
12. Ngo NT, Lampert IA, Naresh KN. Bone marrow trephine morphology and immunohistochemical findings in chronic myelomonocytic leukaemia. Br J Haematol. 2008;141(6):771–81.
13. Orazi A, Chiu R, O'Malley DP, Czader M, Allen SL, An C, et al. Chronic myelomonocytic leukemia: the role of bone marrow biopsy immunohistology. Mod Pathol. 2006;19(12):1536–45.
14. Bennett JM, Catovsky D, Daniel MT, Flandrin G, Galton DA, Gralnick HR, et al. Proposals for the classification of the acute leukaemias. French-American-British (FAB) co-operative group. Br J Haematol. 1976;33(4):451–8.
15. Bain BJ. What is a promonocyte? Am J Hematol. 2013;88(10):919.
16. Goasguen JE, Bennett JM, Bain BJ, Vallespi T, Brunning R, Mufti GJ, et al. Morphological evaluation of monocytes and their precursors. Haematologica. 2009;94(7):994–7.
17. Facchetti F, De Wolf-Peeters C, Kennes C, Rossi G, De Vos R, van den Oord JJ, et al. Leukemia-associated lymph node infiltrates of plasmacytoid monocytes (so-called plasmacytoid T-cells). Evidence for two distinct histological and immunophenotypical patterns. Am J Surg Pathol. 1990;14(2):101–12.
18. Maschek H, Georgii A, Kaloutsi V, Werner M, Bandecar K, Kressel MG, et al. Myelofibrosis in primary myelodysplastic syndromes: a retrospective study of 352 patients. Eur J Haematol. 1992;48(4):208–14.
19. Gur HD, Loghavi S, Garcia-Manero G, Routbort M, Kanagal-Shamanna R, Quesada A, et al. Chronic myelomonocytic leukemia with fibrosis is a distinct disease subset with myeloproliferative features and frequent JAK2 p.V617F mutations. Am J Surg Pathol. 2018;42(6):799–806.
20. Petrova-Drus K, Chiu A, Margolskee E, Barouk-Fox S, Geyer J, Dogan A, et al. Bone marrow fibrosis in chronic myelomonocytic leukemia is associated with increased megakaryopoiesis, splenomegaly and with a shorter median time to disease progression. Oncotarget. 2017;8(61):103274–82.
21. Baddoura FK, Hanson C, Chan WC. Plasmacytoid monocyte proliferation associated with myeloproliferative disorders. Cancer. 1992;69(6):1457–67.
22. Harris NL, Demirjian Z. Plasmacytoid T-zone cell proliferation in a patient with chronic myelomonocytic leukemia. Histologic and immunohistologic characterization. Am J Surg Pathol. 1991;15(1):87–95.
23. Vermi W, Facchetti F, Rosati S, Vergoni F, Rossi E, Festa S, et al. Nodal and extranodal tumor-forming accumulation of plasmacytoid monocytes/interferon-producing cells associated with myeloid disorders. Am J Surg Pathol. 2004;28(5):585–95.
24. Wang HY, Feldman AL. Exuberant nodal proliferation of mature plasmacytoid dendritic cells in a patient with chronic myelomonocytic leukemia. Blood. 2017;130(11):1387.
25. Patnaik MM, Tefferi A. Cytogenetic and molecular abnormalities in chronic myelomonocytic leukemia. Blood Cancer J. 2016;6:e393.

26. Becher R, Carbonell F, Bartram CR. Isochromosome 17q in Ph1-negative leukemia: a clinical, cytogenetic, and molecular study. Blood. 1990;75(8):1679–83.
27. Casalone R, Francesconi D, Pasquali F, Comotti B, Vaccari F. Isochromosome (17q) in Philadelphia chromosome (Ph1)-negative juvenile chronic myelocytic leukemia. Cancer Genet Cytogenet. 1981;3(2):145–8.
28. Kanagal-Shamanna R, Bueso-Ramos CE, Barkoh B, Lu G, Wang S, Garcia-Manero G, et al. Myeloid neoplasms with isolated isochromosome 17q represent a clinicopathologic entity associated with myelodysplastic/myeloproliferative features, a high risk of leukemic transformation, and wild-type TP53. Cancer. 2012;118(11):2879–88.
29. Kanagal-Shamanna R, Luthra R, Yin CC, Patel KP, Takahashi K, Lu X, et al. Myeloid neoplasms with isolated isochromosome 17q demonstrate a high frequency of mutations in SETBP1, SRSF2, ASXL1 and NRAS. Oncotarget. 2016;7(12):14251–8.
30. Lamprianidou E, Kordella C, Papoutselis M, Bezyrgiannidou Z, Nakou E, Papamichos S, et al. Myeloid neoplasms with isolated isochromosome 17q: a yet to be defined entity. Mediterr J Hematol Infect Dis. 2017;9(1):e2017066.
31. Baer MR, Stewart CC, Lawrence D, Arthur DC, Mrozek K, Strout MP, et al. Acute myeloid leukemia with 11q23 translocations: myelomonocytic immunophenotype by multiparameter flow cytometry. Leukemia. 1998;12(3):317–25.
32. Mrozek K, Heinonen K, Lawrence D, Carroll AJ, Koduru PR, Rao KW, et al. Adult patients with de novo acute myeloid leukemia and t(9; 11)(p22; q23) have a superior outcome to patients with other translocations involving band 11q23: a cancer and leukemia group B study. Blood. 1997;90(11):4532–8.
33. Zuo W, Wang SA, DiNardo C, Yabe M, Li S, Medeiros LJ, et al. Acute leukaemia and myelodysplastic syndromes with chromosomal rearrangement involving 11q23 locus, but not MLL gene. J Clin Pathol. 2017;70(3):244–9.
34. Itzykson R, Kosmider O, Renneville A, Gelsi-Boyer V, Meggendorfer M, Morabito M, et al. Prognostic score including gene mutations in chronic myelomonocytic leukemia. J Clin Oncol. 2013;31(19):2428–36.
35. Patnaik MM, Tefferi A. Chronic myelomonocytic leukemia: 2016 update on diagnosis, risk stratification, and management. Am J Hematol. 2016;91(6):631–42.
36. Melo JV, Myint H, Galton DA, Goldman JM. P190BCR-ABL chronic myeloid leukaemia: the missing link with chronic myelomonocytic leukaemia? Leukemia. 1994;8(1):208–11.
37. Elliott MA, Verstovsek S, Dingli D, Schwager SM, Mesa RA, Li CY, et al. Monocytosis is an adverse prognostic factor for survival in younger patients with primary myelofibrosis. Leuk Res. 2007;31(11):1503–9.
38. Tefferi A, Shah S, Mudireddy M, Lasho TL, Barraco D, Hanson CA, et al. Monocytosis is a powerful and independent predictor of inferior survival in primary myelofibrosis. Br J Haematol. 2018;183:835–8.
39. Chapman J, Geyer JT, Khanlari M, Moul A, Casas C, Connor ST, et al. Myeloid neoplasms with features intermediate between primary myelofibrosis and chronic myelomonocytic leukemia. Mod Pathol. 2018;31(3):429–41.
40. Schuler E, Frank F, Hildebrandt B, Betz B, Strupp C, Rudelius M, et al. Myelodysplastic syndromes without peripheral monocytosis but with evidence of marrow monocytosis share clinical and molecular characteristics with CMML. Leuk Res. 2018;65:1–4.
41. Vidholia A, Menon MP. "Cup-like" blasts in acute myeloid leukemia with FLT3 and NPM1 mutations. Blood. 2015;125(5):889.
42. Bennett JM, Pryor J, Laughlin TS, Rothberg PG, Burack WR. Is the association of "cup-like" nuclei with mutation of the NPM1 gene in acute myeloid leukemia clinically useful? Am J Clin Pathol. 2010;134(4):648–52.
43. Jain P, Vega-Vazquez F, Faderl S. "Cup-like" blasts and NPM1 and FLT3 (ITD) mutations in acute myeloid leukemia (AML). Int J Hematol. 2013;98(1):3.
44. Park BG, Chi HS, Jang S, Park CJ, Kim DY, Lee JH, et al. Association of cup-like nuclei in blasts with FLT3 and NPM1 mutations in acute myeloid leukemia. Ann Hematol. 2013;92(4):451–7.
45. Reiter A, Gotlib J. Myeloid neoplasms with eosinophilia. Blood. 2017;129(6):704–14.
46. Deininger MWN, Tyner JW, Solary E. Turning the tide in myelodysplastic/myeloproliferative neoplasms. Nat Rev Cancer. 2017;17(7):425–40.
47. Tefferi A, Skoda R, Vardiman JW. Myeloproliferative neoplasms: contemporary diagnosis using histology and genetics. Nat Rev Clin Oncol. 2009;6(11):627–37.
48. Zukerberg LR, Ferry JA, Conlon M, Harris NL. Plasma cell myeloma with cleaved, multilobated, and monocytoid nuclei. Am J Clin Pathol. 1990;93(5):657–61.
49. Loghavi S, Curry JL, Garcia-Manero G, Patel KP, Xu J, Khoury JD, et al. Chronic myelomonocytic leukemia masquerading as cutaneous indeterminate dendritic cell tumor: expanding the spectrum of skin lesions in chronic myelomonocytic leukemia. J Cutan Pathol. 2017;44(12):1075–9.
50. Julia F, Dalle S, Duru G, Balme B, Vergier B, Ortonne N, et al. Blastic plasmacytoid dendritic cell neoplasms: clinico-immunohistochemical correlations in a series of 91 patients. Am J Surg Pathol. 2014;38(5):673–80.
51. Vitte F, Fabiani B, Benet C, Dalac S, Balme B, Delattre C, et al. Specific skin lesions in chronic myelomonocytic leukemia: a spectrum of myelomonocytic and dendritic cell proliferations: a study of 42 cases. Am J Surg Pathol. 2012;36(9):1302–16.
52. Guru Murthy GS, Dhakal I, Mehta P. Incidence and survival outcomes of chronic myelomonocytic leukemia in the United States. Leuk Lymphoma. 2017;58(7):1648–54.
53. Srour SA, Devesa SS, Morton LM, Check DP, Curtis RE, Linet MS, et al. Incidence and patient survival of myeloproliferative neoplasms and myelodysplastic/myeloproliferative neoplasms in the United States, 2001–12. Br J Haematol. 2016;174(3):382–96.
54. Elena C, Galli A, Such E, Meggendorfer M, Germing U, Rizzo E, et al. Integrating clinical features and genetic lesions in the risk assessment of patients with chronic myelomonocytic leukemia. Blood. 2016;128(10):1408–17.
55. Such E, Germing U, Malcovati L, Cervera J, Kuendgen A, Della Porta MG, et al. Development and validation of a prognostic scoring system for patients with chronic myelomonocytic leukemia. Blood. 2013;121(15):3005–15.
56. Wassie EA, Itzykson R, Lasho TL, Kosmider O, Finke CM, Hanson CA, et al. Molecular and prognostic correlates of cytogenetic abnormalities in chronic myelomonocytic leukemia: a Mayo Clinic-French Consortium Study. Am J Hematol. 2014;89(12):1111–5.
57. Patnaik MM, Wassie EA, Padron E, Onida F, Itzykson R, Lasho TL, et al. Chronic myelomonocytic leukemia in younger patients: molecular and cytogenetic predictors of survival and treatment outcome. Blood Cancer J. 2015;5:e280.
58. Tefferi A, Elliott M, Pardanani A. Chronic neutrophilic leukemia: novel mutations and their impact on clinical practice. Curr Opin Hematol. 2015;22(2):171–6.
59. Patnaik MM, Zahid MF, Lasho TL, Finke C, Ketterling RL, Gangat N, et al. Number and type of TET2 mutations in chronic myelomonocytic leukemia and their clinical relevance. Blood Cancer J. 2016;6(9):e472.
60. Onida F, Kantarjian HM, Smith TL, Ball G, Keating MJ, Estey EH, et al. Prognostic factors and scoring systems in chronic myelomonocytic leukemia: a retrospective analysis of 213 patients. Blood. 2002;99(3):840–9.

61. Germing U, Strupp C, Aivado M, Gattermann N. New prognostic parameters for chronic myelomonocytic leukemia. Blood. 2002;100(2):731–2; author reply 2–3.
62. Kantarjian H, O'Brien S, Ravandi F, Cortes J, Shan J, Bennett JM, et al. Proposal for a new risk model in myelodysplastic syndrome that accounts for events not considered in the original International Prognostic Scoring System. Cancer. 2008;113(6):1351–61.
63. Padron E, Garcia-Manero G, Patnaik MM, Itzykson R, Lasho T, Nazha A, et al. An international data set for CMML validates prognostic scoring systems and demonstrates a need for novel prognostication strategies. Blood Cancer J. 2015;5:e333.
64. Greenberg P, Cox C, LeBeau MM, Fenaux P, Morel P, Sanz G, et al. International scoring system for evaluating prognosis in myelodysplastic syndromes. Blood. 1997;89(6):2079–88.
65. Greenberg PL, Tuechler H, Schanz J, Sanz G, Garcia-Manero G, Sole F, et al. Revised international prognostic scoring system for myelodysplastic syndromes. Blood. 2012;120(12):2454–65.
66. Calvo X, Nomdedeu M, Santacruz R, Martinez N, Costa D, Pereira A, et al. Comparison of three prognostic scoring systems in a series of 146 cases of chronic myelomonocytic leukemia (CMML): MD Anderson prognostic score (MDAPS), CMML-specific prognostic scoring system (CPSS) and Mayo prognostic model. A detailed review of prognostic factors in CMML. Leuk Res. 2015;pii: S0145-2126:30324–6.
67. Solary E, Itzykson R. How I treat chronic myelomonocytic leukemia. Blood. 2017;130(2):126–36.
68. Patnaik MM, Lasho TL, Vijayvargiya P, Finke CM, Hanson CA, Ketterling RP, et al. Prognostic interaction between ASXL1 and TET2 mutations in chronic myelomonocytic leukemia. Blood Cancer J. 2016;6:e385.
69. Patnaik MM, Padron E, LaBorde RR, Lasho TL, Finke CM, Hanson CA, et al. Mayo prognostic model for WHO-defined chronic myelomonocytic leukemia: ASXL1 and spliceosome component mutations and outcomes. Leukemia. 2013;27(7):1504–10.
70. Dao KH, Tyner JW. What's different about atypical CML and chronic neutrophilic leukemia? Hematology Am Soc Hematol Educ Program. 2015;2015:264–71.
71. Gilioli A, Paolini A, Bonacorsi G, Luppi M. A typical atypical chronic myeloid leukemia. Clin Case Rep. 2018;6(5):915–6.
72. Wang SA, Hasserjian RP, Fox PS, Rogers HJ, Geyer JT, Chabot-Richards D, et al. Atypical chronic myeloid leukemia is clinically distinct from unclassifiable myelodysplastic/myeloproliferative neoplasms. Blood. 2014;123(17):2645–51.
73. Vardiman JW, Bennett JM, Bain BJ, Brunning RD, Thiele J. Atypical chronic myeloid leukaemia, BCR-ABL1 negative. In: Swerdlow SH, Campo E, Harris NL, Jaffe ES, Pileri SA, Stein H, et al., editors. WHO classification of tumors of haematopoietic and lymphoid tissues. Lyon: IARC Press; 2008. p. 38–9.
74. Felman P, Bryon PA, Gentilhomme O, Ffrench M, Charrin C, Espinouse D, et al. The syndrome of abnormal chromatin clumping in leucocytes: a myelodysplastic disorder with proliferative features? Br J Haematol. 1988;70(1):49–54.
75. Oscier DG. Atypical chronic myeloid leukaemia, a distinct clinical entity related to the myelodysplastic syndrome? Br J Haematol. 1996;92(3):582–6.
76. Hernandez JM, del Canizo MC, Cuneo A, Garcia JL, Gutierrez NC, Gonzalez M, et al. Clinical, hematological and cytogenetic characteristics of atypical chronic myeloid leukemia. Ann Oncol. 2000;11(4):441–4.
77. Breccia M, Biondo F, Latagliata R, Carmosino I, Mandelli F, Alimena G. Identification of risk factors in atypical chronic myeloid leukemia. Haematologica. 2006;91(11):1566–8.
78. Xubo G, Xingguo L, Xianguo W, Rongzhen X, Xibin X, Lin W, et al. The role of peripheral blood, bone marrow aspirate and especially bone marrow trephine biopsy in distinguishing atypical chronic myeloid leukemia from chronic granulocytic leukemia and chronic myelomonocytic leukemia. Eur J Haematol. 2009;83(4):292–301.
79. Kurzrock R, Kantarjian HM, Shtalrid M, Gutterman JU, Talpaz M. Philadelphia chromosome-negative chronic myelogenous leukemia without breakpoint cluster region rearrangement: a chronic myeloid leukemia with a distinct clinical course. Blood. 1990;75(2):445–52.
80. Gotlib J. How I treat atypical chronic myeloid leukemia. Blood. 2017;129(7):838–45.
81. Dao KT, Tyner JW, Gotlib J. Recent progress in chronic neutrophilic leukemia and atypical chronic myeloid leukemia. Curr Hematol Malig Rep. 2017;12(5):432–41.
82. Patnaik MM, Barraco D, Lasho TL, Finke CM, Reichard K, Hoversten KP, et al. Targeted next generation sequencing and identification of risk factors in World Health Organization defined atypical chronic myeloid leukemia. Am J Hematol. 2017;92(6):542–8.
83. Piazza R, Valletta S, Winkelmann N, Redaelli S, Spinelli R, Pirola A, et al. Recurrent SETBP1 mutations in atypical chronic myeloid leukemia. Nat Genet. 2013;45(1):18–24.
84. Meggendorfer M, Bacher U, Alpermann T, Haferlach C, Kern W, Gambacorti-Passerini C, et al. SETBP1 mutations occur in 9% of MDS/MPN and in 4% of MPN cases and are strongly associated with atypical CML, monosomy 7, isochromosome i(17)(q10), ASXL1 and CBL mutations. Leukemia. 2013;27(9):1852–60.
85. Gotlib J, Maxson JE, George TI, Tyner JW. The new genetics of chronic neutrophilic leukemia and atypical CML: implications for diagnosis and treatment. Blood. 2013;122(10):1707–11.
86. Vardiman JW. Chronic myelogenous leukemia, BCR-ABL1+. Am J Clin Pathol. 2009;132(2):250–60.
87. Elliott MA, Pardanani A, Hanson CA, Lasho TL, Finke CM, Belachew AA, et al. ASXL1 mutations are frequent and prognostically detrimental in CSF3R-mutated chronic neutrophilic leukemia. Am J Hematol. 2015;90(7):653–6.
88. Maxson JE, Gotlib J, Pollyea DA, Fleischman AG, Agarwal A, Eide CA, et al. Oncogenic CSF3R mutations in chronic neutrophilic leukemia and atypical CML. N Engl J Med. 2013;368(19):1781–90.
89. Talati C, Padron E. An exercise in extrapolation: clinical management of atypical CML, MDS/MPN-unclassifiable, and MDS/MPN-RS-T. Curr Hematol Malig Rep. 2016;11(6):425–33.
90. Dhakal P, Gundabolu K, Amador C, Rayamajhi S, Bhatt VR. Atypical chronic myeloid leukemia: a rare entity with management challenges. Future Oncol. 2018;14(2):177–85.
91. Vardiman JW. The World Health Organization (WHO) classification of tumors of the hematopoietic and lymphoid tissues: an overview with emphasis on the myeloid neoplasms. Chem Biol Interact. 2010;184(1–2):16–20.
92. Niemeyer CM, Arico M, Basso G, Biondi A, Cantu Rajnoldi A, Creutzig U, et al. Chronic myelomonocytic leukemia in childhood: a retrospective analysis of 110 cases. European Working Group on Myelodysplastic Syndromes in Childhood (EWOG-MDS). Blood. 1997;89(10):3534–43.
93. Loh ML. Childhood myelodysplastic syndrome: focus on the approach to diagnosis and treatment of juvenile myelomonocytic leukemia. Hematology Am Soc Hematol Educ Program. 2010;2010:357–62.
94. Passmore SJ, Hann IM, Stiller CA, Ramani P, Swansbury GJ, Gibbons B, et al. Pediatric myelodysplasia: a study of 68 children and a new prognostic scoring system. Blood. 1995;85(7):1742–50.
95. Weinberg RS, Leibowitz D, Weinblatt ME, Kochen J, Alter BP. Juvenile chronic myelogenous leukaemia: the only example of truly fetal (not fetal-like) erythropoiesis. Br J Haematol. 1990;76(2):307–10.
96. Stieglitz E, Taylor-Weiner AN, Chang TY, Gelston LC, Wang YD, Mazor T, et al. The genomic landscape of juvenile myelomonocytic leukemia. Nat Genet. 2015;47(11):1326–33.

97. Flotho C, Kratz C, Niemeyer CM. Targeting RAS signaling pathways in juvenile myelomonocytic leukemia. Curr Drug Targets. 2007;8(6):715–25.
98. Moritake H, Ikeda T, Manabe A, Kamimura S, Nunoi H. Cytomegalovirus infection mimicking juvenile myelomonocytic leukemia showing hypersensitivity to granulocyte-macrophage colony stimulating factor. Pediatr Blood Cancer. 2009;53(7):1324–6.
99. Nishio N, Takahashi Y, Tanaka M, Xu Y, Yoshida N, Sakaguchi H, et al. Aberrant phosphorylation of STAT5 by granulocyte-macrophage colony-stimulating factor in infant cytomegalovirus infection mimicking juvenile myelomonocytic leukemia. Leuk Res. 2011;35(9):1261–4.
100. Lorenzana A, Lyons H, Sawaf H, Higgins M, Carrigan D, Emanuel PD. Human herpesvirus 6 infection mimicking juvenile myelomonocytic leukemia in an infant. J Pediatr Hematol Oncol. 2002;24(2):136–41.
101. Herrod HG, Dow LW, Sullivan JL. Persistent epstein-barr virus infection mimicking juvenile chronic myelogenous leukemia: immunologic and hematologic studies. Blood. 1983;61(6):1098–104.
102. Satwani P, Kahn J, Dvorak CC. Juvenile myelomonocytic leukemia. Pediatr Clin N Am. 2015;62(1):95–106.
103. Locatelli F, Niemeyer CM. How I treat juvenile myelomonocytic leukemia. Blood. 2015;125(7):1083–90.
104. Puri K, Singh P, Das RR, Seth R, Gupta R. Diagnostic dilemma of JMML coexisting with CMV infection. Indian J Pediatr. 2011;78(4):485–7.
105. Karow A, Baumann I, Niemeyer CM. Morphologic differential diagnosis of juvenile myelomonocytic leukemia--pitfalls apart from viral infection. J Pediatr Hematol Oncol. 2009;31(5):380.
106. Tartaglia M, Niemeyer CM, Fragale A, Song X, Buechner J, Jung A, et al. Somatic mutations in PTPN11 in juvenile myelomonocytic leukemia, myelodysplastic syndromes and acute myeloid leukemia. Nat Genet. 2003;34(2):148–50.
107. Schubbert S, Zenker M, Rowe SL, Boll S, Klein C, Bollag G, et al. Germline KRAS mutations cause Noonan syndrome. Nat Genet. 2006;38(3):331–6.
108. Kratz CP, Niemeyer CM, Castleberry RP, Cetin M, Bergstrasser E, Emanuel PD, et al. The mutational spectrum of PTPN11 in juvenile myelomonocytic leukemia and Noonan syndrome/myeloproliferative disease. Blood. 2005;106(6):2183–5.
109. Niemeyer CM, Kratz CP. Paediatric myelodysplastic syndromes and juvenile myelomonocytic leukaemia: molecular classification and treatment options. Br J Haematol. 2008;140(6):610–24.
110. Bader-Meunier B, Tchernia G, Mielot F, Fontaine JL, Thomas C, Lyonnet S, et al. Occurrence of myeloproliferative disorder in patients with Noonan syndrome. J Pediatr. 1997;130(6):885–9.
111. Makishima H, Cazzolli H, Szpurka H, Dunbar A, Tiu R, Huh J, et al. Mutations of e3 ubiquitin ligase cbl family members constitute a novel common pathogenic lesion in myeloid malignancies. J Clin Oncol. 2009;27(36):6109–16.
112. Perez B, Mechinaud F, Galambrun C, Ben Romdhane N, Isidor B, Philip N, et al. Germline mutations of the CBL gene define a new genetic syndrome with predisposition to juvenile myelomonocytic leukaemia. J Med Genet. 2010;47(10):686–91.
113. Muramatsu H, Makishima H, Jankowska AM, Cazzolli H, O'Keefe C, Yoshida N, et al. Mutations of an E3 ubiquitin ligase c-Cbl but not TET2 mutations are pathogenic in juvenile myelomonocytic leukemia. Blood. 2010;115(10):1969–75.
114. Niemeyer CM, Kang MW, Shin DH, Furlan I, Erlacher M, Bunin NJ, et al. Germline CBL mutations cause developmental abnormalities and predispose to juvenile myelomonocytic leukemia. Nat Genet. 2010;42(9):794–800.
115. Pathak A, Pemov A, McMaster ML, Dewan R, Ravichandran S, Pak E, et al. Juvenile myelomonocytic leukemia due to a germline CBL Y371C mutation: 35-year follow-up of a large family. Hum Genet. 2015;134(7):775–87.
116. Muraoka M, Okuma C, Kanamitsu K, Ishida H, Kanazawa Y, Washio K, et al. Adults with germline CBL mutation complicated with juvenile myelomonocytic leukemia at infancy. J Hum Genet. 2016;61(6):523–6.
117. Aldrich RA, Steinberg AG, Campbell DC. Pedigree demonstrating a sex-linked recessive condition characterized by draining ears, eczematoid dermatitis and bloody diarrhea. Pediatrics. 1954;13(2):133–9.
118. Sano H, Kobayashi R, Suzuki D, Yasuda K, Nakanishi M, Nagashima T, et al. Wiskott-Aldrich syndrome with unusual clinical features similar to juvenile myelomonocytic leukemia. Int J Hematol. 2012;96(2):279–83.
119. Yoshimi A, Kamachi Y, Imai K, Watanabe N, Nakadate H, Kanazawa T, et al. Wiskott-Aldrich syndrome presenting with a clinical picture mimicking juvenile myelomonocytic leukaemia. Pediatr Blood Cancer. 2013;60(5):836–41.
120. Hoyoux C, Dresse MF, Forget P, Piette C, Rausin L, Villa A, et al. Osteopetrosis mimicking juvenile myelomonocytic leukemia. Pediatr Int. 2014;56(5):779–82.
121. Mazzolari E, Forino C, Razza A, Porta F, Villa A, Notarangelo LD. A single-center experience in 20 patients with infantile malignant osteopetrosis. Am J Hematol. 2009;84(8):473–9.
122. Haroche J, Abla O. Uncommon histiocytic disorders: Rosai-Dorfman, juvenile xanthogranuloma, and Erdheim-Chester disease. Hematology Am Soc Hematol Educ Program. 2015;2015:571–8.
123. Ozono S, Inada H, Nakagawa SI, Ueda K, Matsumura H, Kojima S, et al. Juvenile myelomonocytic leukemia characterized by cutaneous lesion containing Langerhans cell histiocytosis-like cells. Int J Hematol. 2011;93(3):389–93.
124. Gutmann DH, Gurney JG, Shannon KM. Juvenile xanthogranuloma, neurofibromatosis 1, and juvenile chronic myeloid leukemia. Arch Dermatol. 1996;132(11):1390–1.
125. Zvulunov A. Juvenile xanthogranuloma, neurofibromatosis, and juvenile chronic myelogenous leukemia. Arch Dermatol. 1996;132(6):712–3.
126. Zvulunov A, Barak Y, Metzker A. Juvenile xanthogranuloma, neurofibromatosis, and juvenile chronic myelogenous leukemia. World statistical analysis. Arch Dermatol. 1995;131(8):904–8.
127. Campochiaro C, Tomelleri A, Cavalli G, Berti A, Dagna L. Erdheim-Chester disease. Eur J Intern Med. 2015;26(4):223–9.
128. Allen CE, Parsons DW. Biological and clinical significance of somatic mutations in Langerhans cell histiocytosis and related histiocytic neoplastic disorders. Hematology Am Soc Hematol Educ Program. 2015;2015:559–64.
129. Smpokou P, Zand DJ, Rosenbaum KN, Summar ML. Malignancy in Noonan syndrome and related disorders. Clin Genet. 2015;88(6):516–22.
130. Tartaglia M, Gelb BD, Zenker M. Noonan syndrome and clinically related disorders. Best Pract Res Clin Endocrinol Metab. 2011;25(1):161–79.
131. Kratz CP, Schubbert S, Bollag G, Niemeyer CM, Shannon KM, Zenker M. Germline mutations in components of the Ras signaling pathway in Noonan syndrome and related disorders. Cell Cycle. 2006;5(15):1607–11.
132. Tartaglia M, Gelb BD. Noonan syndrome and related disorders: genetics and pathogenesis. Annu Rev Genomics Hum Genet. 2005;6:45–68.
133. Attias D, Grunberger T, Vanek W, Estrov Z, Cohen A, Lau R, et al. B-lineage lymphoid blast crisis in juvenile chronic myelogenous leukemia: II. Interleukin-1-mediated autocrine growth regulation of the lymphoblasts. Leukemia. 1995;9(5):884–8.

134. Lau RC, Squire J, Brisson L, Kamel-Reid S, Grunberger T, Dube I, et al. Lymphoid blast crisis of B-lineage phenotype with monosomy 7 in a patient with juvenile chronic myelogenous leukemia (JCML). Leukemia. 1994;8(5):903–8.
135. Scrideli CA, Baruffi MR, Rogatto SR, Valera ET, Defavery R, Tone LG. B lineage acute lymphoblastic leukemia transformation in a child with juvenile myelomonocytic leukemia, type 1 neurofibromatosis and monosomy of chromosome 7. Possible implications in the leukemogenesis. Leuk Res. 2003;27(4):371–4.
136. Loh ML, Mullighan CG. Advances in the genetics of high-risk childhood B-progenitor acute lymphoblastic leukemia and juvenile myelomonocytic leukemia: implications for therapy. Clin Cancer Res. 2012;18(10):2754–67.
137. Pauli S, Steinemann D, Dittmann K, Wienands J, Shoukier M, Moschner M, et al. Occurrence of acute lymphoblastic leukemia and juvenile myelomonocytic leukemia in a patient with Noonan syndrome carrying the germline PTPN11 mutation p.E139D. Am J Med Genet A. 2012;158A(3):652–8.
138. Ly B, Modi A, Rogers HJ, Makishima H, Hanna R, Cook JR, et al. Concurrent juvenile myelomonocytic leukemia and T-lymphoblastic lymphoma with a shared missense mutation in NRAS. Pediatr Blood Cancer. 2014;61(5):946–8.
139. Raikar SS, Scarborough JD, Sabnis H, Bergsagel J, Wu D, Cooper TM, et al. Early T-cell precursor acute lymphoblastic leukemia in an infant with an NRAS Q61R mutation and clinical features of juvenile myelomonocytic leukemia. Pediatr Blood Cancer. 2016;63(9):1667–70.
140. Maschan AA, Khachatrian LA, Solopova GG, Ossipova EY, Baidun LV, Dmitrieva SV, et al. Development of T-cell acute lymphoblastic leukemia in a patient in very long lasting complete remission of juvenile myelomonocytic leukemia. J Pediatr Hematol Oncol. 2011;33(1):e32–4.
141. Unal S, Cetin M, Kutlay NY, Elmas SA, Gumruk F, Tukun A, et al. Hemophagocytosis associated with leukemia: a striking association with juvenile myelomonocytic leukemia. Ann Hematol. 2010;89(4):359–64.
142. Lo FS, Kuo TT, Wang CJ, Kuo MT, Kuo MC. Hodgkin's lymphoma in a patient with Noonan syndrome with germ-line PTPN11 mutations. Int J Hematol. 2008;88(3):287–90.
143. Passmore SJ, Chessells JM, Kempski H, Hann IM, Brownbill PA, Stiller CA. Paediatric myelodysplastic syndromes and juvenile myelomonocytic leukaemia in the UK: a population-based study of incidence and survival. Br J Haematol. 2003;121(5):758–67.
144. Yoshida N, Yagasaki H, Xu Y, Matsuda K, Yoshimi A, Takahashi Y, et al. Correlation of clinical features with the mutational status of GM-CSF signaling pathway-related genes in juvenile myelomonocytic leukemia. Pediatr Res. 2009;65(3):334–40.
145. Sakashita K, Matsuda K, Koike K. Diagnosis and treatment of juvenile myelomonocytic leukemia. Pediatr Int. 2016;58(8):681–90.
146. Sakaguchi H, Okuno Y, Muramatsu H, Yoshida K, Shiraishi Y, Takahashi M, et al. Exome sequencing identifies secondary mutations of SETBP1 and JAK3 in juvenile myelomonocytic leukemia. Nat Genet. 2013;45(8):937–41.
147. Stieglitz E, Troup CB, Gelston LC, Haliburton J, Chow ED, Yu KB, et al. Subclonal mutations in SETBP1 confer a poor prognosis in juvenile myelomonocytic leukemia. Blood. 2015;125(3):516–24.
148. Niemeyer CM. JMML genomics and decisions. Hematology Am Soc Hematol Educ Program. 2018;2018(1):307–12.
149. Lipka DB, Witte T, Toth R, Yang J, Wiesenfarth M, Nollke P, et al. RAS-pathway mutation patterns define epigenetic subclasses in juvenile myelomonocytic leukemia. Nat Commun. 2017;8(1):2126.
150. Stieglitz E, Ward AF, Gerbing RB, Alonzo TA, Arceci RJ, Liu YL, et al. Phase II/III trial of a pre-transplant farnesyl transferase inhibitor in juvenile myelomonocytic leukemia: a report from the Children's Oncology Group. Pediatr Blood Cancer. 2015;62(4):629–36.
151. Patnaik MM, Tefferi A. Refractory anemia with ring sideroblasts (RARS) and RARS with thrombocytosis (RARS-T): 2017 update on diagnosis, risk-stratification, and management. Am J Hematol. 2017;92(3):297–310.
152. Malcovati L, Della Porta MG, Pietra D, Boveri E, Pellagatti A, Galli A, et al. Molecular and clinical features of refractory anemia with ringed sideroblasts associated with marked thrombocytosis. Blood. 2009;114(17):3538–45.
153. Broseus J, Florensa L, Zipperer E, Schnittger S, Malcovati L, Richebourg S, et al. Clinical features and course of refractory anemia with ring sideroblasts associated with marked thrombocytosis. Haematologica. 2012;97(7):1036–41.
154. Patnaik MM, Lasho TL, Finke CM, Hanson CA, King RL, Ketterling RP, et al. Predictors of survival in refractory anemia with ring sideroblasts and thrombocytosis (RARS-T) and the role of next-generation sequencing. Am J Hematol. 2016;91(5):492–8.
155. Cortelazzo S, Finazzi G, Ruggeri M, Vestri O, Galli M, Rodeghiero F, et al. Hydroxyurea for patients with essential thrombocythemia and a high risk of thrombosis. N Engl J Med. 1995;332(17):1132–6.
156. Huls G, Mulder AB, Rosati S, van de Loosdrecht AA, Vellenga E, de Wolf JT. Efficacy of single-agent lenalidomide in patients with JAK2 (V617F) mutated refractory anemia with ring sideroblasts and thrombocytosis. Blood. 2010;116(2):180–2.
157. Garcia-Manero G. Myelodysplastic syndromes: 2015 update on diagnosis, risk-stratification and management. Am J Hematol. 2015;90(9):831–41.
158. Pardanani A, Lasho TL, Laborde RR, Elliott M, Hanson CA, Knudson RA, et al. CSF3R T618I is a highly prevalent and specific mutation in chronic neutrophilic leukemia. Leukemia. 2013;27(9):1870–3.
159. Voulgarelis M, Giannouli S, Ritis K, Tzioufas AG. Myelodysplasia-associated autoimmunity: clinical and pathophysiologic concepts. Eur J Clin Investig. 2004;34(10):690–700.
160. Elbaek MV, Sorensen AL, Hasselbalch HC. Chronic inflammation and autoimmunity as risk factors for the development of chronic myelomonocytic leukemia? Leuk Lymphoma. 2016;57(8):1793–9.
161. Grignano E, Mekinian A, Braun T, Liozon E, Hamidou M, Decaux O, et al. Autoimmune and inflammatory diseases associated with chronic myelomonocytic leukemia: a series of 26 cases and literature review. Leuk Res. 2016;47:136–41.
162. Jachiet V, Mekinian A, Carrat F, Grignano E, Retbi A, Boffa JJ, et al. Autoimmune manifestations associated with lymphoma: characteristics and outcome in a multicenter retrospective cohort study. Leuk Lymphoma. 2018;59(6):1399–405.
163. Montoro J, Gallur L, Merchan B, Molero A, Roldan E, Martinez-Valle F, et al. Autoimmune disorders are common in myelodysplastic syndrome patients and confer an adverse impact on outcomes. Ann Hematol. 2018;97(8):1349–56.
164. Kosmider O, Itzykson R, Chesnais V, Lasho T, Laborde R, Knudson R, et al. Mutation of the colony-stimulating factor-3 receptor gene is a rare event with poor prognosis in chronic myelomonocytic leukemia. Leukemia. 2013;27(9):1946–9.
165. Ouyang Y, Qiao C, Chen Y, Zhang SJ. Clinical significance of CSF3R, SRSF2 and SETBP1 mutations in chronic neutrophilic leukemia and chronic myelomonocytic leukemia. Oncotarget. 2017;8(13):20834–41.

Plasma Cell Neoplasms (Including Plasma Cell Myeloma)

26

Chuanyi Mark Lu

List of Frequently Asked Questions

1. What is the clinical and pathological spectrum of plasma cell neoplasms?
2. What are the typical morphological findings in plasma cell myeloma and other plasma cell neoplasms?
3. Which diagnostic tests are used to detect monoclonal gammopathy and to quantify monoclonal immunoglobulin produced by plasma cell neoplasms?
4. How to quantify myeloma plasma cells in bone marrow samples?
5. What are the immunophenotypes of reactive and neoplastic plasma cells?
6. How to confirm the monoclonality of neoplastic plasma cells?
7. What additional clinical and radiographic evidence should be obtained in a suspected case of plasma cell myeloma?
8. How to differentiate non-IgM MGUS, asymptomatic (smoldering) myeloma, and symptomatic multiple myeloma?
9. What are the plasma cell myeloma variants, and how to diagnose each variant type?
10. How to define and diagnose solitary plasmacytoma and primary amyloidosis?
11. What is the clinical utility of fluorescent in situ hybridization (FISH) analysis in plasma cell myeloma?
12. What are the mimics of plasma cell neoplasm that could be misinterpreted and mistreated as plasma cell myeloma?
13. What are POEMS syndrome and TEMPI syndrome?
14. How to evaluate and report response to treatment of symptomatic multiple myeloma?

C. M. Lu (✉)
Department of Laboratory Medicine, University of California San Francisco and San Francisco VA Healthcare System, San Francisco, CA, USA
e-mail: mark.lu@va.gov

1. What is the clinical and pathological spectrum of plasma cell neoplasms?

- Plasma cell neoplasms (also known as plasma cell dyscrasias) are diseases in which abnormal clonal plasma cells proliferate and form abnormal infiltrates and sometimes mass lesions in the bones or soft tissue of the body. These neoplastic proliferations of plasma cells produce abnormal monoclonal immunoglobulin (known as monoclonal gammopathy) [1].
- The major subtypes of plasma cell neoplasms include non-IgM monoclonal gammopathy of undetermined significance (MGUS), plasma cell myeloma, plasmacytoma, monoclonal immunoglobulin deposition diseases (e.g., primary amyloidosis), and plasma cell neoplasms with associated paraneoplastic syndrome (Table 26.1).
  - Plasma cell myeloma can be further subclassified as symptomatic plasma cell myeloma (or multiple myeloma), asymptomatic (smoldering) myeloma, nonsecretory myeloma, and plasma cell leukemia. Nonsecretory myeloma and plasma cell leukemia are rare (Table 26.1).
  - With an estimated incidence of 6 cases per 100,000 persons per year, symptomatic multiple myeloma represents the second most common hematologic malignancy and approximately 1% of all cancers. Non-IgM MGUS is present in 3–4% of general population over the age of 50 years and is considered a precursor lesion for plasma cell myeloma (the overall risk of progression to myeloma is about 1% per year) [2].
- Plasma cell neoplasms are characterized by histopathologic evidence of clonal plasma cell proliferation and presence of a monoclonal intact immunoglobulin (monoclonal spike or M spike, or paraprotein) and/or monoclonal free light chain (FLC, not in association with immunoglobulin heavy chains) in serum and/or urine. The monoclonal free light chain (κ or λ type) present in urine is traditionally known as Bence–Jones protein (BJP).

E. Wang, A. S. Lagoo (eds.), *Practical Lymph Node and Bone Marrow Pathology*, Practical Anatomic Pathology,
https://doi.org/10.1007/978-3-030-32189-5_26

Table 26.1 Clinical types of plasma cell neoplasms [1]

Non-IgM monoclonal gammopathy of undetermined significance (MGUS)	– IgG–MGUS – IgA–MGUS – Light chain MGUS – IgD–MGUS (rare)
Plasma cell myeloma	– Symptomatic multiple myeloma – Asymptomatic (smoldering) myeloma – Nonsecretory myeloma (rare) – Plasma cell leukemia (rare)
Plasmacytoma	– Solitary plasmacytoma of bone – Extraosseous (extramedullary) plasmacytoma
Monoclonal immunoglobulin deposition diseases	– Primary amyloidosis – Systemic light or heavy chain deposition disease
Plasma cell neoplasm with associated paraneoplastic syndrome	– POEMS syndrome – TEMPI syndrome (provisional)

- Clinically, plasma cell neoplasms show a spectrum of progressively worse diseases, varying from asymptomatic to overtly symptomatic forms. Patients with MGUS are asymptomatic without organ dysfunction, whereas patients with multiple myeloma have bone marrow involvement and often have immune dysfunction, peripheral cytopenias, lytic bone lesions, and/or organ dysfunction (e.g., renal failure). In contrast, patients with plasmacytoma have well-defined proliferation of clonal plasma cells that occur either inside a bone (solitary bone plasmacytoma) or outside bone (extramedullary or extraosseous plasmacytoma).
- Percentage of plasma cells in bone marrow is <10% in MGUS and typically (but not necessarily) ≥10% in plasma cell myeloma. In plasmacytoma, there is no or only minimal (<10%) clonal plasmacytosis in bone marrow.
- There are also other immunoglobulin-secreting neoplasms that consist of both clonal lymphocytes and plasma cells, including lymphoplasmacytic lymphoma/Waldenstrom macroglobulinemia (LPL/WM) and heavy chain diseases (μ, γ, and α type HCD). Alpha(α) HCD is an immunoproliferative small intestinal disease with features resembling MALT lymphoma. Gamma (γ) HCD has features resembling LPL/WM, while Mu (μ) HCD has features mimicking chronic lymphocytic leukemia (CLL).

2. What are the typical morphological findings in plasma cell myeloma and other plasma cell neoplasms?

- A bone marrow aspirate and trephine biopsy of posterior iliac crest(s) are key components required for the evaluation and diagnosis of plasma cell myeloma and other plasma cell neoplasms. Presence of monoclonal plasma cells in bone marrow is the typical finding in most plasma cell neoplasms, and the estimated percentage of plasma cells among all nucleated bone marrow cells is an important parameter of disease severity.
- On bone marrow biopsy and aspirate clot sections, plasma cells may be scattered interstitially, in small clusters, in focal solid aggregates, or in diffuse sheets. On patient follow-up, there is often progression from interstitial and/or focal disease with areas of preserved hematopoiesis in early plasma cell myeloma to diffuse involvement with large solid plasma cell aggregates in advanced stage of disease.
  - Although coexistence of normal and malignant plasma cells in bone marrow can be demonstrated in all MGUS cases, in plasma cell myeloma, such coexistence is less frequent (<25% of cases) [3].
- The bone marrow plasma cell percentage of total marrow nucleated cells should be estimated individually from all available morphological slides including aspirate smears, core biopsy, and clot sections.
  - Immunohistochemistry is useful in quantifying plasma cells on biopsy and aspirate clot sections, and in confirming a monoclonal proliferation of plasma cells.
  - CD138 staining is often used for quantifying plasma cells, and κ and λ light chain staining can help establish monoclonality (light-chain restriction), respectively. If the plasma cell percentage on aspirate smears and biopsy sections differs, the higher value should be used [4, 5].
  - Flow cytometry analysis of aspirate marrow sample is also used to confirm monoclonality and phenotypic abnormality of the plasma cells, but is unreliable in quantifying plasma cells because it often significantly underestimates the percentage of plasma cells.
- Cytomorphology of abnormal plasma cells: On aspirate smears, malignant plasma cells vary from mature forms (morphologically similar to benign plasma cells), immature or plasmablastic forms, to less commonly seen small-cell variant, and anaplastic or pleomorphic forms.
  - Plasma cells of mature forms are often round or oval shaped, with moderately abundant basophilic cytoplasm and a perinuclear hof (cytoplasmic clearing), a round eccentric nucleus, and mature nuclear chromatin ("spoke-wheel" or "clock-face" like) without nucleoli (Fig. 26.1a).
  - Immature forms have open or dispersed chromatin, high nuclear-to-cytoplasmic (N/C) ratio, and often prominent nucleoli (plasmablastic form) (Fig. 26.1b).
  - The small-cell variant shows a lymphoplasmacytic appearance, with a narrow rim of cytoplasm and occasional perinuclear hof (Fig. 26.1c). Of note, small-cell or lymphoplasmacytic variant is often associated with presence of t(11;14)(q13;q32) involving *CCND1* gene.

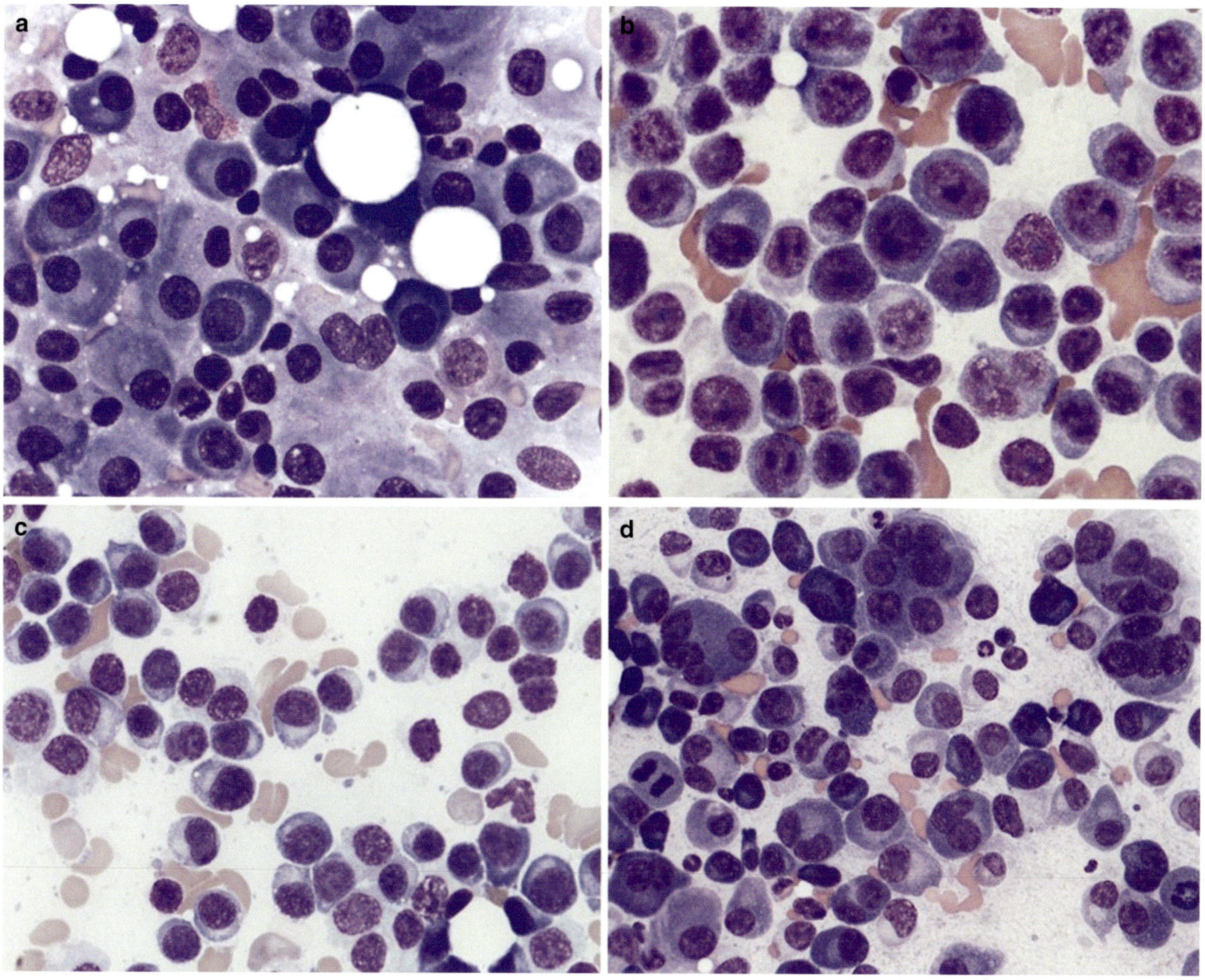

Fig. 26.1 (**a**) Bone marrow aspirate smear from a 53-year-old man shows a focal area with 85% myeloma plasma cells. Giemsa stain. (**b**) Bone marrow aspirate smear from a 68-year-old man shows 90% myeloma plasma cells (plasmablastic morphology). (**c**) Bone marrow aspirate smear from a 68-year-old man shows 85% myeloma plasma cells (small and lymphoplasmacytic variant). Cytogenetic analysis revealed t(11;14) with *CCND1* rearrangement. (**d**) Bone marrow aspirate smear from a 60-year-old man shows 75% myeloma plasma cells (~15% of the plasma cells are large and anaplastic forms). Cytogenetic analysis revealed a very complex karyotype. (**a–d**) Giemsa stain, original magnification ×1000

  - Plasma cells of anaplastic or pleomorphic forms are large and often multinucleated or multilobated, sometimes resembling megakaryocytes on biopsy sections (Figs. 26.1d and 26.2). When present, the proportion of pleomorphic or anaplastic plasma cells in plasma cell myeloma varies from case to case, from less than 5% to 25–50% or higher (higher numbers are often seen in refractory and relapsed cases).
  - In most myeloma cases, binucleated plasma cells are readily identifiable, but by themselves are not indicative of a neoplastic plasma cell population. On the other hand, trinucleation or multinucleation is seen in neoplastic plasma cells.
- Malignant plasma cells have abundant endoplasmic reticulum, which may contain intact or truncated immunoglobulin that is condensed or crystallized, manifesting as a variety of morphological findings in some cases. These include Mott cells (Fig. 26.3a) and morula cells (grape-like cytoplasmic accumulations), Russell bodies (cherry-red refractive round bodies), flame cells (typically IgA myeloma cells with glycogen-rich IgA) (Fig. 26.3b), and crystalline inclusions (Fig. 26.3c). Mott cells and Russell bodies can be prominently present in some cases (Fig. 26.3a). Rarely, plasma cells with Dutcher bodies (Fig. 26.3d) are seen in plasma cell myeloma, which are actually cytoplasmic inclusions that are invaginated into the nucleus (pseudo intranuclear inclusions).
- Amyloid deposition (AL amyloidosis) may be present on bone marrow biopsy sections (interstitial or vascular

Fig. 26.2 Bone marrow biopsy section from a 60-year-old man shows 75% myeloma plasma cells (~15% of the plasma cells are large and anaplastic forms, resembling atypical megakaryocytes). Cytogenetic analysis revealed a very complex karyotype. H/E, original magnification ×1000

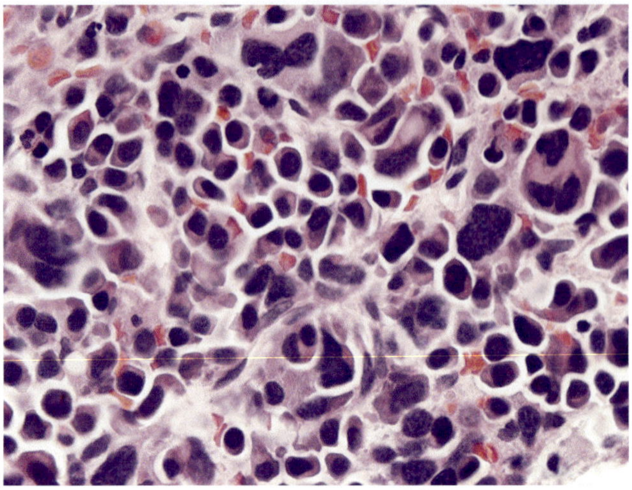

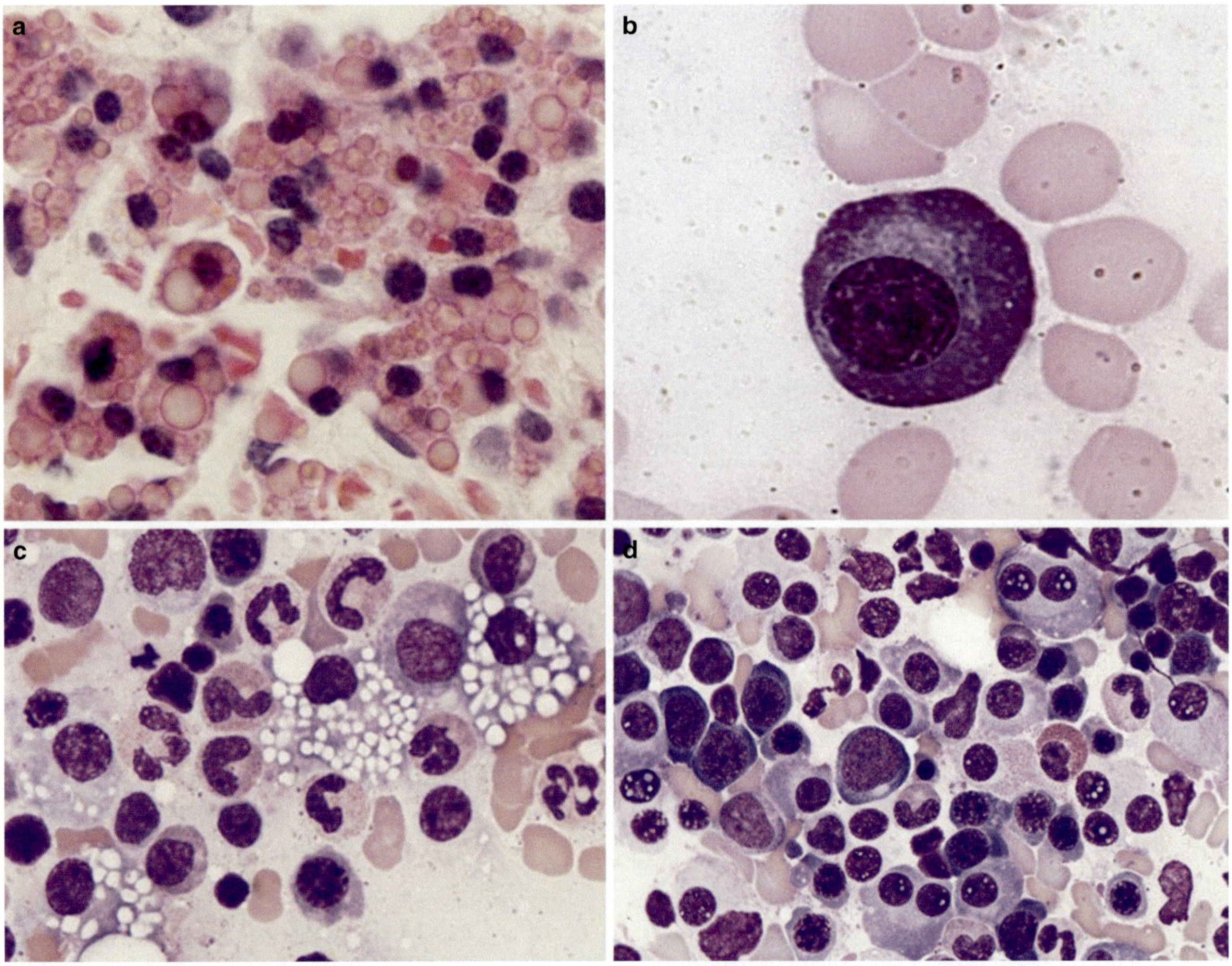

Fig. 26.3 (**a**) Bone marrow biopsy from a 60-year-old man shows 75% myeloma plasma cells, with the majority containing numerous and variably sized Russell bodies in its cytoplasm (so-called Mott cells). There is concomitant myelofibrosis (MF2–3). H/E, original magnification ×1000. (**b**) Flame cells in a bone marrow aspirate smear from a patient with IgA multiple myeloma. Giemsa stain, original magnification ×1000. (**c**) Bone marrow aspirate smear from a 77-year-old man showing a focal area with 25% myeloma plasma cells (approximately 50% of the plasma cells contain crystalline inclusions in its cytoplasm). Giemsa stain, original magnification ×1000. (**d**) Bone marrow aspirate smear from a 61-year-old man shows 35% myeloma plasma cells (approximately 25% of the plasma cells exhibit 1 or 2–4 intranuclear inclusions, so-called Dutcher bodies). Giemsa stain, original magnification ×1000

deposits), and can be confirmed by Congo red staining or electron microscopy. Marked myelofibrosis (MF2–3 on scale of 0–3) is occasionally observed in plasma cell myeloma.

3. Which diagnostic tests are used to detect monoclonal gammopathy and to quantify monoclonal immunoglobulin produced by plasma cell neoplasms?

- Malignant, clonal plasma cells typically produce and secrete a monoclonal protein (M protein), causing monoclonal gammopathy (also known as paraproteinemia). M protein can be detected by serum protein electrophoresis (SPEP) and/or urine protein electrophoresis (UPEP) combined with immunofixation electrophoresis (IFE) and by the serum free light chain (FLC) assays.
  - The M protein in plasma cell neoplasms can be an intact immunoglobulin (i.e., containing both heavy chain and light chains), can be composed of only light chains (e.g., light chain only myeloma), or rarely can consist of heavy chain only (e.g., heavy chain disease).
  - In plasma cell myelomas, approximately 50% serum M proteins are IgG type, 20% IgA, 20% κ or λ light only, 2% bi-clonal, 1% IgD, 1% IgE, <1% IgM, and 1–3% nonsecretory (no detectable M protein). The serum M protein is usually >3.0 g/dL of IgG and >2.0 g/dL of IgA type [1]. Reduction of uninvolved immunoglobulin is seen in 80–90% of patients with plasma cell myeloma.
- Serum protein electrophoresis (SPEP), along with immunofixation electrophoresis (IFE), is used to detect presence or absence of an M protein and to measure the level ("size") of the M protein in serum.
  - SPEP is usually done by the agarose gel method (agarose gel electrophoresis). If an M protein is detected, IFE is then performed to determine the exact heavy and light type of the M protein (so-called immunotyping). Monoclonal band detected can further be quantified using densitometry, in conjunction with the total serum protein concentration.
  - Capillary zone electrophoresis (CZE) (Fig. 26.4), along with immunosubtraction electrophoresis (Fig. 26.5), is an alternative method of performing SPEP. The CZE electrophoretograms are similar to those produced with agarose gel.
  - The relative sensitivities of agarose gel electrophoresis versus CZE for initial screening are comparable. While the specificity of gel-based IFE and capillary electrophoresis-based immunosubtraction for detecting M protein is similar, the latter has slightly lower sensitivity for IgM and light chain types of M protein [6].

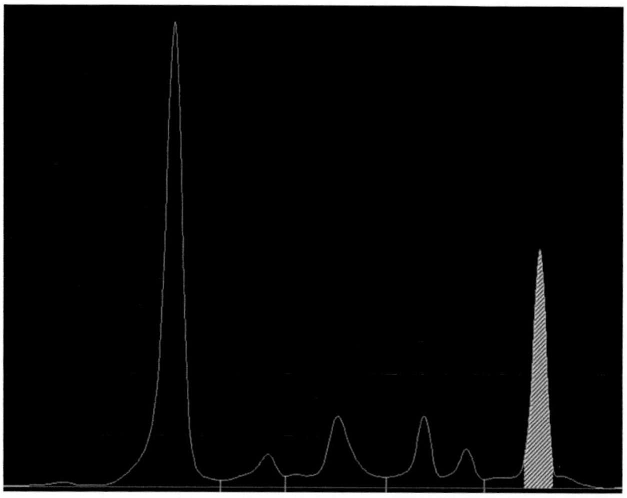

Fig. 26.4 Capillary zone electrophoresis (CZE)-based serum protein electropherogram of a 59-year-old male shows a monoclonal band (M protein) in the gamma region

- Serum free light chain (FLC) assays: The serum FLC assay is a sensitive, antibody-based system that can detect low concentrations of monoclonal free light chains (i.e., κ or λ) in the serum, using polyclonal antibodies directed against "hidden" epitopes on FLC molecules [7, 8].
  - This assay is of particular utility in patients with plasma cell neoplasms which produce only a free light chain that is not bound to a heavy chain (e.g., "light chain only" myeloma). Such abnormal light chains are detectable only in urine samples by traditional methods (called Bence–Jones protein or BJP). The FLC assay can detect low concentrations of monoclonal free light chains in serum.
  - For myelomas secreting intact monoclonal immunoglobulins, an excess of light chains is also produced during immunoglobulin synthesis. In these cases, compared to serum IFE, FLC assays have higher sensitivity for M protein detection (2–4 mg/L by FLC assays versus 100–150 mg/L by IFE).
  - Normal levels of serum FLC in healthy volunteers are as follows (95% confidence intervals): serum free κ light chains 3.3–19.4 mg/L, serum free λ light chains 5.7–26.3 mg/L, and serum free serum κ to λ light chain ratio (sFLC ratio) 0.26–1.65.
  - The diagnostic benefits of sFLC ratio include the following: (1) it provides a quantitative assessment of clonality; and (2) it also reflects the suppression of uninvolved (nontumor) FLC.
  - The serum FLC assay is more sensitive for the detection of monoclonal free light chains than urine IFE [9].

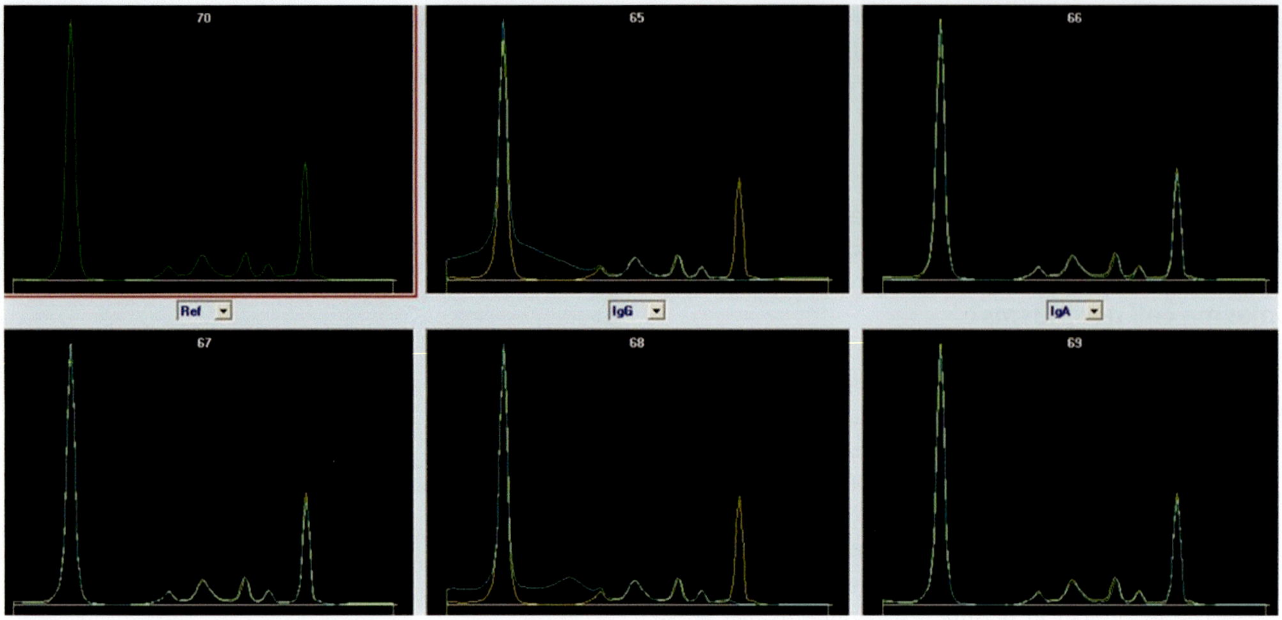

Fig. 26.5 Capillary zone electrophoresis (CZE)-based immunosubtraction electropherograms of a 59-year-old male identify an IgG-kappa paraprotein in patient's serum sample

  The serum FLC assay has essentially eliminated the need for UPEP on a 24-hour urine collection when screening for myeloma and other plasma cell neoplasms, because SPEP/IFE plus serum FLC assay have nearly 100% sensitivity in detecting plasma cell myeloma, and UPEP adds no additional value.
  - The serum FLC assay is also used to assess treatment response in patients with multiple myeloma, and has been incorporated into the criteria of response to treatment of multiple myeloma (see Question #14)
- Urine protein electrophoresis (UPEP): With the availability of serum FLC assay, UPEP is no longer required in the screening for plasma cell myeloma in patients without significant baseline renal insufficiency. Its clinical utility is limited to nephrotoxicity assessment and treatment monitoring in patients with myeloma. Patients with a diagnosis of a plasma cell myeloma should have a baseline UPEP (and IFE if indicated) of an aliquot from a 24-hour urine collection. This test is essential to detect the presence of potentially nephrotoxic concentrations of urinary light chains. UPEP testing can subsequently be used to detect progression and to monitor response to therapy in patients who have urinary monoclonal light chains at baseline.
  - UPEP still has a diagnostic value in patients with baseline renal insufficiency. It has been reported that serum κ light chains are disproportionately increased and the sFLC ratio may increase up to 3.0 in patients with dialysis-dependent renal failure [10]. A sFLC ratio >3.0 is unlikely due to renal insufficiency alone, but it could be difficult to interpret sFLC ratios between 1.65 and 3.0 in the context of renal insufficiency. In such cases, further investigation with UPEP (and IFE if indicated) on a 24-hour urine collection helps to guide interpretation. If UPEP/IFE are normal and the patient has no other findings suggestive of a plasma cell neoplasm, then the slight elevation of sFLC ratio is likely due to the renal insufficiency. Conversely, it should be noted that patients with a λ monoclonal gammopathy and renal insufficiency may have sFLC ratios within normal limits (0.26–1.65) and UPEP/IFE may help in such cases.
- Serum immunoglobulin quantitation: Quantitation of serum immunoglobulins is usually ordered for the detection of hypogammaglobulinemia. It is also a useful adjunct to SPEP, serum FLC assay, and UPEP in following patients with plasma cell myeloma, i.e., to assess response to treatment. When assessing treatment response, SPEP values should only be compared with SPEP values, and quantitative immunoglobulin values only with quantitative immunoglobulin values.
  - It has been observed that immunoglobulins (IgM in particular) are often overestimated by quantitative nephelometry assays. It is recommended that SPEP followed by densitometry (or CZE-based SPEP) is preferable, as these results usually more closely agree with the clinical presentation [11]. In addition, quantitative immunoglobulin assays do not allow an assessment of monoclonality. Increased levels (IgG, IgA, or IgM) can be due to polyclonal or monoclonal eleva-

Table 26.2 Diagnostic criteria for non-IgM MGUS and plasma cell myeloma

Non-IgM MGUS: – Serum M protein (non-IgM) <3.0 g/dL – Bone marrow plasma cells (clonal) <10% – Absence of end-organ damage ("CRAB")[b] and amyloidosis attributable to proliferation of clonal plasma cells *Light-chain MGUS:* – Abnormal serum free light chain ratio – Increased level of the involved free light chain – No Ig heavy chain expression on IFE – Urinary M protein ("BJP") <500 mg/24 hour – Bone marrow plasma cells (clonal) <10% – Absence of end-organ damage ("CRAB") and amyloidosis	*Asymptomatic (smoldering) plasma cell myeloma:* – Serum M protein (IgG or IgA) ≥3.0 g/dL or urinary M protein ("BJP") ≥500 mg/24 hour and/or bone marrow clonal plasma cells 10–60% – Absence of end-organ damage ("CRAB") and amyloidosis – An involved-to-uninvolved serum light chain ratio <100	*Symptomatic plasma cell myeloma (multiple myeloma)*[a]*:* Presence of clonal plasma cells in bone marrow (≥10%) or biopsy-proven plasmacytoma PLUS ≥1 of the following: – End-organ damage attributable to proliferation of clonal plasma cells ("CRAB") – Clonal bone marrow plasma cells ≥60% – An involved-to-uninvolved serum light chain ratio ≥100 (provided involved free light chain is ≥10 mg/dL) – More than one (≥2) focal lesion on MRI (≥5 mm, involving bone or bone marrow)

[a]*In about 5% of cases of symptomatic myeloma, bone marrow plasma cells (clonal) is <10% due to sampling-related underestimation. Approximately 40% of cases of symptomatic myeloma have a serum M protein of <3.0 g/dL. In true nonsecretory myeloma (1–2% of PCM), no M protein is detectable in serum and urine*

[b] "*CRAB*", hyper *C*alcemia, *R*enal insufficiency, *A*nemia, lytic *B*one lesions

tions. Gel-based IFE or capillary electrophoresis-based immunosubtraction has to be used to confirm monoclonality.

- Emerging new laboratory tests for M protein detection and quantitation: The heavy-light chain (HLC) assay is being introduced as an alternative methodology for monoclonal gammopathy evaluation, giving an independent measure of intact Ig-κ and Ig-λ concentrations. HLC assays for IgGκ, IgGλ, IgAκ, IgAλ, IgMκ, and IgMλ are available [12].
  - As the antibodies bind to junctional regions between the κ or λ light chain and its respective heavy chain partner, the combination of κ- and λ-type immunoglobulin measurements allows for the accurate quantification of involved and uninvolved intact immunoglobulins.
  - Clonality is assessed by calculating the ratio of involved immunoglobulin to background uninvolved immunoglobulin concentrations (e.g., IgAκ/IgAλ in an IgAκ myeloma patient).
  - The HLC assay also measures levels of the uninvolved immunoglobulin chain that serves as parameter of suppression, which itself can serve as a biomarker of clinical status.

4. How to quantify myeloma plasma cells in bone marrow samples?

In patients with plasma cell myeloma, the proportion of plasma cells on aspirate smears and biopsy sections varies significantly (typical 10–90% plasma cells), depending on not only the clinical stage but also bone marrow sampling.

- Specimen sampling error is inevitable since bone marrow involvement is often patchy and uneven [13], and the estimated plasma cell percentage from bone marrow samples may not represent actual tumor burden in the body.
- Plasma cell quantification in bone marrow samples is important in the diagnosis and discrimination of various plasma cell neoplasms, especially between MGUS and asymptomatic (smoldering) myeloma as well as between asymptomatic (smoldering) and symptomatic myelomas (Table 26.2). Evaluation of plasma cell number is also used in assessing treatment response and minimal residual disease (MRD) (see Question #14).
- It is generally agreed that plasma cell percentage is best estimated from high-quality aspirate smears stained with Giemsa and biopsy sections immunohistochemically stained for CD138.
  - CD138 is a specific marker for plasma cells in bone marrow samples because all other native bone marrow cells are negative (NB: metastatic epithelial neoplasms of various origins express CD138). CD138 immunostaining allows assessment of plasma cell number and distribution in bone marrow biopsy. Biopsy-based, CD138+ plasma cell percentage is usually higher and more accurate than that of aspirate smears, as aspirate is variably hemodiluted. If the plasma cell percentage estimated from aspirate smears and biopsy differs significantly, the higher value should be used [5].
  - Because plasma cells are typically larger than majority of hematopoietic cells, visual overview CD138 estimates can be influenced by the relatively larger stained area of plasma cells and therefore could overestimate plasma cell percentage.
  - The accuracy of plasma cell estimate may also be influenced by the patchy distribution pattern of

plasma cells within the marrow. Selected area counting technique has been used to help avoid overestimation of CD138+ plasma cells by visual overview [14]. After initial scan of the biopsy section at low and intermediate magnification, an area of 200–300 cells within the section, judged to have approximately the same concentration of plasma cells in the section as a whole, is selected for counting at high magnification. Plasma cells and other nucleated cells in the selected area are individually counted with a differentiation cell counter, and the calculated percentage is reported.
  - Plasma cell percentage cannot be reliably estimated from H&E-stained sections of bone marrow core biopsy, as malignant plasma cells can resemble hematopoietic precursors (e.g., early granulocytic precursors). Although it may be easier to differentiate plasma cells from blasts and granulocytic precursors on Giemsa-stained sections (adopted by some hematopathology groups), underestimation of plasma cell proportion remains a concern.
- Flow cytometry analysis of aspirate sample cannot accurately determine plasma cell percentage [15]. It is well accepted that the percentage of plasma cells is often underrepresented by flow cytometry as compared to morphological methods (e.g., aspirate smears, biopsy section stained for CD138). There are several factors that could be responsible for the observation:
  - Exclusion of lipid phase-associated plasma cell population, as malignant plasma cells are more associated with lipid-enriched marrow spicules in morphology slides, as opposed to lipid-depleted liquid bone marrow analyzed by flow cytometry [16].
  - Significant hemodilution in aspirate samples designated for flow cytometry analysis (and other laboratory tests), as the first aspiration pull is typically used for morphology slides (aspirate smears).
  - Disproportional loss of plasma cells during sample preparation, reportedly due to higher susceptibility of plasma cells for mechanical damage.

High-sensitivity multiparametric flow cytometry (next-generation flow cytometry) has been used for detecting minimal residual disease (MRD) after treatment or autologous stem cell transplant. For MRD detection, highly representative and nonhemodiluted aspirate samples are crucial. It is highly recommended to use the first aspirate pull for flow cytometry-based MRD assessment. The adoption of sample preparation methods that have been validated and has demonstrated superior plasma cell recovery is recommended.

5. What is the immunophenotype of reactive and neoplastic plasma cells?

The immunophenotypic evaluation for plasma cell myeloma is performed with flow cytometry, immunohistochemistry (IHC), or a combination of both. The immunophenotype of malignant plasma cells (myeloma cells) mirrors the immunophenotype of benign reactive plasma cells, but with aberrant antigen expression.

- Normal mature plasma cells typically lack expression of most pan-B cell markers (e.g., CD20, CD22) and surface immunoglobulins but express CD19, CD27, CD38, CD79a, CD81, CD138 (Syndecan-1), CD269 (BCMA), CD319 (SLAMF7), and MUM1/IRF4. The expression of CD45 in benign plasma cells is dim to moderate, while CD56 expression is negative or very weak. Normal plasma cells are variably positive for epithelial membrane antigen (EMA).
- Neoplastic plasma cells express CD38 and CD138, but CD138 expression is brighter than in benign plasma cells. Compared to benign plasma cells, neoplastic plasma cells may aberrantly gain other markers such as CD28 (~40%), CD33 (10–20%), CD52 (8–15%), CD56 (75–80%), CD117 (25–35%), or CD200 (60–75%) and often lose CD27 and CD81. Expression of CD45, CD19, and PAX5 is often negative, and CD20 expression is positive in 10–20% of myeloma cases [17]. Aberrant antigen expression (e.g., CD56, CD117) helps to detect neoplastic (clonal) plasma cells.
- One important immunophenotypic feature of plasma cells is the coexpression of CD38 and CD138. CD38 is expressed on many immune cells, but its intensity is uniquely high on plasma cells, making it a useful marker for plasma cell gating on flow cytometry analysis. Conversely, CD138 is specific to plasma cells within bone marrow cell populations. Combined use of CD38 and CD138 is recommended for the identification of plasma cells by immunohistochemistry and flow cytometry in plasma cell neoplasms (plasma cell enumeration and monoclonality determination) [18]. CD319 has also been used in lieu of CD138 for neoplastic plasma cell isolation on flow cytometry analysis.
- Cyclin D1 is expressed in myeloma plasma cells with t(11;14)(q13;q32)/*IGH/CCND1* and some cases with hyperdiploidy. Overall, up to 30% of myeloma cases are positive for cyclin-D1. MYC expression may be detectable in some myeloma cases. *EBV* is typically negative in myeloma plasma cells.
- Elevated proliferation rate of plasma cells (≥5%) on Ki-67 staining (CD138 co-staining if available) has been correlated with more aggressive clinical course in multiple myeloma [19].

6. How to confirm the monoclonality of neoplastic plasma cells?

The general principles of determining monoclonality of plasma cells are similar to those used in B-cell lymphomas (see Chaps. 1 and 2). Neoplastic plasma cells, like all mature B-cell neoplasms, are characterized by monotypic expression of either κ or λ light chains (light chain restriction), demonstrable by flow cytometry and immunohistochemistry (IHC).

- The normal κ to λ ratio among normal bone marrow plasma cells is about 2:1. A ratio of more than 4:1 or less than 1:2 is used to define κ or λ monoclonality, respectively. This finding distinguishes the monoclonal gammopathies from reactive plasmacytosis (e.g., autoimmune diseases, chronic liver disease, acquired immunodeficiency syndrome, or chronic infection). When using flow cytometry, permeabilization of plasma cells is required because most plasma cells lack surface expression of immunoglobulins. The simultaneous detection of other phenotypic abnormalities (see Question 5) by multiparameter flow cytometry can help avoid missing the occasional bi-clonal plasma cell neoplasm [20].
- Polymerase chain reaction (PCR)-based immunoglobulin (Ig) gene rearrangement analysis can also be used to determine whether a plasma cell population is monoclonal in bone marrow aspirate samples as explained in Chap. 2. It should be noted that the detection of a dominant Ig gene rearrangement is neither 100% sensitive nor 100% specific for the presence of clonal plasma cell proliferation.
- If available, next-generation sequencing (NGS)-based assays can also be used for identifying uniquely rearranged immunoglobulin (Ig) VDJ sequence(s) ("signature" sequences in Ig-heavy, Ig-κ, and/or Ig-λ) in bone marrow samples from patient with plasma cell myeloma. However, the assays are typically used for posttreatment follow-up, not for initial diagnosis. Once the dominant, unique clonotype is identified in a patient's baseline sample, it can be used as molecular marker(s) for future treatment monitoring and minimal residual disease (MRD) measurement [21]. FDA-approved NGS-based test is available.
- As explained in Chap. 2 (Question 13), any of the molecular techniques can potentially show two clonal peaks (or bands) due to nonproductive rearrangement of the first allele followed by rearrangement of the second allele. In such cases, true bi-clonal process can be confirmed by appropriate findings in SPEP, IFE, and/or flow cytometry.

7. What additional clinical and radiographic evidence should be obtained in a suspected case of plasma cell myeloma?

Clinical workup of plasma cell myeloma is comprehensive and multidisciplinary, as listed below:

- Clinical evaluations of bone pain, unexplained anemia and/or weight loss, hypercalcemia, acute renal failure, neuropathy, etc.
- Laboratory testing, including CBC with differential and blood smear review, chemistry panels, SPEP/IFE, serum FLC, UPEP/IFE (only occasionally needed, see Question 3), serum viscosity, serum immunoglobulins, serum β_2-microglobulin, etc.
- Bone marrow examination with ancillary testing as needed, such as immunohistochemistry, flow cytometry, cytogenetics and FISH myeloma panel (see Question 11), and PCR and/or DNA sequencing-based assays (see Question 6)
- Radiographic imaging studies for lytic bone lesions, lymphadenopathy, and isolated tumor mass
- Tissue biopsy as needed (e.g., if solitary plasmacytoma or amyloidosis is suspected)

8. How to differentiate non-IgM MGUS, asymptomatic (smoldering) myeloma, and symptomatic multiple myeloma?

Non-IgM MGUS, asymptomatic (smoldering) myeloma, and symptomatic multiple myeloma fall in a spectrum of overlapping plasma cell neoplasms and may be difficult to differentiate from each other. Since the management strategies and treatment considerations are different for these entities, diagnostic discrimination of multiple myeloma from MGUS and asymptomatic (smoldering) myeloma is critically important.

- Non-IgM MGUS is considered precursor lesion of plasma cell myeloma, in which bone marrow plasma cells are less than 10% and serum M protein is below myeloma level.
- Asymptomatic (smoldering) myeloma is defined as having both of the following findings: (1) 10–59% clonal plasma cells in the marrow and/or an M protein at myeloma levels (i.e., serum IgG or IgA ≥3.0 g/dL or urinary Bence–Jones protein ≥500 mg/24 hours) and (2) no evidence of end-organ damage and amyloidosis. Most patients with asymptomatic (smoldering) myeloma have 10–20% plasma cells in the marrow, and the median level of serum M protein is about 3.0 g/dL. The majority of patients have suppressed normal polyclonal immunoglobulins.

- Symptomatic multiple myeloma is defined as having bone marrow plasma cells and/or M protein levels at myeloma levels, plus at least one of the following findings: (1) end-organ damage that can be clinically attributed to clonal plasma cell proliferation; (2) high numbers of bone marrow plasma cells (≥60%); (3) markedly increased involved-to-uninvolved serum free light chain (sFLC) ratio (≥100); and (4) MRI with more than one focal lesion >5 mm (involving bone or bone marrow) [1, 22].
- It is important to search for evidence of end-organ damage in all patients with a clonal plasma cell proliferation in the marrow, irrespective of the percentage of plasma cells, because end-organ damage is a defining feature that separates the rare cases of plasma cell myeloma with less than 10% marrow plasma cells from MGUS. While approximately 4% of patients diagnosed with symptomatic multiple myeloma have <10% plasma cells in bone marrow, many cases can be attributed to a sampling error related to patchy involvement of the marrow by neoplastic plasma cells [13]. In practice, however, any patient with evidence of end-organ damage but less than 10% bone marrow plasma cells and serum M protein below myeloma level should be carefully evaluated to rule out the possibility that the organ impairment is unrelated to clonal plasma cell proliferation (i.e., the patient actually has MGUS).
- Manifestations of end-organ damage are abbreviated by the acronym "CRAB" [1] and include the following:
  - Hypercalcemia: serum calcium >11 mg/dL (>2.75 mmol/L) or >1.0 mg/dL (>0.25 mmol/L) above the upper limit of normal (laboratory-specific).
  - *R*enal insufficiency: estimated or measured creatinine clearance <40 mL/min or serum creatinine >2.0 mg/dL (>177 μmol/L).
  - *A*nemia: hemoglobulin <10 g/dL (<100 g/L) or >2.0 g/dL (>20 g/L) below the lower limit of normal (laboratory-specific).
  - *B*one lesions: ≥1 osteolytic lesions (≥5 mm in size) on skeletal radiography, low-dose CT or PET/CT, or MRI.
- Manifestations of non-"CRAB" end-organ damage (e.g., hyperviscosity, recurrent bacterial infections, AL amyloidosis, and peripheral neuropathy) are considered nonspecific and not diagnostic of symptomatic multiple myeloma [22].
- The criteria for non-IgM MGUS, asymptomatic (smoldering) myeloma, and symptomatic multiple myeloma are listed in Table 26.2.

9. What are the plasma cell myeloma variants and how to diagnose each variant type?

- Asymptomatic (smoldering) myeloma [23]
  - The diagnostic criteria are listed in Table 26.2. Clinically, asymptomatic (smoldering) myeloma is similar to non-IgM MGUS (see Question 8) in its lack of clinical manifestations (no end-organ damage) but is much more likely to progress to symptomatic multiple myeloma (overall 5–10% per year versus 1% per year, respectively). Although immediate treatment is not indicated, patients with asymptomatic (smoldering) myeloma need more frequent follow-up compared to patients with MGUS: every 3–4 months versus once a year, respectively. Some patients with asymptomatic (smoldering) myeloma can remain stable without treatment over extended periods of time.
  - The cumulative probability of asymptomatic (smoldering) myeloma progression to symptomatic multiple myeloma or amyloidosis is approximately 10% per year for the first 5 years (5% for light chain only type), 2–3% per year for the next 5 years, and 1% per year thereafter.
  - Risk factors for early progression include the following: (1) presence of both ≥10% clonal plasma cells in marrow and ≥3.0 g/dL serum M protein; (2) high percentage of bone marrow plasma cells with an aberrant immunophenotype; (3) an abnormal serum free light chain (FLC) ratio (<0.125 or >8.0); (4) high plasma cell proliferation rate (e.g., ≥5% on Ki-67 staining); (5) presence of circulating plasma cells; (6) IgA isotype; (7) suppression of two uninvolved immunoglobulin isotypes; and (8) certain abnormal karyotype: t(4;14) or del(17p) or 1q gain.
- Nonsecretory myeloma, oligosecretory myeloma, and nonproducer myeloma
  - In about 1–3% of plasma cells, there is absence of an M protein by SPEP/IFE and UPEP/IFE. These rare cases are traditionally classified as nonsecretory myeloma. Acquired mutations in the immunoglobulin light chain variable and/or constant regions have been implicated in the development of nonsecretory state in neoplastic plasma cells. Nonsecretory myeloma must be distinguished from extremely rare IgD and IgE myelomas, as M protein of IgD or IgE isotype is not routinely screened for by IFE.
  - Up to two-thirds of IFE confirmed "nonsecretory" myeloma cases have abnormal serum FLC assay results (e.g., elevated serum free light chains, i.e., the involved FLC is ≥10 mg/dL, and/or abnormal serum FLC ratio). Such cases are now called oligosecretory (minimally secretory) myeloma [24]. Patients with myeloma who have normal serum and urine IFE as well as a normal serum FLC ratio are considered to have true nonsecretory myeloma (about one-third of "nonsecretory" cases). Of these true nonsecretory cases, approximately 85% have cytoplasmic M protein detectable by immunohistochemistry, indicating impaired secretion of immunoglobulin. In the other 15% of cases, no cytoplasmic immunoglobulin is

detectable. Such rare cases are called nonproducer myeloma and most are due to clonal but nonproductive rearrangement of both immunoglobulin alleles (see Question 6).
  - The clinical features, immunophenotype, genetics, and prognosis of nonsecretory myeloma are similar to those of other plasma cell myelomas, although survival appears to be better for patients with a normal baseline serum FLC ratio.
- Plasma cell leukemia
  - Plasma cell leukemia (PCL) is an uncommon but aggressive form of plasma cell myeloma. It is defined by the presence of >20% of plasma cells among total white cells or an absolute plasma cell count of >2.0 x10e9/L based on morphologic evaluation of peripheral blood smears. PCL is further classified as primary if it is an initial presentation of myeloma ("de novo") or as secondary when it is observed as a leukemic transformation in previously diagnosed multiple myeloma (relapsed or refractory myeloma). Both primary and secondary PCL have peripheral plasmacytosis and poor prognosis [25]. Based on published small case series, the median survival is short, ranging from 7 to 13 months, and overall survival rate at 5 years is less than 10%.
  - Phenotypically, compared to typical multiple myeloma, primary PCL is negative for CD56 and CD117 but more often expresses CD20, CD19, and CD45. Chromosome translocations involving 14q32 (IgH locus) are detectable in ~85% PCL cases. In primary PCL with IgH involvement, 11q13 (cyclin D1) is involved almost exclusively. The prevalence of poor risk findings such as del(17p), ampl(1q21), MYC abnormalities, and *RAS* mutations is significantly higher compared to newly diagnosed symptomatic multiple myelomas.
  - The median age of patients with primary PCL is about 10 years younger than the median age of common multiple myeloma and secondary PCL. In PCL, the bone marrow is usually extensively and diffusely infiltrated by neoplastic plasma cells. Plasma cells are also frequently detected in extramedullary sites such as the liver, spleen, body cavity effusions, and cerebral spinal fluid. Lymphadenopathy, organomegaly, and renal failure are more common, and lytic bone lesions and bone pain are less common. A higher proportion of PCL cases are of light chain only, oligosecretory, and IgE or IgD isotype compared to common symptomatic multiple myelomas.
  - At the time of diagnosis and follow-up assessment (e.g., remission status), the following evaluations should be carried out: (1) plasma cell count in peripheral blood; (2) plasma cell count in bone marrow; (3) serologic studies (serum M protein, urinary BJP, serum free light chains); and (4) evaluation of extramedullary involvement.

10. How to define and diagnose solitary plasmacytoma and primary amyloidosis?

- Solitary plasmacytoma
  - Solitary plasmacytoma is an infrequent form of plasma cell neoplasm that presents as a single mass of monoclonal plasma cells, located either extramedullary (extraosseous) or intraosseous [1, 26]. Monoclonality needs to be proven by κ or λ light chain restriction (flow cytometry and/or immunohistochemistry) or by a PCR-based assay. There is typically no or minimal monoclonal plasma cell infiltration in bone marrow. Imaging studies (skeletal survey and MRI or CT) are normal, except for the primary solitary lesion. Clinically there is absence of end-organ damage (i.e., no "CRAB").
  - Solitary bone plasmacytoma (SBP) is defined by the presence of a single lytic bone lesion due to monoclonal plasma cell proliferation, with or without soft-tissue extension. Extramedullary (extraosseous) plasmacytoma (EMP) is defined as localized plasma cell tumor in soft-tissue that is not in contact with bone (e.g., upper respiratory tract, gastrointestinal tract, lymph node).
  - Histomorphology, immunohistochemistry, and flow cytometry typically show no bone marrow plasmacytosis. Nevertheless, minimal bone marrow infiltration by clonal plasma cells (<10%) is still considered consistent with a plasmacytoma diagnosis, if no other lesions are observed (Table 26.3). Among patients with

Table 26.3 Differentiation of solitary plasmacytoma and plasma cell myeloma

	Plasmacytoma	Serum M protein	Bone marrow	"CRAB"	Imaging
Solitary plasmacytoma (SP)					
SP without BM involvement	Present	Not required	Negative	Absent	No other lesions
SP with minimal BM involvement	Present	Not required	<10% clonal PCs	Absent	No other lesions
Plasma cell myeloma					
Macrofocal myeloma	Present	Not required	<10% clonal PCs	Possible	Multiple lesions
Multiple myeloma	Not required	Present	≥10% clonal PCs	Present	Other lesions could be present

BM, bone marrow; *"CRAB"*, hyper *C*alcemia, *R*enal insufficiency, *A*nemia, lytic *B*one lesions; *PC*, plasma cells.

SBP, those with minimal bone marrow involvement have much higher risk of progression to multiple myeloma than those without marrow involvement (60% versus 10% within 3 years of diagnosis, respectively). The rate of progression to myeloma is lower in patients with EMP compared to patients with SBP.

- All patients with suspected plasmacytoma need to have bone marrow aspiration and biopsy to evaluate plasma cell morphology and the degree of plasma cell infiltration. The degree of clonal plasma cell infiltration should be determined by morphologic assessment and flow cytometry on the aspirate, and by immunohistochemistry on the biopsy (e.g., CD138 staining). Whole-body imaging studies (e.g., low-dose CT/PET-CT or MRI) are often required to exclude the presence of additional solitary lesion(s). Presence of multiple lesions of clonal plasma cells is indicative of plasma cell myeloma, with or without bone marrow involvement.
- Differentiation between primary extraosseous plasmacytoma and extraosseous infiltrates of plasma cell myeloma is often straightforward, as the latter is usually seen in patients with advanced or relapsed multiple myeloma. Also, t(11;14) translocation, expression of cyclin D1, and MYC rearrangement are not seen in extraosseous plasmacytoma.

• AL amyloidosis (primary amyloidosis): Primary (amyloid light chain) amyloidosis is a plasma cell neoplasm, characterized by deposition of linear nonbranching fibrils that are derived from misfolded and insoluble monoclonal immunoglobulin light chains (predominantly λ type). The constellation of clinical manifestation is different from that of symptomatic multiple myeloma.
  - The diagnosis of AL amyloidosis should be suspected from typical clinical findings, including macroglossia, malabsorption, nephrotic range proteinuria, and/or restrictive cardiomyopathy, along with a serum or urinary M protein. Tissue biopsy remains the gold standard for diagnosis of amyloidosis (e.g., bone marrow, rectum, and abdominal fat).
  - On H/E sections, amyloid is a pink, amorphous, waxy-looking substance with a cracking artifact, which can be further highlighted using Congo red staining and show typical apple-green birefringence in polarized microscopy. Electron microscopy can also be used to show the presence of amyloid fibrils. Rarely, organ parenchyma may be massively replaced by amyloid (nodular amyloid deposit), and clonal plasma cell infiltrates may be present in adjacent tissues.
  - A diagnosis of AL amyloidosis needs these two findings:
    1. Detection of amyloid deposition on biopsy of the abdominal fat, bone marrow, or the involved organ (e.g., kidney, heart, liver, and sural nerve) if necessary. Mass spectrometry-based proteomic analysis or immunoelectron microscopy can be used to confirm that the amyloid is light chain related.
    2. Evidence of a clonal plasma cell proliferative disorder (e.g., monoclonal gammopathy and/or presence of clonal plasma cells in bone marrow).
  - Bone marrow findings are highly variable, but there is typically only a mild increase in plasma cells. However, overt plasma cell myeloma with extensive marrow involvement may be present. Amyloid deposits in bone marrow are found in about 60% of cases of AL amyloidosis.

11. What is the clinical utility of fluorescent in-situ hybridization (FISH) analysis in plasma cell myeloma?

Cytogenetic abnormalities comprise one of the most important prognostic factors for plasma cell myeloma (Tables 26.4 and 26.5) [27, 28]. For newly diagnosed myeloma, metaphase cytogenetics and interphase FISH analyses using specific panel of probes should be performed. Of note, metaphase cytogenetics often fails to provide reliable information due to the low yield of plasma cells in bone marrow aspirate and the low proliferation rate of plasma cells. FISH panel is therefore an important alternative for evaluating chromosomal abnormalities in CD138 (or CD319)-enriched plasma cells from bone marrow aspirate samples. FISH can reveal abnormalities in >90% of patients. However, FISH analysis only provides information on regions interrogated by the probes used.

Table 26.4 The IMWG molecular cytogenetic classification of plasma cell myeloma [27, 29]

Genetic category	Proportion of cases
Hyperdiploid (gains in 3 or more of the odd-numbered chromosomes 3, 5, 7, 9, 11, 15, 19, and 21)	45%
Nonhyperdiploid	40%
Cyclin D gene translocation	18%
t(11;14)(q13;q32)	16%
t(6;14)(p25;q32)	2%
t(12;14)(p13;q32)	<1%
NSD2 translocation	15%
t(4;14)(p16;q32)	15%
MAF gene translocation	8%
t(14;16)(q32;q23)	5%
t(14;20)(q32;q11)	2%
t(8;14)(q24;q32)	1%
Unclassified (other)	15%

Table 26.5 Cytogenetics-based risk stratification of plasma cell myeloma [28, 29]

Standard risk (60%) t(11;14) t(6;14) Hyperdiploid All others	*Overall survival (OS):* 8–10 years
Intermediate risk (20%) t(4;14) del(13) Hypodiploid	OS: 4–5 years
High risk (20%) del(17p) t(14;16) t(14;20)	OS: 3 years

- The FISH panel at a minimum should include probes for the detection of the most frequent chromosomal aberrations in myeloma [29, 30]: gain(1q21), del(1p), del (13q14), 14q32 rearrangements [translocations t(4;14)(p16;q32), t(11;14) (q13;q32), t(14;16) (q32;q23), t(14;20)(q32;q11)], del (17p13), and trisomy of chromosomes 3, 5, 7, 9, 11, 15, 19, and 21. Note that del(13q) has been considered an adverse prognostic marker for multiple myeloma if it is detected by conventional cytogenetics, not by FISH.

12. What are the mimics of plasma cell neoplasm that could be misinterpreted and mistreated as plasma cell myeloma?

- Reactive polyclonal plasmacytosis
  - Marked reactive bone marrow plasmacytosis (reactive plasma cell hyperplasia) can be seen in a variety of clinical conditions, and should not be misinterpreted as plasma cell myeloma.

    Causes of reactive bone marrow plasmacytosis include cirrhosis, chronic viral and bacterial infections, autoimmune disorders, connective tissue and chronic granulomatous disorders, various solid tumors, multicentric Castleman's disease, status post-intensive chemotherapy, and drug-related agranulocytosis (e.g., levamisole-tainted cocaine and high-dose methimazole) [31].

    In reactive cases, plasma cells usually account for 10–20% of total nucleated bone marrow cells. In some conditions, however, bone marrow plasmacytosis can be massive (>60% of total) and extensively efface the bone marrow interstitium, mimicking multiple myeloma. Furthermore, marked polyclonal plasmacytosis (up to 20% of total) has been reported in multiple myeloma patients on prolonged lenalidomide maintenance therapy [32].

    Morphological features of reactive plasmacytosis include the following: (1) reactive plasma cells typically show normal cell morphology with mature chromatin (note that reactive plasma cells can be binucleated or rarely multinucleated and show cytoplasmic vacuoles) and (2) preservation of normal bone marrow architecture on trephine biopsy sections (i.e., interstitial and perivascular distribution pattern, without forming large solid plasma cell nodule or displacing marrow fat cells). Of note, perivascular plasma cell aggregates are not always benign and can be seen in up to one-third of patients with plasma cell myeloma. Immunophenotyping is the definitive tool to discriminate reactive polyclonal versus neoplastic monoclonal plasmacytosis.

    The pattern, extent, and clonality of bone marrow plasma cell infiltrates are best assessed by immunohistochemistry (CD138, κ, λ). In addition to polyclonal cytoplasmic immunoglobulin, reactive benign plasma cells are typically negative for CD56, whereas myeloma plasma cells often aberrantly express CD56 [33].

    If reactive plasmacytosis is suspected in multiple myeloma patients receiving lenalidomide maintenance therapy, multiparametric flow cytometry can help determine the percentage of malignant plasma cells among all bone marrow plasma cells [32].
- Lymphoplasmacytic lymphoma/Waldenstrom macroglobulinemia (LPL/WM) (see Chap 5 for fuller discussion of LPL/WM)
  - The differentiation between LPL/WM and symptomatic multiple myeloma is typically straightforward since the clinical and morphological features are different, plus the type of M protein seen in WM is rather unique (i.e., IgM, which rarely, if ever, occurs in multiple myeloma).

    In LPL/WM, a substantial lymphocytic component (often with plasmacytoid appearance) is present and expresses a clonal surface immunoglobulin of the same isotype as expressed by the plasma cells in the infiltrate. These cells express pan-B-cell antigens, CD19, CD20, CD22, and PAX5. The plasma cells (and plasmacytoid lymphocytes) do not show aberrant expression of CD56 or cyclin D1.

    Note that patients with multiple myeloma and t(11;14)(q13;q32) often have a lymphoplasmacytic or small mature plasma cell morphology, along with CD20 expression that may resemble LPL/WM. However, the t(11;14)(q13;q32)/*IGH/CCND1* translocation is not seen in LPL/WM.

    Bone marrow involved by LPL/WM often shows increase in background mast cells.

    True myeloma with an IgM paraprotein (IgM multiple myeloma) is extremely rare, comprising only 0.5% of myeloma in large case series. Diagnosis of IgM myeloma and its differentiation from LPL/WM require presence of either lytic bone lesions felt secondary to the plasma cell neoplasm or evidence of the t(11;14) translocation. If available, presence of *MYD88* L265P mutation is strongly indicative of LPL/WM, since the mutation is absent in IgM multiple myeloma. The cell morphology and expression of CD20 may not always be reliable discriminators in differentiation of IgM myeloma versus LPL/WM. Rare case of concomitant LPL/WM (positive for *MYD88* L265P mutation) and small cell variant of multiple myeloma with t(11;14)/*IGH-CCND1* has been reported [34].

- Plasmablastic lymphoma (see Chap. 6 for fuller discussion of this entity)
  - Plasmablastic lymphoma (PBL) is a rare aggressive lymphoma with a diffuse proliferation of large neoplastic cells, mostly resembling B immunoblasts or plasmablasts. It has following characteristics:

    Negative for CD20 and PAX5, but positive for CD138, CD38, and MUM1/IRF4 [1, 35], suggesting an origin from proliferating B cells that have switched to the plasma cell gene expression program.

    Often associated with immunosuppression (e.g., HIV infection, organ transplantation, and iatrogenic immunosuppression).

    The oral cavity is the most common site at presentation (particularly in HIV-infected patients); PBL may be seen in lymph nodes and other extranodal sites including bone marrow.

    Cytoplasmic immunoglobulin is variably present in about 50% of PBL cases. MYC and p53 are commonly overexpressed, and MYC translocations are seen in 50–70% of the cases. Most PBL cases are positive for PRDM1/Blimp1. *EBV* positivity is seen in 50–80% of cases, particularly in patients with HIV infection and other forms of immunosuppression. But *EBV* positivity is not required for diagnosis of PBL.

    The diagnosis of PBL remains a challenge, given its rarity, peculiar morphology, and an immunohistochemical profile similar to plasma cell myeloma. Differentiation between PBL and plasmablastic variant of myeloma is a common problem because of the lack of a distinct phenotype, especially if the phenotype falls in the spectrum of high-grade B-cell lymphoma and plasma cell myeloma. In the absence of immunophenotypic criteria for differentiating between PBL and plasmablastic myeloma, in practice, the distinction frequently depends on clinical correlation.
  - Features favoring plasmablastic lymphoma include clinical background of immunodeficiency, *EBV* positivity, morphologic features resembling B immunoblasts, very high Ki-67 proliferation rate (>90%) and negative marrow involvement.
  - Features favoring plasma cell myeloma include significant level of M protein, significant bone marrow involvement, clinical features of symptomatic myeloma ("CRAB"), positivity for CD56 and cyclin D1, and lower Ki-67 proliferation rate.
  - Rare intermediate cases that show features of both PBL and multiple myeloma do exist, and the diagnostic dilemma should be communicated to clinicians so the optimal treatment regimen can be determined.
- Metastatic carcinoma
  - Bone metastases can arise from many types of solid cancers, especially those arising in the lung, breast, and prostate, and can mimic the lytic lesions of multiple myeloma.

    The presence of lytic bone lesions in a patient with a monoclonal gammopathy suggests the possibility of plasma cell myeloma. However, a subset of patients with metastatic bone disease may have a concomitant, unrelated monoclonal gammopathy (e.g., MGUS). Patients presenting with lytic bone lesions, constitutional symptoms, a small M protein on SPEP/IFE, and <10% clonal plasma cells in bone marrow are more likely to have metastatic carcinoma with an unrelated MGUS rather than multiple myeloma.

    On the other hand, patients with known primary carcinoma and bone lesion(s) cannot be assumed to have bone metastasis as concomitant multiple myelomas can occur and mimic metastasis. The diagnosis should always be confirmed with a biopsy of the bone lesion as well as immunohistochemistry if needed (e.g., metastatic carcinoma versus anaplastic or pleomorphic myeloma). In patients with lytic lesions in whom no M protein is found in the serum or urine, metastatic carcinoma should be excluded before the diagnosis of nonsecretory myeloma is seriously considered, by performing a biopsy of one of the lytic lesions.

13. What are POEMS syndrome and TEMPI syndrome?

- POEMS syndrome
  - POEMS syndrome (osteosclerotic myeloma or Crow–Fukase syndrome: *p*olyneuropathy, *o*rganomegaly, *e*ndocrinopathy, *m*onoclonal protein, *s*kin changes) is a paraneoplastic syndrome associated with plasma cell neoplasm, usually characterized by fibrosis and osteosclerotic changes in trabecular bone, and often with lymph node changes resembling plasma cell variant of Castleman's disease. Patients typically have elevated serum vascular endothelial growth factor (VEGF) levels, which correlate with disease activity [36].

Table 26.6 Diagnostic criteria for POEMS syndrome [1]

Mandatory criteria	– Polyneuropathy (typically demyelinating) – Monoclonal plasma cell proliferative disorder
Major criteria (≥1 required)	– Castleman disease (plasma cell variant) – Osteosclerotic bone lesions – VEGF elevation (serum or plasma)
Minor criteria (≥1 required)	– Organomegaly – Endocrinopathy – Skin changes – Papilloedema – Thrombocytosis – Extravascular volume overload

VEGF vascular endothelial growth factor

The mandatory criteria for diagnosis of POEMS syndrome are (1) a chronic progressive polyneuropathy and (2) a monoclonal plasma cell proliferation disorder. There is usually an M protein of IgG or IgA type, with λ light chain restriction in almost all cases. Organomegaly (hepatomegaly, splenomegaly), endocrinopathy (excluding diabetes mellitus; often hypogonadism or thyroid function abnormality), and skin changes are present in >50%, >65%, and >65% of patients, respectively (Table 26.6). Polyneuropathy is uncommon in classical multiple myeloma and, when present, is usually due to the presence of amyloidosis. The presence of anemia, hypercalcemia, renal failure, pathologic fractures, and a high percent of plasma cells in the bone marrow all serve to distinguish multiple myeloma from POEMS syndrome, since hypercalcemia, renal insufficiency, and pathologic fractures are rarely seen in POEMS syndrome.

- TEMPI syndrome
  - TEMPI syndrome (*t*elangiectasia, *e*levated erythropoietin and erythrocytosis, *m*onoclonal gammopathy, *p*erinephric fluid collection, *i*ntrapulmonary shunt) is a rare paraneoplastic syndrome associated with plasma cell neoplasm [1, 37]. It has an insidious onset with slowly progressive symptoms, which often cause delay in diagnosis. TEMPI syndrome is considered to be an indolent plasma cell neoplasm with low tumor burden.

    TEMPI syndrome should be considered when erythrocytosis and plasma cell dyscrasia coexist. Serum M protein is typically IgG-κ type, and bone marrow plasma cells are often <10%. Peripheral erythrocytosis and bone marrow erythroid hyperplasia is uniformly present, which may be confused with polycythemia vera. Erythropoietin level is markedly increased, and significant decrease in erythropoietin levels correlates with treatment response.

    Vascular endothelial growth factor (VEGF) level is typically normal, and *JAK2* V617F and *JAK2* exon 12 mutations are absent.

14. How to evaluate and report response to treatment of symptomatic multiple myeloma?

The International Myeloma Working Group (IMWG) response criteria are the preferred criteria to determine the patient's response to treatment and to define when a relapse has occurred [38–40]. Whenever applicable (e.g., follow-up bone marrow examination), treatment response assessment should be included in diagnostic comment, based on these following criteria:

- Minimal residual disease (MRD) negative: Absence aberrant clonal plasma cells by next-generation flow cytometry or next-generation sequencing (NGS)-based test on bone marrow aspirates with a sensitivity of 1 in 100,000 nucleated cells or higher.
- Stringent complete response (sCR): In addition to CR criteria (defined below), there is a normal serum FLC ratio and there is no evidence of clonal cell population by bone marrow immunohistochemistry (a κ-to-λ ratio of ≤4:1 and ≥1:2, based on 100 plasma cells or higher).
- Complete response (CR): Absence of M protein in serum and urine by immunofixation with no current evidence of soft tissue plasmacytoma. In addition, bone marrow aspirate and biopsy must demonstrate <5% clonal plasma cells. In patients who lack measurable M proteins in the serum and urine (e.g., nonsecretory myeloma), the definition of CR requires a normalization of the FLC ratio in addition to the above criteria.
- Very good partial response (VGPR): Serum and urine M protein detectable by immunofixation but not on electrophoresis or at least a 90% reduction in serum M protein with a urine M protein <100 mg/24 hours. In patients who lack measurable M proteins in the serum and urine (e.g., nonsecretory myeloma), the definition of VGPR requires >90% decrease in the difference between involved and uninvolved FLC levels.
- Partial response (PR): ≥50% reduction in serum M protein and reduction of 24-hour urinary M protein by 90% or to <200 mg/24 hours. In patients who lack measurable M proteins in the serum and urine (e.g., nonsecretory), the definition of PR requires ≥50% decrease in the difference between involved and uninvolved FLC levels. If the FLC levels were also unmeasurable at baseline, a 50% reduction in bone marrow plasma cells is acceptable as long as the original bone marrow contained at least 30% plasma cells. PR also requires a 50% reduction in size of any soft tissue plasmacytoma if present at baseline.
- Minimal response (MR): ≥25% but ≤49% reduction of serum M protein and reduction in 24-hour urine M protein by 50–89%. If present at baseline, a ≥50% reduction

in the size of soft tissue plasmacytoma is also required for minimal response.
- Stable disease (SD): Does not meet criteria for CR, VGPR, PR, or PD.
- Progressive disease (PD): 25% increase from lowest response value in any of the following: (1) Serum M protein (absolute increase must be ≥0.5 g/dL). A serum M protein increase ≥1 g/dL denotes PD, if the lowest M component was ≥5 g/dL. (2) Urine M protein (absolute increase must be ≥200 mg/24 hours). (3) Difference in the κ and λ FLC (absolute increase must be >10 mg/dL). This FLC criterion should only be used for patients with unmeasurable M protein in the serum and urine (e.g., nonsecretory myeloma). (4) Bone marrow plasma cell percentage (absolute increase must be ≥10%). This criterion should be used for patients without measurable serum and urine M protein levels and without measurable involved FLC levels.
  – PD is also diagnosed when there is a ≥50% increase in the size or development of new bone lesions or soft tissue plasmacytoma. A clinical relapse can be documented based on the development of one or more of the following attributable to the myeloma: a serum calcium >11.5 mg/dL, decrease in hemoglobin of ≥2 g/dL, rise in serum creatinine ≥2 mg/dL, and hyperviscosity related to the serum M protein.

Case Presentations

Learning Objectives

1. To become familiar with the testing algorithm for patients with suspected plasma cell myeloma
2. To become familiar with serum FLC analysis and its utility in the diagnosis and therapeutic monitoring of patients with plasma cell myeloma
3. To recognize the challenge in differentiating plasmablastic variant of plasma cell myeloma and plasmablastic lymphoma

Case 1

Case History

A 57-year-old man sought evaluation of fatigue, lightheadedness, and diffuse body pain. He denied fever, chills, night sweats, and easy bruising. An unintentional weight loss of 30 lb. (13.5 kg) during the past 3 months was noted. His family history was negative for cancer, and he denied illicit drug use, smoking, and alcohol consumption.

Physical examination disclosed tachycardia, with a pulse rate of 105 beats/min. Pallor of the oral mucosa and conjunctival mucous membranes was noted. Cardiac auscultation revealed a grade 3 systolic murmur. Hepatosplenomegaly was absent, and no rashes, petechiae, or purpura was noted on skin examination. Lower extremities showed pitting edema.

Initial Workup and Management

- Initial laboratory results disclosed severe macrocytic anemia (Hgb 7.3 g/dL, MCV 105.6 fL, and MCHC 34.8 g/dL), thrombocytopenia (17,000/uL), and renal dysfunction (BUN 37 mg/dL, creatinine 11.84 mg/dL, and eGFR 5 mL/min/m^2).
- Serum albumin and total calcium were normal at 4.4 g/dL and 10.3 mg/dL, respectively.
- The patient was admitted to the hospital for red blood cell transfusion and hemodialysis and additional diagnostic workup.

Histologic Findings and Additional Workup

- Review of a peripheral blood smear demonstrated pancytopenia with mild anisopoikilocytosis. Few dacrocytes, nucleated red blood cells, immature granulocytes, and rare blasts were present, consistent with peripheral leukoerythroblastosis. No significant rouleaux formation was observed.
- Esophagogastroduodenoscopy and colonoscopy failed to disclose a source of bleeding or malignancy.
- Magnetic resonance imaging of the spine demonstrated diffuse bone marrow abnormality in the visualized vertebral bodies, compatible with infiltrating bone marrow disease.
- A bone marrow aspiration and biopsy was performed. The aspirate was hemodiluted and without spicules; however, it showed medium-to-large plasma cells with a subset of larger forms exhibiting variably distinct nucleoli (plasmablastic feature). Rare multinucleated plasma cells were also seen.
- The biopsy and clot sections revealed a markedly hypercellular marrow for the patient's age (90–95%), composed predominantly of plasma cells in a diffuse, solid pattern of involvement (Fig. 26.6a). A few small foci of residual trilineage hematopoietic elements remained.
- Immunohistochemical stains for CD138, κ, and λ light chains identified a CD138-positive, λ-restricted plasma cell population (Fig. 26.6b, c).
- A reticulin stain of the biopsy specimen demonstrated diffuse reticulin fibrosis (grade 2–3 on a scale of 0–3) (Fig. 26.6d).
- Additional laboratory testing revealed reduced serum immunoglobulin (Ig) G (396 mg/dL), IgA (22 mg/dL), and IgM (<25 mg/dL) levels, markedly elevated β2-microglobulin (26.6 mg/L), and a serum λ free light chain (FLC) level greater than 13,900 mg/L, which is the upper limit of quantitation of the assay. The serum FLC ratio (involved λ to uninvolved κ ratio) was greater than 400.

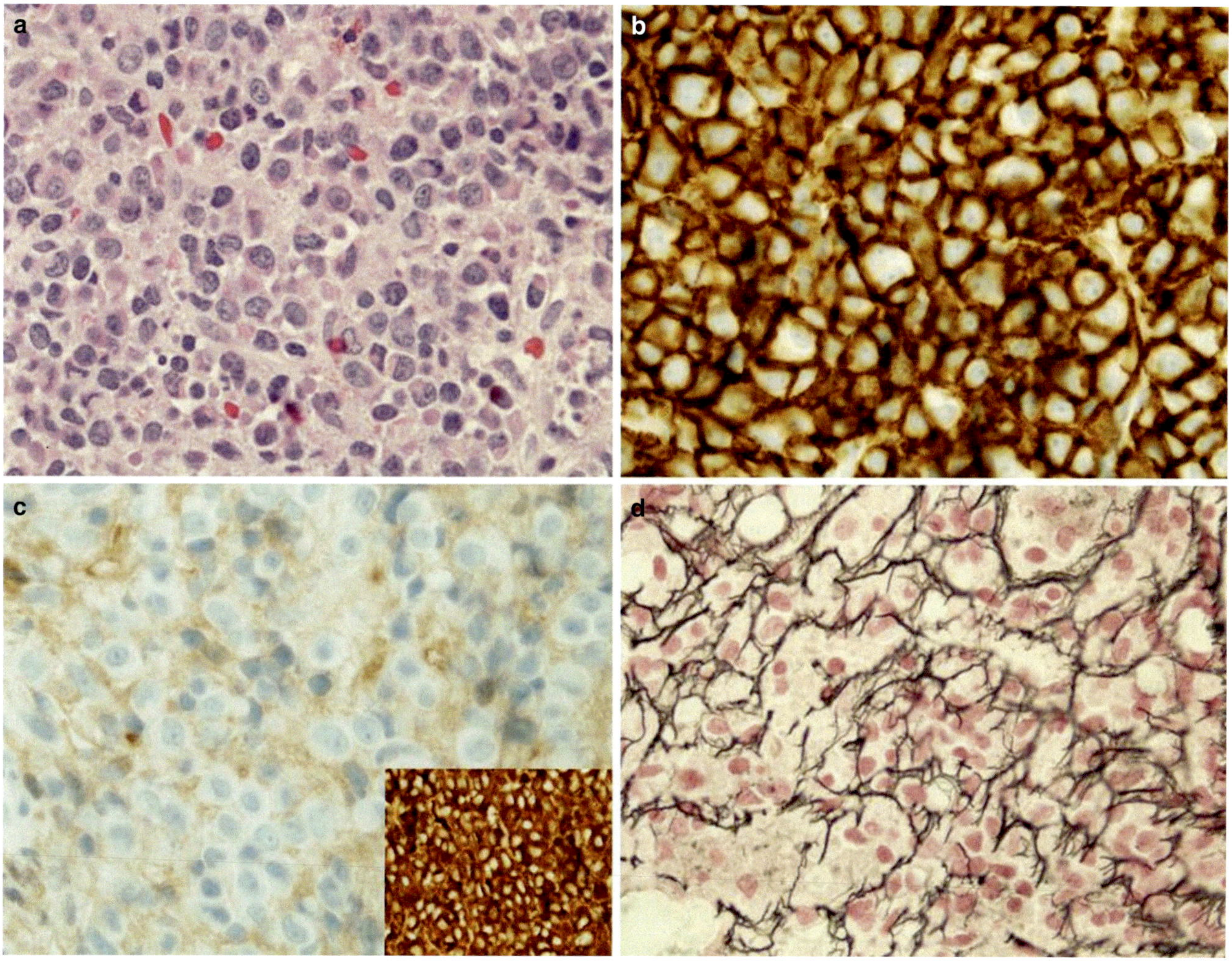

Fig. 26.6 Bone marrow biopsy specimen from a 57-year-old man shows plasma cell myeloma with concomitant myelofibrosis. (**a**) H&E, original magnification ×1000. (**b**) CD138, original magnification ×1000. (**c**) κ light chain (*inset*, λ light chain), original magnification ×1000. (**d**) Reticulin, original magnification ×1000

- Serum protein electrophoresis (SPEP) revealed an elevated γ globulin fraction with a monoclonal spike (1.85 g/dL).
- Immunofixation electrophoresis (IFE) disclosed a monoclonal λ FLC, without an associated heavy-chain component.

Differential Diagnosis

The blood smear findings (pancytopenia, leukoerythroblastosis) are suggestive of primary myelofibrosis, metastatic solid tumor to the marrow, or a hematopoietic or lymphoid tumor with associated myelofibrosis. Results of the bone marrow biopsy and additional laboratory workup indicate a plasma cell neoplasm with associated myelofibrosis.

Final Diagnosis

Symptomatic, light chain only multiple myeloma with associated myelofibrosis

Take-Home Messages

1. The diagnosis of multiple myeloma was based on (A) evidence of end-organ damage: renal failure and anemia; (B) greater than 60% clonal plasma cells in bone marrow; and (C) involved-to-uninvolved serum FLC ratio greater than 100.
2. Besides light chain only plasma cell myeloma, serum FLC analysis is also an important diagnostic tool for identifying patients with "oligo-secretory myeloma."

Case 2

Case History

A 54-year-old man with no significant past medical history presented with 5 days of progressive bilateral lower extremity weakness and back pain. At presentation, patient was found unable to walk and to have loss of sensation from feet to thighs and perineal numbness. A Foley catheter was placed to remove retained urine. Emergent head CT revealed a left retro-orbital lesion (2.7 cm × 1.5 cm × 1.7 cm), and MRI scan showed a large extramedullary thoracic spinal mass lesion (across T5-T7, 8.2 cm × 3.7 cm × 6.9 cm) that was associated with spinal cord compression and disruption of the posteromedial right seventh rib.

Initial Workup and Management

- Laboratory study results disclosed unremarkable CBC except for mild neutrophilic leukocytosis (ANC 11,800/μL, Hgb 13.7 g/dL, and platelets 371,000/μL), normal renal function (BUN 13 mg/dL, creatinine 0.85 mg/dL), normal serum calcium (8.7 mg/dL) and albumin (3.5 g/dL), elevated serum IgG (3760 mg/dL) and suppressed IgM (<25 mg/dL) and IgA (11 mg/dL), abnormal SPEP/IFE (IgG-kappa protein detected at 3.15 g/dL), abnormal serum free light chains (free κ 375 mg/L, free λ 4.1 mg/L, FLC ratio 91), increase in urinary kappa light chain excretion (235 mg/24 hour), and elevated β_2-microglobulin (2.5 mg/L).
- HIV antibody was negative.
- Peripheral blood smear review was unremarkable except for mild reactive neutrophilic leukocytosis and mild Rouleaux formation. No circulating plasma cells or leukoerythroblastosis was observed.
- Emergent decompressive neurosurgery was performed and biopsies of the thoracic spinal lesion were obtained. On frozen sections, the preliminary interpretation was "diffuse large B-cell lymphoma (DLBCL) versus solitary plasmacytoma."

Histologic Findings and Additional Workup

- On immunohistochemistry (IHC), the neoplastic cells from the biopsied large thoracic mass lesion were uniformly positive for CD20 and CD138 and cytoplasmic κ light chain expression and were negative for CD45, CD3, and λ light chain. The tentative diagnosis was "plasmablastic lymphoma" (Fig. 26.7c, d).
- A bone marrow aspiration and biopsy procedure was subsequently performed. The aspirate smears showed mixed trilineage hematopoiesis with approximately 15% plasma cells.
- Most of the plasma cells exhibited immature plasmablastic features (i.e., centrally located nuclei with dispersed chromatin and 1–2 distinct nucleoli) (Fig. 26.7a), and occasional large and multinucleated plasma cells were present (Fig. 26.7b).
- On the biopsy and aspirate clot sections, the marrow cellularity was about 70%, and there was no large solid plasma cell aggregate.
- By IHC CD138 stain, there were about 15% plasma cells that were scattered and intermixed with hematopoietic cell populations.
- Flow cytometry analysis performed on aspirate sample detected a monoclonal plasma cell population (about 7% of total) which was positive for CD45(dim to negative), CD38, CD138, CD117, CD20, and cytoplasmic and surface κ light chains and negative for CD19, CD56, and λ light chain. The S-phase fraction of plasma cells was 27%.
- Cytogenetic analysis revealed a normal male karyotype.
- FISH myeloma panel was not performed at the time.
- An add-on EBER in situ hybridization for Epstein–Barr virus performed on the thoracic lesion biopsies was negative.

Differential Diagnosis

Although DLBCL and solitary plasmacytoma were ruled out, the differential remained challenging because plasmablastic variant of plasma cell myeloma and plasmablastic lymphoma has similar immunophenotype. Features favoring plasma cell myeloma in this case included significant level of IgG-κ paraprotein (>3.0 g/dL) with suppressed IgM and IgA and elevated serum FLC ratio, significant bone marrow involvement (>10% plasma cells), clinical features of symptomatic myeloma (disruption of right seventh rib), negative EBER in the neoplastic plasma cells, and negative HIV testing. Note that CD20 expression can be seen in a small subset (10–20%) of myeloma cases, whereas plasmablastic lymphoma is typically negative for CD20. Nevertheless, the clinical presentation (solid mass lesion with spinal cord compression) and the significant S-phase fraction (~27% among the plasma cells by flow cytometry) suggest a more aggressive clinical course, requiring individualized myeloma treatment decisions.

Final Diagnosis

High-grade plasma cell neoplasm with features favoring plasmablastic variant of plasma cell myeloma

Take-Home Message

1. Due to the absence of immunophenotypic criteria for differentiating between plasmablastic myeloma and plasmablastic lymphoma, the diagnostic interpretation requires clinical correlation (see PBL section in Question 12).

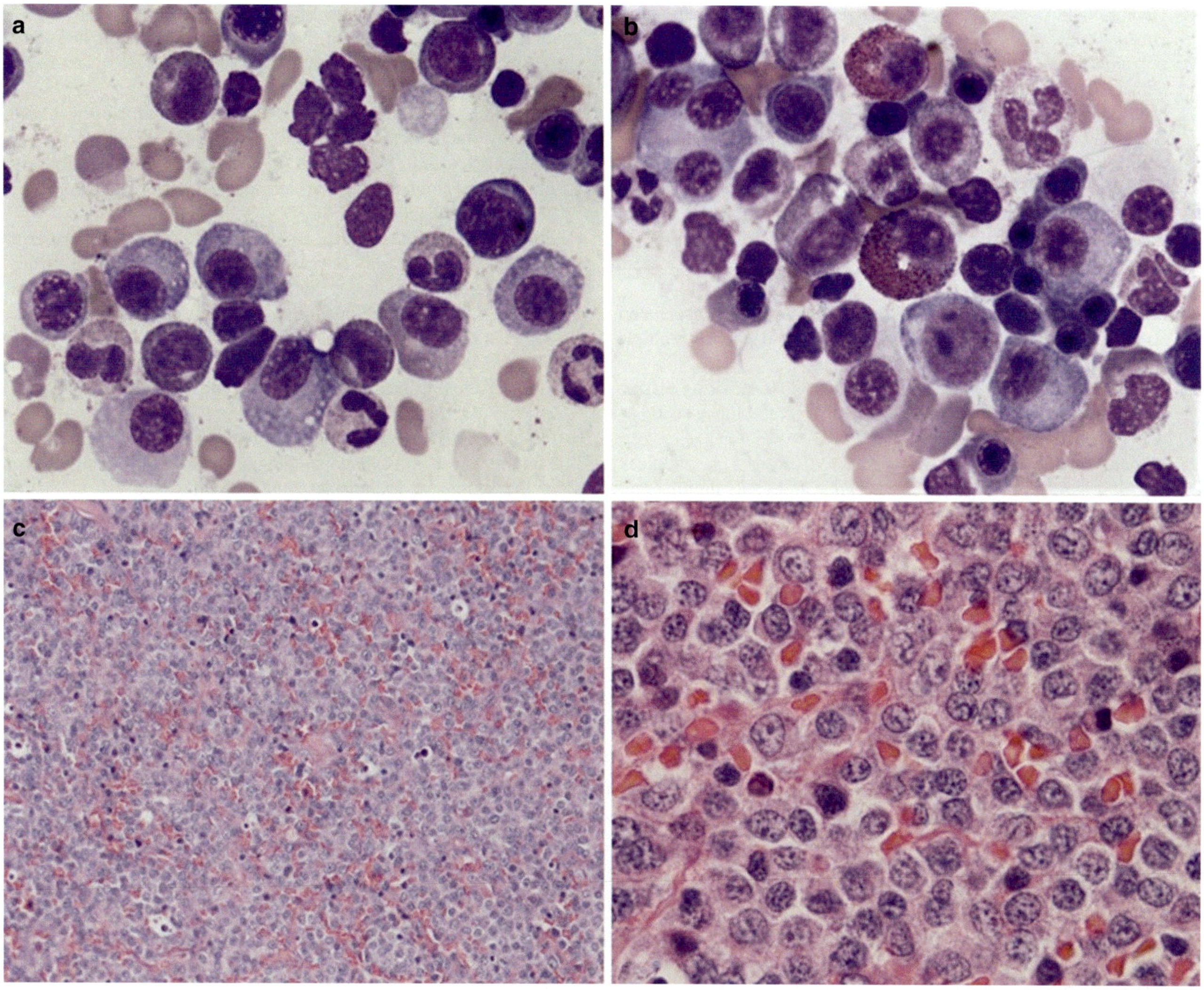

Fig. 26.7 A 54-year-old man with plasmablastic variant of plasma cell myeloma involving bone marrow (~15% plasma cells as shown in **a** and **b**) and forming retro-orbital and thoracic spinal mass (confirmed by biopsy as shown in **c** and **d**). (**a**, **b**) Bone marrow aspirate smear, Giemsa stain, original magnification ×1000. (**c**, **d**) Spinal mass biopsy, H&E, original magnification **c** ×200 & **d** ×1000

References

1. Swerdlow SH, Campo E, Harris NL, Jaffe ES, Pileri SA, Stein H, Thiele J. WHO classification of tumours of haematopoietic and lymphoid tissues (revised 4th edition). IARC: Lyon; 2017.
2. Sant M, Allemani C, Tereanu C, De Angelis R, Capocaccia R, Visser O, et al. HAEMACARE Working Group. Incidence of hematologic malignancies in Europe by morphologic subtype: results of the HAEMACARE project. Blood. 2010;116(19):3724–34.
3. Ocqueteau M, Orfao A, Almeida J, Bladé J, González M, García-Sanz R, et al. Immunophenotypic characterization of plasma cells from monoclonal gammopathy of undetermined significance patients. Implications for the differential diagnosis between MGUS and multiple myeloma. Am J Pathol. 1998;152(6):1655–65.
4. Rajkumar SV, Fonseca R, Dispenzieri A, Lacy MQ, Lust JA, Witzig TE, et al. Methods for estimation of bone marrow plasma cell involvement in myeloma: predictive value for response and survival in patients undergoing autologous stem cell transplantation. Am J Hematol. 2001;68(4):269–75.
5. Lee N, Moon SY, Lee JH, Park HK, Kong SY, Bang SM, et al. Discrepancies between the percentage of plasma cells in bone marrow aspiration and BM biopsy: impact on the revised IMWG diagnostic criteria of multiple myeloma. Blood Cancer J. 2017;7(2):e530.
6. Booth RA, McCudden CR, Balion CM, Blasutig IM, Bouhtiauy I, Rodriguez-Capote K, et al. Candidate recommendations for protein electrophoresis reporting from the Canadian Society of Clinical Chemists Monoclonal Gammopathy Working Group. Clin Biochem. 2018;51:10–20.
7. Milani P, Palladini G, Merlini G. Serum-free light-chain analysis in diagnosis and management of multiple myeloma and related conditions. Scand J Clin Lab Invest Suppl. 2016;245:S113–8.
8. Bradwell AR, Carr-Smith HD, Mead GP, Tang LX, Showell PJ, Drayson MT, et al. Highly sensitive, automated immunoassay for immunoglobulin free light chains in serum and urine. Clin Chem. 2001;47:673–80.
9. Nowrousian MR, Brandhorst D, Sammet C, Kellert M, Daniels R, Schuett P, et al. Serum free light chain analysis and urine immunofixation electrophoresis in patients with multiple myeloma. Clin Cancer Res. 2005;11(24 Pt 1):8706–14.

10. Hutchison CA, Harding S, Hewins P, Mead GP, Townsend J, Bradwell AR, et al. Quantitative assessment of serum and urinary polyclonal free light chains in patients with chronic kidney disease. Clin J Am Soc Nephrol. 2008;3(6):1684–90.
11. Sinclair D, Ballantyne F, Shanley S, Caine E, O'Reilly D, Shenkin A. Estimation of paraproteins by immunoturbidimetry and electrophoresis followed by scanning densitometry. Ann Clin Biochem. 1990;27(Pt 4):335–7.
12. Jacobs JFM, Haagen IA, Lodder A, van der Kroft C, de Kat Angelino CM, Croockewit S, et al. Analytical validation of the Hevylite assays for M-protein quantification. Clin Chem Lab Med. 2018;56(7):1169–75.
13. Kyle RA, Gertz MA, Witzig TE, Lust JA, Lacy MQ, Dispenzieri A, et al. Review of 1027 patients with newly diagnosed multiple myeloma. Mayo Clin Proc. 2003;78(1):21–33.
14. Smith FB, Elnawawi A. A counting strategy for estimating plasma cell number in CD138-stained bone marrow core biopsy sections. Ann Clin Lab Sci. 2008;38(2):138–42.
15. Jelinek T, Bezdekova R, Zatopkova M, Burgos L, Simicek M, Sevcikova T, et al. Current applications of multiparameter flow cytometry in plasma cell disorders. Blood Cancer J. 2017;7(10):e617.
16. Nadav L, Katz BZ, Baron S, Yossipov L, Polliack A, Deutsch V, et al. Diverse niches within multiple myeloma bone marrow aspirates affect plasma cell enumeration. Br J Haematol. 2006;133(5):530–2.
17. Robillard N, Wuillème S, Moreau P, Béné MC. Immunophenotype of normal and myelomatous plasma-cell subsets. Front Immunol. 2014;5:137.
18. Flores-Montero J, de Tute R, Paiva B, Perez JJ, Böttcher S, Wind H, et al. Immunophenotype of normal vs. myeloma plasma cells: toward antibody panel specifications for MRD detection in multiple myeloma. Cytometry B Clin Cytom. 2016;90(1):61–72.
19. Gastinne T, Leleu X, Duhamel A, Moreau AS, Franck G, Andrieux J, et al. Intergroupe francophone du Myelome (IFM). Plasma cell growth fraction using Ki-67 antigen expression identifies a subgroup of multiple myeloma patients displaying short survival within the ISS stage I. Eur J Haematol. 2007;79(4):297–304.
20. Soh KT, Tario JD Jr, Wallace PK. Diagnosis of plasma cell dyscrasias and monitoring of minimal residual disease by multiparametric flow cytometry. Clin Lab Med. 2017;37(4):821–53.
21. Bai Y, Orfao A, Chim CS. Molecular detection of minimal residual disease in multiple myeloma. Br J Haematol. 2018;181(1):11–26.
22. Rajkumar SV, Dimopoulos MA, Palumbo A, Blade J, Merlini G, Mateos MV, et al. International Myeloma Working Group updated criteria for the diagnosis of multiple myeloma. Lancet Oncol. 2014;15(12):e538–48.
23. Rajkumar SV, Landgren O, Mateos MV. Smoldering multiple myeloma. Blood. 2015;125(20):3069–75.
24. Larson D, Kyle RA, Rajkumar SV. Prevalence and monitoring of oligosecretory myeloma. N Engl J Med. 2012;367(6):580–1.
25. Jelinek T, Kryukov F, Rihova L, Hajek R. Plasma cell leukemia: from biology to treatment. Eur J Haematol. 2015;95(1):16–26.
26. Caers J, Paiva B, Zamagni E, Leleu X, Bladé J, Kristinsson SY, et al. Diagnosis, treatment, and response assessment in solitary plasmacytoma: updated recommendations from a European Expert Panel. J Hematol Oncol. 2018;11(1):10.
27. Chan NC, Chan NP. Recurrent cytogenetic abnormalities in multiple myeloma. Methods Mol Biol. 2017;1541:295–302.
28. Joseph NS, Gentili S, Kaufman JL, Lonial S, Nooka AK. High-risk multiple myeloma: definition and management. Clin Lymphoma Myeloma Leuk. 2017;17S:S80–7.
29. Fonseca R, Bergsagel PL, Drach J, Shaughnessy J, Gutierrez N, Stewart AK, et al. International Myeloma Working Group. International Myeloma Working Group molecular classification of multiple myeloma: spotlight review. Leukemia. 2009;23(12):2210–21.
30. Chesi M, Bargsagel PL. Molecular pathogenesis of multiple myeloma: basic and clinical updates. Int J Haematol. 2013;97(3):313–23.
31. Czuchlewski DR, Brackney M, Ewers C, Manna J, Fekrazad MH, Martinez A, et al. Clinicopathologic features of agranulocytosis in the setting of levamisole-tainted cocaine. Am J Clin Pathol. 2010;133(3):466–72.
32. Hassoun H, Roshal M, Sabari J, Nguyen J, Gao Q, Devlin SM, et al. Immunophenotypic evidence for reactive polyclonal marrow plasmacytosis in multiple myeloma patients receiving lenalidomide maintenance. Leuk Lymphoma. 2017;58(12):2962–5.
33. Ioannou MG, Stathakis E, Lazaris AC, Papathomas T, Tsiambas E, Koukoulis GK. Immunohistochemical evaluation of 95 bone marrow reactive plasmacytoses. Pathol Oncol Res. 2009;15(1):25–9.
34. Mansour AT, Shandiz AE, Zimmerman MK, Roth TD, Zhou J. Concomitant lymphoplasmacytic lymphoma and plasma cell myeloma, a diagnostic challenge. Am J Blood Res. 2017;7(2):10–7.
35. Elyamany G, Al Mussaed E, Alzahrani AM. Plasmablastic lymphoma: a review of current knowledge and future directions. Adv Hematol. 2015;2015:315289.
36. Jaccard A. POEMS syndrome: therapeutic options. Hematol Oncol Clin North Am. 2018;32(1):141–51.
37. Rosado FG, Oliveira JL, Sohani AR, Schroyens W, Sykes DB, Kenderian SS, et al. Bone marrow findings of the newly described TEMPI syndrome: when erythrocytosis and plasma cell dyscrasia coexist. Mod Pathol. 2015;28(3):367–72.
38. Kumar S, Paiva B, Anderson KC, Durie B, Landgren O, Moreau P, et al. International myeloma working group consensus criteria for response and minimal residual disease assessment in multiple myeloma. Lancet Oncol. 2016;17(8):e328–46.
39. Rajkumar SV, Harousseau JL, Durie B, Anderson KC, Dimopoulos M, Kyle R, et al. International Myeloma Workshop Consensus Panel 1. Consensus recommendations for the uniform reporting of clinical trials: report of the International Myeloma Workshop Consensus Panel 1. Blood. 2011;117(18):4691–5.
40. Ravi P, Kumar SK, Cerhan JR, Maurer MJ, Dingli D, Ansell SM, et al. Defining cure in multiple myeloma: a comparative study of outcomes of young individuals with myeloma and curable hematologic malignancies. Blood Cancer J. 2018;8(3):26.

Bone Marrow Involvement by Lymphoid Neoplasms

27

Yi Xie

List of Frequently Asked Questions

1. What is the significance of bone marrow examination in the diagnostic work-up of patients with lymphoma?
2. What is the frequency of bone marrow involvement in various lymphoid neoplasms?
3. What is an adequate specimen for staging of lymphoma in bone marrow?
4. What ancillary studies are useful for the diagnosis of lymphoid neoplasms in bone marrow?
5. What are the challenges in the diagnosis of lymphoid neoplasms in bone marrow?
6. What are the pitfalls in the evaluation for residual lymphoid neoplasms in bone marrow during or after treatment?
7. What essential information should be included in the pathology report on bone marrow specimens involved by lymphoma?
8. How does one distinguish reactive lymphoid aggregates from lymphoma?
9. What are the common infiltration patterns of lymphoma in the bone marrow, and what is their significance for classification?
10. What is the definition of discordant bone marrow involvement in non-Hodgkin lymphoma, and what is its significance?
11. What is the significance of detecting a small monoclonal B-cell population in bone marrow in a patient without previously diagnosed lymphoma?
12. What are the distinctive pathologic features of splenic marginal zone lymphoma in bone marrow, and what are the important differential diagnostic considerations?
13. What are the typical pathologic features and caveats in the diagnosis of hairy cell leukemia in bone marrow?
14. What are the main morphologic and immunophenotypic characteristics and challenges in the diagnosis of mature T-/NK-cell neoplasms in the bone marrow?
15. What are the pathologic features of angioimmunoblastic T-cell lymphoma in bone marrow?
16. What are the typical pathologic features of T-cell large granular lymphocytic leukemia in bone marrow, and what are the important differential diagnostic considerations?
17. What are the typical pathologic features of hepatosplenic T-cell lymphoma in the bone marrow, and what are the important differential diagnostic considerations?
18. What are the typical histologic features of classic Hodgkin lymphoma in bone marrow, and what are the important differential diagnostic considerations?

1. What is the significance of bone marrow examination in the diagnostic work-up of patients with lymphoma?

The bone marrow examination is a useful diagnostic and prognostic tool for patients with Hodgkin and non-Hodgkin lymphomas.

- Diagnosis and differential diagnosis: Bone marrow examination can aid in the differential diagnosis and, in some patients, establish a primary diagnosis of lymphoma. For instance, an initial diagnosis is usually made by bone marrow examination in leukemia/lymphomas that primarily involve the bone marrow, such as T-cell large granulocytic leukemia (T-LGL), prolymphocytic leukemia (PLL), Waldenström macroglobulinemia, hairy cell leukemia (HCL), etc. The evaluation of bone marrow (BM) is a key process in the diagnosis of primary bone marrow lymphoma, which is a rare distinct entity with isolated bone marrow infiltration, with no evidence of nodal or extranodal involvement [1]. In lymphoma patients with

Y. Xie (✉)
Department of Laboratory Medicine, University of California San Francisco, San Francisco, CA, USA
e-mail: Yi.Xie@ucsf.edu

E. Wang, A. S. Lagoo (eds.), *Practical Lymph Node and Bone Marrow Pathology*, Practical Anatomic Pathology,
https://doi.org/10.1007/978-3-030-32189-5_27

disseminated disease, splenomegaly, or mass lesions inaccessible for biopsy, bone marrow examination may serve to establish the diagnosis in a subset of the cases.
- Staging and prognosis: Bone marrow biopsy is a well-established staging procedure. In a variety of non-Hodgkin and Hodgkin lymphomas, the presence of bone marrow involvement indicates a high-stage disease and has a significant impact on prognosis [2–5]. For example, bone marrow involvement is associated with significantly worse overall survival in patients with diffuse large B-cell lymphoma (DLBCL). It affects the International Prognostic Index both by increasing the stage of the disease to stage IV and by being assessed as extranodal involvement [3].
- Treatment: The assessment of bone marrow involvement can aid in the selection of appropriate therapeutic approaches in patients with lymphoma [2–5]. Bone marrow examination is also performed to monitor response to treatment or relapse during follow-up.

2. What is the frequency of bone marrow involvement in various lymphoid neoplasms?

The frequency of bone marrow involvement varies according to the subtypes of lymphomas [6].

- Bone marrow almost always involved: primarily leukemic lymphoid neoplasms, such as chronic lymphocytic leukemia (CLL), HCL, PLL, T-LGL, and hepatosplenic T-cell lymphoma (HSTL) (almost 100% of cases).
- Bone marrow often involved: follicular lymphoma (FL), lymphoplasmacytic lymphoma (LPL), splenic marginal zone lymphoma (SMZL) , mantle cell lymphoma (MCL), adult T-cell leukemia/lymphoma (ATLL) , angioimmunoblastic T-cell lymphoma (AITL).
- Bone marrow infrequently involved: DLBCL (10 to 35%), anaplastic large cell lymphoma (ALCL) (10–30%), nodular lymphocyte-predominant Hodgkin lymphoma (<5%). Bone marrow involvement by classic Hodgkin lymphoma (CHL) is rare in immunocompetent patients, occurring in less than 5% in most large clinical series [7], but it is found in 25–50% of cases in patients with HIV infection [8].

3. What is an adequate specimen for staging of lymphoma in bone marrow?

A comprehensive evaluation of bone marrow for lymphoma includes review of peripheral blood smears, bone marrow aspirate smears, clot sections, touch imprints, and core biopsy sections.

- Adequate sampling of the core biopsy is important to detect the frequently focal lymphomatous involvement. It is recommended that an adequate trephine biopsy specimen should be at least 1.5–2 cm in length and contain at least five to six intertrabecular marrow spaces [9]. Bilateral biopsies and step sectioning may be helpful to maximize the detection of lymphoma.
- Samples for ancillary studies such as flow cytometry or cytogenetic and molecular genetic analyses should be obtained for optimal diagnostic yield in patients with non-Hodgkin lymphoma. Because of increased reticulin deposition in infiltrated areas, a dry tap may be observed in 8–10% of bone marrow involved by lymphoma [10]. Additional cores can be obtained for ancillary studies if it is a dry tap.

4. What ancillary studies are useful for the diagnosis of lymphoid neoplasms in bone marrow?

While morphology remains the standard examination technique, various ancillary studies, including immunohistochemistry, flow cytometry, cytogenetic, fluorescent in situ hybridization (FISH), and molecular genetic analysis, can provide valuable complimentary information and have become important adjuncts for diagnosis and subclassification of lymphoma in bone marrow.

- Immunohistochemistry and flow cytometry: Morphology in conjunction with flow cytometry and immunohistochemical examination of the core biopsies allows for classification of lymphoma infiltrates in the majority of the cases. Flow cytometry is especially helpful in detecting small subpopulations with aberrant immunophenotype and/or light chain restriction in a background of reactive cells (but false-negative results can occur; see Question 5 below), while immunohistochemistry on the core biopsy can provide information about quantification, distribution, architecture, and expression of nuclear- or IHC-specific surface markers in the infiltrate. Reticulin stain which highlights stromal changes is helpful in revealing subtle lymphoid infiltration which might be missed in some cases on hematoxylin and eosin (H&E) sections.
- Molecular genetic studies: In some difficult cases, molecular genetic studies to assess B- or T-cell clonality may help to differentiate between benign and neoplastic lymphoid infiltrates. Of note, DNA extracted from decalcified bone marrow trephine biopsies is often degraded and unsuitable for molecular studies when strong acid is used for decalcification. Clot sections and bone marrow biopsies decalcified with EDTA would be acceptable for PCR-based testing.

- Cytogenetic and FISH: With the help of FISH and cytogenetic analyses, specific genetic abnormalities associated with different lymphoma subtypes can be identified. Examples include t(11;14) *CCND1/IGH* for MCL, inv(14)(q11q32) or t(14;14)(q11;q32) for T-cell PLL, and *MYC* rearrangement for Burkitt lymphoma (BL), among others.

Overall, ancillary studies should be employed in a rational and cost-effective manner to aid in the diagnosis of lymphoma in bone marrow.

5. What are the challenges in the diagnosis of lymphoid neoplasms in bone marrow?

Detection and accurate classification of lymphoma on a bone marrow specimen can be difficult even with the help of ancillary studies, especially in patients without a previously established diagnosis. The challenges include:

- Challenges in morphologic examination:
  - Specimen limitations: Bone marrow specimens are often small and do not show the architectural features or may show different architecture than those common to lymphoid tissues [11].
  - While a variety of marrow patterns are described for many lymphoma subtypes (please refer to Question 9 for detailed information), most of the infiltration patterns are nonspecific and may overlap among the different entities and with reactive conditions.
  - Histologic discordance between bone marrow and extramedullary specimens can be observed, most commonly between FLs and DLBCLs [12]. See also Question 10 below.
  - Subtle infiltration patterns such as intrasinusoidal pattern or early interstitial infiltrates may easily be overlooked in standard histological examination. This growth pattern is often seen in certain lymphoma subtypes (see Question 9 below). A high level of suspicion is required; careful examinations of blood and marrow smear and systematic use of flow cytometry and immunohistochemistry in proper clinical context are helpful to avoid this pitfall [13].
- Challenges in interpreting results from ancillary studies:
  - False-negative results by flow cytometric immunophenotyping of bone marrow aspirates: Merli and colleagues reported that in non-Hodgkin lymphomas, false-negative flow cytometry results were recorded more frequently in FL and in LPL, likely due to the paratrabecular pattern in FL in which neoplastic cells are frequently tightly bound to bone trabeculae and to the accompanying reticulin fibrosis in LPL. In addition, the discordance may also be attributed to sampling bias and blood contamination, especially for cases with minimal marrow infiltration [14].
  - Clonality analysis may not be helpful, especially in cases with low tumor cell content. On the other hand, the detection of monoclonality does not equate with a diagnosis of lymphoma.
  - Decalcification and some fixatives may interfere with some IHC/ISH and molecular studies.

Overall, caution should be applied when interpreting results of these ancillary studies. The findings from ancillary studies should be correlated with clinical context and morphology, and the final diagnosis should be based on the integrated information derived from all specimens.

6. What are the pitfalls in the evaluation for residual lymphoid neoplasms in bone marrow during or after treatment?

It is important to have information about the patient's treatment history as therapy-related changes may occur and can potentially lead to diagnostic pitfalls.

- In patients with small B-cell lymphomas, particularly FL, following rituximab immunochemotherapy bone marrow may contain dense T-cell-rich lymphoid nodules morphologically mimicking residual lymphoma.
- Antibody-based immunotherapies may affect results of the ancillary study. For example, rituximab therapy may downregulate CD20 expression for variable length of time, and solitary use of CD20 immunohistochemistry may miss residual B-cell lymphomas in the marrow. To avoid this risk, it is recommended to use a panel that includes alternative B-cell markers like CD79a or PAX5 in such cases. CD20 expression or lack thereof on residual lymphoma provides valuable information to guide additional antibody-based therapy.
- Similarly, CD19-negative relapse in B-cell precursor acute lymphoblastic leukemia is occasionally observed after anti-CD19/CD3 bispecific antibody (blinatumomab) treatment and CD19-directed chimeric antigen receptor (CART19) T-cell immunotherapy. In rare patients with anaplastic large cell lymphoma following brentuximab therapy, loss of CD30 expression has been reported [15, 16].

7. What essential information should be included in the pathology report on bone marrow specimens involved by lymphoma?

- It is recommended that an integrated report be issued that summarizes the morphologic findings from all specimens and the results of all relevant ancillary studies including flow cytometric analysis, immunohistochemistry, and molecular and genetic studies, if possible. The current World Health Organization (WHO) Classification should be used.
- When the marrow examination is performed for staging, the bone marrow findings should be compared to the lymphoma in the primary site. Concurrent review and cross-referencing of other relevant specimens may be required [17].
- The extent of the involvement should be estimated, which will provide clinically significant information regarding the patient's baseline involvement prior to therapy or response to the treatment.
- It is also important to report the quality of the specimen, cellularity, hematopoietic elements, and additional significant findings such as hemophagocytosis, etc.
- If a definite diagnosis cannot be made or there are remaining questions that cannot be resolved, the specific problem should be addressed in the report, and the pathologist's recommendation for further work-up should be included.

8. How does one distinguish reactive lymphoid aggregates from lymphoma?

A common diagnostic problem that pathologists encounter in evaluation of bone marrow biopsies is the distinction of reactive lymphoid infiltrates from infiltrates of malignant lymphomas.

- Reactive lymphoid aggregates are frequently seen in older individuals, in association with infection, inflammation, autoimmune disorders (Fig. 27.1), and myelodysplastic syndromes/myeloproliferative neoplasms, as well as in post therapy bone marrow specimens.
- The morphologic features that are helpful for distinguishing reactive from neoplastic lymphoid aggregates in the bone marrow are listed in Table 27.1 [18]. Familiarity with these features can aid in forming a differential diagnosis and guiding the selection of appropriate ancillary studies for further work-up.

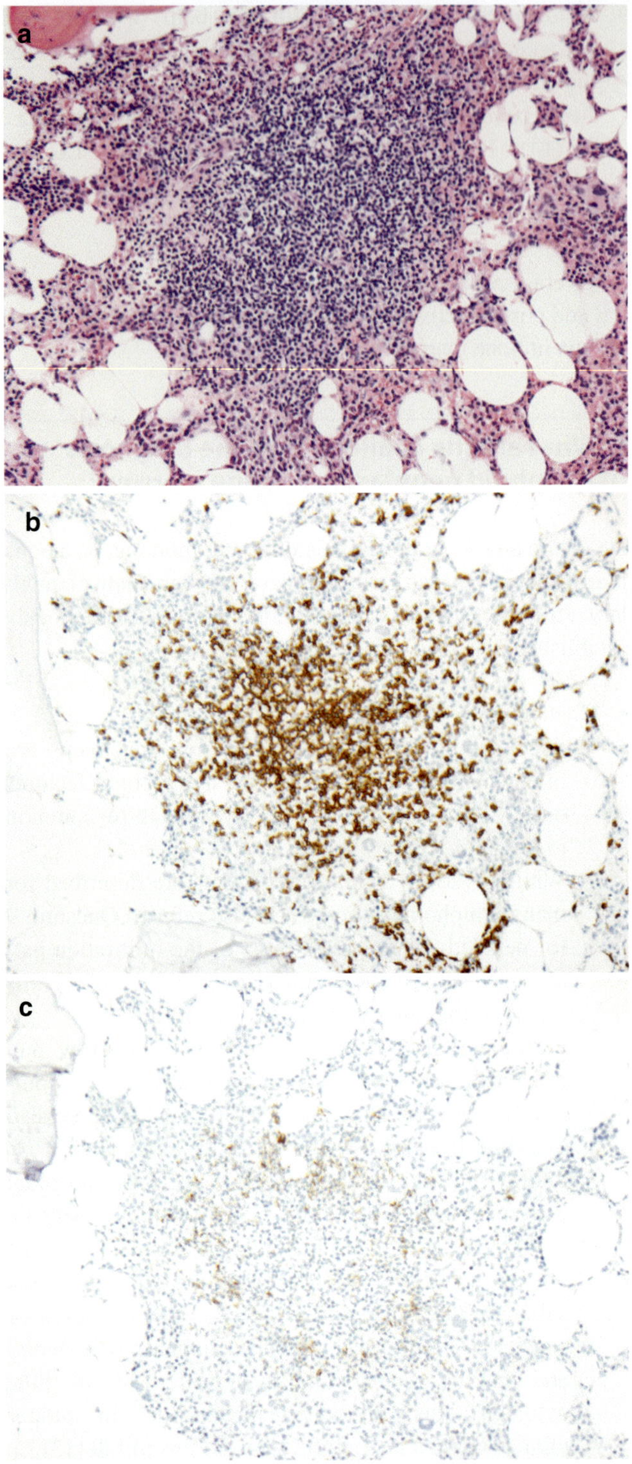

Fig. 27.1 Benign lymphoid aggregate in the bone marrow of a patient with systemic lupus erythematosus. (**a**) The lymphoid aggregate is small, well circumscribed, present in the intertrabecular region, and composed of small mature lymphocytes. (**b**) Immunohistochemical staining for CD3 highlights numerous small T cells in the aggregate. (**c**) Immunohistochemical staining for CD20 highlights a few small B cells

Table 27.1 Features that are helpful for distinguishing reactive from neoplastic lymphoid aggregates in bone marrow biopsies

Reactive	Neoplastic
Usually few in number	Variable and may be multiple
Intertrabecular or perivascular localization	Paratrabecular aggregates may be present
Round, with smooth borders	Irregular, with infiltrative borders
Polymorphous cellular composition	Usually monomorphous
No morphologically abnormal lymphoid cells	Morphologically abnormal lymphoid cells may be present
Immunostains show mixed B and T cells, often with T-cell predominance	Immunostains may show predominance of B or T cells
No monotypic B-cell population or immunophenotypically abnormal T-cell population by flow cytometry	Light chain restriction or aberrant phenotype may be identified by flow cytometry
No clonal *IG* or *TCR* gene rearrangement by molecular analysis	Monoclonal *IG* or *TCR* gene rearrangement may be identified by molecular analysis

9. What are the common infiltration patterns of lymphoma in the bone marrow, and what is their significance for classification?

Previous studies have shown that different lymphoma subtypes often demonstrate characteristic patterns of bone marrow involvement, and pattern analysis may help in the classification [11, 19]. The main histologic features of various mature B-cell neoplasms involving bone marrow are summarized in Table 27.2.

- The typical pattern of involvement includes paratrabecular, nodular non-paratrabecular, interstitial, diffuse, intrasinusoidal, and mixed.
- In general, the nodular pattern and mixed pattern are most common but least specific and can be seen in virtually all lymphoma subtypes.
- While it is well known that the paratrabecular pattern is characteristic of FL (Fig. 27.2) [20], it is not specific to FL and can be seen in a wide variety of lymphoma types, including MCL, marginal zone lymphoma (MZL), LPL, etc. [11, 19], although it is not usually seen in CLL/SLL as the only pattern of involvement.
- A diffuse pattern appears to be associated with more aggressive lymphomas such as DLBCL and BL. Notably, marrow necrosis is also more commonly associated with high-grade diseases such as lymphoblastic lymphoma/leukemia, DLBCL, or BL [19, 21].
- Granulomas and fibrosis are uncommon in small cell B-cell lymphomas (with the notable exception of paratrabecular deposits of FL), but frequently seen in classic Hodgkin lymphoma and nodular lymphocyte-predominant Hodgkin lymphoma. A histiocyte-rich infiltrate in T-cell histiocyte-rich DLBCL and in "Lennert-type" T-cell lymphoma may be mistaken for a reactive granuloma, unless appropriate IHC staining is used based on clinical history. See also Question 18 below.

Table 27.2 Histologic features of mature B-cell neoplasms involving bone marrow

Lymphoma subtype	Patterns of marrow involvement	Comments
Follicular lymphoma	Predominantly paratrabecular	Patients with DLBCL may have discordant, low-grade follicular lymphoma in the bone marrow
Chronic lymphocytic leukemia/small lymphocytic lymphoma	Nodular, interstitial, or diffuse	Paratrabecular infiltrates usually exclude CLL/SLL
Mantle cell lymphoma	Nodular, interstitial, or diffuse	Focal paratrabecular infiltrates may be present
Lymphoplasmacytic lymphoma	Nodular, interstitial, or diffuse	Spectrum of small lymphocytes, plasmacytoid lymphocytes, and plasma cells
Splenic marginal zone lymphoma	Diffuse, sinusoidal, or nodular	Reactive germinal centers may be present
Hairy cell leukemia	Diffuse or interstitial	Cases may be misdiagnosed as MDS or aplastic anemia
Diffuse large B-cell lymphoma	Nodular, diffuse, or interstitial	The infiltrate may contain many T cells
Burkitt lymphoma	Nodular or diffuse	The "starry sky" pattern may not be present

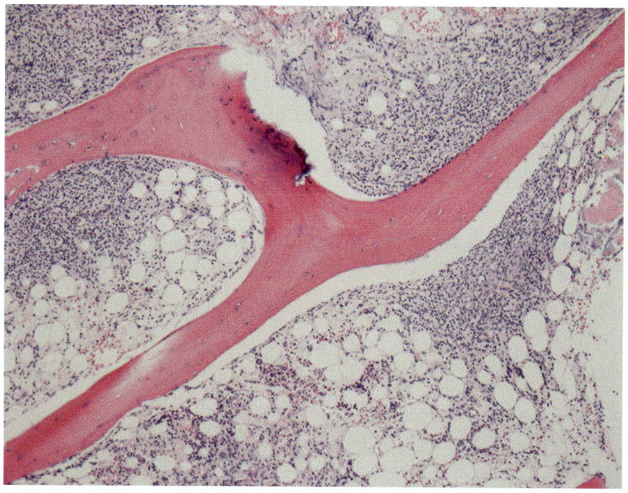

Fig. 27.2 Follicular lymphoma in the bone marrow. Note the paratrabecular infiltration pattern

- Though not absolutely specific, an intrasinusoidal infiltration pattern is most often associated with MZL, intravascular large B-cell lymphoma, ALCL, and HSTL, while an interstitial pattern is most often associated with LPL, CLL, MCL, etc.
- Of note, patterns can change during the course of the disease. While the patterns of bone marrow involvement may provide clues to the diagnosis, they are not specific. It is essential to correlate morphologic findings with ancillary studies and clinical history to achieve a definitive diagnosis.

10. What is the definition of discordant bone marrow involvement in non-Hodgkin lymphoma, and what is its significance?

- Discordance refers to those lymphoma cases where the histology is distinctly different between the bone marrow and other sites of involvement [12].
- Discordant bone marrow involvement typically happens when an aggressive lymphoma, usually DLBCL, is found in a lymph node biopsy with an indolent lymphoma, usually FL, in a bone marrow biopsy (Fig. 27.3).
- Only few previous reports assessed the clonal relationship of discordant lymphomas and have shown that histologically discordant bone marrow infiltrates may be either clonally related, suggesting transformation of the original indolent neoplasm, or clonally unrelated, suggesting unrelated B-cell neoplasms presenting synchronously at different locations [22].
- Patients with DLBCL and discordant bone marrow involvement have been reported to have better prognosis than those having concordant marrow involvement [12].
- These data reinforce the importance of correlation of bone marrow findings with extramedullary sites and evaluation of lymphoma involvement of lymph nodes or other sites if diagnosis is based on the bone marrow alone and discordance is suspected.

11. What is the significance of detecting a small monoclonal B-cell population in bone marrow in a patient without previously diagnosed lymphoma?

- Small clonal B-cell populations also known as monoclonal B-cell lymphocytosis (MBL) have been well characterized in peripheral blood. It is defined as less than 5.0×10^9/L monoclonal B cells in the blood of otherwise healthy subjects and is detected with an estimated frequency between 3.5% and 12.0% [23].
- Three subcategories have been identified based on the immunophenotypic features: CLL type, atypical CLL type, and CD5- MBL.
- Bone marrow examination is not required for the establishment of MBL diagnosis; therefore there is limited data on bone marrow findings in MBL [24].
  - Randen et al. studied 26 patients with MBL and showed most patients with MBL also have bone marrow lymphoid infiltration [25].
  - The pattern of infiltration and immunophenotype is indistinguishable from that of limited infiltration with lymphoma, especially CLL or marginal zone lymphoma [25, 26].
  - There was no correlation between the extent of BM infiltration and the absolute number of peripheral blood monoclonal B cells [24], and current WHO criteria for CLL/SLL do not include extent of bone marrow involvement as a disease-defining feature.

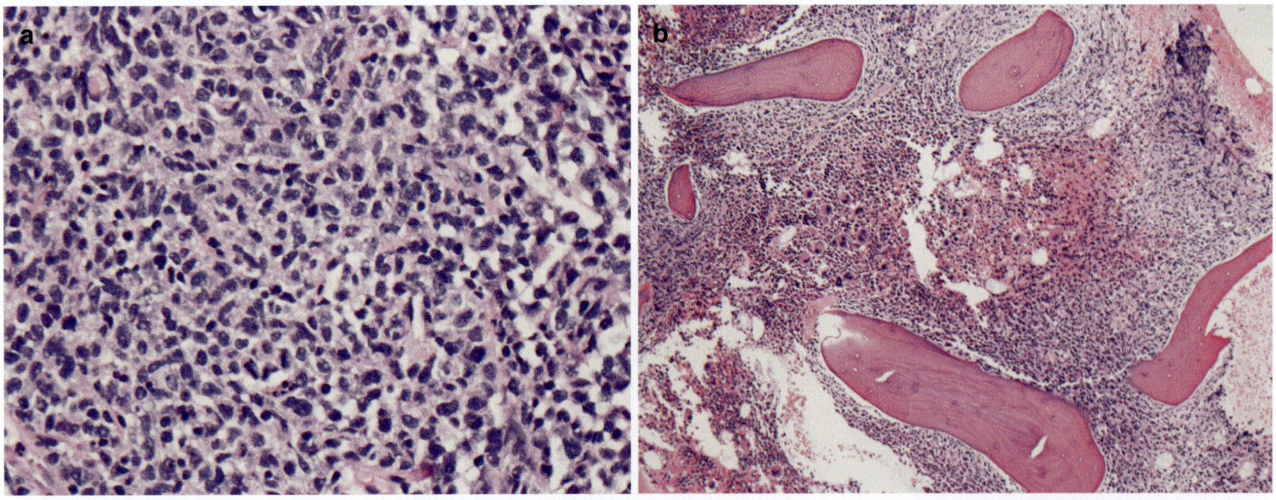

Fig. 27.3 Lymphoma with discordant morphology in lymph node and bone marrow. (**a**) The lymph node biopsy shows diffuse large B-cell lymphoma. (**b**) The bone marrow core biopsy shows low-grade follicular lymphoma

It is important to note that the mere presence of small monoclonal B-cell populations detected in the bone marrow by flow cytometry is not diagnostic of involvement by lymphoma. Monoclonal B-cell populations should always be interpreted in the clinical context and correlated with other laboratory findings.

Characteristic Features of Specific Lymphomas Involving the Bone Marrow

12. What are the distinctive pathologic features of splenic marginal zone lymphoma in bone marrow, and what are the important differential diagnostic considerations?

Splenic marginal zone lymphoma (SMZL) is an indolent small B-cell lymphoma that regularly involves the spleen and bone marrow (see also Chap. 5). For practical reasons, bone marrow examination is almost always the primary (and often the only) diagnostic tissue available. The characteristic clinical and pathologic features of splenic marginal zone lymphoma include:

- Clinically, patients usually present with massive splenomegaly. Splenic hilar lymph nodes may be involved, but peripheral lymphadenopathy and extranodal infiltration are extremely uncommon.
- Lymphoma cells with short polar villi, so-called villous lymphocytes, may be detected in peripheral blood (Fig. 27.4a) [27, 28].
- In the bone marrow, SMZLs typically exhibit nodular interstitial and intrasinusoidal infiltration patterns. Occasionally, reactive germinal centers may be present (Fig. 27.4b). Plasmacytic differentiation can be seen in a subset of the cases.
- Immunophenotypically SMZLs express B-cell markers CD20, CD79a, and surface IgM and usually IgD as well. CD5 may be positive in 10–25% of the cases. They are usually negative for the immunophenotypic markers that are typical of other small B-cell lymphomas, such as CD10 and BCL6 in FL, LEF1 in CLL, cyclin D1 and SOX11 in MCL, and CD103 and annexin A1 in hairy cell leukemia, respectively.

Differential diagnosis among SMZL, LPL, nodal marginal zone lymphoma (NMZL), and extranodal marginal zone lymphoma of mucosa-associated lymphoid tissue (MALT) may be difficult due to the overlapping morphologic and immunophenotypic features. Detailed clinical information is crucial; additionally, cytogenetic and molecular markers may be helpful.

- Clinically, patients with SMZL may have a small paraprotein, but marked hyperviscosity and hypergammaglobulinemia are uncommon.
- A subset of SMZL shows cytogenetic abnormalities such as gains of 3q and deletions of 7q. The t(11;18)(q21;q21), t(14;18)(q32;q21), and t(1;14)(p22;q32) seen in MALT lymphomas are not reported in SMZL [29].

Another useful marker is *MYD88* L265P mutation that is frequent in LPL (90–100%) and rare in SMZL (6%) [30, 31].

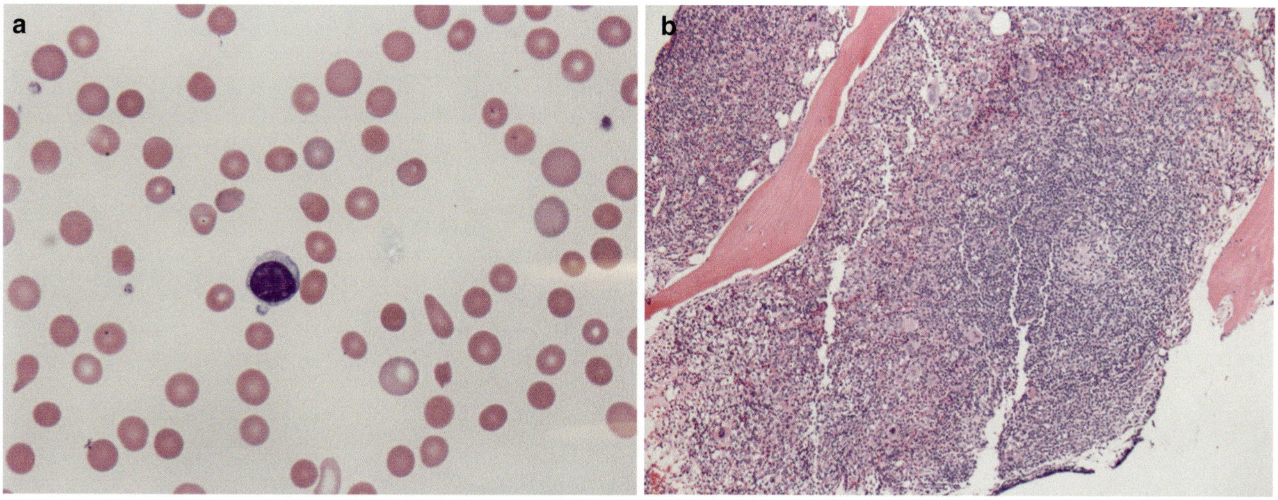

Fig. 27.4 Splenic marginal zone lymphoma in the peripheral blood and bone marrow. (**a**) A lymphoma cell with polar villi is present in the peripheral blood. (**b**) Bone marrow biopsy shows a large lymphoid aggregate with a small residual germinal center

13. What are the typical pathologic features and caveats in the diagnosis of classic hairy cell leukemia in bone marrow?

Hairy cell leukemia (HCL) is a mature B-cell neoplasm with distinct clinical, cytologic, immunophenotypic, and molecular features. It should be differentiated from hairy cell leukemia variant (vHCL) which is more aggressive and resistant to conventional HCL therapy with purine nucleoside analogs.

- HCL usually involves the blood, bone marrow, and spleen. The diagnosis is established from blood and bone marrow examination, and the spleen is submitted for pathological examination in rare cases when splenectomy is performed for therapeutic purposes.
- Most patients present with splenomegaly and cytopenia particularly monocytopenia. Lymphocytosis is usually quite limited or absent in classic hairy cell leukemia (cHCL).
- Generally, only few circulating hairy cells are seen on peripheral blood smears. The cells show a characteristic appearance with an oval or kidney-shaped nucleus and abundant pale cytoplasm with circumferential projections (Fig. 27.5a). A bone marrow biopsy, in addition to an aspirate, is advised for the initial diagnosis of HCL as the bone marrow is often difficult or impossible to aspirate (dry tap) due to tumor-associated reticulin fibrosis.
- In the bone marrow, HCL typically shows a diffuse or subtle patchy interstitial infiltrate composed of "boringly" monotonous lymphoid cells with widely spaced oval or indented nuclei and abundant clear cytoplasm, imparting a "fried-egg" appearance.
- Although usually hypercellular, in some cases the bone marrow may exhibit hypoplastic features with only

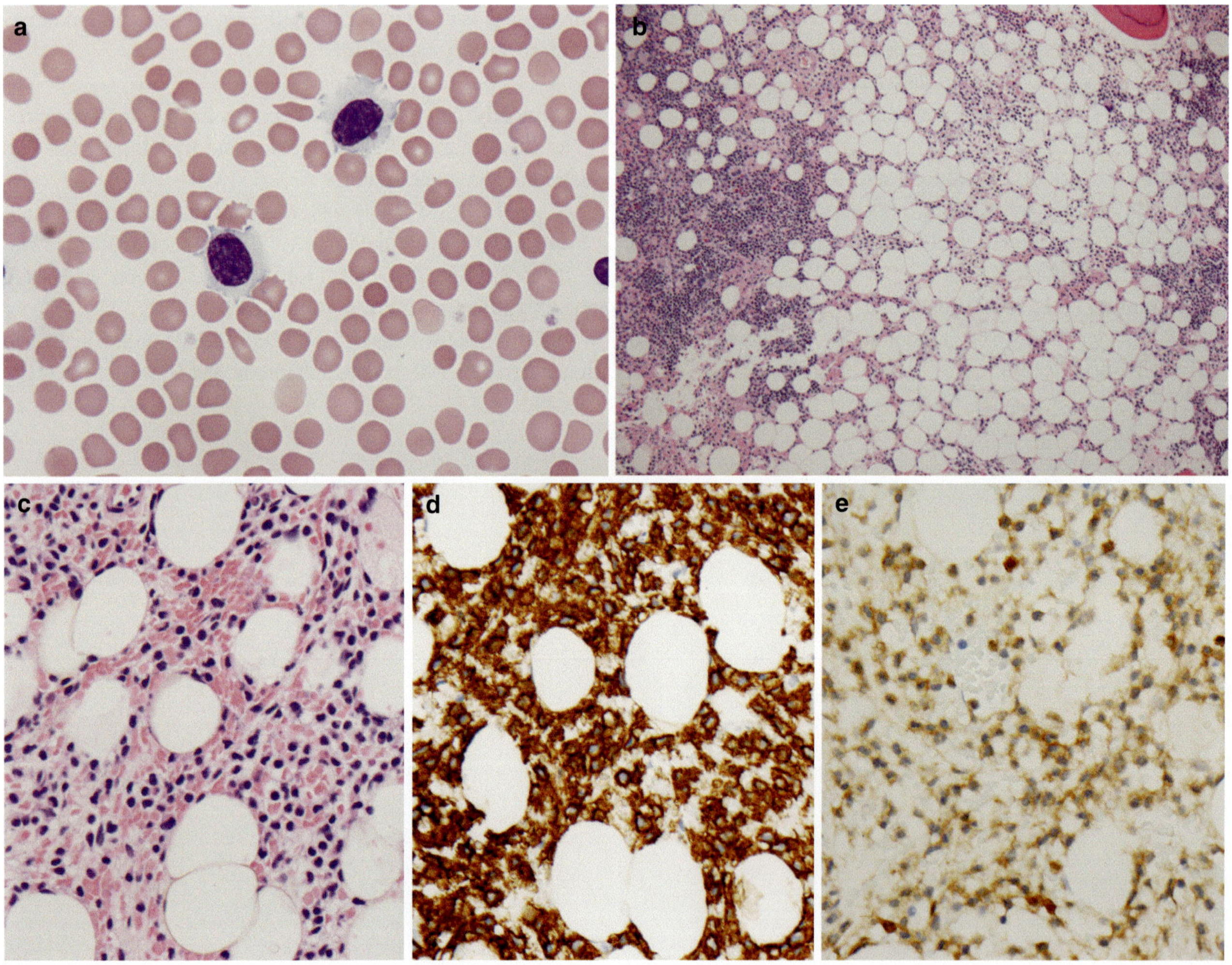

Fig. 27.5 Hairy cell leukemia in the peripheral blood and bone marrow. (**a**) Two hairy cells with typical morphologic features are present in the peripheral blood. (**b**) Bone marrow biopsy shows a subtle interstitial infiltration by hairy cell leukemia. (**c**) High-magnification view shows hairy cells with widely spaced oval or indented nuclei. (**d**) Immunohistochemical staining for CD20 highlights hairy cells. (**e**) Immunohistochemical staining for annexin A1 highlights hairy cells

small numbers of hairy cells infiltrating around fat cells, resembling aplastic anemia (Fig. 27.5b, c). Some cases may show atypical morphologic features mimicking dysplastic changes and can be misdiagnosed as myelodysplastic syndrome. It is important to be aware of these pathologic variations and to perform immunohistochemical assays to aid in the diagnosis.

- In cHCL, hairy cells express pan-B-cell antigens including CD19, CD20, and CD22 and characteristically express CD11c, CD25, CD103, CD123 (bright), cyclin D1 (usually weak), TRAP, DBA44, T-bet, and annexin A1. They usually lack expression of CD5, CD10, and CD23 but cases with atypical phenotypes are described.
- Annexin A1 is considered to be the most specific marker for HCL. However, it must be interpreted in conjunction with staining for a B-cell antigen because it is also expressed by myeloid cells and some T cells (Fig. 27.5d, e). For this reason, its utility in the diagnosis of minimal residual disease is limited.
- Although less specific, T-bet consistently displays homogeneous strong nuclear staining in HCL and is suggested to be an effective marker of minimal residual disease in follow-up biopsies [32].
- In addition, virtually all cHCL is positive for *BRAF* V600E mutation, and immunohistochemical staining for *BRAF* V600E mutant protein may be useful for detecting residual disease [33].

HCL treatment differs from other B-cell lymphomas, and therefore it must be distinguished from other indolent B-cell lymphoproliferations with predominant bone marrow and splenic involvement, such as HCL-variant (vHCL), SMZL, and splenic diffuse red pulp small B-cell lymphoma (SDRPL). Generally, these entities can be excluded based on morphologic and immunophenotypic features.

- Unlike cHCL, patients with vHCL commonly present with lymphocytosis with higher numbers of circulating neoplastic cells. Morphologically, the cells also have circumferential cytoplasmic projections but often a prominent nucleolus.
- In contrast to HCL, the marrow infiltration tends to be predominantly sinusoidal in HCL-v and SDRPL. As mentioned previously, SMZL shows a distinct nodular and intrasinusoidal infiltration pattern in bone marrow, different from cHCL.
- Immunophenotyping is an important tool for diagnosis. The tumor cells in SMZL, vHCL, and SDRPL typically do not express several key HCL antigens such as annexin A1, CD25, and CD123.
- Furthermore, molecular analysis for the *BRAF* V600E mutation is positive in essentially all cases of cHCL but not in vHCL or other B-cell lymphomas.

14. What are the main morphologic and immunophenotypic characteristics and challenges in the diagnosis of mature T-/NK-cell neoplasms in the bone marrow?

Bone marrow involvement by T-/NK-cell neoplasms can be challenging to diagnose, particularly in patients without known history of lymphoma. See Chap. 8 for diagnostic features of these lymphomas outside the bone marrow. Subtle infiltration is more frequent in T- than in B-cell lymphomas, and bone marrow may show nonspecific histological features which differ from those of nodal biopsy specimens. Furthermore, various secondary changes, such as hyperplasia of the hematopoietic precursors, eosinophilia, polyclonal plasmacytosis, hemophagocytosis, etc., may obscure the neoplastic infiltrate. The main morphologic and immunophenotypic characteristics of bone marrow involvement in different mature T-/NK-cell neoplasms are summarized in Table 27.3. It is important to recognize the characteristic infiltration patterns and misleading features and integrate morphologic findings, ancillary studies, and clinical information in the diagnosis.

Table 27.3 Histologic features of mature T-/NK-cell neoplasms involving bone marrow

Lymphoma subtype	Patterns of marrow involvement	Comments
T-LGL	Interstitial or intrasinusoidal	Small T lymphocytes positive for CD3, CD8, CD57, and TIA1
AITL	Patchy, ill-defined nodular, or diffuse	Polymorphous infiltrates with increased plasma cells and eosinophils. Neoplastic cells often have clear cytoplasm
ALCL	Patchy, intrasinusoidal, sparse	Immunostaining for CD30 or ALK1 aids in detecting the neoplastic cells
Hepatosplenic T-cell lymphoma	Intrasinusoidal, interstitial	Monomorphic small- to medium-sized lymphocytes. Isochromosome 7q is common
ATLL	Nodular, patchy loose aggregates	Osteolytic bone resorption is common
PTCL, NOS	Nodular or diffuse	Polymorphous infiltrate may be present, containing lymphoma cells intermixed with reactive cells
Aggressive NK-cell leukemia	Interstitial, intrasinusoidal, or diffuse	Variably sized atypical lymphoid cells. In situ hybridization for EBER highlights the neoplastic cells

15. What are the pathologic features of angioimmunoblastic T-cell lymphoma in bone marrow?

Angioimmunoblastic T-cell lymphoma (AITL) is a peripheral T-cell lymphoma of T-follicular helper cell origin and is characterized by a polymorphous infiltrate involving lymph node with a prominent proliferation of high endothelial venules and follicular dendritic cells. AITL typically presents with advanced-stage disease and is known to frequently involve bone marrow. The histological changes of bone marrow often mimic features seen in the peripheral lymph nodes. A few reports have described pathologic findings of AITL in bone marrow [34–36], which are summarized below.

- The infiltrate is often multifocal and may show a paratrabecular or intertrabecular distribution and a vaguely nodular or interstitial pattern.
- Most cases contain poorly defined lymphoid or lymphohistiocytic aggregates composed of small- to medium-sized lymphoid cells, scattered large transformed cells, occasional eosinophils, and increased plasma cells.
- Atypical lymphocytes with clear or pale cytoplasm, so-called clear cells, are detectable only in a small subset of the cases (Fig. 27.6a).
- In some cases, plasma cells may be markedly increased, mimicking a plasma cell neoplasm. B-immuno blasts can also be seen, some resembling Reed-Sternberg cells.

In the bone marrows suspicious for involvement by AITL, immunohistochemical studies are very helpful for establishing the diagnosis.

- The neoplastic T cells are positive for pan-T-cell markers CD2, CD3, and CD5 and are mostly positive for CD4 and PD1 (Fig. 27.6b, c).
- Of note, CD10 and CXCL13, which are expressed by neoplastic T cells in the lymph node involved by AITL, are rarely expressed by the tumor cells infiltrating the marrow [35].
- In addition, in contrast to lymph node, CD21+ or CD35+ follicular dendritic cells are usually not present in AITL infiltrates in bone marrow.

16. What are the typical pathologic features of T-cell large granular lymphocytic (T-LGL) leukemia in bone marrow, and what are the important differential diagnostic considerations?

- T-cell large granular lymphocytic (T-LGL) leukemia is a chronic, indolent, clonal proliferation of T-LGLs characterized by a persistent (>6 months) increase in the number of peripheral blood T-cell LGLs, usually to 2–20 × 10^9/l without a clearly identified cause.
- Patients with T-LGL frequently present with splenomegaly, neutropenia, and autoimmune diseases like rheumatoid arthritis. Although lymphocyte counts often exceed 2 × 10^9/l, a subset of patients may lack lymphocytosis or increased LGLs in the peripheral blood.
- The bone marrow cellularity in patients with T-LGL leukemia varies from hypocellular to mildly hypercellular. The neoplastic T cells show mainly interstitial infiltration, but an intrasinusoidal component may also be present (Fig. 27.7a, b). Interestingly, reactive intertrabecular lymphoid aggregates are also frequently present containing polyclonal B-cell centers surrounded by a rim of CD4+ T cells.
- Most cases of T-LGL leukemia demonstrate a CD3+, CD8+, CD4-, CD57+, CD16+, TCRαβ+ phenotype and express cytotoxic markers, TIA1 and/or granzyme B. Rare cases of T-LGL leukemia have variant phenotypes such as CD8+/TCR γδ+, CD4+/TCRαβ+, or CD4-/CD8- phenotype.
- The interstitial and intrasinusoidal infiltration of neoplastic T cells may be subtle on H&E-stained sections. Ancillary studies including immunohistochemistry, flow cytometric analysis, and PCR for *TCR* gene rearrangement are helpful to confirm the diagnosis.

The differential diagnosis of T-LGL leukemia includes reactive large granular lymphocytosis, T-cell PLL, HSTL, chronic lymphoproliferative disorders of NK cells, among others. Increased large granular lymphocytes may be seen in various reactive conditions including autoimmune disorders, infectious diseases, post-bone marrow transplant states, non-Hodgkin lymphomas, etc. The reactive LGL lymphocytosis is often transient and is generally a non-clonal process. However, clonal or oligoclonal T-cell gene rearrangements can be detected in nonneoplastic conditions such as in chronic inflammatory states or following allogeneic bone marrow transplantation; thus they are not entirely specific for T-LGL leukemia. Previous study has shown that the combined identification of a T-cell clone and a CD8 + (dim)/CD57+ T-cell population and/or loss of CD5 on T cells is a more reliable predictor of T-LGL leukemia.

17. What are the typical pathologic features of hepatosplenic T-cell lymphoma in the bone marrow, and what are the important differential diagnostic considerations?

Hepatosplenic T-cell lymphoma (HSTL) is a rare, aggressive T-cell lymphoma usually affecting young male patients. Patients often have systemic symptoms, hepatosplenomegaly, bone marrow involvement, and peripheral

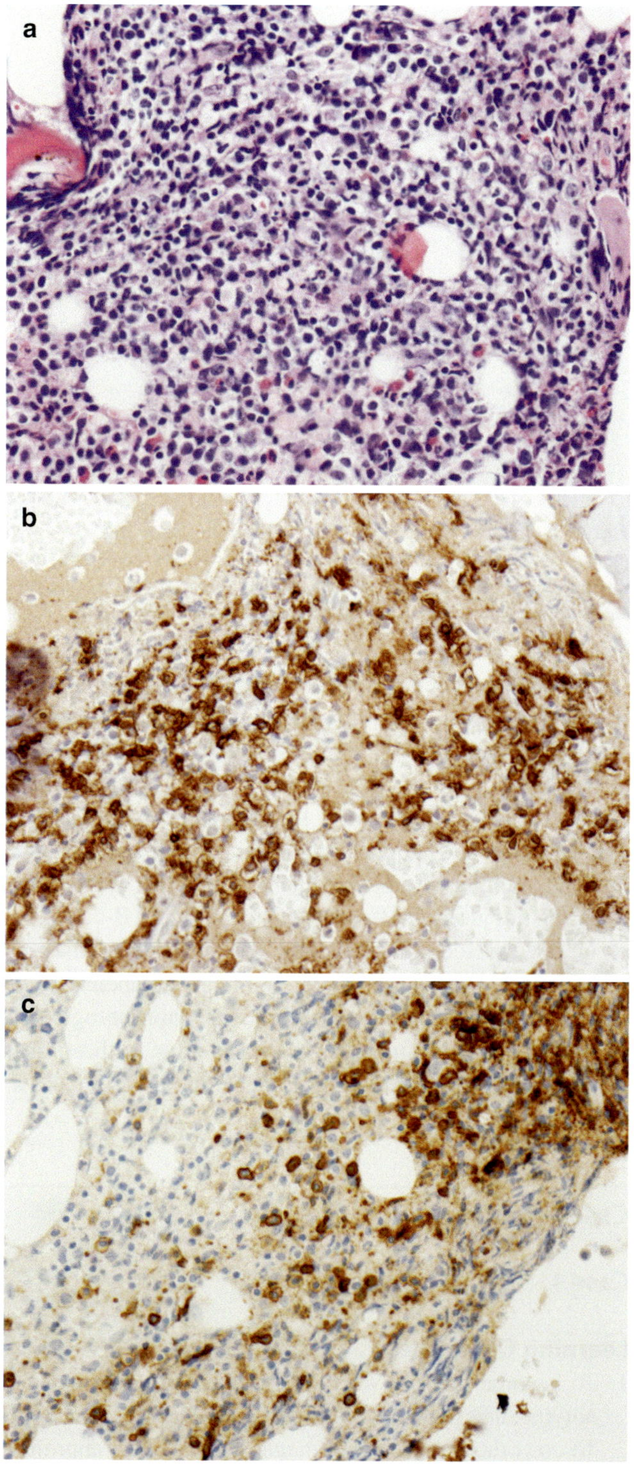

Fig. 27.6 Angioimmunoblastic T-cell lymphoma involving the bone marrow. (**a**) Bone marrow biopsy shows an abnormal lymphoid infiltrate consisting of lymphocytes, histiocytes, plasma cells, and eosinophils. Atypical lymphocytes with clear cytoplasm are present. (**b**) Immunohistochemical staining for CD3 highlights small- to medium-sized T cells. (**c**) Immunohistochemical staining for PD1 is positive in the neoplastic cells

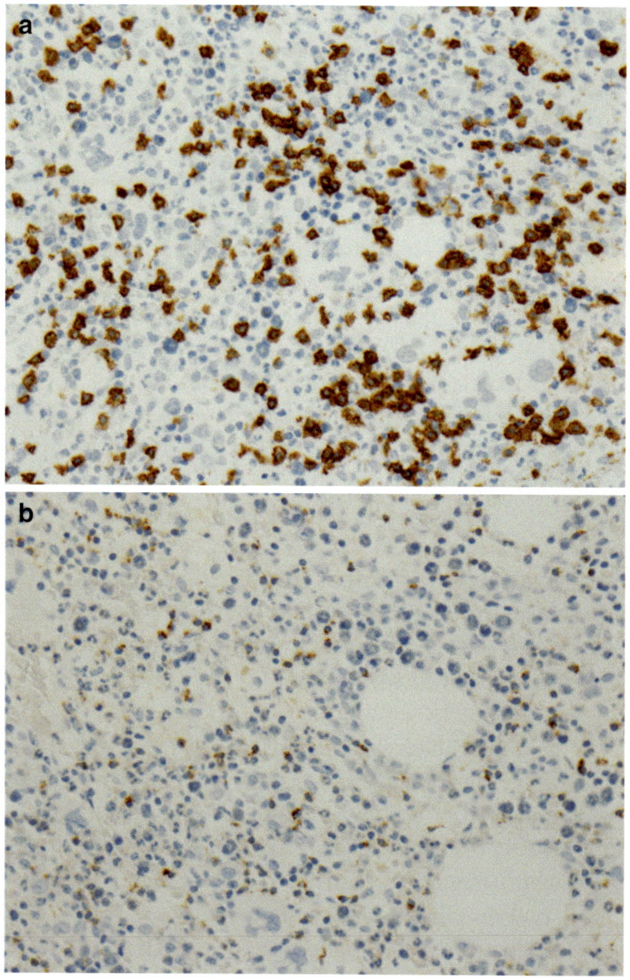

Fig. 27.7 T-cell large granular lymphocytic leukemia involving the bone marrow. (**a**) Immunohistochemical staining for CD8 highlights the T-cell LGL with interstitial and intrasinusoidal infiltration. (**b**) Immunohistochemical staining for TIA1 highlights the neoplastic T cells

blood cytopenias particularly thrombocytopenia. The characteristic pathologic features of HSTL include:

- The neoplastic T cells of HSTL are nonactivated cytotoxic T cells that usually express CD2, CD3, and TCRγδ and lack CD4, CD5, and CD8, although a minority of cases is of alpha beta type [37]. CD56 is frequently expressed and CD16 is positive in a subset of the cases.
- The bone marrow core biopsies are often hypercellular with a frequently subtle, predominantly sinusoidal infiltrate of atypical small- to medium-sized lymphoid cells. With progression, the pattern of HSTL in bone marrow biopsy specimens became increasingly interstitial [38].

- The differential diagnosis of HSTL includes T-LGL and aggressive NK-cell leukemia/lymphoma, etc.
- The clinical setting, immunophenotype, and neoplastic lymphocytes devoid of cytoplasmic azurophilic granules help to distinguish HSTCL from T-LGL [39].
- The presence of i(7q) and/or trisomy 8 was also significantly correlated with the diagnosis of HSTL [40].
- Aggressive NK-cell leukemia/lymphoma typically has a fulminant clinical course. Although the neoplastic cells share some of the immunophenotypic features of HSTL (CD2+, CD56+, CD16+), they express all cytotoxic protein markers (granzyme B and perforin) and lack surface CD3 and TCR. In addition, in situ hybridization for EBER highlights the neoplastic cells. The *TCR* genes are in the germline configuration [38].

18. What are the typical histologic features of Hodgkin lymphoma (HL) in bone marrow, and what are the important differential diagnostic considerations?

See Chap. 9 for diagnostic features of HL outside the bone marrow. It is uncommon to encounter nodular lymphocyte-predominant HL in BM. When present, the morphologic features usually resemble those in lymph node but may mimic marrow involvement by classic HL. A high degree of suspicion based on clinical history and use of appropriate IHC stains to identify the abnormal "popcorn" cells with increased follicular T-helper cells in the surrounding infiltrate are necessary for accurate diagnosis.

Bone marrow involvement by CHL is usually focal but can be diffuse. Ample sampling is important and step sections may be required to detect small patchy infiltrates. The typical features of CHL in bone marrow include:

- The lymphoma infiltrate resembles a poorly formed granuloma and is polymorphic, consisting of small lymphocytes, histiocytes, and various numbers of plasma cells, eosinophils, and occasional Hodgkin Reed-Sternberg (HRS) cells (Fig. 27.8).
- The infiltrate often evokes a certain degree of fibrosis. Atypical cells may not be easily identified on routine staining, but lesions rich in histiocytes and/or fibrillary matrix in a patient with a history of HL should raise the suspicion of bone marrow involvement.
- Immunohistochemical stains and/ or step sections may be required to establish the diagnosis.
- HRS cells are only rarely detected in aspirate smears. They may be sparse in the infiltrate and many of the HRS cells may not show prototypical RS cell morphology. Immunohistochemical stains for CD30, CD15, and PAX5 greatly aid in the identification of HRS cells in bone marrow core biopsy.

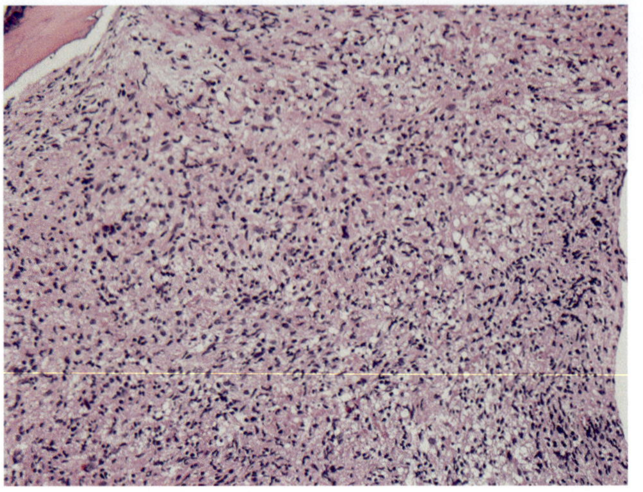

Fig. 27.8 Classic Hodgkin lymphoma involving bone marrow. Bone marrow biopsy demonstrates an abnormal infiltrate containing rare large atypical cells in a background of numerous histiocytes, scattered small lymphocytes, and occasional plasma cells and eosinophils

Bone marrow involvement by CHL can be simulated by many reactive or neoplastic conditions, including ALCL, nodular lymphocyte-predominant Hodgkin lymphoma, T-cell/histiocyte-rich B-cell lymphoma, large B-cell lymphoma with Hodgkin-like cells, granulomatous diseases and histiocytes disorders, etc. Immunohistochemistry is essential in differentiating these entities. Morphologic and immunophenotypic findings, in combination with clinical information, usually allow achieving a definitive diagnosis.

Case Presentations

Case 1

Learning Objectives

1. To become familiar with the morphologic, immunophenotypic, and molecular features of the entity
2. To construct a differential diagnosis and select appropriate diagnostic tests in the work-up

Case History

A 75-year-old male presented with progressive sensory neuropathy, fatigue, drenching night sweats, and 10 lb weight loss over the last 1–2 years. He was found to have IgM kappa paraprotein 1.9 g/dL.

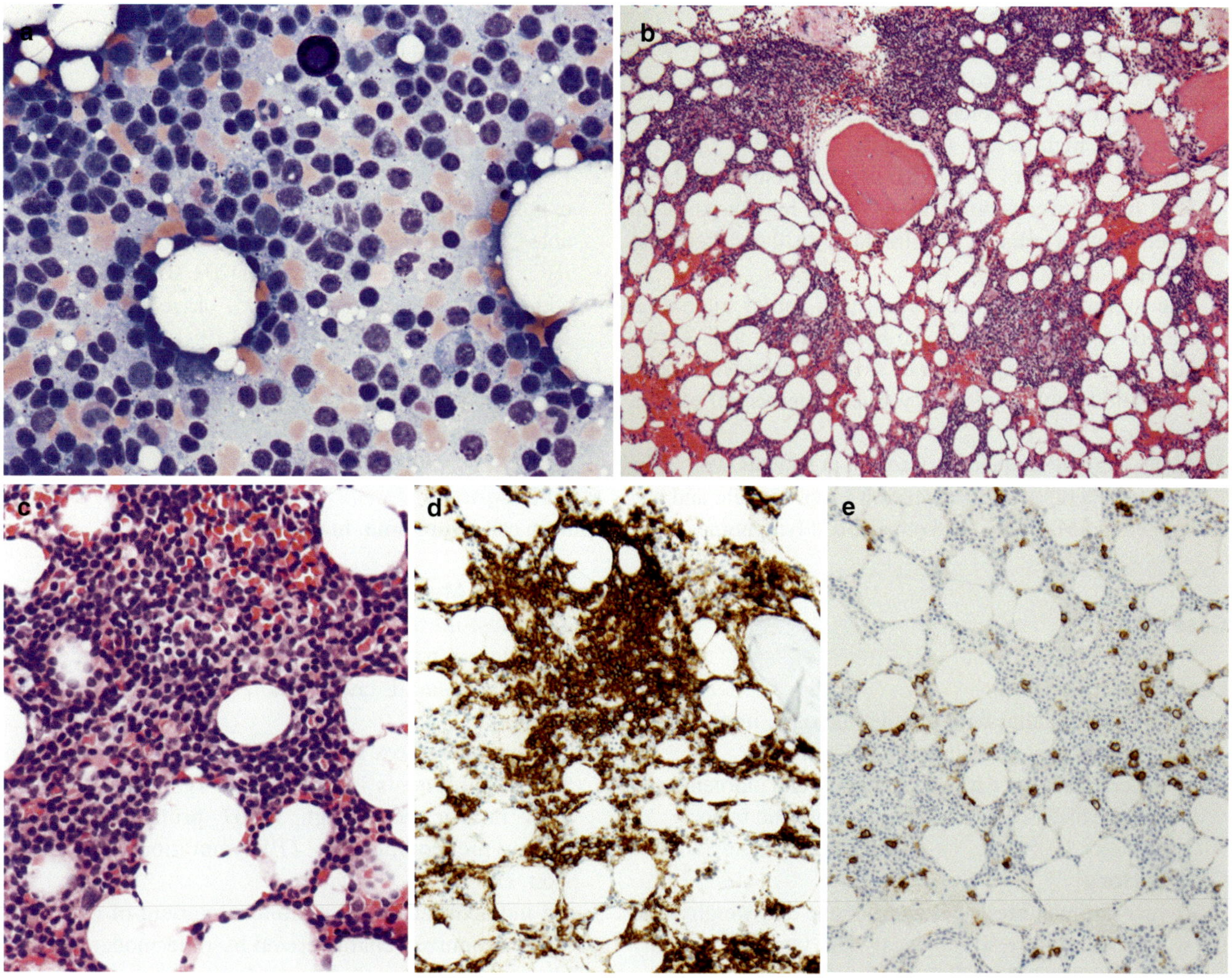

Fig. 27.9 Waldenström macroglobulinemia involving bone marrow. (**a**) Bone marrow aspirate smear demonstrates an increase in small lymphocytes, plasmacytoid lymphocytes, and plasma cells. (**b**) Bone marrow biopsy demonstrates multiple lymphoid aggregates and an increase in interstitial lymphocytes. (**c**) High-magnification view shows a mixture of small lymphocytes and plasma cells. (**d**) Immunohistochemical staining for CD20 highlights numerous small B cells. (**e**) Immunohistochemical staining for CD138 highlights scattered plasma cells

Histologic Findings

- Aspirate: focal areas with many small lymphocytes, plasmacytoid lymphocytes, and frequent plasma cells (Fig. 27.9a)
- Core biopsy: multiple non-paratrabecular lymphoid aggregates, scattered interstitial lymphocytes, and occasional plasma cells (Fig. 27.9b, c)

Differential Diagnosis

- Marginal zone lymphoma
- Waldenström macroglobulinemia/LPL
- CLL/SLL
- Reactive lymphocytosis
- Plasma cell dyscrasia

IHC and Other Ancillary Studies (Fig. 27.9d, e)

- Flow cytometry: kappa-restricted B-cell population without co-expression of CD5 or CD10.
- IHC: CD20 and PAX5 highlight scattered small B cells and B-cell aggregates comprising approximately 50% of marrow cellularity. CD138, kappa, and lambda stain approximately 5% plasma cells with marked kappa predominance.
- FISH study: positive for gain of FGFR3 (4p16) (41.0%).
- Molecular study: *MYD88* L265P mutation detected.

Final Diagnosis

Waldenström macroglobulinemia

Take-Home Messages

1. IgM paraproteinemia is associated most commonly with LPL/WM but can also occur in patients with other lymphoid neoplasms, such as CLL/SLL or MZL, etc. Although high levels (>3 g/dL) of serum IgM are strongly in favor of LPL/WM, many patients with LPL/WM have lower serum levels. Serum IgM paraprotein level is not a reliable discriminator in the differential diagnosis [41].
2. The infiltrate shows nodular, diffuse, and/or interstitial pattern of involvement in the bone marrow and is usually composed of spectrum of small lymphocytes, plasmacytoid lymphocytes, and variable numbers of plasma cells.
3. *MYD88* L265P mutation is frequent in patients with LPL/WM (~90%) [30, 42]. However, it is not specific and can be seen in SMZL (6%) and other B-cell lymphomas [31].

Case 2

Learning Objectives

1. To become familiar with the morphologic, immunophenotypic, and genetic features of the entity
2. To become familiar with the aggressive and indolent variants of the disease and significant prognostic factors

Case History

A 70-year-old man presented with fatigue and weight loss. He was found to have splenomegaly and lymphadenopathy on physical exam. His CBC was remarkable for anemia (HGB 8.7 g/dl) and atypical lymphocytosis (lymphocytes 27.64 ×10^9/L).

Histologic Findings

- Peripheral blood and aspirate: numerous small atypical lymphocytes with irregularly folded or cleaved nuclei, finely dispersed chromatin, prominent nucleoli, and scant basophilic cytoplasm (Fig. 27.10a)
- Core biopsy: hypercellular bone marrow with nodular and diffuse interstitial lymphoid infiltrates composed of small lymphocytes (Fig. 27.10b)

Differential Diagnosis

- Mantle cell lymphoma
- CLL/SLL
- Prolymphocytic leukemia
- Lymphoblastic leukemia/lymphoma

IHC and Other Ancillary Studies (Fig. 27.10c–e)

- Flow cytometry: Lambda-restricted B-cell population expressing weak CD5, CD19, CD20, weak CD22, variable CD23, and HLA-DR.
- IHC: The lymphoid cells are CD20+ B cells which are additionally positive for dim CD5, variable CD23, cyclin D1, and SOX11, but negative for LEF-1.
- Cytogenetic study: 43–47, XY, t(11;14)(q13;q32), +der(14)t(11;14),inc[3]/46, XY[17].

Final Diagnosis

Mantle cell lymphoma, blastoid variant

Take-Home Messages

1. The blastoid and pleomorphic variants of MCL are considered to be more aggressive variants [43], while the small cell variant appears to be more indolent.
2. The other features that have been associated with an adverse prognosis in mantle cell lymphoma include high mitotic rate, high Ki-67 proliferation rate, karyotypic complexity, *TP53* mutation/overexpression, etc.
3. An indolent leukemic, extranodal variant of MCL has been recognized characterized by mild-moderate lymphocytosis, lack of lymphadenopathy and hepatosplenomegaly, low-level (usually <5%) interstitial bone marrow involvement, kappa light chain expression, lack of SOX11 expression, and a simple karyotype [44].

Case 3

Learning Objectives

1. To recognize the challenges in the diagnosis of this entity in the bone marrow
2. To become familiar with the characteristic morphologic and immunohistochemical findings and the differential diagnosis

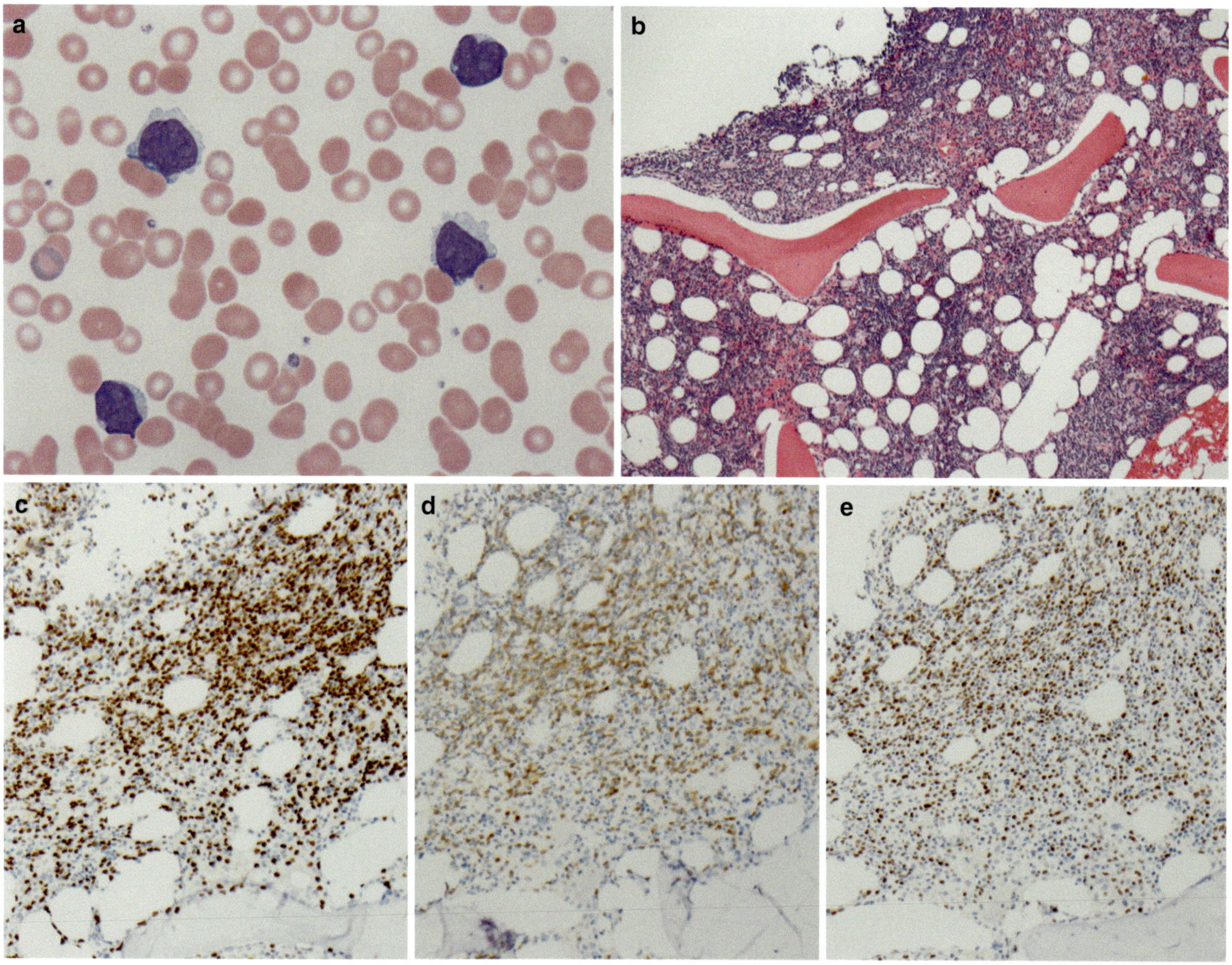

Fig. 27.10 Mantle cell lymphoma involving bone marrow. (**a**) Tumor cells resembling lymphoblasts are present in the peripheral blood. (**b**) Bone marrow biopsy demonstrates nodular and diffuse interstitial lymphoid infiltrates. (**c**) Immunohistochemical staining for PAX5 highlights the neoplastic B cells. (**d**) Immunohistochemical staining for cyclin D1 is positive in the neoplastic cells. (**e**) Immunohistochemical staining for SOX11 is positive in the neoplastic cells

Case History

A 26-year-old male presented with fever and pancytopenia. He was found on imaging studies to have mild mediastinal lymphadenopathy.

Histologic Findings

- The marrow space is almost completely replaced by a diffuse lymphohistiocytic infiltrate (Fig. 27.11a)
- Scattered large atypical lymphoid cells with monolobated or multilobated nuclei and relatively abundant eosinophilic cytoplasm are identified. Rare mummified cells are seen. Many small lymphocytes, histiocytes, scattered plasma cells, and rare eosinophils are present in the background (Fig. 27.11b)

Differential Diagnosis

- Classic Hodgkin lymphoma
- T-cell/histiocyte-rich large B-cell lymphoma
- Granulomatous inflammation
- Atypical histiocytic infiltrate

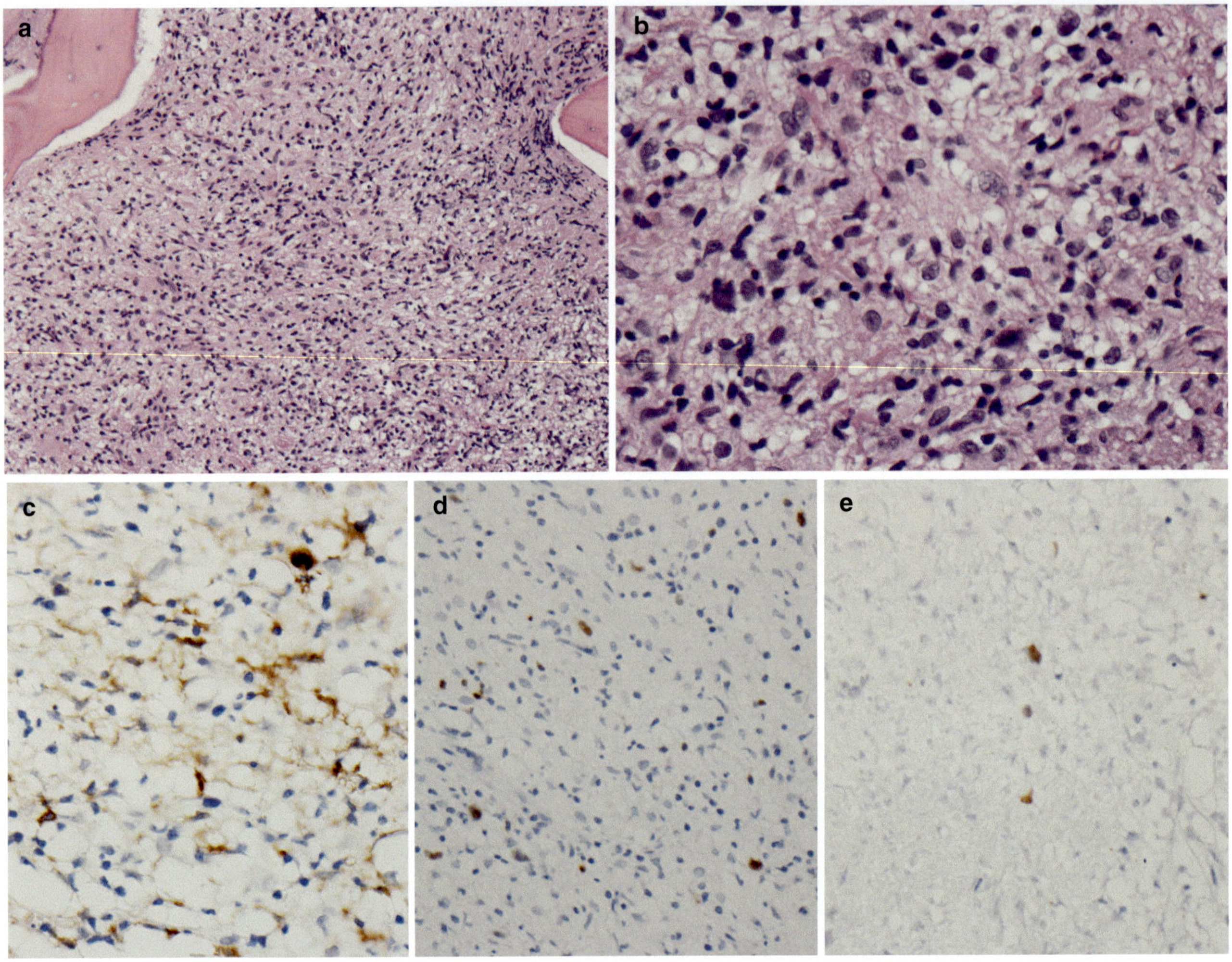

Fig. 27.11 Classic Hodgkin lymphoma involving bone marrow. (**a**) Bone marrow biopsy demonstrates a diffuse lymphohistiocytic infiltrate. (**b**) High-magnification view shows scattered large lymphoid cells with lobated nuclei in a background of small lymphocytes and numerous histiocytes. (**c**) Immunohistochemical staining for CD30 highlights the Hodgkin Reed-Sternberg (HRS) cells. (**d**) Immunohistochemical staining for PAX5 labelled the nuclei of the HRS cells weakly and the background small B cells strongly. (**e**) *EBV*-encoded small RNA (EBER) in situ hybridization is positive in the HRS cells

IHC and Other Ancillary Studies (Fig. 27.11c–e)

- IHC: The large atypical cells are positive for CD30, CD15 (dim and variable), PAX5 (dim and variable), and MUM1, but are negative for CD20, CD3, ALK1, and CD138.
- EBER ISH stains scattered large atypical nuclei.
- AFB and GMS stains were negative for microorganisms.

Final Diagnosis

Classic Hodgkin lymphoma, *EBV* positive

Take-Home Messages

1. Bone marrow may be the primary diagnostic tissue in rare cases of CHL, especially in HIV-positive patients.
2. The infiltrates are polymorphic and are frequently associated with fibrosis, granulomas, and/or necrosis.
3. Reed-Sternberg-like cells can also be seen in non-Hodgkin lymphomas such as peripheral T-cell lymphoma and *EBV*-associated lymphoproliferative disorders.
4. CHL is not subclassified in bone marrow.

Case 4

Learning Objectives

1. To recognize the challenges in the diagnosis of this entity in the bone marrow

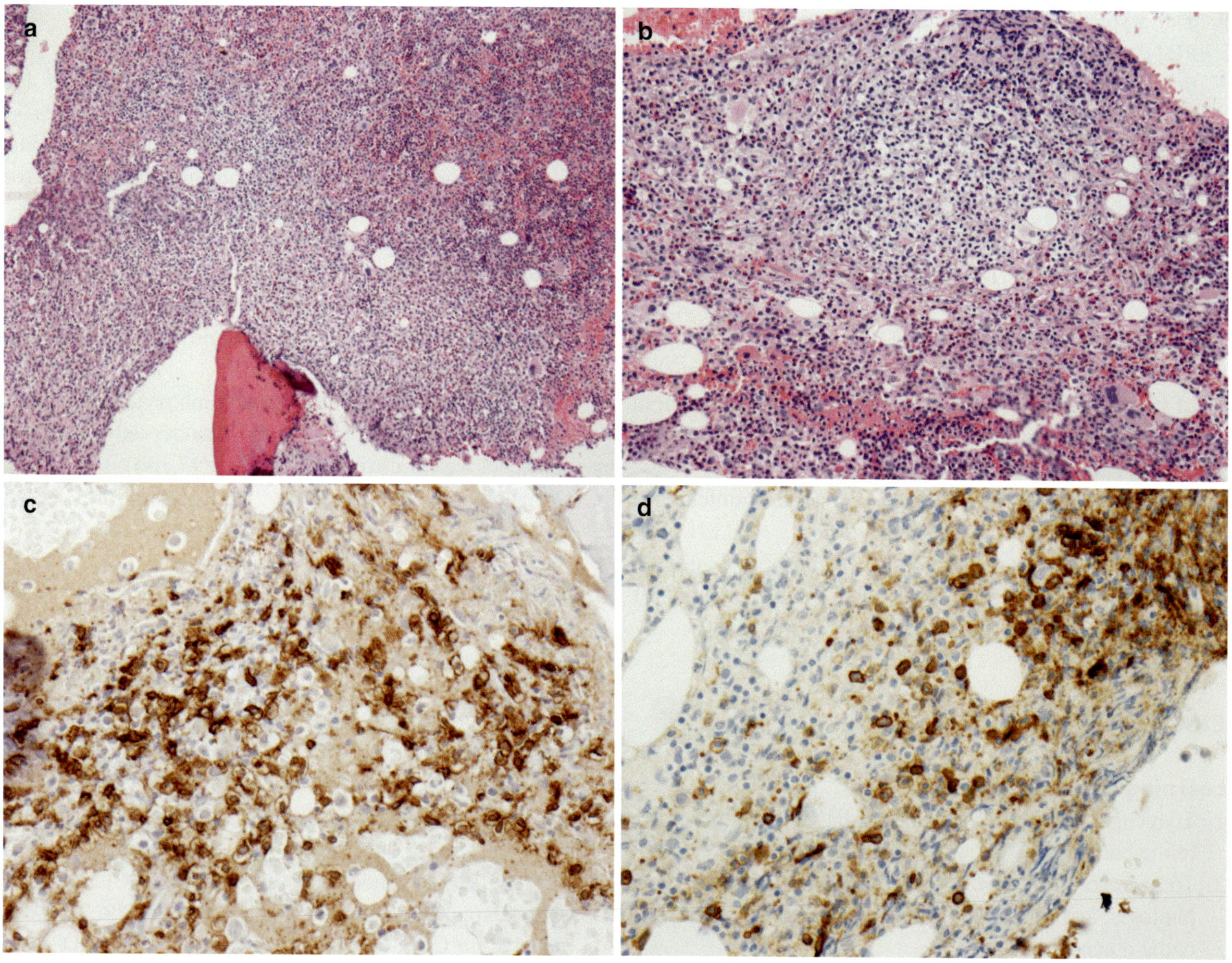

Fig. 27.12 Angioimmunoblastic T-cell lymphoma involving bone marrow. (**a**) Bone marrow biopsy shows an ill-defined polymorphous lymphoid infiltrate. (**b**) High-magnification view shows small to medium lymphoid cells with abundant clear cytoplasm. (**c**) Immunohistochemical staining for CD3 highlights neoplastic T cells. (**d**) The neoplastic cells show strong immunoreactivity for PD1

2. To become familiar with the characteristic morphologic and immunohistochemical findings and the differential diagnosis

Case History

A 60-year-old woman with history of Sjögren's syndrome presented with fatigue and weight loss. She was found to have diffuse lymphadenopathy and splenomegaly. Laboratory testing showed anemia, thrombocytopenia, and elevated total protein with serum electrophoresis revealing both elevated kappa and lambda light chains with a kappa/lambda ratio of 2.55.

Histologic Findings

- Multiple ill-defined, polymorphic lymphoid aggregates are present composed of small- to medium-sized lymphocytes with oval or mildly irregular nuclei and relatively abundant clear cytoplasm (Fig. 27.12a).
- Frequent eosinophils and plasma cells are intermixed in the filtrate (Fig. 27.12b)

Differential Diagnosis

- Peripheral T-cell lymphoma
- Angioimmunoblastic T-cell lymphoma
- Small B-cell lymphoma
- Reactive lymphoid aggregates

IHC and Other Ancillary Studies (Fig. 27.12c, d)

- CD3 highlights many small- to medium-sized atypical T lymphocytes with clear cytoplasm in the lymphoid infiltrates.

- The atypical T cells are additionally positive for CD4, PD1, and CXCL13.
- Scattered CD30+ cells are present.
- CD138, kappa, and lambda highlight many polytypic plasma cells.

Final Diagnosis

Angioimmunoblastic T-cell lymphoma

Take-Home Messages

1. The infiltrate of AITL is often heterogeneous and consists of variable numbers of small- to medium-sized lymphoid cells, scattered large transformed cells, occasional eosinophils, and increased plasma cells.
2. Plasma cells may be markedly increased, mimicking a plasma cell neoplasm or plasmacytosis.
3. In patients without previously established diagnosis, biopsy of the involved lymph node or tumor is needed for accurate classification.

Case 5

Learning Objectives

1. To recognize the challenges in the diagnosis of this entity in the bone marrow
2. To become familiar with the characteristic clinical, morphologic, and immunophenotypic findings and the differential diagnosis

Case History

A 70-year-old Asian man with no prior medical history presented with fever, chills, fatigue, and 15lb weight loss. He was found to have hepatosplenomegaly, pancytopenia, coagulopathy, acute liver injury, and acute renal failure. In addition, he had high titer *EBV* viral load, meeting criteria for hemophagocytic lymphohistiocytosis.

Histologic Findings

- Hypercellular bone marrow with large areas of necrosis and multifocal vaguely nodular and subtle interstitial lymphoid infiltrates (Fig. 27.13a).
- Atypical small- to medium-sized lymphocytes are present with pleomorphic, irregular nuclei, condensed chromatin, and scant basophilic cytoplasm (Fig. 27.13b).
- Occasional hemophagocytic histiocytes are noted (Fig. 27.13c).

Differential Diagnosis

- T-cell leukemia/lymphoma
- NK-cell leukemia/lymphoma
- Chronic active *EBV* infection
- Acute *EBV*-associated hemophagocytic lymphohistiocytosis

IHC and Other Ancillary Studies (Fig. 27.13d–g)

- The atypical lymphoid cells are positive for CD2, CD3 (cytoplasmic staining), CD56, TIA1, and EBER. They are negative for CD5, CD7, CD4, CD8, CD57, and CD30.

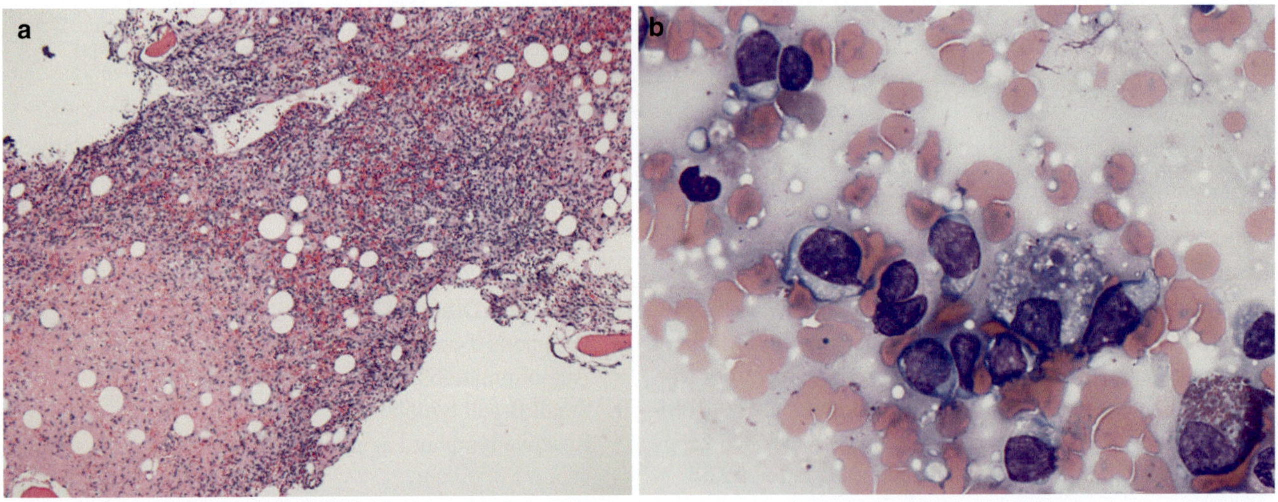

Fig. 27.13 Aggressive NK-cell leukemia/lymphoma involving bone marrow. (**a**) Bone marrow biopsy shows massive infiltration by the neoplastic cells and large areas of necrosis. (**b**) The neoplastic cells have irregular nuclei and distinct nucleoli.

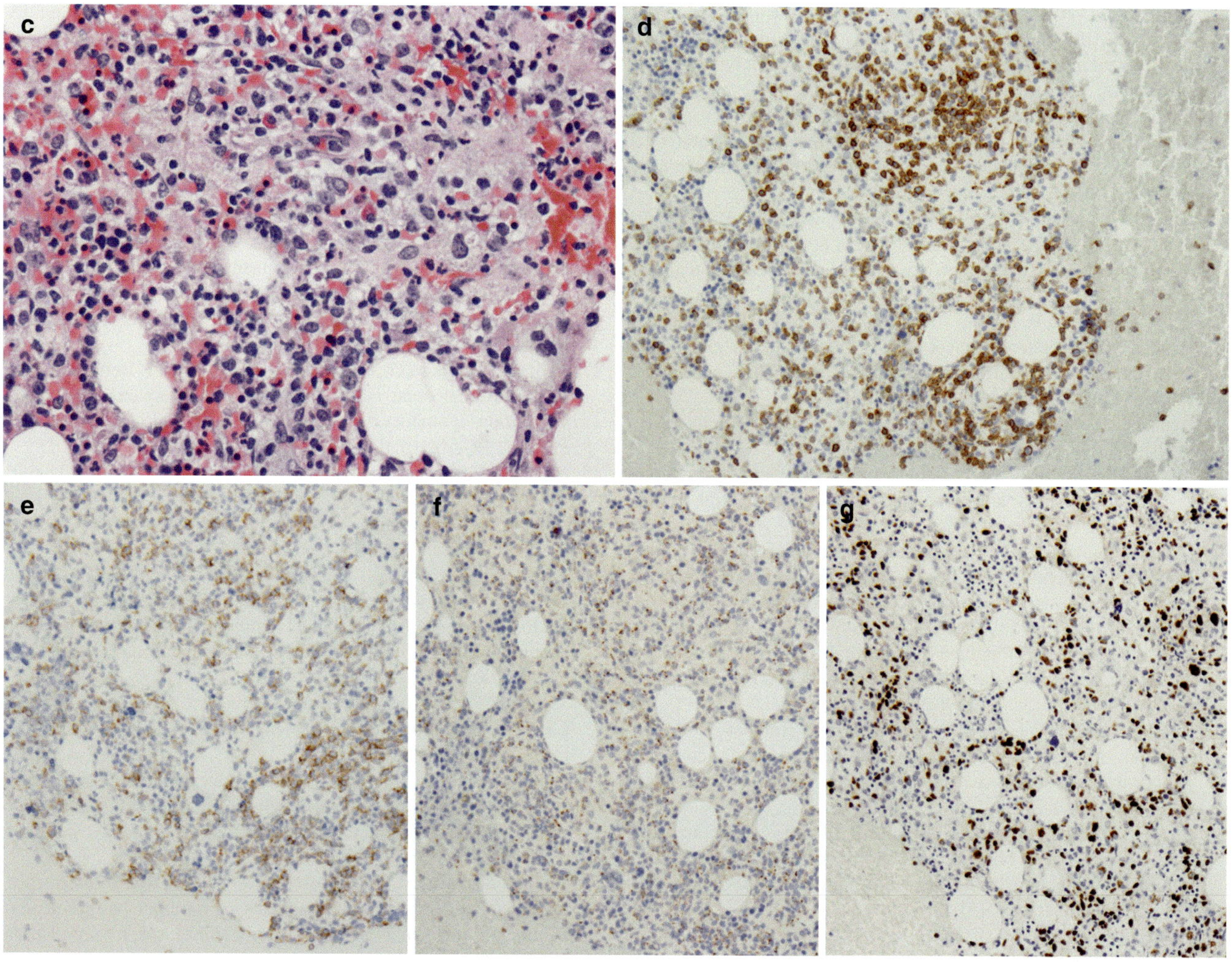

Fig. 27.13 (continued) (**c**) The neoplastic cells are admixed with hematopoietic cells and hemophagocytic histiocytes. (**d**) Immunohistochemical staining for CD3 highlights neoplastic cells. Note the cytoplasmic staining pattern. (**e**) The neoplastic cells show immunoreactivity for CD56. (**f**) The neoplastic cells show immunoreactivity for TIA1. (**g**) EBER in situ hybridization is positive in the neoplastic cells

Final Diagnosis

Aggressive NK-cell leukemia/lymphoma

Take-Home Messages

1. The number of neoplastic cells may be limited in peripheral blood and bone marrow. The diagnosis of early aggressive NK-cell leukemia can be challenging and may be delayed.
2. Necrosis is common.
3. Distinction between aggressive NK-cell leukemia and end-stage extranodal NK−/T-cell lymphoma can be difficult [45].

References

1. Martinez A, Ponzoni M, Agostinelli C, Hebeda KM, Matutes E, Peccatori J, et al. Primary bone marrow lymphoma: an uncommon extranodal presentation of aggressive non-Hodgkin lymphomas. Am J Surg Pathol. 2012;36(2):296–304.
2. Fend F, Kremer M. Diagnosis and classification of malignant lymphoma and related entities in the bone marrow trephine biopsy. Pathobiology. 2007;74(2):133–43.
3. Shipp MA. Prognostic factors in aggressive non-Hodgkin's lymphoma: who has "high-risk" disease? Blood. 1994;83(5):1165–73.
4. McKenna RW, Hernandez JA. Bone marrow in malignant lymphoma. Hematol Oncol Clin North Am. 1988;2(4):617–35.

5. Yan Y, Chan WC, Weisenburger DD, Anderson JR, Bast MA, Vose JM, et al. Clinical and prognostic significance of bone marrow involvement in patients with diffuse aggressive B-cell lymphoma. J Clin Oncol. 1995;13(6):1336–42.
6. Lambertenghi-Deliliers G, Annaloro C, Soligo D, Oriani A, Pozzoli E, Quirici N, et al. Incidence and histological features of bone marrow involvement in malignant lymphomas. Ann Hematol. 1992;65(2):61–5.
7. Howell SJ, Grey M, Chang J, Morgenstern GR, Cowan RA, Deakin DP, et al. The value of bone marrow examination in the staging of Hodgkin's lymphoma: a review of 955 cases seen in a regional cancer centre. Br J Haematol. 2002;119(2):408–11.
8. Levy R, Colonna P, Tourani JM, Gastaut JA, Brice P, Raphael M, et al. Human immunodeficiency virus associated Hodgkin's disease: report of 45 cases from the French Registry of HIV-Associated Tumors. Leuk Lymphoma. 1995;16(5–6):451–6.
9. Bain BJ. Bone marrow trephine biopsy. J Clin Pathol. 2001; 54(10):737–42.
10. Navone R, Colombano MT. Histopathological trephine biopsy findings in cases of 'dry tap' bone marrow aspirations. Appl Pathol. 1984;2(5):264–71.
11. Arber DA, George TI. Bone marrow biopsy involvement by non-Hodgkin's lymphoma: frequency of lymphoma types, patterns, blood involvement, and discordance with other sites in 450 specimens. Am J Surg Pathol. 2005;29(12):1549–57.
12. Brudno J, Tadmor T, Pittaluga S, Nicolae A, Polliack A, Dunleavy K. Discordant bone marrow involvement in non-Hodgkin lymphoma. Blood. 2015;127(8):965–70.
13. Costes V, Duchayne E, Taib J, Delfour C, Rousset T, Baldet P, et al. Intrasinusoidal bone marrow infiltration: a common growth pattern for different lymphoma subtypes. Br J Haematol. 2002;119(4):916–22.
14. Merli M, Arcaini L, Boveri E, Rattotti S, Picone C, Passamonti F, et al. Assessment of bone marrow involvement in non-Hodgkin's lymphomas: comparison between histology and flow cytometry. Eur J Haematol. 2010;85(5):405–15.
15. Al-Rohil RN, Torres-Cabala CA, Patel A, Tetzlaff MT, Ivan D, Nagarajan P, et al. Loss of CD30 expression after treatment with brentuximab vedotin in a patient with anaplastic large cell lymphoma: a novel finding. J Cutan Pathol. 2016;43(12):1161–6.
16. Nielson C, Fischer R, Fraga G, Aires D. Loss of CD30 expression in anaplastic large cell lymphoma following Brentuximab therapy. J Drugs Dermatol. 2016;15(7):894–5.
17. Wilkins BS. Pitfalls in bone marrow pathology: avoiding errors in bone marrow trephine biopsy diagnosis. J Clin Pathol. 2011;64(5):380–6.
18. Thiele J, Zirbes TK, Kvasnicka HM, Fischer R. Focal lymphoid aggregates (nodules) in bone marrow biopsies: differentiation between benign hyperplasia and malignant lymphoma--a practical guideline. J Clin Pathol. 1999;52(4):294–300.
19. Sovani V, Harvey C, Haynes AP, McMillan AK, Clark DM, O'Connor SR. Bone marrow trephine biopsy involvement by lymphoma: review of histopathological features in 511 specimens and correlation with diagnostic biopsy, aspirate and peripheral blood findings. J Clin Pathol. 2014;67(5):389–95.
20. Torlakovic E, Torlakovic G, Brunning RD. Follicular pattern of bone marrow involvement by follicular lymphoma. Am J Clin Pathol. 2002;118(5):780–6.
21. Wool GD, Deucher A. Bone marrow necrosis: ten-year retrospective review of bone marrow biopsy specimens. Am J Clin Pathol. 2015;143(2):201–13; quiz 306.
22. Kremer M, Spitzer M, Mandl-Weber S, Stecker K, Schmidt B, Hofler H, et al. Discordant bone marrow involvement in diffuse large B-cell lymphoma: comparative molecular analysis reveals a heterogeneous group of disorders. Lab Investig. 2003;83(1):107–14.
23. Rawstron AC, Green MJ, Kuzmicki A, Kennedy B, Fenton JA, Evans PA, et al. Monoclonal B lymphocytes with the characteristics of "indolent" chronic lymphocytic leukemia are present in 3.5% of adults with normal blood counts. Blood. 2002;100(2):635–9.
24. Kalpadakis C, Pangalis GA, Sachanas S, Vassilakopoulos TP, Kyriakaki S, Korkolopoulou P, et al. New insights into monoclonal B-cell lymphocytosis. Biomed Res Int. 2014;2014:258917.
25. Randen U, Tierens AM, Tjonnfjord GE, Delabie J. Bone marrow histology in monoclonal B-cell lymphocytosis shows various B-cell infiltration patterns. Am J Clin Pathol. 2013;139(3):390–5.
26. Nelson BP, Abdul-Nabi A, Goolsby C, Winter J, Peterson L. Characterization of tissue findings in bone marrow biopsy specimens with small monoclonal B-cell populations. Am J Clin Pathol. 2014;141(5):687–96.
27. Labouyrie E, Marit G, Vial JP, Lacombe F, Fialon P, Bernard P, et al. Intrasinusoidal bone marrow involvement by splenic lymphoma with villous lymphocytes: a helpful immunohistologic feature. Mod Pathol. 1997;10(10):1015–20.
28. Mollejo M, Menarguez J, Lloret E, Sanchez A, Campo E, Algara P, et al. Splenic marginal zone lymphoma: a distinctive type of low-grade B-cell lymphoma. A clinicopathological study of 13 cases. Am J Surg Pathol. 1995;19(10):1146–57.
29. Remstein ED, Kurtin PJ, James CD, Wang XY, Meyer RG, Dewald GW. Mucosa-associated lymphoid tissue lymphomas with t(11;18)(q21;q21) and mucosa-associated lymphoid tissue lymphomas with aneuploidy develop along different pathogenetic pathways. Am J Pathol. 2002;161(1):63–71.
30. Treon SP, Xu L, Yang G, Zhou Y, Liu X, Cao Y, et al. MYD88 L265P somatic mutation in Waldenstrom's macroglobulinemia. N Engl J Med. 2012;367(9):826–33.
31. Swerdlow SH, Kuzu I, Dogan A, Dirnhofer S, Chan JK, Sander B, et al. The many faces of small B cell lymphomas with plasmacytic differentiation and the contribution of MYD88 testing. Virchows Arch. 2016;468(3):259–75.
32. Johrens K, Stein H, Anagnostopoulos I. T-bet transcription factor detection facilitates the diagnosis of minimal hairy cell leukemia infiltrates in bone marrow trephines. Am J Surg Pathol. 2007;31(8):1181–5.
33. Sherman MJ, Hanson CA, Hoyer JD. An assessment of the usefulness of immunohistochemical stains in the diagnosis of hairy cell leukemia. Am J Clin Pathol. 2011;136(3):390–9.
34. Dogan A, Morice WG. Bone marrow histopathology in peripheral T-cell lymphomas. Br J Haematol. 2004;127(2):140–54.
35. Khokhar FA, Payne WD, Talwalkar SS, Jorgensen JL, Bueso-Ramos CE, Medeiros LJ, et al. Angioimmunoblastic T-cell lymphoma in bone marrow: a morphologic and immunophenotypic study. Hum Pathol. 2010;41(1):79–87.
36. Cho YU, Chi HS, Park CJ, Jang S, Seo EJ, Huh J. Distinct features of angioimmunoblastic T-cell lymphoma with bone marrow involvement. Am J Clin Pathol. 2009;131(5):640–6.
37. Weidmann E. Hepatosplenic T cell lymphoma. A review on 45 cases since the first report describing the disease as a distinct lymphoma entity in 1990. Leukemia. 2000;14(6):991–7.
38. Vega F, Medeiros LJ, Bueso-Ramos C, Jones D, Lai R, Luthra R, et al. Hepatosplenic gamma/delta T-cell lymphoma in bone marrow. A sinusoidal neoplasm with blastic cytologic features. Am J Clin Pathol. 2001;116(3):410–9.
39. Yabe M, Medeiros LJ, Tang G, Wang SA, Ahmed S, Nieto Y, et al. Prognostic factors of hepatosplenic T-cell lymphoma: clinicopathologic study of 28 cases. Am J Surg Pathol. 2016;40(5):676–88.
40. Wang CC, Tien HF, Lin MT, Su IJ, Wang CH, Chuang SM, et al. Consistent presence of isochromosome 7q in hepatosplenic T gamma/delta lymphoma: a new cytogenetic-clinicopathologic entity. Genes Chromosomes Cancer. 1995;12(3):161–4.

41. Lin P, Hao S, Handy BC, Bueso-Ramos CE, Medeiros LJ. Lymphoid neoplasms associated with IgM paraprotein: a study of 382 patients. Am J Clin Pathol. 2005;123(2):200–5.
42. Poulain S, Roumier C, Decambron A, Renneville A, Herbaux C, Bertrand E, et al. MYD88 L265P mutation in Waldenstrom macroglobulinemia. Blood. 2013;121(22):4504–11.
43. Viswanatha DS, Foucar K, Berry BR, Gascoyne RD, Evans HL, Leith CP. Blastic mantle cell leukemia: an unusual presentation of blastic mantle cell lymphoma. Mod Pathol. 2000;13(7):825–33.
44. Ondrejka SL, Lai R, Smith SD, Hsi ED. Indolent mantle cell leukemia: a clinicopathological variant characterized by isolated lymphocytosis, interstitial bone marrow involvement, kappa light chain restriction, and good prognosis. Haematologica. 2011;96(8):1121–7.
45. Wong KF, Chan JK, Cheung MM, So JC. Bone marrow involvement by nasal NK cell lymphoma at diagnosis is uncommon. Am J Clin Pathol. 2001;115(2):266–70.

Bone Marrow Involvement by Metastases and Granulomatous Conditions

28

Ashley S. Hagiya and Cleandrea Williams

Abbreviations

BCG	Bacillus Calmette-Guerin
BM	Bone marrow
CMV	Cytomegalovirus
EBV	Epstein-Barr virus
GCDFP-15	Gross cystic disease fluid protein-15
GMS	Gomori Methenamine-Silver
HCV	Hepatitis C virus
HIV	Human immunodeficiency virus
IHC	Immunohistochemistry
ILCA	Invasive lobular carcinoma
LDH	Lactate dehydrogenase
MAC	*Mycobacterium avium-intracellulare*
MAHA	Microangiopathic hemolytic anemia
NST	No special type
PNET	Primitive neuroectodermal tumor

List of Frequently Asked Questions

1. What are typical peripheral blood findings in patients with metastatic disease involving the bone marrow (BM)?
2. What are common clinical findings present when metastatic disease involves the BM?
3. What is the appropriate BM specimen to detect metastatic disease?
4. What are the major non-hematopoietic adult malignancies that metastasize to the BM?
5. What are the major non-hematopoietic pediatric malignancies that metastasize to the BM?
6. What is the differential diagnosis for metastatic disease to the BM?
7. What is the differential diagnosis for the etiology of BM granulomas?
8. What is the appropriate work-up for granulomas in the BM?

1. What are typical peripheral blood findings in patients with metastatic disease involving the bone marrow (BM)?

The peripheral blood findings of patients with metastatic involvement of the bone marrow (BM) are nonspecific [1].

- The most common abnormality is anemia, followed by thrombocytopenia [1, 2]. Other findings include leukocytosis, thrombocytosis, and pancytopenia. The CBC may also be normal [3, 4].
- Some patients develop microangiopathic hemolytic anemia (MAHA) characterized by anemia with schistocytes [5].
- Circulating tumor cells are rarely identified on the peripheral blood smear, a phenomenon termed carcinocythemia [6, 7].
- Earlier studies reported that leukoerythroblastosis, defined as circulating normoblasts and immature granulocytes in the peripheral blood, is always a sign of BM metastasis in patients with known malignancy [8] (Fig. 28.1). However, more recent studies show that this is not a specific finding, as it can be seen in a wide range of illnesses [9]. Leukoerythroblastosis likely occurs late in the disease course [2]. The mechanism is unclear, but invasion of cancer cells may cause the early release of certain cytokines leading to the development of a myelophthisic blood picture even before the BM is entirely replaced by tumor [10]. Absence of leukoerythroblastosis does not exclude BM involvement.

A. S. Hagiya (✉) · C. Williams
Department of Pathology, Keck Medical Center of the University of Southern California, Los Angeles, CA, USA
e-mail: Ashley.Hagiya@med.usc.edu; cleandrea.williams@med.usc.edu

E. Wang, A. S. Lagoo (eds.), *Practical Lymph Node and Bone Marrow Pathology*, Practical Anatomic Pathology,
https://doi.org/10.1007/978-3-030-32189-5_28

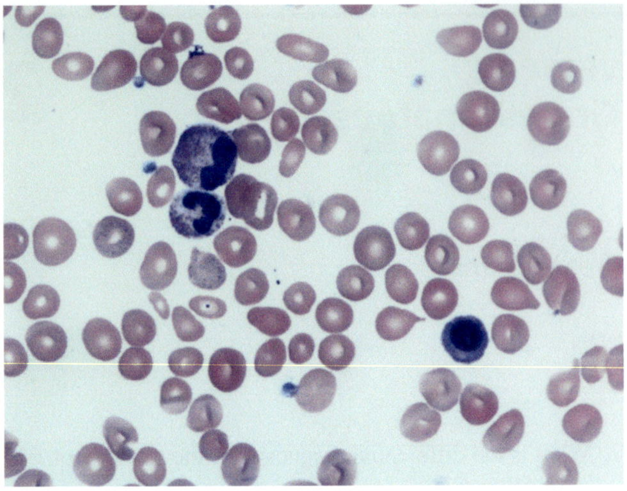

Fig. 28.1 Peripheral blood smear demonstrating leukoerythroblastic anemia with nucleated red blood cells and immature granulocytes

2. What are common clinical findings present when metastatic disease involves the BM?

There is no single specific indicator of BM infiltration.

- Clinically, patients present with constitutional symptoms and bone pain [1, 11].
- Abnormal laboratory studies can include elevated lactate dehydrogenase (LDH), hypercalcemia, elevated alkaline phosphatase, cytopenias, elevated serum uric acid, or elevated BUN [1, 11, 12]. In the presence of MAHA, there is an increase in haptoglobin, alkaline phosphatase, LDH, and bilirubin [5].
- Treatment may alter the laboratory findings. As such, these parameters should be interpreted with caution in patients who have received therapy [12].

3. What is the appropriate BM specimen to detect metastatic disease?

BM aspiration and biopsy are complementary in evaluating metastatic carcinoma [11, 13–15].

- The aspirate smears allow one to evaluate cytologic features, while the trephine biopsy is used to assess cellularity, fibrosis, and infiltrative disease.
- Fibrosis and sclerosis may prevent aspiration of tumor cells leading to a "dry tap." Trephine biopsies are especially useful in these cases [16, 17].
- Bilateral biopsies also increase the diagnostic yield by about 1/3 in non-hematopoietic neoplasms [1, 18].
- In addition, examining serial sections of the biopsy may increase the rate of detection [4, 14, 17].

4. What are the major non-hematopoietic adult malignancies that metastasize to the BM?

Almost any malignant tumor has the potential to metastasize, including carcinomas, sarcomas, and melanomas. In adults, the most common malignancies are breast, prostate, lung, and gastrointestinal cancers [19]. Systemic disease does not often present with BM involvement alone, even though BM metastases are common. As such, it is unusual to make a first time diagnosis of a non-hematopoietic malignancy in the BM [10]. When it does occur, the use of immunohistochemistry (IHC) combined with morphology can aid in determining tumor origin.

- Lung
  The frequency of lung cancer metastasis differs with histologic subtype. Small cell carcinoma is the most frequent, followed by adenocarcinoma. Squamous cell carcinoma is the least likely to metastasize to the BM [20].
  - Small cell carcinoma
    BM metastases are present in 20–25% of patients with small cell carcinoma at diagnosis [21]. On aspirate smears or touch preparations, the cells are often clustered with nuclear molding. They have hyperchromatic nuclei with granular chromatin, inconspicuous or absent nucleoli, and scant cytoplasm [22]. Tumor cells can occasionally show basophilic cytoplasm with cytoplasmic vacuoles, mimicking hematopoietic malignancy [23]. The trephine biopsy typically exhibits focal involvement with tumor cells arranged in nests [19]. The cells are intermediate in size with hyperchromatic nuclei and scant cytoplasm and are prone to crush artifact [20]. Osteoblastic reaction and fibrosis are frequent [22]. By IHC, TTF-1 is positive; however, this is not specific for lung, as it is seen in neuroendocrine carcinomas at other sites [24]. Synaptophysin and chromogranin A are useful neuroendocrine markers, with the latter being a more sensitive marker of small cell carcinoma [25] (Fig. 28.2).
  - Adenocarcinoma
    Adenocarcinomas display a variety of morphologies. The tumor cells can form glands, sheets, or papillae with mucin formation. A desmoplastic reaction, bone remodeling, osteolysis, or necrosis may be present [26]. By IHC, adenocarcinomas are positive for CK7, TTF-1, and napsin A and negative for CK20 [24] (Fig. 28.3).
  - Squamous cell carcinoma
    Squamous cell carcinoma rarely metastasizes to the BM [20]. Tumor is uniformly and strongly positive for p63 and p40 [27]. CK5/6 also shows uniform staining [28]. CK7 and CK20 are negative.

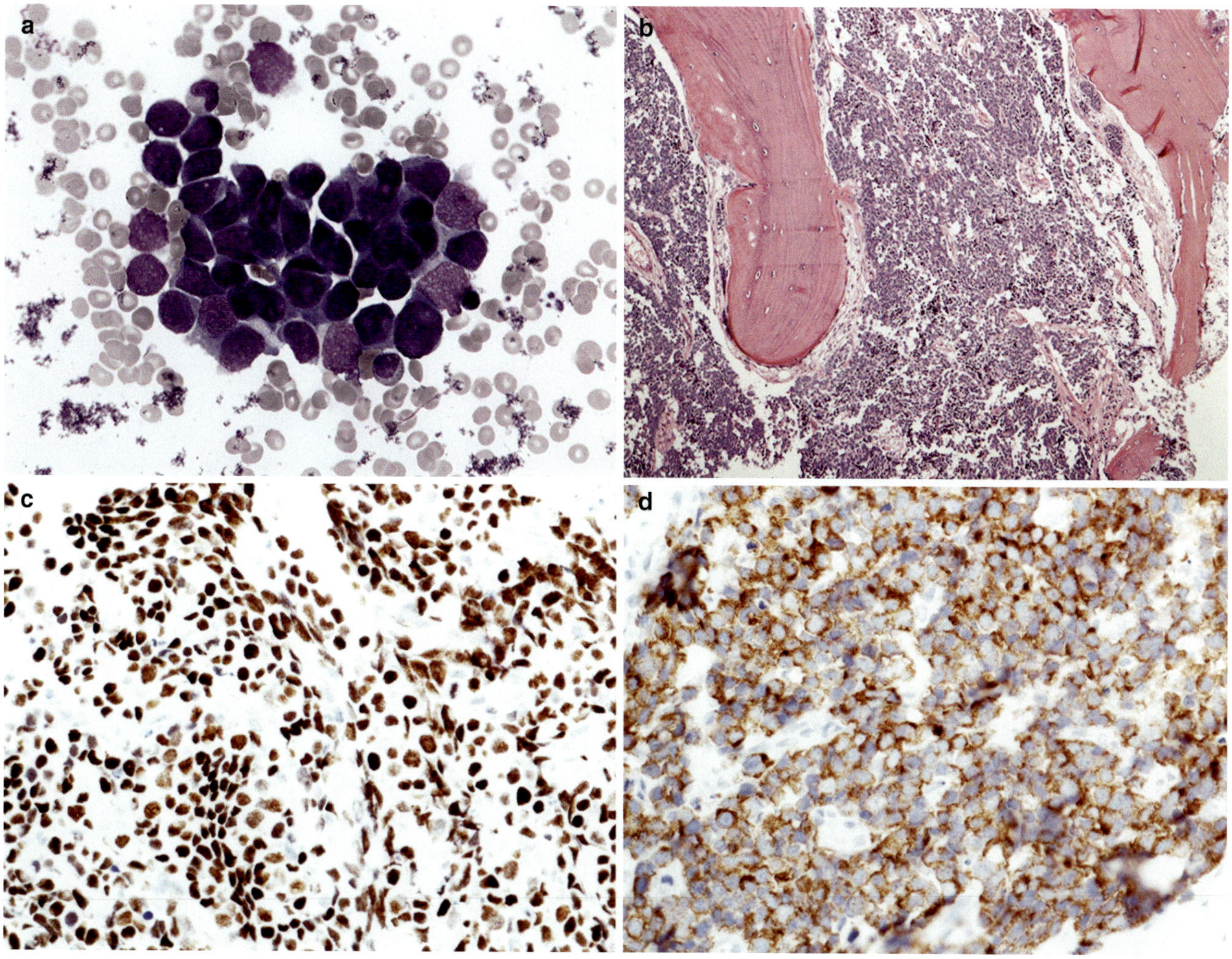

Fig. 28.2 Metastatic small cell carcinoma of the lung present in an aspirate smear (**a**) as cohesive clusters of large cells with scant cytoplasm and as sheets in the trephine biopsy (**b**). The tumor cells are positive for TF1-1 (**c**) and synaptophysin (**d**)

- Breast
  - Invasive breast carcinoma of no special type (NST; formerly known as invasive ductal carcinoma) comprises most of the cases of metastasis to the BM, with invasive lobular carcinoma (ILCA) accounting for a much smaller subset of cases [26, 29].
  - Circulating carcinoma cells are rarely seen in peripheral blood smears. The cells are larger than blasts and may show intracytoplasmic mucin [7, 30].
  - The trephine biopsy often demonstrates a prominent desmoplastic reaction with large cells arranged in cords or trabeculae [19] (Fig. 28.4).
  - Individually scattered infiltrates of lobular can also be seen, but this is more common in ILCA [26]. ILCA can be difficult to identify, as the tumor cells are more discohesive, with individually dispersed cells or cells in a single file.
  - The effect on bone may be osteolytic or osteoblastic [31].
  - Breast carcinomas are positive for CK7 and negative for CK20 [24]. Traditionally, mammaglobin and gross cystic disease fluid protein-15 (GCDFP-15) are the IHC stains used to detect breast cancer. Mammaglobin is a more sensitive marker than GCDFP-15 for breast carcinoma, but GCDFP-15 has greater specificity [32]. GATA3 is a newer marker which is significantly more sensitive than mammaglobin and GCDFP-15 [33]. Use of ER has only a limited role, as not all breast cancers are ER positive [24]. E-cadherin expression is lost in ILCA [26].
- Prostate
  - Prostatic adenocarcinoma often metastasizes to the BM [19]. The tumor characteristically causes osteoblastic changes.
  - On smears, the tumor cells are cohesive and may sometimes give the impression of acini formation. Nucleoli are frequently large and prominent or

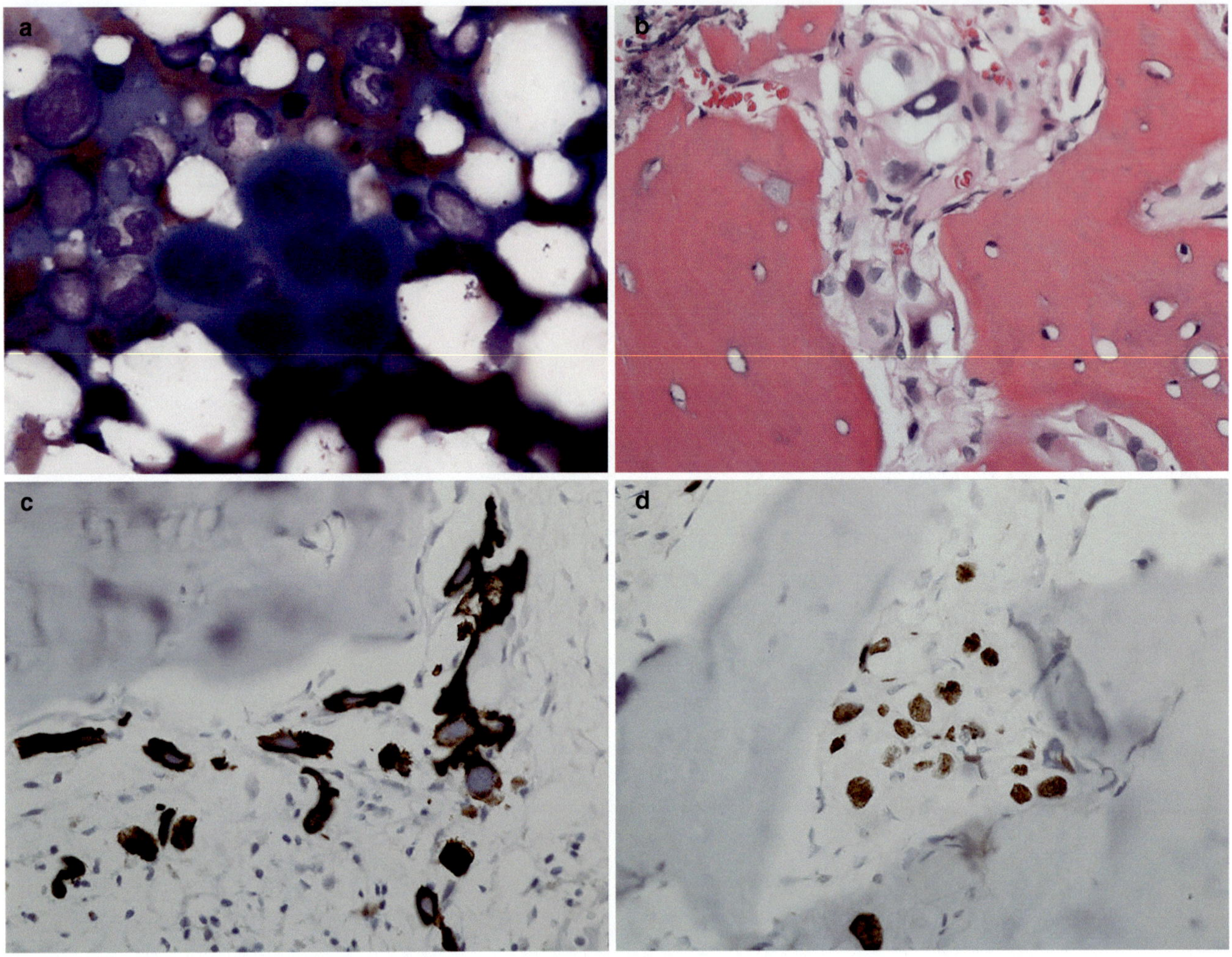

Fig. 28.3 Metastatic adenocarcinoma of the lung present in an imprint smear (**a**) and focally in a trephine biopsy (**b**) as a cohesive cluster of large cells with irregular nuclear contours and intracytoplasmic mucin. The tumor cells are positive for CK7 (**c**) and TTF-1 (**d**)

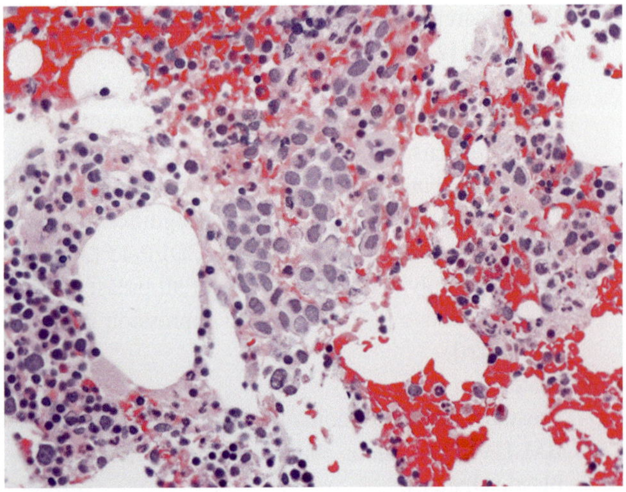

Fig. 28.4 Clot biopsy section of metastatic breast carcinoma present as a cohesive cluster of large cells with irregular nuclear contours and abundant cytoplasm, distinct from the surrounding hematopoietic cells

multiple. The cytoplasm is often abundant with poorly delineated cell boundaries [34].

  - Prostatic adenocarcinoma typically shows extensive involvement of the trephine biopsy and may cause fibrosis [19].
  - Higher grade tumors have a greater tendency to metastasize [35].
  - PSA and NKX3.1 are highly sensitive and specific markers for prostatic adenocarcinoma [36] (Fig. 28.5). CK7 and CK20 are negative [24].
- Gastrointestinal cancer
  - Gastrointestinal cancers metastasize to the BM less frequently than lung, breast, and prostate cancer. Gastric and colonic tumors are the most common [19].
  - Most gastric cancers with BM dissemination are poorly differentiated adenocarcinomas [16]. Squamous cell carcinomas and neuroendocrine tumors also rarely metastasize to the BM [26].

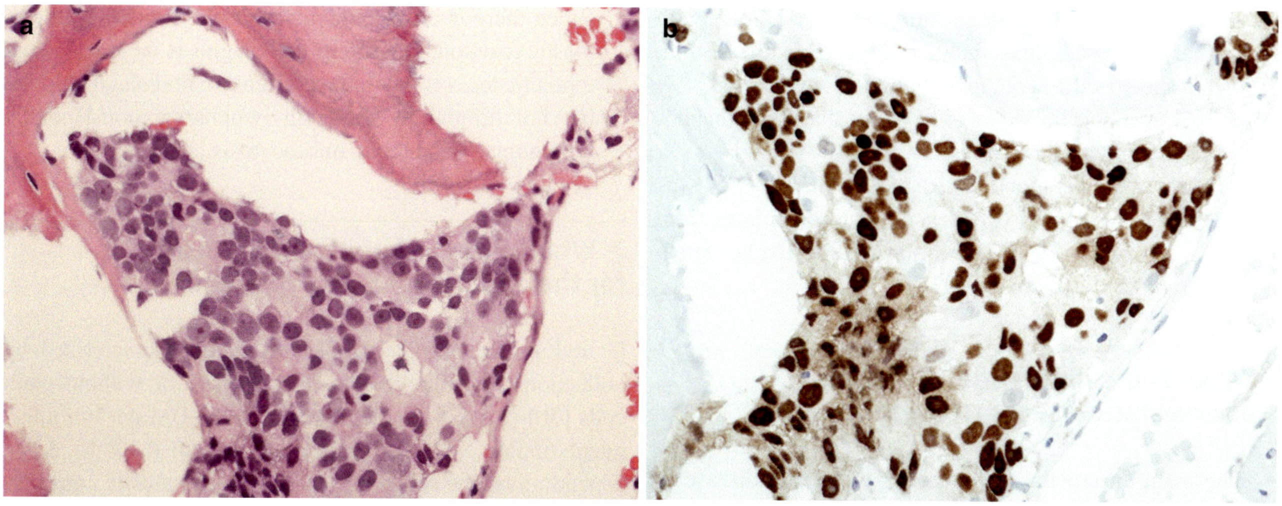

Fig. 28.5 Metastatic prostatic adenocarcinoma present in a trephine biopsy (**a**); the cells are cohesive with prominent central nucleoli. The tumor is positive for NKX3.1 (**b**)

- Colorectal adenocarcinomas are often CK7 negative and CK20 positive, while expression is variable in gastric adenocarcinomas. CDX2 is expressed in the majority of colorectal adenocarcinomas, and in some gastric adenocarcinomas, especially those of intestinal type [37]. Villin expression is greatest in tumors of colorectal origin, but lower levels are seen in gastric cancer [24].

5. What are the major non-hematopoietic pediatric malignancies that metastasize to the BM?

Small round blue cell tumors comprise most of the non-hematopoietic malignancies that metastasize to the BM in children, with neuroblastoma being the most common [38]. Rhabdomyosarcoma, tumors of the central nervous system (medulloblastoma and retinoblastoma), osteosarcoma, and Ewing sarcoma/primitive neuroectodermal tumor (PNET) less frequently demonstrate BM metastasis [19, 26, 38].

- Neuroblastoma
  - Neuroblastomas arise from the sympathetic ganglia and show varying degrees of maturation [39]. Metastases are present in about 50% of patients at diagnosis, and the BM is one of the most common sites [40]. It is often bilateral or multifocal [26].
  - The tumor cells are usually larger than small lymphocytes with round to oval nuclei, finely granular chromatin, and scant cytoplasm, which is rarely vacuolated (Fig. 28.6). In a subset of cases, Homer Wright rosettes are identified, which are composed of tumor cells in a ring surrounding central neuropil. Involvement varies from focal to almost complete replacement of the normal BM elements [41, 42].

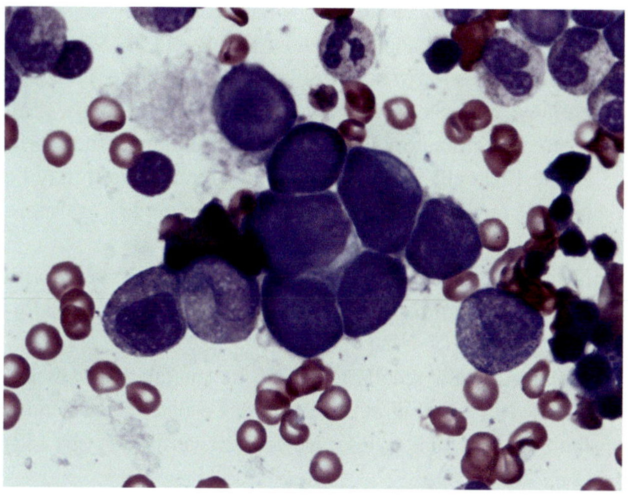

Fig. 28.6 Cohesive cluster of neuroblastoma tumor cells present in an aspirate smear. The cells are larger than the adjacent normal bone marrow cells. (Courtesy of Dr. Russell K. Brynes)

  - By IHC, synaptophysin and chromogranin A are positive; however, they are not specific. Other positive markers include PHOX2B, tyrosine hydroxylase, and NB84 [39, 43]. GATA3 may also be useful [44].
- Rhabdomyosarcoma
  - Rhabdomyosarcoma is usually seen in those younger than 20 years of age. It can rarely occur as widely disseminated disease without any obvious primary site [45].
  - The tumor cells are large with round nuclei, fine chromatin, one or more nucleoli, and moderate amounts of agranular basophilic cytoplasm. The cells can be discohesive with occasional cytoplasmic vacuoles, mimicking blasts [46, 47].

- IHC is helpful in distinguishing between the two, with rhabdomyosarcomas showing expression of desmin, muscle-specific actin, myogenin, and myoD1 [48, 49]. However, it is important to be aware that some rhabdomyosarcomas may express PAX5 [50].
- Many alveolar rhabdomyosarcomas harbor a *PAX3-FOXO1* or *PAX7-FOXO1* gene fusion resulting from t(2;13) or t(1;13) translocations, respectively, which portend a worse prognosis [51].

6. What is the differential diagnosis for metastatic disease to the BM?

- The main differential diagnosis for metastatic disease to the BM includes hematopoietic malignancies. Non-hematopoietic malignancies, such as neuroblastoma, rhabdomyosarcoma, breast carcinoma, small cell carcinoma, and medulloblastoma, can mimic leukemia or lymphoma, especially when circulating tumor cells are seen in the peripheral blood and cytopenias are present [7, 52–54].
- BM aspirates may show singly dispersed, large, undifferentiated, vacuolated cells with blast-like chromatin [52]. These non-hematopoietic tumor cells are larger than most of the BM cells and are usually clustered, which may be helpful in distinguishing the two. Single cells are more difficult to differentiate [55].
- Necrosis is not a specific finding as it can be seen with leukemias, lymphomas, and non-hematopoietic malignancies [26].
- Metastatic tumor cells may also be mistaken for megakaryocytes, plasma cells, osteoblasts, osteoclasts, endothelial cells, monocytes, and connective tissue cells [42] (Fig. 28.7).

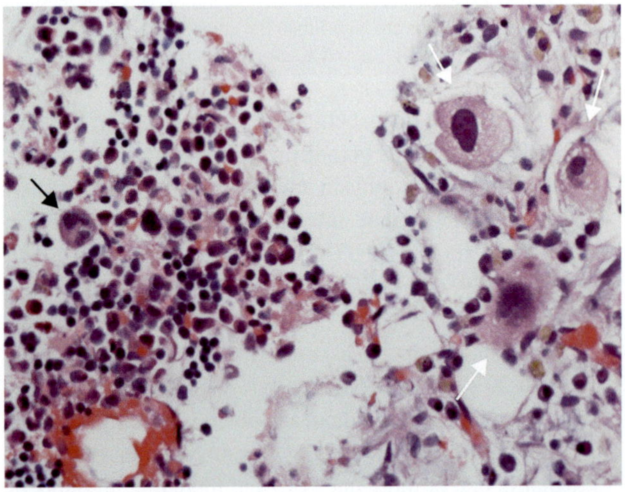

Fig. 28.7 Tumor cells (*white arrows*) can be mistaken for megakaryocytes (*black arrow*); in this case the tumor cells are much larger and contain abundant cytoplasm with mucin

- When there is obvious tumor with fibrosis and a desmoplastic reaction, the differential diagnosis includes hematopoietic lesions that induce extensive fibrosis, including, but not limited to, Hodgkin lymphoma, non-Hodgkin lymphoma, or systemic mastocytosis [26].

7. What is the differential diagnosis for the etiology of BM granulomas?

Granulomas are inflammatory responses characterized by collections of epithelioid histiocytes with or without giant cells [56] (Fig. 28.8). Granulomas in the BM are not a frequent finding. The incidence ranges from 0.3% to 2.2%, depending on the series [57]. The main diagnostic considerations are malignancy, infection, autoimmune disease, drugs, and sarcoidosis. Most studies show a prevalence of infections, sarcoidosis, and malignancy as the causes of BM granulomas. A more recent study showed that B-cell lymphomas, sarcoidosis, and autoimmune disease were the most common causes, with infections accounting for very few cases, which may be due to varying geographic locations [56].

- Malignancy
  - Malignant neoplasms have been reported as the cause of BM granulomas in 20–25% of cases, most commonly Hodgkin and non-Hodgkin lymphomas [58].
  - Many other malignancies have been associated with BM granulomas including plasma cell dyscrasias, myeloid neoplasms, carcinomas, sarcomas, and neuroblastomas.
  - The granulomas are seen both at the time of active disease prior to treatment and after treatment in remission. Involvement is minimal when the marrow shows the presence of malignancy [56].
- Infectious Disease
  - There are a wide range of infectious causes including tuberculosis, Mycobacterium avium-intracellulare (MAC), histoplasmosis, Epstein-Barr virus (*EBV*), cytomegalovirus (CMV), human immunodeficiency virus (HIV), brucellosis, typhoid fever, Q fever, tularemia, Mycoplasma species, bacillus Calmette-Guerin (BCG), leprosy, rickettsiosis, syphilis, cryptococcosis, coccidioidomycosis, aspergillosis, blastomycosis, and hepatitis C virus (HCV).
  - In one study, special stains were helpful only when tuberculosis and histoplasmosis were the causative agents [59].
- Sarcoidosis
  - Sarcoidosis is one of the most common causes of BM granulomas. However, it is rare for sarcoidosis to present as a granuloma in the BM. The diagnosis is established by clinical and radiologic findings, bronchoalveolar lavage, and ACE levels [57, 58].

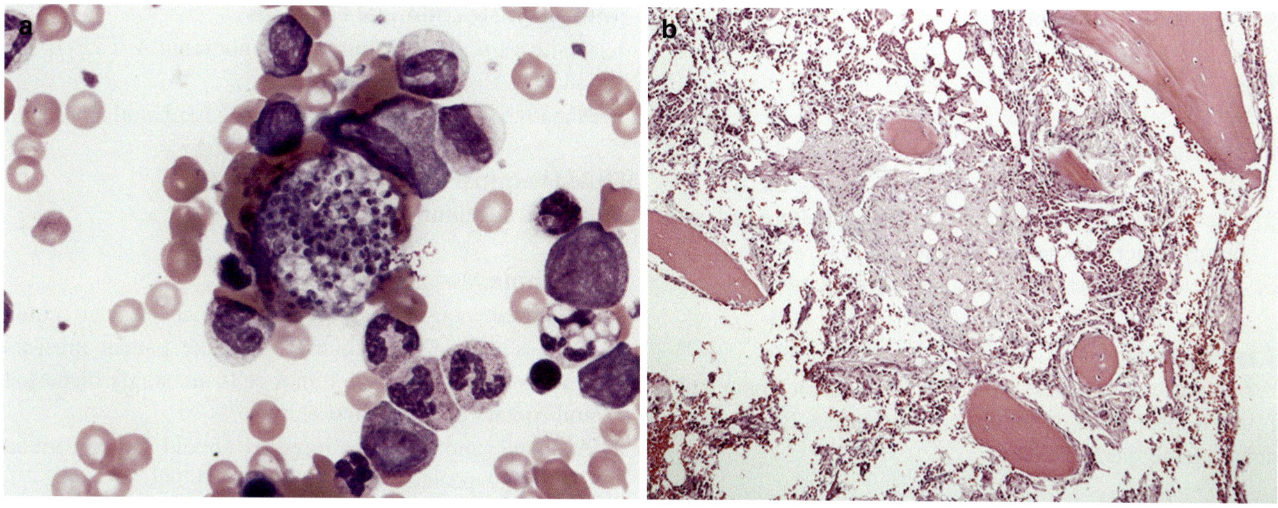

Fig. 28.8 Aspirate smear (**a**) showing histiocytes filled with *Histoplasma* organisms. The trephine biopsy (**b**) shows a non-necrotizing granuloma. (Courtesy of Dr. Russell K. Brynes)

- Drugs
  - BM granulomas have been reported with a number of medications such as procainamide and sulfonamide.
  - Rare cases have also been described with chlorpropamide, phenylbutazone, phenytoin, methyldopa, allopurinol, ibuprofen, penicillamine, and tolmetin sodium [58, 59].
- Autoimmune Disease
  - Autoimmune diseases have been associated with BM granulomas, including rheumatoid arthritis, primary biliary cirrhosis, Felty's syndrome, and systemic lupus erythematosus, to name a few. However, most are isolated cases [58].
- No Definitive Cause
  - Sometimes there will be no definitive cause for the BM granulomas. Brackers de Hugo et al. studied 48 cases and found no underlying diagnosis in 21% of the patients [60]. Except for one patient who died of an unrelated cause, the remaining patients were alive and well without treatment after a median of 30-month follow-up. These findings suggest that BM granulomas of undetermined origin have good prognosis and are not associated with the development of underlying disease.

Although some specific pathologic findings can point to a certain diagnosis (i.e., caseation in tuberculosis), these findings are uncommonly seen in the BM, and there is no association with the qualitative histologic features and the cause of the granulomas. BM granulomas should be seen as a nonspecific indicator of inflammation or malignancy, with the source potentially being outside the marrow. A search for any underlying cause should only be initiated and directed by the clinical features [57]. Unless a specific organism can be identified in a granulomatous lesion, the diagnosis cannot be made solely on pathologic criteria; rather, it will have to be based on epidemiologic, clinical, laboratory, and radiologic data [58, 61].

8. What is the appropriate work-up for granulomas in the BM?

- Review of serial sections is important [61]. In addition, both clot and trephine biopsy sections should be evaluated [62].
- In a study by Bhargava et al., BM culture was rarely submitted from patients with hematologic disorders or nonhematopoietic malignancies [57]. In these cases, granulomas were an unexpected finding which did not correlate with clinical evidence of infection. If not done initially, repeat biopsy for culture may not be necessary in an immunocompetent patient. However, immunocompromised patients may have a wide variety of unsuspected marrow infections, and in this setting repeat biopsy for culture is probably warranted.
- Although stains for organisms have a low yield, including Ziehl-Neelsen and Gomori Methenamine-Silver (GMS), they should be done.
- Most importantly, clinical findings, including a medication history, should direct further work-up. If an infectious etiology is suspected, more targeted testing is required.

Case Presentations

Case 1

Learning Objectives

1. Recognize non-hematopoietic neoplasms of the BM
2. Recognize the morphologic and IHC features of non-hematopoietic neoplasms of the BM
3. Develop a differential diagnosis based on morphology

Case History

A 68-year-old man presents with worsening back pain and is found to be anemic and thrombocytopenic. A BM biopsy is subsequently performed.

Morphologic Findings

- The aspirate smear is aparticulate with singly dispersed large cells with irregular nuclear contours, fine chromatin, inconspicuous nucleoli, and scant cytoplasm with occasional vacuoles (Fig. 28.9a).
- There is extensive involvement of the BM trephine biopsy by sheets and nests of large cells with oval nuclei, granular chromatin, inconspicuous nucleoli, and scant cytoplasm (Fig. 28.9b).

Differential Diagnosis

- Metastatic non-hematopoietic malignancy, i.e., small cell carcinoma
- Acute leukemia
- Lymphoma

Immunohistochemical Findings

- Positive for synaptophysin, chromogranin A, TTF-1, and CK7
- Negative for CD45 and myeloid and lymphoid markers

Final Diagnosis

Small cell carcinoma

Take-Home Messages

1. Metastatic non-hematopoietic malignancies can mimic acute leukemia, particularly when the patient presents with cytopenias and the tumor cells are singly dispersed and contain cytoplasmic vacuoles.
2. Aspirates and trephine biopsies should be performed together, especially when there is a dry tap.

Case 2

Learning Objectives

1. Recognize non-hematopoietic neoplasms of the BM
2. Recognize the morphologic and IHC features of non-hematopoietic neoplasms of the BM
3. Develop a differential diagnosis based on morphology

Case History

A 48-year-old woman is admitted for a cholecystectomy for presumed gallstone pancreatitis and is found to be markedly anemic and thrombocytopenic. She is also found to have a small monoclonal protein (0.1 g/dL; IgM/kappa). A BM biopsy is subsequently performed.

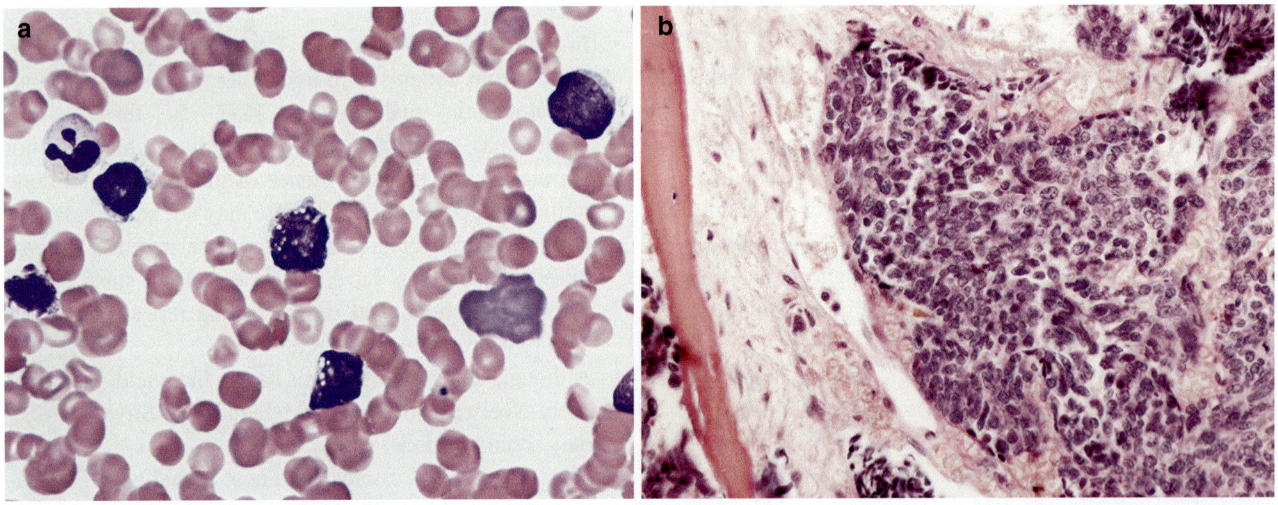

Fig. 28.9 The aspirate smear (**a**) demonstrates singly dispersed large cells with irregular nuclear contours, fine chromatin, inconspicuous nucleoli, and scant cytoplasm with occasional vacuoles. The trephine biopsy (**b**) shows tumor cells arranged in sheets and nests. (Courtesy of Dr. Russell K. Brynes)

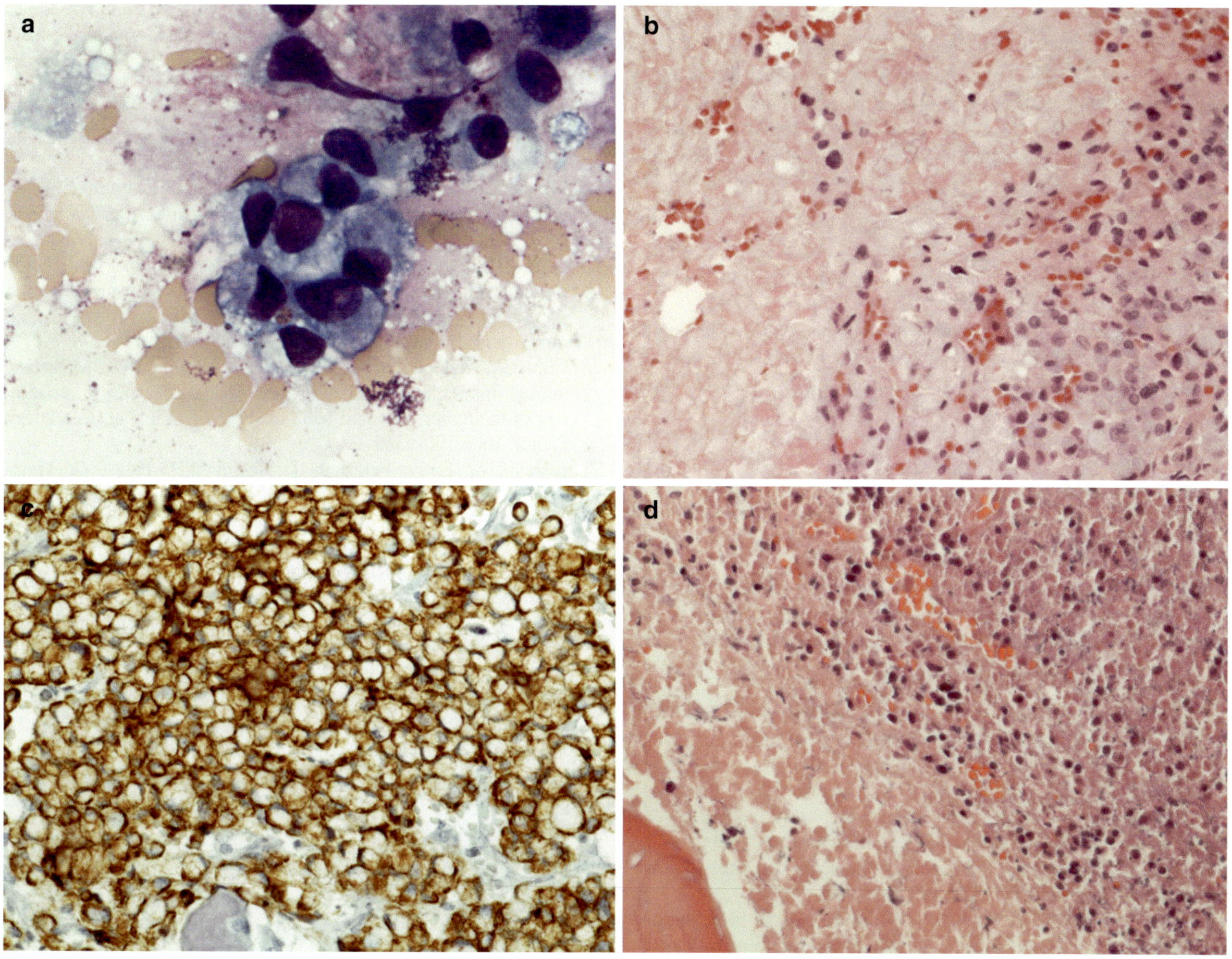

Fig. 28.10 The aspirate smear (**a**) demonstrates clusters of large cells with eccentric nuclei and abundant cytoplasm. The trephine biopsy (**b**) shows necrosis with the viable areas consisting of sheets of large cells with mucin displacing the nuclei to the side. The tumor is positive for AE1/AE3 (**c**). Hematopoietic malignancies, such as lymphoma, can also show necrosis (**d**)

Morphologic Findings

- The aspirate smears show large cells, arranged singly and in clusters, with round eccentric nuclei and dispersed chromatin (Fig. 28.10a).
- The BM trephine biopsy shows extensive necrosis. The viable areas demonstrate large cells with displaced nuclei (Fig. 28.10b). The cells have a signet ring appearance, with intracytoplasmic mucin.

Differential Diagnosis

- Metastatic adenocarcinoma
- Plasma cell myeloma

Immunohistochemical Findings

- Positive for AE1/AE3 (Fig. 28.10c), CK20, and villin
- Negative for CD138, CK7, TTF1, napsin A, ER, and GATA3

Final Diagnosis

Adenocarcinoma with signet ring features, favor lower gastrointestinal primary

Take-Home Messages

1. Clinical features are nonspecific, and similar findings may be seen in both metastatic non-hematopoietic malignancies and hematopoietic tumors.
2. Necrosis is not a specific finding. It can be seen with any type of malignancy, including leukemias and lymphomas (Fig. 28.10d).
3. IHC is helpful in determining the primary origin of non-hematopoietic malignancies.

References

1. Papac RJ. Bone marrow metastases. A review. Cancer. 1994;74(9):2403–13.
2. Contreras E, Ellis LD, Lee RE. Value of the bone marrow biopsy in the diagnosis of metastatic carcinoma. Cancer. 1972;29(3):778–83.
3. Roeckel IE. Diagnosis of metastatic carcinoma by bone marrow biopsy versus bone marrow aspiration. Ann Clin Lab Sci. 1974;4(3):193–7.
4. Brochamer WL Jr, Keeling MM. The bone marrow biopsy, osteoscan, and peripheral blood in non-hematopoietic cancer. Cancer. 1977;40(2):836–40.
5. Shin SY, Park H, Chae SW, Woo HY. Microangiopathic hemolytic anemia as the first manifestation of metastatic signet ring cell carcinoma of unknown origin: a case report and review of literature. Korean J Lab Med. 2011;31(3):157–61.
6. Rowan DJ, Logunova V, van Tuinen P, Olteanu H, Peterson JF. Circulating breast carcinoma cells mimicking therapy-related acute myeloid leukemia. Int J Surg Pathol. 2017;25(1):87–93.
7. Carey RW, Taft PD, Bennett JM, Kaufman S. Carcinocythemia (carcinoma cell leukemia). An acute leukemia-like picture due to metastatic carcinoma cells. Am J Med. 1976;60(2):273–8.
8. Delsol G, Guiu-Godfrin B, Guiu M, Pris J, Corberand J, Fabre J. Leukoerythroblastosis and cancer frequency, prognosis, and physiopathologic significance. Cancer. 1979;44(3):1009–13.
9. Brigden ML, Page N. Leukoerythroblastosis: a much maligned phenomenon? CMAJ. 1987;137(9):785–6.
10. Ozkalemkas F, Ali R, Ozkocaman V, Ozcelik T, Ozan U, Ozturk H, et al. The bone marrow aspirate and biopsy in the diagnosis of unsuspected nonhematologic malignancy: a clinical study of 19 cases. BMC Cancer. 2005;5:144.
11. Ellman L. Bone marrow biopsy in the evaluation of lymphoma, carcinoma and granulomatous disorders. Am J Med. 1976;60(1):1–7.
12. Chernow B, Wallner SF. Variables predictive of bone marrow metastasis. Cancer. 1978;42(5):2373–8.
13. Grann V, Pool JL, Mayer K. Comparative study of bone marrow aspiration and biopsy in patients with neoplastic disease. Cancer. 1966;19(12):1898–900.
14. Bearden JD, Ratkin GA, Coltman CA. Comparison of the diagnostic value of bone marrow biopsy and bone marrow aspiration in neoplastic disease. J Clin Pathol. 1974;27(9):738–40.
15. Garrett TJ, Gee TS, Lieberman PH, McKenzie S, Clarkson BD. The role of bone marrow aspiration and biopsy in detecting marrow involvement by nonhematologic malignancies. Cancer. 1976;38(6):2401–3.
16. Moid F, DePalma L. Comparison of relative value of bone marrow aspirates and bone marrow trephine biopsies in the diagnosis of solid tumor metastasis and Hodgkin lymphoma: institutional experience and literature review. Arch Pathol Lab Med. 2005;129(4):497–501.
17. Singh G, Krause JR, Breitfeld V. Bone marrow examination: for metastatic tumor: aspirate and biopsy. Cancer. 1977;40(5):2317–21.
18. Brunning RD, Bloomfield CD, McKenna RW, Peterson LA. Bilateral trephine bone marrow biopsies in lymphoma and other neoplastic diseases. Ann Intern Med. 1975;82(3):365–6.
19. Krishnan C, George TI, Arber DA. Bone marrow metastases: a survey of nonhematologic metastases with immunohistochemical study of metastatic carcinomas. Appl Immunohistochem Mol Morphol. 2007;15(1):1–7.
20. Hansen HH, Muggia FM, Selawry OS. Bone-marrow examination in 100 consecutive patients with bronchogenic carcinoma. Lancet. 1971;2(7722):443–5.
21. Tritz DB, Doll DC, Ringenberg QS, Anderson S, Madsen R, Perry MC, et al. Bone marrow involvement in small cell lung cancer. Clinical significance and correlation with routine laboratory variables. Cancer. 1989;63(4):763–6.
22. Ihde DC, Simms EB, Matthews MJ, Cohen MH, Bunn PA, Minna JD. Bone marrow metastases in small cell carcinoma of the lung: frequency, description, and influence on chemotherapeutic toxicity and prognosis. Blood. 1979;53(4):677–86.
23. Iguchi T, Awaya N, Kobayashi K, Okamoto S. Bone marrow metastases of small cell carcinoma of the lung mimicking Burkitt lymphoma/leukaemia. Br J Haematol. 2005;130(5):652.
24. Kandalaft PL, Gown AM. Practical applications in immunohistochemistry: carcinomas of unknown primary site. Arch Pathol Lab Med. 2016;140(6):508–23.
25. Lyda MH, Tetef M, Carter NH, Ikle D, Weiss LM, Arber DA. Keratin immunohistochemistry detects clinically significant metastases in bone marrow biopsy specimens in women with lobular breast carcinoma. Am J Surg Pathol. 2000;24(12):1593–9.
26. Cotta CV, Konoplev S, Medeiros LJ, Bueso-Ramos CE. Metastatic tumors in bone marrow: histopathology and advances in the biology of the tumor cells and bone marrow environment. Ann Diagn Pathol. 2006;10(3):169–92.
27. Bishop JA, Teruya-Feldstein J, Westra WH, Pelosi G, Travis WD, Rekhtman N. p40 (ΔNp63) is superior to p63 for the diagnosis of pulmonary squamous cell carcinoma. Mod Pathol. 2012;25(3):405–15.
28. Mukhopadhyay S, Katzenstein AL. Subclassification of non-small cell lung carcinomas lacking morphologic differentiation on biopsy specimens: utility of an immunohistochemical panel containing TTF-1, napsin A, p63, and CK5/6. Am J Surg Pathol. 2011;35(1):15–25.
29. Sinn HP, Kreipe H. A brief overview of the WHO classification of breast tumors, 4th edition, focusing on issues and updates from the 3rd edition. Breast Care (Basel). 2013;8(2):149–54.
30. Myerowitz RL, Edwards PA, Sartiano GP. Carcinocythemia (carcinoma cell leukemia) due to metastatic carcinoma of the breast: report of a case. Cancer. 1977;40(6):3107–11.
31. Ridell B, Landys K. Incidence and histopathology of metastases of mammary carcinoma in biopsies from the posterior iliac crest. Cancer. 1979;44(5):1782–8.
32. Bhargava R, Beriwal S, Dabbs DJ. Mammaglobin vs GCDFP-15: an immunohistologic validation survey for sensitivity and specificity. Am J Clin Pathol. 2007;127(1):103–13.
33. Sangoi AR, Shrestha B, Yang G, Mego O, Beck AH. The novel marker GATA3 is significantly more sensitive than traditional markers mammaglobin and GCDFP15 for identifying breast cancer in surgical and cytology specimens of metastatic and matched primary tumors. Appl Immunohistochem Mol Morphol. 2016;24(4):229–37.
34. Rundles RW, Jonsson U. Metastases in bone marrow and myelophthisic anemia from carcinoma of the prostate. Am J Med Sci. 1949;218(3):241–50.
35. Bubendorf L, Schöpfer A, Wagner U, Sauter G, Moch H, Willi N, et al. Metastatic patterns of prostate cancer: an autopsy study of 1,589 patients. Hum Pathol. 2000;31(5):578–83.
36. Gurel B, Ali TZ, Montgomery EA, Begum S, Hicks J, Goggins M, et al. NKX3.1 as a marker of prostatic origin in metastatic tumors. Am J Surg Pathol. 2010;34(8):1097–105.
37. Bayrak R, Haltas H, Yenidunya S. The value of CDX2 and cytokeratins 7 and 20 expression in differentiating colorectal adenocarcinomas from extraintestinal gastrointestinal adenocarcinomas: cytokeratin 7−/20+ phenotype is more specific than CDX2 antibody. Diagn Pathol. 2012;7:9.
38. Mishra P, Das S, Kar R, Jacob SE, Basu D. Non-haematopoietic malignancies metastasing to the bone marrow: a 5 year record-based descriptive study from a tertiary care centre in South India. Indian J Cancer. 2014;51(1):30–4.
39. Parham DM. Modern diagnosis of small cell malignancies of children. Surg Pathol Clin. 2010;3(3):515–51.

40. Tolbert VP, Matthay KK. Neuroblastoma: clinical and biological approach to risk stratification and treatment. Cell Tissue Res. 2018;372(2):195–209.
41. Burchill SA, Beiske K, Shimada H, Ambros PF, Seeger R, Tytgat GA, et al. Recommendations for the standardization of bone marrow disease assessment and reporting in children with neuroblastoma on behalf of the International Neuroblastoma Response Criteria Bone Marrow Working Group. Cancer. 2017;123(7):1095–105.
42. Delta BG, Pinkel D. Bone marrow aspiration in children with malignant tumors. J Pediatr. 1964;64:542–6.
43. Hung YP, Lee JP, Bellizzi AM, Hornick JL. PHOX2B reliably distinguishes neuroblastoma among small round blue cell tumors. Histopathology. 2017;71(5):786–94.
44. Wiles AB, Karrs JX, Pitt S, Almenara J, Powers CN, Smith SC. GATA3 is a reliable marker for neuroblastoma in limited samples, including FNA Cell Blocks, core biopsies, and touch imprints. Cancer Cytopathol. 2017;125(12):940–6.
45. Hayashi Y, Kikuchi F, Oka T, Itoyama S, Mohri N, Usuki K, et al. Rhabdomyosarcoma with bone marrow metastasis simulating acute leukemia. Report of two cases. Acta Pathol Jpn. 1988;38(6):789–98.
46. Kern JB, Hii A, Kruse MJ, Szabo Z, Argani P, Hibbard MK, et al. A leukemic presentation of alveolar rhabdomyosarcoma in a 52-year-old woman without an identifiable primary tumor. Int J Surg Pathol. 2015;23(1):75–7.
47. Morandi S, Manna A, Sabattini E, Porcellini A. Rhabdomyosarcoma presenting as acute leukemia. J Pediatr Hematol Oncol. 1996;18(3):305–7.
48. Parham DM, Webber B, Holt H, Williams WK, Maurer H. Immunohistochemical study of childhood rhabdomyosarcomas and related neoplasms. Results of an Intergroup Rhabdomyosarcoma study project. Cancer. 1991;67(12):3072–80.
49. Cessna MH, Zhou H, Perkins SL, Tripp SR, Layfield L, Daines C, et al. Are myogenin and myoD1 expression specific for rhabdomyosarcoma? A study of 150 cases, with emphasis on spindle cell mimics. Am J Surg Pathol. 2001;25(9):1150–7.
50. Sorensen PH, Lynch JC, Qualman SJ, Tirabosco R, Lim JF, Maurer HM, et al. PAX3-FKHR and PAX7-FKHR gene fusions are prognostic indications in alveolar rhabdomyosarcoma: a report from the children's oncology group. J Clin Oncol. 2002;20(11):2672–9.
51. Hanna JA, Garcia MR, Lardennois A, Leavey PJ, Maglic D, Fagnan A, et al. PAX3-FOXO1 drives miR-486-5p and represses miR-221 contributing to pathogenesis of alveolar rhabdomyosarcoma. Oncogene. 2018;37(15):1991–2007.
52. Taetle R, Wohl H. Oat cell carcinoma mimicking acute leukemia. West J Med. 1978;129(6):497–500.
53. Chu JY. Metastatic medulloblastoma simulating acute leukemia. J Pediatr. 1979;94(6):921–3.
54. Parry TE. Proceedings: two cases of neuroblastoma with marrow findings mimicking acute leukemia. Arch Dis Child. 1974;49(6):497.
55. Tasleem RA, Chowdhary ND, Kadri SM, Chowdhary QA. Metastasis of solid tumours in bone marrow: a study from Kashmir, India. J Clin Pathol. 2003;56(10):803.
56. Crispin P, Holmes A. Clinical and pathological feature of bone marrow granulomas: a modern Australian series. Int J Lab Hematol. 2018;40(2):123–7.
57. Bhargava V, Farhi DC. Bone marrow granulomas: clinicopathologic findings in 72 cases and review of the literature. Hematol Pathol. 1988;2(1):43–50.
58. Eid A, Carion W, Nystrom JS. Differential diagnoses of bone marrow granuloma. West J Med. 1996;164(6):510–5.
59. Bodem CR, Harmory BH, Taylor HM, Kleopfer L. Granulomatous bone marrow disease. A review of the literature and clinicopathologic analysis of 58 cases. Medicine (Baltimore). 1983;62(6):372–83.
60. Brackers de Hugo L, Ffrench M, Broussolle C, Sève P. Granulomatous lesions in bone marrow: clinicopathologic findings and significance in a study of 48 cases. Eur J Intern Med. 2013;24(5):468–73.
61. Pease GL. Granulomatous lesions in bone marrow. Blood. 1956;11(8):720–34.
62. Vilalta-Castel E, Valdés-Sanchez MD, Guerra-Vales JM, Teno-Esteban C, Garzón A, López JI, et al. Significance of granulomas in bone marrow: a study of 40 cases. Eur J Haematol. 1988;41(1):12–6.

Bone Marrow Findings in Congenital/ Hereditary Conditions

29

Juehua Gao and Shunyou Gong

List of Frequently Asked Questions

1. What is the role of a hematopathologist in diagnosing congenital/hereditary conditions by evaluating peripheral blood and/or bone marrow findings?
2. What is "bone marrow failure syndrome," and what are the common inherited bone marrow failure syndromes?
3. What is the general approach in diagnosing bone marrow failure syndromes?
4. What are the major findings in patients with Fanconi anemia?
5. What are the abnormalities of hematopoietic system seen in patients with Down syndrome?
6. What are the broad categories and the overall frequency of myeloid neoplasm with germline predisposition?
7. What are the distinguishing features of the major entities under "myeloid neoplasms with germline predisposition without a preexisting disorder or organ dysfunction"?
8. What are the major entities under "myeloid neoplasms with germline predisposition and preexisting platelet disorders"? What are the clinical and morphologic features of these entities?
9. What are the major entities under "myeloid neoplasms with germline predisposition and other organ dysfunction"? What are the clinical and morphologic features of these entities including germline *GATA2* deficiency?
10. What could be a potential pitfall for diagnosing myeloid neoplasms in the setting of underlying germline condition?
11. When and which tissue should be tested to confirm the presence of a germline condition in patients with myeloid neoplasms?
12. What are the bone marrow features of common variable immunodeficiency (CVID)?
13. What is familial hemophagocytic lymphohistiocytosis (FHL)? What are the peripheral blood and bone marrow findings in FHL?
14. How is FHL diagnosed and what are the diagnostic pitfalls?
15. What is autoimmune lymphoproliferative syndrome (ALPS), and what are the peripheral blood and bone marrow findings in ALPS?
16. What are the peripheral blood and bone marrow findings in the major entities of lysosomal storage diseases?

J. Gao (✉)
Department of Pathology, Northwestern University Feinberg School of Medicine, Chicago, IL, USA
e-mail: j-gao@northwestern.edu

S. Gong
Hematology and Hematopathology, Department of Pathology, Ann & Robert H. Lurie Children's Hospital, Northwestern University Feinberg School of Medicine, Chicago, IL, USA

1. What is the role of a hematopathologist in diagnosing congenital/ hereditary conditions by evaluating peripheral blood and/or bone marrow findings?

Although many congenital or hereditary conditions can indirectly affect the bone marrow hematopoiesis and cause numerical or morphologic changes in peripheral blood and/ or bone marrow, in this chapter we will consider only selected conditions with direct, constant, and/ or characteristic effects on bone marrow or blood cells.

- Congenital/hereditary conditions primarily affecting the hematopoietic system are rare. However, correct identification of these conditions is critical for appropriate management of affected individuals to avoid progressive harm to the patients and to provide genetic counseling. The pathologist must consider these congenital/hereditary conditions in the differential diagnosis when the more common acquired etiologies fail to explain the observed bone marrow and blood findings. This is particularly true

E. Wang, A. S. Lagoo (eds.), *Practical Lymph Node and Bone Marrow Pathology*, Practical Anatomic Pathology,
https://doi.org/10.1007/978-3-030-32189-5_29

Table 29.1 Indications to prompt genetic counseling and germline testing

Family history	Family history of myeloid neoplasm (2 or more) or unexplained cytopenias Early onset (<50) of hematologic malignancy Multiple (2 or more) close relatives with cancer
Personal history	History of bleeding episodes or preexisting platelet disorders Lymphedema or monocytopenia or atypical infection Skin pigmentation or nail abnormalities Leukopenia and pulmonary fibrosis Bone marrow failure syndrome
Somatic mutations detected in myeloid neoplasm	Biallelic *CEBPA* mutation Deleterious *GATA2* mutation Deleterious *RUNX1* mutation Frameshift *DDX41* mutation

when these conditions do not have significant systemic manifestations outside the blood and marrow or when they manifest in adult life. Other clinical and pathological indications where prompt germline testing may be indicated are given in Table 29.1.

- In other cases, the pathologist may be asked to rule in or rule out one of these conditions suspected on the basis of clinical findings including cutaneous or other systemic lesions. In such cases, the pathologist must be familiar with morphological findings in the marrow and know the appropriate molecular or genetic tests, the correct sample required for these tests, and the diagnostic specificity and sensitivity of each test.
- The underlying mechanisms of these conditions, their effects on bone marrow and blood cells, and extent and type of systemic involvement outside the hematopoietic system are diverse. From the perspective of a practicing hematopathologist, these conditions are best categorized according to their effect on bone marrow morphology and peripheral blood findings:
  - Suspected bone marrow failure based on peripheral blood cytopenia (Questions 2–4)
  - Suspected myeloid neoplasm (Questions 5–11)
  - Suspected immune dysregulation, immune deficiency, autoimmunity or lymphoid neoplasm (Questions 12–15)
  - Suspected storage diseases (Question 16)
  - Rare conditions with characteristic morphologic findings in the marrow
- In these categories, there are some conditions which primarily affect the hematopoietic system, with or without involvement of other organs, while some conditions primarily have multi-organ manifestation, including the hematopoietic system. Several case studies are presented at the end to highlight these clinical, pathological, and molecular properties of many of these interesting, though rare conditions.
- Even though various red cell membrane defects, thalassemia or hemoglobinopathies, constitute hereditary conditions affecting the erythroid cells, these entities are often diagnosed on the peripheral blood smear review. Presence of characteristic features such as increased number of elliptocytes and spherocytes and presence of sickle cells sometimes trigger additional laboratory studies such as osmotic fragility test, EMA binding test by flow cytometry, SDS-PAGE analysis, or hemoglobin electrophoresis, which are helpful for establishing the diagnosis. However, more often, the conditions are suspected from family history and prenatal or neonatal testing coupled with presence of anemia. Bone marrow biopsy, if performed, may show erythroid hyperplasia in response to hemolytic anemia.

2. What is "bone marrow failure syndrome," and what are the common inherited bone marrow failure syndromes?

- Bone marrow failure syndrome is a group of disorders that manifest as single cytopenia or pancytopenias due to decreased bone marrow production. They can generally be classified as acquired or inherited.
- Acquired bone marrow failure syndrome develops later in life and may be associated with toxin, medication, viral infection, or immune-mediated destruction. Inherited cases occur early in life and are often associated with one or more genetic abnormalities and manifested as cytopenias, some with physical abnormalities and increased risks of cancer.
- Inherited bone marrow failure syndrome can generally be classified according to the main presenting hematological abnormality such as those present as pancytopenias or as single lineage cytopenias. See Table 29.2.
  - Multilineage failure is seen in conditions such as Fanconi anemia (see Question 4 and Case 1) and dyskeratosis congenita (see Case 2).
  - Diamond-Blackfan anemia is characterized by red cell aplasia or hypoplasia with relatively preserved granulocytic and megakaryocytic lineages (see Case 3); congenital sideroblastic anemia is associated with reticulocytopenia, ineffective erythropoiesis, and secondary iron overload (see Case 4).
  - Severe congenital neutropenia (see Case 5) or cyclic neutropenia manifests predominantly as granulocytic hypoplasia. Shwachman-Diamond syndrome also primarily affects neutrophils (Case 6). Rarely, peripheral neutropenia may be due to the congenital condition called myelokathexis in which neutrophil are unable to exit the bone marrow (see Case 7).
  - Reduced megakaryocytes with relatively preserved erythroid and granulocytic lineages raise the possibility of thrombocytopenia with absent radii (TAR) syndrome (see Case 8) and congenital amegakaryocytic thrombocytopenia (see Case 9). Thrombocytopenia with small

platelets is an isolated blood abnormality in Wiskott-Aldrich syndrome, but characteristic skin manifestations are often the presenting symptom (see Case 9).

3. What is the general approach in diagnosing bone marrow failure syndromes?

- The etiology of cytopenias often differs in children and adults; inherited bone marrow failure syndromes more likely occur in younger patients. Family history and constitutional symptoms should be carefully evaluated. Clinical correlation is necessary to identify acquired etiology such as drugs, toxin, and viral infection or evaluate response to GCSF or immunosuppression treatment.
- Patient's specific clinical features and bone marrow findings may help to narrow the differential diagnosis among these entities (see Table 29.2). Genetic testing for relevant genes listed in the table is becoming available for patients with clinical suspicion of bone marrow failure syndromes [1, 2].
- Many bone marrow failure syndromes are associated with increased risks of developing hematologic or solid organ malignancies.

Table 29.2 Characteristic clinical and morphologic features in bone marrow failure syndromes

Disorders	Entities	Clinical features	Peripheral blood or bone marrow morphology	Common mutations
Multilineage failure	Fanconi anemia	Progressive bone marrow failure during childhood, congenital abnormalities, increased risk for AML/MDS, solid tumors arise in adulthood	Gradual development of single or multilineage aplasia	Fanconi anemia genes *FANCA*, *FANCC*, etc.
	Dyskeratosis congenita	Nail dystrophy, abnormal skin pigmentation, oral leukoplakia, pulmonary fibrosis, bone marrow failure	Gradual development of pancytopenias	*DKC1*, *TERT*, *TERC*, etc.
	Telomere biology disorder	Bone marrow failure, idiopathic pulmonary fibrosis, predispose to AML/MDS, and a variety of solid tumors	Aplasia, increased bone marrow reticulin fibrosis, dysplasia in myeloid and megakaryocytic lineages	*TERT*, *TERC*, etc.
Red cell disorders	Diamond-Blackfan anemia	Congenital hypoplastic anemia	Complete red cell aplasia or loss of earliest erythroid precursors; granulocytic and megakaryocytic lineages are preserved	Ribosome biogenesis genes *RPS19*, *RPL5*, *RPL10*, etc. and *GATA1*
	Congenital dyserythropoietic anemia	Variable anemia, splenomegaly, hepatomegaly, intermittent jaundice, and cholelithiasis	Erythroid hyperplasia and dyserythropoiesis; thin chromatin bridges between paired erythroblasts; binucleated or multinucleated erythroblasts	*CDAN1*, *C15ORF41*, *SEC23B*, *KIF23*, *KIF1*
	Congenital sideroblastic anemia	Variable anemia, rarely occurs as part of genetic syndrome with metabolic or neuromuscular manifestation	Anemia with dimorphic red cell morphology; ring sideroblasts on Prussian blue-stained bone marrow aspirate smears	*ALAS2*, *SLC25A38*, *TRNT1* [36]
Granulocyte disorders	Shwachman-Diamond syndrome	Pancreatic dysfunction, bone abnormalities and cytopenias, failure to thrive	Variable cellularity with granulocytic hypoplasia and shift to immaturity, variably preserved erythroid and megakaryocytic maturation	*SBDS*
	Severe congenital neutropenia	Infection, severe neutropenia and dysmorphic features; Kostmann syndrome represents autosomal recessive form of severe congenital neutropenia	Left-shifted granulocytic hypoplasia or granulocytic aplasia; cases of Kostmann syndrome may show binucleated or multinucleated promyelocytes	*ELANE (ELA2)*, *HAX1*
	Cyclic neutropenia	21 days periodicity of neutropenia followed by counts rebound	Granulocytic hypoplasia followed by hyperplasia and full maturation	*ELANE(ELA2)*
Megakaryocytic disorders	Thrombocytopenia with absent radii (TAR)	Constitutional thrombocytopenia with bone anomaly	Reduced megakaryocytes	1q21.1 microdeletion
	Congenital amegakaryocytic thrombocytopenia	Constitutional thrombocytopenia	Reduced megakaryocytes	*MPL*
	Wiskott-Aldrich syndrome	Thrombocytopenia, eczema, and immunodeficiency	Small platelet volume	*WAS*

4. What are the major findings in patients with Fanconi anemia?

- Fanconi anemia is the most common type of inherited bone marrow failure syndromes. According to National Organization of Rare Disorders (NORD) data, the incidence of Fanconi anemia is estimated to be about 1 in 136,000 births (https://rarediseases.org/rare-diseases/fanconi-anemia/).
- The patients are characterized by pancytopenias, physical abnormalities including short stature, thumb anomalies, microcephaly, developmental delay, hyperpigmentation, and café au lait spots. There are also significantly increased risks for developing myeloid neoplasms and solid tumors.
- Fanconi anemia patients have inherited genomic instability as a result of impaired response to DNA damage. In clinically suspected cases, a screening chromsome breakage test may be considered. This is a phenotypic assay that examines chromosome breakage after culturing peripheral blood T cells in the presence of DNA cross-linkers. The presence of a large number of chromosome breakages and rearrangements indicates defects in DNA damage repair and is a typical finding in Fanconi anemia.
- Fanconi anemia gene sequencing is recommended for all patients with a positive result from chromosome breakage testing. There are at least 17 different FA gene subtypes identified. The most commonly mutated genes are *FANCA*, *FANCC*, and *FANCG*, accounting for 80 to 90% of Fanconi anemia [3] (see Case 1).

5. What are the abnormalities of hematopoietic system seen in patients with Down syndrome?

- Transient abnormal myelopoiesis (TAM) is a unique phenomenon occurring in approximately 4–10% of infants with Down syndrome [4–6]. The majority of TAM can resolve spontaneously usually by the age of 6 months. Therefore, caution is advised to diagnose acute myeloid leukemia in Down syndrome infant less than 1 year old. However, approximately 10% of neonates with TAM may develop subsequent acute myeloid leukemia.
- TAM is characterized by leukocytosis, thrombocytopenia, and circulating blasts with the feature of megakaryoblasts (see Case 10). These blasts are medium to large in size with basophilic cytoplasm, coarse granules and cytoplasmic blebs.
  - The typical blasts are positive for CD34, CD117, CD13, CD33, and CD36 and negative for MPO, CD14, CD15, and hemoglobin A. The blasts express the megakaryocytic markers CD41, CD42, and CD61 and with aberrant expression of CD7 and dim CD4 [7, 8].
  - Cytogenetic analysis for trisomy 21 should be performed to confirm the diagnosis.
- Children with Down syndrome have increased risks of developing lymphoid and myeloid leukemia, especially acute megakaryoblastic leukemia (see Case 11). The incidence of acute leukemia is significantly higher (almost 50 times) in individuals with Down syndrome compared to those without Down syndrome. More than half of the AMLs are acute megakaryoblastic leukemia. AML may develop after an MDS-like phase.
  - Both MDS and overt AML are classified under the category of "myeloid leukemia associated with Down syndrome" as there is no biological difference between MDS and AML in this setting.
  - Somatic *GATA1* mutation is associated with most TAM cases and Down syndrome-related megakaryoblastic leukemia, indicating a biologic continuum in these two entities [9].

6. What are the broad categories and the overall frequency of myeloid neoplasm with germline predisposition?

- The WHO classification of myeloid neoplasm with germline predisposition disorders, along with the salient features of each, is presented in Table 29.3. Broadly speaking, these disorders can be categorized based on whether or not they occur:
  - Without a preexisting disorder or organ dysfunction (see Question 7)
  - With preexisting platelet disorder (see Question 8)
  - With other organ dysfunction (see Question 9)
- Myeloid neoplasms with germline predisposition were considered to be very rare in the past; however, the frequency may have been underestimated.
  - Among these rare entities, myeloid neoplasm with germline *CEBPA* mutations appears to be the most common (see Case 12). Studies of large series of normal-karyotype AML have reported an overall frequency of *CEBPA* mutation of 8% to 13% [10–12]; among these, 7–11% have germline *CEBPA* mutations [10, 11].
  - Somatic mutations of *RUNX1* have been reported in 10–33% of de novo AML and MDS [13–16]; however, the prevalence of germline *RUNX1* mutation is unknown; there are fewer than 70 pedigrees reported in the literature [17]. The exact frequency of other germline mutations associated with myeloid neoplasm is largely unknown. Based on limited studies, germline *DDX41* mutation is approximately 1–3% of myeloid neoplasm [15–19], germline *ETV6* mutation is present in 5% (7 out of 130) families with inherited thrombocytopenia of unknown etiology [20], and germline *ANKRD26* mutation is identified in 11% (23 of 215) of individuals in the inherited thrombocytopenia registry [21].

Table 29.3 WHO classification of myeloid neoplasms with germline predisposition

Category	Entity	Morphology	Genetic features
Myeloid neoplasm with germline predisposition without a preexisting disorder or organ dysfunction	Acute myeloid leukemia with germline *CEBPA* mutation	AML with minimal differentiation or without maturation; blasts with frequent Auer rods and aberrant CD7 expression by flow cytometry	Normal karyotype; biallelic *CEBPA* mutations with an N-terminal frameshift or nonsense mutation and a somatic C-terminal in-frame on the other allele [10, 37]
	Myeloid neoplasms with germline *DDX41* mutation	Acute erythroid leukemia (AML) or high-grade MDS	*DDX41* somatic mutation with N-terminal frameshift p. D140Gfs*2 and acquired somatic mutation p.R525H
Myeloid neoplasm with germline predisposition and preexisting platelet disorder	Myeloid neoplasms with germline *RUNX1* mutation	Thrombocytopenia with normal platelet size	Missense, nonsense, frameshift mutations, or large deletions in *RUNX1* [17]
	Myeloid neoplasms with germline *ANKRD26* mutation	Thrombocytopenia with normal platelet size; dysmegakaryopoiesis	Single-nucleotide substitutions in 5′ untranslated region of *ANKRD26* [38, 39]
	Myeloid neoplasms with germline *ETV6* mutation	Thrombocytopenia with normal platelet size; megakaryocytic dysplasia; increased bone marrow reticulin fibrosis	Deleterious *ETV6* mutations clustered in the DNA-binding and central domains [20, 26]
Myeloid neoplasm with germline predisposition and other organ dysfunction	Myeloid neoplasms with germline *GATA2* mutation	Neutropenia, monocytopenia, B/NK/dendritic cell deficiencies, atypical infections, lymphedema	Deleterious *GATA2* mutation including stopgain, indel, or splice site abnormalities, less frequent missense mutations
	Myeloid neoplasms associated with bone marrow failure syndromes	AML/MDS is often preceded by a hypoplastic/aplastic phase	Mutations in various genes associated with inherited bone marrow failure syndromes
	Myeloid neoplasms associated with telomere biology disorders	Increased bone marrow reticulin fibrosis, dysplasia in myeloid and megakaryocytic lineages	Mutations in *TERT* and *TERC*
	Juvenile myelomonocytic leukemia associated with neurofibromatosis, Noonan syndrome, or Noonan syndrome-like disorder	Peripheral blood with neutrophilia and monocytosis; hypercellular bone marrow with myeloid predominance	Mutations involving *PTPN11*, *SOS1*, *RAF1*, and *KRAS*
	Myeloid neoplasm associated with Down syndrome	AML particularly acute megakaryoblastic leukemia	Constitutional trisomy 21; *GATA1* mutation

– Germline mutation involving *GATA2* is also rare (see Case 13), however, appears more common in pediatric MDS (7%) and particularly in those with monosomy 7 (~72%) [22].

7. What are the distinguishing features of the major entities under "myeloid neoplasms with germline predisposition without a preexisting disorder or organ dysfunction"?

- There are two major entities in this subtype: acute myeloid leukemia (AML) with *CEBPA* mutation and myeloid neoplasm with *DDX41* mutation.
- Morphologically, AML with mutated *CEBPA* often presents as acute myeloid leukemia with minimal differentiation or acute myeloid leukemia without maturation (see Case 12). The blasts may show frequent Auer rods and express aberrant CD7 by flow cytometry. The majority of AML with germline *CEBPA* mutation has mutations on different alleles and is often associated with normal karyotype.
- Myeloid neoplasms with germline *DDX41* mutation have variable morphology including acute myeloid leukemia of erythroid lineage, high-grade MDS with erythroid dysplasia, or chronic myeloid leukemia.

8. What are the major entities under "myeloid neoplasms with germline predisposition and preexisting platelet disorders"? What are the clinical and morphologic features of these entities?

- There are three major entities in this subtype: myeloid neoplasms with germline *RUNX1*, *ANKRD26*, and *ETV6* mutations.

  - The entities share the clinical features of long-standing mild to moderate thrombocytopenia, mild bleeding tendency, and an increased lifetime risk of developing MDS or AML.
  - One common morphologic feature of these entities is megakaryocytic dysplasia, which can be seen in asymptomatic carriers due to the underlying germline mutations.
  - Patients developing myeloid neoplasms may present with new anemia and/or leukopenia in addition to thrombocytopenia, multilineage dysplasia, increased blasts or presence of an additional clonal event either a cytogenetic or a molecular aberration [23].
- Some mutation specific morphologic findings include:
  - Bone marrow biopsies from patients with germline *ANKRD26* mutation show increased reticulin fibrosis, in addition to increased micromegakaryocytes and/or hypolobated megakaryocytes [21, 24, 25].
  - Some cases of germline *ETV6* mutation also show mild dyserythropoiesis [26].
- Carriers with isolated thrombocytopenia could be mistaken as immune thrombocytopenic purpura (ITP). Megakaryocytic dysplasia may also pose a diagnostic challenge to differentiate thrombocytopenia in the setting of germline mutation versus MDS.

9. What are the major entities under "myeloid neoplasms with germline predisposition and other organ dysfunction"? What are the clinical and morphologic features of these entities including germline *GATA2* mutation?

- Myeloid neoplasms arising in the setting of germline *GATA2* mutation (see Case 13), inherited bone marrow failure syndromes, telomere biology disorders, and other genetic disorders such as neurofibromatosis, Noonan syndrome, or Down syndrome are classified into this category. These entities present with other organ manifestations such as skin lesions, neurologic or immunologic disorders, and hematologic abnormalities as listed in Table 29.3.
- Features of Down syndrome associated myeloid neoplasms are discussed in Question 5.
- Neurofibromatosis (NF) is an autosomal dominant genetic disorder with clinical features characterized by *café au lait* macules, neurofibromas, and Lisch nodules. NF is associated with multiple malignancies including juvenile myelomonocytic leukemia (JMML).
- Children with Noonan syndrome have increased risks for developing JMML or JMML-like disorder in the first few weeks of life. JMML is a rare type of myelodysplastic/myeloproliferative neoplasm of infancy and early childhood, which usually requires aggressive treatment; JMML-like myeloproliferative disorder in Noonan syndrome is an indolent disorder that may resolve without treatment. See Case 14 for a case of JMML-like myeloproliferative disorder in the setting of Noonan syndrome.
- Germline *GATA2* mutation: Patients with germline *GATA2* mutation have a broad spectrum of clinical presentations.
  - Severe infections, most commonly viral or non-tuberculosis mycobacterial infection, respiratory problems such as pulmonary fibrosis and alveolar proteinosis, leg swelling, and increased risks for hematologic disease can occur.
  - *GATA2* mutation is shown as the unifying genetic abnormality underlying several distinct entities including monoMAC syndrome characterized by monocytopenia and non-tuberculosis mycobacterial infection, DCML (dendritic cells, monocyte and lymphocyte) deficiency with vulnerability to viral infections, familial MDS/AML, and Emberger syndrome characterized by primary lymphedema with MDS [27].
  - The patients may or may not display any prior hematologic abnormalities or infection before developing myeloid neoplasm. The age at onset of myeloid neoplasm is also variable, even within the same family.

10. What could be a potential pitfall for diagnosing myeloid neoplasms in the setting of underlying germline condition?

- The diagnosis of MDS could be challenging in patients with germline condition, as these patients often have cytopenias. Some studies also described bone marrow dysplastic changes due to the underlying genetic abnormalities in asymptomatic carriers without obvious progression [23, 25].
- Currently, there are no consensus diagnostic criteria to address this unique challenge. Limited studies recommended that additional morphologic or genetic evidence is needed to diagnose disease progression to MDS or AML in the setting of underlying germline conditions. These may include cytopenias or dysplasia in multiple cell lineages, increased blasts, and presence of additional clonal event either by cytogenetic or molecular studies [23].

11. When and which tissue should be tested to confirm the presence of a germline condition in patients with myeloid neoplasms?

- Germline analysis is recommended in any newly diagnosed myeloid neoplasm with biallelic *CEBPA* mutation, a deleterious *GATA2* mutation, or a deleterious *RUNX1* mutation [28].
- If clinical or pathological findings suggest an underlying germline condition, it is necessary to identify the genetic variants in non-hematopoietic tissue or in multiple generations of the affected families.
  - Molecular testing on uninvolved tissue such as skin biopsy, buccal swab/saliva, or cultured mesenchymal cells is required to confirm the germline nature of the genetic alteration. Caution is advised that the uninvolved tissue may contain hematopoietic cells, such as lymphocytes carrying the somatic mutations.
  - Although testing of blood or bone marrow during complete remission from AML may suggest germline nature of variants, as residual leukemic cells are negligible in these samples, these results should be confirmed with testing in non-hematopoietic tissue.

12. What are the bone marrow features of common variable immunodeficiency (CVID)?

- CVID is the most common, but poorly understood, primary humoral immunodeficiency in adults, with an incidence between 1/10000 and 1/50000 in Caucasians; it is rarely described in Asian and African populations [29]. It can occur as a congenital or acquired condition in which hypogammaglobulinemia is the common feature, and other specific causes of hypogammaglobulinemia are excluded. It is considered to be caused by mutations in genes involved in the survival and maturation of B cells (Table 29.4), but the genetic cause in up to 90% of the cases remains elusive [30].
- By definition, patients present with variable degrees of phenotypes most commonly increased susceptibility to

Table 29.4 Common gene mutations in common variable immune deficiency disorders

Gene	Location	Protein function	Estimated share	Clinical spectrum	Immunologic spectrum
ICOS	2q33.2	Ig-like co-stimulatory molecule on T cells, essential for germinal center formation	3.74%	Recurrent infections, rheumatologic disorders, hepatosplenomegaly, granulomata, malignancy	Decrease in serum Ig Secretion, absent memory B cells, absent bone marrow plasma cells, low-circulating T-helper cells, low CTLA-4 expression
TACI (*TNFRSF13b*)	17p11.2	Tumor necrosis factor (TNF) receptor superfamily member, receptor for BAFF APRIL, induces class-switch recombination events in B cells	5–10%	Highly variable from no infection to very severe infections, autoimmune manifestations, lymphoma, and other cancers	Low IgG, defect in antibody responses to polysaccharide vaccines, low memory B cells
CD19	16p11.2	Member of BCR co-receptor complex	3.74%	Recurrent infections, intermittent microscopic hematuria, postinfectious glomerulonephritis, IgA nephropathy	Decrease in serum Ig Secretion, defect in response to T-cell-dependent antigens
BAFFR (*TNFRSF13c*)	22q13.2	Member of the TNF receptor family that specifically binds BAFF, required for B-cell maturation and survival	Unknown	Recurrent infections, splenomegaly, granulomata, chronic diarrhea with weight loss, failure to thrive	Decrease in serum Ig Secretion, defect in antibody responses to polysaccharide vaccines, low total B cells, low memory B cells
CD20	11q12.2	Part of a B-cell surface complex involved in transmembrane Ca^{2+} transport, important in B-cell signal transduction, proliferation, and differentiation	0.53%	Recurrent bronchopneumonia and respiratory tract infections	Decrease in serum Ig Secretion, decreased antibody responses to polysaccharide vaccines, decrease in memory B-cell count

(continued)

Table 29.4 (continued)

Gene	Location	Protein function	Estimated share	Clinical spectrum	Immunologic spectrum
CD81	11p15.5	Forms a complex that signals in conjunction with the B-cell antigen receptor	0.53%	Recurrent infections, glomerulonephritis with progression to end-stage renal disease, undefined systemic inflammatory syndrome	Decrease in serum Ig Secretion, defect in antibody responses to protein and polysaccharide vaccines, low memory B cells, low BCR signaling, absent CD19 and CD21 expression
CD21	1q32	Complement receptor type 2, B-cell membrane protein to which the Epstein-Barr virus binds and infect cells, a member of B-cell co-receptor and enhances antigen specific B lymphocyte responses	1.07%	Recurrent infections, chronic diarrhea with weight loss, splenomegaly	Decrease in serum Ig Secretion, defect in antibody response to polysaccharide vaccines, low memory B cells, low BCR signaling
CTLA-4	2q33	Inhibitory T-cell receptor that negatively regulates immune responses, competes with the co-stimulatory protein CD28 for binding to CD80/CD86, thereby preventing excessive T-cell activation and maintaining immune tolerance	6.42%	Severe autoimmune disorders, severe *EBV*-induced lymphoproliferation, granulomata, recurrent infections, hepatosplenomegaly, malignancy, failure to thrive	Decrease in serum Ig Secretion, defect in antibody responses to polysaccharide vaccines, variably decreased total B cells, memory B cells, total lymphocytes, total T cells, CD4+/CD8+ T cells, CD4+/CD8+ naive T cells, variably increased double negative T cells and Treg cells, hyperactivity in effector T cells
Lipopolysaccharide-responsive beige-like anchor protein (*LRBA*)	4q31	A cytosolic protein localized in endoplasmic reticulum, trans-Golgi apparatus, endocytosis vesicles and lysosomes, functions in polarized vesicle trafficking and polarized responses of immune effector cells, autophagy, and positive regulation of cell survival	26.74%	Severe autoimmune disorders, severe *EBV*-induced lymphoproliferation, granulomata, recurrent infections, growth hormone deficiency	Decrease in serum Ig Secretion, defect in antibody responses to protein and/or polysaccharide vaccines, variably decreased total B cells, memory B cells, plasmablasts, total lymphocytes, CD4+/CD8+ naive T cells, Treg cells, variably increased double-negative T cells, Tfh cells, variably decreased in vitro T-cell proliferation responses, Fas-mediated apoptosis, CTLA-4 surface expression
PIK3CD	1p36	Functions as PI3K catalytic subunit p110δ, mutations result in overactivity of the PI3K signaling pathway, enhanced p110δ membrane association and kinase activity	26.74%	Recurrent infections, failure to thrive, autoimmune disorders, *EBV*-induced lymphoproliferation, hepatosplenomegaly, malignancy (mainly lymphoma)	Decrease in serum Ig Secretion, defect in antibody responses to protein and/or polysaccharide vaccines, variably decreased total B cells, memory B cells, naive B cells, total lymphocytes, total/CD4+/CD8+ T cells, CD4+/CD8+ naive T cells, NK-cell cytotoxicity, variably increased CD4+/CD8+ memory T cells, T cell activation-induced cell death

infections, autoimmune disorders due to disturbed immune homeostasis, and predisposition to development of malignancies particularly lymphoma.

- Bone marrow biopsy is sometimes performed due to suspicion of lymphoma, which may develop secondarily in CVID patients. The bone marrow in CVID patients may show diffuse or nodular lymphocytic infiltrate composed of predominantly CD3+ T lymphocytes [28] (see Case 15).
- Bone marrow B cells may demonstrate development blockage at the pre-B stage. Bone marrow plasma cells are either absent or significantly reduced.
  - Immunodeficiency due to B-cell defects is sometimes associated with other hematopoietic cell abnormalities. For example, see Case 15.
- The lymphocytic infiltrate in CVID bone marrow may be very intense and focally replace normal hematopoietic components but usually still maintains a composition of mixed CD4 and CD8 T cells and/or immunophenotypically normal B cells, distinguishing from T- or B-cell lymphoma.

13. What is familial hemophagocytic lymphohistiocytosis (FHL)? What are the peripheral blood and bone marrow findings in FHL?

- Hemophagocytic lymphohistiocytosis (HLH) is a clinicopathological entity characterized by systemic immune activation leading to lymphohistiocytic infiltration of tissues and destruction of vital organs. The central mechanism of HLH is dysfunctional cytolytic responses of NK cells and/or cytotoxic T cells. Although most of HLH cases are secondary to infectious, autoimmune, or oncologic processes, a subset of them are familial HLH and caused by genetic defects affecting NK or cytotoxic T-cell function, most commonly perforin (PRF). See Table 29.5 for a list of genes implicated in FHL.
- FHL affects around 1:50,000 live-born children and typically has its onset during infancy or early childhood. It has very poor prognosis, with median survival of less than 2 months if untreated.
- Blood and bone marrow findings in FHL include:
  - Cytopenia in at least two of three lineages.
  - Depletion of myeloid and erythroid precursors and/or megakaryocytes.
  - Bone marrow infiltration by small mature lymphocytes and histiocytes.
  - Hemophagocytosis, most remarkably erythrophagocytosis, may be present (see Case 16).

14. How is FHL diagnosed and what are the diagnostic pitfalls?

- Non-familial hemophagocytic lymphohistiocytosis (HLH) is a common presentation of many infectious and oncologic processes. Extensive work-up must be performed to rule out secondary HLH before FLH is considered.
- Detection of pathogenic mutation in one of the genes (Table 29.5) satisfies a diagnosis of FHL [31]. However, not all FHLs have identifiable gene mutations. For example, an unknown gene located on 9q21.3–22 is involved in FHL1.
- According to HLH-2004 consensus [32], in cases before a genetic diagnosis is available or where a specific mutation cannot be demonstrated but causes of acquired HLH are thoroughly ruled out, many patients meet five of eight following clinical and/or laboratory abnormalities.
  - Fever
  - Splenomegaly

Table 29.5 Mutated genes, protein functions, and disease types in familial hemophagocytic lymphohistiocytosis

Gene	Location	Protein	Function	Disease
PRF1	10q21-22	Perforin	Vesicle content	FHL2
UNC13D	17q25	Munc13-4	Vesicle priming	FHL3
STX11	6q24	Syntaxin	Vesicle docking and fusion	FHL4
STXBP2	19p13	Syntaxin-binding protein 2	Vesicle docking and fusion	FHL5
LYST	1q42.1-42.2	Lysosomal trafficking regulator	Vesicle trafficking	Chediak-Higashi syndrome
RAB27a	15q21	Ras-related protein Rab-27A	Vesicle fusion or fission	Griscelli syndrome
AP3B1	5q14.1	AP-3 complex subunit beta-1	Vesicle trafficking	Hermansky-Pudlak II
SH2D1A	Xq24-26	SLAM-associated protein (SAP)	Multiple effects including CD8 T/NK-cell cytotoxicity	X-linked lymphoproliferative syndrome 1 (XLP1)
XIAP	Xq25	X-linked inhibitor of apoptosis protein	Multiple signaling pathways	XLP2/X-linked HLH
Unknown	9q21.3-22	Unknown	Unknown	FHL1

- Cytopenias (affecting two of three lineages in the peripheral blood):
  Hemoglobin <90 g/L (in infants <4 weeks: hemoglobin <100 g/L)
  Platelets <100 K/uL
  Neutrophils <1 K/uL
- Hypertriglyceridemia and/or hypofibrinogenemia:
  Fasting triglycerides >265 mg/dl
  Fibrinogen <150 mg/dL
- Hemophagocytosis in bone marrow or spleen or lymph nodes
- Low or absent NK-cell function
- Ferritin >50 mg/dL
- Soluble CD25 (i.e., soluble IL-2 receptor) >2400 U/ml

• Note that these clinical/laboratory criteria are not strictly required for familial cases with confirmed mutation of genes listed above, but nevertheless one or more of these features are present in familial cases. Morphologic evidence of hemophagocytosis may not be present, so a high level of suspicion should be maintained, and relevant work-up should be initiated for unexplained five or more laboratory and/or clinical abnormalities listed in HLH-2004.

15. What is autoimmune lymphoproliferative syndrome (ALPS), and what are the peripheral and bone marrow findings in ALPS?

• ALPS is an autoimmune disorder characterized by proliferation of T cells and B cells harboring gene mutations in the Fas-FasL signaling pathway, leading to lymphocytosis in peripheral blood bone marrow, and/or tissue/organ infiltration and damage.
• Clinical presentation of ALPS may include [33]:
  - Lymphadenopathy (>95%).
  - Splenomegaly (>90%).
  - Hepatomegaly (40–50%).
  - Increased IL-10, IL-18, vitamin B12, soluble FAS ligand (sFASL), and IgG in plasma.
  - Median age at presentation is 11.5 months, but adult presentation is not uncommon.
• Blood findings include:
  - Single or multilineage cytopenias, most commonly anemia and thrombocytopenia.
  - A proportion of patients (22% in one study, [34]) may have lymphocytosis.
• Characteristic circulating T-cell population termed "double negative T cells" (DNTs), which express CD3 and the alpha/beta T-cell receptor (TCRα/β) but lack CD4 and CD8, detectable by flow cytometry.
• Bone marrow biopsy may show:
  - Lymphocytosis: present in majority of cases, which may demonstrate several distribution patterns: lymphoid aggregates comprising T cells in most cases, B cells, and a mixture of T and B cells in fewer cases (see Case 16).
  - Double negative T cells were detected by immunohistochemistry in a minority of cases, but these cases usually demonstrate prominent T-cell aggregates, which may variably replace the normal hematopoietic elements.

16. What are the peripheral and bone marrow findings in the major entities of lysosomal storage diseases?

• Many of these diseases are systemic and may have manifestations in non-hematopoietic organs/systems, but bone marrow may be the presenting site and first specimen leading to a diagnosis of a lysosomal storage disease.
• All these disorders are rare. Moreover, underlying genetic defects are greatly heterogeneous, involving the enzymes of lysosomal lipid/carbohydrate metabolism or amino acid/peptide transporters of lysosome (Table 29.6). The relatively more common storage diseases and deficient enzymes/proteins diagnosed in the bone marrow are:
  - Gaucher's disease: Acid β-glucosidase
  - Niemann-Pick disease: Sphingomyelinase
  - Cystinosis [35]: Cystinosin (a cystine transport protein on the lysosomal membrane), see Case 17
  - Cytopenia is common due to infiltration of bone marrow by storage disease histiocytes; vacuolated lymphocytes in peripheral blood may be seen in certain types of diseases such as sialidosis and sphingolipidosis
• Bone marrow aspiration and biopsy may show patchy and diffuse infiltration by characteristic disease histiocytes as follows (Fig. 29.1):
  - Gaucher cells: histiocytes with voluminous crinkly, eosinophilic cytoplasm
  - Niemann-Pick cells: foamy histiocytes with voluminous cytoplasm packed with uniform vacuoles
  - Sea-blue histiocytosis: histiocytes with cytoplasmic deep blue granules
  - Cystinosis: Clear (non-staining on Wright-Giemsa stained marrow aspirate slides) crystals with straight edges and hexagonal shape

Table 29.6 Gene mutations and clinicopathological findings in selected lysosomal storage diseases

Disease	Gene affected	Protein function	Involved organs	Bone marrow findings
Gaucher's disease	β-Glucocerebrosidase (*GBA*)	Degradation of glucosylceramide	Brain, bone, joints, liver, spleen, bone marrow	Infiltration by histiocytes with voluminous crinkly, eosinophilic cytoplasm (Gaucher cells)
Niemann-Pick disease	Sphingomyelinase (*SMPD*)	Degradation of sphingomyelin	Brain, liver, spleen, lung, bone marrow	Infiltration by histiocytes with voluminous cytoplasm packed with uniform vacuoles (Niemann-Pick cells), or histiocytes with cytoplasmic deep blue granules (sea-blue histiocytes)
Cystinosis	Cystinosin (*CTNS*)	Transport cystine out of lysosome	Kidneys, liver, eyes, bone marrow	Infiltration by histiocytes laden with clear crystals of straight edges and hexagonal shape

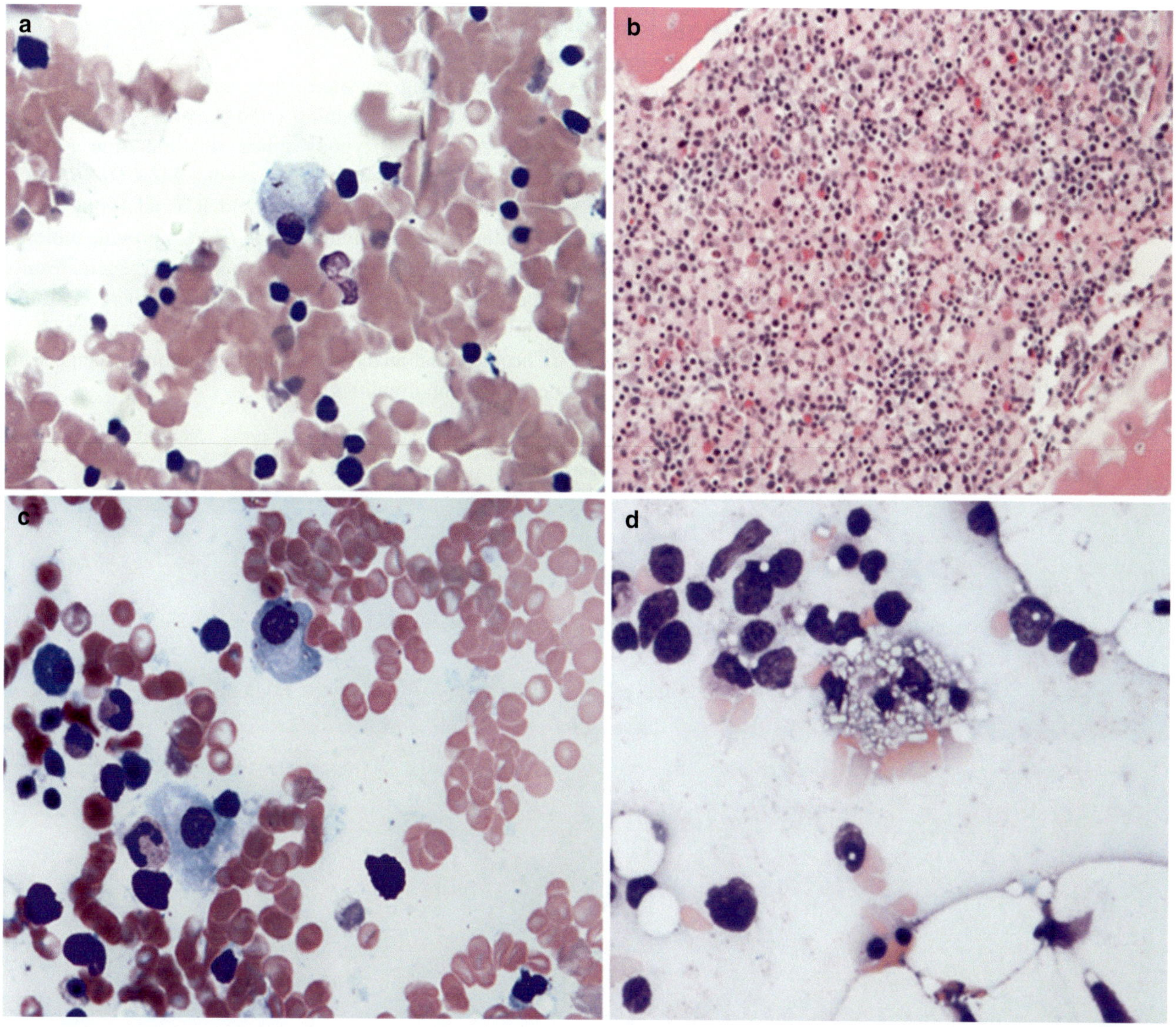

Fig. 29.1 Bone marrow findings of selected lysosomal storage diseases. (**a**) The bone marrow aspirate of a patient with Gaucher's disease revealed a Gaucher cell, with voluminous cytoplasm demonstrating classic "wrinkled tissue paper" sign (Wright-Giemsa, ×1000). (**b**) The bone marrow biopsy of the same patient as in A revealed infiltration by numerous foamy histiocytes with abundant eosinophilic cytoplasm (hematoxylin-eosin, ×200). (**c**) The bone marrow aspirate showed many sea-blue histiocytes, which can be seen in variants of Niemann-Pick disease and also a variety of bone marrow disorders with rapid cell turnover rate, such as myelodysplastic syndrome, idiopathic thrombocytopenic purpura, and hemophagocytic lymphohistiocytosis (Wright-Giemsa, ×1000). (**d**) The bone marrow aspirate of a patient with systemic cystinosis revealed a crystal-laden macrophage (Wright-Giemsa, ×400)

Case Presentations

Case 1 (Fig. 29.2)

Learning Objectives

1. To be aware of increased risks for myeloid neoplasms in patients with Fanconi anemia
2. To understand the role of genetic testing in the diagnosis of Fanconi anemia

Case History

This is an 8-year-old boy who presented with pancytopenia in the setting of failure to thrive and short stature. The boy's mother died from breast cancer 5 years ago. CBC reported WBC 2.5 K/uL, Hb 3.9 g/dL, HCT 11.0%, MCV 103 fl, RDW 17.2%, and PLT 89 k/uL.

Histologic Findings

- The peripheral blood smear reveals pancytopenia.
- The bone marrow aspirate smears show increased blasts and dysplastic megakaryocytes with hypolobated nuclei or separate nuclear lobes.
- The bone marrow core biopsy is hypercellular with increased blasts.
- A CD34 immunohistochemical stain confirms increased number of blasts, comprising ~10% of the bone marrow cellularity.

Differential Diagnosis

- Myelodysplastic syndrome with germline disposition associated with Fanconi anemia
- Myelodysplastic syndrome with germline disposition associated with another bone marrow failure syndrome
- Myelodysplastic syndrome with germline predisposition
- Bone marrow failure syndrome
- Acute myeloid leukemia with germline predisposition
- Myelodysplastic syndrome without identifiable germline predisposition

Ancillary Studies

- Genetic testing revealed a heterozygous *FANCA* c.(?_-42)_(586 +?)del spanning coding exon 1–6 within the *FANCA*, a heterozygous splice site alteration *FANCA* c.1369 + 1G > C, and a heterozygous *FANCD1 (BRCA2)* frameshift mutation c.5722_5723delCT, p.L1908Rfs∗2.
- The findings of two mutations in *FANCA* provide molecular confirmation of Fanconi anemia FA-A (genetic results courtesy of Dr. Robert Liem, Ann& Robert H. Lurie Children's Hospital of Chicago).
- Chromosomal analysis demonstrated clonal change with complex abnormalities.

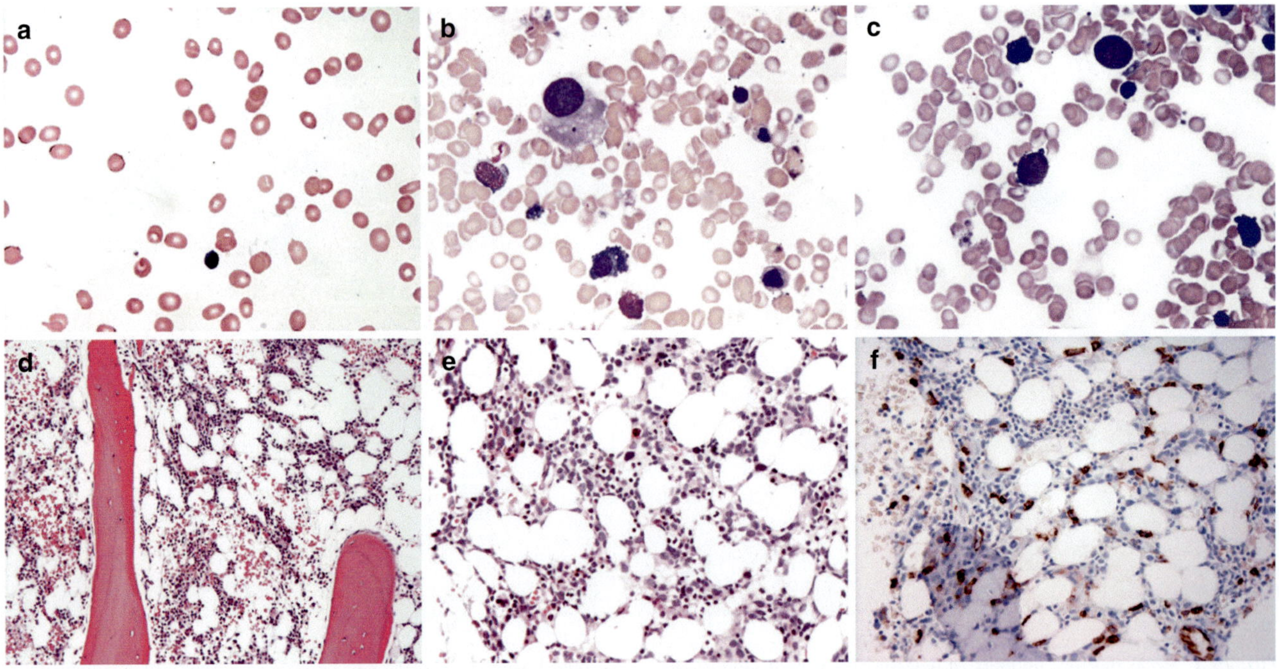

Fig. 29.2 Myelodysplastic syndrome with excess blasts arising in the setting of Fanconi anemia with biallelic *FANCA* mutations. (**a**) Peripheral blood smear reveals pancytopenia (Wright-Giemsa, ×600). (**b**, **c**) Bone marrow aspirate smears show increased blasts and dysplastic megakaryocytes with hypolobated nuclei or separate nuclear lobes (**b**, **c**: Wright-Giemsa, ×600). (**d**, **e**) Bone marrow core biopsy is hypercellular with increased blasts (**d**, hematoxylin-eosin, ×200; **e**, hematoxylin-eosin, ×400). (**f**) A CD34 immunohistochemical stain confirms increased number of blasts, comprising ~10% of the bone marrow cellularity (peroxidase, ×400)

Final Diagnosis

Myelodysplastic syndrome with excess blasts arising in the setting of Fanconi anemia with biallelic *FANCA* mutations

Take-Home Messages

1. Fanconi anemia is a bone marrow failure syndrome with increased risks for developing myeloid neoplasm and solid tumors.
2. Mutations involving Fanconi complementation groups (*FANC*) have been implicated in the pathogenesis of Fanconi anemia and can be used to confirm the diagnosis.

Case 2 (Fig. 29.3)

Learning Objectives

1. To be familiar with the clinical and pathological features of dyskeratosis congenita.
2. To be aware of the role of genetic testing in the diagnosis of dyskeratosis congenita.

Case History

The patient is an 8-year-old boy with a clinical suspicion of dyskeratosis congenita. CBC reported WBC 3.74 k/uL, Hb 11.9 g/dL, HCT 35.0%, MCV 100 fl, and PLT 170 k/uL.

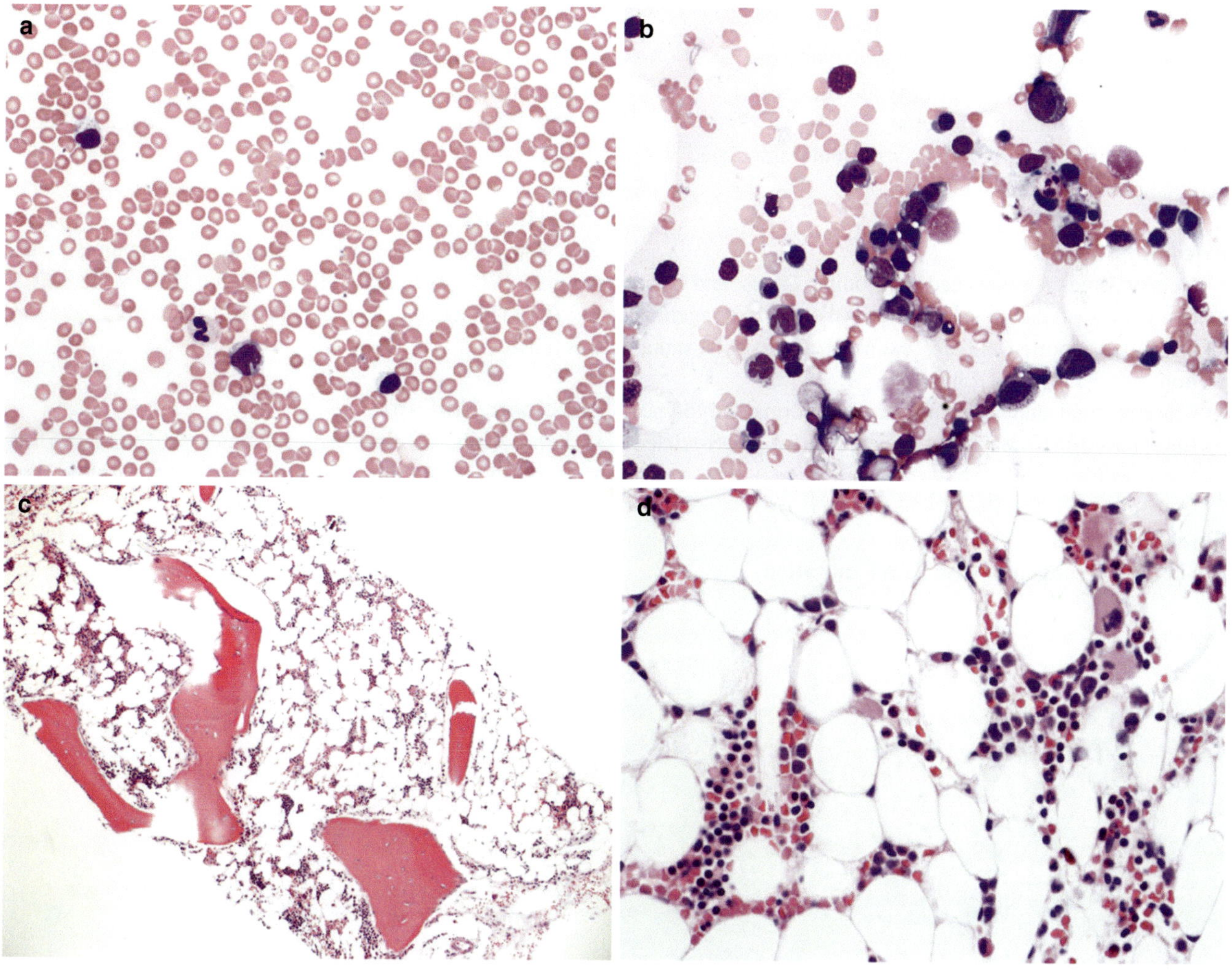

Fig. 29.3 Dyskeratosis congenita with *TERT* mutation. (**a**) The peripheral blood smear shows mild macrocytosis and mild neutropenia (Wright-Giemsa, ×600). (**b**) The bone marrow aspirate smear contains rare hypocellular particle with myeloid and erythroid precursors demonstrating orderly maturation with no apparent dysplastic features. Rare megakaryocytes show unremarkable morphology (Wright-Giemsa, ×600). (**c**, **d**) The bone marrow core biopsy contains hypocellular marrow with a cellularity of 10–20%. Myeloid and erythroid precursors are decreased but show progressive maturation. Megakaryocytes are present with unremarkable morphology (**c**, hematoxylin-eosin, ×100; **d**, hematoxylin-eosin, ×600). A CD34 immunostain reveals no increased blasts (not shown). A CD61 immunostain reveals decreased number of megakaryocytes with unremarkable morphology (not shown)

Histologic Findings

- The peripheral blood smear shows mild macrocytosis and mild neutropenia.
- The bone marrow aspirate smear contains rare hypocellular particle with myeloid and erythroid precursors demonstrating orderly maturation with no apparent dysplastic features. Rare megakaryocytes show unremarkable morphology.
- The bone marrow core biopsy contains hypocellular marrow with a cellularity of 10–20%. Myeloid and erythroid precursors are decreased but show progressive maturation. Megakaryocytes are present with unremarkable morphology.
- A CD34 immunostain reveals no increased blasts.

Differential Diagnosis

- Evolving aplastic anemia
- Hypoplastic myelodysplastic syndrome
- Bone marrow failure syndrome
- Hypoplastic myelodysplastic syndrome associated with bone marrow failure syndrome

Ancillary Studies

- Genetic studies sequenced all coding exons and exon boundaries of the genes on the dyskeratosis congenital panel and reported a *TERT* exon 2 heterozygous mutation: c.416 T > G, p.L139R.
- Chromosomal analysis demonstrated a normal karyotype.
- Interphase FISH analysis was negative for MDS-related abnormalities.

Final Diagnosis

Dyskeratosis congenita with *TERT* mutation

Take-Home Messages

1. Dyskeratosis congenita is an inheritable telomere disorder with multi-organ manifestations including bone marrow failure, pulmonary fibrosis and typical mucocutaneous triad of abnormal skin pigmentation, nail dystrophy, and leukoplakia of the oral mucosa.
2. Multiple genes including *DKC1*, *TERT*, and *TERC* have been reportedly associated with dyskeratosis congenita.

Case 3 (Fig. 29.4)

Learning Objectives

1. To be familiar with the clinical and pathologic features of Diamond-Blackfan anemia
2. To understand the role of genetic testing in the diagnosis of Diamond-Blackfan anemia

Case History

This 8-week-old baby girl presented with anemia. CBC reported WBC 6.1 k/uL, Hb 3.2 g/dL, HCT 9.5%, MCV 112 fL, RDW 16.1%, and PLT 381 k/uL. Reticulocyte count was 0.3%.

Histologic Findings

- The peripheral blood smear shows profound slightly macrocytic anemia with adequate neutrophils and platelets.
- The bone marrow aspirate smear shows marked erythroid hypoplasia with relative myeloid hyperplasia, scattered

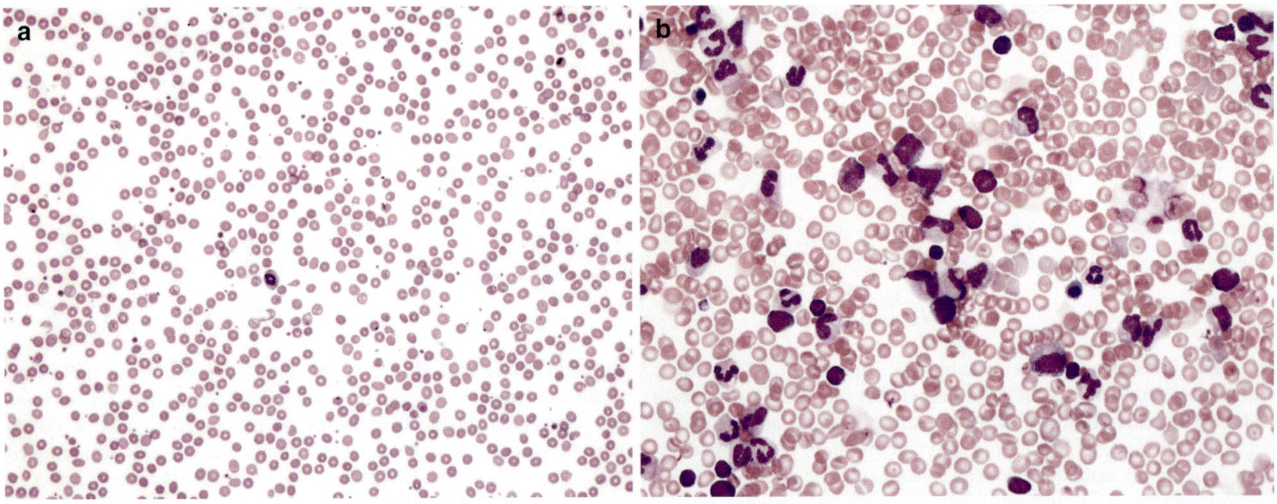

Fig. 29.4 Diamond-Blackfan anemia with *RPS19* mutation. (**a**) The peripheral blood smear shows profound slightly macrocytic anemia with adequate neutrophils and platelets (Wright-Giemsa, ×400). (**b**) The bone marrow aspirate smear shows marked erythroid hypoplasia with relative myeloid hyperplasia, scattered hematogones, and reduced megakaryocytes (Wright-Giemsa, ×600). Erythroid precursors are less than 5% based on a 500 cell differential counts

hematogones, and reduced megakaryocytes. Erythroid precursors are less than 5% based on 500 cell differential counts.

Differential Diagnosis

- Diamond-Blackfan anemia
- Congenital parvovirus B19 infection
- Pure red cell aplasia due to other etiologies

Ancillary Studies

- Molecular studies for *RPS19* gene analysis reported a heterozygous mutation c.178A > C, p.T60P.

Final Diagnosis

Diamond-Blackfan anemia with *RPS19* mutation

Take-Home Messages

1. Diamond-Blackfan anemia is characterized by congenital anemia with erythroid hypoplasia.
2. Mutations in ribosomal protein genes have been reported in approximately half of the cases.
3. Identification of ribosomal protein gene mutations helps to confirm the diagnosis and to differentiate from other etiology of erythroid failure such as transient erythroblastopenia of childhood and parvovirus B19 infection.

Case 4 (Fig. 29.5)

Learning Objective

Sideroblastic anemia is a heterogeneous group of acquired and inherited disorders of erythropoiesis characterized by the presence of ring sideroblasts in the bone marrow

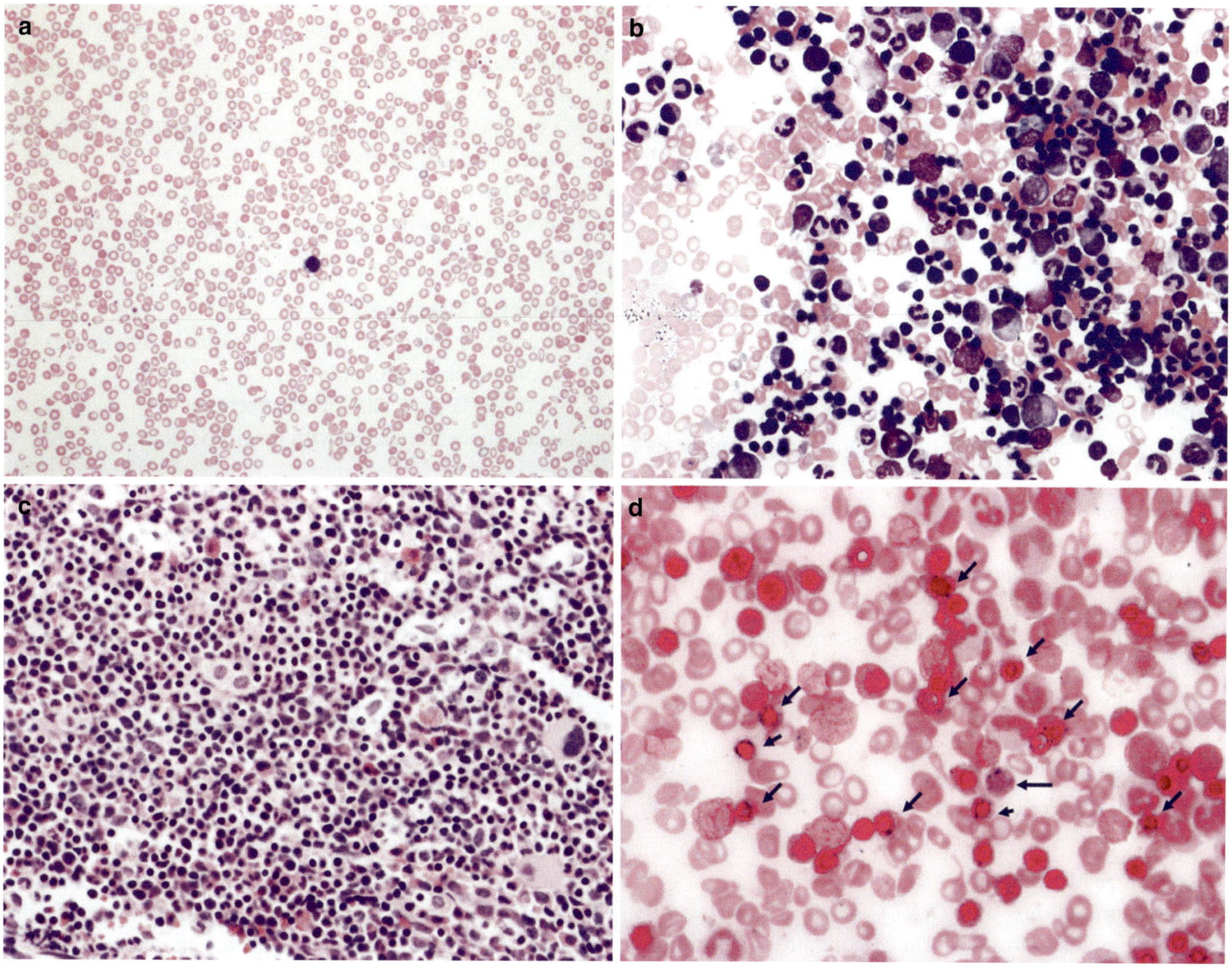

Fig. 29.5 Congenital sideroblastic anemia with *TRNT1* mutation. (**a**) The peripheral blood smear shows marked microcytic anemia, anisopoikilocytosis with frequent ovalocytes, and occasional target cells (Wright-Giemsa, ×400). (**b**) The bone marrow aspirate smear shows erythroid predominance but with maturation and occasional nuclear budding or irregular forms (Wright-Giemsa, ×600). Granulocytic precursors show progressive maturation. (**c**) The bone marrow core biopsy shows hypercellular marrow with erythroid predominance (hematoxylin-eosin, ×200). (**d**) Iron stain reveals numerous ring sideroblasts (Prussian blue, ×1000)

Case History

This 1-year-old male presented with developmental delay, hypotonia, abnormal movements, GERD, decreased cardiac function and microcytic anemia, and recurrent febrile episodes associated with fever. CBC reported WBC 3.75 k/uL, Hb 10.2 g/dL, HCT 32.9%, MCV 58.5 fL, RDW 23.1%, and PLT 225 k/uL.

Histologic Findings

- The peripheral blood smear shows marked microcytic anemia and anisopoikilocytosis with frequent ovalocytes and occasional target cells. There is mild absolute lymphopenia with occasional reactive lymphocytes. Neutrophils are adequate with unremarkable morphology. Platelets are adequate.
- The bone marrow aspirate smear shows erythroid predominance but with maturation and occasional nuclear budding or irregular forms. Granulocytic precursors show progressive maturation. Iron stain reveals numerous ring sideroblasts.
- The bone marrow core biopsy shows hypercellular marrow with erythroid predominance. Myeloid precursors are relatively decreased but with progressive maturation. Megakaryocytes are present in adequate number with normal distribution.

Differential Diagnosis

- Congenital sideroblastic anemia
- Myelodysplastic syndrome with ring sideroblasts

Ancillary Studies

- Cytogenetic analysis reported a normal male karyotype: 46, XY [20].
- Whole exome sequencing performed on the DNA obtained from the blood specimen of this patient identified compound heterozygous Thr49fs and Ile122Thr variants in the *TRTN1* gene.
- Parental studies demonstrated that the Thr49fs variant was maternally inherited and the Ile122Thr variant was paternally inherited.

Final Diagnosis

Congenital sideroblastic anemia with *TRNT1* mutation

Take-Home Message

Biallelic mutations in *TRNT1* have been recently described as a syndromic form of congenital sideroblastic anemia associated with B-cell immunodeficiency, periodic fevers, and developmental delay (SIFD)

Case 5 (Fig. 29.6)

Learning Objectives

1. To be familiar with the clinical and pathological features of congenital neutropenia
2. To understand the role of genetic testing in the diagnosis of congenital neutropenia

Case History

This 9-month-old male infant presented with neutropenia, recurrent viral and bacterial infections, recurrent pneumonia, ear infections, and sinusitis. CBC reported WBC 13.85 k/uL, Hb 11.1 g/dL, HCT 34.6%, MCV 74 fl, and PLT 275 k/uL.

Histologic Findings

- The peripheral blood smear shows neutropenia with very rare neutrophils and myelocytes noted upon scan. Differential reported lymphocytes 76%, monocytes 22%, and 2% neutrophils.
- The bone marrow aspirate smears reveal granulopoiesis with maturation arrest. But the eosinophilic granulocytes show progressive maturation to segmented forms. Occasional myeloid cells show enlargement with rare binucleated promyelocytes.
- The bone marrow core biopsy shows granulopoiesis with maturation arrest, adequate erythropoiesis, and megakaryocytes.

Differential Diagnosis

- Severe congenital neutropenia (Kostmann syndrome)
- Autoimmune neutropenia
- Neutropenia associated with infections
- Neutropenia associated with medications

Ancillary Studies

- Cytogenetic analysis performed on the bone marrow aspirate reported a normal male karyotype.
- Molecular studies revealed a heterozygous mutation *ELA2* c.170C > T, p.A57V.

Final Diagnosis

Congenital neutropenia with *ELA2* mutation

Take-Home Messages

1. Congenital neutropenia is characterized by severe neutropenia starting in infancy due to a primary bone marrow failure syndrome primarily involving the myeloid lineage.
2. Bone marrow biopsy shows myeloid maturation arrest at the promyelocyte/myelocyte stage, often with atypical nuclei.
3. Heterozygous mutation of *ELA2* gene is identified in 50–60% of congenital neutropenia.

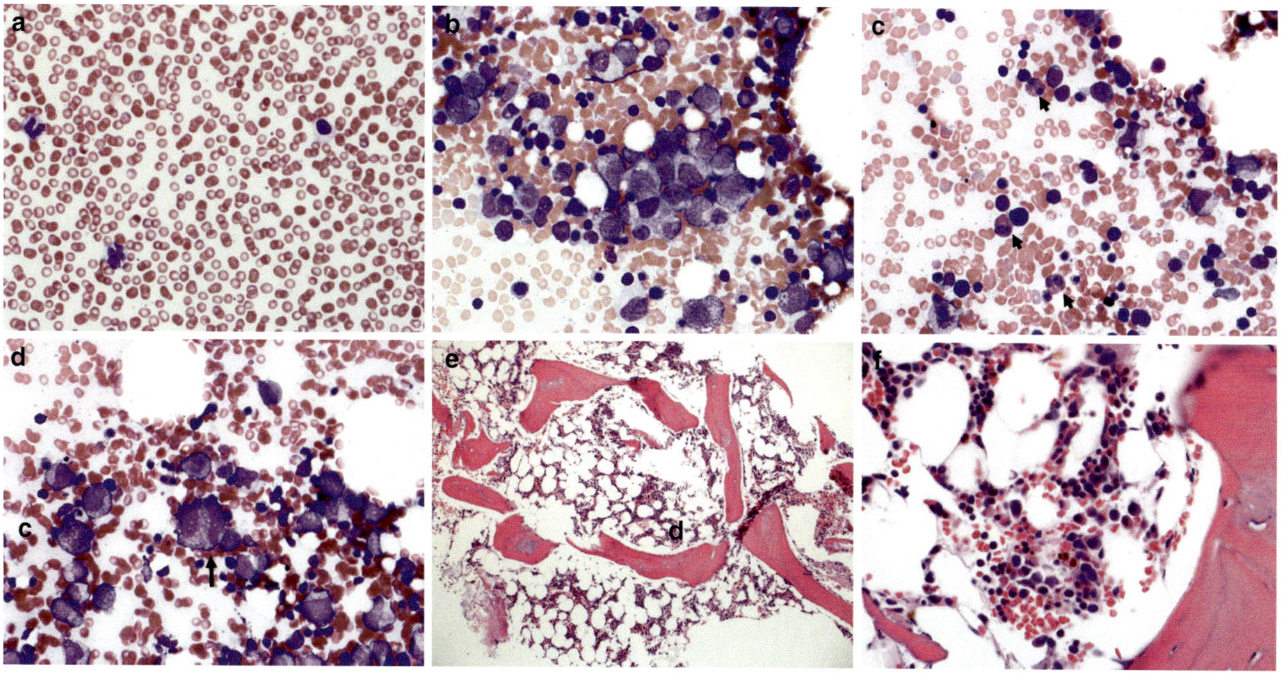

Fig. 29.6 Congenital neutropenia with *ELA2* mutation. (**a**) Peripheral blood smear shows neutropenia with very rare neutrophils and myelocytes noted upon scan. Differential reported lymphocytes 76%, monocytes 22%, and 2% neutrophils (**a**: Wright-Giemsa, ×600). (**b**) The bone marrow aspirate smears reveal granulopoiesis with maturation arrest (**b**: Wright-Giemsa, ×600). (**c**) Eosinophilic granulocytes show progressive maturation to segmented forms (arrow) (**c**: Wright-Giemsa, ×600) (**d**) Myeloid cells show enlargement with rare binucleated promyelocytes (*arrow*) (**d**: Wright-Giemsa, ×600). (**e**, **f**) The bone marrow core biopsy shows granulopoiesis with maturation arrest, adequate erythropoiesis, and megakaryocytes (**e**, hematoxylin-eosin, ×200; **f**, hematoxylin-eosin, ×600)

4. *HAX-1* mutation is reported in autosomal recessive severe congenital neutropenia.

Case 6 (Fig. 29.7)

Learning Objectives

1. To be aware of increased risks for myeloid neoplasms in patients with Shwachman-Diamond syndrome
2. To understand the role of genetic testing in the diagnosis of Shwachman-Diamond syndrome

Case History

This is an 18-year-old male with a long history of pancreatic dysfuntion, anemia and thrombocytopenia since birth. CBC reported WBC 11.09 k/uL, Hb 10.4 g/dL, HCT 31.7%, MCV 82 fl, and PLT 24 k/uL.

Histologic Findings

- The peripheral blood smear shows mild anemia with circulating nucleated red blood cells, mild neutropenia with a shift to immaturity, marked thrombocytopenia, and ~10% blasts.
- The bone marrow aspirate smear shows myeloid shift to immaturity with 13% blasts and mild dyserythropoiesis.
- The bone marrow core biopsy is hypercellular with increased immature cells present in patchy distribution.

Differential Diagnosis

- Myelodysplastic syndrome associated with Shwachman-Diamond syndrome
- Myelodysplastic syndrome with germline disposition associated with another bone marrow failure syndrome
- Myelodysplastic syndrome with germline predisposition
- Acute myeloid leukemia with germline predisposition
- Myelodysplastic syndrome without identifiable germline predisposition

Ancillary Studies

- Flow cytometry confirms a myeloid blast population that is CD34+, CD117+, dim MPO+, CD13+, CD33+, and HLADR+, negative for all lymphoid and monocytic markers tested.
- Cytogenetic analysis reported an abnormal complex male karyotype including loss of chromosomes 5 and 7 and trisomy 8.
- Molecular studies for common bone marrow failure disorders reported double heterozygosity in *SBDS* genes (c.183_184delTAinsCT, p.K62X and c.258 + 2 T > C, IVS + 2 T > C).

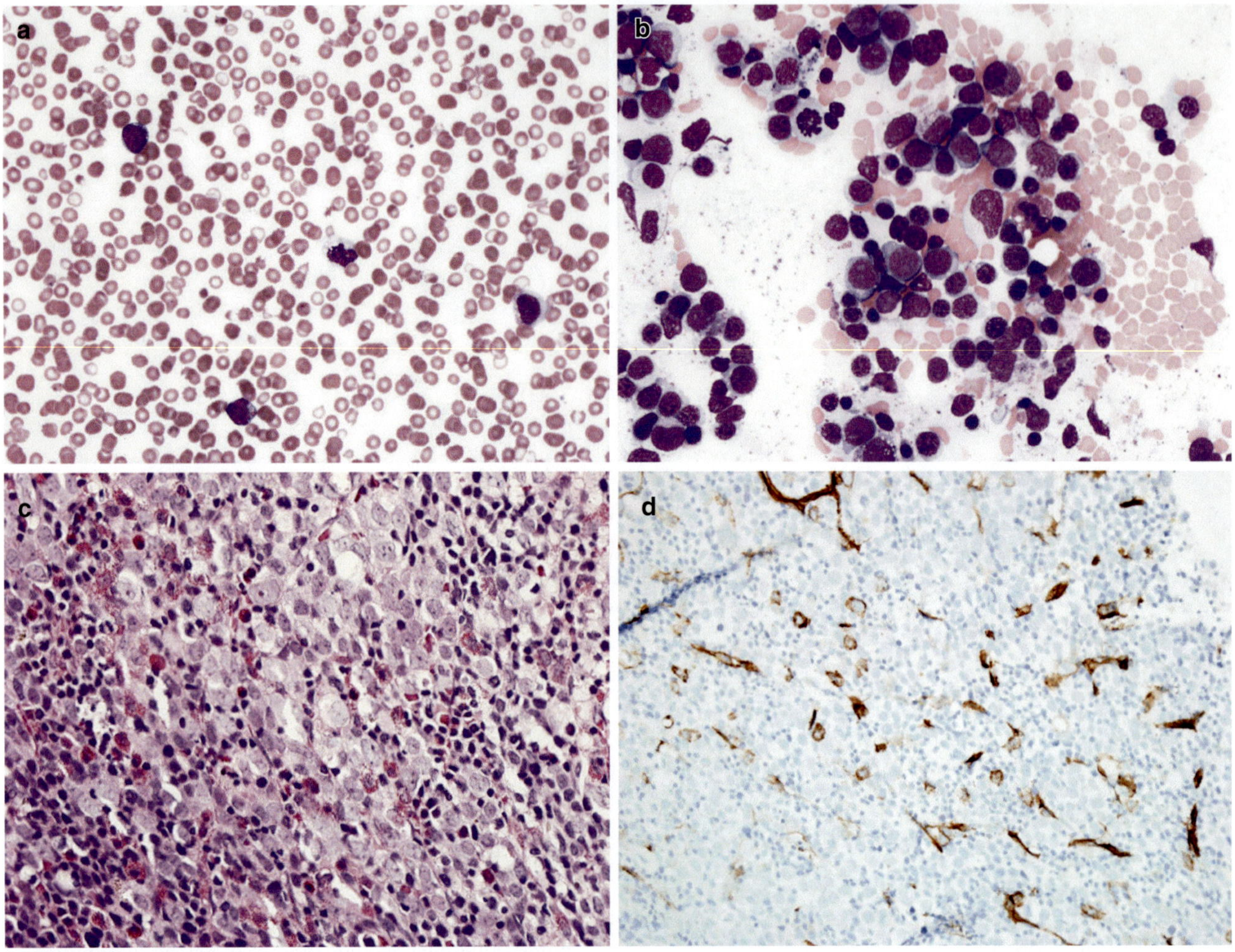

Fig. 29.7 Myeloid neoplasm, consistent with myelodysplastic syndrome with excess blasts 2 (MDS-EB2), arising from Shwachman-Diamond syndrome with *SBDS* mutation. (**a**) The peripheral blood smear shows mild anemia with circulating nucleated red blood cells, mild neutropenia with a shift to immaturity, marked thrombocytopenia, and ~10% blasts (Wright-Giemsa, ×600). (**b**) The bone marrow aspirate smear shows myeloid shift to immaturity with 13% blasts, mild dyserythropoiesis (Wright-Giemsa, ×600). (**c**) The bone marrow core biopsy is hypercellular with increased immature cells present in patchy distribution (**c**: hematoxylin and eosin, ×400). (**d**) A CD34 immunostain highlights increased blasts (peroxidase, ×400)

Final Diagnosis

Myeloid neoplasm, consistent with myelodysplastic syndrome with excess blasts 2 (MDS-EB2), arising from Shwachman-Diamond syndrome with *SBDS* mutation

Take-Home Messages

1. Shwachman-Diamond syndrome is characterized by pancreatic dysfunction, cytopenias, and susceptibility to myelodysplastic syndrome or acute myeloid leukemia.
2. The diagnosis of Shwachman-Diamond syndrome relies on the clinical features and could be confirmed by detection of biallelic pathogenic variants in *SBDS*.

Case 7 (Fig. 29.8)

Learning Objective

Myelokathexis is characterized by retention of granulocytes in the bone marrow and peripheral neutropenia.

Case History

This is a 4-year-old female with hypogammaglobinemia and immunodeficiency and persistent leukopenia. CBC reported WBC 0.97 k/uL, Hb 12.1 g/dL, HCT 34.9%, MCV 75.2 fL, RDW 15.7%, and PLT 243 k/uL.

Histologic Findings

- The peripheral blood smear shows marked neutropenia and mild lymphopenia. There is no evidence of overt dys-

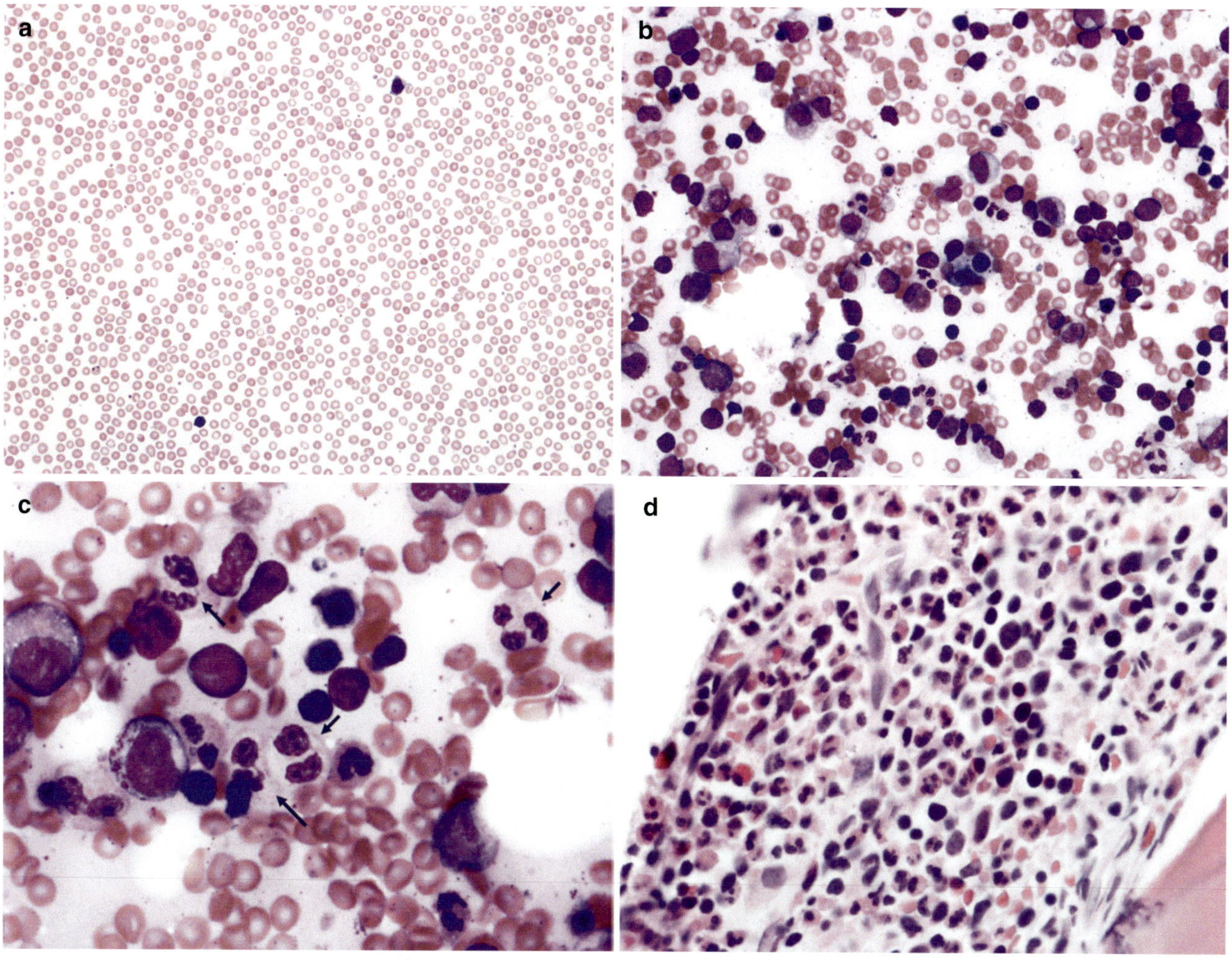

Fig. 29.8 Myelokathexis in WHIM syndrome with *CXCR4* mutation. (**a**) The peripheral blood smear shows marked neutropenia without overt dysplasia (Wright-Giemsa, ×400). (**b**, **c**) The bone marrow aspirate smear shows myeloid and erythroid precursors with orderly maturation with no overt dysplasia. Some neutrophils demonstrate widely spaced lobules with long intersegmental filaments or hypersegmented lobes (**b**, Wright-Giemsa, ×400; **c**, Wright-Giemsa, ×1000). (**d**) The bone marrow core biopsy shows hypercellular marrow with granulocytic hyperplasia. The granulocytic precursors show progressive maturation but with occasional abnormal nuclear segmentation or intersegmental filaments (hematoxylin-eosin, ×600)

plasia or any circulating blasts identified. Red blood cells and platelets are adequate and unremarkable.
- The bone marrow aspirate smear shows myeloid and erythroid precursors with orderly maturation with no overt dysplasia. Some neutrophils demonstrate widely spaced lobes with long intersegmental filaments or hypersegmented lobes.
- The bone marrow core biopsy shows hypercellular marrow with granulocytic hyperplasia. The granulocytic precursors show progressive maturation but with occasional abnormal nuclear segmentation or intersegmental filaments.

Differential Diagnosis

- Myelodysplastic syndrome with germline predisposition.
- Myelokathexis (WHIM syndrome)
- Autoimmune neutropenia
- Neutropenia associated with infections
- Neutropenia associated with medications

Ancillary Studies

- Cytogenetic analysis reported a normal male karyotype: 46, XY [20].
- Next-generation sequencing of a comprehensive panel of immunodeficiency-associated genes reported a heterozygous pathogenic variant in the *CXCR4* gene which is known to be associated with WHIM syndrome (warts, hypogammaglobinemia, infection and myelokathexis).

Final Diagnosis

Peripheral blood with marked neutropenia and hypercellular bone marrow with granulocytic hyperplasia, fea-

tures that are consistent with myelokathexis found in patients with WHIM syndrome

Take-Home Messages

1. WHIM syndrome is a rare autosomal dominant disorder characterized by warts, hypogammaglobulinemia, infections, and myelokathexis.
2. WHIM syndrome harbors a mutation in the *CXCR4* receptor, resulting in retention and apoptosis of aging granulocytes in the bone marrow and peripheral neutropenia.

Case 8 (Fig. 29.9)

Learning Objectives

1. To be familiar with the clinical features of thrombocytopenia-absent radius (TAR) syndrome
2. To be aware that hematologic malignancy in the setting of TAR syndrome has been reported

Case History

The patient is an 11-year-old female with a history of thrombocytopenia-absent radius (TAR) syndrome presented with pancytopenia. CBC reported WBC 4.36 k/uL, Hb 9.5 g/dL, HCT 28.2%, MCV 83 fL, RDW 18.3%, and PLT 72 k/uL. X-ray showed absence of the long, thin bones of the forearms (radii).

Histologic Findings

- The peripheral blood smear shows mild neutropenia with a shift to immaturity and 2% circulating blasts, normochromic normocytic anemia with rare nucleated red blood cells, and thrombocytopenia.
- The bone marrow aspirate smear shows myeloid precursors with marked shift to immaturity with 14% blasts, mild dyserythropoiesis, and frequent dysplastic megakaryocytes.
- The core biopsy shows slightly hypocellular marrow with myeloid and erythroid precursors and dysplastic

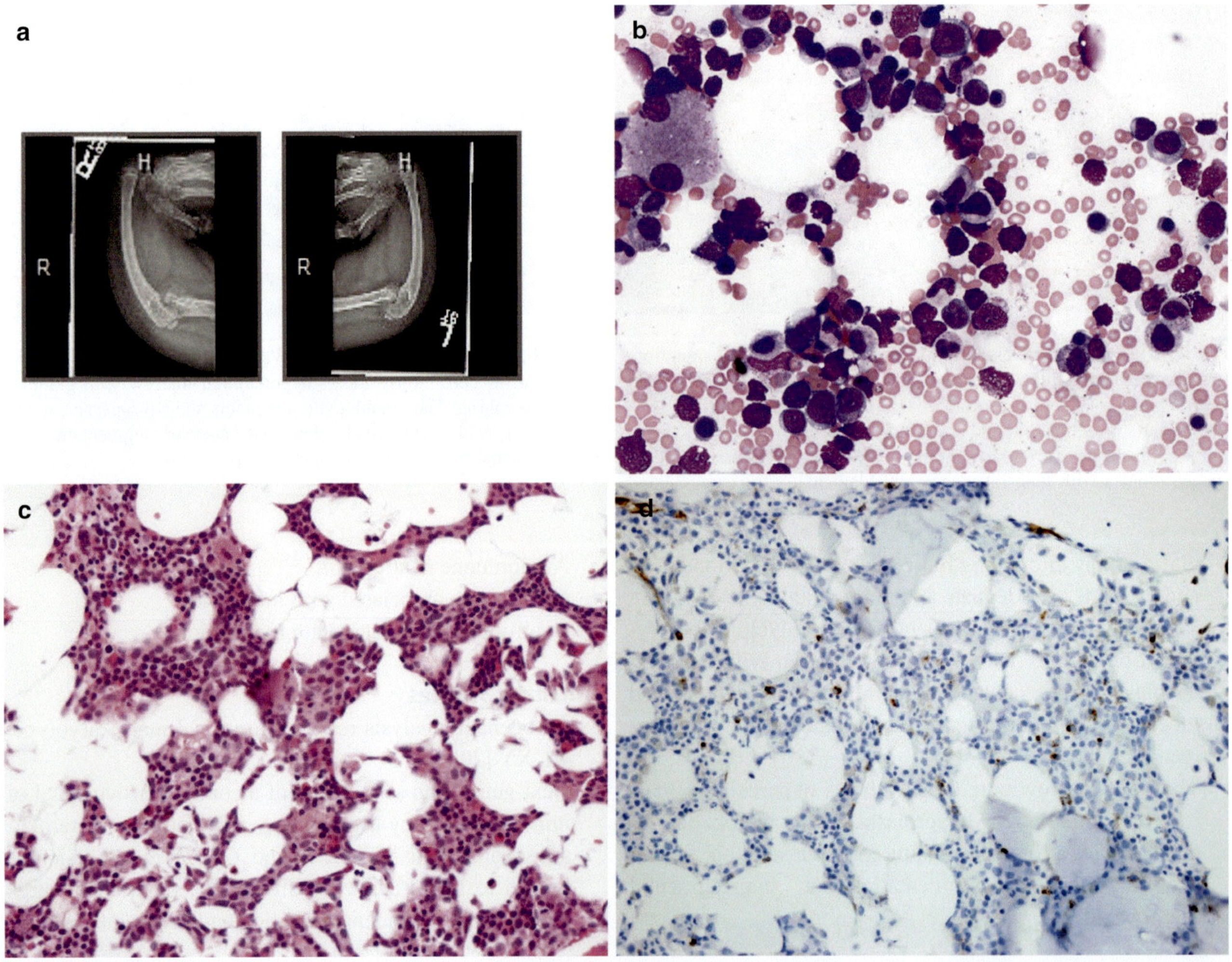

Fig. 29.9 Myelodysplastic syndrome in a patient with thrombocytopenia-absent radius (TAR) syndrome. (**a**) X-ray showed absence of the long, thin bones of the forearms (radii) (courtesy of Dr. Joanna Weinstein, Ann& Robert H. Lurie Children's Hospital of Chicago). (**b**) The bone marrow aspirate smear shows myeloid precursors with marked shift to immaturity with 14% blasts, mild dyserythropoiesis and frequent dysplastic megakaryocytes (Wright-Giemsa, ×600). (**c**) The core biopsy shows slightly hypocellular marrow with myeloid and erythroid precursors and dysplastic megakaryocytes (hematoxylin-eosin, ×400). (**d**) A CD34 immunostain highlights increased blasts (~10%)

megakaryocytes. Blasts appear increased, and this was confirmed by a CD34 immunostain which highlights ~10% blasts.

Differential Diagnosis

- Myelodysplastic syndrome in a patient with thrombocytopenia-absent radius (TAR) syndrome
- Myelodysplastic syndrome associated with other congenital disorders
- Myelodysplastic syndrome with germline predisposition

Ancillary Studies

- Flow cytometric analysis reported a myeloblast population that is CD34+, CD117+, MPO+, HLA-DR+, CD13+, and CD33+, negative for lymphoid and monocytic markers assayed.
- Cytogenetic analysis reported a normal female karyotype.

Final Diagnosis

Myelodysplastic syndrome in a patient with thrombocytopenia-absent radius (TAR) syndrome

Take-Home Messages

1. TAR syndrome has two essential features, hypomegakaryocytic thrombocytopenia and bilateral radial aplasia.
2. Limited data suggest TAR syndrome may be associated with predisposition to the development of hematologic malignancies.

Case 9 (Fig. 29.10)

Learning Objectives

1. To be familiar with the clinical symptoms of Wiskott-Aldrich syndrome
2. To understand the role of genetic testing in the diagnosis of Wiskott-Aldrich syndrome

Case History

The patient is a 3-year-old boy with a history of thrombocytopenia. CBC reported WBC 8.5 k/uL, Hb 12.4 g/dL, HCT 36.6%, MCV 78 fL, RDW 14.4%, and PLT 26 k/uL.

Histologic Findings

- The peripheral blood smear shows thrombocytopenia but no anemia and leukopenia. Few platelets present are small in size.
- The bone marrow aspirate smears show multilineage hematopoiesis with slightly increased blasts and atypical megakaryocytes that are frequently hypolobated.
- The bone marrow core biopsy is hypercellular with scattered atypical megakaryocytes.
- CD34 immunostain highlights slightly increased blasts.

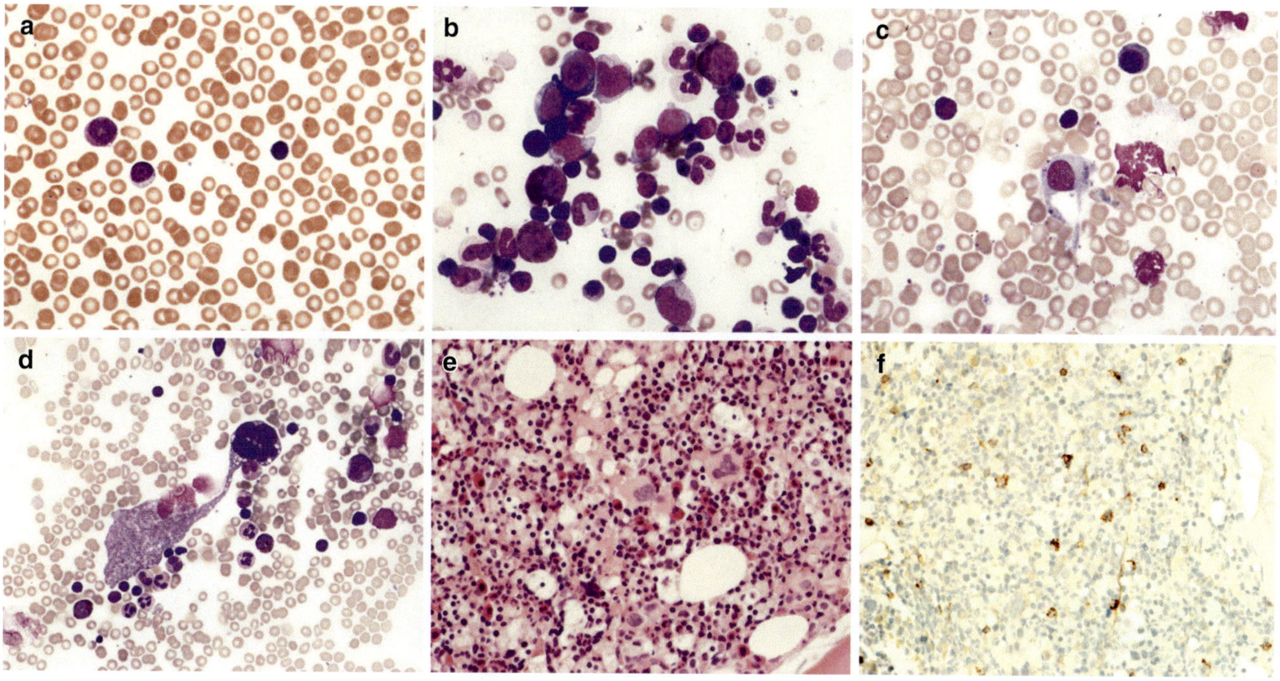

Fig. 29.10 Myelodysplastic syndrome arising from X-linked thrombocytopenia with germline *WAS* mutation. (**a**) Peripheral blood smear shows thrombocytopenia. Few platelets present are small in size (Wright-Giemsa, ×1000). (**b**, **d**) Bone marrow aspirate smears show multilineage hematopoiesis with slightly increased blasts (**b**: Wright-Giemsa, ×1000) and atypical megakaryocytes (**c**, Wright-Giemsa, ×1000; **d**, Wright-Giemsa, ×600). (**e**) The bone marrow core biopsy is hypercellular with scattered atypical megakaryocytes (hematoxylin-eosin, ×400). (**f**) A CD34 immunostain highlights slightly increased blasts (peroxidase, ×400)

Differential Diagnosis

- Myelodysplastic syndrome with germline predisposition
- Myelodysplastic syndrome in the setting of bone marrow failure syndrome
- Immune thrombocytopenic purpura (ITP)

Ancillary Studies

- Cytogenetic analysis performed on the bone marrow aspirate reported a normal male karyotype.
- Molecular studies revealed a hemizygous pathogenic variant in the *WAS* gene c.223G > A, p.V75 M.

Final Diagnosis

Myelodysplastic syndrome arising from X-linked thrombocytopenia with germline *WAS* mutation

Take-Home Messages

1. Wiskott-Aldrich syndrome is characterized by microthrombocytopenia, eczema and immune deficiency.
2. A diagnosis of Wiskott-Aldrich syndrome can be made on clinical and pathologic features and confirmed by the detection of *WAS* mutation.
3. Patients with Wiskott-Aldrich syndrome have predisposition for malignancies including myeloid neoplasm.

Case 10 (Fig. 29.11)

Learning Objectives

1. To be aware of transient abnormal myelopoiesis (TAM) as a rare and unique disorder affecting newborns with Down syndrome
2. To understand the difference between TAM and acute myeloid leukemia particularly acute megakaryoblastic leukemia

Case History

This is a newborn with trisomy 21 delivered at 31 weeks of gestational age. CBC reported WBC 169.1 k/uL, Hb 13.2 g/dL, HCT 39.2%, MCV 110 fL, RDW 29.3%, and PLT 308 k/uL.

Histologic Findings

- The peripheral blood smear shows marked neutrophilia with a shift to immaturity including many blasts (67%), normochromic normocytic anemia with circulating nucleated red blood cells, and frequent large and degranulated platelets.

Differential Diagnosis

- Transient abnormal myelopoiesis associated with Down syndrome
- Acute myeloid leukemia associated with Down syndrome

Final Diagnosis

Transient abnormal myelopoiesis associated with Down syndrome

Take-Home Messages

1. The characteristic hematologic changes in transient abnormal myelopoiesis include leukocytosis, thrombocytopenia, and circulating blasts, often with features of megakaryoblasts.

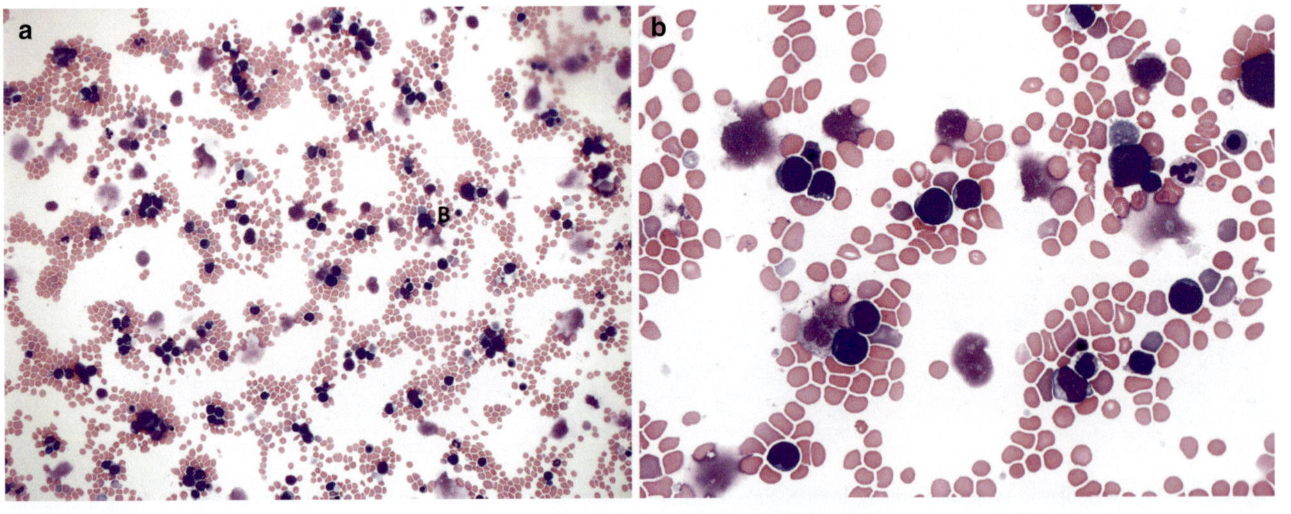

Fig. 29.11 Transient abnormal myelopoiesis associated with Down syndrome. (**a**, **b**). The peripheral blood smear shows marked neutrophilia with a shift to immaturity including many blasts (67%), normochromic normocytic anemia with circulating nucleated red blood cells, frequent large and degranulated platelets (**a**, Wright-Giemsa, ×200; **b**, Wright-Giemsa, ×600)

2. Most cases of TAM occur in neonate, in contrast to myeloid leukemia that often occurs in later life.
3. In addition to constitutional trisomy 21, somatic *GATA1* mutations are present.
4. TAM is a self-limiting process; but a subset of infants with TAM may develop acute myeloid leukemia 1–3 years later.

Case 11 (Fig. 29.12)

Learning Objective

To be aware of increased risks for AML particularly acute megakaryoblastic leukemia in patients with Down syndrome

Case History

This is a 2-year old boy with Down syndrome and newly diagnosed acute myeloid leukemia.

Histologic Findings

- The peripheral blood smear shows moderate thrombocytopenia, mild anemia, and 5% circulating blasts.
- The bone marrow aspirate smear shows 32% blasts. The blasts are medium to large in size, many with deeply basophilic cytoplasm and cytoplasmic projections. Scattered hypolobated megakaryocytes are also present.
- The bone marrow core biopsy contains hypercellular marrow with increased blasts and frequent dysplastic megakaryocytes with monolobated and hyperchromatic nuclei. Immunostains performed on the core biopsy revealed the blasts are CD34+, CD117+, and subset CD61 + .

Differential Diagnosis

- Acute myeloid leukemia associated with Down syndrome
- Acute megakaryoblastic leukemia associated with Down syndrome
- Transient abnormal myelopoiesis associated with Down syndrome

Ancillary Studies

- Flow cytometric analysis reported a myeloid blast population that is dim CD45+, partial CD34+, CD117+, CD13+, CD33+, CD36+, MPO-, CD14-, HLA-DR-, CD41-, CD61-, CD7+, and negative for other T- and B-cell markers assayed.
- Cytogenetic analysis reported a male karyotype with a constitutional abnormality consistent with Down syndrome: 47, XY, +21c [21].

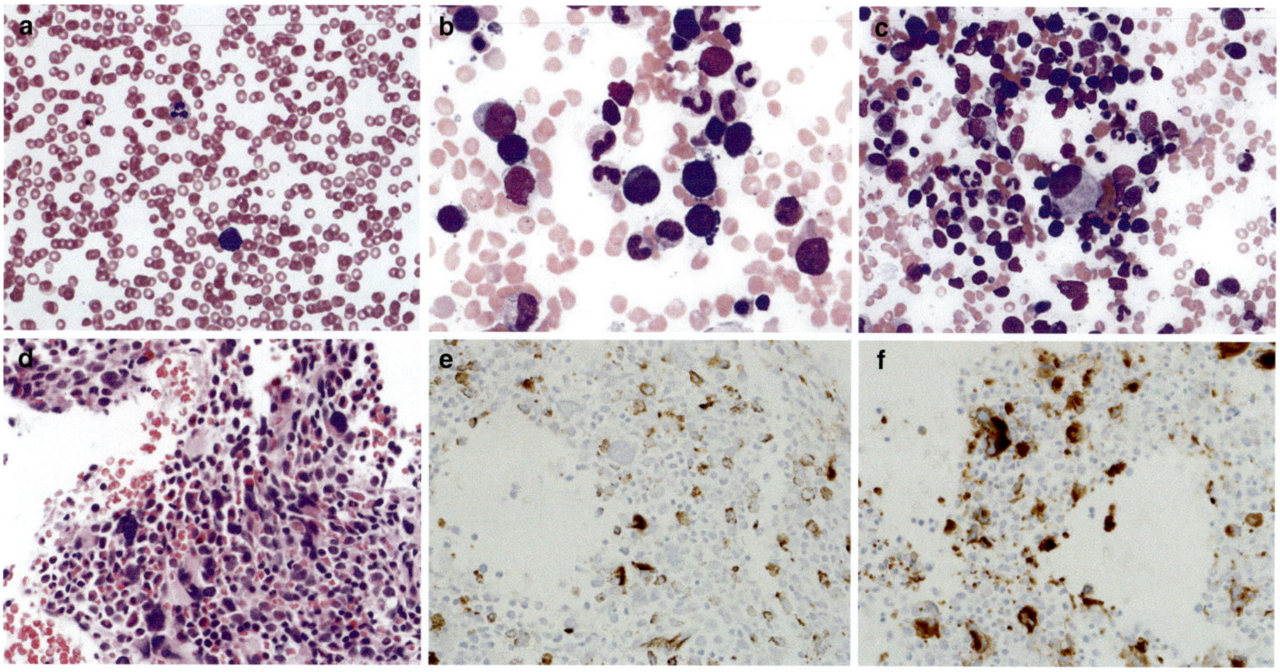

Fig. 29.12 Acute myeloid leukemia associated with Down syndrome. (**a**) The peripheral blood smear shows moderate thrombocytopenia, mild anemia, and 5% circulating blasts (Wright-Giemsa, ×600). (**b**) The bone marrow aspirate smear shows 32% blasts. The blasts are medium to large in size, many with deeply basophilic cytoplasm and cytoplasmic projections (Wright-Giemsa, ×1000). (**c**) Scattered hypolobated megakaryocytes are also present (Wright-Giemsa, ×600). (**d**) The bone marrow core biopsy contains hypercellular marrow with increased blasts and frequent dysplastic megakaryocytes with monolobated and hyperchromatic nuclei (hematoxylin-eosin, ×600). (**e** and **f**) The blasts are CD34+ (**e**: peroxidase, ×600), CD117+ (not shown), and subset CD61+ (**f**: peroxidase, ×600)

Final Diagnosis

Acute megakaryoblastic leukemia associated with Down syndrome

Take-Home Messages

1. Down syndrome patients are associated with increased risks for AML, particularly acute megakaryoblastic leukemia.
2. Similar to TAM, somatic mutations in *GATA1* are present in MDS or AML associated with Down syndrome.

Case 12 (Fig. 29.13)

Learning Objective

To become familiar with the genetic features of myeloid neoplasm with germline *CEBPA* mutations

Case History

The patient is a 35-year-old female with newly diagnosed acute myeloid leukemia. Family history is significant for maternal aunt died from breast cancer in her 50s.

Histologic Findings

- Bone marrow aspirate smears reveal increased blasts with frequent Auer rods.
- Bone marrow core biopsy contains hypercellular bone marrow replaced by sheets of blasts.

Differential Diagnosis

- Acute myeloid leukemia with germline predisposition
- Acute myeloid leukemia without germline predisposition

Ancillary Studies

- Next-generation sequencing identified the presence of both N-terminal frameshift mutation (*CEBPA*

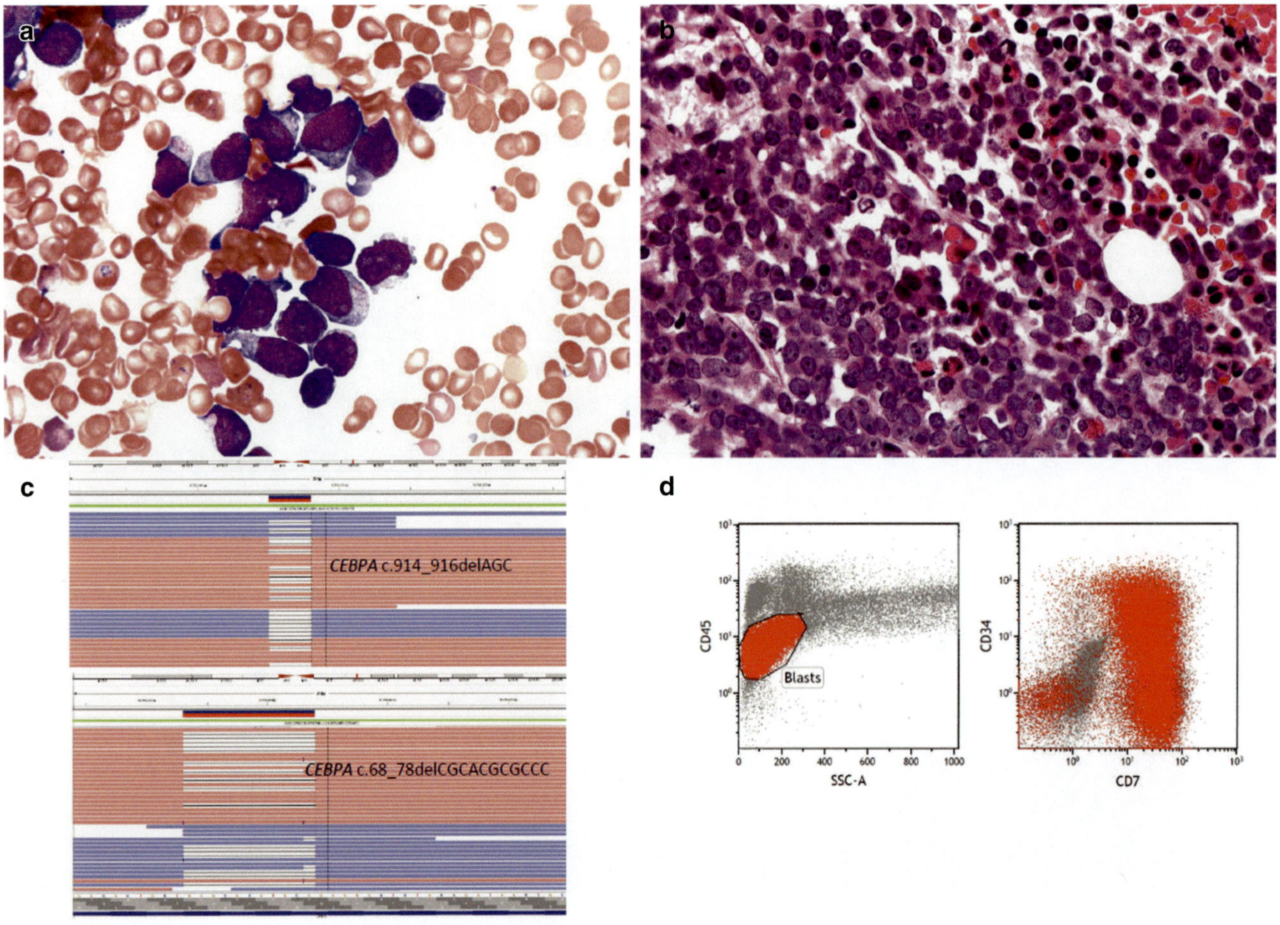

Fig. 29.13 Acute myeloid leukemia with germline *CEBPA* mutations. (**a**) Bone marrow aspirate smears reveal increased blasts with frequent Auer rods. (**b**) Bone marrow core biopsy contains hypercellular bone marrow replaced by sheets of blasts. (**c**) Next-generation sequencing identified the presence of both N-terminal frameshift mutation (*CEBPA* c.68_78delCGCACGCGCCC, p.Pro23fs; variant allele fraction 47%) and C-terminal in-frame deletion (*CEBPA* c.914_916delAGC, p. Gln305del; variant allele fraction 32%) (**d**) Flow cytometric analysis reveals myeloid blasts with aberrant CD7 expression)

c.68_78delCGCACGCGCCC, p.Pro23fs; variant allele fraction 47%) and C-terminal in-frame deletion (*CEBPA* c.914_916delAGC, p.Gln305del; variant allele fraction 32%).

- Flow cytometric analysis reveals a large myeloid blast population with aberrant CD7 expression.
- The patient was referred to cancer geneticist for further work up and later was determined the N terminal *CEBPA* mutation was germline.

Final Diagnosis

Acute myeloid leukemia with germline *CEBPA* mutations

Take-Home Message

The finding of biallelic *CEBPA* mutations in any newly diagnosed acute myeloid leukemia should prompt further investigation of the possibility of germline *CEBPA* mutation.

Case 13 (Fig. 29.14)

Learning Objectives

1. To appreciate the wide spectrum of clinical presentations for germline *GATA2* mutations
2. To become familiar with the genetic features of myeloid neoplasm with germline *GATA2* mutations

Case History

The patient is a 50-year-old Caucasian woman with a 25-year history of thrombocytopenia who presented with abnormal CBC with circulating blasts. CBC reported Hb 9.5 g/dL, WBC 8.7 K/uL including 25% blasts, and PLT 55 K/uL. Family history is significant for thrombocytopenia affecting her mother, siblings and their children, as well as her own children. Both her mother and maternal aunt died from MDS.

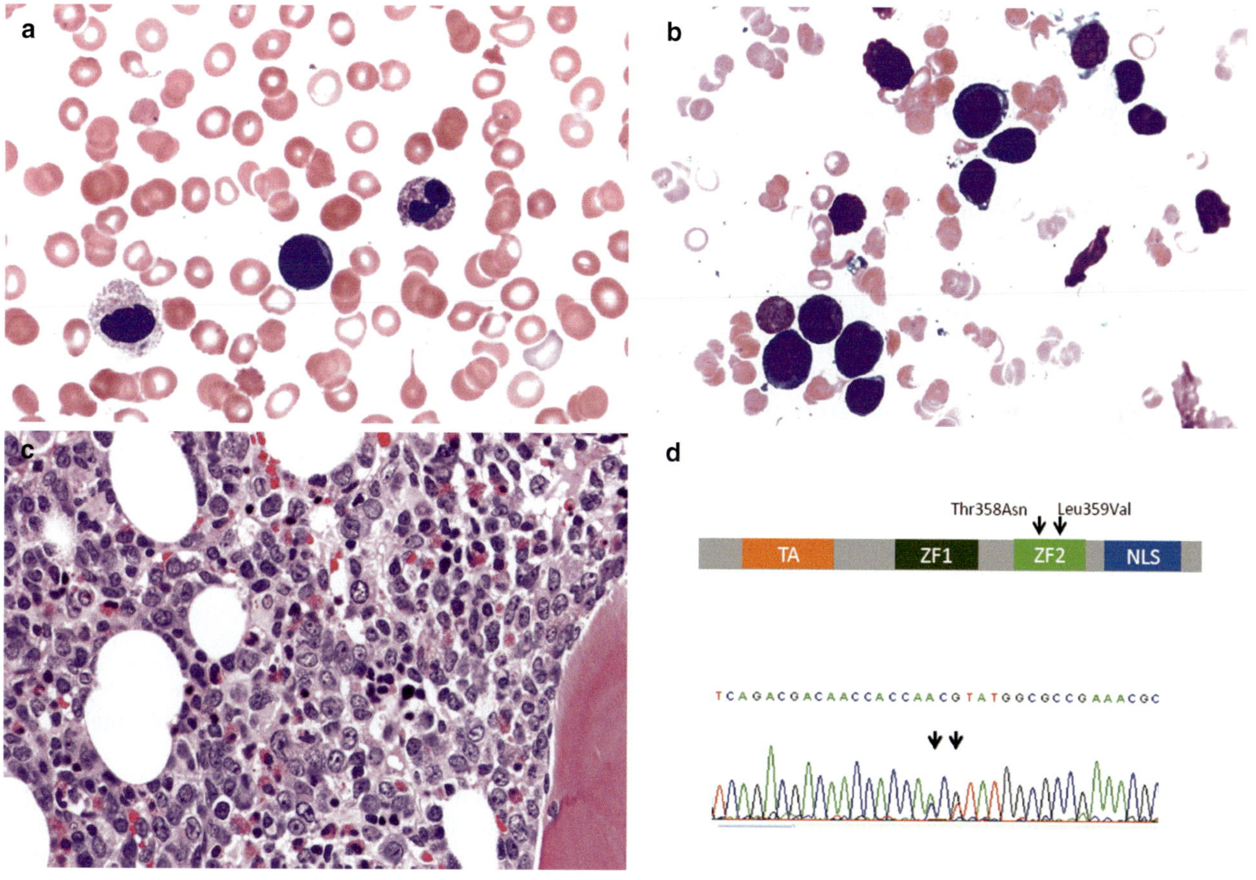

Fig. 29.14 Acute myeloid leukemia with *GATA2* mutation. (**a**) Peripheral blood smear revealed increased number of blasts, occasional dysplastic neutrophils with hyposegmented nuclei, and platelets with abnormal morphology (Wright-Giemsa, ×400). (**b**) Bone marrow aspirate smears contain occasional blasts with fine chromatin, round nuclei, and scant cytoplasm (Wright-Giemsa, ×1000). (**c** and **d**) The bone marrow core biopsy sections showed a markedly hypercellular bone marrow with significantly increased numbers of blasts (**c**, hematoxylin and eosin, ×200; **d**: hematoxylin and eosin, ×600)

Histologic Findings

- The peripheral blood smear revealed increased number of blasts, occasional dysplastic neutrophils with hyposegmented nuclei, and platelets with abnormal morphology.
- The bone marrow aspirate smears contain occasional blasts with fine chromatin, round nuclei, and scant cytoplasm.
- The bone marrow core biopsy sections showed a markedly hypercellular bone marrow with significantly increased numbers of blasts.

Differential Diagnosis

- Myelodysplastic syndrome
- Acute myeloid leukemia with germline predisposition
- Acute myeloid leukemia arising from preexisting myelodysplastic syndrome

Ancillary Studies

- Flow cytometric analysis demonstrated 23% myeloid blasts.
- Cytogenetic analysis performed on the bone marrow aspirate revealed 46,XX,del(7)(q22q36) [20].
- Molecular studies identified two heterozygous mutations in the 2nd zinc finger domain of *GATA2* gene, p. Thr358Asn (c.1074C > A), and p.Leu359Val (c.1076 T > G).

Final Diagnosis

Acute myeloid leukemia with *GATA2* mutation

Follow-Up

The patient later received double-cord stem cell transplant with disease remission. The patient's posttransplant history was complicated by multiple infections and eventually died from infection. Family members seeked genetic studies. One of the *GATA2* mutations was confirmed to be inherited.

Take-Home Messages

1. Patients with germline *GATA2* mutation can have a broad spectrum of clinical presentations including immunodeficiency, lymphedema, and increased risks for hematologic disease.
2. Any deleterious *GATA2* mutation in newly diagnosed AML or MDS should prompt further investigation of the possibility of germline *GATA2* mutation.

Case 14 (Fig. 29.15)

Learning Objectives

1. To be aware of predisposition to juvenile myelomonocytic leukemia (JMML) or JMML-like myeloproliferative disorders in infants with Noonan syndrome
2. To be aware of the role of genetic testing in the diagnosis of Noonan syndrome

Case History

This patient is a 2-month-old boy presented with leukocytosis and thrombocytopenia. CBC reported WBC 49.79 k/uL, Hb 9.9 g/dL, HCT 31.5%, MCV 86 fl, and PLT 36 k/uL.

Histologic Findings

- The peripheral blood smear shows neutrophilia and monocytosis, anemia, and thrombocytopenia. The neutrophils show a shift to immaturity including myelocytes, promyelocytes, and 4% blasts.
- The bone marrow aspirate smears are very cellular and demonstrate a myeloid predominance with a myeloid to erythroid ratio of 7:1. The myeloid precursors show progressive maturation with a slight increase in blasts (8%).
- The core biopsy contains markedly hypercellular marrow approaching 100% in cellularity. The cellular composition is similar to that seen in the aspirate smears.
- CD34 immunostain shows mildly increased blasts (5%).

Differential Diagnosis

- Juvenile myelomonocytic leukemia
- Juvenile myelomonocytic leukemia-like myeloproliferative disorder associated with Noonan syndrome
- Reactive monocytosis and myeloid hyperplasia

Ancillary Studies

- Chromosomal analysis demonstrated a normal karyotype.
- The patient had development disorder concerning for Noonan syndrome. Genetic testing confirmed the diagnosis of Noonan syndrome with a germline heterozygous *PTPN11* mutation (exon 3, p.Thr73Ile).
- FISH for *BCR/ABL1* was negative.

Final Diagnosis

Juvenile myelomonocytic leukemia-like myeloproliferative disorder associated with Noonan syndrome

Take-Home Messages

1. The diagnosis of Noonan syndrome is based on the person's clinical symptoms and the presence of mutations involving *PTPN11*, *SOS1*, *RAF1*, and *KRAS*.
2. Infants with Noonan syndrome are predisposed to developing juvenile myelomonocytic leukemia (JMML) or JMML-like myeloproliferative disorders.

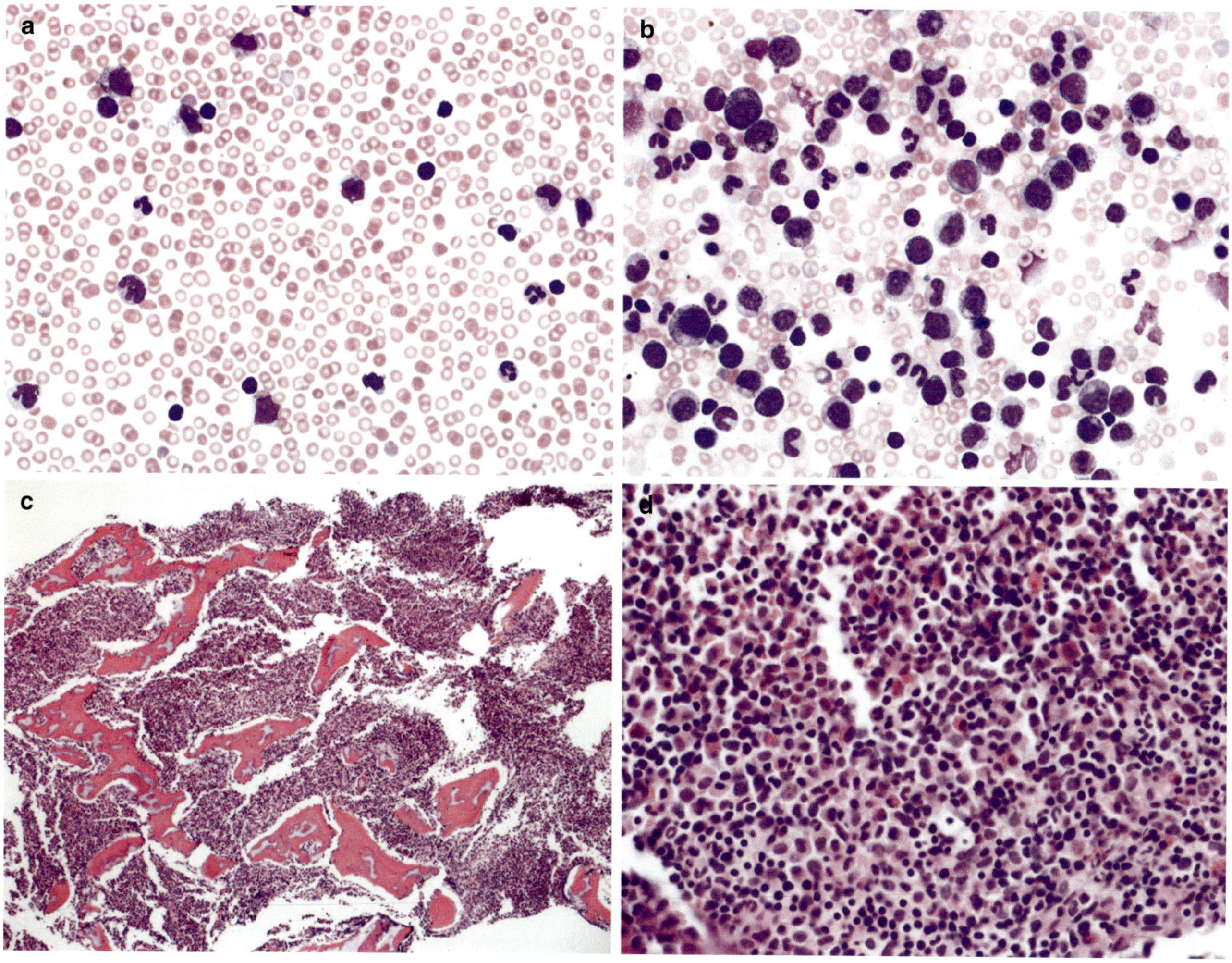

Fig. 29.15 Juvenile myelomonocytic leukemia-like myeloproliferative disorder associated with Noonan syndrome. (**a**) The peripheral blood smear shows neutrophilia and monocytosis, anemia, and thrombocytopenia. The neutrophils show a shift to immaturity including myelocytes, promyelocytes, and 4% blasts (Wright-Giemsa, ×600). (**b**) The bone marrow aspirate smears are very cellular and demonstrate a myeloid predominance with a myeloid to erythroid ratio of 7:1. The myeloid precursors show progressive maturation with a slight increase in blasts (8%) (Wright-Giemsa, ×600). (**c, d**) The core biopsy contains markedly hypercellular marrow approaching 100% in cellularity. The cellular composition is similar to that seen in the aspirate smears. A CD34 immunostains show mildly increased blasts (5%) (not shown)

Case 15 (Fig. 29.16)

Learning Objective

Common variable immune deficiency (CVID) patients have severe dysregulation of the immune system including immunodeficiency and accumulation of immune cells

Case History

This is a 21-year-old man with a history of common variable immune deficiency (CVID) presented with anemia and thrombocytopenia at 6 years of age. CBC reported WBC 12.47 k/uL, Hb 8.4 g/dL, HCT 25.7%, MCV 88.7 fL, RDW 17.5%, and PLT 5/uL.

Histologic Findings

- The peripheral blood smear shows marked thrombocytopenia, moderate anemia, and rare spherocytes.
- The bone marrow aspirate smear shows myeloid and erythroid precursors with progressive maturation. Megakaryocytes are easily identified. Lymphocytes are focally increased and are mature appearing.
- The bone marrow core biopsy shows hypercellular marrow with several large lymphoid aggregates, some with reactive appearing germinal centers. Myeloid and erythroid precursors are present with progressive maturation. Megakaryocytes are increased with unremarkable morphology.

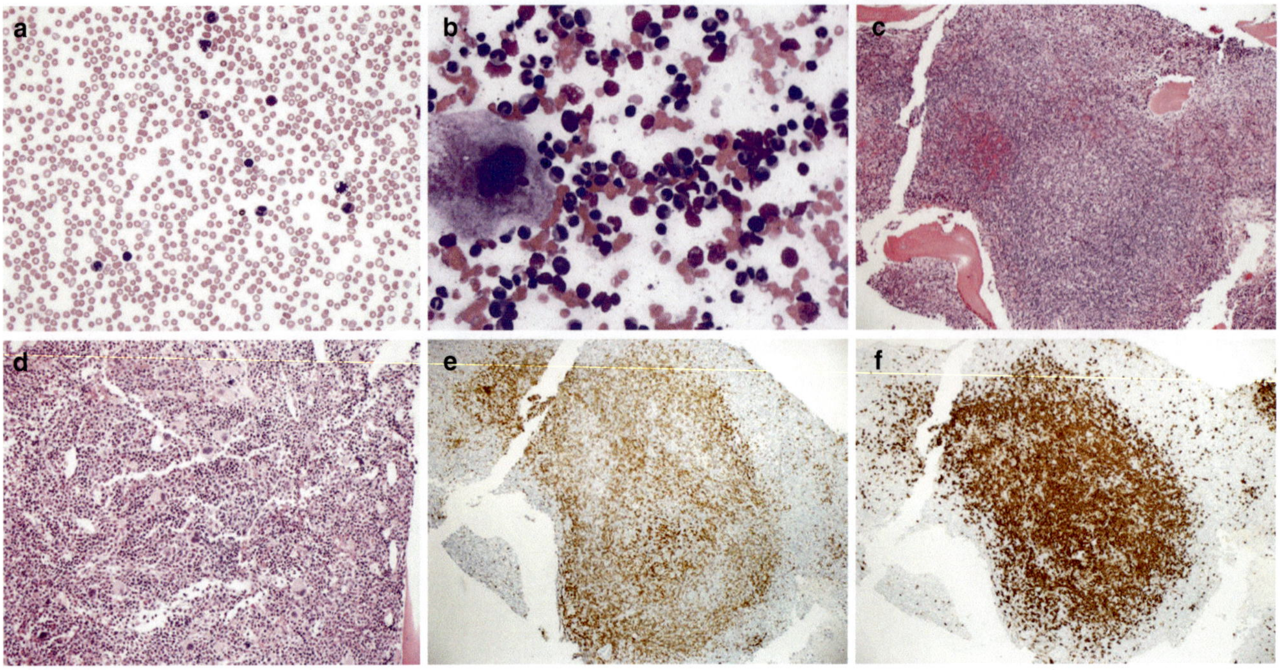

Fig. 29.16 CVID bone marrow. (**a**) The peripheral blood smear shows marked thrombocytopenia, moderate anemia, and rare spherocytes (Wright-Giemsa, ×200). (**b**) The bone marrow aspirate smear shows myeloid and erythroid precursors with progressive maturation. Megakaryocytes are easily identified. Lymphocytes are focally increased and are mature appearing (Wright-Giemsa, ×600). (**c** and **d**) The bone marrow core biopsy shows hypercellular marrow with several large lymphoid aggregates, some with reactive appearing germinal centers. Myeloid and erythroid precursors are present with progressive maturation. Megakaryocytes are increased with unremarkable morphology (hematoxylin-eosin, ×100). (e and f) Immunostains performed on the core biopsy sections reveal the lymphoid aggregates consist of a mixture of T and B cells (**e**, CD3, peroxidase, ×100; **f**, CD20, peroxidase, ×100)

- Immunostains performed on the core biopsy sections reveal the lymphoid aggregates consist of a mixture of T and B cells. BCL2 is negative in the increased number of CD20+ B cells within and between the lymphoid follicles.

Differential Diagnosis

- Immune-mediated anemia and thrombocytopenia
- Lymphoproliferative disease associated with CVID
- B cell lymphoma

Ancillary Studies

- *EBV* in situ hybridization (EBER) is negative on the section of bone marrow biopsy.
- Flow cytometric analysis reported immunophenotypically unremarkable T cells and polytypic B cells.
- Cytogenetic analysis reported a normal male karyotype: 46, XY.

Final Diagnosis

Bone marrow with benign lymphoid aggregates, increased megakaryocytes in the setting of CVID and immune thrombocytopenic purpura

Take-Home Messages

1. CVID is an autoimmune disorder and may show accumulation of immune cells in multiple organs including bone marrow.
2. CVID patients have increased risks for autoimmune hemolytic anemia and/or immune thrombocytopenia purpura.

Case 16 (Fig. 29.17)

Learning Objectives

1. Primary or familial hemophagocytic lymphohistiocytosis (fHLH) harbors inherited defects in cytolytic immune function.
2. Mutations in genes needed for cytolytic immune function serve as part of the HLH diagnostic criteria.

Case History

This is a 3-week-old female with a clinical history of pancytopenia with hepatosplenomegaly who underwent a bone marrow evaluation. CBC reported WBC 1.58 k/uL, Hb 11.3 g/dL, HCT 31.3%, MCV 84.5 fL, RDW 15.6%, and PLT 12/uL.

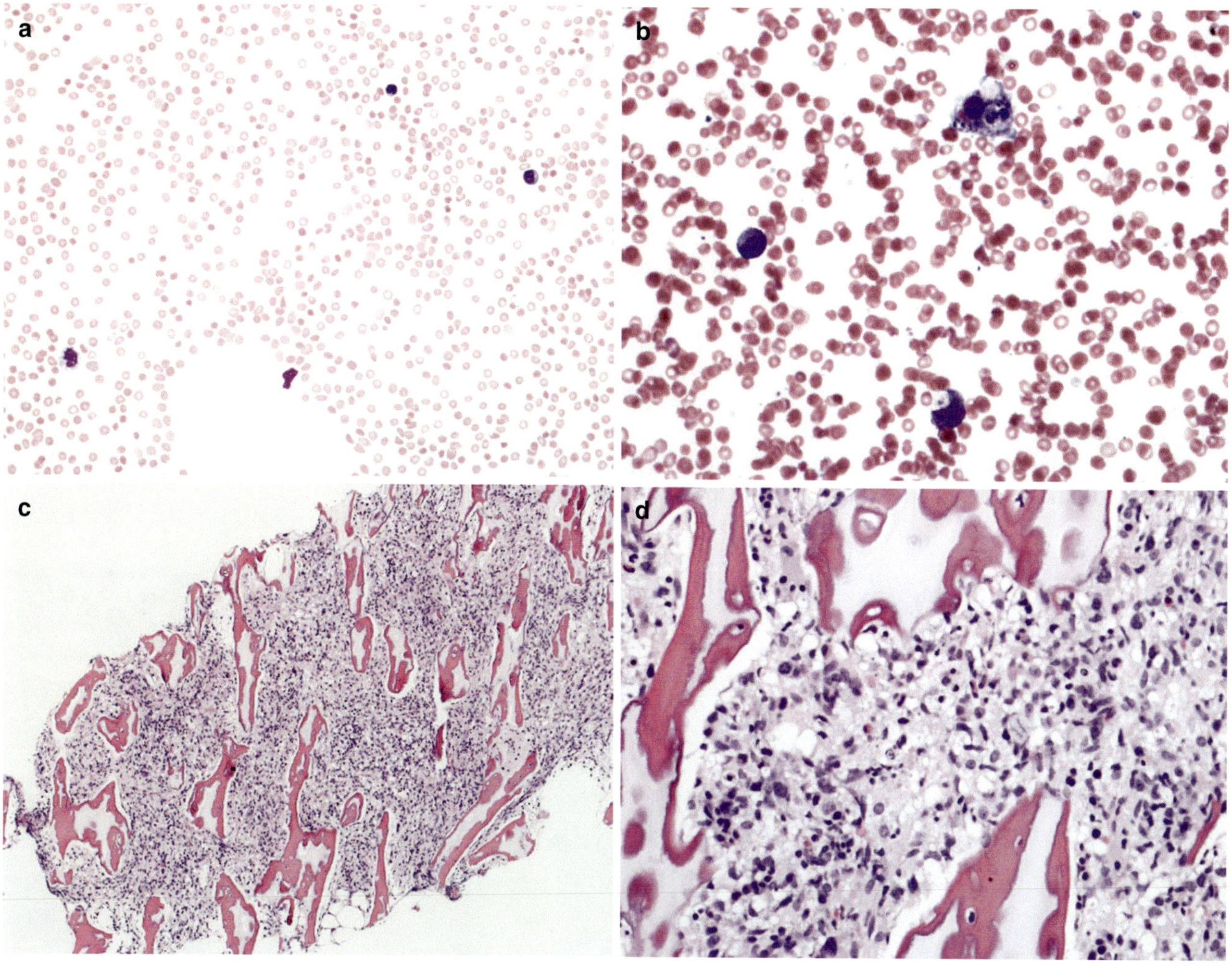

Fig. 29.17 Hemophagocytic lymphohistiocytosis. (**a**) The peripheral blood smear shows pancytopenia characterized by mild anemia, marked neutropenia, and thrombocytopenia. No blasts are identified. Most of the lymphocytes are reactive appearing. Monocytes are not increased and have abundant and occasionally vacuolated cytoplasm (Wright-Giemsa, ×400). (**b**) The bone marrow aspirate are paucicellular with no particles but scattered single marrow cells for evaluation. There are increased small mature-appearing lymphocytes. Numerous histiocytes with abundant vacuolated cytoplasm are noted; some display prominent hemophagocytosis (Wright-Giemsa, ×600). (**c** and **d**) The bone marrow core biopsy shows marked lymphohistiocytosis and overall reduced hematopoiesis (hematoxylin-eosin, ×100). Immunohistochemical stains show numerous CD68+ histiocytes throughout the marrow (not shown). T cells are increased and show a mixed population of CD4+ and CD8+ T lymphocytes (not shown). Myeloperoxidase, glycophorin, and CD61 stain reduced number of granulocytic, erythroid, and megakaryocytic cells (not shown)

Histologic Findings

- The peripheral blood smear shows pancytopenia characterized by mild anemia, marked neutropenia, and thrombocytopenia. No blasts are identified. Most of the lymphocytes are reactive appearing. Monocytes are not increased and have abundant and occasionally vacuolated cytoplasm.
- The bone marrow aspirates are paucicellular with no particles but scattered marrow cells for evaluation. There are increased small mature appearing lymphocytes. Numerous histiocytes with abundant vacuolated cytoplasm are noted; some display prominent hemophagocytosis.
- The bone marrow core biopsy shows marked lymphohistiocytosis and overall reduced hematopoiesis.
- Immunohistochemical stains show numerous CD68+ histiocytes. T cells are increased and show a mixed population of CD4+ and CD8+ T lymphocytes. Myeloperoxidase, glycophorin, and CD61 stain reduced number of granulocytic, erythroid, and megakaryocytic cells.

Differential Diagnosis

- Familial hemophagocytic lymphohistiocytosis
- Hemophagocytic lymphohistiocytosis associated with primary immunodeficiency
- Infectious mononucleosis
- Secondary hemophagocytic lymphohistiocytosis associated with other infectious etiologies
- T-cell lymphoproliferative disorder

- NK-cell lymphoproliferative disorder
- Immune-mediated pancytopenia

Ancillary Studies

- A peripheral blood sample was sent to Cincinnati Children's Hospital for hemophagocytic lymphohistiocytosis panel by next-generation sequencing.
- No mutations were found in the coding region and exon/intron boundaries of *PRF1*, *STX11*, *STXBP2*, *RAB27A*, *SH2D1A*, and *BIRC4*.
- A heterozygous 4 bp deletion mutation in *MUNC13–4* gene c.2346_2349 del GGAG, p. R782fsX793 is identified.

Final Diagnosis

Lymphohistiocytic proliferation and hemophagocytosis, consistent with hemophagocytic lymphohistiocytosis

Take-Home Messages

1. Peripheral blood and bone marrow findings such as pancytopenia and hemophagocytosis, in the appropriate clinical setting, can assist in the diagnosis of HLH.
2. Mutations involving perforin gene 1 (*PRF1*) or other genes involved in the perforin pathway are often detected in familial HLH.

Case 17 (Fig. 29.18)

Learning Objective

Autoimmune disorders or B lymphoproliferative process due to mutations of genes affecting B-cell proliferation, apoptosis, or homeostasis may involve bone marrow.

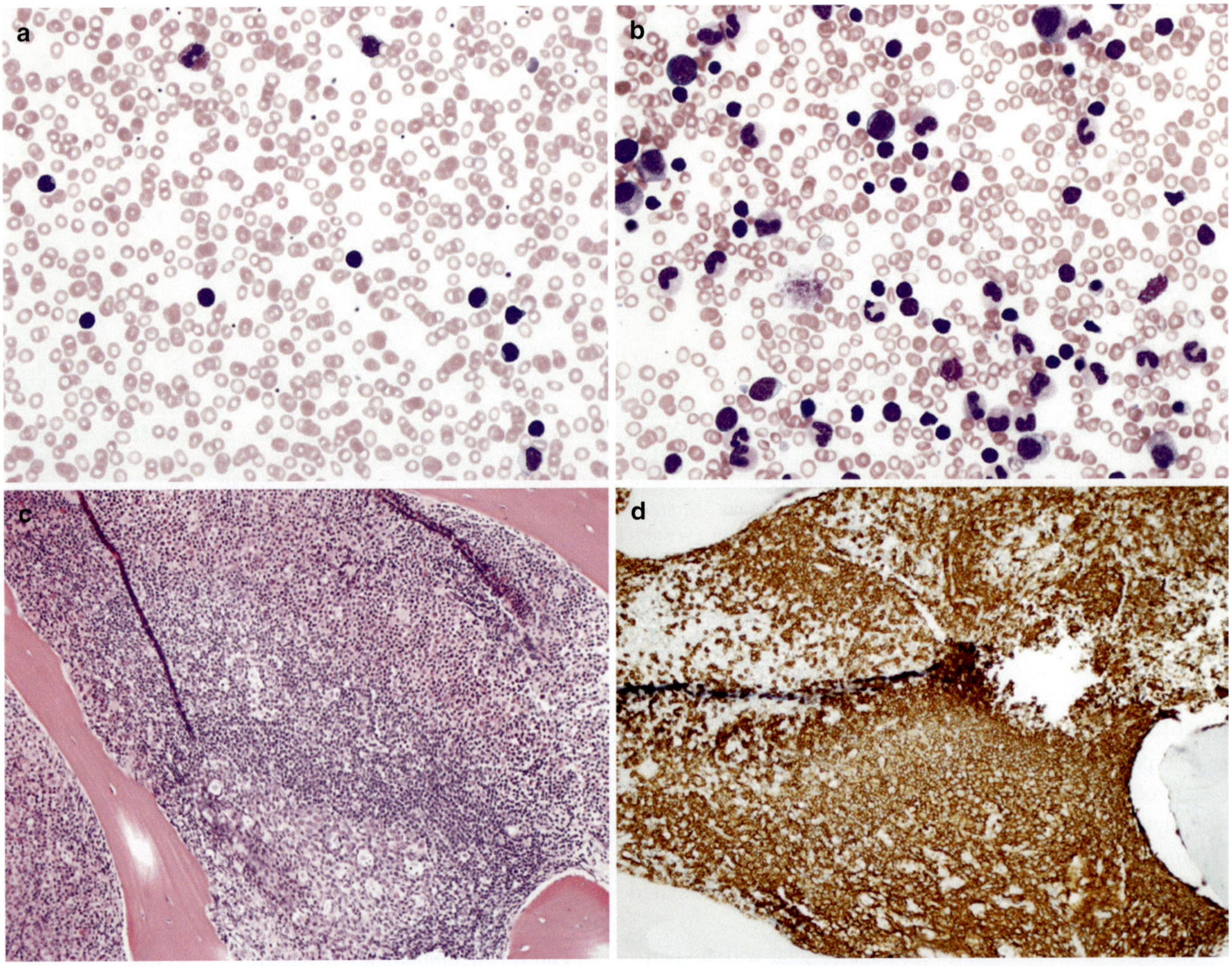

Fig. 29.18 Polytypic B-cell expansion due to *CARD11* mutations. (**a**) The peripheral blood smear shows mild anemia, thrombocytopenia, adequate neutrophils, and absolute lymphocytosis (15.2 k/uL). The lymphocytes are predominantly small mature appearing with scant cytoplasm and mature chromatin (Wright-Giemsa, ×400). (**b**) The bone marrow aspirate smear shows myeloid and erythroid precursors with orderly maturation and increased small mature lymphocytes (Wright-Giemsa, ×400). (**c**) The bone marrow core biopsy shows hypercellular marrow with multiple large lymphoid aggregates in both paratrabecular and interstitial patterns. Some lymphoid aggregates contain reactive appearing germinal centers consistent with reactive follicular hyperplasia (hematoxylin-eosin, ×200). (**d**) Immunostains performed on the core biopsy sections reveal increased number of CD20+ B cells within and between the lymphoid follicles (peroxidase, ×200)

Case History

This is a 1-year old boy infant with diffuse marked lymphadenopathy, splenomegaly, and peripheral blood lymphocytosis. CBC reported WBC 25.13 k/uL, Hb 9.3 g/dL, HCT 31.8%, MCV 67.3 fL, RDW 19.9%, and PLT 81/uL.

Histologic Findings

- The peripheral blood smear shows mild anemia, thrombocytopenia, and adequate neutrophils with a mild shift to immaturity and absolute lymphocytosis (15.2 k/uL). The lymphocytes are predominantly small mature appearing with scant cytoplasm and mature chromatin.
- The bone marrow aspirate smear shows myeloid and erythroid precursors with orderly maturation and increased small mature lymphocytes.
- The bone marrow core biopsy shows hypercellular marrow with multiple large lymphoid aggregates in both paratrabecular and interstitial patterns. Some lymphoid aggregates contain reactive appearing germinal centers consistent with reactive follicular hyperplasia.
- Immunostains performed on the core biopsy sections reveal increased number of CD20+ B cells within and between the lymphoid follicles. The follicles are CD10+, BCL6+, and BCL2-. CD21 stains the follicular dendritic cell meshwork within the follicles. Many of the B cells are weakly CD5 + .

Differential Diagnosis

- Reactive lymphoid hyperplasia associated with infectious etiology
- Lymphoproliferative disorder associated with primary immunodeficiency
- Lymphoproliferative disorder associated with primary autoimmune disease
- B cell lymphoma

Ancillary Studies

- Flow cytometric analysis reported increased mature B cells comprising 21% of the total cellular events. The B cells are CD5+ with a kappa to lambda ratio of 1:1.
- Molecular studies reported a heterozygous likely pathogenic variant in *CARD11* c.377G > A, p.Gly126Asp.
- Cytogenetic analysis reported a normal male karyotype: 46, XY [20].

Final Diagnosis

Bone marrow with increased CD5+ polytypic B cells in the setting of an autoimmune disorder with *CARD11* deficiency

Take-Home Message

B-cell expansion in the peripheral blood and bone marrow may be driven by mutations of genes affecting B-cell proliferation, apoptosis, or homeostasis.

Case 18 (Fig. 29.19)

Learning Objective

To be aware of bone marrow involvement can be an uncommon manifestation of cystinosis, a congenital lysosomal storage disease.

Case History

This is a 17-year-old female with cystinosis status kidney transplant presented with anemia and leukopenia. CBC reported WBC 1.61 k/uL, Hb 8.7 g/dL, HCT 25.7%, MCV 84.7 fL, RDW 18.7%, and PLT 222 k/uL.

Histologic Findings

- The peripheral blood smear shows leukopenia including marked lymphopenia, moderate neutropenia, and moderate normocytic anemia.
- The bone marrow aspirate smear shows myeloid precursors with a shift to immaturity and erythroid precursors with progressive maturation. Many histiocytes are enlarged and filled with crystals, consistent with cystine crystals.
- The bone marrow core biopsy is mildly hypocellular for age with multilineage hematopoiesis and patchy aggregates of histiocytes with abundant foamy cytoplasm.

Differential Diagnosis

- Gaucher's disease
- Niemann-Pick disease
- Cystinosis
- Other storage diseases

Ancillary Studies

- Many hexagonal colorless crystals consistent with cystine crystals were identified in urine precipitate.
- Tandem mass spectrometry demonstrated high level of cystine in white blood cells.
- Flow cytometric analysis reported reduced hematogones, but no immunophenotypic evidence of leukemia or lymphoid neoplasm.
- Cytogenetic analysis reported a normal male karyotype: 46, XX [20].

Final Diagnosis

Bone marrow with crystal deposition, consistent with systemic cystinosis

Take-Home Messages

1. Congenital storage disease, such as systemic cystinosis, can involve multiple organs including bone marrow, besides kidney.
2. The diagnosis relies on morphologic examination of the crystals within macrophages and other laboratory evaluations.

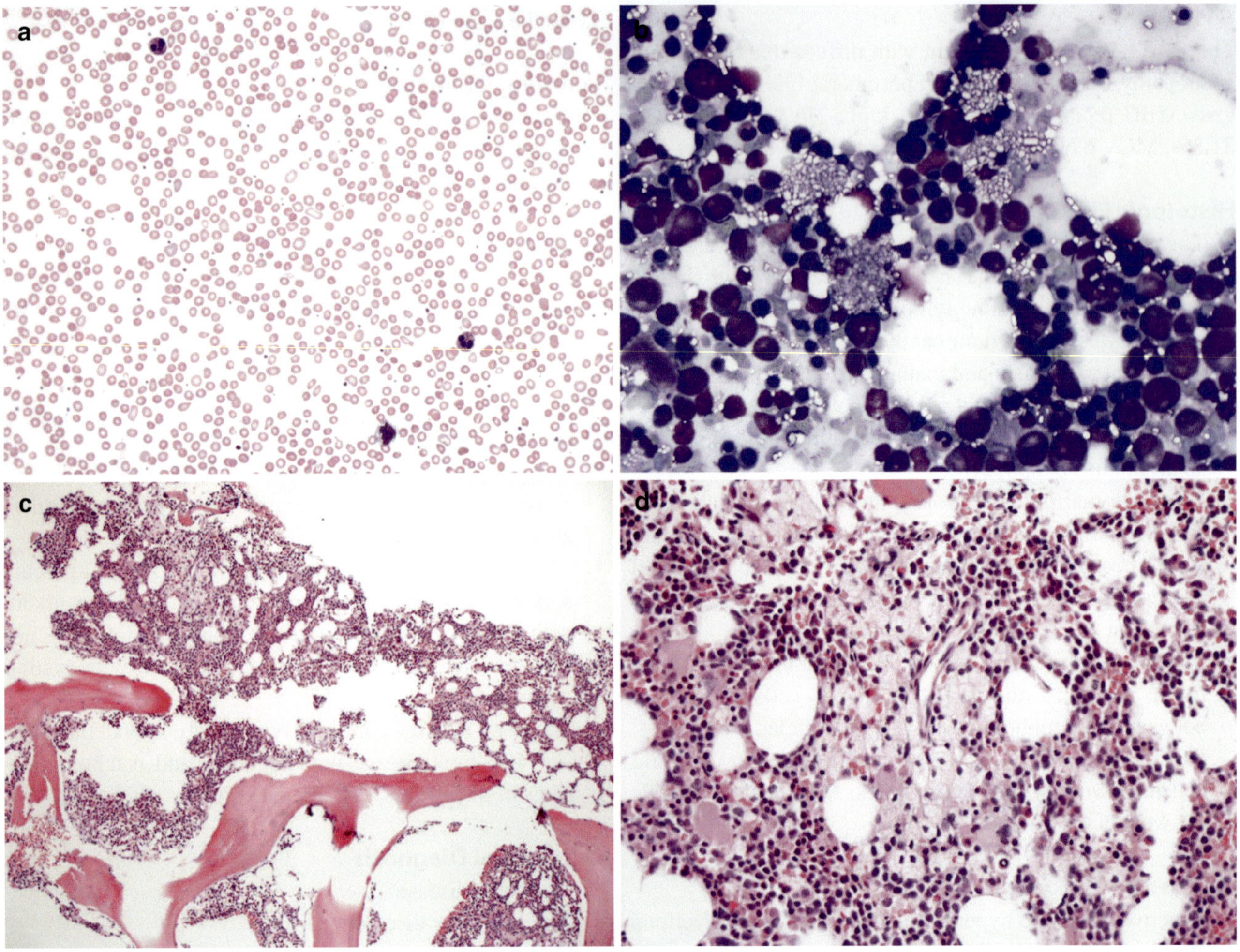

Fig. 29.19 Bone marrow involvement by systemic cystinosis. (**a**) The peripheral blood smear shows leukopenia including marked lymphopenia, moderate neutropenia, and moderate normocytic anemia (Wright-Giemsa, ×400). (**b**) The bone marrow aspirate smear shows myeloid precursors with a shift to immaturity and erythroid precursors with progressive maturation. Many histiocytes are enlarged and filled with crystals, consistent with cystine crystals (Wright-Giemsa, ×600). (**c**, **d**) The bone marrow core biopsy is mildly hypocellular for age with multilineage hematopoiesis and patchy aggregates of histiocytes with abundant foamy cytoplasm (**c**, hematoxylin-eosin, ×200; **d**, hematoxylin-eosin, ×600)

References

1. DeZern AE, Brodsky RA. Genetic panels in young patients with bone marrow failure: are they clinically relevant? Haematologica. 2016;101(11):1275–6.
2. Dokal I, Vulliamy T. Inherited bone marrow failure syndromes. Haematologica. 2010;95(8):1236–40.
3. Peffault de Latour R, Soulier J. How I treat MDS and AML in Fanconi anemia. Blood. 2016;127(24):2971–9.
4. Henry E, Walker D, Wiedmeier SE, Christensen RD. Hematological abnormalities during the first week of life among neonates with Down syndrome: data from a multihospital healthcare system. Am J Med Genet A. 2007;143A(1):42–50.
5. Pine SR, Guo Q, Yin C, Jayabose S, Druschel CM, Sandoval C. Incidence and clinical implications of GATA1 mutations in newborns with Down syndrome. Blood. 2007;110(6):2128–31.
6. Gamis AS, Alonzo TA, Gerbing RB, Hilden JM, Sorrell AD, Sharma M, et al. Natural history of transient myeloproliferative disorder clinically diagnosed in Down syndrome neonates: a report from the Children's Oncology Group Study A2971. Blood. 2011;118(26):6752–9; quiz 996.
7. Karandikar NJ, Aquino DB, McKenna RW, Kroft SH. Transient myeloproliferative disorder and acute myeloid leukemia in Down syndrome. An immunophenotypic analysis. Am J Clin Pathol. 2001;116(2):204–10.
8. Yumura-Yagi K, Hara J, Kurahashi H, Nishiura T, Kaneyama Y, Osugi Y, et al. Mixed phenotype of blasts in acute megakaryocytic leukaemia and transient abnormal myelopoiesis in Down's syndrome. Br J Haematol. 1992;81(4):520–5.
9. Greene ME, Mundschau G, Wechsler J, McDevitt M, Gamis A, Karp J, et al. Mutations in GATA1 in both transient myeloproliferative disorder and acute megakaryoblastic leukemia of Down syndrome. Blood Cells Mol Dis. 2003;31(3):351–6.
10. Pabst T, Eyholzer M, Haefliger S, Schardt J, Mueller BU. Somatic CEBPA mutations are a frequent second event in families with germline CEBPA mutations and familial acute myeloid leukemia. J Clin Oncol. 2008;26(31):5088–93.
11. Taskesen E, Bullinger L, Corbacioglu A, Sanders MA, Erpelinck CA, Wouters BJ, et al. Prognostic impact, concurrent genetic muta-

tions, and gene expression features of AML with CEBPA mutations in a cohort of 1182 cytogenetically normal AML patients: further evidence for CEBPA double mutant AML as a distinctive disease entity. Blood. 2011;117(8):2469–75.
12. Preudhomme C, Sagot C, Boissel N, Cayuela JM, Tigaud I, de Botton S, et al. Favorable prognostic significance of CEBPA mutations in patients with de novo acute myeloid leukemia: a study from the Acute Leukemia French Association (ALFA). Blood. 2002;100(8):2717–23.
13. Cancer Genome Atlas Research Network, Ley TJ, Miller C, Ding L, Raphael BJ, Mungall AJ, et al. Genomic and epigenomic landscapes of adult de novo acute myeloid leukemia. N Engl J Med. 2013;368(22):2059–74.
14. Chen CY, Lin LI, Tang JL, Ko BS, Tsay W, Chou WC, et al. RUNX1 gene mutation in primary myelodysplastic syndrome—the mutation can be detected early at diagnosis or acquired during disease progression and is associated with poor outcome. Br J Haematol. 2007;139(3):405–14.
15. Tang JL, Hou HA, Chen CY, Liu CY, Chou WC, Tseng MH, et al. AML1/RUNX1 mutations in 470 adult patients with de novo acute myeloid leukemia: prognostic implication and interaction with other gene alterations. Blood. 2009;114(26):5352–61.
16. Schnittger S, Dicker F, Kern W, Wendland N, Sundermann J, Alpermann T, et al. RUNX1 mutations are frequent in de novo AML with noncomplex karyotype and confer an unfavorable prognosis. Blood. 2011;117(8):2348–57.
17. Sood R, Kamikubo Y, Liu P. Role of RUNX1 in hematological malignancies. Blood. 2017;129(15):2070–82.
18. Polprasert C, Schulze I, Sekeres MA, Makishima H, Przychodzen B, Hosono N, et al. Inherited and somatic defects in DDX41 in myeloid neoplasms. Cancer Cell. 2015;27(5):658–70.
19. Lewinsohn M, Brown AL, Weinel LM, Phung C, Rafidi G, Lee MK, et al. Novel germ line DDX41 mutations define families with a lower age of MDS/AML onset and lymphoid malignancies. Blood. 2016;127(8):1017–23.
20. Melazzini F, Palombo F, Balduini A, De Rocco D, Marconi C, Noris P, et al. Clinical and pathogenic features of ETV6-related thrombocytopenia with predisposition to acute lymphoblastic leukemia. Haematologica. 2016;101(11):1333–42.
21. Noris P, Favier R, Alessi MC, Geddis AE, Kunishima S, Heller PG, et al. ANKRD26-related thrombocytopenia and myeloid malignancies. Blood. 2013;122(11):1987–9.
22. Wlodarski MW, Hirabayashi S, Pastor V, Stary J, Hasle H, Masetti R, et al. Prevalence, clinical characteristics, and prognosis of GATA2-related myelodysplastic syndromes in children and adolescents. Blood. 2016;127(11):1387–97; quiz 518.
23. Kanagal-Shamanna R, Loghavi S, DiNardo CD, Medeiros LJ, Garcia-Manero G, Jabbour E, et al. Bone marrow pathologic abnormalities in familial platelet disorder with propensity for myeloid malignancy and germline RUNX1 mutation. Haematologica. 2017;102(10):1661–70.
24. Noris P, Perrotta S, Seri M, Pecci A, Gnan C, Loffredo G, et al. Mutations in ANKRD26 are responsible for a frequent form of inherited thrombocytopenia: analysis of 78 patients from 21 families. Blood. 2011;117(24):6673–80.
25. Tsang HC, Bussel JB, Mathew S, Liu YC, Imahiyerobo AA, Orazi A, et al. Bone marrow morphology and disease progression in congenital thrombocytopenia: a detailed clinicopathologic and genetic study of eight cases. Mod Pathol. 2017;30(4):486–98.
26. Noetzli L, Lo RW, Lee-Sherick AB, Callaghan M, Noris P, Savoia A, et al. Germline mutations in ETV6 are associated with thrombocytopenia, red cell macrocytosis and predisposition to lymphoblastic leukemia. Nat Genet. 2015;47(5):535–8.
27. Spinner MA, Sanchez LA, Hsu AP, Shaw PA, Zerbe CS, Calvo KR, et al. GATA2 deficiency: a protean disorder of hematopoiesis, lymphatics, and immunity. Blood. 2014;123(6):809–21.
28. University of Chicago Hematopoietic Malignancies Cancer Risk T. How I diagnose and manage individuals at risk for inherited myeloid malignancies. Blood. 2016;128(14):1800–13.
29. Yazdani R, Hakemi MG, Sherkat R, Homayouni V, Farahani R. Genetic defects and the role of helper T-cells in the pathogenesis of common variable immunodeficiency. Adv Biomed Res. 2014;3:2.
30. Bogaert DJ, Dullaers M, Lambrecht BN, Vermaelen KY, De Baere E, Haerynck F. Genes associated with common variable immunodeficiency: one diagnosis to rule them all? J Med Genet. 2016;53(9):575–90.
31. Jordan MB, Allen CE, Weitzman S, Filipovich AH, McClain KL. How I treat hemophagocytic lymphohistiocytosis. Blood. 2011;118(15):4041–52.
32. Weitzman S. Approach to hemophagocytic syndromes. Hematology Am Soc Hematol Educ Program. 2011;2011:178–83.
33. Bride K, Teachey D. Autoimmune lymphoproliferative syndrome: more than a FAScinating disease. F1000Res. 2017;6:1928.
34. Xie Y, Pittaluga S, Price S, Raffeld M, Hahn J, Jaffe ES, et al. Bone marrow findings in autoimmune lymphoproliferative syndrome with germline FAS mutation. Haematologica. 2017;102(2):364–72.
35. Abdulsalam AH, Khamis MH, Bain BJ. Diagnosis of cystinosis from a bone marrow aspirate. Am J Hematol. 2013;88(2):151.
36. Mariani R, Gong S. Bone marrow histopathologic findings in SIFD syndrome: beyond the erythroid lineage. Blood. 2018;132(13):1459.
37. Tawana K, Wang J, Renneville A, Bodor C, Hills R, Loveday C, et al. Disease evolution and outcomes in familial AML with germline CEBPA mutations. Blood. 2015;126(10):1214–23.
38. Bluteau D, Balduini A, Balayn N, Currao M, Nurden P, Deswarte C, et al. Thrombocytopenia-associated mutations in the ANKRD26 regulatory region induce MAPK hyperactivation. J Clin Invest. 2014;124(2):580–91.
39. Pippucci T, Savoia A, Perrotta S, Pujol-Moix N, Noris P, Castegnaro G, et al. Mutations in the 5' UTR of ANKRD26, the ankirin repeat domain 26 gene, cause an autosomal-dominant form of inherited thrombocytopenia, THC2. Am J Hum Genet. 2011;88(1):115–20.

Bone Marrow Involvement by More Than One Entity of Hematolymphoid Neoplasm

30

Yue Zhao, Anand Shreeram Lagoo, and Endi Wang

List of Frequently Asked Questions

1. What are the common combinations of concurrent hematolymphoid neoplasms in bone marrow?
2. What are the common clinical and diagnostic settings in which dual hematolymphoid neoplasms may be identified? Can such dual populations be appreciated on aspirate smear or H&E stained core biopsy?
3. What are the potential diagnostic errors in the presence of coexisting neoplasms, and what is the clinical relevance of misinterpretation with reference to mistreatment and/or wrong prognosis?
4. Which morphological findings in the bone marrow biopsy are reliably diagnostic of dual involvement? Which ones suggest the diagnosis? Which is (are) unreliable for diagnosis? Which findings rule out the diagnosis?
5. What is the minimal and optimal ancillary work-up required to ensure correct diagnosis and accurate classification of both malignancies involving the marrow?
6. Which ancillary test results are diagnostic, suggestive of diagnosis, unreliable for diagnosis, or rule out the diagnosis?
7. How to distinguish small mature B-cell leukemia/lymphoma with plasmacytoid differentiation from concurrent small B-cell leukemia/lymphoma and plasma cell neoplasm? How to dissect the two B-cell neoplasms in order to determine biclonality or monoclonality?
8. Which subtypes of marrow involvement by more than one entity are clinically relevant and which are morphologically defined but have unproven/minimal clinical relevance?
9. What is an adequate specimen for this condition?
10. What information can be conveyed to the clinician during each stage of the work-up?
11. What should be the approach to provide maximum, but defensible information, from limited specimen or work-up? What is a descriptive diagnosis appropriate in such situations?
12. When is it appropriate to seek external consultation for this condition?

1. What are the common combinations of concurrent hematolymphoid neoplasms in bone marrow?

- Only infrequently, bone marrow biopsies demonstrate simultaneous presence of more than one hematolymphoid neoplasms. In a majority of cases, the second neoplastic entity is suspected based on morphological findings or ancillary test results obtained on bone marrows being examined for a known or suspected hematolymphoid neoplasm and the second process is discovered unexpectedly. There are several possible combinations of dual neoplastic components simultaneously involving the bone marrow but most are rare and described as case reports [1–14]. The relatively common combinations, reported as case series, consist of a myeloid neoplasm, most commonly myelodysplastic syndrome (MDS) or myeloproliferative neoplasm (MPN), seen together with either plasma cell neoplasm (PCN) [15, 16], chronic lymphocytic leukemia (CLL) [17, 18], other CLL-like mature, B-cell leukemia/lymphoma, or T-cell large

Y. Zhao (✉)
Department of Pathology, College of Basic Medical Sciences and the First Affiliated Hospital, China Medical University, Shenyang, P. R. China

Department of Pathology, Duke University School of Medicine, Durham, NC, USA
e-mail: yue.zhao197@duke.edu; zhaoyue@cmu.edu.cn

A. S. Lagoo · E. Wang
Department of Pathology, Duke University School of Medicine and Duke Health System, Durham, NC, USA

E. Wang, A. S. Lagoo (eds.), *Practical Lymph Node and Bone Marrow Pathology*, Practical Anatomic Pathology,
https://doi.org/10.1007/978-3-030-32189-5_30

granular lymphocytic leukemia (T-LGL) [19]. Also described in the literature are combinations like PCN with CLL [20], PCN with lymphoplasmacytic lymphoma (LPL) [21], CLL with T-LGL [22], CLL with B-lymphoblastic leukemia [23, 24], etc.

- The co-occurrence of a myeloid and lymphoid neoplasm in the same patient is clinically quite rare, reported in less than 0.5% of the nearly 10,000 patients presenting with a hematologic malignancy at one center [25]. An important exception noted recently is the presence of a monoclonal gammopathy of undetermined significance (MGUS) in a high proportion of patients (nearly 14%) with non-*BCR/ABL* myeloproliferative neoplasms (MPNs) [26]. Importantly, this concurrence is associated with a worse outcome. On the other hand, coexistence of MPNs with CLL apparently does not adversely affect prognosis of either disease [27].
- Concurrency of three different hematolymphoid neoplasms in a bone marrow biopsy has been described [28], but that is extremely rare.
- Presence of systemic mastocytosis with non-mast cell clonal processes as well as eosinophilia and mutations in *PDGFR/FGFR* genes are designated as distinct entities and are considered further in Chap. 24.

2. What are the common clinical and diagnostic settings in which dual hematolymphoid neoplasms may be identified? Can such dual populations be appreciated on aspirate smear or H&E stained core biopsy?

- Second neoplasm induced by treatment for first: Most commonly, a patient with one type of hematolymphoid neoplasm demonstrates a second hematolymphoid neoplasm in a follow-up bone marrow examination after treatment for first neoplasm. For instance, patients receiving chemotherapy for CLL or plasma cell myeloma (PCM) may later develop a myeloid neoplasm, either MDS or acute myeloid leukemia (AML), while the residual CLL or PCN is still present in the bone marrow biopsy. (See also Chap. 32 for additional features of therapy-induced myeloid neoplasms.)
- Second neoplasm unmasked by treatment for first: A previously "hidden" small population of clonal plasma cells or B-cells may be revealed after treatment of acute myeloid leukemia. As leukemic blasts decrease due to treatment, the second clonal population may expand to some extent.
- Simultaneous occurrence of both neoplasms at diagnosis: Less commonly, patient presents with anemia or cytopenia, and bone marrow examination demonstrates coexisting neoplasms. As mentioned above, a relatively high proportion of patients with MPNs can have an MGUS, but significant plasmacytosis is not seen in the marrow of most patients (median marrow plasma cells ~1%) [26]. Even when untreated, CLL and follicular lymphoma increase the risk of a second malignancy, but in many cases, these second cancers are not of hematolymphoid origin [29].
- Metachronous occurrence of apparently unrelated neoplasms: Rarely, a patient with an indolent hematolymphoid neoplasm observed without specific treatment may demonstrate another unrelated hematolymphoid neoplasm in a subsequent biopsy together with the first neoplasm. For instance, a patient with MGUS or low stage CLL may be diagnosed years later with a myeloid neoplasm, either MDS or AML [15, 17, 18, 30].

3. What are the potential diagnostic errors in the presence of coexisting neoplasms, and what is the clinical relevance of misinterpretation with reference to mistreatment and/or wrong prognosis?

- Missed diagnosis: In setting of coexisting hematolymphoid neoplasms in bone marrow, one component may be missed, depending on type of neoplasm and its proportion in the bone marrow biopsy.
  - In case of PCN or CLL with subsequent or concurrent low risk MDS, the component of MDS could potentially be overlooked, especially when PCN or CLL is overwhelming in number, thus masking the MDS component.
  - In contrast, PCN or CLL with coexisting AML is hard to miss because of morphologic distinction and routine flow cytometric detection of both components.
  - A diagnosis of PCN/CLL without identification of concurrent MDS would result in delayed treatment for MDS, which will eventually progress to AML and often prevail over PCN/CLL in determining the clinical outcome. MGUS is relatively common in MPNs and has detrimental effect on prognosis of underlying MPN, but ancillary studies such as serum immunofixation electrophoresis (IFE) are required to detect this clonal process due to the low number of plasma cells in the marrow [26].
- Underdiagnosis: The distinction between high- and low-grade MDS and AML depends on precise quantification of blasts.
  - Carefully identify blasts in the presence of atypical mononuclear cells such as large cell lymphoma cells, plasmablasts, etc.

  - When conducting a differential count from an aspirate to calculate blast percentage, plasma cells and lymphocytes are not excluded from the total count.
  - Reticulin fibrosis is not usual for AML, PCM, and CLL. If there are suspicious areas with spindle cells in marrow biopsy and/or if reticulin fibrosis is detected, particularly in paratrabecular location, appropriate immunostains should be performed to rule out one or more of the following conditions as appropriate – osteosclerotic myeloma, megakaryoblastic leukemia, involvement by lymphomas other than CLL (particularly follicular lymphoma and hairy cell leukemia), systemic mastocytosis, Langerhans cell histiocytosis, and MPNs.

    Flow cytometry may be negative if the lymphoma cells are "trapped" in the fibrosis and are not aspirated.
- Overdiagnosis:
  - When patients have received chemotherapy for an established hematolymphoid neoplasm, atypia in erythroid cells or pelgeroid changes in neutrophils should not be interpreted as evidence of myelodysplasia. See also Chap. 32 for further discussion of the morphological findings in this setting.

    Overdiagnosis of MDS in such cases may lead to inappropriate treatment.
  - Myeloid hyperplasia and left shift consequent to growth factor administration should not be overdiagnosed as MPN.
  - Plasma cell proportion may be high in bone marrow rendered hypocellular by chemotherapy for myeloid neoplasm. Binucleate plasma cells and Russell bodies may be present. These should not be over-interpreted as a plasma cell dyscrasia without obtaining histological confirmation of marrow cellularity from a core biopsy.
  - In some bone marrow biopsies with isolated CLL, focal myeloid hyperplasia with increased megakaryocytes may be seen, possibly due to cytokine produced by CLL cells and paracrine stimulation. Presence of suspected chronic myeloid leukemia (CML) or other MPN could be confirmed by cytogenetic analysis and/or molecular diagnostic tests such as *JAK2* V617F mutation analysis (see below for the details).
- Misdiagnosis:
  - Poorly differentiated carcinoma and other solid tumors, as well as some histiocytes, may mimic plasma cells. Megaloblastoid erythroid precursors, some AML blasts, and plasma cells may be difficult to distinguish on morphological examination alone. Index of suspicion should be high when the clinical finding is not straightforward and/or the patient has received multiple modalities of treatment. Ancillary studies should be used in such cases when in doubt.
  - Paratrabecular spindle-shaped cells may represent myeloma cells, mast cells, dendritic cells, or lymphoma cells.

4. Which morphological findings in the bone marrow biopsy are reliably diagnostic of dual involvement? Which ones suggest the diagnosis? Which is (are) unreliable for diagnosis? Which findings rule out the diagnosis?

A 500 cell differential count on high-quality aspirate smear conducted by someone unbiased by prior history is an important safeguard against wrong interpretation of marrow findings. Please see the appropriate earlier chapters for the morphological findings in the individual diseases affecting the marrow. Following sections emphasize additional points for the more common dual disease scenarios:

- PCN with AML: In case of previously diagnosed and treated PCN with subsequent therapy-related AML, the increased blasts in bone marrow are hard to miss when the AML has evolved fully. However, evolution of AML from MDS can be a long process, and some cases may go through a hypocellular phase or remain hypocellular. Lack of obvious increase of plasma cells should not be interpreted as absence of residual plasma cell neoplasm.
- In case of the concurrent diagnosis of AML and PCN, the latter component may be overlooked if its level is low (MGUS), plasma cells lack cytological atypia, and/or laboratory evidence is absent. When at a low level, such as 5% or lower, PCN often shows no striking light chain restriction by immunohistochemistry for kappa and lambda light chains, but high proportion of CD56 or cyclin D1 expression in plasma cells is more convincing evidence of PCN.
- PCN with MDS: In most cases, patients have history of PCN, either treated (myeloma) or untreated (MGUS). Presence of MDS is potentially overlooked, if residual PCN is relatively high so as to mask the neoplastic myeloid component, blasts are not increased, and myelodysplasia is subtle. In this combination, MDS is often detected by ancillary tests, particularly cytogenetic studies, and in some cases without increased blasts or significant myelodysplasia, diagnosis of MDS is not in consideration until unexpected identification of clonal cytogenetic abnormality suggestive of myeloid origin (see below for details).
- PCN with small B-cell lymphoma: Small mature B-cell leukemia/lymphoma, such as CLL or marginal zone

lymphoma (MZL), may occasionally show plasmacytoid or plasmacytic differentiation and exhibit significant number of plasma cells in the bone marrow, but the two components are the same clone. Therefore, the presence of monotypic plasma cells or plasmacytoid cells along with a significant population of monotypic small, mature B-cells needs careful evaluation to determine if there is only a single entity or two separate neoplasms involving the marrow. While some morphological clues favor certain scenarios, in practice, ancillary studies are required to determine the true process(es).

- The single entity can be either LPL or MZL with plasmacytic differentiation. The small lymphocytes are usually (but not always) predominant over the plasma cells, and the latter component is often mixed into the former components.
- Two separate entities can be a PCN, and a small B-cell lymphoma concurrently involves the marrow. Focal collection of exclusively plasma cells, as opposed to mixed infiltration of plasma cell and small mature lymphocytes, suggests a separate PCN in addition to a B-cell lymphoma. Since the two neoplasms are clonally unrelated, the relative proportions of each component in bone marrow biopsy can vary widely, depending on the growth rate and survival potential of each neoplastic component.
- When the light chain restriction of the plasma cell component and the B-cell component is different, it effectively rules out the possibility of a single entity. In these situations, the B-cell lymphoma is further classified based on the immunophenotype and cytogenetic profile (see Chap. 5) and the plasma cell component by the ancillary studies as detailed in Chap. 26.
- When the plasma cells and B-cells have the same light chain restriction: it is critical to determine if it is a single lympho plasmacytic neoplasm or two separate neoplasms. A single neoplasm implies a lymphoma and must be treated as such. Two separate neoplasms potentially require separate treatments for a PCM and a B-cell lymphoma.
  - In this situation, additional immunophenotypic features of abnormal plasma cells determined by immunohistochemistry (IHC) and flow cytometry (aberrant expression of CD56, Cyclin D1, and/or CD117 and/or loss of CD19 and other antigens) and the immunophenotype of the abnormal B-cells (CD5, CD10, CD23, CD103 or CD123 expression, intensity of antigen expression, Cyclin D1 and SOX11 expression) are necessary to distinguish between the two possibilities. See Alley et al. [20] for additional discussion.
- CLL with AML: The increased number of CLL cells may hamper accurate determination of M:E ratio. CLL with large proportion of prolymphocytes or paraimmunoblasts may confound the blast count. CLL usually demonstrates circulating abnormal lymphocytes, and flow cytometric detection of CLL is easier than that of PCN.
- CLL with MDS: The evaluation for this combination is similar to that of PCN with MDS. In particular, MDS is often retrospectively diagnosed after unexpected finding of clonal cytogenetic abnormality suggestive of myeloid origin (see below for details).
- CLL with CML: Cytology and flow cytometry easily separate CLL cells and chronic phase CML cells. Increased prolymphocytes or Richter transformation of CLL should not be interpreted as accelerated or blast phase of CML. The possibility of a lymphoid blast phase of CML should be excluded in cases where only B-cells are detected by IHC on the marrow. The blasts of B-ALL (i.e., lymphoid blast phase of CML) are usually easily distinguished from typical CLL cells. But in cases with poor morphology, flow cytometry and IHC stains on core biopsy or clot section for CD19, CD10, CD5, PAX5, CD34, TdT, Ki-67, etc., may be required.

References [15, 17, 18, 20, 21, 30–33]

5. What is the minimal and optimal ancillary work up required to ensure correct diagnosis and accurate classification of both malignancies involving the marrow?

In most laboratories, the repertoire of ancillary studies is dictated by the known or suspected diagnosis (the "primary" diagnosis), and studies are directed to confirm the primary diagnosis and refine its classification. The occurrence of the second neoplasm (the "secondary" diagnosis) may be suspected based on an unexpected morphological findings or an unexpected result of an ancillary test. The extra work-up is required, at a minimum, to confirm that the secondary process is indeed clonal (neoplastic) and not reactive. Optimally, the extra work-up should classify the second neoplasm and provide guidance for treatment targets and prognosis. Please see the preceding chapters on myeloid and lymphoid neoplasms for ancillary studies performed in individual diseases. Here we emphasize only the additional ancillary tests required by the dual involvement of the marrow. For this purpose, these cases can be divided according to the "primary" diagnosis into myeloid, lymphoid, and plasmacytic.

- Myeloid "primary" diagnosis:
  - PCN suspected as the "secondary" diagnosis. Minimum work-up: IHC for CD138 for accurate enumeration of plasma cells, kappa and lambda stain for light chain restriction, CD56 and Cyclin D1 stains to confirm atypical nature of plasma cells. Optimal work-up: Flow

Table 30.1 Diagnostic utility of ancillary studies in evaluating coexisting hematolymphoid neoplasms in bone marrow

	IHC	Flow cytometry	Chromosomal analysis	FISH	Molecular testing	Other lab tests
AML	++	+++	+++	+++		
MDS	+	+	+++	+++		
MPN			+++	+++	*JAK2*, *MPL*, *CALR*	
CML			+++ (Ph)	+++ (*BCR/ABL*)	*BCR/ABL1*	
B-ALL	+++	+++	+++	+++	PCR-*IGH/K*	
PCN	+++	++	++	+++	PCR-*IGH/K*	SPEP, IFE, FLC
CLL	+++	+++	++	+++	PCR-*IGH/K*	
LPL	+++	+++	++		PCR-*IGH/K*, *MYD88*	SPEP, IFE, FLC
T-LGL	++	+++	++		PCR-*TCR*	

+, ++, and +++ indicate levels of usefulness in separating coexisting hematolymphoid neoplasms, which represent only the authors' own experience/opinion

cytometry to define immunophenotype of plasma cells (for future reference to detect minimal residual disease), Congo red stain, plasma cell FISH panel, serum protein electrophoresis (SPEP) and IFE, serum free light chain analysis (FLC), radiographic skeletal survey to define the extent of the plasma cell neoplasm.
  - Lymphoid malignancy suspected as the "secondary" diagnosis. Minimum work-up: Flow cytometry to examine monotypicality and expression of antigens defining the type of B-cell lymphoma (CD5, CD10, CD23, CD103, CD123). Also IHC for Kappa, lambda, IgM, IgG, and IgA if plasmacytoid cells are detected. Optimal work-up: IHC for BCL2, BCL6, CD3, CD20, CD138, cMYC, Cyclin D1, Ki-67, MUM1, SOX11 to define the subtype of lymphoma, lymphoma FISH panel to examine the possibility of high-grade lymphoma, *MYD88* mutation to rule out LPL.
- Lymphoid "primary" diagnosis: It is of utmost importance to determine what was the subtype of original lymphoma and what treatment was given. Obtain the diagnostic material for review if primary was diagnosed outside your facility. If both malignancies are discovered simultaneously, history of non-hematolymphoid neoplasms and their treatment is important.
  - PCN suspected as "secondary" diagnosis: If the underlying lymphoma is of T-cell origin, the work-up to characterize the plasma cells is similar to the above. However, additional studies are required when the lymphoma is of B-cell origin and in particular when the B-cells and plasma cells have the same light chain restriction. See Question #7 for more discussion on handling such cases.
- Lymphoid or PCN "primary" diagnosis:
  - Myeloid neoplasms suspected as "secondary" diagnosis. Minimum work-up: History of growth factor administration must be ruled out. Laboratory tests to rule out dietary deficiencies, heavy metal poisoning, viral and bacterial infections, autoimmune processes, etc., which can mimic changes of myeloproliferative or myelodysplastic neoplasms. The optimal work-up includes flow cytometry, specific FISH tests or myeloid FISH panel (MDS panel, AML panel, or other depending on suspected myeloid neoplasm), specific mutation analysis, and myeloid NGS panel.
- Sensitivity and utility of ancillary studies: While flow cytometry and chromosomal analysis are performed on almost every bone marrow obtained; tier 2 tests such as immunohistochemistry, FISH, B-cell and T-cell receptor gene rearrangement analysis, PCR-based mutation analysis, NGS analysis, and SPEP/IFE/FLC, etc., are employed based on the morphologic evaluation and the results of flow cytometry or other ancillary tests. Sensitivity of each individual test varies with type of neoplasms. For instance, flow cytometry is sensitive and specific for detecting lymphoid neoplasm, particularly B-cell non-Hodgkin lymphomas, and increase in blasts, while it is less so for detecting Hodgkin lymphoma (HL), MDS, or MPN. The applications of commonly used ancillary tests in evaluating concurrent hematolymphoid neoplasms are summarized in Table 30.1.

References [15, 17, 19–21, 23, 30, 32, 33]

6. Which ancillary test results are diagnostic, suggestive of diagnosis, unreliable for diagnosis, or rule out the diagnosis?

Please refer to the individual chapters on various lymphomas in Part 2 and chapters on acute leukemia, MDS, MPN, and PCN in Part 3 for discussion of the reliability and specificity of ancillary tests to confirm or rule out a particular diagnosis. Here we emphasize additional points related to coexistence of two neoplasms:

- B-cell clonality assay:
  - Molecular assays, of immunoglobulin heavy chain or light chain clonality, either PCR-based or NGS-based, do *not* distinguish between B-cell lymphoma and PCN. Similarly, presence of two clonal peaks by PCR (or equivalent in NGS) does not guarantee two separate clones as these can be derived from two rearrangements of the maternal and paternal chromosomes in the same clone. Flow cytometry and IHC staining are necessary to identify two suspected B-cell clonal processes.

    Presence of B-cell clone(s) does not equate a B-cell lymphoma or plasma cell myeloma. The size of the clonal expansion and its effects on the patient are important for diagnosis.
  - A B-cell component may be suggested by serum paraprotein detected by SPEP/IFE or FLC, if the B-cell neoplasm has plasmacytoid differentiation and secrets paraprotein. Quantitative assessment and time course of these abnormal results are valuable adjuncts to correct diagnosis.
- Blasts and blast equivalents: Flow cytometry is sensitive and specific for detecting myeloid and lymphoid blasts, but the percentage of blasts detected by flow cytometry may be an overestimation. This may happen if the erythroid or plasmacytic component in the marrow is high. Because these cells can be sensitive to the RBC lysis step of flow cytometry, the blast percentage is inflated in the residual cells. Manual count on bone marrow smears is the gold standard for blast percentage, but if these smears are paucicellular, IHC for CD34 or similar antigen on core biopsy is recommended.
  - Promonocytes are counted as blast equivalents. While flow cytometry can suggest an immature monocytic phenotype, these findings are inconsistent and morphological identification is required.
  - Extra care must be taken when counting blasts if a concurrent high-grade lymphoma or plasmablastic myeloma is present.
- In cases of myeloid neoplasms, either MDS or MPN, immunohistochemical analysis and flow cytometry are usually less informative, particularly in cases without increased blasts. Clonal cytogenetic abnormality is often the only defining factor for the diagnosis of MDS or MPN, particularly in cases without hyperplastic hematopoiesis or other morphologic atypia. In many cases of CLL or PCN with concurrent MDS or MPN, the component of myeloid neoplasm is often overlooked due to overwhelming CLL or PCN, and the diagnosis of myeloid neoplasm is not rendered until unexpected finding of cytogenetic abnormalities. More than half of the concurrent myeloid neoplasms in dual hematolymphoid neoplasms have clonal cytogenetic abnormalities detected by karyotyping.
  - Relatively myeloid specific cytogenetic abnormalities include −7, +8, −5q, etc. There is no cytogenetic change currently considered specific for CLL or LPL. However, clonal cytogenetic abnormalities detected in unstimulated culture are usually suggestive of myeloid origin of neoplasm, while those detected in mitogen stimulated culture are considered lymphoid origin rather than myeloid.

References [15, 17, 19–21, 23, 30, 32, 33]

7. How to distinguish small mature B-cell leukemia/lymphoma with plasmacytoid differentiation from concurrent small B-cell leukemia/lymphoma and plasma cell neoplasm? How to dissect the two B-cell neoplasms in order to determine biclonality or monoclonality?

- It is easier to confirm the presence of two separate neoplastic proliferations when there is flow cytometric evidence of biclonality (two separate kappa and lambda restricted populations), but the presence of same light chain restriction by two morphologically or phenotypically different processes does not prove that they are clonally related. If flow cytometry and/or IHC can demonstrate discordant light chain restriction, then it is safe to assume that two separate clonal processes are present. It is theoretically possible (and has been demonstrated very rarely) that a B-cell clone with kappa chain restriction can subsequently rearrange and express lambda chain. However, for all practical purposes, discordant light chain restriction can be assumed to indicate two clonal processes.
  - In most cases, these two B-cell neoplasms can be highlighted by IHC by their lineage defining antigens (CD20 for B-cells and CD138 for plasma cells, etc.) and/or by their separate geographic distributions in the core biopsy.
- When the B-cell lymphoma and PCN (or two separate B-cell lymphomas or PCNs) share the same light chain restriction, discordant heavy chain restriction may be used to demonstrate the two separate neoplasms. While discordant heavy chain restriction can sometimes be seen on immunohistochemical section, particularly for poorly differentiated PCN, SPEP/IFE provides more reliable evidence of biclonal processes (see Fig. 30.4 in Case 3).
- Perhaps most challenging is to dissect the simultaneous presence of a small mature B-cell neoplasm which can have significant (but highly variable) plasmacytic differentiation, such as CLL or LPL with concurrent PCN. In such cases, expression of either CD56 or cyclin D1 in

plasma cells suggests a separate PCN, in addition to CLL or LPL which can be detected by flow cytometry.

- Plasma cell component in small mature B-cell lymphoma with plasmacytoid differentiation is often negative for these aberrant antigens seen in PCN. Small mature B-cell component in this combination can be demonstrated by B-cell antigen stains such as CD20 and PAX5, presence of surface light chain restriction by flow cytometry, and absence of plasma cell specific antigen such as CD138.

- Cytogenetic study (FISH) for myeloma panel is now routinely performed on CD138 enriched sample. If cytogenetic abnormality, for instance, presence of del(13q), is detected in plasma cell enriched specimen, it can be compared with the result of the test performed on unsorted sample to determine whether the two components are related or not.
- As indicated above, two B-cell neoplasms with same light chain or heavy chain restriction are not necessarily clonally related. Additionally, a significant fraction of PCN does not express aberrant antigens such as CD56 or cyclin D1. In theory, immunoglobulin gene rearrangement analysis performed on microdissected tissues to compare amplicon sizes from the two morphologic components can determine their clonal relationship. However, in most case of small B-cell neoplasm with plasmacytic/plasmacytoid differentiation, and even in a majority of cases of concurrent small B-cell lymphoma and plasma cell neoplasm, plasma cells are often intermingled with the mature B-cell component without forming exclusive aggregates. Therefore, it is difficult to isolate or sort one component without contamination by the other.
  - In practice, if the plasma cells are well to moderately differentiated, positive for CD19, negative for CD56 and cyclin D1, and are a minor population admixed with many more small mature lymphocytes without forming exclusive aggregates, and IFE demonstrates a single clonal paraprotein, it is safe to assume the presence of a B-cell lymphoma with plasmacytic differentiation rather than two separate processes (Table 30.2).

References [20, 21, 34, 35]

Table 30.2 Distinction between B-cell leukemia/lymphoma with plasmacytic differentiation (clonal B-cell neoplasm) and concurrent B-cell neoplasm and plasma cell neoplasm (biclonal B-cell neoplasm)

	Single clonal B-cell neoplasm	Biclonal B-cell neoplasms
Geographic separation	–	+
Plasmablastic morphology	–	+
CD56 in plasma cells	–	+
Cyclin D1 in plasma cells	–	+
CD117 in plasma cells	–	+
Loss of CD19 in plasma cells	–	+
Retention of CD19 in plasma cells	+	–
Discordant light chain	–	++
Discordant heavy chain	–	+
Biclonality by SPEP/IFE	–	+
Positive for myeloma FISH	–	+

+ and ++ indicate the rated level of suggestion for the clonal relationship between neoplastic B-cells and neoplastic plasma cells, which represents the authors' own experience/opinion

8. Which subtypes of marrow involvement by more than one entity are clinically relevant and which are morphologically defined but have unproven/minimal clinical relevance?

- The clinical relevance of detecting two hematolymphoid neoplasms simultaneously in the marrow pertains to:
  - Treatment decisions: The requirement for treating both neoplasms separately and possible impediments in treatment of one due to the presence of the other neoplasm.
  - Prognosis: The relative prognostic impact of the two neoplasms and possible worsening of overall prognosis beyond that predicted for either process due to the simultaneous presence of both.
  - Marrow function: Long-term sequela of these processes and their treatment on bone marrow function.
- Treatment decisions: Treatment protocol for concurrent hematolymphoid neoplasms has not been established yet. The literature is limited to the experience of single case reports or small series, but the major strategy is to target the more aggressive component, for instance, treating myeloid neoplasm in CLL or PCM with AML. Otherwise, it is advocated that the cases should be handled on a case-by-case basis, and the component that causes clinical symptoms and signs should be targeted.
  - Since treatment of PCM and low-grade B-cell lymphomas differs significantly, distinction between plasma cell myeloma and B-cell lymphomas with marked plasmacytic differentiation is important. A small plasma cell component in MGUS or a small monoclonal B-cell component in monoclonal B-cell lymphocytosis of undetermined significance (MBLUS) does not need specific treatment.
  - Treatment-related myeloid neoplasms, primarily MDS and AML, due to prior chemoradiation, for lymphoma, PCM, or other malignant or non-malignant conditions, may require specific treatment such as demethylating agents or proteasome inhibitors. Such patients usually demonstrate "new" cytogenetic abnormalities in the myeloid clone. Even if active treatment is not instituted, the patients need close follow-up to monitor disease progression.

  - Cumulative toxicities from prior chemotherapy for one condition may preclude subsequent potentially curative treatment such as stem cell transplantation contemplated for the second condition.
- Prognosis: If the "primary" diagnosis suspected clinically has substantially worse prognosis than the incidentally determined second tumor, the latter will be clinically insignificant.
  - It is well documented that the presence of systemic mastocytosis along with another clonal hematolymphoid process worsens the prognosis for both conditions taken separately. The concurrent occurrence of myeloid and lymphoid neoplasms predicts a worse prognosis than either isolated neoplasm, due to additive morbidity and mortality.
  - Immune dysregulation due to overt or subclinical B-cell neoplasm may be etiologically relevant in cases of simultaneous discovery of B-cell and myeloid neoplasms and cases in which a myeloid neoplasm precedes the B-cell lymphoma. The clinical outcome of myeloid neoplasms in this group is similar to that of de novo diseases in general. While this group of myeloid neoplasms is considered unrelated to therapy, whether or not preexisting condition or concomitant condition facilitates the development of myeloid neoplasm is unclear. Literatures suggest that patients with indolent B-cell neoplasm may have an intrinsic predisposition to development of another hematolymphoid neoplasm. This group of the disease demonstrates that the proportion of MPN is significantly higher than the other related to therapy or de novo myeloid neoplasm in general, suggesting a unique pathogenesis in the group.
- Marrow function: The development of a myeloid neoplasm secondary to the presence of a small cell B-cell lymphoma, without history of chemotherapy for the lymphoma, is likely related to the immunodeficiency or immune dysregulation associated with the lymphoma [15] and may lead to marrow failure of variable severity in the future. This scenario may also explain cases of simultaneous diagnosis of CLL/PCN and myeloid neoplasm and cases of reversed sequence of the two hematolymphoid neoplasms, i.e., myeloid neoplasm diagnosed before CLL or PCN.

References [15, 17, 18, 23, 24, 32]

9. What is an adequate specimen for this condition?

- An adequate bone marrow biopsy for morphologic evaluation of concurrent hematolymphoid neoplasms should include a peripheral blood smear, aspirate smear, touch imprint, core biopsy, and clot section. In addition, aliquot of aspirate sample should be sent for flow cytometric analysis and cytogenetic studies.

10. What information can be conveyed to the clinician during each stage of the work up?

- When morphological findings suggest the possibility of marrow involvement by two hematolymphoid neoplasms, possible history suggesting one neoplasm or the other should be discussed with treating clinicians. If prior history of one neoplasm is confirmed, the treatment received by the patient for the primary malignancy should be verified from the treating clinician. The secondary neoplasm would be classified differently, depending on presence or absence of relevant history and corresponding treatment, particularly for the cases where the secondary neoplasm is myeloid.
- Cases of concurrent hematolymphoid neoplasms in bone marrow are rare, and clinicians do not usually expect identification of a second neoplasm. Therefore, in cases of known CLL or PCN, any unexpected identification of AML or MDS should elicit a communication with the treating clinician to emphasize the relationship of AML or MDS to prior therapy. As indicated above, therapy-related myeloid neoplasm predicts a poor clinical outcome compared with de novo counterpart (those without exposure to treatment).
- In case of CLL or PCN with low-risk MDS, the MDS portion may be overlooked until the cytogenetic analysis identified a clonal abnormality, usually few days to a week after completion of histopathologic evaluation. In this case, an addendum should be issued to report the diagnosis of MDS in addition to CLL or PCN, and the treating physicians should be contacted directly.
- The diagnosis, particularly of CLL or LPL with PCN, should be conveyed to clinician emphasizing biclonal nature of the neoplasms, and exclusion of clonal evolution of single clonal process. It should be indicated that after treatment, one neoplasm may persist as residual disease or may relapse, while the other neoplasm is completely in control, given their different biology and sensitivity to certain treatment.
- In case of concurrent CLL or PCN with myeloid neoplasm, or CLL or LPL with PCN, uncertain underlying pathogenesis should be emphasized, even though natural immunodeficiency may be the cause of secondary neoplasm.

References [15, 23, 24, 32]

11. What should be the approach to provide maximum, but defensible information, from limited specimen or work-up? What is a descriptive diagnosis appropriate in such situations?

- In case of CLL or PCN with MDS, the diagnosis of MDS may not be made definitely, due to absence of increased blasts and prominent dysplasia. At the moment, it may be adequate to make a descriptive diagnosis indicating suggestive evidence such as hypercellularity or mild dysplasia, and comments about suspicion for MDS and pending cytogenetic analysis to document the clonality. Of note, a significant number of cases won't be able to have the diagnosis established until supportive cytogenetic evidence, or the diagnosis is retrospectively rendered after supportive cytogenetic result. If cytogenetic study detects a clonal abnormality, the diagnosis of MDS is confirmed. Otherwise, clinician may need a close follow-up of the patient for possible disease evolution.
- In some cases of CLL or LPL with PCN, biclonal processes cannot be ultimately determined, due to minor PCN population without forming aggregates, absence of CD56 and cyclin D1, and absence of dual clonal paraproteins by SPEP/IFE. At this time, you may issue a descriptive diagnosis with comment suggestive of either small mature B-cell leukemia/lymphoma with plasmacytoid differentiation versus small B-cell neoplasm with concurrent PCN (MGUS).

References [15, 20, 21, 24]

12. When is it appropriate to seek external consultation for this condition?

- Bone marrow involvement by two separate neoplastic entities is rare, and one neoplastic component may potentially be overlooked. As with other areas in hematopathology, when morphology, ancillary studies, and clinical findings are not congruent, and the alternative interpretations have vastly different outcome for the patient or require substantially different treatments, an outside consultation should be obtained. In particular, persistent morphological features which suggest therapy-induced MDS/AML but which do not show any molecular or cytogenetic abnormalities may warrant outside consultation. Conversely, isolated cytogenetic or molecular abnormality, without morphological abnormalities, also need outside verification.

Case Presentations

Case 1

Learning Objectives

1. To become familiar with typical clinical scenario of AML in setting of PCM
2. To become familiar with the morphologic presentation, immunohistochemical features, flow cytometric findings, and cytogenetic studies of the disease
3. To discuss the clinical significance of AML or other myeloid neoplasm related to therapy for PCM in distinction from AML concurrent with PCN

Case History

A 64-year-old male patient with history of PCM was treated with chemotherapy followed by autologous stem cell transplant. He responded to therapy and underwent clinical remission. He had since received maintenance therapy with lenolidomide for 6 years. He recently presented with pancytopenia. Laboratory evaluation demonstrated serum paraprotein of the same type.

Bone Marrow Morphology and Immunohistochemical Findings

- A few circulating blasts in peripheral blood film.
- Increased blasts and myelodysplasia in aspirate smear (Fig. 30.1a).
- Hyperplastic bone marrow with increased blasts and atypical megakaryocytes on core biopsy section (Fig. 30.1b).
- Clusters of abnormal plasma cells highlighted by CD138 (Fig. 30.1c) and CD56 (Fig. 30.1d).
- CD117 stain highlights increased blasts and abnormal plasma cells (Fig. 30.1e).

Differential Diagnosis

- Acute myeloid leukemia, therapy-related, and residual plasma cell myeloma
- Acute leukemia of another cell lineage, therapy-related, and residual plasma cell myeloma
- High-grade myelodysplastic syndrome, therapy-related, and residual plasma cell myeloma

Ancillary Studies

- Flow cytometric findings
  - 23% myeloid blasts (Fig. 30.2a-d)
  - 1% phenotypically abnormal plasma cells with CD56 and CD117

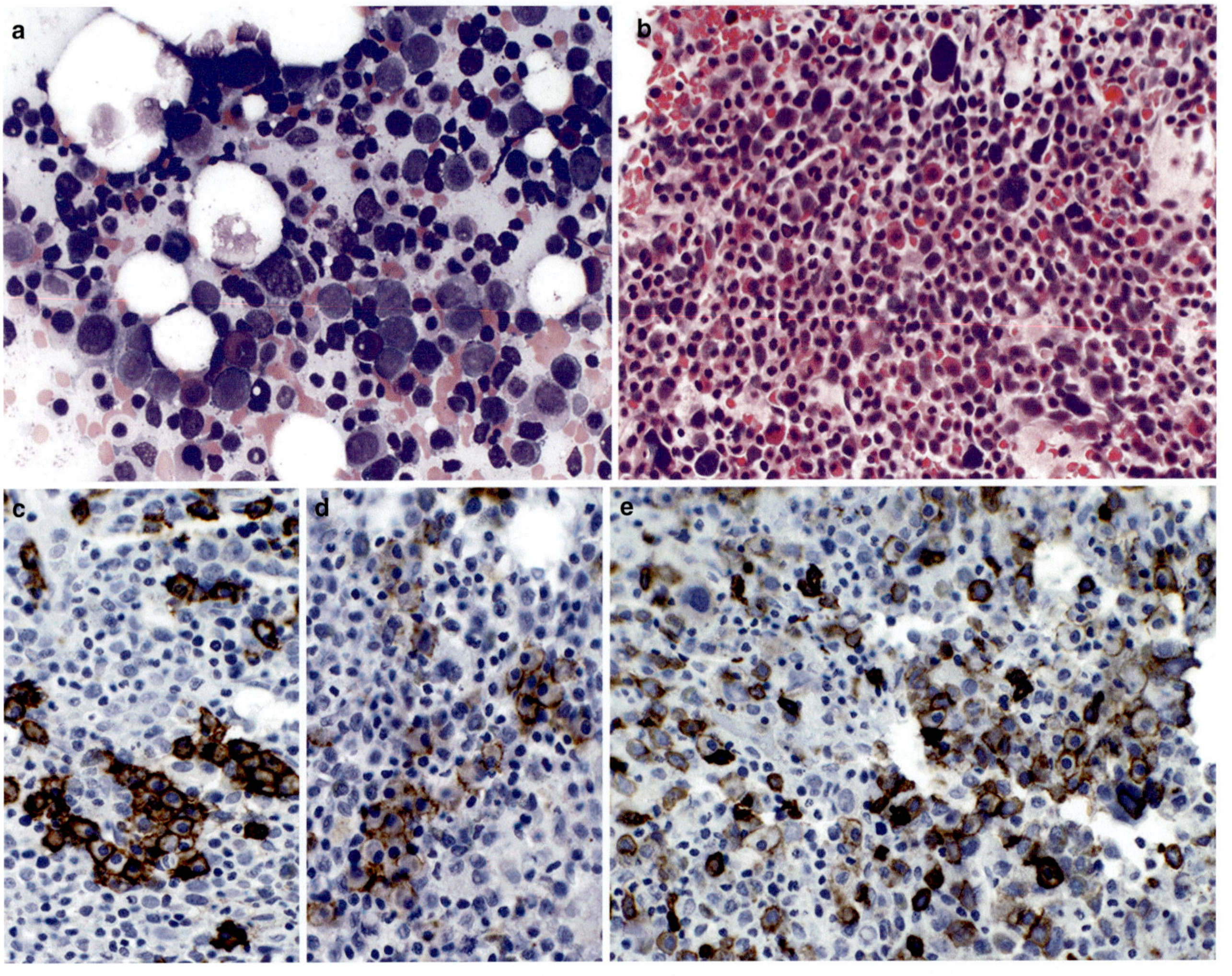

Fig. 30.1 Bone marrow examination of Case 1 with concurrent myeloid neoplasm and plasma cell neoplasm. (**a**) Bone marrow aspirate smear. Note small megakaryocytes, dysplastic erythroid precursors, and scattered blasts (Wright Giemsa stain). (**b**) Bone marrow core biopsy (H&E stain). Note hypercellularity, small megakaryocytes with hyperchromatic nuclei, and scattered increased blasts. (**c**) Clusters of plasma cells highlighted by CD138. (**d**) Plasma cells are positive for CD56. (**e**) Plasma cells are positive for CD117. In addition, the stain highlights scattered myeloid precursors with blastic morphology. **a**–**e**, ×400

- Cytogenetic analysis
  - Karyotype: 41~53,X,-Y,-4,der(5;17)(p10;q10)add(5)(p14),del(7)(q22),-13,-14,add(18)(p11.3),-19,-21,-22,+r,+2~10mar[cp20]
  - FISH on CD138 enriched plasma cells: del(17p13) in 81% of the total interphase nuclei

Final Diagnosis

1. **Acute myeloid leukemia, likely therapy-related (28% blasts)**
2. **Residual plasma cell myeloma (11% abnormal plasma cells)**

Take-Home Messages

1. Given the history of plasma cell myeloma and corresponding treatment, AML in this case is likely therapy-related.
2. Complex karyotypic abnormality with chromosome 7 or 5 change is more frequently seen in therapy-related myeloid neoplasm
3. Although regimens and doses used in myeloma chemotherapy are less mutagenic than chemotherapy for large B-cell lymphoma or acute leukemia, risk for AML and MDS does increase, especially with melphalan-containing protocol, compared with cases without exposure to

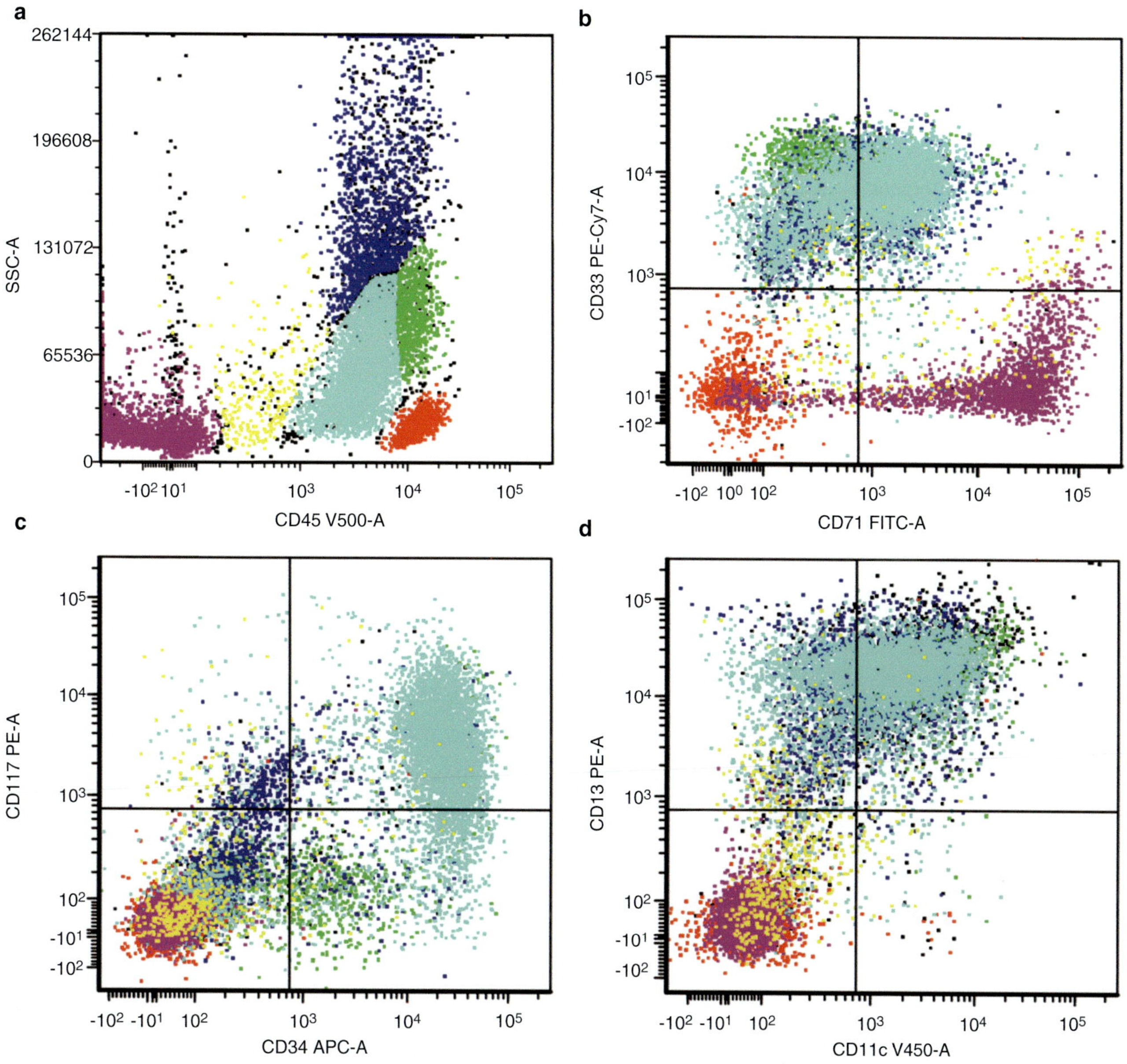

Fig. 30.2 Flow cytometric analysis demonstrating increased myeloid blasts in concurrent myeloid neoplasm and plasma cell neoplasm. (**a**) CD45 versus SSC plot shows increased events in blast window (*blue events*). The blasts are positive for CD33 (**b**), CD34, CD117 (**c**), and CD13 (**d**)

chemotherapy or radiotherapy, such as myeloid neoplasm in setting of MGUS.

Reference [15]

Case 2

Learning Objectives

1. To become familiar with typical clinical scenario of MDS in setting of CLL
2. To become familiar with morphologic presentation, immunohistochemical features, and flow cytometric findings of MDS in setting of CLL
3. To become familiar with diagnostic significance of cytogenetic findings in establishing the diagnosis of low-grade MDS
4. To discuss the clinical significance of MDS, AML, or other myeloid neoplasms related to therapy for CLL in distinction from each counterpart without prior exposure to chemotherapy

Case History A 59-year-old male patient with history of CLL was treated with chemotherapy followed by autologous stem cell transplant. He responded to therapy and underwent clinical remission. Five years after treatment, he presented with profound anemia and thrombocytopenia.

Bone Marrow Morphology and Immunohistochemical Findings

- Relative lymphocytosis with monotonous small- to medium-sized lymphocytes with clumped chromatin in peripheral blood film.
- Increase in small lymphocytes and myelodysplasia in aspirate smear and increase in blasts that are counted for 10 to 15% of the total nucleated cells.
- Interstitial lymphocytic infiltrate and myeloid hyperplasia with atypical megakaryocytic proliferation on core biopsy section (Fig. 30.3a).
- Small lymphocytes are positive for CD79a on core section (Fig. 30.3b).
- Dysplastic megakaryocytes (Fig. 30.3c) and increased myeloid blasts (Fig. 30.3d and e) on the core biopsy.

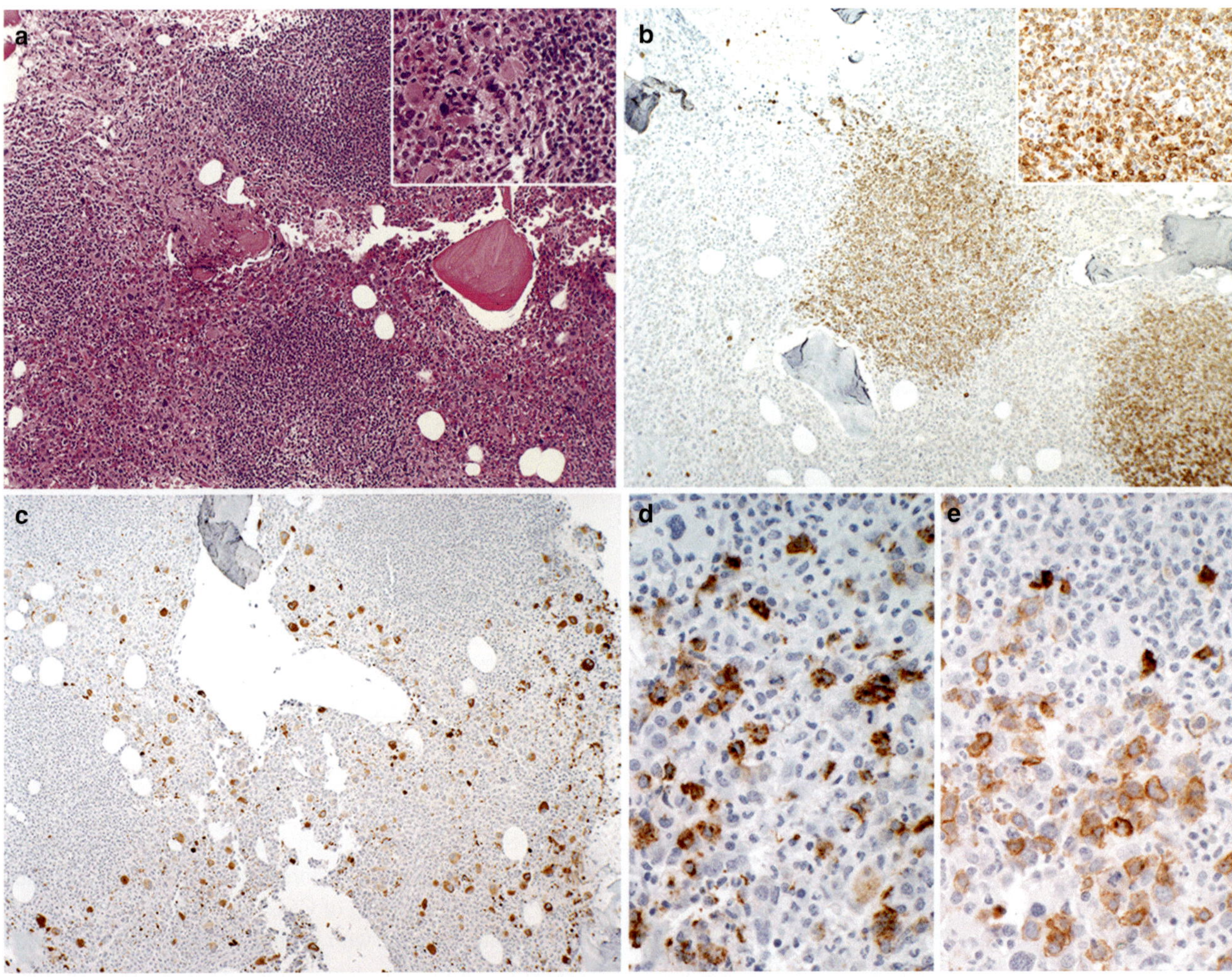

Fig. 30.3 Bone marrow examination of Case 2 with concurrent myeloid neoplasm and chronic lymphocytic leukemia. (**a**) Bone marrow core biopsy shows hypercellularity with nodular lymphoid aggregates and intervening hyperplastic hematopoietic elements. Note increased small hyperchromatic megakaryocytes. H&E stain, ×100. Inset shows a high magnification of the border between lymphoid nodules and adjacent hyperplastic hematopoiesis with increased megakaryocytes. H&E stain, ×400. (**b**) Nodular lymphoid aggregates are positive for CD79a. ×100. The inset shows small- to medium-sized lymphoid cells with cytoplasmic CD79a. ×400. (**c**) CD61 stain highlights increased small megakaryocytes between the lymphoid nodules. ×100. (**d**) CD34 stain shows increased blastic hematopoietic precursors adjacent to a lymphoid nodule. ×400. (**e**) CD117 stain highlights increased hematopoietic precursors adjacent to a lymphoid nodule (upper right corner). ×400

Differential Diagnosis

- Myelodysplastic syndrome, therapy-related, and residual chronic lymphocytic leukemia
- Residual chronic lymphocytic leukemia and reactive myeloid hyperplasia

Ancillary Studies

- Flow cytometric findings (data not shown):
  - 27% monoclonal B-cell population with CD5 and CD23
  - Aberrant CD56 in monocytes and granulocytic cells
  - 14% abnormal myeloid blasts
- Cytogenetic analysis:
  - Karyotype: 43–45,XY,add(1)(q?31),-3,add(5)(q31),-7,+8,-12,-15,-18,1-3mar[cp4]/47,XY,+3,add(9)(p13),-1,?del(17)(p11.2),?add(18)(q21),+mar[cp3]/46,XY [12]
  - FISH: del(13q) in 27% of the total interphase nuclei

Final Diagnosis

1. **High-grade myelodysplastic syndrome, likely therapy-related**
2. **Chronic lymphocytic leukemia (25% neoplastic B-cells)**

Take-Home Messages

1. Given the history of CLL and corresponding treatment, MDS in this case is likely therapy-related.
2. Complex karyotypic abnormality with monosomy 7 is more frequently seen in therapy-related myeloid neoplasm. Other cytogenetic changes related to therapy include monosomy 7, −7q, −5/−5q, and 11q23 rearrangement. In significant number of cases without prominent dysplasia or increased blasts, diagnosis of MDS cannot be established before identification of myeloid-related cytogenetic abnormalities, and in others, diagnosis of MDS is made retrospectively after an abnormal cytogenetic result.
3. Although regimens and doses used in CLL chemotherapy are less mutagenic than chemotherapy for large B-cell lymphoma or acute leukemia, risk for MDS, AML, and other myeloid neoplasms does increase, especially with fludarabine and cyclophosphamide-containing protocol, compared with cases without exposure to chemotherapy, such as myeloid neoplasm in setting of untreated CLL.

Case 3

Learning Objectives

1. To become familiar with typical clinical scenario of LPL in setting of PCN
2. To become familiar with morphologic presentation, immunohistochemical features, flow cytometric findings, and cytogenetic/molecular profile of LPL concurrent with PCN
3. To become familiar with laboratory features of LPL and PCN
4. To discuss the clinical significance of LPL with concurrent PCN

Case History

A 51-year-old female patient with history of pancytopenia. Laboratory evaluation demonstrated serum paraprotein of both IgM kappa and IgA kappa (Fig. 30.4).

Bone Marrow Morphology

- A few circulating plasmacytoid lymphocytes in peripheral blood film
- Increase in small mature lymphocytes and plasma cells in aspirate smear
- Lymphoid aggregates with clusters of plasma cells on core biopsy section (Fig. 30.5a)

Immunohistochemical Findings

- B-cells in lymphoid aggregates highlighted by PAX5 stain (Fig. 30.5b)
- Clusters of plasma cells highlighted by CD138, Cyclin D1, and CD56 stains (Fig. 30.5c, d, d- inset)

Differential Diagnosis

- Lymphoplasmacytic lymphoma and concurrent plasma cell myeloma
- Non-LPL type B-cell lymphoma and concurrent plasma cell myeloma

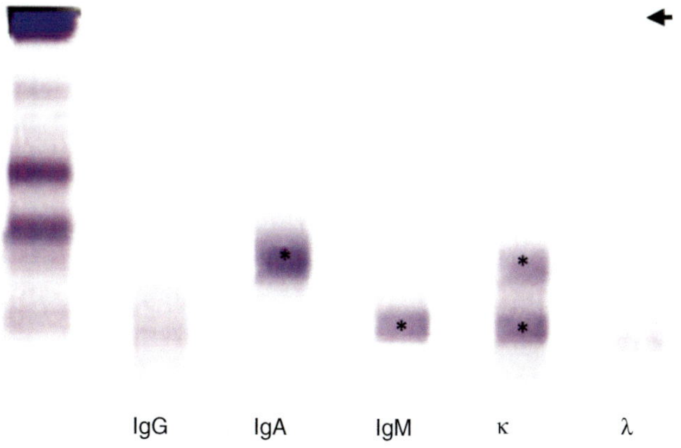

Fig. 30.4 Immunofixation serum protein electrophoresis of Case 3 with concurrent lymphoplasmacytic lymphoma and plasma cell neoplasm. Biclonal bands are identified, IgA kappa and IgM kappa (the bands marked by asterisk). The arrow indicates the application point of the sample, and the migration is from the top to the bottom

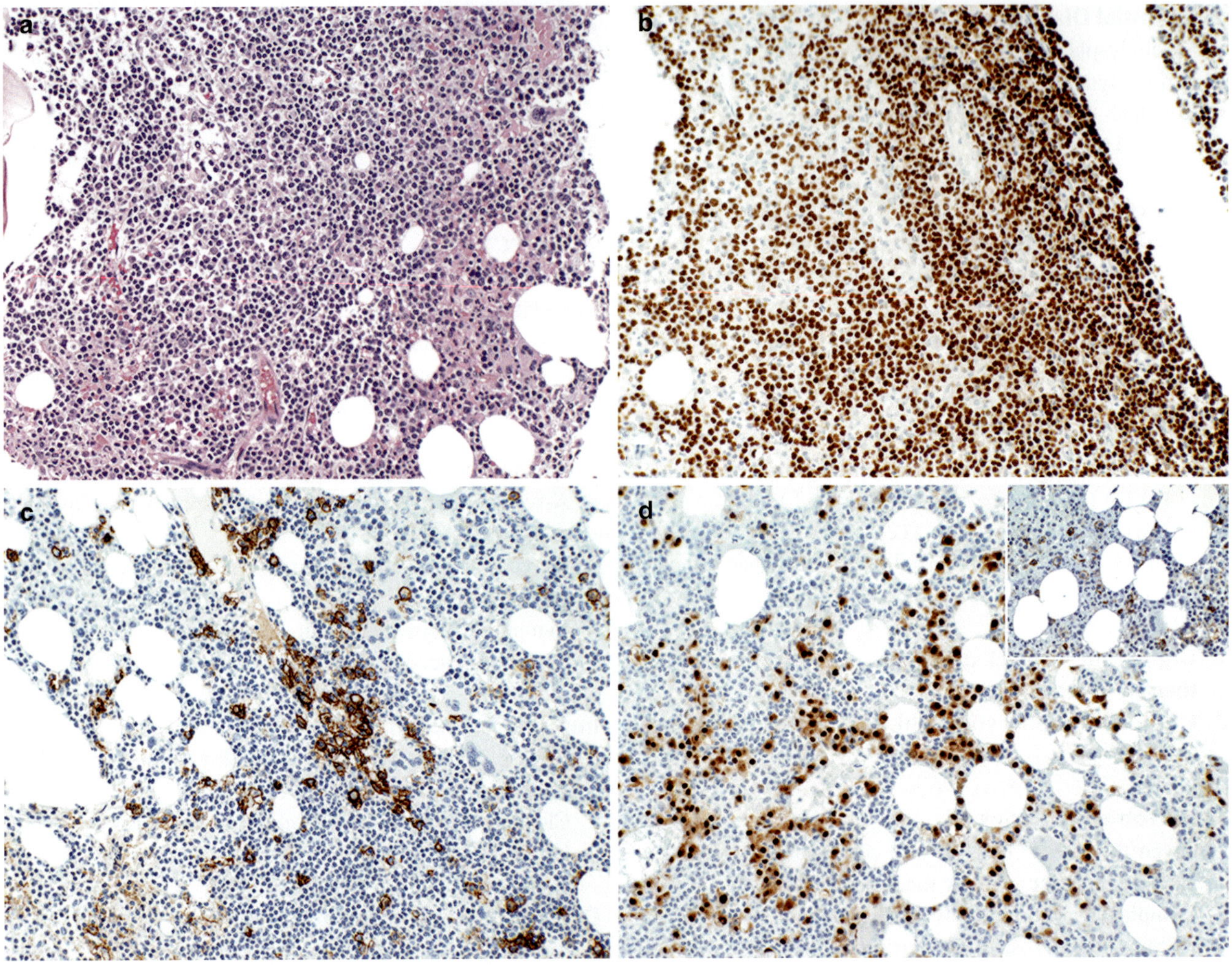

Fig. 30.5 Bone marrow examination of concurrent lymphoplasmacytic lymphoma and plasma cell neoplasm in Case 3. (**a**) Bone marrow core biopsy shows interstitial lymphoplasmacytic infiltrate (H&E stain). (**b**) These lymphocytes are positive for PAX5. (**c**) CD138 stain highlights clusters of plasma cells admixed with lymphoid cells. (**d**) Plasma cells are positive for cyclin D1 with nuclear staining. Inset shows CD56 staining in plasma cells. **a–d**, ×200

- Isolated lymphoplasmacytic lymphoma
- Isolated marginal zone lymphoma

Ancillary Studies

- Flow cytometric findings:
  - 29% monoclonal B-cell population with negative CD5 and negative CD10
  - 2% abnormal plasma cell population with aberrant CD56
- Cytogenetic analysis:
  - Karyotype : 46,XY [20]
  - FISH on CD138 enriched plasma cells: *CCND1/IGH* in 89% of interphase nuclei
- Molecular diagnosis:
  - Positive for *MYD88* L265P mutation in bone marrow aspirate sample

Final Diagnosis

1. **Lymphoplasmacytic lymphoma (30% lymphoma cells)**
2. **Plasma cell neoplasm (10% abnormal plasma cells)**

Take-Home Messages

1. LPL concomitant with PCN often manifests as biclonal paraprotein, with discordant light chain restriction and/or discordant heavy chain restriction.
2. Plasma cell component could show aggregates or clusters, and demonstrate aberrant expression of CD56, CD117, and/or cyclin D1, and be negative for CD19. While flow cytometry could detect both neoplastic populations, dual neoplastic components are best highlighted by immunohistochemistry because of their

distinct geographic distributions and aberrant expression of certain antigens on PCN.

3. FISH on plasma cell enriched sample may detect plasma cell specific abnormality, confirming the presence of PCN in addition to LPL.
4. *MYD88* L265P mutation occurs more frequent in LPL than other mature B-cell lymphoma, including MZL.

Case 4

Learning Objectives

1. To become familiar with typical clinical scenario of CLL and concurrent CML
2. To become familiar with morphologic presentation, immunohistochemical features, flow cytometric findings, and cytogenetic/molecular profile of CLL concurrent with CML
3. To discuss the clinical significance of CLL with concurrent CML

Case History

A 58-year-old female patient with history of leukocytosis. Laboratory evaluation demonstrated increased lymphocytes. She was diagnosed with chronic lymphocytic leukemia by flow cytometry and bone marrow examination. Due to low stage of the disease, the patient was observed without therapeutic intervention until her leukocytosis became worse 5 years later. She was found to have marked thrombocytosis (772×10^9/L) in addition to leukocytosis (30.2×10^6/L). Her blood hemoglobin level was 15.4 gram/dL.

Bone Marrow Morphology

- Increased abnormal lymphocytes, immature granulocytes, and increased basophils in peripheral blood film (Fig. 30.6a)
- Increase in small mature lymphocytes, myeloid hyperplasia, and increased small megakaryocytes in aspirate smear
- Interstitial lymphoid infiltrate and small megakaryocytic hyperplasia with clustering on core biopsy section (Fig. 30.6b)

Differential Diagnosis

- Chronic lymphocyticleukemia and concurrent chronic myeloid leukemia
- Chronic lymphocyticleukemia and concurrent non-CML type myeloproliferative neoplasm
- Chronic lymphocyticleukemia with reactive hematopoietic hyperplasia

Ancillary Studies

- Flow cytometric findings:
  - 35% monoclonal B-cell population with aberrant CD5 (Fig. 30.7a), dim lambda light chain restriction (Fig. 30.7b) and CD23
  - No increase in blasts
- Cytogenetic analysis:
  - Karyotype: 46,XX,t(9;22)(q34;q11.2) [13]/46,XX [6].
  - FISH: *BCR/ABL1* fusion in 47% of the total interphase nuclei; CLL panel including *TP53* (17p13.1), *ATM* (11q22.3), Trisomy 12, del(13q), monosomy 13 and t(11;14) is negative.

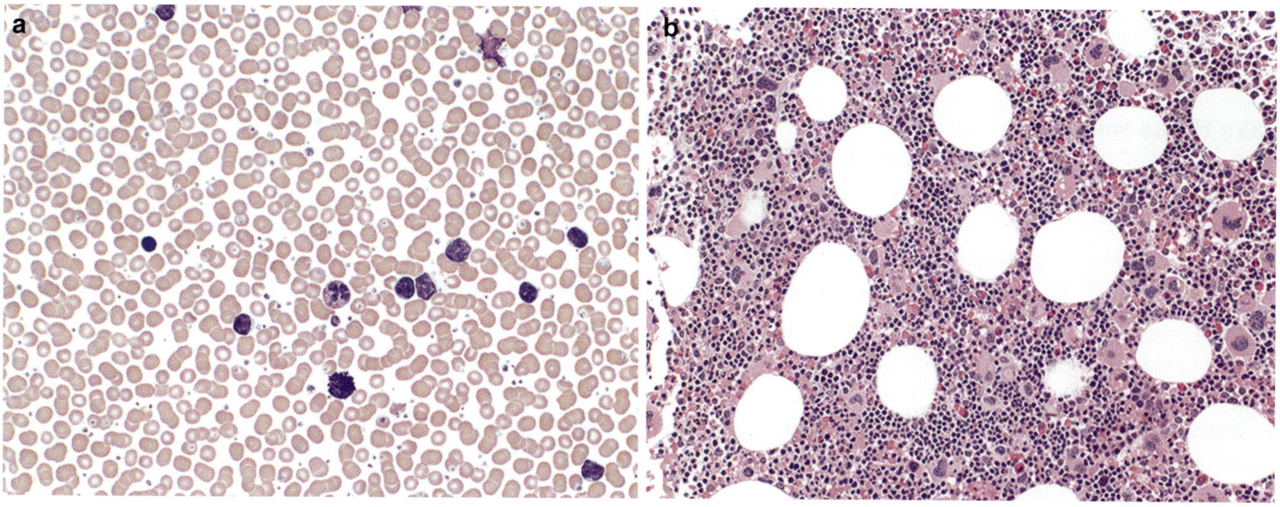

Fig. 30.6 Bone marrow examination of Case 4 with concurrent chronic lymphocytic leukemia and chronic myeloid leukemia. (**a**) Peripheral blood film shows circulating abnormal lymphocytes and abnormal basophils. Note the monotonous small lymphocytes with clumped chromatin characteristic of chronic lymphocytic leukemia. Wright Giemsa stain, ×400. (**b**) Bone marrow core biopsy demonstrates hypercellular bone marrow with interstitial lymphocytosis and small megakaryocytic hyperplasia. H&E stain, ×200

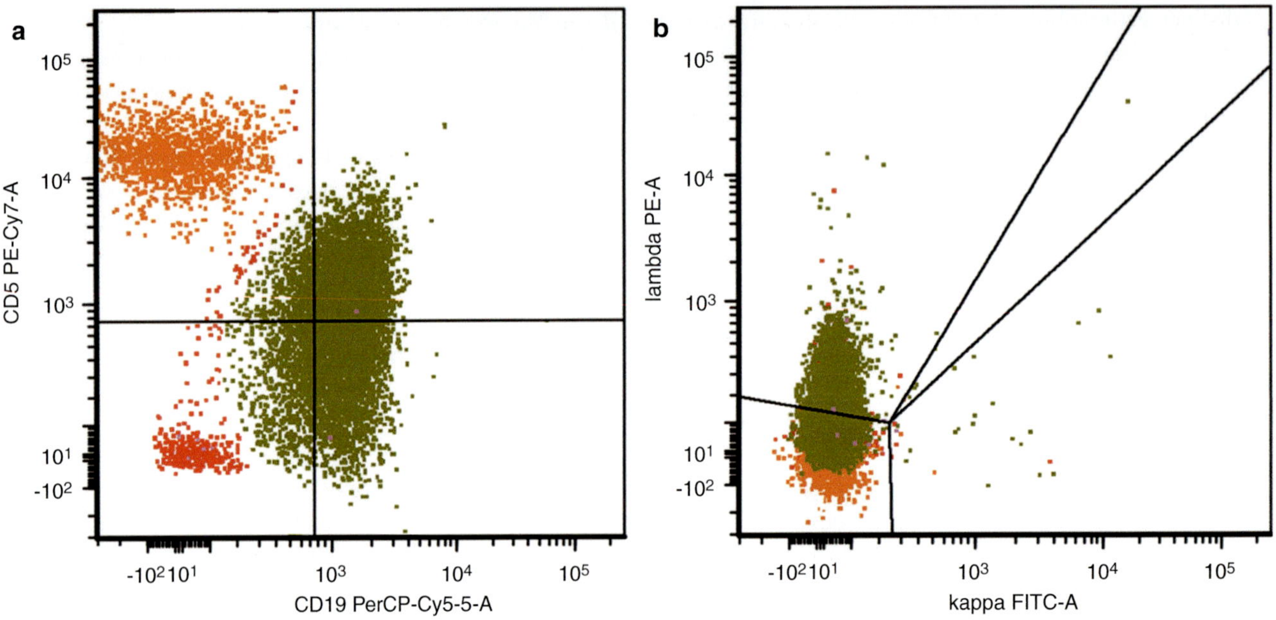

Fig. 30.7 (**a**, **b**) Flow cytometric analysis of bone marrow aspirate sample of Case 4. Note an abnormal B-cell population with aberrant CD5 that is dimmer than T-cells (*orange events*), and restricted lambda light chain (*dim staining)*

- Molecular diagnosis:
  - Positive for p210 *BCR/ABL1* fusion transcripts with International Scale (IS) % = 39.2541% in bone marrow aspirate sample
  - The detected *IGH* clone with a productive rearrangement shows a mutated status with 91.6–91.9% homology to the *IGHV4*–34∗01 or *IGHV4*–34∗04 gene germline sequence

Final Diagnosis

1. **Chronic myeloid leukemia (47%)**
2. **Chronic lymphocytic leukemia (40%)**

Take-Home Messages

1. In addition to MDS and AML, MPN including CML occurs in setting of untreated CLL. The pathogenesis of CML secondary to CLL is unknown, but the considerations are given to diminished immunity, underlying genomic defect, damaged microenvironment, etc.
2. Both neoplastic components could be visible on peripheral blood film, bone marrow aspirate smear and core section, but confirmation of each component needs ancillary tests. On section, CLL could show lymphoid aggregates or interstitial infiltrate and demonstrate aberrant expression of CD5 and CD23, while CML often displays atypical megakaryocytic hyperplasia and myeloid hyperplasia. Flow cytometry could detect CLL, but not CML.
3. Chromosomal analysis and FISH for *BCR/ABL1* can confirm the diagnosis of CML. Interphase FISH analysis can quantify CML components and CLL as well, if it harbors cytogenetic abnormalities.
4. While Q-RT-PCR for *BCR/ABL1* fusion transcripts can quantify the CML component, it could be diluted by CLL component, as in this case.

References

1. Akashi K, Harada M, Shibuya T, Fukagawa K, Kimura N, Sagawa K, et al. Simultaneous occurrence of myelomonocytic leukemia and multiple myeloma: involvement of common leukemic progenitors and their developmental abnormality of "lineage infidelity". J Cell Physiol. 1991;148(3):446–56.
2. Esteve J, Cervantes F, Rives S, Rozman M, Zarco MA, Montserrat E. Simultaneous occurrence of B-cell chronic lymphocytic leukemia and chronic myeloid leukemia with further evolution to lymphoid blast crisis. Haematologica. 1997;82(5):596–9.
3. Friesenbichler W, Schumich A, Simonitsch-Klupp I, Panzer-Grumayer R, Haas O, Mann G, et al. Concurrent acute myelofibrosis and acute lymphoblastic leukemia in childhood: case report and review of the literature. J Pediatr Hematol Oncol. 2018;40(3):235–7.
4. Abuelgasim KA, Rehan H, Alsubaie M, Al Atwi N, Al Balwi M, Alshieban S, et al. Coexistence of chronic myeloid leukemia and diffuse large B-cell lymphoma with antecedent chronic lymphocytic leukemia: a case report and review of the literature. J Med Case Rep. 2018;12(1):64.
5. Yin G, Xiao Z, He G, Miao K. Concurrent Epstein-Barr virus associated NK/T cell lymphoma after immunosuppressive therapy for aplastic anemia: report of a case and review of literature. Int J Clin Exp Pathol. 2015;8(6):7588–93.
6. Xiao Z, Ni Y, Yin G, Wu H, Li J, Miao K. Mantle cell lymphoma concurrent with T-large granular lymphocytic leukemia:

report of a case and review of literature. Int J Clin Exp Pathol. 2015;8(3):3365–9.
7. Xu J, Tang Y, Zhao S, Zhang W, Xiu Y, Liu T, et al. Angioimmunoblastic T-cell lymphoma with coexisting plasma cell myeloma: a case report and review of the literature. Tohoku J Exp Med. 2015;235(4):283–8.
8. Alomari A, Hui P, Xu M. Composite peripheral T-cell lymphoma not otherwise specified, and B-cell small lymphocytic lymphoma presenting with hemophagocytic lymphohistiocytosis. Int J Surg Pathol. 2013;21(3):303–8.
9. Perifanis V, Diamantidis MD, Chalvatzi K, Kaloutsi V, Markala D, Voulgaridou V, et al. Concurrent presentation of nodal myeloid sarcoma and bone marrow chronic lymphocytic leukemia/small lymphocytic lymphoma: a unique association. Int J Hematol. 2014;99(4):508–12.
10. Kishimoto W, Shirase T, Chihara D, Maeda T, Arimoto-Miyamoto K, Takeoka T, et al. Double-hit lymphoma with a feature of follicular lymphoma concurrent with clonally related B lymphoblastic leukemia: a preference of transformation for the bone marrow. J Clin Exp Hematop. 2012;52(2):113–9.
11. Huppmann AR, Liu ML, Nava VE. Concurrent diagnoses of Hodgkin lymphoma and biclonal myeloma in the bone marrow. Ann Diagn Pathol. 2010;14(4):268–72.
12. Starr AG, Jonna SR, Chahine JJ, Kallakury BV, Ujjani CS. Concurrent diagnosis of chronic myeloid leukemia and follicular lymphoma: an unreported presentation. Case Rep Hematol. 2018;2018:7493601.
13. Nair V, Prajapat D, Talwar D. Sarcoidosis and multiple myeloma: concurrent presentation of an unusual association. Lung India. 2016;33(1):75–8.
14. Kishimoto W, Takiuchi Y, Nakae Y, Tabata S, Fukunaga A, Matsuzaki N, et al. A case of AITL complicated by EBV-positive B cell and monoclonal plasma cell proliferation and effectively treated with lenalidomide. Int J Hematol. 2019;109:499.
15. Reddi DM, Lu CM, Fedoriw G, Liu YC, Wang FF, Ely S, et al. Myeloid neoplasms secondary to plasma cell myeloma: an intrinsic predisposition or therapy-related phenomenon? A clinicopathologic study of 41 cases and correlation of cytogenetic features with treatment regimens. Am J Clin Pathol. 2012;138(6):855–66.
16. Malhotra J, Kremyanskaya M, Schorr E, Hoffman R, Mascarenhas J. Coexistence of myeloproliferative neoplasm and plasma-cell dyscrasia. Clin Lymphoma Myeloma Leuk. 2014;14(1):31–6.
17. Chavez JC, Dalia S, Sandoval-Sus J, Kharfan-Dabaja MA, Al-Ali N, Komrokji R, et al. Second myeloid malignancies in a large cohort of patients with chronic lymphocytic leukemia: a single institution experience. Clin Lymphoma Myeloma Leuk. 2015;15(Suppl):S14–8.
18. Lai R, Arber DA, Brynes RK, Chan O, Chang KL. Untreated chronic lymphocytic leukemia concurrent with or followed by acute myelogenous leukemia or myelodysplastic syndrome. A report of five cases and review of the literature. Am J Clin Pathol. 1999;111(3):373–8.
19. Huh YO, Medeiros LJ, Ravandi F, Konoplev S, Jorgensen JL, Miranda RN. T-cell large granular lymphocyte leukemia associated with myelodysplastic syndrome: a clinicopathologic study of nine cases. Am J Clin Pathol. 2009;131(3):347–56.
20. Alley CL, Wang E, Dunphy CH, Gong JZ, Lu CM, Boswell EL, et al. Diagnostic and clinical considerations in concomitant bone marrow involvement by plasma cell myeloma and chronic lymphocytic leukemia/monoclonal B-cell lymphocytosis: a series of 15 cases and review of literature. Arch Pathol Lab Med. 2013;137(4):503–17.
21. Wang E, Kulbacki E, Stoecker M. Concomitant Waldenstrom macroglobulinemia and IgA plasmablastic myeloma in a patient with untreated IgM paraproteinemia: sequential development of biclonal B-cell neoplasms over a 10-year period in a single individual. Hum Pathol. 2012;43(7):1135–41.
22. Lesesve JF, Feugier P, Lamy T, Bene MC, Gregoire MJ, Lenormand B, et al. Association of B-chronic lymphocytic leukaemia and T-large granular lymphocyte leukaemia. Clin Lab Haematol. 2000;22(2):121–2.
23. Chakhachiro Z, Yin CC, Abruzzo LV, Aladily TN, Barron LL, Banks HE, et al. B-lymphoblastic leukemia in patients with chronic lymphocytic leukemia: a report of four cases. Am J Clin Pathol. 2015;144(2):333–40.
24. Wu B, Ingersoll K, Rehder C, Wang E. B-lymphoblastic leukemia in a patient with chronic lymphocytic leukemia: sequential development of biclonal B-cell neoplasms over a 23-year period in a single individual. Pathol Res Pract. 2016;212(11):1089–93.
25. Masarova L, Newberry KJ, Pierce SA, Estrov Z, Cortes JE, Kantarjian HM, et al. Association of lymphoid malignancies and Philadelphia-chromosome negative myeloproliferative neoplasms: clinical characteristics, therapy and outcome. Leuk Res. 2015;39(8):822–7.
26. Le Clech L, Sakka M, Meskar A, Kerspern H, Eveillard JR, Berthou C, et al. The presence of monoclonal gammopathy in Ph-negative myeloproliferative neoplasms is associated with a detrimental effect on outcomes. Leuk Lymphoma. 2017;58(11):2582–7.
27. Laurenti L, Tarnani M, Nichele I, Ciolli S, Cortelezzi A, Forconi F, et al. The coexistence of chronic lymphocytic leukemia and myeloproliperative neoplasms: a retrospective multicentric GIMEMA experience. Am J Hematol. 2011;86(12):1007–12.
28. Garrido P, Jimenez P, Sanchez C, Valero F, Balanzategui A, Almagro M, et al. Molecular and flow cytometry characterization during the follow-up of three simultaneous lymphoproliferative disorders: hairy cell leukemia, monoclonal B-cell lymphocytosis, and CD4(++) /CD8(+/− dim) T-large granular lymphocytosis--a case report. Cytometry B Clin Cytom. 2011;80(3):195–200.
29. Morton LM, Curtis RE, Linet MS, Bluhm EC, Tucker MA, Caporaso N, et al. Second malignancy risks after non-Hodgkin's lymphoma and chronic lymphocytic leukemia: differences by lymphoma subtype. J Clin Oncol. 2010;28(33):4935–44.
30. Smith MR, Neuberg D, Flinn IW, Grever MR, Lazarus HM, Rowe JM, et al. Incidence of therapy-related myeloid neoplasia after initial therapy for chronic lymphocytic leukemia with fludarabine-cyclophosphamide versus fludarabine: long-term follow-up of US Intergroup Study E2997. Blood. 2011;118(13):3525–7.
31. Arber DA, Orazi A, Hasserjian R, Thiele J, Borowitz MJ, Le Beau MM, et al. The 2016 revision to the World Health Organization classification of myeloid neoplasms and acute leukemia. Blood. 2016;127(20):2391–405.
32. Zhou Y, Tang G, Medeiros LJ, McDonnell TJ, Keating MJ, Wierda WG, et al. Therapy-related myeloid neoplasms following fludarabine, cyclophosphamide, and rituximab (FCR) treatment in patients with chronic lymphocytic leukemia/small lymphocytic lymphoma. Mod Pathol. 2012;25(2):237–45.
33. D'Arena G, Gemei M, Luciano L, D'Auria F, Deaglio S, Statuto T, et al. Chronic lymphocytic leukemia after chronic myeloid leukemia in the same patient: two different genomic events and a common treatment? J Clin Oncol. 2012;30(32):e327–30.
34. Mansour AT, Shandiz AE, Zimmerman MK, Roth TD, Zhou J. Concomitant lymphoplasmacytic lymphoma and plasma cell myeloma, a diagnostic challenge. Am J Blood Res. 2017;7(2):10–7.
35. Carulli G, Ciancia EM, Azzara A, Ottaviano V, Grassi S, Ciabatti E, et al. Simultaneous presentation of Waldenstrom macroglobulinemia and multiple myeloma: multidisciplinary diagnosis, treatment and 30-month follow-up. J Clin Exp Hematop. 2013;53(1):29–36.

Detection of Minimal Residual Disease

31

Yi Zhou

List of Frequently Asked Questions

1. What is minimal residual disease?
2. Why is minimal residual disease testing clinically important?
3. Which methods are commonly used in minimal residual disease detection and how do they work?
4. What are the strengths and limitations of next-generation-sequencing applied in MRD testing?
5. Are there standard antibody panels used in MFC-based MRD testing?
6. How is MRD identified in the MFC data analysis?
7. Which pre-analytic factors should be considered in MRD testing?

1. What is minimal residual disease?

Minimal residual disease (MRD) is the presence of low-level disease detected in bone marrow or peripheral blood using high sensitivity ancillary technics in patients with hematopoietic malignancies in complete remission. Complete remission (CR) in general is defined as the absence of morphologic evidence of disease and the recovery of complete blood counts after treatment. In some patients, however, tumor cells with the abnormal immunophenotype or genetic abnormality associated with the neoplasm can still be detected in CR by multiparameter flow cytometry (MFC) or molecular testing, respectively. These ancillary technics are much more sensitive than morphologic evaluation. Disease can be detected typically at a level of $1{:}10^3$ (= 0.1%) to $1{:}10^6$ (= 0.0001%) of total nucleated cells, compared with 1:20 (=5%) cells by morphology [1, 2].

Y. Zhou (✉)
Pathology and Laboratory Medicine, University of Miami Miller School of Medicine, Miami, FL, USA
e-mail: yxz1599@miami.edu

MRD has been extensively studied in acute lymphoblastic leukemia (ALL) [3, 4], acute myeloid leukemia (AML) [5, 6], chronic lymphocytic leukemia (CLL) [7, 8], and multiple myeloma (MM) [9, 10]. All of these diseases predominantly occur as bone marrow diseases.

2. Why is minimal residual disease testing clinically important?

- Prognosis: presence of MRD in CR is a significant risk factor for relapse [11–26]. More importantly, the prognostic significance of MRD is independent of other clinical and genetic risk factors, which are typically identified before starting treatment. MRD testing provides an objective assessment of the quality of remission (Fig. 31.1). In fact, patients with AML who are in morphologic remission (≤5% blasts) but have MRD detected by MFC demonstrate similar outcomes to those who do not achieve morphologic remission [26, 27]. On the other hand, patients who appear to have persistent disease (≥5% blasts by morphology) but are negative for MRD have similar outcomes to those who are in morphologic remission and negative for MRD [28–31]. It is worth noting that clinical significance of MRD varies depending on the clinical context, such as type of treatment and sampling time during or after treatment.
- Guidance for additional treatment: MRD-positive patients may receive therapy intensification, novel therapy, or hematopoietic stem cell transplants to eradicate MRD, whereas MRD negative patients may receive less therapy to minimize therapy-related morbidity and mortality. The MRD-guided treatment has proven beneficial in some prospective trials in acute lymphoblastic leukemia [32–34] and subtypes of acute myeloid leukemia [35, 36].
- Clinical trials of novel treatments: Good correlation between MRD status at CR and the clinical outcome suggests MRD status may be a suitable surrogate end-point

E. Wang, A. S. Lagoo (eds.), *Practical Lymph Node and Bone Marrow Pathology*, Practical Anatomic Pathology,
https://doi.org/10.1007/978-3-030-32189-5_31

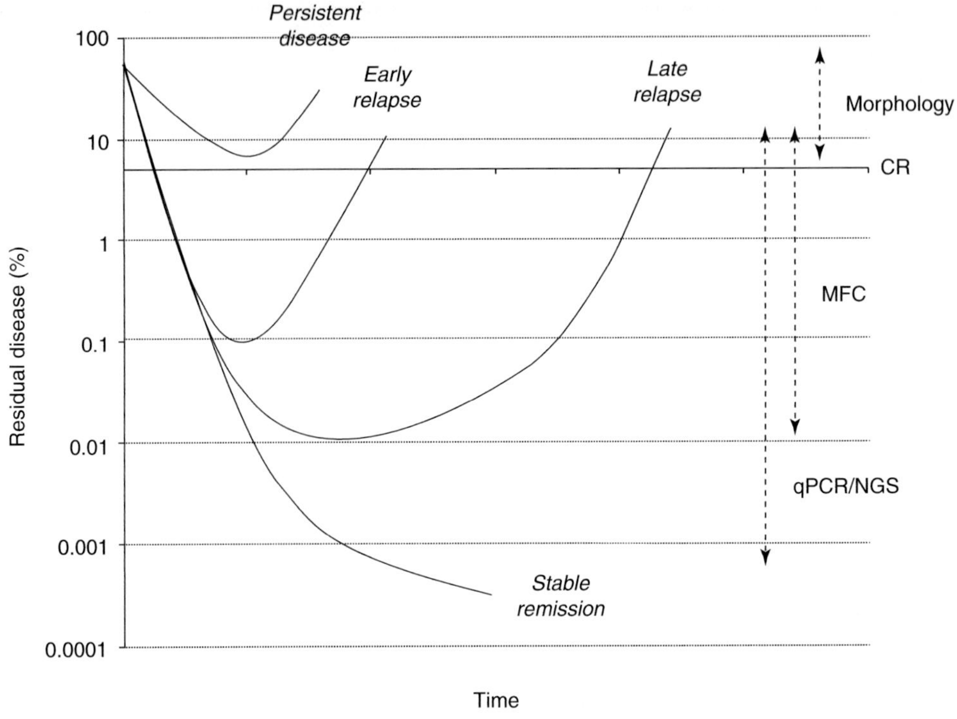

Fig. 31.1 MRD testing and duration of remission. MRD testing after induction therapy can provide independent risk assessment for relapse. The lower the level of the MRD is, the longer the duration of remission may be. Absence of MRD detected by sensitive MRD assay, typically with limit of detection below 0.01% (less than 1 in 104 leukocytes), may predict stable remission

Table 31.1 Comparison of MRD detection methods

	FISH	MFC	ASO-qPCR	RT-qPCR	NGS
Analyte	Chromosomes (translocations, deletions, or additions)	Abnormal protein expression	DNA (clonal *IG or TCR* rearrangement)	RNA (recurrent fusion genes or *NPM1* mutation)	DNA and RNA (mutations, copy number variations, or fusion genes)
Disease indication	Lymphoid and myeloid neoplasm	Lymphoid and myeloid neoplasm	Lymphoid neoplasm	Lymphoid and myeloid neoplasm	Lymphoid and myeloid neoplasm
Applicability	Small subset	>90%	90–95%	~40%	90–95%
Limit of detection	10^{-2}	10^{-3} to 10^{-4}	10^{-4} to 10^{-5}	10^{-5} to 10^{-6}	10^{-3} to 10^{-6}
Advantage	Standardized test	Fast, low cost, may not require pre-treatment data	Sensitive, specific, standardized	Sensitive, specific and standardizable	Sensitive, specific, standardizable, multiplexing
Disadvantage	Low sensitivity and applicability	Variable sensitivity, requiring extensive experience, limited standardization	Requiring personalized ASO design and validation, time consuming with high cost	Low applicability	Variable sensitivity, high cost, requiring pre-treatment sequencing

in clinical trials, which will significantly shorten the clinical trial cycle and accelerate drug-development. But well-controlled prospective clinical trials are still needed to prove this concept.

- Current application of MRD: In addition to lymphoblastic leukemia [37], recent recommendations for treatment of acute myeloid leukemia [38], chronic lymphocytic leukemia [39], and multiple myeloma [40] have included MRD status as a category in the assessment of treatment response. MRD testing is especially important in clinical trials aimed at maximizing the depth of remission.

3. Which methods are commonly used in minimal residual disease detection and how do they work?

- MRD testing relies on the detection of tumor-associated immunophenotypes and/or genetic abnormalities. Multiparameter flow cytometry (MFC) and real time quantitative polymerase chain reaction (qPCR) have been the most commonly used testing methods since the early 1990s [41, 42]. Next-generation-sequencing (NGS) has recently been explored in MRD detection (Table 31.1).

- MFC detects binding of fluorescently labeled antibodies against selected protein markers that collectively distinguish a neoplastic population from normal hematopoietic populations. MRD is typically identified as a discrete cell population comprising of more than 20–50 cells with an immunophenotype clearly different from its normal counterparts. Using 8 or 10 color MFC, an abnormal population can be detected at a level of 0.01% (10^{-4}) of total nucleated cells. Assay sensitivity depends on the tested antibodies (antibody panel), sample processing, number of analyzed events, and operator's knowledge of immunophenotypic pattern of normal hematopoietic populations and their reactive changes.
- Some genetic markers associated with hematopoietic malignancies can be detected by qPCR. These markers include clonal immunoglobulin and/or T-cell receptor gene (*IG-TR*) rearrangements, recurrent gene fusion, or gene mutations. Clonal *IG or TCR* rearrangement in ALL [43], CLL [44], or MM [45, 46] can be detected by allele-specific oligonucleotide quantitative PCR (ASO-qPCR), which detects a specific *IG or TCR* rearrangement using personalized primers in qPCR reaction. A similar approach has also been used in the detection of mutated *NPM1* in AML [47]. Recurrent gene fusions in ALL or AML can be detected by reverse transcription qPCR (RT-qPCR) [12, 48]. Quantitative PCR-based MRD testing is highly sensitive, specific, and standardizable and thus is considered the gold standard in MRD testing. On the other hand, ASO-PCR requires DNA sequencing at the time of initial diagnosis. The complexity and high cost of personalized primer design and validation limits its application to centralized laboratories. False negatives occur if the sequence of a pre-determined genetic marker changes after therapy.

4. What are the strengths and limitations of next-generation-sequencing applied in MRD testing?

- Compared to ASO-PCR, the NGS approach does not require laborious ASO design and validation, thus simplifying the MRD testing workflow. One application is immunosequencing to detect low-level clonal *IG or TCR* clonal rearrangement [19, 22, 49–51]. NGS also avoids false positives due to nonspecific ASO binding and false negatives due to clonal evolution with sequence changes [52].
- NGS provides a platform for parallel sequencing of a panel of hotspot mutations. Approximately 90% of acute myeloid leukemias carry at least one mutation in a panel of genes commonly mutated in myeloid neoplasm (i.e., hotspot mutations) [53–55]. With sufficient sequencing coverage, NGS can detect rare mutation(s) associated with residual AML. This application is best demonstrated in the detection of mutated *NPM1* at a level of 0.01% with a linear dynamic range compatible with qPCR [56–58]. NGS panel based MRD testing was first tested in 2015 [55] and has since been confirmed in larger studies of AML patients [53, 59].
- Challenges in NGS-based mutation detection include (1) To distinguish low-level mutation from random errors generated in the sequencing reaction can be challenging. It is estimated that the sequencing error rate in NGS is up to 1%, with 2% variant allele frequency (VAF) being the commonly accepted limit of detection. This error rate, however, can be reduced through in silico correction or the use of molecular barcoding [60]. (2) The other challenge is to distinguish mutations associated with acute leukemia from mutation present in non-leukemic clonal proliferation. A recent study has shown that the presence of mutations associated with clonal hematopoiesis, including *TET2*, *DNMT3A*, and *ASXL1*, does not have significant prognostic value as compared to the presence of other mutations [53].

5. Are there standard antibody panels used in MFC- based MRD testing?

Antibodies used in MRD testing are selected to maximally separate a neoplastic population from its normal counterparts. This usually requires one to three testing tubes, each containing 8–10 antibodies. Typically, an MRD testing panel includes lineage identification markers, maturation markers (for acute leukemia), and markers that are aberrantly expressed on neoplastic cells. In practice, the selection of the antibody panel depends on clinical utility, flow cytometer, cost, operator experience, and diagnostic approach used to identify leukemic blasts. Some of the well-validated antibody panels used in MRD detection are summarized in Table 31.2.

Table 31.2 Antibody panels used in MRD detection

B-lymphoblastic leukemia
CD9, CD10, CD13/CD33, CD19, CD20, CD34, CD38, CD45, CD58 [66]
CD10, CD19, CD20, CD38, CD45, CD81, CD66c, CD73, CD123, CD304 [67]
Chronic lymphocytic leukemia
CD3, CD5, CD19, CD20, CD22, CD43, CD79b, CD81 [22]
Multiple myeloma
CD19, CD27, CD38, CD45, CD56, CD81, CD117, CD138, cIgK, cIgλ [68, 69]
Acute myeloid leukemia
CD4, CD5, CD7, CD13, CD14, CD15, CD16, CD19, CD33, CD34, CD38, CD45, CD56, CD64, CD117, CD123, HLA-DR [70]
CD2, CD4, CD7, CD11b, CD13, CD14, CD15, CD19, CD33, CD34, CD38, CD45, CD56, CD64, CD117, HLA-DR [64]
CD45RA, CLL-1, TIM-3, CD7, CD11b, CD22, CD34, CD38, CD56, CD123, CD33, CD44 (AML leukemic stem cell) [64]

6. How is MRD identified in the MFC data analysis?

In general, neoplastic cells are identified by two related approaches in MFC analysis (Table 31.3).

- LAIP approach requires identification of leukemia-associated-immunophenotypes (LAIPs) before treatment; selected antibody combinations best representing LAIPs are used in MRD testing after therapy [61]. The limit of detection of tested LAIP can be determined by the background expression in non-leukemic specimens. The LAIP approach has a pre-defined limit-of-detection for each tested LAIP and provides consistency in MRD detection, but it requires highly harmonized testing protocols. More importantly, this approach is not effective if LAIPs or normal background populations change significantly after therapy.
- Different-from-normal approach (DfN) identifies blast populations with an immunophenotype significantly differing from regenerative hematopoietic cell populations after therapy [62, 63]. DfN uses the same antibody panel for diagnosis and MRD testing. This approach takes population density and distribution into consideration to distinguish background noise from a true abnormal population (see case studies). Since pre-treatment LAIPs are not required, DfN is resilient to immunophenotypic change after therapy and can be applied in laboratories where pre-treatment LAIPs are not available. On the other hand, DfN heavily relies on the operator's knowledge of the immunophenotypic pattern of normal hematopoietic populations; therefore, inter-observer discrepancies may be higher. In addition, DfN does not distinguish acute leukemia from pre-leukemic clonal hematopoiesis that may exhibit immunophenotypic aberrancies.
- Using higher-level multicolor flow cytometer (>= 8 simultaneous antigens), LAIP and DfN can be integrated in a LAIP-based-DfN approach [64]. The ELN MRD Working Party recommends characterizing phenotypic abnormalities observed in MRD testing into three categories: DfN and identical to LAIPs detected at diagnosis, DfN but different from LAIPs, and DfN without diagnostic LAIPs.

Table 31.3 Comparison of two MRD detection approaches in MFC data analysis

Leukemia-associated immunophenotypes (LAIPs)	Different-from-normal (DfN)
Pre-treatment specimen required	Pre-treatment specimen NOT required
LAIPs identified before treatment	LAIPs identified at any time
Predetermined sensitivity for each LAIP	Sensitivity varies between patients and specimens
Simple analysis procedure	Requires extensive knowledge of normal immunophenotypes
Complex workflow in LAIP identification and validation	Standardized work flow
Vulnerable to changes in LAIP	Robust to changes in LAIP

7. Which pre-analytic factors should be considered in MRD testing?

- Specimen type: MRD testing on bone marrow is approximately 10 times more sensitive than testing on peripheral blood. Bone marrow aspirate is typically tested in the assessment of treatment response at the time of remission. Collecting peripheral blood is much less invasive than collecting bone marrow, however. Therefore, peripheral blood can be more frequently tested. If detection sensitivity is sufficient, peripheral blood may be more suitable for disease surveillance [65] and provide better prognostic stratification [24, 35].
- Sample quality. Adequate sample quality is a prerequisite in MRD detection. Hemodilution is a major factor that reduces detection sensitivity in bone marrow aspirate. To minimize hemodilution, it is strongly recommended that MRD is tested using the first pull of marrow aspirate without excessive volume (less than 10 ml) [64]. Bone marrow aspirate remains adequate for 48 hours after collection at room temperature without excessive temperature change. Hemolysis, clotting, and large aspirate volumes should be avoided. Less than 85% of viability suggests compromised sample quality.
- Total number cells analyzed. In MFC MRD testing, 2×10^5 to 5×10^6 leukocytes per tube are analyzed to reach detection sensitivity at a level of 10^{-4}. In molecular MRD testing, if RNA is tested for gene fusion or mutated genes, 1 μg RNA is used for cDNA synthesis, and cDNA equivalent to 0.1 μg RNA (approximately 2×10^5 cells) is tested per reaction; if genomic DNA is tested, 0.1 to 1 μg DNA (approximately 1.5×10^4 to 1.5×10^5 diploid cells) is tested per reaction.
- Reporting MRD results should include: (1) the absolute number of abnormal cells detected and the percentage of abnormal cells in total analyzed leukocytes, (2) the status of the detected abnormality in pre-treatment specimen, (3) MRD status according to a pre-determined clinical threshold, (4) the analytical limit of detection of abnormal cells, (5) comments on sample quality in terms of viability, regenerative hematopoiesis, and, for bone marrow, presence of hemodilution artifact.

Case Presentations

Case 1

Learning Objective
Understand the principles in distinguishing B-lymphoblasts from regenerative immature B cells by flow cytometry.

Case History
A 27-year-old male was treated for B-lymphoblastic leukemia. Bone marrow aspirate was collected on day 29 after induction for assessment of treatment response.

Findings (Fig. 31.2)
- Immature B cells have a characteristic immunophenotype, including low side scatter with expression of CD10, CD19, variable CD20, and moderate CD45.
- Normal immature B cells (in blue) have uniform CD38 expression and gradual increase in CD20 expression.
- Residual B-lymphoblastic leukemia (in red) represents 0.01% of nucleated mononuclear cells. Compared to the normal immature B cells, the residual leukemia has abnormal expression of CD10 (increased), CD38 (decreased), and CD58 (increased).

Differential Diagnosis
- Presence versus absence of residual B-lymphoblastic leukemia

Final Diagnosis
Residual/recurrent B-lymphoblastic leukemia/lymphoma, representing 0.01% of nucleated mononucleated cells

Take-Home Messages
1. Neoplastic B-lymphoblasts usually have an immunophenotype that is different from regenerative immature B-cell precursors.
2. The most common immunophenotype aberrancies on B-lymphoblasts include increase in CD10 and/or CD58, and loss or decrease in CD38 and/or CD45.

Case 2

Learning Objective
Know the application of flow cytometry and quantitative PCR in detection of B-lymphoblasts associated with *BCR-ABL1*

Case History
A 75-year-old female was treated for Ph^+ B-lymphoblastic leukemia. Bone marrow aspirate was collected after consolidation for assessment of treatment response.

Findings
- Normal B-cell precursors (in blue) have uniform CD38 expression and two levels of CD9 expression without expression of CD13/CD33 (Fig. 31.3).

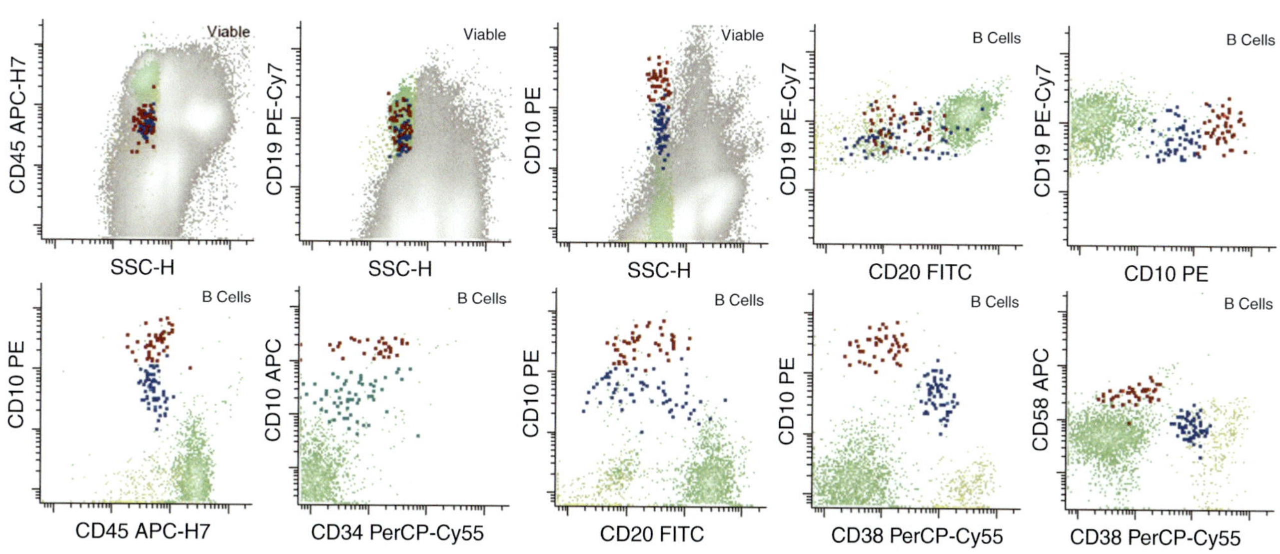

Fig. 31.2 Detection of B-lymphoblasts in regenerative bone marrow with normal immature B cells in the background, example 1. Normal immature B cells in blue. Leukemic B-lymphoblasts in red. In the background, the mature B-cell population is highlighted in green and plasma cell population is highlighted in yellow

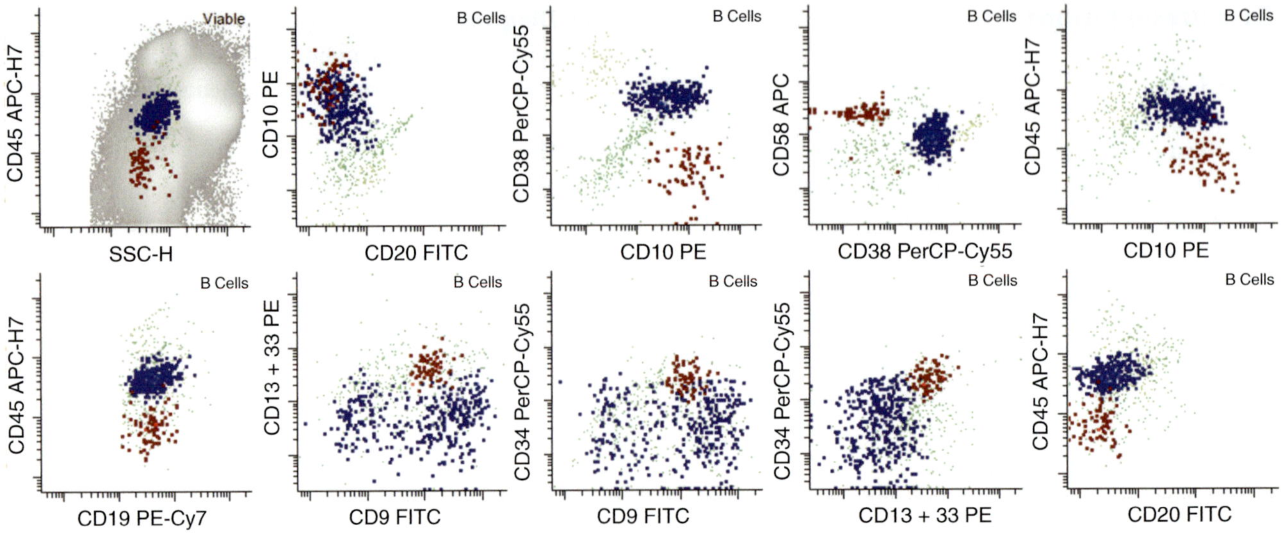

Fig. 31.3 Detection of B-lymphoblasts in regenerative bone marrow with normal immature B cells in the background, example 2. Normal immature B cells in blue. Leukemic B-lymphoblasts in red

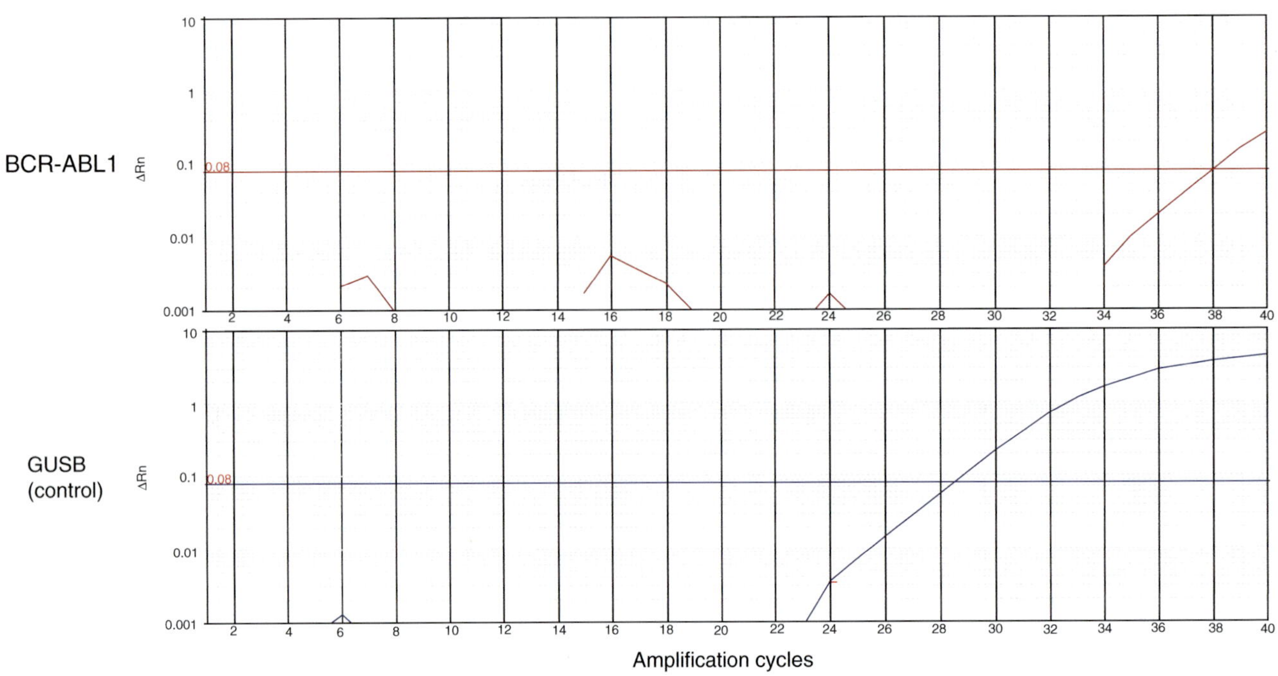

Fig. 31.4 Detection of *BCR-ABL1* fusion transcripts (p190) by real-time quantitative RT-PCR. The number of amplification cycles at which fluorescent signal reaching a detection threshold reflects the quantity of the tested molecules in the reaction. *BCR-ABL1* fusion transcripts are the tested target. GUSB is a methodology control

- Residual B-lymphoblastic leukemia (in red) represents 0.02% of nucleated mononuclear cells. The leukemic blasts have abnormal expression of CD9 (uniform), CD10 (slightly increased), CD34 (increased), CD38 (decreased), CD45 (decreased), and CD58 (increased).
- Despite of CD13/CD33 expression, lymphoblasts can be distinguished from regenerative myeloid blasts based on their expression of CD10, CD19, and decreased CD45.
- The concurrent RT-PCR testing for *BCR/ABL1* p190 fusion transcripts was positive at a level of 0.03% (Fig. 31.4).

Differential Diagnosis

- Presence versus absence of residual B-lymphoblastic leukemia

Final Diagnosis

Residual/recurrent B-lymphoblastic leukemia/lymphoma, representing 0.02% of nucleated mononucleated cells

Take-Home Message

Minimal residual B-lymphoblastic leukemia/lymphoma associated with recurrent genetic abnormalities can be detected by either quantitative PCR or flow cytometry. Quantitative PCR can be analytically more sensitive than flow cytometry but has limited application.

Case 3

Learning Objective

Recognize leukemic myeloid blasts after induction therapy

Case History

A 67-year-old male was treated for secondary acute myeloid leukemia transformed from chronic myelomonocytic leukemia. Bone marrow was collected on day 28 after induction for assessment of treatment response.

Findings (Fig. 31.5)

- Two populations of CD34-positive myeloid blasts are highlighted: blue represents regenerative myeloid blasts (0.4% of total white cells) and red represents leukemic blasts (0.11% of total white cells).
- Regenerative myeloid blasts include $CD34^+/CD38^{neg\ or\ dim}$ stem cells and $CD34^+/CD38^+$ progenitors. The stem cells usually have bright CD34, higher-level CD45, and dim to absent CD13, CD33, CD38, CD117, and HLA-DR without expression of lymphoid markers (there are few normal stem cells detected in this specimen).
- The leukemic blasts mimic stem cells with bright CD34 and dim CD38 but have abnormal expression of CD7 (uniform), CD13 (increased), CD56 (uniform), and CD71 (increased).

Differential Diagnosis

- Presence versus absence of residual acute myeloid leukemia

Final Diagnosis

Residual/recurrent acute myeloid leukemia, representing 0.1% of total white cells

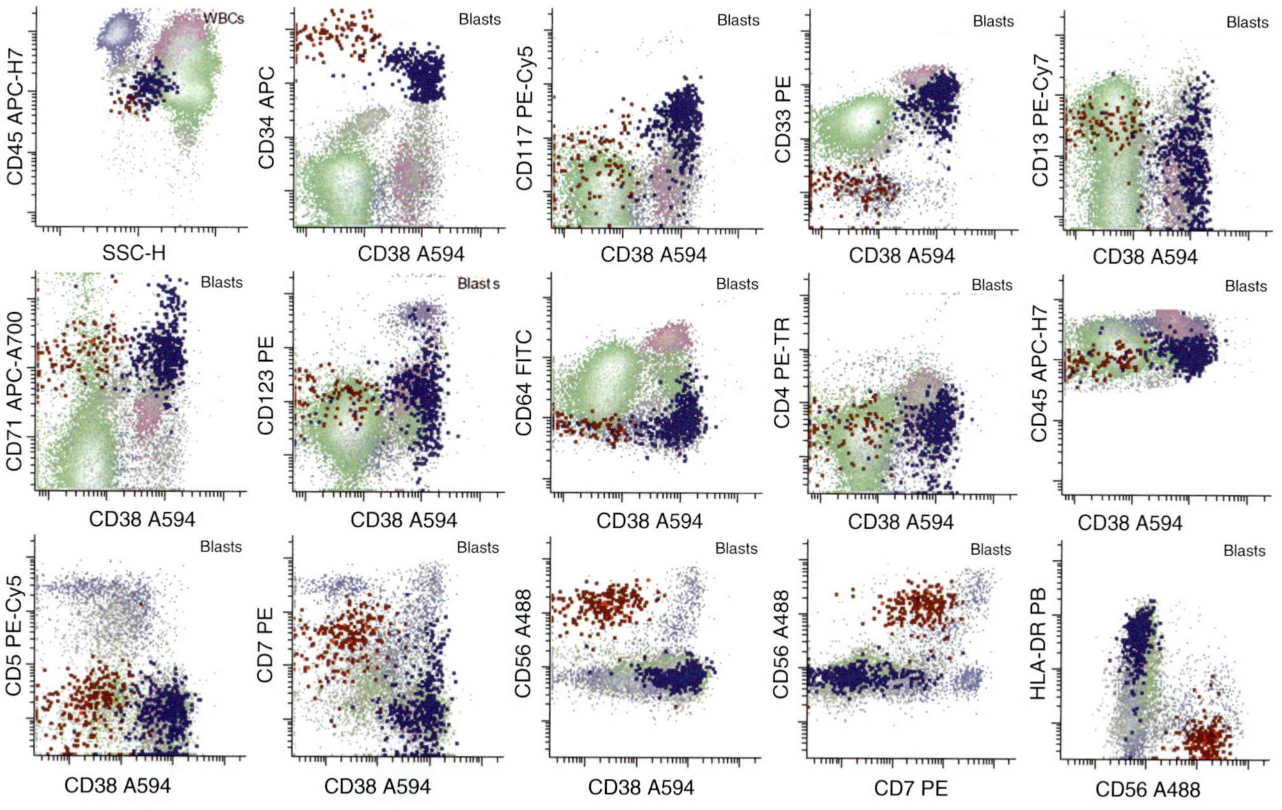

Fig. 31.5 Detection of leukemic myeloid blasts in regenerative bone marrow with regenerative myeloid blasts in the background, example 1. Regenerative myeloid blasts are in blue. Leukemic myeloid blasts are in red. Regenerative granulocytes and monocytes are in green and pink, respectively

Take-Home Messages

1. Regenerative myeloid blasts have different subsets with immunophenotypic pattern according to their differentiation.
2. Leukemic myeloid blasts may have an immunophenotype that is different from that of regenerative myeloid blasts subsets.

Case 4

Learning Objective

Know the immunophenotypic characteristics of myeloid blasts in acute myeloid leukemia associated with mutated NPM1

Case History

A 64-year-old male was treated for relapsed acute myeloid leukemia with mutated *NPM1*. Bone marrow aspirate was collected on day 28 for assessment of treatment response.

Findings (Fig. 31.6)

- Regenerative promyelocytes (in green) are CD117-positive, CD34-negative, and HLA-DR-negative and have bright CD13 with co-expression of CD15 and CD64.
- The leukemic blasts (in red), similar to promyelocytes, express CD117 with decreased to absent CD34 and HLA-DR. In contrast to regenerative promyelocytes, leukemic blasts express moderate CD13 and absent CD15 or CD64. In addition, the leukemic blasts express bright CD33 and increased CD123.
- The immunophenotype of myeloid blasts in acute myeloid leukemia associated with mutated *NPM1* is different from that of regenerative myeloid blasts, promyelocytes, or immature monocytes and thus can be recognized in a background of regenerative bone marrow.
- Acute myeloid leukemia with mutated *NPM1* can morphologically present as acute myeloid leukemia with monocytic differentiation. In contrast to leukemic myeloid blasts, leukemic monocytes do not have immunophenotypic abnormalities that can be consistently distinguished from their regenerative counterparts. Thus, in most cases, MRD detection in acute myeloid leukemia with monocytic differentiation relies on identifying abnormal myeloid blasts with CD34 or CD117 expression.

Differential Diagnosis

- Presence versus absence of residual acute myeloid leukemia

Final Diagnosis

Residual acute myeloid leukemia, representing 0.1% of total white cells

Take-Home Messages

1. Leukemic myeloid blasts in acute myeloid leukemia associated with mutated *NPM1* are usually negative, at least partially, for CD34, but positive for CD117. This immunophenotype mimics regenerative promyelocytes.
2. The leukemic myeloid blasts can be distinguished from regenerative promyelocytes or immature monocytes in their dyssynchronous expression of CD13 and HLA-DR and absence of CD15 and CD64.

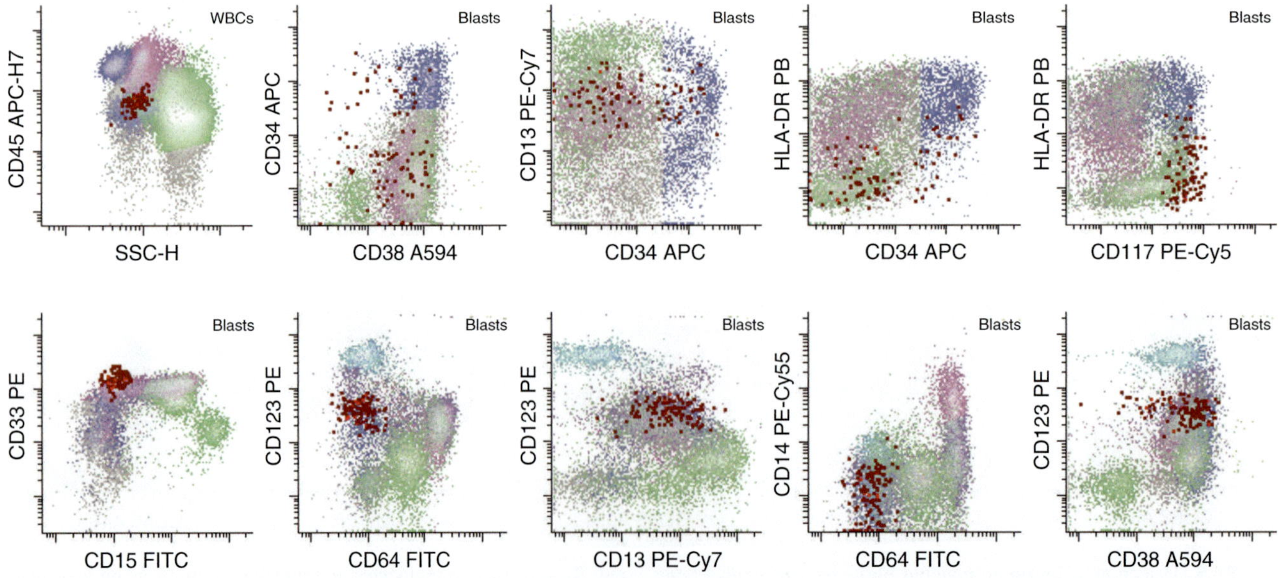

Fig. 31.6 Detection of leukemic myeloid blasts in regenerative bone marrow with regenerative myeloid blasts in the background, example 2. Leukemic blast population is highlighted in red, comprising 0.1% of total white cells. The background population in blue, green, pink, and aqua represents regenerative myeloid blasts and granulocytic, monocytic, and plasmacytoid dendritic cells, respectively

References

1. Cheson BD, Bennett JM, Kopecky KJ, Buchner T, Willman CL, Estey EH, et al. Revised recommendations of the International Working Group for Diagnosis, standardization of response criteria, treatment outcomes, and reporting standards for therapeutic trials in acute myeloid leukemia. J Clin Oncol. 2003;21(24):4642–9.
2. Harousseau JL, Attal M, Avet-Loiseau H. The role of complete response in multiple myeloma. Blood. 2009;114(15):3139–46.
3. van Dongen JJ, van der Velden VH, Bruggemann M, Orfao A. Minimal residual disease diagnostics in acute lymphoblastic leukemia: need for sensitive, fast, and standardized technologies. Blood. 2015;125(26):3996–4009.
4. Berry DA, Zhou S, Higley H, Mukundan L, Fu S, Reaman GH, et al. Association of minimal residual disease with clinical outcome in pediatric and adult acute lymphoblastic leukemia: a meta-analysis. JAMA Oncol. 2017;3(7):e170580.
5. Hourigan CS, Gale RP, Gormley NJ, Ossenkoppele GJ, Walter RB. Measurable residual disease testing in acute myeloid leukaemia. Leukemia. 2017;31(7):1482–90.
6. Grimwade D, Freeman SD. Defining minimal residual disease in acute myeloid leukemia: which platforms are ready for "prime time"? Blood. 2014;124(23):3345–55.
7. Thompson M, Brander D, Nabhan C, Mato A. Minimal residual disease in chronic lymphocytic leukemia in the era of novel agents: a review. JAMA Oncol. 2018;4(3):394–400.
8. Ghia P, Rawstron A. Minimal residual disease analysis in chronic lymphocytic leukemia: a way for achieving more personalized treatments. Leukemia. 2018;32(6):1307–16.
9. Kumar S, Paiva B, Anderson KC, Durie B, Landgren O, Moreau P, et al. International Myeloma Working Group consensus criteria for response and minimal residual disease assessment in multiple myeloma. Lancet Oncol. 2016;17(8):e328–e46.
10. Harousseau JL, Avet-Loiseau H. Minimal residual disease negativity is a new end point of myeloma therapy. J Clin Oncol. 2017;35(25):2863–5.
11. Borowitz MJ, Devidas M, Hunger SP, Bowman WP, Carroll AJ, Carroll WL, et al. Clinical significance of minimal residual disease in childhood acute lymphoblastic leukemia and its relationship to other prognostic factors: a Children's Oncology Group study. Blood. 2008;111(12):5477–85.
12. Yin JA, O'Brien MA, Hills RK, Daly SB, Wheatley K, Burnett AK. Minimal residual disease monitoring by quantitative RT-PCR in core binding factor AML allows risk stratification and predicts relapse: results of the United Kingdom MRC AML-15 trial. Blood. 2012;120(14):2826–35.
13. Bottcher S, Ritgen M, Fischer K, Stilgenbauer S, Busch RM, Fingerle-Rowson G, et al. Minimal residual disease quantification is an independent predictor of progression-free and overall survival in chronic lymphocytic leukemia: a multivariate analysis from the randomized GCLLSG CLL8 trial. J Clin Oncol. 2012;30(9):980–8.
14. Paiva B, Gutierrez NC, Rosinol L, Vidriales MB, Montalban MA, Martinez-Lopez J, et al. High-risk cytogenetics and persistent minimal residual disease by multiparameter flow cytometry predict unsustained complete response after autologous stem cell transplantation in multiple myeloma. Blood. 2012;119(3):687–91.
15. Garand R, Beldjord K, Cave H, Fossat C, Arnoux I, Asnafi V, et al. Flow cytometry and IG/TCR quantitative PCR for minimal residual disease quantitation in acute lymphoblastic leukemia: a French multicenter prospective study on behalf of the FRALLE, EORTC and GRAALL. Leukemia. 2013;27(2):370–6.
16. Rawstron AC, Child JA, de Tute RM, Davies FE, Gregory WM, Bell SE, et al. Minimal residual disease assessed by multiparameter flow cytometry in multiple myeloma: impact on outcome in the Medical Research Council Myeloma IX Study. J Clin Oncol. 2013;31(20):2540–7.
17. Terwijn M, van Putten WL, Kelder A, van der Velden VH, Brooimans RA, Pabst T, et al. High prognostic impact of flow cytometric minimal residual disease detection in acute myeloid leukemia: data from the HOVON/SAKK AML 42A study. J Clin Oncol. 2013;31(31):3889–97.
18. Beldjord K, Chevret S, Asnafi V, Huguet F, Boulland ML, Leguay T, et al. Oncogenetics and minimal residual disease are independent outcome predictors in adult patients with acute lymphoblastic leukemia. Blood. 2014;123(24):3739–49.
19. Martinez-Lopez J, Lahuerta JJ, Pepin F, Gonzalez M, Barrio S, Ayala R, et al. Prognostic value of deep sequencing method for minimal residual disease detection in multiple myeloma. Blood. 2014;123(20):3073–9.
20. Rawstron AC, Gregory WM, de Tute RM, Davies FE, Bell SE, Drayson MT, et al. Minimal residual disease in myeloma by flow cytometry: independent prediction of survival benefit per log reduction. Blood. 2015;125(12):1932–5.
21. Borowitz MJ, Wood BL, Devidas M, Loh ML, Raetz EA, Salzer WL, et al. Prognostic significance of minimal residual disease in high risk B-ALL: a report from Children's Oncology Group study AALL0232. Blood. 2015;126(8):964–71.
22. Rawstron AC, Fazi C, Agathangelidis A, Villamor N, Letestu R, Nomdedeu J, et al. A complementary role of multiparameter flow cytometry and high-throughput sequencing for minimal residual disease detection in chronic lymphocytic leukemia: an European Research Initiative on CLL study. Leukemia. 2016;30(4):929–36.
23. Kwok M, Rawstron AC, Varghese A, Evans PA, O'Connor SJ, Doughty C, et al. Minimal residual disease is an independent predictor for 10-year survival in CLL. Blood. 2016;128(24):2770–3.
24. Ivey A, Hills RK, Simpson MA, Jovanovic JV, Gilkes A, Grech A, et al. Assessment of minimal residual disease in standard-risk AML. N Engl J Med. 2016;374(5):422–33.
25. Gupta S, Devidas M, Loh ML, Raetz EA, Chen S, Wang C, et al. Flow-cytometric vs. -morphologic assessment of remission in childhood acute lymphoblastic leukemia: a report from the Children's Oncology Group (COG). Leukemia. 2018;32(6):1370–9.
26. Freeman SD, Hills RK, Virgo P, Khan N, Couzens S, Dillon R, et al. Measurable residual disease at induction redefines partial response in acute myeloid leukemia and stratifies outcomes in patients at standard risk without NPM1 mutations. J Clin Oncol. 2018;36(15):1486–97.
27. Araki D, Wood BL, Othus M, Radich JP, Halpern AB, Zhou Y, et al. Allogeneic hematopoietic cell transplantation for acute myeloid Leukemia: time to move toward a minimal residual disease-based definition of complete remission? J Clin Oncol. 2016;34(4):329–36.
28. Inaba H, Coustan-Smith E, Cao X, Pounds SB, Shurtleff SA, Wang KY, et al. Comparative analysis of different approaches to measure treatment response in acute myeloid leukemia. J Clin Oncol. 2012;30(29):3625–32.
29. Loken MR, Alonzo TA, Pardo L, Gerbing RB, Raimondi SC, Hirsch BA, et al. Residual disease detected by multidimensional flow cytometry signifies high relapse risk in patients with de novo acute myeloid leukemia: a report from Children's Oncology Group. Blood. 2012;120(8):1581–8.
30. Ouyang J, Goswami M, Tang G, Peng J, Ravandi F, Daval D, et al. The clinical significance of negative flow cytometry immunophenotypic results in a morphologically scored positive bone marrow in patients following treatment for acute myeloid leukemia. Am J Hematol. 2015;90(6):504–10.
31. O'Connor D, Moorman AV, Wade R, Hancock J, Tan RM, Bartram J, et al. Use of minimal residual disease assessment to redefine induction failure in pediatric acute lymphoblastic leukemia. J Clin Oncol. 2017;35(6):660–7.
32. Vora A, Goulden N, Mitchell C, Hancock J, Hough R, Rowntree C, et al. Augmented post-remission therapy for a minimal residual disease-defined high-risk subgroup of children and young people

with clinical standard-risk and intermediate-risk acute lymphoblastic leukaemia (UKALL 2003): a randomised controlled trial. Lancet Oncol. 2014;15(8):809–18.
33. Pieters R, de Groot-Kruseman H, Van der Velden V, Fiocco M, van den Berg H, de Bont E, et al. Successful therapy reduction and intensification for childhood acute lymphoblastic leukemia based on minimal residual disease monitoring: study ALL10 from the Dutch Childhood Oncology Group. J Clin Oncol. 2016;34(22):2591–601.
34. Pui CH, Pei D, Raimondi SC, Coustan-Smith E, Jeha S, Cheng C, et al. Clinical impact of minimal residual disease in children with different subtypes of acute lymphoblastic leukemia treated with response-adapted therapy. Leukemia. 2017;31(2):333–9.
35. Balsat M, Renneville A, Thomas X, de Botton S, Caillot D, Marceau A, et al. Postinduction minimal residual disease predicts outcome and benefit from allogeneic stem cell transplantation in acute myeloid leukemia with NPM1 mutation: a study by the acute Leukemia French Association Group. J Clin Oncol. 2017;35(2):185–93.
36. Zhu HH, Zhang XH, Qin YZ, Liu DH, Jiang H, Chen H, et al. MRD-directed risk stratification treatment may improve outcomes of t(8;21) AML in the first complete remission: results from the AML05 multicenter trial. Blood. 2013;121(20):4056–62.
37. Schultz KR, Pullen DJ, Sather HN, Shuster JJ, Devidas M, Borowitz MJ, et al. Risk- and response-based classification of childhood B-precursor acute lymphoblastic leukemia: a combined analysis of prognostic markers from the Pediatric Oncology Group (POG) and Children's Cancer Group (CCG). Blood. 2007;109(3):926–35.
38. Dohner H, Estey E, Grimwade D, Amadori S, Appelbaum FR, Buchner T, et al. Diagnosis and management of AML in adults: 2017 ELN recommendations from an international expert panel. Blood. 2017;129(4):424–47.
39. Hallek M, Cheson BD, Catovsky D, Caligaris-Cappio F, Dighiero G, Dohner H, et al. Guidelines for diagnosis, indications for treatment, response assessment and supportive management of chronic lymphocytic leukemia. Blood. 2018;
40. Paiva B, van Dongen JJ, Orfao A. New criteria for response assessment: role of minimal residual disease in multiple myeloma. Blood. 2015;125(20):3059–68.
41. Campana D, Coustan-Smith E, Janossy G. The immunologic detection of minimal residual disease in acute leukemia. Blood. 1990;76(1):163–71.
42. van Dongen JJ, Breit TM, Adriaansen HJ, Beishuizen A, Hooijkaas H. Detection of minimal residual disease in acute leukemia by immunological marker analysis and polymerase chain reaction. Leukemia. 1992;6(Suppl 1):47–59.
43. van der Velden VH, Cazzaniga G, Schrauder A, Hancock J, Bader P, Panzer-Grumayer ER, et al. Analysis of minimal residual disease by Ig/TCR gene rearrangements: guidelines for interpretation of real-time quantitative PCR data. Leukemia. 2007;21(4):604–11.
44. Farina L, Carniti C, Dodero A, Vendramin A, Raganato A, Spina F, et al. Qualitative and quantitative polymerase chain reaction monitoring of minimal residual disease in relapsed chronic lymphocytic leukemia: early assessment can predict long-term outcome after reduced intensity allogeneic transplantation. Haematologica. 2009;94(5):654–62.
45. Ladetto M, Ferrero S, Drandi D, Festuccia M, Patriarca F, Mordini N, et al. Prospective molecular monitoring of minimal residual disease after non-myeloablative allografting in newly diagnosed multiple myeloma. Leukemia. 2016;30(5):1211–4.
46. Puig N, Sarasquete ME, Balanzategui A, Martinez J, Paiva B, Garcia H, et al. Critical evaluation of ASO RQ-PCR for minimal residual disease evaluation in multiple myeloma. A comparative analysis with flow cytometry. Leukemia. 2014;28(2):391–7.
47. Schnittger S, Kern W, Tschulik C, Weiss T, Dicker F, Falini B, et al. Minimal residual disease levels assessed by NPM1 mutation-specific RQ-PCR provide important prognostic information in AML. Blood. 2009;114(11):2220–31.
48. Gabert J, Beillard E, van der Velden VH, Bi W, Grimwade D, Pallisgaard N, et al. Standardization and quality control studies of 'real-time' quantitative reverse transcriptase polymerase chain reaction of fusion gene transcripts for residual disease detection in leukemia - a Europe against cancer program. Leukemia. 2003;17(12):2318–57.
49. Faham M, Zheng J, Moorhead M, Carlton VE, Stow P, Coustan-Smith E, et al. Deep-sequencing approach for minimal residual disease detection in acute lymphoblastic leukemia. Blood. 2012;120(26):5173–80.
50. Ladetto M, Bruggemann M, Monitillo L, Ferrero S, Pepin F, Drandi D, et al. Next-generation sequencing and real-time quantitative PCR for minimal residual disease detection in B-cell disorders. Leukemia. 2014;28(6):1299–307.
51. Wu D, Sherwood A, Fromm JR, Winter SS, Dunsmore KP, Loh ML, et al. High-throughput sequencing detects minimal residual disease in acute T lymphoblastic leukemia. Sci Transl Med. 2012;4(134):134ra63.
52. Wood B, Wu D, Crossley B, Dai Y, Williamson D, Gawad C, et al. Measurable residual disease detection by high-throughput sequencing improves risk stratification for pediatric B-ALL. Blood. 2018;131(12):1350–9.
53. Jongen-Lavrencic M, Grob T, Hanekamp D, Kavelaars FG, Al Hinai A, Zeilemaker A, et al. Molecular minimal residual disease in acute myeloid leukemia. N Engl J Med. 2018;378(13):1189–99.
54. Cancer Genome Atlas Research N, Ley TJ, Miller C, Ding L, Raphael BJ, Mungall AJ, et al. Genomic and epigenomic landscapes of adult de novo acute myeloid leukemia. N Engl J Med. 2013;368(22):2059–74.
55. Klco JM, Miller CA, Griffith M, Petti A, Spencer DH, Ketkar-Kulkarni S, et al. Association between mutation clearance after induction therapy and outcomes in acute myeloid leukemia. JAMA. 2015;314(8):811–22.
56. Thol F, Kolking B, Damm F, Reinhardt K, Klusmann JH, Reinhardt D, et al. Next-generation sequencing for minimal residual disease monitoring in acute myeloid leukemia patients with FLT3-ITD or NPM1 mutations. Genes Chromosomes Cancer. 2012;51(7):689–95.
57. Salipante SJ, Fromm JR, Shendure J, Wood BL, Wu D. Detection of minimal residual disease in NPM1-mutated acute myeloid leukemia by next-generation sequencing. Mod Pathol. 2014;27(11): 1438–46.
58. Zhou Y, Othus M, Walter RB, Estey EH, Wu D, Wood BL. Deep NPM1 sequencing following allogeneic hematopoietic cell transplantation improves risk assessment in adults with NPM1-mutated AML. Biol Blood Marrow Transplant. 2018;24(8):1615–20.
59. Morita K, Kantarjian HM, Wang F, Yan Y, Bueso-Ramos C, Sasaki K, et al. Clearance of somatic mutations at remission and the risk of relapse in acute myeloid leukemia. J Clin Oncol. 2018;36(18):1788–97.
60. Salk JJ, Schmitt MW, Loeb LA. Enhancing the accuracy of next-generation sequencing for detecting rare and subclonal mutations. Nat Rev Genet. 2018;19(5):269–85.
61. Feller N, van der Velden VH, Brooimans RA, Boeckx N, Preijers F, Kelder A, et al. Defining consensus leukemia-associated immunophenotypes for detection of minimal residual disease in acute myeloid leukemia in a multicenter setting. Blood Cancer J. 2013;3:e129.
62. Kussick SJ, Wood BL. Using 4-color flow cytometry to identify abnormal myeloid populations. Arch Pathol Lab Med. 2003;127(9):1140–7.
63. Loken MR. Residual disease in AML, a target that can move in more than one direction. Cytometry B Clin Cytom. 2014;86(1):15–7.

64. Schuurhuis GJ, Heuser M, Freeman S, Bene MC, Buccisano F, Cloos J, et al. Minimal/measurable residual disease in AML: a consensus document from the European LeukemiaNet MRD Working Party. Blood. 2018;131(12):1275–91.
65. Zeijlemaker W, Kelder A, Oussoren-Brockhoff YJ, Scholten WJ, Snel AN, Veldhuizen D, et al. Peripheral blood minimal residual disease may replace bone marrow minimal residual disease as an immunophenotypic biomarker for impending relapse in acute myeloid leukemia. Leukemia. 2016;30(3):708–15.
66. Keeney M, Wood BL, Hedley BD, DiGiuseppe JA, Stetler-Stevenson M, Paietta E, et al. A QA program for MRD testing demonstrates that systematic education can reduce discordance among experienced interpreters. Cytometry B Clin Cytom. 2018; 94:239–249
67. Denys B, van der Sluijs-Gelling AJ, Homburg C, van der Schoot CE, de Haas V, Philippe J, et al. Improved flow cytometric detection of minimal residual disease in childhood acute lymphoblastic leukemia. Leukemia. 2013;27(3):635–41.
68. Stetler-Stevenson M, Paiva B, Stoolman L, Lin P, Jorgensen JL, Orfao A, et al. Consensus guidelines for myeloma minimal residual disease sample staining and data acquisition. Cytometry B Clin Cytom. 2016;90(1):26–30.
69. Flores-Montero J, Sanoja-Flores L, Paiva B, Puig N, Garcia-Sanchez O, Bottcher S, et al. Next generation flow for highly sensitive and standardized detection of minimal residual disease in multiple myeloma. Leukemia. 2017;31(10):2094–103.
70. Wood BL. Flow cytometric monitoring of residual disease in acute leukemia. Methods Mol Biol. 2013;999:123–36.

Therapy-Induced Marrow Changes

32

Parul Bhargava and Jeffrey D. Whitman

List of Frequently Asked Questions

1. What are the major patterns of drug-induced bone marrow changes?
2. What are the typical morphological findings in various patterns of therapy-induced marrow changes?
3. What are the mimics of therapy-induced marrow changes? What is the clinical relevance of misinterpretation between the true diagnosis and mimics?
4. Which morphological findings in the peripheral blood and bone marrow are reliably diagnostic? Which ones suggest the diagnosis? Which findings rule out the diagnosis?
5. What is the minimal and optimal ancillary workup for diagnosis and subclassification in these cases? Which test results are specific, and which should be interpreted with caution?
6. Which findings in these cases identify clinically relevant entities and which ancillary tests can provide prognostic and therapeutic target information for subsequent management?
7. What is an adequate marrow specimen in previously treated patients?
8. What information should be conveyed to the clinician during each stage of the workup and/or when the specimen is limited?
9. When is a diagnostic comment necessary, and what should be discussed in the comment in these cases?
10. When is it appropriate to seek external consultation in these cases?

P. Bhargava (✉) · J. D. Whitman
Department of Laboratory Medicine, University of California, San Francisco, San Francisco, CA, USA
e-mail: Parul.Bhargava@ucsf.edu; Jeffrey.Whitman@ucsf.edu

Introduction

Hematopoietic and lymphoid cells comprise some of the most active and dynamic tissues in the human body. As such, they are particularly susceptible to modulation from therapies that can stimulate, disrupt, or damage activation, metabolism, and replicative processes. The effects of therapies on the hematopoietic system may be direct or indirect. They range from development of aggressive therapy-related secondary neoplasms, to transient morphologic changes, to more subtle changes detected only via immunophenotyping, cytogenetic analyses, or molecular testing. Disease progression or transformation that is not secondary to therapy is described in prior chapters. In particular, see Chap. 5 (transformation of small B-cell lymphomas, particularly CLL/SLL), Chap. 22 (CML accelerated phase and blast phase transformation), Chap. 23 (other MPNs with transformation or progression to fibrotic stage), Chap. 25 (MDS and MDS/MPN with progression to acute leukemia), and Chap. 26 (progression of plasma cell dyscrasia from MGUS to plasma cell leukemia).

Herein, we concentrate on the examination of bone marrow and blood findings after treatment, primarily for hematological conditions, but also others that affect the bone marrow and blood in a significant manner.

1. What are the major patterns of drug induced bone marrow changes?

Therapeutic interventions may lead to significant intended and unintended changes in hematopoietic cells. The changes may be in hematopoietic cell morphology, immunophenotype, or genetics. The exact type of therapeutic agent used, duration of use, and latency between agent usage and biopsy timing all impact the types of changes observed. Such iatrogenic changes can be broadly divided into the following six morphologic categories:

E. Wang, A. S. Lagoo (eds.), *Practical Lymph Node and Bone Marrow Pathology*, Practical Anatomic Pathology,
https://doi.org/10.1007/978-3-030-32189-5_32

A. Marrow hypocellularity and/or cytopenias
B. Marrow hypercellularity and cytoses
C. Maturation of malignant cells
D. Dysplastic changes in hematopoietic cells
E. Therapy-induced secondary neoplasms
F. Miscellaneous

The therapies inducing each of these patterns of changes and the possible mechanisms are discussed below. See Question 2 for detailed morphological findings in each type of change.

A. *Therapy-associated marked marrow hypocellularity or cytopenias:*

The marrow findings may include acute cell dropout/ablation from cytotoxic/cytolytic therapies, marrow aplasia from non-cytotoxic therapies, serous atrophy or necrosis.

- Cytotoxic/cytolytic therapy: Along with targeted neoplastic cells, normal marrow cells may be damaged by chemotherapeutic drugs and radiotherapy leading to myeloablation.
- Drug-induced cytopenias may be uni-lineage or multi-lineage; a list of some agents and the hematopoietic cell lines affected is provided in Table 32.1.
  - Most drugs cause direct myelotoxicity, which is reversible upon drug discontinuation. However, immune-mediated idiosyncratic drug reactions can occur, leading to cytopenias, which may be irreversible [1]. This was seen with some earlier formulations of recombinant erythropoietin (rEPO). Susceptible patients developed progressive anemia, reticulocytopenia, and sometimes thrombocytopenia due to anti-rEPO IgG antibody development and cross-inhibition of native erythropoietin.
  - Isolated thrombocytopenia may similarly be the result to direct marrow suppression, or production of drug-dependent antibodies with increased platelet clearance.
- Serous fat atrophy has been described classically in patients with anorexia nervosa [2], but also other systemic disorders associated with malnutrition and cachexia including AIDS, alcoholism, scurvy, malignancies (lymphomas, carcinomas, myelodysplasia, etc.). More recently, reports of gelatinous transformation in imatinib-treated chronic myeloid leukemia patients [3] and ATRA-treated acute promyelocytic leukemia patients [4] have also been published.

B. *Marrow hypercellularity and/or peripheral blood cytoses from growth factor or other therapies:*

- Physiologic hematopoietic growth factor proteins include granulocyte colony stimulating factor (G-CSF), erythropoietin (EPO), and thrombopoietin (TPO), which primarily affect myeloid progenitors, erythroid progenitors, and megakaryocytes, respectively. Recombinant forms of these proteins are used therapeutically and are often structurally modified to prolong their effects (Table 32.2).
- In patients of small lymphocytic lymphoma/chronic lymphocytic leukemia (SLL/CLL) treated with the Bruton tyrosine kinase inhibitor, Ibrutinib, there is a paradoxical rise in peripheral blood lymphocyte count due to mobilization of abnormal cells from involved lymph nodes [5]. Similar lymphocytosis may be seen in other lymphomas treated with this agent [6].

C. *Differentiation of malignant hematologic cells from agents such as all-trans retinoic acid (ATRA) or IDH 1/2 inhibitors:*

- The excessive and abnormal proliferative signaling characteristic of cancer cells may occur via arrest of normal maturation to promote persistence of immature forms, or dedifferentiation into a more proliferative state.
  - A well-characterized example of maturation arrest is acute promyelocytic leukemia (APL) in which the abnormal gene product PML-RARA prevents

Table 32.1 Agents implicated in iatrogenic cytopenias

Effect on hematopoiesis	Drug class
Aplastic anemia	Cytotoxic drugs, radiation, drug reaction (anti-seizure agents like carbamazepine, phenytoin, antibiotics like sulfonamides, chloramphenicol, non-steroidal anti-inflammatory drugs, anti-thyroid medications, gold, arsenicals), toxic chemicals (benzene, solvents, glue vapors)
Agranulocytosis/neutropenia	Anti-thyroid, anti-inflammatory, psychotropic drugs, gastrointestinal (sulfasalazine, H2 antagonists), cardiovascular (tocainide, procainamide, flecainide, ticlopidine, enalapril, captopril, propranolol, dipyridamole, digoxin), dermatologic (Dapsone, Isotretinoin), antibiotics, antifungals, antimalarial, anticonvulsants, diuretics, sulfonylureas, iron chelators
Pure red cell aplasia	Recombinant erythropoietin, phenytoin, trimethoprim-sulfamethoxazole, zidovudine, chlorpropamide, mycophenolate mofetil
Isolated thrombocytopenia	Abciximab, beta-lactam antibiotics, carbamazepine, eptifibatide, gold, heparin, linezolid, MMR vaccine, phenytoin, Piperacillin, quinidine, quinine, rifampin, sulfonamides, tirofiban, trimethoprim-sulfamethoxazole, valproic acid, vancomycin
Lymphopenia	Immunosuppressive agents (e.g., glucocorticoids, antilymphocyte globulin, alemtuzumab, rituximab), chemotherapy (e.g., fludarabine, cladribine), hematopoietic cell transplantation, radiation therapy (e.g., total body irradiation, radiation injury)

Table 32.2 Hematopoietic growth factor therapies

Common hematopoietic stimulatory drugs	Class	Physiologic growth factor mimic	Drug type	Modifications to increase half-life
Filgrastim (Neupogen)	Myeloid growth factor	Granulocyte – colony-stimulating factor	Recombinant protein	
Pegfilgrastim (Neulasta)	Myeloid growth factor	Granulocyte –colony-stimulating factor	Recombinant protein	PEGylated
Sargramostim (Leukine)	Myeloid growth factor	Granulocyte-macrophage colony-stimulating factor	Recombinant protein	
Epoetin alfa (Epogen, Procrit)	Erythroid growth factor	Erythropoietin	Recombinant protein	
Darbepoetin alfa (Aranesp)	Erythroid growth factor	Erythropoietin	Recombinant protein	Additional sialic acid moieties
Romiplostim (Nplate)	Thrombopoietic growth factor	Thrombopoietin	Small polypeptide	Linked to IgG1 heavy chain
Eltrombopag (Promacta, Revolade)	Thrombopoietic growth factor	Thrombopoietin	Small molecule	

Data from: Kuter et al. 2016 [33]

transcription of key differentiation genes [7]. See Chaps. 2 and 21 for details of molecular mechanisms involved.
  - Dedifferentiation in malignancy arises from dysregulation of key differentiation genes in mature cells with epigenetic mechanisms, specifically with DNA hypermethylation increasingly implicated. This is observed in malignancies with mutations in genes associated with regulating DNA methylation including *TET2* and *IDH1/IDH2* [8]. Global DNA hypermethylation causing epigenetic silencing may lead to tumorigenesis [9–11]. *TET2* mutations act by decreasing the normal demethylation activity of this gene product while *IDH1/IDH2* mutations are indirect mediators of DNA hypermethylation acting through a neomorphic product, 2-hydroxyglutarate (2-HG) [12].
- The following established and emerging therapies induce differentiation in the malignant cells in hematologic malignancies, which may be mistaken for regenerating marrow:
  - All-trans retinoic acid (ATRA), used in APL treatment, is a potent ligand of retinoic acid receptor and induces maturation by allowing normal gene transcription to resume.
  - A new class of small molecule inhibitors of mutant *IDH1* and *IDH2* (ivosidenib and enasidenib, respectively) has emerged for treatment of mutated *IDH* acute myeloid leukemia (mIDH AML) and other *IDH* mutated malignancies [13, 14] with morphologic and immunophenotypic maturation of myeloid blasts noted in the initial clinical trials.

D. *Therapy-associated dysmorphology and dysplastic changes:*

A variety of medications effect the morphologic appearance of hematopoietic cells without causing any clonal genetic change or neoplasm. Such dysmorphologies are temporally related to initiation of therapy and are reversible upon discontinuation of medication. Some examples of such changes are described below.

- Mild irregularity of nuclear shapes and megaloblastoid change in erythroid precursors are not uncommon in bone marrows regenerating after myeloablative chemotherapy and may persist for up to 6 months.
- Dysmorphic changes in myeloid cells can occur due to various types of therapy, including sulphonamides [15], anti-inflammatory agents, and immunosuppressive drugs. This effect may be particularly prominent in the chronic and complex immunosuppression used in solid organ and hematopoietic stem cell transplantation (Table 32.3).
  - True Pelger-Huët anomaly (PHA) is due to an autosomal dominant mutation of the lamin B receptor gene that produces characteristic hypolobate granulocytes with heterochromatic clumped nuclear features [16–18].
  - Pseudo-Pelger-Huët anomaly (PPHA) change is noted to have many of the same features of PHA, including hyposegmented neutrophils and clumped chromatin; however, the true mechanism is largely unknown [19–21]. This is a reversible morphologic change seen in patients receiving drugs like mycophenolate mofetil and tacrolimus (Table 32.3).
- Methotrexate therapy leads to hypersegmentation of neutrophils due to its anti-metabolite properties.

E. *Secondary neoplasms: Therapy-associated myeloid neoplasms and immunodeficiency-associated lymphoproliferative disorders:*

A variety of secondary neoplasms, including solid tumor, may develop after exposure to radiotherapy, chemotherapy, or after autologous or allogeneic bone

Table 32.3 Pseudo-Pelger-Huët anomaly-associated medications

Drug	Class	Mechanism	Indication
mycophenolate mofetil	Immunosuppressant	Inhibitor of guanine synthesis	Organ transplant
Tacrolimus	Immunosuppressant	Calcineurin inhibitor/IL-2 production inhibitor	Organ transplant
Valproate	Anti-seizure	GABA transaminase inhibitor	Seizure, psychiatric disorders
Sulfisoxazole	Antibiotic	Inhibitor of bacterial folic acid synthesis	Bacterial infection
Ganciclovir	Antiviral	Viral DNA polymerase inhibitor	Viral (CMV) infection
Fluconazole	Antifungal	Fungal cell wall inhibitor	Fungal infection
D-Penicillamine	Chelating agent	Non-specific chelator	Heavy metal poisoning, rheumatic conditions
Paclitaxel	Antimitotic	Microtubule stabilization	Cancer
Docetaxel	Antimitotic	Microtubule stabilization	Cancer
Colchicine	Antimitotic	Microtubule depolarization	Gout
Ibuprofen	Anti-inflammatory	COX inhibitor	Inflammation
G-CSF	Myeloid growth factor	G-CSF receptor activation.	Neutropenia

Data from Wang et al. 2011 [21]

Table 32.4 Differences in therapy-associated myeloid neoplasms (tMN) in different classes of chemotherapeutic agents

Chemotherapeutic agent	Alkylating agents or ionizing radiation	Topoisomerase II inhibitors
Age	Risk of t-MN increases with age	Risk similar across all ages
Latency	5–10 years after exposure	1–5 years after exposure
Presentation	Most commonly tMDS	Most commonly tAML
Cytogenetics	Complex karyotypes, unbalanced loss of genetic material, abnormalities in chromosomes 5, 7, mutations or deletions of *TP53*	Balanced translocations, often involving chromosome 11q23, may have t(8;21) or t(3;21), t(15;17) or inv 16

marrow transplantation. Therapy-associated hematopoietic neoplasms that may present in the marrow include:

- Therapy-related myeloid neoplasms: This category includes myelodysplastic syndromes, acute myeloid leukemias, and hybrid myelodysplastic/myeloproliferative neoplasms that occur after treatment with cytotoxic chemotherapy and/or radiotherapy (Table 32.4).
- Post-transplant lymphoproliferative disorders and other immunodeficiency-associated lymphoproliferative disorders
  - Post-transplant lymphoproliferative disorders (PTLD) are a group of disorders with proliferations of lymphocytes or plasma cells occurring after a solid organ or allogenic stem cell transplant. While many of these present as mass lesions outside of the marrow (discussed separately in Chaps. 10 and 11), this chapter will focus on marrow changes occurring in this setting.
  - Patients with autoimmune disorders (e.g., rheumatoid arthritis, systemic lupus erythematosus, Crohn disease, therapy-induced bone marrow changes: inflammatory bowel disease, psoriasis) treated with immunosuppressive agents (e.g., methotrexate, TNF antagonists, etc.) may develop lymphoproliferative disorders [22]. These include B-non-Hodgkin lymphomas, T-non-Hodgkin lymphomas, classic Hodgkin lymphoma, Hodgkin-like lesions, or *EBV*(+) mucocutaneous ulcers.

F. *Miscellaneous:*

- Therapeutic agents may lead to more subtle changes that may only be detected via specialized testing such as immunophenotyping, cytogenetics, or molecular studies. Examples include antigenic shifts/drifts in acute leukemia post therapy [23], downregulation of an antigen following immunotherapies (e.g., *CD20* downregulation/loss following anti-*CD20* therapy), development of clonal hematopoiesis post radiation therapy, etc.

2. What are the typical morphological findings in various patterns of therapy induced marrow changes?

A. *Therapy-associated marked marrow hypocellularity or cytopenias:*

- Myeloablative chemotherapy leads to destruction of most dividing cells in the marrow particularly granulocytic precursors, erythroid precursors, and megakaryocytes, with the sparing of plasma cells and lymphocytes [24].

- Peripheral blood shows pancytopenia, with marked neutropenia and a relative lymphocytosis initially. A relative monocytosis is observed transiently before neutrophil counts recover [25].
- Marrow aspirate samples have markedly hypocellular particles comprised mainly of stromal cells, small capillaries, histiocytes, plasma cells, and lymphocytes.
- In the core biopsy, therapy-induced acute cell dropout leads to presence of acellular background eosinophilic stroma, along with scattered elongated nuclei of stromal cells (Fig. 32.1a). Intervening sinusoids may appear widely patent, and on reticulin staining, a reactive mild increase in reticulin fibrosis may be seen. Occasional histiocytes with variable hemosiderin deposits and ingested cellular debris may be noted. Residual lymphocytes in highly variable numbers may be seen singly or in occasional clusters. Plasma cells are easily seen, particularly in perivascular areas. Rarely, in older patients, an underlying plasma cell dyscrasia may be uncovered when the myeloid cells are cleared.
- If sample is obtained past the nadir of 14 days, the acellular eosinophilic stroma begins to resorb with lobulated fat deposition. Signs of early marrow recovery including small megakaryocytic clusters, early erythroid islands, and clusters of early myeloid progenitors may be noted [26].

• Serous atrophy or gelatinous transformation is characterized by the following findings:
  - Focal loss of hematopoietic cells with patchy hypocellularity (Fig. 32.1b), fat atrophy and deposition of extracellular gelatinous substances.
  - The extracellular substances are mucopolysaccharides rich in hyaluronic acid [27]. The latter is weakly periodic acid-Schiff positive and stains with Alcian blue at pH 2.5.

• Necrosis: This may be seen in marrows extensively infiltrated by a tumor that is undergoing necrosis or in marrow infarction.
  - Many malignancies involving the marrow, most commonly acute leukemias, high-grade lymphomas, and certain carcinomas, may undergo necrosis. Combination chemotherapies (e.g., CHOP) induce rapid necrosis of malignant cells and one may observe areas of geographic necrosis with possible peripheral rim of residual malignant cells. Areas of necrosis may demonstrate ghost outlines of mononuclear cells (Fig. 32.1c) or eosinophilic granular material with karyorrhectic debris [28].
  - In bone marrow infarction on the other hand, there is necrosis of normal hematopoietic elements in the inter-trabecular space, as well as empty lacunae within bony trabeculae due to death of osteocytes [29].

• Aplastic anemia may be drug-induced, but the implicated drug is not primarily a cytotoxic agent. This condition must be differentiated from marked hypocellularity induced by cytotoxic chemotherapy or radiation (see question 3 for differentiating features).

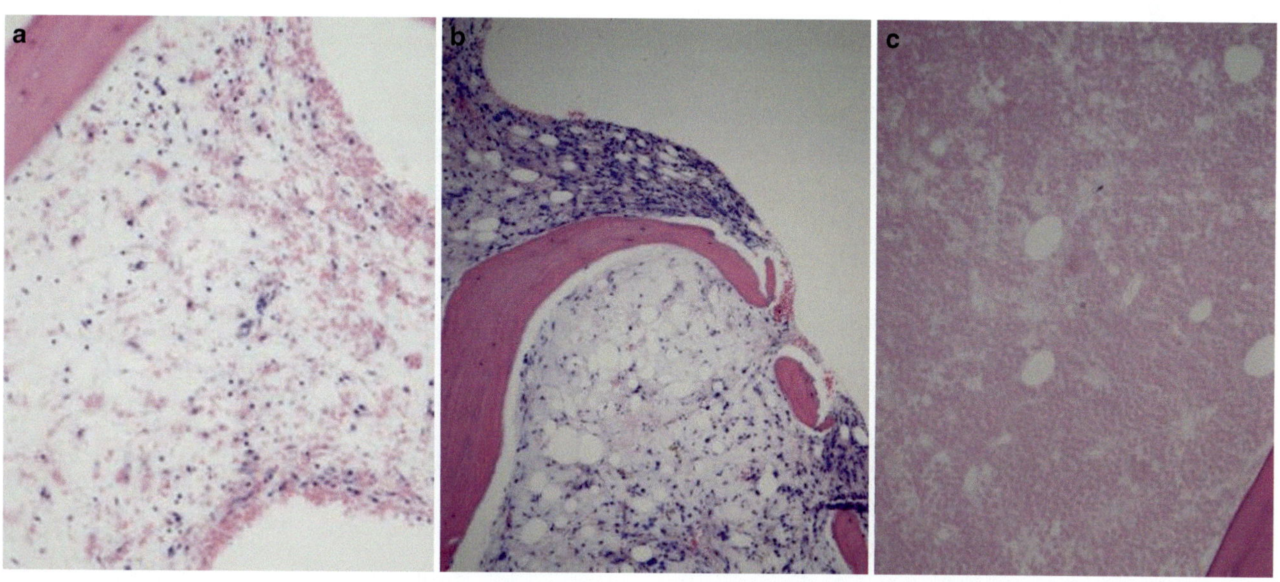

Fig. 32.1 (**a**) Bone marrow obtained on day 14 post chemotherapeutic ablation (H&E, 200×) showing marked hypocellularity, scattered interstitial lymphocytes, and few mainly perivascular plasma cells. (**b**) Bone marrow with gelatinous transformation (H&E, 100×), with patchy hypocellularity, and (**c**) Bone marrow with extensive necrosis (H&E, 200×) with ghost outlines of cells

- When aplasia is drug-induced, the temporal sequence of cytopenias is generally neutropenia (in hours to days), followed by thrombocytopenia (days to weeks), and finally anemia (weeks to months) [1].
- Aplastic marrows are generally markedly hypocellular. Patchy areas of granulopoiesis of erythropoiesis with cells in similar stages of maturation may be seen. Morphologic changes suggesting myelotoxicity may include maturation arrest in granulocytic lineage with near complete absence of granulocytes beyond the myelocyte stage, or left-shifted erythropoiesis with dysplastic changes or multinucleation [30–32]. Lymphocytes, plasma cells, mast cells, and histiocytes including some with hemophagocytosis may be seen. Peripheral blood shows pancytopenia with lack of polychromasia.

B. *Marrow hypercellularity and/or peripheral blood cytoses from growth factor or other therapies:*

In general, hematopoietic growth factor therapies are homologs of physiologic single-lineage hematopoietic stimulators. Therefore, the peripheral blood and bone marrow findings will vary depending on each class of therapy, be it myeloid, erythroid, or thrombopoietic growth factor. Additionally, their physiologic effects can vary in their hyperplastic and activating capacities. Myeloid growth factors tend to exhibit increased production and reactive morphology, while erythroid and thrombopoietic growth factors are predominantly hyperplastic/proliferative [33, 34].

- Granulocytic stimulating factors (G-CSF, GM-CSF, etc.) include the following features.
  - Bone marrow: hypercellularity, myeloid hyperplasia with left-shift and increased granulation in the myeloid lineage.

    Based on limited pathologic studies, bone marrow cellularity increases by ~50–80% [34]. Among the myeloid precursors, promyelocytes and myelocytes increased by 50–60%, while metamyelocytes, bands, and neutrophils tend to increase by a lesser degree (25–50%) compared to the normal proportion of the respective precursors. While there is a left shift, mature forms should still be the most abundant. Occasionally, such therapy may cause an alarming but transient increase in blasts [35].

    Secondary granulation in all non-blast precursor forms is increased, with a striking increase in promyelocyte/myelocyte stages.

    In addition, less prominent morphologic findings may include ringed neutrophils or more plump nuclei of band cells.
  - Peripheral blood: May also show leukocytosis [36], left-shifted myeloid lineage cells, and signs of activation. Depending on the dose, in adult patients a spectrum of maturity is seen with about 85–90% mature neutrophils/band forms, <10% immature granulocytes (promyelocytes to metamyelocytes), and <5% blasts.

    Reactive changes include toxic granulation and Döhle bodies present in more mature forms (Fig. 32.2).

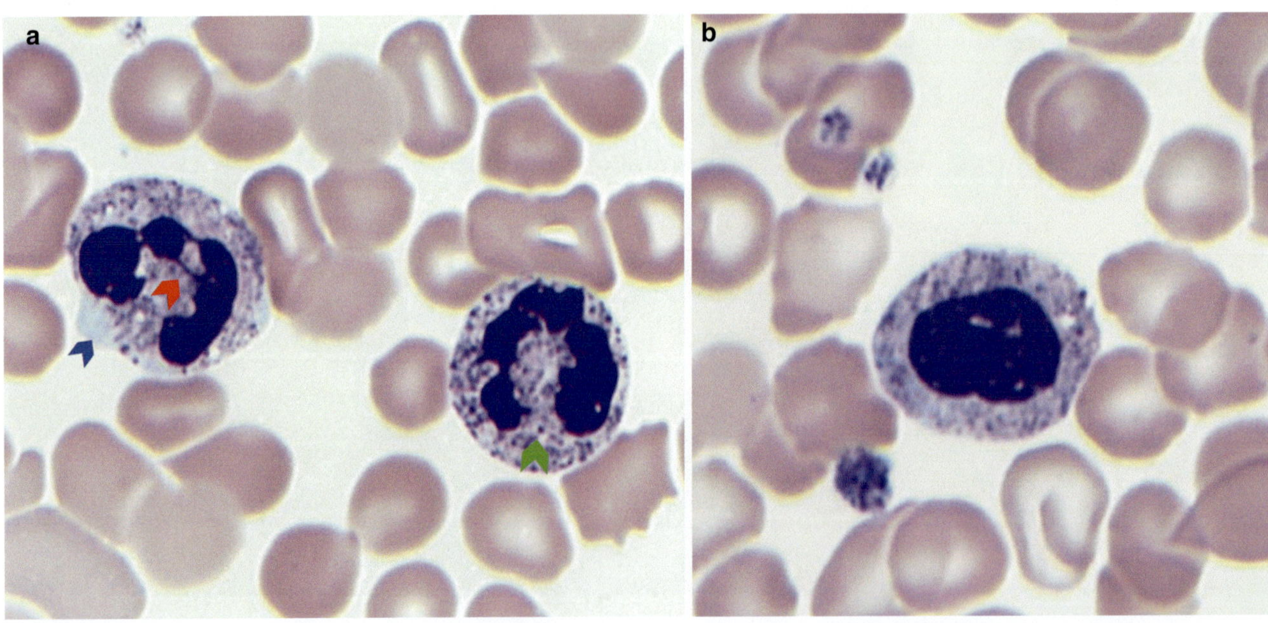

Fig. 32.2 G-CSF effect on neutrophils, 400× Objective. (**a**) Characteristic reactive neutrophils are observed with abundant secondary granules (toxic granulation) (*green arrow*), Döhle material (blue arrow), and some dysplastic morphology seen by nuclear threading (*red arrow*). (**b**) Dysmorphic hypolobated neutrophil from G-CSF, which can be mistaken for or confound evaluation of true myeloid dysplasia

Dysplastic morphology may also be observed in a subset of mature neutrophils including hypogranulation, hyper- or hypolobation, and ringed nuclei; however, these changes are not related to molecular or chromosomal abnormalities.

Other lineages may show signs of activation, including vacuolated monocytes, large granular lymphocytes, and plasmacytoid lymphocytes.

Myeloid growth factors induce demarginalization of neutrophils from vascular endothelium, release of neutrophil reserves from the bone marrow, and increased/accelerated production, accounting for the leukocytosis in 1 hour, up to 36 hours, and greater than 36 hours after starting therapy, respectively [33].

- Erythroid growth factors:
  - Bone marrow shows left-shifted erythroid hyperplasia. EPO receptors are present on pronormoblasts, basophilic normoblasts, polychromatophilic, and orthochromatophilic normoblasts, but not reticulocytes or mature red cells.

    Dysplastic morphology may be observed in a subset of erythroid cells (<10%) including megaloblastic change, asymmetric nuclear budding, and internuclear threading. These findings are reflective of accelerated proliferation and not a clonal process.
  - Peripheral blood findings may include polychromasia and possibly leukoerythroblastic change. Reticulocyte counts rise around day 3 and peak around day 10 [33].
- Thrombopoietic growth factors: promote maturation from megakaryocyte colony forming units and mitosis/endomitosis in megakaryocytic precursors. The morphologic effects of this therapy include:
  - Bone marrow: greatly increased numbers of mature megakaryocytes (early) and apparently "dysplastic" morphology including small mature megakaryocytes, hypo or hyperlobated, and/or hyperchromatic nuclei.
  - Increased transient reticulin fibrosis with occasional findings of osteosclerosis and new bone formation [37]. After cessation of therapy, reticulin fibrosis usually resolves over approximately 1 month.
  - Peripheral blood: thrombocytosis and possibly rare circulating megakaryocytes may be seen. Platelet morphology may show variability in size with large and possibly rare giant forms due to acceleration of platelet production.
  - The time course of changes after thrombopoietic growth factors: megakaryocyte hyperplasia and platelet production are observable in the bone marrow and peripheral blood within 5 days of initiation, peak at 10–15 days, and taper to baseline over ~30 days [33, 37].

C. *Differentiation of malignant hematologic cells from agents such as all-trans retinoic acid (ATRA) or IDH 1/2 inhibitors:*

Morphologic features of these therapies include progressive maturation of myeloid precursors to mature neutrophils, observed simultaneously in both the peripheral blood and bone marrow (Fig. 32.3).

- Significant leukocytosis may be observed in both diseases and respective therapies in the days to weeks following initiation, representing the drug-induced maturation of blast forms and pro-inflammatory signaling from maturing cells [38, 39].
- Such therapy-induced maturing cells may not follow the usual recognizable sequence from promyelocytes, myelocytes, metamyelocytes, band forms, to segmented polymorphonuclear (PMN) cells, and are sometimes referred to as "intermediate" cells. In some cases of ATRA treated APL, PMNs with cytoplasmic Auer rods may be observed [40].
- Subsequently, as normal hematopoiesis resumes, the leukocytosis will decline over approximately 1 month, in line with white blood cell lifespan [38, 41, 42]. These findings may be confounded by additional cytotoxic chemotherapy given in the treatment of these leukemias.

D. *Therapy-associated dysmorphology and dysplastic changes:*

- See also Chap. 24 for detailed discussion of mimics of myelodysplasia.
- After various forms of chemotherapy, normal regenerating marrow may show atypia, particularly of the erythroid precursors. This takes the form of irregular nuclear shape or excessively clumped chromatin in most cases but rarely nuclear budding, binucleation, or internuclear bridging may also occur. In occasional patients, presence of numerous ring sideroblasts may lead to an erroneous diagnosis of therapy-induced myeloid neoplasm [43].
- Therapy-induced Pelgeroid change in neutrophilic cells manifests as hypolobation and coarsely clumped chromatin in a proportion of cells; Wang et al. (2011) [21] reported Pelgeroid change in an average of 33% of neutrophils, with a range of 11–94% in patients with therapy-induced changes.
- Of the circulating Pelgeroid neutrophils, the majority has unilobate or ovoid nuclei, while others may have "coffee bean," "peanut"-shaped, or bilobed nuclei. Occasionally, other forms can be observed including detached round nuclear fragments.

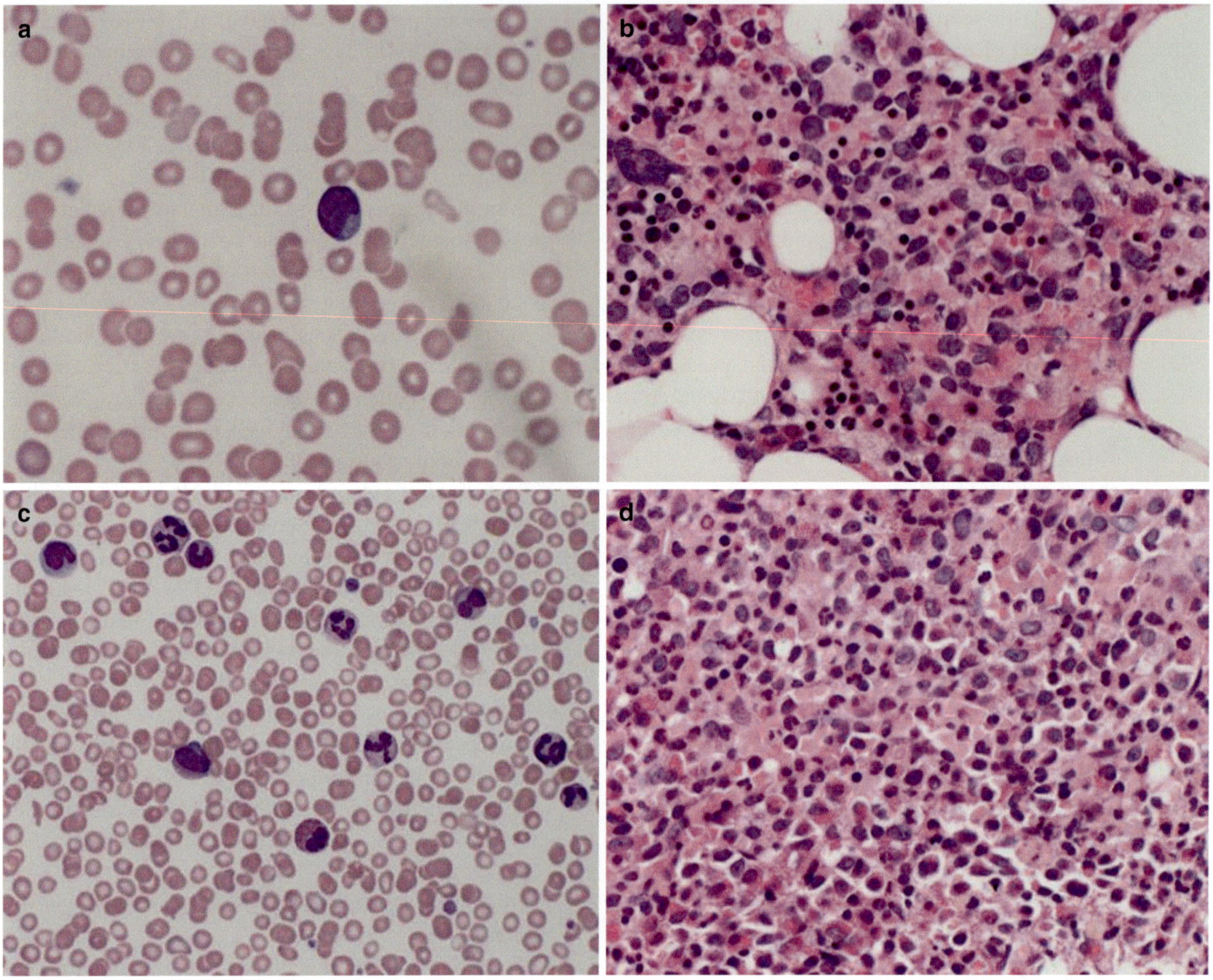

Fig. 32.3 Peripheral smear and marrow core biopsy findings in a patient with acute myeloid leukemia with mIDH treated with AG-120 (Ivosidenib). Pre-treatment (**a**) Peripheral blood smear (Wright stained, 1000×) with pancytopenia (WBC 2.3 k/uL) and circulating blasts with Auer rods, and (**b**) bone marrow core biopsy (H&E, 600×) with increased interstitial blasts. Patient received mutant IDH1 Inhibitor treatment. (**c**) Peripheral blood smear obtained 2 months later, and post AG-120 therapy shows leukocytosis (WBC 37.3 k/uL) with immature granulocytes and neutrophils with abnormal lobation. (**d**) Bone marrow core biopsy (H&E, 600×) is hypercellular with myeloid predominant maturing hematopoiesis and eosinophilia

- Another characteristic feature is the coarse and densely clumped chromatin, which can make the nuclei seem chunky or curdled (Fig. 32.4).

E. *Therapy-associated hematolymphoid neoplasms including therapy-associated MDS/AML and immunodeficiency-associated lymphoproliferative disorders:*

1. Therapy related myeloid neoplasms (tMN)
   - In t-MDS, the peripheral blood smear shows cytopenias of one or more lineages. Anemia is common with macrocytosis. Dysplastic neutrophils with abnormal nuclear segmentation and hypogranularity may be seen and basophilia is frequent.
   - The marrow is variably cellular, with trilineage dysplasia and increased reticulin fibrosis. The morphologic features of dysplasia are similar to those seen in primary MDS (see Chap. 24).
     - Dyserythropoiesis: asymmetric nuclear budding, irregular nuclear contours, multinucleation, chromatin bridging, satellite nuclei, and nuclear-cytoplasmic dyssynchrony may be seen (Fig. 32.5b, c). Ringed sideroblasts may be seen in Prussian blue stained aspirate smears (Fig. 32.5d).
     - Dysgranulopoiesis: forms with abnormally large or small nuclei, nuclear segmentation abnormalities (hyposegmentation, hypersegmentation, etc.), granulation abnormalities (hypogranularity, pseudo-Chediak-Higashi granules), Döhle bodies, or Auer rods may be seen (Fig 32.5a, e).

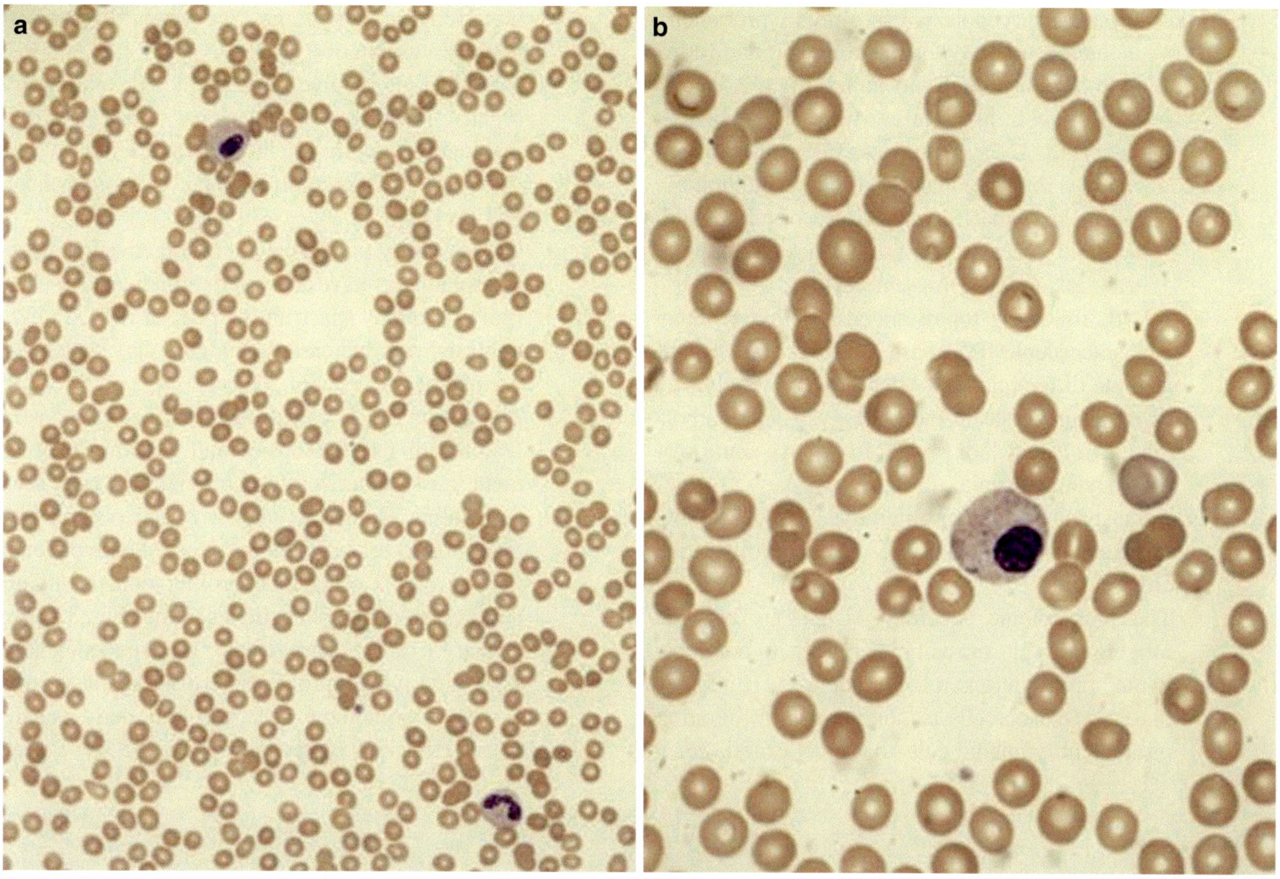

Fig. 32.4 Peripheral smear findings in a patient receiving tacrolimus. Monolobated neutrophils with coarsely condensed chromatin in keeping with pseudo-Pelger-Huët anomaly are seen. (**a**) Wright stain, 400×, and (**b**) Wright stain 600×

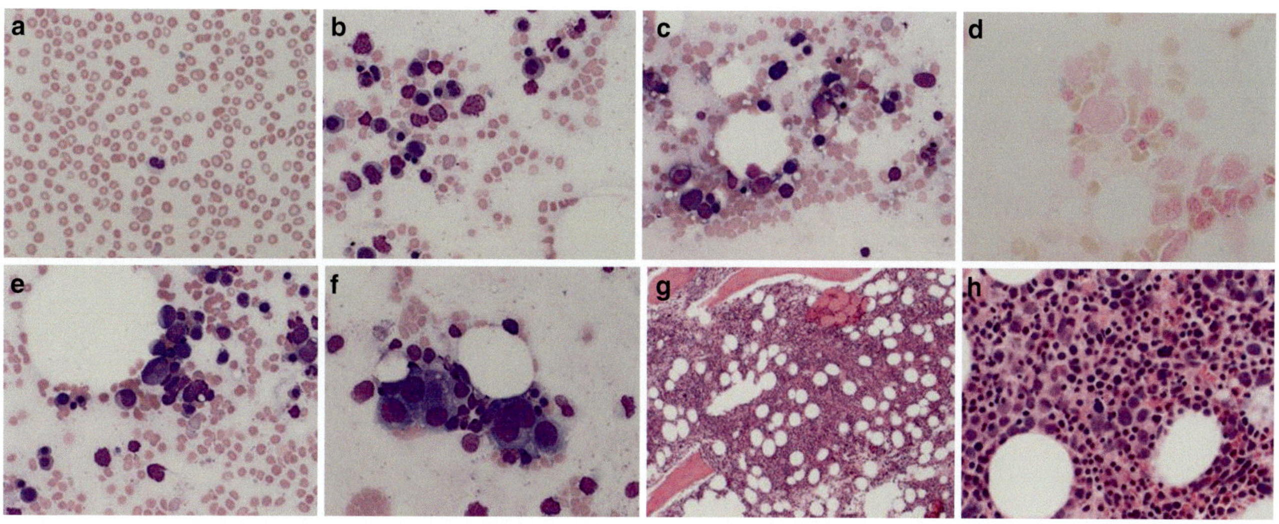

Fig. 32.5 Therapy-related myelodysplastic syndrome occurring in a patient who received alkylators 7 years prior. (**a**) Peripheral smear (Wright stain, 600×) with pancytopenia. A hypogranular and hypolobated neutrophil is noted along with coarse basophilic stippling in RBCs. (**b**) Bone marrow aspirate smear (Wright stained, 600×) with asymmetric nuclear budding and nuclear-cytoplasmic dys-synchrony in erythroid precursors. (**c**) Touch imprint (Wright stained, 600×) with satellite nuclei in erythroid precursors. (**d**) Aspirate smear (Prussian blue stain, 1000×) with ringed sideroblasts. (**e**) Aspirate smear (Wright-stain, 600×) with abnormal nuclear lobation in a granulocytic precursors. (**f**) Aspirate (Wright stain, 600×) with hypolobated small megakaryocytes. (**g**) Core biopsy (H&E stained, 100×) with hypercellularity and (**h**) core biopsy (H&E stained, 1000×) showing hypercellularity, left-shifted maturation, erythroid predominance, and trilineage dysplasia

  - Dysmegakaryopoiesis is often prominent, including small hypolobated nuclei, and forms with disjointed multiple nuclei (Fig. 32.5f).
  - Marrow core biopsies are generally hypercellular (Fig. 32.5g, h), and less frequently normo- or even hypocellular. Disorderly maturation, with abnormal localization of immature myeloid precursors present away from bony trabeculae may be present [44].
- t-AML following topoisomerase II therapy may lack antecedent MDS phase. Blasts exceed 20% of aspirate differential and often have a monoblastic or myelomonoblastic morphology. Those harboring t(15;17) may look similar to de novo acute promyelocytic leukemia.

2. Post-transplant lymphoproliferative disorders and immunodeficiency associated lymphoproliferative disorders
   - The morphologic spectrum of PTLDs is wide ranging from plasma cell hyperplasia, to polymorphous proliferations of lymphocytes, immunoblasts and plasma cells, to monotonous proliferation of atypical lymphoid cells that meet criteria for a non-Hodgkin lymphoma. See Chap. 10 for primary discussion of PTLD.
   - Most PTLDs involve lymph nodes or other solid organs forming mass lesions. Bone marrow involvement is rare in plasmacytomas, but present in 15–20% of polymorphous and monomorphous PTLDs [22].
   - Occasionally, patients with *EBV* activation post-transplant may have characteristic activated B-cells (polymorphous spectrum of plasma cells, immunoblasts, and increased smudge cells) present in peripheral smears (Fig. 32.6a).
   - The major PTLD categories, their key diagnostic features in tissue biopsies and marrow involvement are summarized in Table 32.5 below. Cases resembling Hodgkin lymphoma and plasma cell myeloma have also been described. Some patients may develop T-cell lymphoproliferations including large granular lymphocytic leukemia (Fig. 32.6b).
   - Primary and iatrogenic immunodeficiency-associated lymphoproliferative disorders also have a wide morphologic spectrum and may include B-non-Hodgkin lymphomas (Fig. 32.7), T-non-

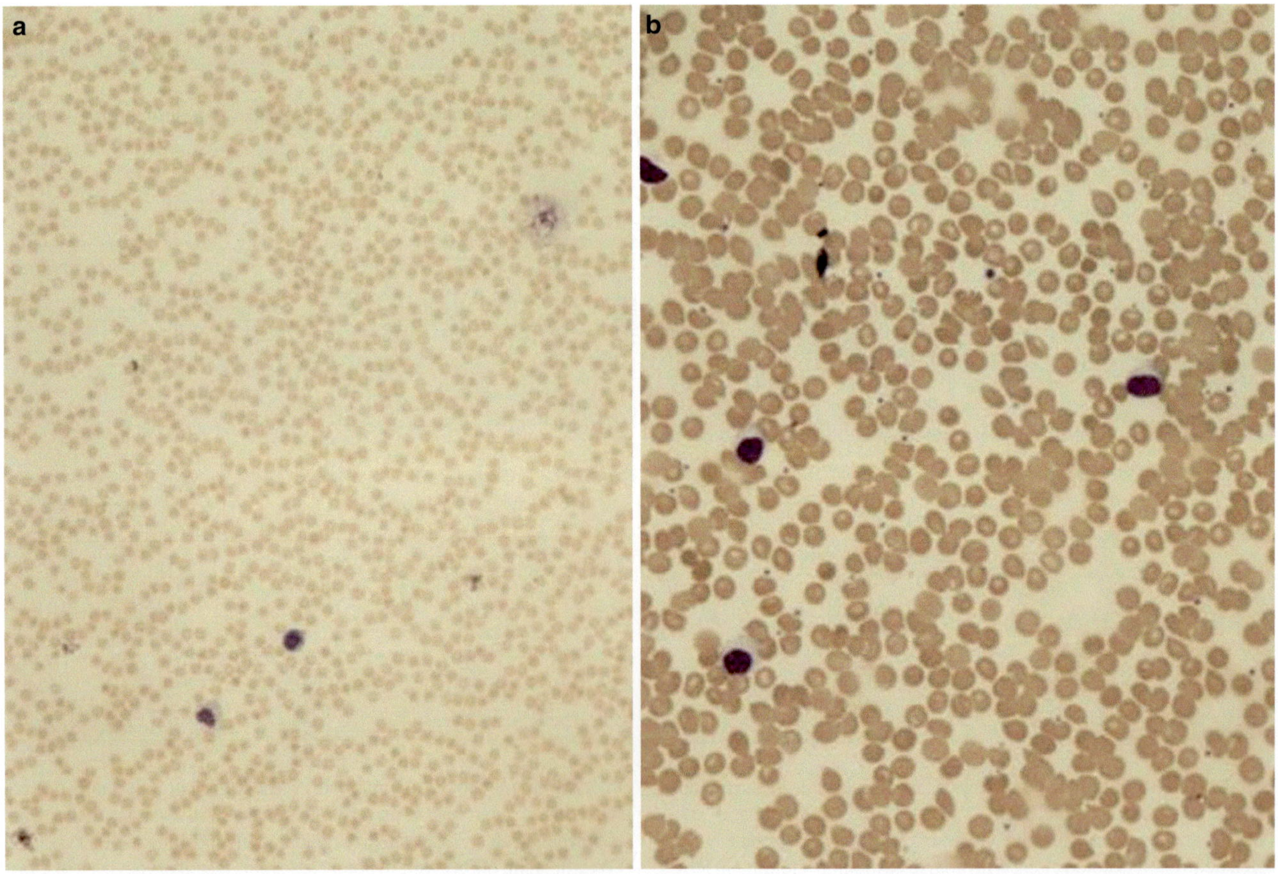

Fig. 32.6 (**a**) Post-transplant lymphoproliferative disorder, *EBV*(+), with circulating atypical plasmacytoid lymphocytes and smudge cells (peripheral smear, Wright stained, 200×). (**b**) Post bone –marrow transplant large granular lymphocytic leukemia (Peripheral smear, Wright stained, 400×)

Table 32.5 Key features of PTLDs in tissue and marrow biopsies

	Tissue involvement	Bone marrow involvement
Non-destructive PTLDs [plasma cell hyperplasia (PH), follicular hyperplasia (FH), infectious mononucleosis (IM) like]	PH: Numerous plasma cells, lymphocytes, infrequent immunoblasts; IM: paracortical expansion with numerous immunoblasts, T-cells, plasma cells. *EBV*+ and polyclonal with occasional small clones	Generally not seen
Polymorphic PTLD	Effaced architecture, spectrum of B-cells from immunoblasts to plasma cells, admixed numerous T-cells, Reed-Sternberg like cells (CD30+, CD20+, CD15-), mitoses, necrosis Generally *EBV*+	Variably sized lymphoid aggregates with or without plasma cells
Monomorphic PTLD	Generally high-grade B-LPD (DLBCL, Burkitt, plasmacytoma, and rarely myeloma) Low-grade B-LPD very rare (e.g., *EBV*+ MALT) Rare T/NK LPD (PTCL-NOS, hepatosplenic TCL, T-LGL, etc.)	Marrow involvement, if present, has features similar to the de novo counterpart
Classic Hodgkin lymphoma	Mixed cellularity (CD30+, CD15+, *EBV*+ Reed Sternberg cells)	Paratrabebular infiltrates with background fibrosis, mixed inflammation and rare Reed-Sternberg cells

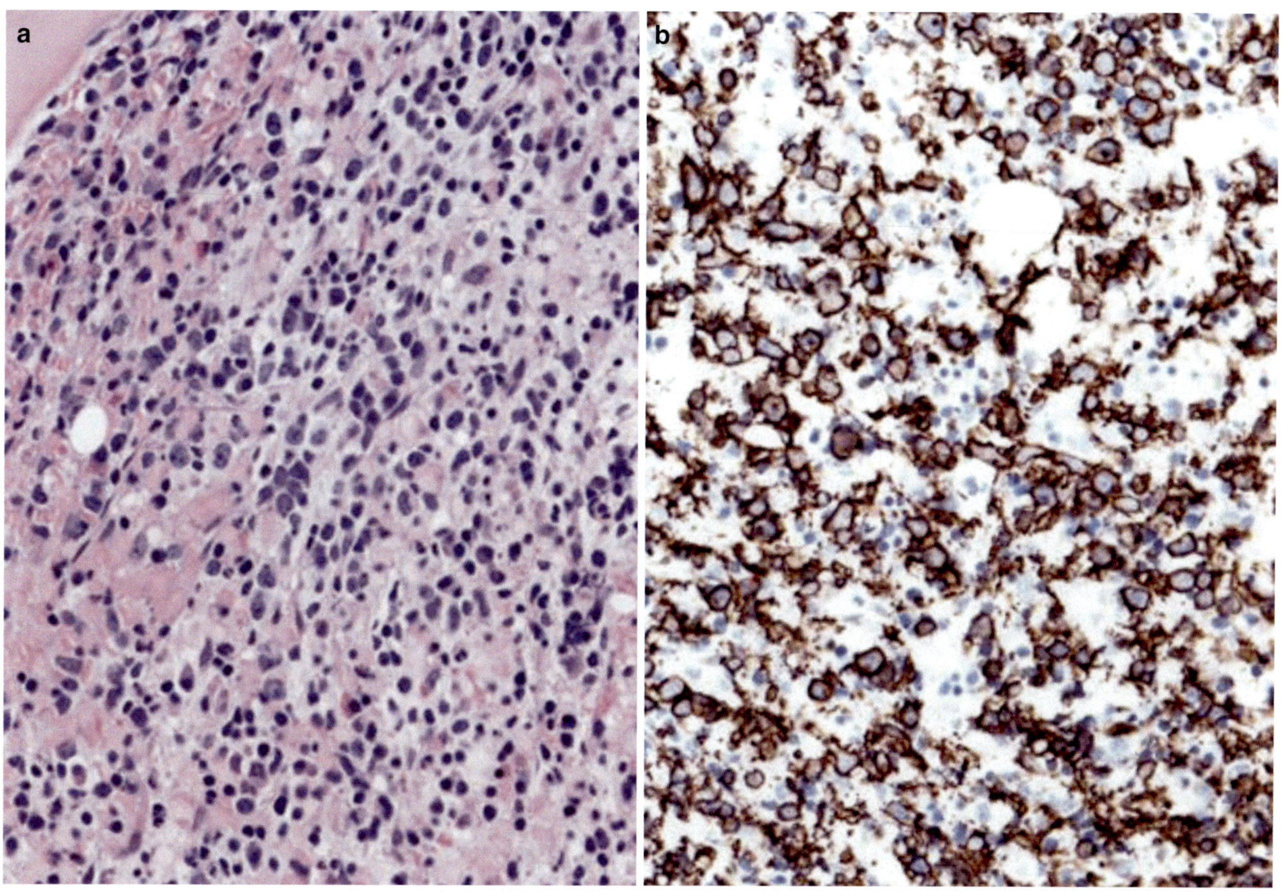

Fig. 32.7 Methotrexate-induced lymphoproliferative disorder with extensive marrow involvement. Bone marrow core (**a**) H&E, 400× and (**b**) CD20 immunostaining, 400×) with a diffuse infiltrate of atypical B-cells

Hodgkin lymphomas, classic Hodgkin lymphoma, Hodgkin-like lesions, or *EBV*(+)mucocutaneous ulcers (see also Chap. 11).

F. *Miscellaneous:*

Clonal hematopoiesis post radiotherapy: Detection of clonal hematopoiesis post radiotherapy or chemotherapy exposure has been reported [45]. Such changes are not discernable on routine morphologic examination of blood or marrow and require sophisticated molecular analyses such as deep sequencing.

3. What are the mimics of therapy induced marrow changes? What is the clinical relevance of misinterpretation between the true diagnosis and mimics?

In following situations, the patterns of drug-induced bone marrow changes may morphologically closely resemble other conditions with vastly different management and prognosis. Knowledge of prior treatment, along with blood and marrow findings before the treatment was initiated, are crucial for correct interpretation. Thus:

A. *Marked marrow hypocellularity or cytopenia(s) can occur due to:*
   - Myeloablation in a patient with acute leukemia receiving induction chemotherapy. The nadir of cytopenias and maximal marrow hypocellularity is generally reached on day 14 of initiation of therapy.
   - Gelatinous transformation and marrow edema: These findings point towards malnutrition, and are reversible with nutritional supplementation. However, a similar marrow injury effect is seen after induction chemotherapy.
   - Aplastic anemia may require an extensive workup of secondary (e.g., medications, immune, etc.) or primary causes
   - Amyloid deposition, confirmed by special stain, indicates a plasma cell dyscrasia.
   - Extensive marrow necrosis may point towards a neoplasm packing the marrow that has undergone necrosis.
   - Other disorders which may present with pancytopenia and marrow hypocellularity include infections, nutritional deficiencies, hypoplastic myelodysplastic syndrome, paroxysmal nocturnal hemoglobinuria, certain lymphoproliferative disorders, and rarely even plasma cell myeloma [46, 47]. These mimics have their own specific therapies.

B. *Therapy-associated marrow hypercellularity and/or peripheral blood cytoses:*

- The following conditions may show morphologically overlapping features with hematopoietic growth factor-induced changes:
  - Sepsis/inflammatory changes
  - Primary hematologic malignancies
  - Drug or toxicant related (other than hematopoietic growth factor)
  - Infiltrative bone marrow processes
- Be aware that growth factor therapies are often given in the setting of hematologic malignancy, including myelodysplastic syndrome (MDS), aplastic anemia, or post-induction chemotherapy from acute myeloid leukemia (AML).
  - Interpretation of therapy-related dysplastic morphology may confound the microscopic assessment of residual disease.
  - The regeneration may be accelerated and appear synchronized when growth factors are administered after myeloablative therapy. The bone marrow aspirate may be highly cellular and may contain high proportion of apparent promyelocytes with prominent granulation induced by the growth factors. If subsequent maturation stages are sparse, the morphological findings can mimic APL. In such cases, a careful search for Auer rods and correlation with immunophenotype of marrow cells provides clues to the correct diagnosis.

C. *Apparent differentiation of malignant hematologic cells: ATRA, IDH 1/2 inhibitors:*
   - Differentiation inducing agents may lead to transient leukocytosis [48]. The presence of a spectrum of blasts, immature granulocytes, and mature myeloid cells observed during differentiation therapy may overlap morphologically with leukemoid reaction in inflammatory response. Thus, therapy-induced morphologic changes may coincide with or mask infection.
   - "Intermediate cells" with cytomorphologic features that are in between blasts and mature neutrophils appear after treatment with differentiating agents. These cells often do not follow the systematic progression from promyelocytes to neutrophils, but should not be regarded as blasts or blast equivalents.
   - Dysmorphic features may appear in maturing cells: nuclear-cytoplasmic dyssynchrony, abnormal nuclear lobation, presence of Auer rods in mature neutrophils, etc. These should not be interpreted as indicators of underlying myelodysplasia.

D. *Therapy-associated dysmorphology and dysplastic changes:*
   - The major differential diagnoses to be considered when hypolobate myeloid cells are seen in peripheral blood or bone marrow should be PHA, PPHA, and underlying myeloid malignancy (Fig. 32.8). While true PHA and immunosuppressant-induced

PPHA are benign conditions, their presence may confound assessment of dysplasia in the evaluation of myeloid malignancy, especially in the post-chemotherapy and/or post-stem cell transplant setting. In an algorithm proposed in Wang et al. (2011), PPHA should be suggested if the patient has had prior normal neutrophilic segmentation, is currently on PPHA-associated medications (Table 32.6), and is without cytopenias. If cytopenias are present, or hypogranulation is seen along with hypolobation, a workup for myelodysplastic syndrome may be warranted.

E. *Therapy-related secondary hematolymphoid neoplasms:*
   - Therapy-related myelodysplasia and therapy-related acute leukemias may be morphologically indistinguishable from their de novo counterparts. Knowledge of antecedent radiotherapy and/or chemotherapy is required to make this diagnosis. Therapy-related myeloid neoplasms generally have a worse prognosis, especially in younger individuals [49].
   - The early lesions of post-transplant lymphoproliferative disorders (e.g., follicular hyperplasia, plasma cell hyperplasia) may be misinterpreted as reactive hyperplasias. A diagnosis of immunodeficiency-associated lymphoproliferative disorder requires reduction of immunosuppression, without which, these may progress or, in the case of infectious-mononucleosis like lesions [50], may even be fatal.

F. *Miscellaneous:*

With increasing use of ancillary testing, one needs to be aware of changes of immunophenotype or genetics that may occur over time after treatment. Tumor heterogeneity and emergence of new/resistant clones may be seen post-therapy which may make diagnosing minimal residual disease challenging [23].

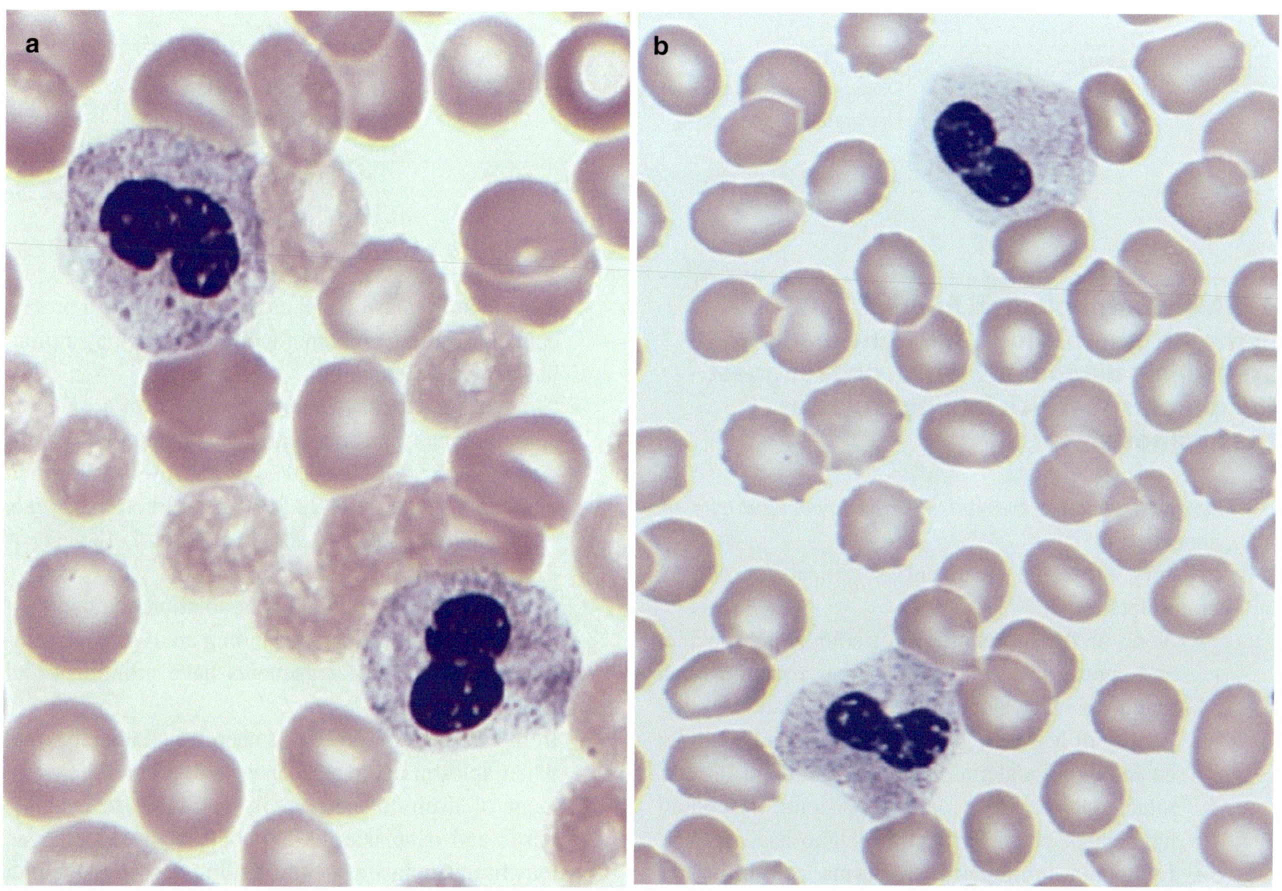

Fig. 32.8 Comparison of pseudo-Pelger-Huët anomaly and Pelger-Huët anomaly, 400×. (**a**) Neutrophils of a solid organ transplant patient on mycophenolate mofetil and tacrolimus displaying pseudo-Pelger-Huët anomaly with "peanut"- and "bean"-shaped morphology and clumped chromatin. (**b**) Pelger-Huët anomaly in an infant with cytogenetic abnormality of 1q41–43 deletion

Table 32.6 Bone marrow conditions that morphologically mimic growth factor therapy

Confounding process	Pathology	Etiopathogenesis	Therapeutic mimic
Reactive changes			
	Infection	Immune response to pathogen-associated molecular patterns (PAMP)/cytokine effect	Myeloid growth factor
	Rheumatologic disease	Primary dysfunctional immune signaling, secondary damage-associated molecular patterns (DAMP) immune activation/cytokine effect	Myeloid growth factor
	Neoplasm	Immune response to transformed/malignant cells	Myeloid growth factor
	Non-specific allergic/inflammatory	Cytokine effect	Myeloid growth factor
Myeloid neoplasm			
	Chronic myeloid leukemia (CML)	t(9;22)/*BCR-ABL1* gene fusion mitogenic signaling	Myeloid growth factor
	Polycythemia Vera (PV)	Mutated *JAK2*, *MPL*, or *CALR* mitogenic signaling	Erythroid growth factor; myeloid growth factor (if granulocytosis present)
	Essential thrombocythemia (ET)	Mutated *JAK2*, *MPL*, or *CALR* mitogenic signaling	Thrombopoietic growth factor
	Primary myelofibrosis (PMF)	Mutated *JAK2*, *MPL*, or *CALR* mitogenic signaling	Thrombopoietic growth factor; myeloid growth factor (if granulocytosis present)
	Myelodysplastic syndrome	Mutations or chromosomal abnormalities causing dysplastic/ineffective hematopoiesis	Dysplastic changes associated with myeloid, erythroid, and thrombopoietic growth factors
Medications/toxicants			
	Glucocorticoids	Demarginalization/release from the bone marrow	Myeloid growth factor
	Catecholamines (epinephrine)	Demarginalization	Myeloid growth factor
	Lithium	Increased myeloid production and mobilization	Myeloid growth factor

4. Which morphological findings in the peripheral blood and bone marrow are reliably diagnostic? Which ones suggest the diagnosis? Which findings rule out the diagnosis?

A. *Therapy-associated marked marrow hypocellularity or cytopenias:*
   - History of recent treatment is critical for correct interpretation.
     - None of the morphological findings are specific, and appropriate clinical context is required for a diagnosis of myeloablation. A combination of cellularity of less than 5%, with background acellular eosinophilic material, hemosiderin deposits and intact plasma cells, and occasional lymphoid aggregates, characterizes this diagnosis.
     - Lymphoid infiltrates and plasma cell infiltrates may appear unusually prominent in such biopsies and generally do not require extensive workup for a lymphoproliferative disorder. Plasma cells localized perivascularly with few scattered interstitially generally denote normal reactive plasma cells.
   - Regenerating marrows in children may have a prominent population of hematogones which may mimic blasts morphologically.
     - Per a recent flow cytometry-based study of morphologically normal marrows, hematogones comprised 15.5% (2.2–32.9%) of marrow cellularity in infants, 9.0% (1.3–22.8%) in children 1–7 years old, and 2.0% (0.2–4.9%) in children 7–18 years of age [51].
   - In serous atrophy, unlike myeloablation, the hypocellularity is patchy with surrounding areas of normocellular marrow. The fat vacuoles have prominent and irregular outlines.
   - In the absence of history of chemo/radiotherapy, and when aplastic anemia is suspected, a careful assessment of aspirate material is warranted to evaluate blasts and dysplasia, as hypoplastic myelodysplasia may mimic aplastic anemia. Cellularity assessment in the core biopsy together with absolute neutrophil count (ANC) is used to clinically grade the severity of aplasia [46].

B. *Therapy-associated marrow hypercellularity and/or peripheral blood cytoses:*

Leukocytosis induced by G-CSF therapy is difficult to distinguish morphologically from leukemoid reactions due to infection/inflammation.

- Morphological features that help distinguish leukemoid reactions from clonal myeloproliferative disorders are described below:
  - Leukemoid reactions typically evolve over days, have toxic changes in neutrophils, typically do not have basophilia, dysplasia is not prominent, and generally have a paucity of circulating blasts with <5% blasts in the bone marrow.
  - Myeloproliferative neoplasms generally evolve over months, and patients may have splenomegaly. Morphologically, neutrophils lack toxic changes. Basophilia, eosinophilia, and blasts may be easily seen.

    Ancillary laboratory studies, such as cytogenetics/FISH, flow cytometry, and molecular studies to assess for genetic abnormalities would be more specific considering they should only be present in hematologic disease.

C. *Therapeutic differentiation of malignant hematologic cells: ATRA, IDH 1/2 inhibitors:*
- The maturing myeloid forms induced by these drugs may still appear morphologically abnormal, demonstrate aberrant immunophenotype, and harbor pathognomonic genetic/molecular changes (t(15;17) or *IDH* mutations) [52–54].
- In APL treated with ATRA, FISH or molecular methods are required to conclusively rule out residual disease [55].

D. *Therapy-associated dysmorphology and dysplastic changes in blood and marrow:*
- History of prior therapy known to cause pseudo Pelger – Huët changes is important, but even in these cases, concomitant therapy-induced myeloid neoplasm and primary MDS must be excluded. Morphological findings favoring chronic immunosuppression induced pseudo-Pelger-Huët change over Pelger-Huët anomaly (PHA) include:
  - Hypolobated nuclei and clumped chromatin in PPHA are restricted to only a subset of neutrophils, while PHA affects other myeloid cells, including monocytes and eosinophils (though not always readily apparent), and 50% to 90% neutrophils.
  - Neutrophil nuclei in PHA have uniform lobes and generally have a characteristic "pince-nez" shape, while in PPHA the nuclei are variable from cell to cell, and have shapes ranging from pince-nez, band form, rod-like, or irregularly oval [18].
  - MDS-related hypolobation is generally accompanied by hypogranularity and the changes are seen in fewer circulating cells (average 12%, median 9%, range 2–28% in MDS compared to average 47%, median 33%, range 11–94% in immunosuppression related cases) [21]. In true PHA, hypolobated neutrophils generally comprise a range of 50–90% of circulating neutrophils [18].

E. *Therapy-related secondary hematolymphoid neoplasms:*
- Therapy-related myeloid neoplasms often have multilineage dysplasia. However, cytologic dysplasia is not specific for this diagnosis and a clinical history of exposure to alkylators or radiation is critical in making the diagnosis. In patients treated with topoisomerase inhibitors, the latency of myelodysplasia is short and they may present with a high blast count making assessing dysplasia difficult. In these situations, absence of cytologic dysplasia does not rule out this diagnosis.
- Post-transplant lymphoproliferative disorders and immunodeficiency-associated lymphoproliferations: clinical history of an antecedent transplant and presence of a mass lesion are critical for making a diagnosis. Morphologic findings are not specific with significant overlap with both reactive proliferations (plasma cell hyperplasia, follicular hyperplasia, infectious-mononucleosis like lesions) and other de novo lymphomas. Most early lesions show evidence of *EBV* but late occurring lesions may be *EBV* negative. Blood and marrow involvement is seen only in a minority of cases. One may see reactive lymphocytes on peripheral smears while marrow, when involved, may only have small lymphoid and/or plasma cell infiltrates in early lesions.

5. What is the minimal and optimal ancillary work up for diagnosis and sub-classification in these cases? Which test results are specific and which should be interpreted with caution?

A. *Therapy-associated marked marrow hypocellularity or cytopenias:*
- In the context of recent chemotherapy, a myeloablated marrow (cellularity <5%) without any overt clusters of immature cells typically does not require any further workup. Selected immunohistochemical stains (e.g., CD34, CD117), flow cytometry, cytogenetics, etc. may sometimes be used to distinguish residual disease from regenerating normal blasts and is essential for pediatric age patients with treated precursor B acute lymphoblastic leukemia (B-ALL). See also Chap. 31 for additional discussion of minimal residual disease.

- In the case of marrow necrosis, immunohistochemical stains may suggest possible origin of ghost cells, but these need to be interpreted with caution as both false negative and false positive results occur.
- A diagnosis of serous fat atrophy is generally made on light microscopy without any ancillary workup. If special stains are performed, the fibrinous depositions in serous fat atrophy are PAS weak positive, Alcian Blue strong positive and Congo red negative.
- In aplastic anemia, flow cytometric assessment of peripheral blood to exclude paroxysmal nocturnal hemoglobinuria or other causes of cytopenia such as large granular lymphocytic leukemia may be useful. Cytogenetic analysis with karyotype and possible FISH studies should be performed to rule out hypoplastic MDS.
  – A limited immunohistochemical panel may be performed to evaluate for blasts (CD34, CD117) or micromegakaryocytes (CD61) if a differential diagnosis of hypoplastic AML or MDS is being considered.
  – Ancillary studies employed in cases of peripheral blood cytopenias which may be investigated with focused immunohistochemical studies on the marrow based on clinical and histopathologic findings include evaluation for certain infectious causes (e.g., parvovirus), for certain lymphoproliferative disorders (e.g., hairy cell and large granular lymphocytic leukemia) and rarely for plasma cell dyscrasias.

B. *Growth factor and other therapy-associated peripheral blood cytoses or marrow hypercellularity:*
- For initial evaluation of cytoses after initiation of growth factor therapy, a complete blood count (CBC) with differential and peripheral blood smear review is used to ensure appropriate therapeutic effect and a full spectrum of maturation.
- Serial CBCs are often obtained to assess adequate therapeutic effect. Serial peripheral blood smear reviews are unnecessary if the patient has a history of growth factor therapy with expected fluctuations in CBC parameters.
- Generally speaking, marrow biopsies immediately following growth factor administration should be avoided. However, if assessing a specimen post growth factor administration, note that the underlying disease may be "masked" or underestimated due to extreme myeloid and/or erythroid hyperplasia.

C. *Therapy-induced differentiation of malignant hematologic Cells: ATRA, IDH 1/2 inhibitors:*
- Immunophenotyping by flow cytometry is routine in initial diagnosis and after treatment; however, these studies are generally used to assess abnormal blast populations and not the degree of cellular maturation [53, 56]. Notably, differentiating myeloid precursors may continue to show some immunophenotypic abnormalities.
- Molecular studies for pathognomonic APL and *IDH* mutations are required at defined points after cytotoxic chemotherapy for assessment of minimal residual disease.
- Differentiated marrow cells after therapy may still harbor genetic abnormalities, despite being functionally mature [55].
- One major complication of these therapies is differentiation syndrome (see Question 6 below), and CBC data can support this diagnosis with an elevated, myeloid predominant leukocytosis; however, no exact white blood cell count is predictive [41].

D. *Therapy-associated dysmorphology and dysplastic changes in blood and marrow:*
- No ancillary testing is needed to confirm medication-related pseudo Pelger-Huët change in neutrophils when temporally-associated with therapies known to cause such changes (see Table 32.6).
- However, this does not rule out the co-existence of a clonal hematologic process. Particularly in patients with prior history of chemo–/radiotherapy and/or if there is significant clinical concern for a clonal process (e.g., unexplained cytopenias), bone marrow biopsy and ancillary laboratory testing, including cytogenetics, flow cytometry, and molecular testing, may be warranted.

E. *Therapy-related secondary hematolymphoid neoplasms*
Therapy-associated myeloid neoplasms (tMN):
- At a minimum iron stain on aspirate smears (Prussian blue) is needed (in addition to the routine stains on aspirate and biopsy) to workup myelodysplasia and / or leukemia.
- Immunophenotyping may aid blast enumeration; however, there are no specific immunophenotypic findings that can distinguish tMN from de novo MDS/AML.
- Some common antigenic aberrations that are seen in therapy-associated myeloid neoplasms include aberrant expression of CD56 and/or CD7 on myeloid cells.
- Flow cytometric assessment is useful to exclude other possible causes of cytopenias (e.g., large granular lymphocytosis, paroxysmal nocturnal hemoglobinuria, etc.).
- Cytogenetic analysis often shows a complex karyotype with unbalanced translocations involving chromosomes 5, 7, 20, or balanced translocations involving 11q23, 21q22, and others. Again, none are specific for therapy-associated MN.

Post-transplant and immunodeficiency (iatrogenic)-associated lymphoproliferations:

- For suspected PTLD with non-destructive lesions, *EBV* immunoreactivity is critical for establishing the diagnosis even in the appropriate clinical context. In-situ hybridization for *EBV* encoded RNA, or EBER is the preferred test as it has the highest sensitivity. *EBV* negative lesions are extremely difficult to identify as PTLD given their non-specific histologic appearance. On the other hand, *EBV* expression is not specific for PTLD and approximately one-third of B-cell PTLDs and two-thirds of T-cell PTLDs may be *EBV* negative.
- Workup of suspected PTLD also requires a panel of immunohistochemical stains including B-cell markers (CD20, PAX5), T-cell markers (CD3), CD30, CD15, proliferation marker Ki-67, and *EBV* IHC stains (EBNA2, LMP1), if EBER in-situ hybridization test is not available.
- It is important to distinguish Hodgkin lymphoma from lymphomas with Hodgkin-like features and the B-cell or T-cell origin of other PTLDs [22]. Monomorphic B-PTLDs often express CD30 and are of post-germinal center origin (expressing MUM1, BCL6); however, these immunophenotypic findings are neither specific nor sensitive for a diagnosis of PTLD. See also Chap. 10 for detailed workup for PTLD.

6. Which findings in these cases identify clinically relevant entities and which ancillary tests can provide prognostic and therapeutic target information for subsequent management?

A. *Therapy-associated marked marrow hypocellularity or cytopenias:*

- Per NCCN guidelines, marrow assessment to document hypocellularity (<5% cellularity) and blasts less than 5% is recommended at 14–21 days post initiation of myeloablative induction therapy in AML. Re-induction is recommended if residual disease is present. Differentiating regenerating blasts from residual disease blasts has therapeutic implications. Post-chemotherapeutic myeloablated marrows are not the optimal source for prognostic and therapeutic target information, which is generally obtained through ancillary studies (e.g., flow cytometry, cytogenetics, molecular) performed on the pre-treatment diagnostic marrow.
- Recent literature suggests that day 14 marrows in adults with Philadelphia negative acute lymphoblastic leukemia (ALL) may also have prognostic value [57, 58].
- A marrow with extensive necrosis warrants deeper sectioning to assess for viable tumor. Ability to derive prognostic and therapeutic target information is generally limited in poorly viable material.
- Serous atrophy often requires a clinical assessment for underlying causes.
- A diagnosis of aplastic anemia is made in patients with cytopenias with a reduced marrow cellularity of less than 25%. Further risk stratification is done based on degree of cytopenias, with severe AA being presence of at least two of the following: ANC of less than 500 per microliter, platelets less than 20 per microliter, or reticulocyte count of less than 20 per microliter. Very severe AA is ANC less than 200 per microliter. Patients without severe AA may be observed [59], while those with severe AA require treatment generally involving bone marrow transplant and immunosuppression.
- Although 40–50% of cases of aplastic anemia may have PNH clones, PNH specific therapy is generally considered only if there is associated hemolysis and thrombosis and/or the PNH clone is large (exceeding 50%) [59]. Additionally, in many patients with acquired aplastic anemia, an antecedent exposure to an offending chemical, infectious or other agent is difficult to establish and differentiating this from other inherited syndromes may be difficult. Since some inherited syndromes, e.g., telomeropathies, may present later in life and may not have other overt clinical features, some experts recommend testing for blood leukocyte telomerase length in all patients with aplastic anemia [59].

B. *Therapy-associated marrow hypercellularity or peripheral blood cytoses:*

No specific workup other than monitoring blood counts for therapeutic effect is required. Studies on erythroid growth factor administration have demonstrated an approximately two-fold increase in thromboembolism; however, the significant benefits of reducing transfusion may outweigh this risk depending on the clinical scenario [60]. Thrombopoietic agents on the other hand have yet to demonstrate clear associations with increased thrombotic risk; however, these findings may be confounded by the prothrombotic potential of idiopathic thrombocytopenic purpura, which is one of the major indications for this therapy [33, 61].

C. *Therapy-associated differentiation of malignant hematologic cells: ATRA, IDH 1/2 inhibitors:*

- The prognostic risk assessment for APL is based on clinical and CBC parameters [55].
- Prognostic significance of mutant *IDH* in AML is still debated; current studies suggest adverse prognosis to standard chemotherapy [62].

- The degree of differentiation induced by these agents is not known to affect prognosis.
- Differentiation syndrome is observed in a subset (<10%) of patients who receive arsenic trioxide or ATRA for APL and mIDH inhibitors. This adverse entity is characterized by an elevated white count, fever, pulmonary signs and symptoms (dyspnea, respiratory distress, pulmonary infiltrates, pulmonary edema or pleural effusions), weight gain, headaches, bone pain, congestive heart failure, hepatotoxicity, and renal failure.
  - Early recognition and management are essential to reduce mortality. Risk factors include a high baseline WBC count, high body mass index, sequential (instead of concurrent) chemotherapy [63].

D. *Therapy-associated dysmorphology and dysplastic changes:*

The most relevant step in working up these cases is to ensure that a clonal hematopoietic process is not over- or underdiagnosed on the basis of morphological atypia.

E. *Therapy-related secondary hematolymphoid neoplasms:*

- tMN are associated with a poor prognosis with a median survival of 8–14 months [64, 65]. Although tMN can be categorized as tMDS or tAML based on blast counts of under 20% of 20% or higher, both categories are essentially similar clinically, with poor prognosis.
  - Factors that worsen prognosis include unfavorable karyotype (complex karyotypes, deletions in chromosome 5, deletion in chromosome 7 and trisomy 8) [66].
  - Therapy-related MN patients tend to have more comorbidities, worse performance status, and high-risk karyotypes compared to their de novo counterparts. If these factors are balanced, the prognosis of patients older than 60 years with tMN approaches that of de novo MN in the elderly; however, tMN is an independent adverse prognostic indicator in younger patients [67].
- In PTLD, various combinations of reduction of immunosuppression, rituximab, chemotherapy, regional radiotherapy, surgery and in select cases, other developing strategies like immune checkpoint blockade, adoptive cell therapies including unselected donor lymphocyte infusion and *EBV*-specific cytotoxic T lymphocyte infusion are utilized [68].
  - Reduction/withdrawal of immunosuppression may be sufficient in non-destructive PTLDs (early lesions) but in a lesser proportion of polymorphous PTLDs and only a small proportion of monomorphous PTLDs. Pathologic workup to assess potential therapeutic targets is still investigational, but may include assessment of PD1/PDL-1 [69] as well as *EBV*.
  - Withdrawal of methotrexate often results in regression of the methotrexate-associated lymphoproliferations, but the hepatosplenic gamma delta T-cell lymphomas associated with TNF-blocking agents often require aggressive therapy and allogenic bone marrow transplantation.

7. What is an adequate marrow specimen in previously treated patients?

- The adequacy of specimen depends somewhat on the type of prior treatment since the information sought from a repeat blood and marrow examination is somewhat different in each case. In hypocellular marrows, it is particularly important to have an adequately long core biopsy to ensure sampling beyond the subcortical area. See Chap. 20 and Question 8 below for additional discussion about variation in cellularity in different locations in the marrow. In patients treated with growth factors, peripheral blood counts and smear evaluation are generally adequate. Bone marrow examination is considered only if there is concern for new, persistent, or recurrent myeloid neoplasm.
- In patients receiving differentiation-inducing therapy (ATRA, IDH1/2 inhibitors), peripheral blood counts, smear, and post- treatment bone marrow biopsies at standard intervals are performed. If new cytopenias or Pelgeroid changes or other evidence of dysplasia are observed on peripheral blood counts and smears, good-quality bone marrow aspirate is usually the most informative specimen.
  - Archived smears or previous CBC results and peripheral blood smear comments in the medical history are helpful for evaluating duration of changes and temporal association with offending medications.
- For suspected tMN, assessment of peripheral blood, marrow aspirate, core biopsy, iron-stained aspirate smears and ancillary workup including flow cytometry, and cytogenetics is generally required. Molecular analysis is also generally performed for prognosis and increasingly to assess candidacy for newer targeted therapies.
- For post-transplant and other iatrogenic lymphoproliferations, a bone marrow biopsy may not be the optimal specimen for establishing the diagnosis and an excisional biopsy of the mass lesion with viable tissue that is adequate for histologic and immunohistochemical workup is needed. For cutaneous and mucosal sites, the biopsy should be deep enough to allow adequate assessment [70]. An unfixed sample for flow cytometric immunophenotyping to assess clonality is also helpful.

8. What information should be conveyed to the clinician during each stage of the work up and/ or when the specimen is limited?

A. *Therapy-associated marked marrow hypocellularity or cytopenia(s):*
   - Specimen from patients after cytotoxic/cytolytic therapy: Evaluation of day 14 marrows performed to assess chemotherapeutic ablation in AML is often time sensitive. It is advisable to convey presence of residual blasts, either on peripheral smear, bone marrow aspirate smear, or flow cytometry to the treating clinician. In the absence of overt disease, reporting of aspirate findings should include a comment regarding specimen adequacy, and defer the definitive assessment of cellularity to the core biopsy.
   - If aplastic anemia is a clinical consideration, caution should be exercised in providing interpretation in limited marrow biopsies. Subcortical marrow is often hypocellular, and a diagnosis of AA should not be rendered in either short biopsies or longer but tangential biopsies that may possibly have sampled only subcortical marrow. Furthermore, AA is a diagnosis of exclusion, and an adequate sample to exclude other differential diagnostic considerations, including ancillary studies such as flow cytometry and cytogenetics, is crucial.
     - Nearly 20% of MDS may be hypoplastic; morphologic and/or immunohistochemical finding of small micromegakaryocytes and karyotypic abnormalities characteristic of MDS help distinguish this from AA. In limited samples without adequate morphologic assessment, and/or available cytogenetics, this distinction cannot be made reliably.
   - In marrows replaced by necrotic/non-viable tissues, a morphologic description stating presence of non-viable ghost outlines of mononuclear cells can be provided. A suggestion to evaluate the patient clinically and via imaging to identify any other mass lesions is appropriate. Biopsy of such lesions can be requested for definitive diagnosis.

B. *Therapy-associated marrow hypercellularity and/or peripheral blood cytoses:*
   - Expected cytoses or marrow hypercellularity from growth factor therapies do not need to be communicated verbally. However, a concern for recurrent disease such as persistent cytopenias/inadequate response to growth factors and presence of abnormal blasts (e.g., with Auer rods or of disease phenotype) should be communicated promptly.
   - Reactive and dysplastic morphology that may be observed in the setting of myeloid growth factors (see Question 2 above) should be described with a disclaimer that these findings reflect cytokine effect that can arise from a number of etiologies including infection, inflammation, direct or indirect drug effects, or potentially myeloid neoplasm.

C. *Therapy-associated malignant cell differentiation (ATRA, IDH 1/2 inhibitors,* etc.*):*
   - During therapeutic differentiation, significant leukocytosis may occur as the malignant cells mature into functional granulocytes. The kinetics of this change and the degree of resulting leukocytosis can vary widely.
     - Peak ATRA-induced leukocytosis often occurs over the first 30 days of therapy, with a median time to peak count after 10 days [21].
     - Initial data from the first clinical trials of IDH1 and IDH2 inhibitors (ivosidenib and enasidenib, respectively) report leukocytosis occurring during the first 60 days of treatment [13, 14].
     - The prolonged time course of the leukocytosis and the lack of clear relationship between the level of leukocyte count and development of differentiation syndrome should be pointed out to the clinician along with any evidence of secondary infection or cytokine effects.

D. *Therapy-associated dysmorphology and dysplastic changes:*
   - Presence of dysmorphology should always be documented in cases whether or not there is clinical concern for a hematologic malignancy. In this manner, the patient's dysmorphology can be temporally-associated with medication administration from medical record or monitored over time if there is concern for an underlying myeloid malignancy.
     - Additional helpful information may include increase or decrease in the proportion of cells displaying dysmorphology from previous sample and/ or any lineages disproportionately affected by this morphology.

E. *Therapy-related neoplasms:*
   - When morphologic features are diagnostic of tMN, the findings can be conveyed to the clinical team. A complete assessment requires karyotypic analysis. A request for a repeat marrow biopsy is appropriate if the marrow sample is aparticulate and hemodilute. If circulating blasts are present above the diagnostic threshold of 20%, then in the appropriate clinical context the possibility of a tAML can be raised. Rarely, the diagnosis of tMN is made via a tissue biopsy of an extramedullary myeloid sarcoma. In such cases, request for a bone marrow biopsy is appropriate.
   - The clinical presentation of PTLDs can vary widely, and while many present as mass lesions, others may have non-specific systemic symptoms, or viral septic shock like picture. The clinical differential diagnosis

in many such cases may include PTLD versus an infection. If histologic features of a PTLD are seen, it is desirable to convey the preliminary pathologic diagnosis to the clinical team, pending availability of immunohistochemical stains. If the sample is limited, or a complete immunohistochemical workup is not available, differential diagnostic possibilities may be raised. In some situations, e.g., lesions involving mucosa or skin, a deep biopsy allowing visualization of base of the ulcer is important for an accurate diagnosis of *EBV*-associated mucocutaneous ulcer.

9. When is a diagnostic comment necessary and what should be discussed in the comment in these cases?

A. *Therapy-associated marked marrow hypocellularity or cytopenias:*
   - In day 14 myeloablated marrows, the presence of few blasts in an otherwise markedly hypocellular marrow may be indicative of recovering marrow versus minimal residual disease. This should be discussed in the diagnostic comment. Options for further assessment may include correlation with ancillary studies, if any, to detect any previously detected abnormalities or, alternatively, clinical monitoring with a re-biopsy after 2–3 days.
   - For patients with an aplastic marrow, the diagnostic comment should mention specimen adequacy, especially if there is a concern that the sample is subcortical and the observed hypocellularity may not be representative. Also, any concern for differential diagnostic considerations such as hypoplastic myelodysplastic syndrome should be mentioned.
   - A diagnostic comment for marrows with serous fat atrophy should include possible relevant etiologies of this finding, to direct clinical investigation. This is a finding seen in malnutrition including from severe chronic illnesses. In young adults, anorexia nervosa, acute febrile illnesses, AIDS, while in older adults alcoholism, lymphoma, and chronic heart failure are common associations [27].
   - In necrotic marrows, the diagnostic comment should include differential diagnostic concerns, as well as a comment on unreliability of immunohistochemical workup on non-viable tissue.

B. *Therapy-associated marrow hypercellularity and/or peripheral blood cytoses:*
   - The source of information confirming growth factor therapy, e.g., electronic patient records, discussion with clinician, etc., should be documented so that the morphological changes can be correlated with this information.
   - Reactive and dysplastic morphology that may be observed in the setting of myeloid growth factors (see section 2B above) should be described with a disclaimer that these findings reflect cytokine effect that can arise from a number of etiologies including infection, inflammation, direct or indirect drug effects, or potentially myeloid neoplasm.

C. *Therapy-associated differentiation of malignant hematologic cells:*
   - In the presence of "intermediate cells," a comment stating that the findings are compatible with ATRA or mIDH inhibitor therapy is warranted, especially as the therapy-induced changes can often be dramatic both in speed (maturation over a matter of days) and degree of leukocytosis (neutrophilia may exceed 10 k cells/μL).
   - Where appropriate, a differential diagnosis, including conditions such as infection and cytokine effect, should be included.

D. *Therapy-associated dysmorphology and dysplastic changes:*
   - When the morphological changes are borderline or not readily explained by available clinical information, the comment should draw attention to the changes and request clinical correlation with prior therapy, etc.
   - When appropriate, alternative differential diagnostic considerations should be discussed.

E. *Therapy-related secondary hematolymphoid neoplasms*
   - tMN: The diagnostic comment should emphasize that this is a clinicopathological diagnosis and include known antecedent therapies that are being implicated. The necessity for correlation with any pending ancillary studies to confirm the diagnosis should be mentioned.
   - Post-transplant and other immunodeficiency-associated lymphoproliferative disorders: This diagnosis should include the implicated therapy that led to the immunosuppressed state (e.g., post-transplant, methotrexate-associated, etc.), as well as any viral association (e.g., *EBV*, HHV8) [70]. Diagnostic comments are often utilized for the following:
     - To reiterate information available to the pathologist regarding antecedent transplant or other immunosuppressants, based on which this diagnosis was made.
     - To discuss differential diagnosis, when treatment history is less clear, or in *EBV*-negative cases occurring post-transplant after a long latency.
     - To discuss rationale of classifying the lymphoma within a particular subtype. For example, a PTLD with Reed-Sternberg like cells not definitively meeting criteria for classic Hodgkin lymphoma is best regarded as a polymorphous or monomorphous PTLD, with RS like cells.
     - To highlight pertinent characteristics of clinical course and/or prognosis.

10. When is it appropriate to seek external consultation in these cases?

A large proportion of post-therapy bone marrow biopsies are examined at academic centers conducting stem cell transplantation and other advanced therapies for these conditions. Novel molecular or immune-based therapies are being introduced rapidly, and their morphological effects are largely undocumented. If the pathologist has limited experience in handling such biopsies or if the morphological findings are not typical and/or the repertoire of ancillary studies available is limited, it would be appropriate to request external consultation. More specific situations are listed below.

A. *Therapy-associated marked marrow hypocellularity or cytopenias:*

Cases showing presence of immature cells in blood or marrow, discrepant results in blood and marrow, grossly unbalanced survival of different hematopoietic lineages, excessive or atypical lymphoid cells, plasma cells or histiocytes, and fibrosis or bone changes which are not readily explained by prior clinical history may be appropriate for external consultation.

B. *Therapy-associated marrow hypercellularity and/or peripheral blood cytoses:*

If there is clinical concern for continued disease or if results of ancillary studies are discordant with morphological findings, the possibility that growth factor induced cellular proliferation is masking the pathology should be considered. In case a definitive diagnosis is difficult, it may be appropriate to seek external consultation.

- Presence of disproportionate number (>10%) of dysplastic cells in peripheral blood or bone marrow, an unbalanced spectrum of myeloid maturation with >10% immature granulocytes, or increased blasts warrant further workup. Myeloid growth factors generally have the least effect on blast counts [34, 35]. If discontinuation of therapy does not correct these findings or if therapy cannot be discontinued for clinical reasons, it may be appropriate to seek external consultation.

C. *Therapy-associated differentiation of malignant hematologic cells:*

If marrow cellularity does not decrease as expected after routine chemotherapy of acute myeloid leukemia and the surviving cells cannot be clearly classified or if morphologic assessment is challenging due to the wide spectrum of abnormally differentiating cells with background abnormal diseased marrow, external consult may be obtained. Apparently, mature cells may harbor genetic changes of the leukemic clone though are not blast equivalents [8, 53, 71].

D. *Therapy-associated dysmorphology and dysplastic changes:*

- A thorough clinical review to rule out any autoimmune, infectious, dietary, or toxic causes of apparent dyspoiesis and medication history is necessary. External pathology consultation is appropriate when the dysplasia cannot be attributed to any known causes.

E. *Therapy-related secondary hematolymphoid neoplasms*

- tMN: External consultation should be sought whenever a complete workup is not available at your facility. The recommended initial workup for MDS, including therapy-related MDS, includes a morphologic review of peripheral smear and review of marrow aspirate, biopsy, and iron stain. Cytogenetic analysis by standard karyotyping should be done, and if a karyotype cannot be obtained, then an MDS FISH panel needs to be done. Molecular testing to evaluate somatic mutations should be considered. Additional cytogenetic and molecular testing may sometimes be needed, particularly in younger patients, to evaluate hereditary mutations that predispose to hematologic malignancies (e.g., Diamond-Blackfan anemia, Fanconi anemia, Shwachman-Diamond syndrome, telomere biology disorders, congenital neutropenia, Down syndrome), congenital sideroblastic anemias, and other familial genetic disorders associated with MDS (e.g., RUNX1, *GATA2*, etc.). Flow cytometry, particularly to evaluate for large granular lymphocytic leukemias, and/or aplastic anemias, and HLA typing in patients who are considering bone marrow transplantation may be necessary.
- Post-transplant or immunodeficiency-associated lymphoproliferative disorders: The morphological overlap of early lesions of PTLD with reactive processes, the presence of prior diagnosis of lymphoma, an apparent low-grade lymphoma occurring as possible PTLD, discrepancies between engraftment studies and bone marrow findings, and suspicion of donor-derived disease are confounding factors which may warrant external consultation.

Case Presentations

Case 1

Learning Objectives

1. Understand the temporal development of marrow suppression and recovery.
2. Expand the differential diagnostic considerations of a leucoerythroblastic smear.
3. Review a spectrum of therapy-related marrow suppression and recovery.

Case History

A 78-year old male with a past medical history of benign prostatic hypertrophy, psoriatic arthritis (on weekly methotrexate 2.5 mg), diabetes mellitus type 2, ischemic cardiomyopathy treated with CABG 15 years prior (on Coumadin), and coronary artery disease with carotid endarterectomy, presents with pancytopenia of unclear etiology discovered after a syncopal episode. CBC at presentation was WBC 2.3, Hgb 11.1, Plt 104, INR 2.5, AST 80/ALT 127, with a WBC nadir of 0.8 within a few days. A broad infectious workup was negative, without localizing signs. Pancytopenia was thought to be from methotrexate (MTX)-induced marrow suppression; MTX was held, patient administered B12, and referred to hematology service.

One week after stopping MTX, patient continued to be pancytopenic (WBC 1.3, RBC 3.10, HgB 8.9, HCT 26.4, MCV 85 fL, MCH 28.7 pg, MCHC 33.7 g/dL, Plt 95). Differential count shows neutropenia, circulating nucleated RBCs, and new appearance of 6% blasts.

Differential Diagnosis

- Marrow recovery following MTX cessation
- Myelodysplastic syndrome or acute myeloid leukemia
- Unrelated marrow infiltrative process with leukoerythroblastosis

Histologic Findings

- Bone marrow aspirate was aparticulate, with an M:E ratio of 10:1. Granulocytes were markedly left-shifted and comprised of blasts (5%), promyelocytes, and myelocytes. A few unremarkable megakaryocytes are seen. No dysplasia or metastatic disease seen (Fig. 32.9).
- Bone marrow core biopsy has variable cellularity, ranging from less than 5% to patchy areas with 50% cellularity. Cellularity is myeloid predominant with marked left-shift (Fig. 32.10).

Ancillary Studies Performed on the Bone Marrow

- Flow cytometry: Myeloid blasts mildly increased in number (5.7% of total events). The immunophenotype of the blasts was mildly atypical with weaker-than-normal expression of CD71 and CD117. The significance of this finding is unclear since myeloid blasts can be increased in both neoplastic and reactive conditions.
- Karyotype: A normal male karyotype was detected in 5 of 20 cells analyzed. The remaining 15 cells showed clonal loss of the Y chromosome, which is a common finding in elderly males with little known diagnostic and prognostic significance.
- FISH: No evidence of common AML-related chromosome abnormalities was detected by interphase FISH analysis

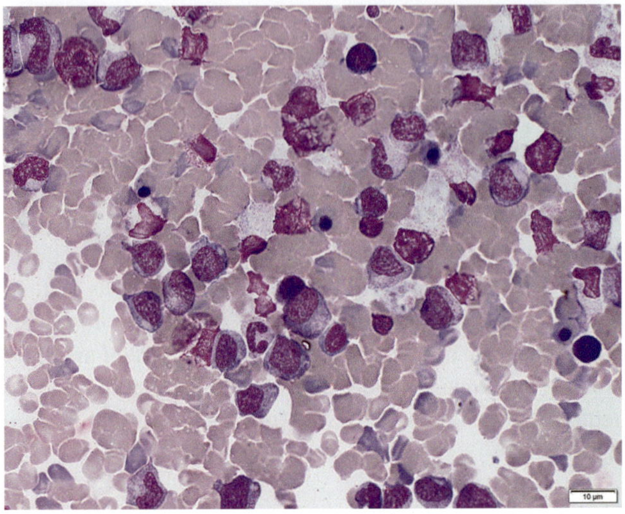

Fig. 32.9 Case 1. Bone marrow aspirate (Wright-Giemsa stained, 600× magnification): Granulocytic predominance with marked left-shift. A majority of the granulocytes are at the myelocyte stage of differentiation with rare metamyelocytes and bands. A few erythroid precursors are seen without significant dyspoiesis

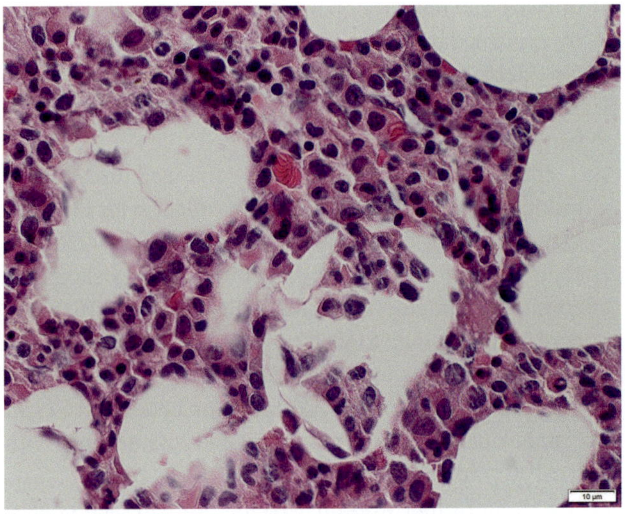

Fig. 32.10 Case 1. Bone marrow core biopsy (H&E stained, 600× magnification): Granulocytic predominant hematopoiesis with marked left-shift

Final Diagnosis

Left-shifted granulopoiesis most compatible with regenerating marrow

Take-Home Messages

1. Marrow suppressant medications can present with significant pancytopenia. Myelosuppression is a major dose-limiting side effect of high-dose methotrexate requiring serial monitoring of CBC (monthly for the first 3 months and every 2–3 months thereafter).

2. After offending agent is removed, there can be brisk marrow recovery, sometimes with blasts in peripheral blood.
3. Marrow biopsies performed in early marrow recovery may have early myeloid precursors at similar stages of maturation that can mimic acute leukemia. Normal cytomorphology, recovering peripheral counts, absence of aberrant markers on blasts, and lack of cytogenetic abnormalities are clues that help in the differential diagnosis.

Case 2

Learning Objectives

1. Assessment of leukocytosis in a myeloid leukemia patient after differentiating therapy
2. Appropriate ancillary testing for monitoring mIDH myeloid leukemia on mIDH inhibitors

Case History

The patient is a 60-year-old male with a recent history of acute myeloid leukemia harboring an *IDH1* R132C mutation, now undergoing cycle 4 of ivosidenib therapy (mIDH1 inhibitor).

Laboratory Findings (Fig. 32.11)

- CBC; WBC 37.3, Hgb 10.7, MCV 87, Plt – 103
  - WBC Differential; ANC 21.3, Monocytes (Abs) 4.1, immature granulocytes (Abs) 4.1, Blasts (Abs): 0.37

Histologic Findings (Fig. 32.12)

- Bone marrow core biopsy; cellularity: 100%, M:E ratio: 6–7:1.
  - Differential (%); Blasts <1, promyelocytes: 1, myelocytes 5, metamyelocytes 15, granulocytes 68, eosinophils 4, basophils <1, lymphocytes 2, erythroid 5

Differential Diagnosis

- Differentiation of myeloid blasts
- Reactive leukocytosis

Ancillary Studies

- Flow cytometry: Atypical myeloid blasts (2%), mature granulocytes (~65%)
- Molecular studies: Mutated *IDH* R132C; 50% allelic burden

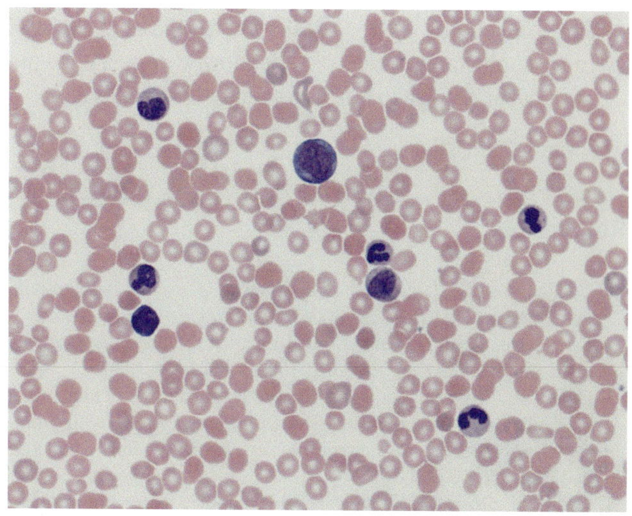

Fig. 32.11 Case 2. Peripheral blood smear (400×)

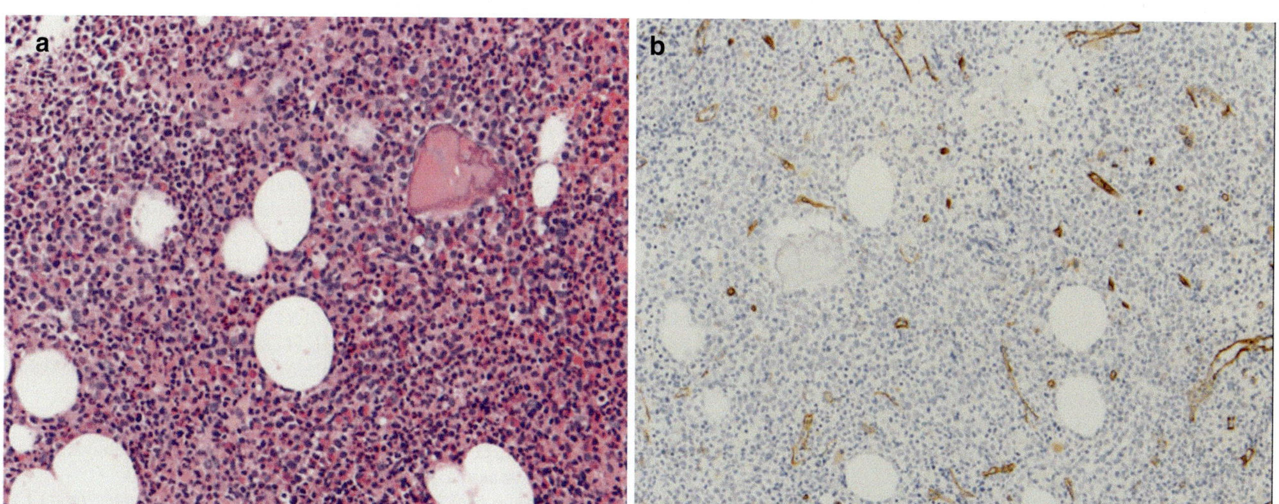

Fig. 32.12 Case 2. Bone marrow biopsy Core. (**a**) Hematoxylin and eosin staining (200×), (**b**) CD34 immunohistochemistry (200×)

Final Diagnosis

Hypercellular myeloid-predominant marrow with features of treated acute leukemia and persistent population of abnormal blasts (~2%)

Take-Home Messages

1. Differentiation therapies (mIDH inhibitors and all-trans retinoic acid) for certain myeloid malignancies (mIDH AML, acute promyelocytic leukemia) promote differentiation of myeloid blasts into mature, functioning granulocytes.
2. Granulocytosis can be a sign of treatment efficacy if differentiation therapy is initiated. However, monitoring for clinical signs of differentiation syndrome is warranted.
3. Despite maturation, disease cells retain the same genetic composition and can harbor a leukemic mutational burden depending on additional cytotoxic therapy. Immunophenotypic analysis by flow cytometry is the most accurate way to assess residual disease blasts.

References

1. Vandendries ER, Drews RE. Drug-associated disease: hematologic dysfunction. Crit Care Clin. 2006;22(2):347–55, viii
2. Schafernak KT. Gelatinous transformation of the bone marrow from anorexia nervosa. Blood. 2016;127(10):1374.
3. Chang E, Rivero G, Jiang B, Yellapragada S, Thiagarajan P. Gelatinous marrow transformation associated with imatinib: case report and literature review. Case Rep Hematol. 2017;2017:1950724.
4. Goyal M, Gupta A, Yarlagadda S, Handoo A. Fatty but starving marrow! Gelatinous transformation of bone marrow secondary to plasma cell disorder and all-trans-retinoic acid therapy: a report of two cases. South Asian J Cancer. 2017;6(1):40–1.
5. Barrientos JC, Burger JA, Byrd JC, Hillmen P, Zhou C, Ninomoto J, et al. Characterizing the kinetics of lymphocytosis in patients with chronic lymphocytic leukemia treated with single-agent ibrutinib. Leuk Lymphoma. 2019;60:1000–5.
6. Chang BY, Francesco M, De Rooij MF, Magadala P, Steggerda SM, Huang MM, et al. Egress of CD19(+)CD5(+) cells into peripheral blood following treatment with the Bruton tyrosine kinase inhibitor ibrutinib in mantle cell lymphoma patients. Blood. 2013;122(14):2412–24.
7. de The H, Chen Z. Acute promyelocytic leukaemia: novel insights into the mechanisms of cure. Nat Rev Cancer. 2010;10(11):775–83.
8. de The H. Differentiation therapy revisited. Nat Rev Cancer. 2018;18(2):117–27.
9. Lu C, Ward PS, Kapoor GS, Rohle D, Turcan S, Abdel-Wahab O, et al. IDH mutation impairs histone demethylation and results in a block to cell differentiation. Nature. 2012;483(7390):474–8.
10. Chaturvedi A, Araujo Cruz MM, Jyotsana N, Sharma A, Yun H, Gorlich K, et al. Mutant IDH1 promotes leukemogenesis in vivo and can be specifically targeted in human AML. Blood. 2013;122(16):2877–87.
11. Losman JA, Looper RE, Koivunen P, Lee S, Schneider RK, McMahon C, et al. (R)-2-hydroxyglutarate is sufficient to promote leukemogenesis and its effects are reversible. Science. 2013;339(6127):1621–5.
12. Figueroa ME, Abdel-Wahab O, Lu C, Ward PS, Patel J, Shih A, et al. Leukemic IDH1 and IDH2 mutations result in a hypermethylation phenotype, disrupt TET2 function, and impair hematopoietic differentiation. Cancer Cell. 2010;18(6):553–67.
13. Stein EM, DiNardo CD, Pollyea DA, Fathi AT, Roboz GJ, Altman JK, et al. Enasidenib in mutant IDH2 relapsed or refractory acute myeloid leukemia. Blood. 2017;130(6):722–31.
14. DiNardo CD, Stein EM, de Botton S, Roboz GJ, Altman JK, Mims AS, et al. Durable remissions with ivosidenib in IDH1-mutated relapsed or refractory AML. N Engl J Med. 2018;378(25):2386–98.
15. Kaplan JM, Barrett O Jr. Reversible pseudo-Pelger anomaly related to sulfisoxazole therapy. N Engl J Med. 1967;277(8):421–2.
16. Hoffmann K, Dreger CK, Olins AL, Olins DE, Shultz LD, Lucke B, et al. Mutations in the gene encoding the lamin B receptor produce an altered nuclear morphology in granulocytes (Pelger-Huet anomaly). Nat Genet. 2002;31(4):410–4.
17. Speeckaert MM, Verhelst C, Koch A, Speeckaert R, Lacquet F. Pelger-Huet anomaly: a critical review of the literature. Acta Haematol. 2009;121(4):202–6.
18. Colella R, Hollensead SC. Understanding and recognizing the Pelger-Huet anomaly. Am J Clin Pathol. 2012;137(3):358–66.
19. Etzell JE, Wang E. Acquired Pelger-Huet anomaly in association with concomitant tacrolimus and mycophenolate mofetil in a liver transplant patient: a case report and review of the literature. Arch Pathol Lab Med. 2006;130(1):93–6.
20. Dusse LM, Moreira AM, Vieira LM, Rios DR, Silva RM, Carvalho M. Acquired Pelger-Huet: what does it really mean? Clin Chim Acta. 2010;411(21–22):1587–90.
21. Wang E, Boswell E, Siddiqi I, Lu CM, Sebastian S, Rehder C, et al. Pseudo-Pelger-Huet anomaly induced by medications: a clinicopathologic study in comparison with myelodysplastic syndrome-related pseudo-Pelger-Huet anomaly. Am J Clin Pathol. 2011;135(2):291–303.
22. Swerdlow SHWS, Chadburn A, Ferry JA. Post transplant lymphoproliferative disorders. In: Swedlow SH, Campo E, Harris NL, Jaffe ES, Pileri SA, Stein H, Thiele J, Arber DA, Hasserjian RP, Le Beau MM, Siebert AOR, editors. WHO classification of tumours of hematopoietic and lymphoid tissues. World Health Organization Classification of Tumours. Revised 4th edition. Lyon: International Agency for Research on Cancer (IARC); 2017. p. 453–7.
23. Zeijlemaker W, Gratama JW, Schuurhuis GJ. Tumor heterogeneity makes AML a "moving target" for detection of residual disease. Cytometry B Clin Cytom. 2014;86(1):3–14.
24. Wittels B. Bone marrow biopsy changes following chemotherapy for acute leukemia. Am J Surg Pathol. 1980;4(2):135–42.
25. Ouyang W, Liu Y, Deng D, Zhou F, Xie C. The change in peripheral blood monocyte count: a predictor to make the management of chemotherapy-induced neutropenia. J Cancer Res Ther. 2018;14(Supplement):S565–S70.
26. Islam A, Catovsky D, Galton DA. Histological study of bone marrow regeneration following chemotherapy for acute myeloid leukaemia and chronic granulocytic leukaemia in blast transformation. Br J Haematol. 1980;45(4):535–40.
27. Bohm J. Gelatinous transformation of the bone marrow: the spectrum of underlying diseases. Am J Surg Pathol. 2000;24(1):56–65.
28. Li KD, Salama ME. Therapy effect: impact on bone marrow morphology. Surg Pathol Clin. 2016;9(1):177–87.
29. Janssens AM, Offner FC, Van Hove WZ. Bone marrow necrosis. Cancer. 2000;88(8):1769–80.
30. Marsh JC, Ball SE, Cavenagh J, Darbyshire P, Dokal I, Gordon-Smith EC, et al. Guidelines for the diagnosis and management of aplastic anaemia. Br J Haematol. 2009;147(1):43–70.
31. de Planque MM, van Krieken JH, Kluin-Nelemans HC, Colla LP, van der Burgh F, Brand A, et al. Bone marrow histopathology of patients with severe aplastic anaemia before treatment and at follow-up. Br J Haematol. 1989;72(3):439–44.

32. Frisch B, Lewis SM. The bone marrow in aplastic anaemia: diagnostic and prognostic features. J Clin Pathol. 1974;27(3):231–41.
33. Kuter DJ. Hematopoietic growth factors. In: Toby L, Simon JM, Snyder EL, Solheim BG, Strauss RG, editors. Rossi's principle of transfusion medicine. 5th ed: NJ. Wiley Blackwell; 2016. p. 418–29.
34. Tegg EM, Tuck DM, Lowenthal RM, Marsden KA. The effect of G-CSF on the composition of human bone marrow. Clin Lab Haematol. 1999;21(4):265–70.
35. Meyerson HJ, Farhi DC, Rosenthal NS. Transient increase in blasts mimicking acute leukemia and progressing myelodysplasia in patients receiving growth factor. Am J Clin Pathol. 1998;109(6):675–81.
36. Brandt SJ, Peters WP, Atwater SK, Kurtzberg J, Borowitz MJ, Jones RB, et al. Effect of recombinant human granulocyte-macrophage colony-stimulating factor on hematopoietic reconstitution after high-dose chemotherapy and autologous bone marrow transplantation. N Engl J Med. 1988;318(14):869–76.
37. Douglas VK, Tallman MS, Cripe LD, Peterson LC. Thrombopoietin administered during induction chemotherapy to patients with acute myeloid leukemia induces transient morphologic changes that may resemble chronic myeloproliferative disorders. Am J Clin Pathol. 2002;117(6):844–50.
38. Montesinos P, Bergua JM, Vellenga E, Rayon C, Parody R, de la Serna J, et al. Differentiation syndrome in patients with acute promyelocytic leukemia treated with all-trans retinoic acid and anthracycline chemotherapy: characteristics, outcome, and prognostic factors. Blood. 2009;113(4):775–83.
39. Luesink M, Jansen JH. Advances in understanding the pulmonary infiltration in acute promyelocytic leukaemia. Br J Haematol. 2010;151(3):209–20.
40. Luu HS, Rahaman PA. Mature neutrophils with Auer rods following treatment with all-trans retinoic acid for acute promyelocytic leukemia. Blood. 2015;126(1):121.
41. Tallman MS, Andersen JW, Schiffer CA, Appelbaum FR, Feusner JH, Ogden A, et al. Clinical description of 44 patients with acute promyelocytic leukemia who developed the retinoic acid syndrome. Blood. 2000;95(1):90–5.
42. Martin S, Tallman JKA. How I treat acute promyelocytic leukemia. Blood. 2009;114(25):5126–35.
43. Ok CY, Medeiros LJ, Hu Y, Bueso-Ramos CE, Wang SA. Transient/reversible ring sideroblasts in bone marrow of patients post cytotoxic therapies for primary malignancies. Leuk Res. 2011;35(12):1605–10.
44. Orazi A, Cattoretti G, Soligo D, Luksch R, Lambertenghi-Deliliers G. Therapy-related myelodysplastic syndromes: FAB classification, bone marrow histology, and immunohistology in the prognostic assessment. Leukemia. 1993;7(6):838–47.
45. Coombs CC, Zehir A, Devlin SM, Kishtagari A, Syed A, Jonsson P, et al. Therapy-related clonal hematopoiesis in patients with non-hematologic cancers is common and associated with adverse clinical outcomes. Cell Stem Cell. 2017;21(3):374–82.e4.
46. Peslak SA, Olson T, Babushok DV. Diagnosis and treatment of aplastic anemia. Curr Treat Options in Oncol. 2017;18(12):70.
47. Riccardi A, Ucci G, Luoni R, Castello A, Coci A, Magrini U, et al. Bone marrow biopsy in monoclonal gammopathies: correlations between pathological findings and clinical data. The Cooperative Group for Study and Treatment of Multiple Myeloma. J Clin Pathol. 1990;43(6):469–75.
48. Birendra KC, DiNardo CD. Evidence for clinical differentiation and differentiation syndrome in patients with acute myeloid leukemia and IDH1 mutations treated with the targeted mutant IDH1 inhibitor, AG-120. Clin Lymphoma Myeloma Leuk. 2016;16(8):460–5.
49. Granfeldt Ostgard LS, Medeiros BC, Sengelov H, Norgaard M, Andersen MK, Dufva IH, et al. Epidemiology and clinical significance of secondary and therapy-related acute myeloid leukemia: a National Population-Based Cohort Study. J Clin Oncol. 2015;33(31):3641–9.
50. Hauke R, Smir B, Greiner T, Bierman P, Tarantolo S, Anderson J, et al. Clinical and pathological features of posttransplant lymphoproliferative disorders: influence on survival and response to treatment. Ann Oncol. 2001;12(6):831–4.
51. Pont J, Souvignet A, Campos L, Plesa A, Bulabois B, Pernollet M, et al. Accurate quantification of fourteen normal bone marrow cell subsets in infants to the elderly by flow cytometry. Cytometry B Clin Cytom. 2018;94(5):627–36.
52. Warrell RP Jr, Frankel SR, Miller WH Jr, Scheinberg DA, Itri LM, Hittelman WN, et al. Differentiation therapy of acute promyelocytic leukemia with tretinoin (all-trans-retinoic acid). N Engl J Med. 1991;324(20):1385–93.
53. Amatangelo MD, Quek L, Shih A, Stein EM, Roshal M, David MD, et al. Enasidenib induces acute myeloid leukemia cell differentiation to promote clinical response. Blood. 2017;130(6):732–41.
54. Glasser L, Fiederlein RL, Shamdas GJ, Brothman AR. Functional characteristics of in vivo induced neutrophils after differentiation therapy of acute promyelocytic leukemia with all-trans-retinoic acid. Cancer. 1994;73(4):1206–12.
55. Cicconi L, Lo-Coco F. Current management of newly diagnosed acute promyelocytic leukemia. Ann Oncol. 2016;27(8):1474–81.
56. Horna P, Zhang L, Sotomayor EM, Lancet JE, Moscinski LC. Diagnostic immunophenotype of acute promyelocytic leukemia before and early during therapy with all-trans retinoic acid. Am J Clin Pathol. 2014;142(4):546–52.
57. Short NJ, Kantarjian HM, Sasaki K, Cortes JE, Ravandi F, Thomas DA, et al. Prognostic significance of day 14 bone marrow evaluation in adults with Philadelphia chromosome-negative acute lymphoblastic leukemia. Cancer. 2016;122(24):3812–20.
58. Park HS, Kim DY, Choi EJ, Lee JH, Lee JH, Jeon M, et al. Blast percentage of bone marrow aspirate on day 14 of induction chemotherapy predicts adult acute lymphoblastic leukemia treatment outcomes. Acta Haematol. 2018;139(4):220–7.
59. Scheinberg P, Young NS. How I treat acquired aplastic anemia. Blood. 2012;120(6):1185–96.
60. Bohlius J, Wilson J, Seidenfeld J, Piper M, Schwarzer G, Sandercock J, et al. Erythropoietin or darbepoetin for patients with cancer. Cochrane Database Syst Rev. 2006;(3):CD003407.
61. Rodeghiero F. ITP and thrombosis: an intriguing association. Blood Adv. 2017;1(24):2280.
62. Medeiros BC, Fathi AT, DiNardo CD, Pollyea DA, Chan SM, Swords R. Isocitrate dehydrogenase mutations in myeloid malignancies. Leukemia. 2017;31(2):272–81.
63. Rogers JE, Yang D. Differentiation syndrome in patients with acute promyelocytic leukemia. J Oncol Pharm Pract. 2012;18(1):109–14.
64. Smith SM, Le Beau MM, Huo D, Karrison T, Sobecks RM, Anastasi J, et al. Clinical-cytogenetic associations in 306 patients with therapy-related myelodysplasia and myeloid leukemia: the University of Chicago series. Blood. 2003;102(1):43–52.
65. Fianchi L, Pagano L, Piciocchi A, Candoni A, Gaidano G, Breccia M, et al. Characteristics and outcome of therapy-related myeloid neoplasms: report from the Italian network on secondary leukemias. Am J Hematol. 2015;90(5):E80–5.
66. Schoch C, Kern W, Schnittger S, Hiddemann W, Haferlach T. Karyotype is an independent prognostic parameter in therapy-related acute myeloid leukemia (t-AML): an analysis of 93 patients with t-AML in comparison to 1091 patients with de novo AML. Leukemia. 2004;18(1):120–5.
67. McNerney ME, Godley LA, Le Beau MM. Therapy-related myeloid neoplasms: when genetics and environment collide. Nat Rev Cancer. 2017;17(9):513–27.

68. Liu L, Zhang X, Feng S. Epstein-Barr virus-related post-transplantation lymphoproliferative disorders after allogeneic hematopoietic stem cell transplantation. Biol Blood Marrow Transplant. 2018;24(7):1341–9.
69. Goodman A, Patel SP, Kurzrock R. PD-1-PD-L1 immune-checkpoint blockade in B-cell lymphomas. Nat Rev Clin Oncol. 2017;14(4):203–20.
70. Natkunam Y, Gratzinger D, Chadburn A, Goodlad JR, Chan JKC, Said J, et al. Immunodeficiency-associated lymphoproliferative disorders: time for reappraisal? Blood. 2018;132(18):1871–8.
71. Dalal BI, Bruyere H, Barnett MJ. Significance of persistent Auer rods and cytogenetic abnormality after first cycle of therapy for acute promyelocytic leukaemia. Br J Haematol. 2007;137(5):385.

Index

E. Wang, A. S. Lagoo (eds.), *Practical Lymph Node and Bone Marrow Pathology*, Practical Anatomic Pathology,
https://doi.org/10.1007/978-3-030-32189-5

D

E

F

I

N

O

P

MIX
Papier aus verantwortungsvollen Quellen
Paper from responsible sources
FSC® C105338

If you have any concerns about our products,
you can contact us on
ProductSafety@springernature.com

In case Publisher is established outside the EU,
the EU authorized representative is:
Springer Nature Customer Service Center GmbH
Europaplatz 3, 69115 Heidelberg, Germany

Printed by Libri Plureos GmbH
in Hamburg, Germany